THE PRACTICE OF EMERGENCY CARE

JAMES H. COSGRIFF, JR., M.D.

Assistant Clinical Professor of Surgery, School of Medicine, State University of New York at Buffalo;
Attending Surgeon, Chief of Trauma Service, Sisters of Charity Hospital, Buffalo, New York;
Chairman, New York State Committee on Trauma, American College of Surgeons

DIANN LADEN ANDERSON, R.N., M.N

Coordinator, Department of Health Sciences, San Jose City College, San Jose, California

Philadelphia J. B. LIPPINCOTT COMPANY

London · Mexico City · New York · St. Louis · São Paulo · Sydney

THE PRACTICE OF EMERGENCY CARE

SECOND EDITION

Sponsoring Editor: Jeanne H. Wallace
Manuscript Editor: Don Shenkle
Indexer: Kathleen Garcia
Art Director: Tracy Baldwin
Designer: Adrianne Onderdonk Dudden
Production Supervisor: Tina Rebane
Production Coordinators: Field & Squibb
Compositor: TAPSCO, Inc.
Printer/Binder: The Murray Printing Company
Cover Photo: Bob Desabaye, courtesy of The
  Graduate Hospital, Philadelphia, Pennsyl-
  vania

Second Edition

6 5 4 3 2 1

The authors and publisher have exerted every effort to ensure that drug selection and dosage set forth in this text are in accord with current recommendations and practice at the time of publication. However, in view of ongoing research, changes in government regulations, and the constant flow of information relating to drug therapy and drug reactions, the reader is urged to check the package insert for each drug for any change in indications and dosage and for added warnings and precautions. This is particularly important when the recommended agent is a new or infrequently employed drug.

Library of Congress Cataloging in Publication Data
Main entry under title:

The Practice of emergency care.

  Rev. ed. of: The Practice of emergency nursing. 1975.
  Bibliography: p.
  Includes index.
    1. Emergency nursing. I. Cosgriff, James H.
II. Anderson, Diann, Laden. III. Practice of emergency
nursing. [DNLM: 1. Emergencies.   2. Emergency medical
services.   3. Emergency service, Hospital.   4. Allied
health personnel.   5. Crisis intervention. WX 215 P895]
RT120.E4P73 1984   616'.025   83-22230
ISBN 0-397-54357-3

To
Mary Louise, Nancy, Maribeth, and Jim

To
Carl, Kirsten, and Eric

CONTRIBUTORS

Carl Anderson, P.T., M.A.
Independent Physical Therapist Contractor,
Willow Glen Physical Therapy,
San Jose, California

Diann Laden Anderson, R.N., M.N.
Coordinator, Department of Health Sciences, San Jose
City College, San Jose, California

John D. Bartels, M.D., F.A.C.O.G.
Associate Clinical Professor of Obstetrics and
Gynecology, State University of New York at Buffalo
School of Medicine; Attending Obstetrician and
Gynecologist, Sisters of Charity Hospital, Buffalo, New
York; Kenmore Mercy Hospital, Kenmore, New York

Paula Bauda, R.N., B.S.
Staff Nurse, Intensive Care Unit, Buffalo Veterans
Administration Medical Center, Buffalo, New York

Jo Ann Cahill, R.N., B.S.N.
Director, Division of Hospital Services, The Fischer
Mangold Group, Pleasanton, California

Rita E. Caughill, R.N., M.S.
Associate Professor Emeritus, Department of Graduate
Education, School of Nursing, State University of New
York at Buffalo, Buffalo, New York

Louis C. Cloutier, M.D., F.A.C.S.
Clinical Instructor in Surgery, School of Medicine,
State University of New York at Buffalo; Chief of
Ambulatory Care Services, Sisters of Charity Hospital;
Director of Burn Unit, Sheehan Memorial Emergency
Hospital, Buffalo, New York

James H. Cosgriff, Jr., M.D., F.A.C.S.
Assistant Clinical Professor of Surgery, School of
Medicine, State University of New York at Buffalo;
Attending Surgeon, Chief of Trauma Service, Sisters of
Charity Hospital, Buffalo, New York; Chairman New
York State Committee on Trauma, American College
of Surgeons

Florence Dziekan, R.N.
Former Supervisor, Burn Treatment Center, Sheehan
Memorial Emergency Hospital, Buffalo, New York

Joseph P. Gambacorta, M.D.
Attending Surgeon (Urology), Sisters of Charity
Hospital, St. Joseph's Intercommunity Hospital and
Sheehan Memorial Emergency Hospital, Buffalo,
New York

Judith Stoner Halpern, R.N., M.S., C.E.N.
Clinical Nursing Specialist, Bronson Methodist
Hospital, Kalamazoo, Michigan; formerly Clinical
Instructor, Emergency Department, Santa Clara
Valley Medical Center, San Jose, California

Jill D. Holmes, R.N., B.S., M.S.
Continuing Education Coordinator, Intensive Care
Unit; Scripps Clinic, Green Hospital, La Jolla,
California

Patrick J. Kelly, M.D.
Associate Professor of Neurosurgery, School of
Medicine, State University of New York Buffalo; Chief
of Neurosurgery, Sisters of Charity Hospital, Buffalo,
New York

Ambrose A. Macie, M.D., F.A.C.O.G.
Chief, Department of Obstetrics and Gynecology,
Sisters of Charity Hospital, Buffalo, New York

Albert D. Menno, M.D., F.A.C.S.
Assistant Clinical Professor of Surgery, School of
Medicine, State University of New York at Buffalo;
Transplant Surgeon, Attending Surgeon, Sisters of
Charity Hospital, Deaconess Hospital, Buffalo,
New York

Camille Ratajczyk, R.N., M.S.
Surgical Nurse Practitioner, Sisters of Charity
Hospital, Buffalo, New York

M. Kathleen Rose-Grippa, R.N., M.S.
Associate Professor and Interim Chairperson,
Department of Nursing, San Jose State University, San
Jose, California

Mary C. Sand, R.N.
Certified Urologic Nurse, Sisters of Charity Hospital,
Buffalo, New York

Arthur J. Schaefer, M.D., F.A.C.S.
Associate Clinical Professor of Surgery
(Ophthalmology), School of Medicine, State University
of New York at Buffalo; Chief of Ophthalmology, Sisters
of Charity Hospital and St. Joseph's Intercommunity
Hospital, Buffalo, New York; Director, Ophthalmic
Plastic and Reconstructive Surgery Clinic, Erie
County Medical Center, Buffalo, New York

Mark Schiffman, M.D.
Associate Director, Emergency Department,
Eisenhower Medical Center, Rancho Mirage,
California

Joseph C. Serio, M.D.
Chief of Otolaryngology, Sheehan Memorial
Emergency Hospital; Attending Surgeon (ENT) Sisters
of Charity Hospital, Buffalo, New York

Boyd G. Stephens, M.T., A.S.C.P., M.D., F.F.A.F.S.
Assistant Clinical Professor of Pathology, University of
San Francisco; Chief Medical Examiner/Coroner, City
and County of San Francisco; Teaching Consultant,
Forensic Pathology and Forensic Medicine

Barbara Secord-Pletz, R.N., M.I.C.N.
Consultant, Emergency Medical Services

James S. Williams, M.D., F.A.C.S.
Chief, Department of Surgery, Millard Fillmore
Hospital, Buffalo, New York

William D. Ziter, D.M.D.
Associate Professor of Oral Surgery, State University of
New York at Buffalo, School of Dentistry, and Chief,
Department of Oral Surgery, Erie County Medical
Center, Buffalo, New York

PREFACE

Many readers of the first edition of THE PRACTICE OF EMERGENCY NURSING will consider the second edition of this text a completely new book. In fact, much of the second edition of *The Practice of Emergency Care is* new, including its title, scope, focus, and format. Yet, the best of the first edition, content that has stood the test of time in the rapidly changing field of emergency care, has been retained.

During the writing of the first edition, emergency nursing was in its infancy. There was a need to identify emergency nursing philosophy, goals, and specialized skills and to develop its body of knowledge. (This trend was also occurring in emergency medicine and within disciplines in prehospital emergency care at that time.) Thus, the first edition focused on identifying and developing the body of knowledge germane to emergency nursing, especially as it was and should be practiced in emergency department settings.

Now, emergency nursing has become an established specialty in nursing with a comprehensive curriculum and certification examinations. Emergency medicine has been similarly recognized as a specialty. Roles and responsibilities of prehospital emergency care providers, EMTs, and paramedics are becoming well-defined, and their training programs and competency examinations are becoming standardized.

The dawning of specialization in emergency care has generated new goals to be attained. In our view, these goals include:

- Providing optimal emergency care wherever emergencies occur, outside *and* within the hospital setting
- Ensuring the delivery of high-quality emergency care to all individuals by:
  - Working together as a team, even though physical locations where care is given may be diverse
  - Understanding and appreciating the abilities and contributions of other team members
  - Sharing our body of knowledge of emergency care with others so that they, too, can deliver capable, skilful emergency care to those in need
  - Maintaining competency in a rapidly changing health field

With these goals in mind, the scope and focus of the second edition have been broadened to facilitate application of emergency care concepts not only in the emergency department, but in other in-patient hospital departments and in the field, the community, and other health care settings. The second edition will be a comprehensive resource to many health care professionals practicing in a variety of patient care settings.

The text is divided into three units. Unit I addresses the more general concepts of emergency care that are applicable to many situations. Unit II focuses on psychosocial aspects of emergency care. These considerations can underlie or cause an infinite variety of emergency problems and can affect the assessment and the nature of care rendered. Unit III deals with procedures and management, proceeding from general to specific subject areas.

This edition has been expanded from 29 to 35 chapters. Nine new chapters cover forensic aspects, sexual assault, domestic violence, laboratory studies, parenteral fluid therapy, resuscitation, obstetric emergencies, bites and stings, and environmental trauma. Much new material was added to chapters on pediatric emergencies, cardiac emergencies, poisoning and drug overdose, and legal aspects of emergency care.

All chapters from the first edition were carefully reviewed and revised to conform to present standards of practice.

Contributions have been sought from professionals with exceptional expertise in their fields to provide current, comprehensive information in their subject areas. Careful editing has been done throughout the text to ensure consistency and to avoid redundancy.

Content reflecting "pearls of practice," principles, procedures, and sequential actions of importance have been highlighted. Charts summarizing prehospital and hospital assessment and care are outlined throughout the text as appropriate to provide ready reference guides to assessment and care.

Our goal in preparing this new edition is to bring safe, knowledgeable, appropriate, and caring assessment and treatment to persons who encounter unexpected acute illness or injury. This is an objective we all share in administering patient care; hopefully, this text will make reaching this goal a little easier.

Diann Anderson
James H. Cosgriff, Jr.

ACKNOWLEDGMENTS

This volume is an amalgam of ideas and experiences gleaned from a number of our friends and colleagues and brought to fruition by the talented staff of J. B. Lippincott Company. We are deeply grateful to David T. Miller, Vice President and Editor, Nursing Department, who has given the benefit of his experience and personal support in this endeavor. Diana Intenzo, sponsoring editor, provided us with a new outlook and new goals by developing a unique format for a text that will appeal to many health disciplines. Jeanne Wallace, development editor, implemented these ideas in a practical way to enhance the meaning of the chapters by putting the authors' material in a concise, consistent, organized manner, highlighted by the use of bulleted lists, charts, and summaries. Her attention to detail and refinement of the manuscript and her patience and demeanor in difficult and sometimes stressful circumstances has been a rewarding experience for us. Don Shenkle, manuscript editor, reviewed the freshly edited manuscript and molded it into a readable, flowing form that accents the essential elements of the subject matter, thus stressing the important points to the reader. While he was a tough taskmaster, his ensuring our conformance to a rigid schedule of review of the galley and page proofs allowed us to complete the last important portion of the work effort on time. We are most appreciative of his understanding and advice.

Stephanie Wong, Eleonore Barlog, and Geraldine Brady spent many hours typing, editing, and retyping the manuscript and attending to detail while responding to our need for promptness and continued progress in the preparation of the copy.

Bobbie Phillips, Judy Stoner Halpern, Phyllis Harding and Ron Mock, professional nurses, gave freely of their clinical expertise and personal and professional assistance. Camille Ratajczyk, a surgical nurse practitioner, proofread a large number of complicated chapters while providing a penetrating, unique view of the material and making suggestions for major alterations. In addition, she co-authored three other chapters. To each of these nurses, we owe an immeasurable debt of gratitude.

Special thanks are due to the library staffs of Sisters of Charity Hospital and San Jose City College for their unrelenting efforts in the search for essential, often obscure reference materials. Anne Cohen, the medical librarian at Sisters Hospital and Hilda Borrer of San Jose City College Library were particularly helpful in securing needed information with minimal delay. Dr. Hyan Sung of the Department of Radiology of Sisters Hospital kindly made available a number of the new radiographs presented throughout the text. Dr. Nang Van Ta, a surgeon and accomplished medical illustrator, provided a singular approach to the new illustrations in the text. Dennis Atkinson, Chief Biomedical photographer at the State University of New York at Buffalo, took many of the photographs for both the initial volume and this. His commitment to photographic excellence has enhanced the text greatly.

To our families we owe the warmest appreciation for their continued support and gift of time required for the preparation of the manuscript. Last, we wish to recognize with all our humility our colleagues, teachers, students, and patients, who have provided us with an educational experience beyond their realization.

CONTENTS

Contents

UNIT ONE

GENERAL CONCEPTS IN EMERGENCY CARE

1

THE EMS SYSTEM AND THE EMERGENCY CARE TEAM: CONCEPTS OF PREHOSPITAL AND HOSPITAL CARE

DIANN ANDERSON and JAMES H. COSGRIFF, JR.

The unique requirements of emergency health care call for a high degree of coordination and cooperation as well as individual competence, judgment, and dedication. The emergency medical services (EMS) system is a still evolving response to the need for the assessment and coordination of regional facilities, patient flow, and standards of care. The emergency care team concept involves the meshing of independent roles in an interdependent team effort to provide optimal care to the patient.

EMERGENCY MEDICAL SERVICES SYSTEMS

The principle and standard set forth in the following statements by the Joint Commission on Accreditation of Hospitals (JCAH) concisely express the current view on the broad subject of emergency medical services (EMS).[10]

> Any individual who comes to the hospital for emergency medical evaluation or initial treatment shall be properly assessed by qualified individuals, and appropriate services shall be rendered within the defined capability of the hospital.*
> A well defined plan for emergency care, based on community need and on the capability of the hospital, shall be implemented by every hospital.†

SCOPE OF EMERGENCY MEDICAL SERVICES

Hospital emergency departments have been in existence for many years. However, they have undergone significant evolutionary changes since the historic monograph prepared by the National Academy of Sciences/National Research Council (NAS/NRC) "Accidental Death and Disability: The Neglected Disease of Modern Society" and the passage of The National Highway Safety Act in 1966.[11]

For decades, the emergency department (ED) served as a focal point for the acutely ill and injured. In the last 30 years, however, a major change has occurred. The emergency department now serves an estimated 70 million patient visits annually, of which approximately 85% are not medical or surgical emergencies. Perhaps only 5% to 10% of patient visits constitute life-threatening episodes. The reasons for this tremendous expansion are many; they include population mobility, improvements in transportation, inability or lack of interest on the part of patients to establish a professional relationship with a physician, fiscal intermediaries, and government intervention.

This expansion has brought about many problems and has prompted federal legislation, notably the Emergency Medical Services Act (PL 93-154) of 1973. This act was amended in 1976 to provide for the inclusion of 15 system-operating components and the identification of major areas of concern for the acute medical and surgical emergency patient. Monies were appropriated with the bills to support emergency medical technician (EMT) training, hospital-to-ambulance communications, EMS systems development, and regional categorization of hospital facilities and services.

---

* Principle elucidated by The Joint Commission on Accreditation of Hospitals, 1980.
† Emergency Medical Services, Standard I, 1980.

More than 300 EMS regions were designated throughout the country to establish "wall-to-wall" contiguous coverage for all EMS services.

Scope of Clinical Coverage

Clinical areas of special concern include the following:
- Multiply-injured patient
- Acute cardiac patient
- High-risk maternal patient
- High-risk neonate
- Acutely psychotic patient
- Drug overdose patient
- Alcoholic intoxication
- Patient with spinal cord injury
- Burned patient

CARE DELIVERY SYSTEMS

If one accepts the premise that every patient is entitled to, or should have, whatever level of care is necessary to treat him, a *system* must be developed to provide this care. It is neither economically feasible nor practically possible to provide a full range of necessary services in every hospital in the country. By using a systems approach, regionalization of special services and special care units can be established and a mechanism developed by which the patient can be treated in an appropriate facility.

A system involves a complexity of individuals and activities that must be coordinated, function efficiently, and provide continuity of care beginning with the prehospital phase and progressing to full rehabilitation. It is not a simple task to establish a system. Local laws or ambulance ordinances must be enacted or existing ones amended to allow patients to be taken to the appropriate emergency facility.[7]

Many hospitals fear loss of revenue if an EMS system is developed. It must be kept in mind, however, that 85% of patients can be handled locally, while 10% need further care or an intensive care unit (ICU) setting. Only 5% need specialized care in a designated center. In spinal cord injury, these figures may be reversed.[6]

With respect to local needs, it is interesting to note that in the United States there are extensive rural areas in which, individually, accidents occur infrequently, but which collectively account for 80% of highway-related deaths.

Trauma Centers

In a California study of trauma care, 100 trauma deaths in San Francisco and a like number in Orange County were reviewed.[13] In Orange County, which had no established EMS system, the patient was taken to a local hospital; in San Francisco the patient was transferred to a trauma center. The authors concluded from this retrospective study that in Orange County, one-third of the deaths were clearly preventable. In San Francisco, there were no preventable deaths. It was their opinion that the availability of a trauma center does make a difference in survival. Inappropriate care is a leading factor contributing to morbidity and mortality.[8]

The development of spinal cord injury centers has had a significant impact on morbidity, mortality, ultimate rehabilitation, and cost effectiveness in the management of this dread injury.

Mobile Units

A significant decrease in morbidity and mortality has been demonstrated with the use of a mobile coronary care unit.[12] The mobile unit allows acute cardiac patients to receive emergency treatment and resuscitation in the home or at the incident site and to be moved to the hospital when stabilized.

Systems Planning and Development

Systems development must start at the grass roots level in the community with a lead agency, an individual, or a group that will provide direction in coordinating both lay and professional activities. Representatives of medicine, nursing, and the health-related professions, consumers, and public agencies with an interest in health care must be included in the process.[11]

The essential elements of systems planning and development are the following:
- Assessment of needs in the area
- Identification and inventory of existing services
- Recommendation and implementation of an appropriate plan of action

COORDINATION OF FACILITIES AND PATIENT FLOW

Both the prehospital and hospital phases of care must be considered in a coordinated manner to provide continuity. An integral part of such a system consists of *categorization* and *designation* of facilities and development of patient flow patterns that will allow for "matching" the patient with the appropriate facility.

Categorization of Facilities

Hospitals have been categorized according to a number of criteria and methods, which to some extent has been confusing. The following three types of categorization are currently in use.
1. *Horizontal,* which addresses the emergency department personnel and equipment needs for *all* types of emergency services. The hospital's capability is measured by the presence of general and specialty physicians, nurses, critical care units, operating suites, laboratory and blood banking services, etc. on a 24-hour, 7-days-a-week basis.
2. *Vertical,* which addresses the specific clinical areas of emergency services mentioned earlier in this chapter and assesses the capability of the hospital to provide definitive care in each of these areas. Thus, a hospital may be limited to the care of certain types of patients (drug overdose, acute psychotic, burned patient, multiply-injured patient) and provide a full range of services for the total care of such patients. An example is the Shriners Burn Institute in Boston, which limits its care to burn victims. Similarly,

the Maryland Institute of Emergency Medical Services Systems (MIEMSS) in Baltimore receives only trauma patients.
3. *Circular,* which addresses emergency care needs and response on a regional basis.

The categorization criteria developed by the JCAH are presented in Chart 1-1.

Uniform Guidelines

Whichever system is used, it should be uniform throughout an entire region and coordinated with systems of contiguous regions. Treatment protocols for the prehospital phase of care should be developed along with interhospital agreements that allow for the orderly transfer of patients to appropriate facilities.

Guidelines for the triage and management of critically ill or injured patients may be devised, but must clearly be no more than that. They are designed to help the physician make decisions involving patient flow through an EMS system. The decision to treat or transfer a patient must remain within the province of the physician. A suggested transfer form including a transfer agreement is shown in Figure 1-1.

With respect to the injured patient, The American College of Surgeons Committee on Trauma has developed a field categorization of patients which is devised to rate the severity of injury at the incident site (Chart 1-2). The purpose is to get the right trauma patient to the appropriate hospital at the proper time. In addition, a Hospital Trauma Index was developed in an effort to standardize and quantitate the degree of injury in patients. An example of this is shown in Figure 10-3. Both of these indices are intended only as guidelines for health professionals. They may also serve as a basis for a similar effort in other areas of emergency care.[1]

Boyd has conceptualized a regional EMS system consisting of three models: urban/suburban, rural/metropolitan, and wilderness/metropolitan.[6] The rural/metropolitan model is diagrammed in Figure 1-2.

COORDINATION OF CARE

Prehospital Phase

As an absolute minimum, those providing care at the scene of the incident must be trained to provide basic life support and standard emergency care. This level of performance corresponds to that of the EMT-1 or EMT-A. More highly trained personnel, capable of providing advanced life support at the scene, under the direction of a physician by radio or in accord with established protocols, are now commonplace in the United States. Paramedics are trained to fill this role in the delivery of prehospital care.

Although ground ambulances are the most common mode of transport of the acutely ill or injured, other means may be required because of geographic location or terrain. Water vehicles, snowmobiles, and fixed-wing aircraft or helicopters serve admirably in such situations. The same rules and regulations that apply to ground ambulances also apply to these other emergency vehicles.

Chart 1-1

CATEGORIZATION CRITERIA FOR HOSPITAL EMERGENCY SERVICE CAPABILITIES*

It is recognized that hospitals may offer critical therapeutic services in specialized clinical areas such as spinal cord injury, burns, trauma, and so forth. Such hospitals shall be considered as providing comprehensive (Level I) services for the specific clinical focus of care, while the emergency services otherwise provided shall be evaluated at the appropriate level.

Level I

A Level I emergency department/service offers comprehensive emergency care 24 hours a day, with at least one physician experienced in emergency care on duty in the emergency care area. There shall be in-hospital physician coverage for at least medical, surgical, orthopedic, obstetric/gynecologic, pediatric, and anesthesiology services by members of the medical staff or by senior-level residents, with other specialty consultation available within approximately 30 minutes, as needed. Initial consultation through two-way voice communication is acceptable. The hospital's scope of services shall include in-house capabilities for managing physical and related emotional problems on a definitive basis. The above requirements apply to a comprehensive-level emergency department/service provided by a hospital offering care only to a limited group of patients, such as pediatric, obstetric, ophthalmologic, and orthopedic.

Level II

A Level II emergency department/service offers emergency care 24 hours a day, with at least one physician experienced in emergency care on duty in the emergency care area, and specialty consultation available within approximately 30 minutes by members of the medical staff or by senior-level residents. Initial consultation through two-way voice communication is acceptable. The hospital's scope of services shall include in-house capabilities for managing physical and related emotional problems, with provision for patient transfer to another facility when needed.

Level III

A Level III emergency department/service offers emergency care 24 hours a day, with at least one physician available to the emergency care area within approximately 30 minutes through a medical staff call roster. Initial consultation through two-way voice communication is acceptable. Specialty consultation shall be available by request of the attending medical staff member or by transfer to a designated hospital where definitive care can be provided.

Level IV

A Level IV emergency service offers reasonable care in determining whether an emergency exists, renders lifesaving first aid, and makes appropriate referral to the nearest facilities that have the capability of providing needed services. The mechanism for providing physician coverage at all times shall be defined by the medical staff.

(Accreditation Manual for Hospitals, 1981. Chicago, Joint Commission on Accreditation of Hospitals, 1981)

Hospital Phase

Hospitals and their medical staffs that choose to participate in a regional EMS system must be dedicated to the task. Acceptable care of the acutely ill or injured patient requires adequate facilities and equipment and well-trained personnel at all levels to ensure prompt, appropriate treatment. The entire medical and nursing staff with its many disciplines must play a role in the planning and implementation of an optimal response for the care of emergency patients. The ultimate responsibility, however, rests with the hospital administration.

SECTION A
TRANSFER FORM

A. Patient's Name _____

Address _____

Age _____ Sex _____ Weight _____

Next of kin _____

Address _____

Phone _____

B. History of Injury or Illness:
History of previous conditions and medications:

C. Condition on admission.

Blood pressure _____ / _____ Pulse _____ Temperature _____

D. Initial impressions:

E. Diagnostic Studies:
  1. Laboratory
      a. Complete blood count
      b. Urinalysis
      c. Electrolytes
      d. Arterial blood gases
  2. Radiological

F. Treatment rendered to patient.
  1. Medications given with amount and time.
  2. Intravenous (IV) fluids with type and amount.
  3. Other

G. Status of patient when transferred:
H. Management during transport:

I. Name of physician transferring patient _____

Phone _____

J. Name of physician and hospital contacted _____

_____

SECTION B

SUGGESTED TRANSFER AGREEMENT

Memorandum of Agreement between _____ Hospital and _____ Hospital relative to the transfer of trauma patients.

The parties below have reviewed the data contained in "Interhospital Transfer of Patients" and "How to Transfer a Patient" and have approved their use.

In the event that a situation arises where specialized trauma care is required and the attending physician requests the transfer of a patient to another hospital, and that other hospital and its physicians accept such patient, the material contained in Interhospital Transfer of Patients and in How to Transfer a Patient will serve as a guide for such movement.

It is understood by all parties that guidelines are "guides" only to assist physicians in making medical decisions.

Figure 1-1 Transfer form and agreement. (Bulletin of the American College of Surgeons, February 1980)

Chart 1-2

FIELD CATEGORIZATION OF TRAUMA PATIENTS

System	Category 1	Category 2	Category 3
Soft tissue	Avulsion type injuries, severe uncontrolled bleeding	Soft-tissue injuries with stabilized bleeding	Soft-tissue injuries of moderate degree
Fractures	Open fractures, pelvic fractures, severe maxillofacial injuries	Single open or closed fractures	Uncomplicated fractures
Abdomen	Blunt or penetrating abdominal injuries especially when associated with hypotension	Blunt abdominal or penetrating trauma not producing hypotension	No abdominal injuries
Chest	Unstable chest injuries, respiratory rate >30 or <10	Multiple rib fractures without flailed segments, respiratory rate >20 or <10	No respiratory distress, respiratory rate 10–20
Head and neck, upper respiratory	Severe maxillofacial injuries, open penetrating and blunt trauma to face, neck, and cervical spine, multiple facial fractures and injuries affecting vision	Facial trauma with single facial fractures, (without airway or major cervical vascular or cervical spine involvement)	Simple contusions of the head and neck, nasal fractures
Neurologic	Prolonged loss of consciousness, posturing, lateralizing signs, open cranial injuries, paralysis	Transient loss of consciousness, oriented to time, place, and person	No neurologic injuries
Vital signs	BP < 90 systolic P > 100 or <60, skin cool, ashen, pale	BP > 90 systolic P = 60–100, skin warm to slightly cool	BP > 100 systolic P = 60–100, skin dry, warm

(Bulletin of the American College of Surgeons, February, 1980)

Special expertise in any of the aforementioned clinical areas requires a commitment of funds and personnel on the part of the hospital and the nursing and medical staffs to achieve and maintain a level of professional excellence. The latter implies ongoing educational programs for all levels of the staff, medical and nursing care evaluation, and chart review and audit procedures for emergency care and all ED deaths. Multidisciplinary conferences involving nurses, physicians, EMTs, and other health professionals in emergency care are useful not only from the teaching standpoint, but also in supporting the concept of the team approach to patient care and continuity of care. Such conferences also provide a forum for the discussion of problems inherent in each

discipline.[2,3,4,5] In addition, research studies of a clinical or basic scientific nature are important adjuncts to better care.

DISASTER PREPAREDNESS

Disaster planning is one of the 15 components defined in the Emergency Medical Service Systems Act of 1973 and is essential to regional emergency medical care systems. A disaster has been defined as any situation requiring resources beyond those readily available. This definition may apply to a community-wide problem such as an earthquake, train

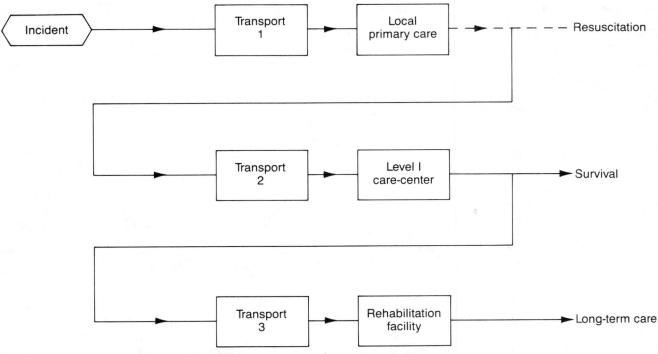

Figure 1-2 *Rural/metropolitan "Systems Operation Design." (After Boyd DR: J Trauma 20:14–24, 1980)*

wreck, or airplane crash or to a problem that arises in a single hospital emergency department when several critically injured patients are brought in from a multiple-car accident. Whatever the cause, a disaster is unpredictable, unscheduled, and unplanned. The response to a disaster, *i.e.,* disaster preparedness, should be planned, scheduled, and predictable. This goal is difficult to achieve because it involves abandoning daily routines and switching rapidly to an alternate system.

The JCAH has formulated standards for disaster preparedness that call for written plans for the timely care of casualties and documentation of rehearsals of these plans. Disasters are classified as external (occurring outside of the hospital) and internal (occurring inside the hospital).

External Disaster

External disasters vary in scope. In some, very few medical casualties are involved, and the main concern is the evacuation of large numbers of people from the area—for example, the accident at Three Mile Island, Pennsylvania, or a freight train wreck in which potentially explosive or volatile chemicals are released. In other incidents, such as school bus accidents or passenger train wrecks, large numbers of injured casualties require medical attention.

An external disaster response requires community-wide planning. Representatives of civic and professional groups such as the following are usually included.
- Local and regional government(s)
- Hospital association
- Regional EMS council
- Public safety

- Medical society
- Nursing association
- Dental society
- Local and regional law enforcement agencies
- Organized commercial and volunteer ambulance and first-aid agencies
- Local and regional health department
- Consumer advocate groups
- Local and regional fire agencies

The above list is not necessarily all-inclusive and may be modified according to specific needs in the area under consideration. For example, in a region with a nuclear power plant, in which radiation injury is a potential danger, a person familiar with radiation and its hazards may be an important member of the community committee.

Whatever its size, capability, or limitations, each hospital in the community must play a role in disaster response. Roles may range from providing simple first-aid and preparing casualties for transfer to administering definitive care. Hospital resources should be identified and categorized, then coordinated into the community effort.

Ambulance organizations, whether land- or air-based or water evacuation groups must also be assessed and coordinated to provide optimum response. A radio communication system linking hospital, ambulances, police, and other public agencies is essential as an alternative to telephone communications, which may be overtaxed or damaged in the disaster and thus unusable.

Implementation of the disaster plan requires a unified medical command. In incidents involving many casualties, appropriate triage calls for life-and-death decisions. Therefore, there must be a qualified physician in charge at the scene and in each of the hospitals involved in the disaster response. Triage, emergency treatment, casualty identification and evacuation, and hospital readiness are key considerations in an appropriate plan.

The specific responsibilities of the hospital are clearly stated in the JCAH manual, which is updated at regular intervals. The reader is referred to this source for a more detailed account of these obligations. Further information should be sought from the office of disaster planning of the local government, area EMS Council, or health department.

Internal Disaster

For the purposes of this chapter, there are two types of internal disaster: (1) an acute incident that affects the lives and/or property of persons in the hospital, for example, a fire, explosion, or bomb threat, and (2) the sudden overburdening of a hospital's emergency facility by the arrival of several critically ill or injured victims.

Incidents involving danger to hospital property and/or personnel and patients require a coordinated plan developed by experts (fire, safety, engineers, nuclear medicine) both within the hospital and in the community who may be called upon to respond in the event of such a disaster. The important details of such planning are described in the JCAH manual. Interhospital transfer agreements allowing the evacuation of certain patients to other hospitals in the area are an important element of such a plan.

Sudden overcrowding of a hospital emergency department by the arrival of a number of critically ill or injured patients may tax the facility beyond its resources. In such an instance, portions of the disaster plan may have to be implemented to provide adequate personnel, space, equipment, supplies, and auxiliary services (laboratory, blood bank, x-ray) to respond to the sudden, unexpected influx of patients. Additional nursing department personnel may be summoned to duty, medical staff personnel are alerted to be available, and special care areas such as the operating room, x-ray department, and critical care unit must be alerted and prepared to cancel or delay elective procedures until the emergency situation has ended. The effectiveness of such a plan depends on a close working relationship among all individuals and groups concerned.

THE EMERGENCY CARE TEAM

In recent years, the numbers, types, and roles of various emergency care personnel have been adjusted to meet the increasing need of the general public for services. Emergency medical technicians (EMT-1A or EMT-A), the EMT-II, paramedics, emergency nurses, and emergency physicians have witnessed vast changes within their respective disciplines. These changes represent a response to the increasing number of patients and the wide variety of medical problems seen in emergency medical services settings today.

The purpose of this section is to survey the scope of practice and training standards for emergency care personnel

and to discuss the interacting roles of these colleagues in emergency care.

HOSPITAL EMERGENCY CARE PERSONNEL

The capabilities of the emergency department in the daily routine of caring for patients depend largely on the staff. Continuous patient traffic flow, without delay in treatment or admission, is the responsibility of the personnel who work day to day in the emergency department, for it is they who know best how the department is geared to function.

There are many considerations involved in selecting the type of personnel for a hospital emergency department. What may be adequate, even recommended for one department may not be at all suitable for another. The geographic location, the proximity of other area hospitals, the local population, the medical services offered and, in general, the particular hospital's concept of the function of its emergency department determines staffing.

The Emergency Nurse

Emergency nurses are usually described as nurses who work in emergency department settings. Their practice is a specialty within nursing that traces its beginnings to dedicated emergency *department* nurses. As health care has become increasingly community based, so has the delivery of emergency care, and now emergency nursing care is given in many settings—in fact, wherever emergencies commonly occur—in industrial plants, jails, schools, mobile emergency care units, and community clinics. Nurses teach in emergency care training programs, provide inservice education and continuing education to emergency care personnel, and administer and manage EMS projects in cities and counties across the country.

Scope of Emergency Nursing Practice. In terms of the *nature* and scope of the practice, emergency nurses can be best described as generalists in episodic acute nursing care whose expertise must encompass the basic nursing specialty areas of obstetrics and gynecology, pediatrics, community health, medical-surgical, and psychiatric nursing and other specialty areas such as rehabilitation, orthopedics, critical care, and others.

Emergency nurses must possess an understanding of all kinds of health problems in all age groups, from the neonate to the elderly person, and they must be thoroughly familiar with the physical and emotional developmental tasks of each age group, especially as they relate to presenting health needs.

Emergency nursing is unique in that it involves care of patients with health problems that (1) are undiagnosed and (2) are perceived by the patient as sufficiently acute to warrant seeking emergency care. These two characteristics require astute patient evaluation and many capably administered dependent and independent nursing interventions.

Because patients present with signs and symptoms rather than medical diagnoses, refined assessment skills are crucially important. Like technical skills, assessment skills can be perfected only through practice; unlike many technical skills, nursing assessment must be based on a wide foundation of knowledge that serves as a guide in collecting information, making observations, and evaluating data. This foundation enables the nurse to sort and analyze relevant information, to communicate it to the patient's physician, and to develop the nursing care plan, and is useful in interpreting medical and nursing diagnoses to the patient and his family. Because assessment is such an important element of emergency care, subsequent chapters provide detailed information on the evaluation of patients with selected complaints, signs, and symptoms and on related anatomy, physiology, and pathophysiology.

In many instances the emergency nurse is the first professional to see an acutely ill or injured patient, and measures usually thought within the scope of the physician must be instituted. Thus, the emergency nurse functions independently, interdependently, and collaboratively. Emergency nurses possess a unique body of knowledge and a set of skills that can be mobilized on short notice. They work cooperatively with prehospital emergency personnel, physicians, and other health-related personnel and agencies in the community to provide optimal care for the patient. Their duties in the ED include expediting patient flow, triage, hands-on care, implementing the physician's medical orders, providing emotional support during crises, preparing adequate documentation, and arranging for continuity of care, admission to the hospital, transfer to another health care facility, or discharge into the community.

Physician coverage of emergency departments varies tremendously—from 24-hour physician coverage exclusively devoted to the emergency department to physicians on dual assignment, both in the emergency department and the remainder of the hospital, to on-call, off-premises coverage. One recent study revealed that the vast majority of smaller hospitals provide the latter coverage.[41] In emergency departments lacking 24-hour physician coverage, nurses function in expanded roles, preferably with guidance from established protocols, in directing care of patients both within and outside the hospital setting.

The Specialty of Emergency Nursing. A growing awareness of the uniqueness of emergency department nursing practice and of the need to organize for the purpose of improving emergency health care delivery prompted a group of concerned and dedicated nurses to form the Emergency Department Nurses Association (EDNA) in 1970. Since its modest beginnings, the association has grown to over 12,000 members; it has become a member of the Federation of Specialty Nursing Organizations (1973) and publishes its own journal, The Journal of Emergency Nursing (1975).

The Standards of Emergency Nursing Practice were jointly developed by EDNA and the American Nurses Association (ANA) and published in 1975. This document identified the criteria by which emergency nursing practice is measured. These standards have recently been expanded and published. Also, the Continuing Education Core Curriculum for emergency nursing was published.* The curriculum serves as a

guide for developing courses in emergency nursing; moreover, it specifies the knowledge and skills needed by emergency nurses. The Standards and Curriculum describe the clinical specialty of emergency nursing and provide the foundation for the certifying examinations.

Certification. The first certifying examination for emergency nurses was given in July 1980; 1274 nurses became certified and received the designation Certified Emergency Nurse (CEN).

The certifying examination evaluates the nurse's knowledge and skills by measuring them against accepted standards of emergency nursing practice. Certification motivates the emergency nurse to pursue excellence and provides some assurance to the public and to the administration of the employing agencies that standards of competency have been met. Finally, certification recognizes and rewards the nurse who has achieved a level of excellence in practice.

The Mobile Intensive Care Nurse (MICN). Extended roles for emergency department nurses have evolved to keep pace with developments in emergency medical services. One such role is that of the MICN, an experienced, ED-registered nurse who has additional knowledge and training in prehospital emergency care, recognition and management of arrhythmias (advanced cardiac life support), and hospital-mobile unit communications. Though the term *MICN* suggests a mobile assignment, the MICN typically works in a hospital emergency department designated as a base-station that directs the patient care activities of one or more paramedic or advanced life-support field units.

The major function of the MICN is to provide instructions to paramedics according to specific criteria and protocols. However, though MICNs typically practice within the base-station setting, they may also function in the field situation and in air or ground transport units providing advanced life support (ALS). They may also be involved in training programs for paramedics or other MICNs or in implementing paramedic-MICN programs within their counties.

Preparation for the MICN role varies from informal in-service sessions and on-the-job training to formal comprehensive courses that are more than 80 hours long. Continuing education and experience are needed to prepare for this role, since the nurse's usual exposure to field management, biotelemetry, and radio communications is limited. Many states or counties require documentation of continued competency through recertifying examinations at 2- to 3-year intervals.

The Nurse Practitioner. It is estimated that one-half to two-thirds of all ED visits fall into nonurgent, non-acute care categories.[29] It is not surprising then, that the nurse-practitioner* has become a valuable manpower resource in caring

---

* The Standards and Curriculum are available from the Emergency Department Nurses Association, 666 North Lake Shore Drive, Chicago, Illinois 60611.

* Although there is much variation in the educational programs that prepare nurses in this expanded role, generally nurse practitioners share these qualities: (1) they are registered professional nurses and graduates of basic nursing programs; (2) they have nursing and medical skills, notably history-taking and physical assessment; (3) they employ independent judgments within their own areas of competence; and (4) they participate in patient care directly or in consultation with the physician; the final responsibility for medical care rests with the physician.

for this patient population, freeing the emergency physician and staff for the care of patients with urgent or life-threatening problems. In many emergency departments, a "walk-in" or ambulatory care clinic is provided where the nurse practitioner assesses and treats patient problems according to established protocols and does health screening, referral, patient and family teaching, and counseling.

The Emergency Nurse Practitioner. The emergency nurse practitioner has acquired expanded skills in primary care and, in addition, has developed the capability to manage critical patients when necessary. Use of the emergency nurse practitioner depends on the philosophy and goals of the training curriculum, the employing instituion, and the community it serves. Underlying effective use of the nurse practitioner is acceptance by patients, physicians, and nurses within the employing institution and the community and the development of mechanisms to evaluate the quality of care.

Preparation for this expanded role may be acquired in programs leading to a certificate or a masters degree. A few programs specifically prepare the emergency nurse practitioner; others provide a core nurse practitioner curriculum after which the candidate specializes in one area, such as primary care, adult health, rural care, pediatrics, emergency/ambulatory care, surgery, gerontology, etc., through additional coursework and/or clinical perceptorships.

The Physician's Assistant

The physician's assistant (PA) is a recent addition to the health care team. The PA role has developed partly because of a decrease in the number of primary-care physicians and partly because of the availability of a large pool of hospital corpsmen who had been trained in the military medical corps and had returned to civilian life. Military hospital corpsmen received extensive training and many functioned independently in providing health care to military personnel and their dependents. Since the initial experience in training PAs at Duke University, there has been a significant change in the educational background required of students entering such programs. More than one-third have baccalaureate or masters degrees.

A number of PAs trained in specialties have entered the health care work force. Specific training in emergency care is received by the emergency services physician's assistant (ESPA) or emergency physician's assistant (EPA).

The ESPA in the emergency department performs a number of tasks previously carried out by physicians. These include:
- Patient assessment
- Collection of laboratory data and other data
- Interpretation of laboratory results
- Minor surgical procedures
- Assisting in integrating multidisciplinary care
- Patient education

PAs can function according to established protocols. Their use depends on a defined need in a community and may not be applicable to all ED settings.

The PA is not meant to replace the physician, but to extend the capability of the physician. Physicians and nurses have not wholeheartedly accepted the PA concept. In some cases, this may be based on serious concern for the quality of care, but in others it is founded on biases, lack of understanding, and unclear definition of roles. Often differences resulting from personality conflicts have been resolved as each discipline has recognized and accepted the merits of the other. Patient acceptance is another concern and generally has been positive.

The scope of practice of the PA and nurse practitioner should not be confused. Although their roles and functions overlap, the PA's focus in practice relates to patient evaluation and to the technical skills relating to minor surgical procedures, diagnostic studies, and laboratory procedures. The nurse practitioner's focus is geared toward patient counseling and teaching, psychosocial care, and development of a health maintenance plan. Both professionals have become valuable members of the emergency care team in some locales.

The Emergency Physician

As demands on emergency departments have increased and changes in emergency care have developed, a new area of specialty practice has evolved within the medical profession—emergency medicine. The decade of the 1970s was a time of significant change in emergency medical care, partly in response to the Highway Safety Act of 1966 and partly because of the availability of physicians and the development of new ideas on graduate medical education. Residency training programs in emergency medicine of 2 and 3 years were established and at the beginning of 1981 numbered 52 across the United States.

The American College of Emergency Physicians (ACEP), chartered in 1968, has served as the advocate for recognition of this new specialty. This goal was achieved in 1979, when the American Medical Association (AMA) granted recognition to the specialty of emergency medicine. The American Board of Emergency Medicine (ABEM) was established and gave its first examinations in 1980. Several hundred applicants successfully completed the examination.

Although the number of emergency physicians is increasing annually and the JCAH has established numerous guidelines and regulations pertaining to emergency medical services in hospitals, the majority of hospital EDs are not staffed by specialists in emergency medicine. Rather, physicians currently working in hospital EDs represent very varied backgrounds. This is particularly true of smaller city hospitals and those in suburban areas. The tasks and procedures relating to the patient care that emergency physicians may perform are often guided and limited by the hospital administration and the by-laws of the medical staff.

In an effort to upgrade the capability of the physicians staffing hospital EDs, the American College of Surgeons Committee on Trauma in 1980 developed and promoted a course entitled Advanced Trauma Life Support (ATLS). This course, directed toward second career emergency physicians and rural physicians, has generated a tremendous amount of national interest.

Essential to a good emergency department is the availability of adequate, qualified physician coverage at all times. Specialty back-up must be accessible for consultation and definitive management of the seriously ill or the critically injured patient.

The trauma patient with multiple-system injury presents a unique challenge to emergency personnel. The availability of a general surgeon, trained and dedicated to the care of such patients is essential. The general surgeon in this instance assesses the patient, initiates or continues resuscitative measures, coordinates requests for appropriate specialty consultation, and provides continuity of care. Similarly, the internist and/or cardiologist may act in the same capacity with respect to the critically ill patient.

ROLES IN PREHOSPITAL EMERGENCY CARE

Significant growth and change have occurred in the area of prehospital care during the past decade. With the commitment of federal monies to programs designed to improve the delivery of emergency medical services, quality care has become more readily available to patients. Public education and the training of lay persons to respond appropriately to medical emergencies has improved, reducing mortality and morbidity.

Trends in Public Education

Crucial to the implementation of any emergency medical services plan is education of the public in how to gain access to the EMS system and what to do until help arrives. Considering the numbers of people to be educated and their varying degrees of motivation to learn this information, this task is monumental. Some activities that have helped to achieve these goals are:

- *Assessing public awareness.* Surveys by telephone, mail, and public service and information booths at fairs provide data on community awareness of the EMS system and what to do in an emergency. In some communities the availability of these data has provided the basis for formulating and implementing a public education plan.

- *Disseminating information to the public through the media.* Telephone books, TV spots, motivational films, and brochures have helped spread the word about whom to call and what to do in case of a medical emergency. In some communities, aggressive programs providing basic and advanced first aid courses and cardiopulmonary resuscitation (CPR) training have been singled out as a major factor in reducing mortality and morbidity. Some communities offer CPR in the high school curriculum, and some initially expose children to CPR techniques at the elementary school level.

- *Continuing education courses.* The American Red Cross, adult education programs, community colleges, and various interest groups provide courses on what to do in a variety of emergency situations.

The emergency medical technician (EMT) was trained initially to give care to the sick and injured at the scene and en route to a medical facility, primarily in an ambulance. Recently, training in emergency care to this level has become a desirable or required prerequisite for work in a variety of occupations, including firefighting, police work, occupational health programs in industry, community health clinics, ski patrols, and many others.

The Emergency Medical Technician (EMT-1)

Standards for the training of EMTs have varied widely from state to state and, in some areas, from county to county; but the emergency medical technician training program introduced in 1967 has resulted in the upgrading of training programs and in some degree of standardization. Most jurisdictions recognize the Basic Training Course for Emergency Medical Technicians (the 81-hour curriculum prepared for the U.S. Department of Transportation) as the standard. Although these programs are primarily designed to prepare the EMT for ambulance work, firemen, peace officers, industrial safety personnel, and many others have applied EMT training to their own work, which frequently involves them as first responders.

It is important for hospital-based emergency personnel to be aware of what the EMT-1 can and cannot do, so that their expectations of them are realistic. The certified EMT-1 should be able to:

- Recognize the nature and seriousness of a patient's condition or the extent of his injuries in order to determine needs for emergency care. He should be able to carry out triage of multiple victims in an accident as well as set priorities for the care of the multiply injured victim. One must be sensitive to the adverse conditions in which EMTs conduct their assessments—darkness, extreme cold, restrictive spaces, such as underneath dashboards or other vehicles, etc. Mistakes can be made—and are—that are not noted until the patient arrives at the well-lit ED and is further assessed by trained professionals with more sophisticated assessment skills. Participating in the field with the EMT is an informative and sensitizing experience for hospital-based emergency care personnel.

- Administer appropriate emergency care to stabilize the patient's condition. The skills of the EMT-1 are limited yet inclusive. They are sufficient to provide life support until definitive care can be given at the hospital. The skills one can expect all EMTs to have include the following:

  1. *Physical assessment,* including measurement of temperature, pulse, respiration, blood pressure, and pupil response

  2. *Cardiopulmonary resuscitation* of infants, children, and adults according to the standards of the American Heart Association or the American Red Cross

  3. *Maintenance of an open airway:* positioning; insertion of an oropharyngeal airway; suction devices and techniques; anti-choking maneuvers

  4. *Use of mechanical aids to breathing:* oxygen tanks, regulators, nasal cannulas, and masks; bag-valve-mask resuscitators; mechanical resuscitators

  5. *Techniques to control bleeding*

  6. *Application of dressings, bandages, and slings*

  7. *Immobilization techniques:* application of inflatable, rigid, and traction splints; cervical collars; short and long backboards

  8. *Lifting and moving techniques*

9. Techniques of *simple extrication* from entrapment
10. *Emergency childbirth* assistance

Because the EMT is a trained lay person, he must recertify periodically according to the regulations in the state in which he practices. This typically involves taking a refresher course and successfully completing a theory and skills examination.

The EMT-Paramedic

The EMT may acquire advanced training in specific areas and may be known by various other titles across the country, such as EMT-P or MICP (paramedic), EMT-C (cardiac) EMT-T (trauma), EMT II and so forth. Preparation and certification of personnel for the role of EMT paramedic are not yet standardized. Wide variation exists from state to state and, in some states, from county to county. To complicate matters more, various communities have developed programs to train EMTs to a level somewhere between the EMT-1 and paramedic, and these emergency care providers are given yet another title. As an example, the paramedic, or MICP, represents the highest level of EMT training in California; however, the EMT II can provide some paramedic level procedures, but not all of them. Such labels are confusing, not only to a community's citizens, but to other professionals in emergency care.

A standard curriculum for paramedic training—the National Training Course–has been developed for the U.S. Department of Transportation, which should help to standardize the training and certification of these persons across the country. Upon completion of this curriculum, the EMT-paramedic should be competent to do the following:

- Recognize a medical emergency, assess the situation, manage emergency care and light extrication, and direct and coordinate paramedic efforts with those of other agencies at the scene
- Make an appropriate assessment, assign priorities of emergency treatment, and record and communicate data to the designated medical command authority or other responsible physician
- Initiate and continue emergency medical care under medical telecommunications control, including (1) recognizing and initiating appropriate invasive and noninvasive treatments for conditions such as life-threatening arrhythmias, shock, psychological crises, airway and respiratory problems, and trauma, and (2) assessing and reporting the response of the patient to this treatment and initiating appropriate changes as required under physician direction
- Function according to standing orders when telecommunications equipment cannot be used and exercise personal judgment in treating or stabilizing the patient based on usual and customary practice in the community
- Direct and coordinate patient transport by selecting the best available method(s) after approval of medical command authority
- Record details of the incident and the patient's emergency care
- Direct the maintenance and preparation of emergency care equipment and supplies.

(National Training Course, Emergency Medical Technician: Paramedic Course Guide. Washington, D.C., U.S. Department of Transportation, pp 2–3)

The distinguishing features of advanced EMT preparation consist in the paramedic's ability to do the following:
1. Monitor and interpret cardiac arrhythmias and treat them with appropriate medications and defibrillation
2. Use esophageal airways and/or endotracheal intubation for airway management

3. Perform venipuncture and begin intravenous infusions with selected solutions
4. Administer selected medications
5. Assume control of medical care at the scene of an emergency with approval of medical care authority

The training program extends 120 to 180 hours beyond EMT-1 training. Many training programs are much longer. Training should include classroom instruction in theory, clinical instruction with supervised practice of emergency medical skills, and a field internship in which the candidate's performance is critically evaluated. Recertification must occur periodically, usually every 2 to 3 years, according to the criteria determined by the community or state in which the paramedic is employed. This usually involves continuing education activities, continuous service as a paramedic, and successful performance on examinations of theoretical competence and practical skills.

COORDINATING ROLES OF EMS PROFESSIONALS

Communications

Basic to the function of any activity involving more than one person is the effective exchange of information—in other words, good communications. Emergency personnel within and outside of the hospital setting have specific obligations regarding communications, which may be described as follows:

1. *Hospital personnel should seek information from prehospital personnel.* This conveys the following messages:
   - Prehospital personnel are important and you value their assessments and care of the patients.
   - You expect adequate assessments and appropriate care to be given in the field.
   - What has happened prior to the patient's arrival is important baseline information.
   - Mutual learning and sharing of experiences promote growth in each professional and ultimately better team function and patient care.

2. *Hospital personnel should expect good verbal and written reports from prehospital personnel.* Communication skills must be nurtured and developed. Communicating assessment information and interpreting what has been said over a two-way radio is not easy; doing so consistently well represents a challenge. These skills require much practice and frequent discussions between the transmitter and receiver after the patient is received by the hospital. Moreover, it is worthwhile to ride with the ambulance personnel and transmit patient assessment information to the hospital ED.

3. *Prehospital personnel must be assertive in obtaining information* needed for optimal patient care during transport. Diligence in acquiring information from family, friends, and bystanders can be of great help to the EMT and to the receiving hospital personnel. In transfer situations, patient information must be obtained from hospital personnel in order to give appropriate care during transport. If this information is not volunteered, it must be sought.

4. *All personnel should become comfortable with telecommunications equipment and the communications vocabulary used in the community.* It is human nature to avoid anything one is not comfortable with—telecom-

munications equipment is commonly avoided by staff members.

5. *Communications responsibilities include discharge teaching and conveying information to the persons receiving the patient.* In addition to receiving and interpreting information, staff members must also *convey* relevant information clearly.

Discharge planning and teaching require instructional, communication, and interviewing skills, awareness of community and hospital resources, appreciation of socioeconomic and cultural influences on the patient, and knowledge of how to use patient and/or family feedback to determine whether instructions are understood and can be followed. Determining whether the patient understands what has been taught is often neglected. To verify this, note whether the patient can do the following:

- Tell in his own words what you have explained to him about his illness
- Tell how he plans to carry out his medical regime
- Identify secondary problems that may affect his ability to implement the medical regime
- Show that he sees the value of follow-up care and is committed to making and keeping follow-up appointments.

If the patient is able to do the above, discharge teaching has been effective.

Conveying information clearly to personnel who will be assuming the care of the patient is necessary to provide continuity of care. The patient who is transferred from the mobile unit to the hospital or from one facility to another should be accompanied by well-documented records. Presenting a concise report of the patient's status and the treatment received while in your care eases the transition from one place to another and promotes good public relations.

Prior to discharge from the ED, the nonadmitted patient should be given specific information in the form of verbal or written instructions pertinent to further care. Appropriate referral to his private physician or clinic must be made to ensure continuity of care.

Follow-up hospital visits are an excellent means for evaluating the care the patient received while in your care and for building relationships with the staff who commonly receive emergency patients.

Related Activities

Activities that can contribute to preventing "burn-out," broadening interdisciplinary understanding, maintaining

skills, facilitating care, and improving relations with the community should be encouraged.

Clinical and Field Rotation. Working in other patient care settings that relate to the ED enables hospital personnel to develop an appreciation and respect for what others do; to establish rapport; to learn how to make others' work easier; and to broaden their own knowledge and skills. Some staff members resist rotation because of their own insecurities about functioning in new or unfamiliar patient care areas. Others welcome the change—as an authorized time-out from a situation that can produce burn-out. In base-station hospitals, MICN candidates and emergency physicians may be required to participate in patient care in mobile emergency care units. Extending patient care beyond the walls of the ED has resulted in better, more comprehensive patient care and improved relationships with prehospital personnel.

Continuing Education. Participation in continuing education and in-service programs is a mandate for many because of state regulations tied to relicensure and recertification. Educational programs should involve nurses, physicians, and staff as well as prehospital emergency personnel and should be geared to broaden the knowledge and sharpen the technical skills of all. Both patients and staff benefit from a well-informed, challenged emergency care team, and staff members feel more competent and content when they are growing with their jobs.

Community Service. It is important to serve on community committees and in organizations that help improve the delivery of emergency medical care. Often decisions about emergency care are made without any input from the professionals primarily affected. This is not intentional but occurs because their opinions are neither sought nor offered. Representatives from all parts of the emergency care team must be involved at the community level when decisions are made that affect them and their patients. It is also essential to know your community's resources and use them. No one person or facility can be everything to everyone. Certainly, some institutions provide a large number of services, but none to the extent that it completely serves its community. Volunteer self-help organizations, crisis hotlines, community clinics, nonacute transport services, all-night drug stores—the list of resources that emergency patients need is endless. In addition, when you've run out of appropriate available resources, know whom to call for help.

BIBLIOGRAPHY

EMERGENCY MEDICAL SERVICES SYSTEMS

1. American College of Surgeons Committee on Trauma: Field categorization of trauma patients and hospital trauma index. Bull Am Coll Surg 65:28, 1980
2. American College of Surgeons Committee on Trauma: Hospital resources for optimal care of the injured patient. Bull Am Coll Surg 64, 1979
3. American College of Surgeons Committee on Trauma: Interhospital transfer of patients. Bull Am Coll Surg 65:13, 1980
4. American College of Surgeons Committee on Trauma: Quality assurance and education in the emergency department. Bull Am Coll Surg 65:23, 1980

5. American College of Surgeons Committee on Trauma: Verification program for hospital. Bull Am Coll Surg 65:23, 1980
6. Boyd DR: Trauma: A controllable disease in the 1980s. J Trauma 20:14, 1980
7. Cosgriff JH Jr: Response to the crisis in emergency care. NY State J Med 73:2366, 1973
8. Dove DB, Stahl WM, DelGuercio LRM: A five-year review of deaths following urban trauma. J Trauma 20:760, 1980
9. Gann DS et al: Panel: Current status of emergency medical services. J Trauma 21:196, 1981
10. Joint Commission on Accreditation of Hospitals: Emergency

Services. Accreditation Manual for Hospitals '81. Chicago, Joint Commission on Accreditation of Hospitals, 1980

11. National Academy of Sciences/National Research Council: Accidental Death and Disability: The Neglected Disease of Modern Society. Washington, D.C., National Academy of Sciences/National Research Council, 1966
12. Pantridge JF: Mobile coronary care. Chest 58:229, 1970
13. West JG, Trunkey DD, Lim RC: Systems of trauma care: A study of two counties. Arch Surg 114:455, 1979

DISASTER PREPAREDNESS

14. Accreditation Manual for Hospital, 1981, p 46–7. Chicago, Joint Commission on Accreditation of Hospital, 1981
15. Crooks L, Corn M, DeAtley C: Disaster planning: A team effort. AORN J 28:395–410, 1978
16. Eiseman B, Bond V: Surgical Care of Nuclear Casualties. Surg Gynecol Obstet 146:877–883, 1978
17. Evans RF: Major disasters: The patient with multiple injuries. Br J Hosp Med 4:329–332, 1979
18. Hargreaves A et al: Blizzard '78: Dealing with disaster. Am J Nurs pp 268–271, 1979
19. Henry S: Mississauga Hospital: Largest evacuation in Canada's history. CMA Journal 122:582–586, 1980
20. Holloway RD, Steliga JF, Ryan CT: The EMS system and disaster planning: Some observations. JACEP 7:2, 1978
21. Patterson C., Rowbottom B: Explosion! A case study in disaster drills. 3:9–19, 1977
22. Yates DW: Major disasters: Surgical triage. Br J Hosp Med 4:323–328, 1979

THE EMERGENCY CARE TEAM

23. Standards of Emergency Nursing Practice. American Nurses' Association and EDNA, 1975

24. Anwar RAH: Trends in training: Focus on emergency medicine. Ann Emerg Med 9:60–71, 1980
25. Brown LL: The emergency department at the bedside? A case for crisis follow-up. RN pp 48–58, 1977
26. Chapman A, Harvey A: Making sure the patient understands discharge planning: Nurse in the emergency department. J Emerg Nurs pp 33–36, 1976
27. Continuing Education Core Curriculum. EDNA, 1980
28. Finke MK: Emergency nursing: The backbone of the emergency department. In Warner CG: Emergency Care: Assessment and Intervention, 2nd ed. St Louis, CV Mosby, 1978
29. Gibson G: States of urban services. Hospitals 45:49–54, 1971
30. Goldfrank L et al: The emergency services physician assistant: Result of two years' experience. Ann Emerg Med 9:96–99, 1980
31. Greenfield S et al: Efficiency and cost of primary care by nurses and physicians' assistants. N Engl J Med 298:305–309, 1978
32. Hardy VGS: The emergency nurse practitioner: The role and training of an emergency health professional. JACEP 7:372–376, 1978
33. Krome R: The emergency physician. Emerg Med Services 6:109, 1977
34. Levinson D: Sounding board: Roles, tasks and practitioners. N Engl J Med 296:1291–1293, 1977
35. Lowry JW, Lauro AJ: A general EMS curriculum for residency training. Ann Emerg Med 9:250–252, 1980
36. McDade JP: The ABEM certification examination: A brief review. Ann Emerg Med 9:276, 1980
37. National Training Course, Emergency Medical Technician: Paramedic Course Guide. Washington, D.C., U.S. Department of Transportation/National Highway Traffic Safety Administration (DOT HS 802 437)
38. Page JR: The physician and EMS. Ann Emerg Med 10:64, 1981
39. Perry HB III: An analysis of the professional performance of physician's assistant. J Med Educ 52:639–647, 1977
40. Podgorny G: Emergency physician assistants: An important adjunct. Ann Emerg Med 9:109, 1980
41. Wackerle JF et al: The emergency nurse as a primary health care provider: A retrospective study. J Emerg Nurs 3:21–25, 1977

2
LEGAL ASPECTS OF EMERGENCY MEDICAL CARE

JO ANN CAHILL

Emergency personnel practice in an environment that is in a state of continual change. This mutability is in fact the nature of emergency care and the reason why many have chosen it for their careers. As roles expand and change, emergency personnel are becoming increasingly aware of the legal implications of emergency care.

With few exceptions, each step of emergency intervention is associated in some way with a legal precept. However, rather than approach the patient as a potential legal problem, one should view the situation as one in which the objective is intervention resulting in the reversal of disease processes and the maintenance of health. With this as the ultimate objective, legal implications become peripheral factors addressed in the normal course of patient care.

This chapter begins with a discussion of general principles and fundamentals of law that are essential to an understanding of more specific issues. These concepts have application in all areas of practice and form the basis of the legal implications of patient care. Adherence to these basic principles, irrespective of one's knowledge in the more specific area of emergency care, will be a most important factor when legal liability is considered. The major portion of the chapter is devoted to the legal aspects of direct patient care. In conclusion, the legal issues relating to emergency department management and personnel supervision are briefly discussed.

The concepts presented in this chapter relate to *general* legal considerations encountered in emergency care. Individual states and localities have specific laws and regulations that have an impact on the delivery of emergency care, and these should be familiar to the personnel affected by them.

GENERAL PRINCIPLES AND FUNDAMENTALS OF LAW

Throughout the discussion of the legal implications of emergency care, the yardstick against which actions are to be measured is *reasonable care*. It is only when one does not adhere to principles of patient care that are reasonable that legal difficulties may arise. Emergency care personnel are legally liable for harm resulting from their negligent acts or failure to meet a standard of reasonable care and competence. Their status as employees of a hospital or other agency does not relieve them of individual legal responsibility for their actions.[1]

STANDARD OF CARE

The index that the law has developed is called the standard of care. The standard of care is determined by deciding what a reasonably prudent professional acting under similar circumstances would have done.

Negligence. A professional who fails to adhere to the standard of care may be open to a charge of negligence. *Negligence* can be defined as the failure to do something that

a reasonable person, guided by the considerations that ordinarily regulate human affairs, would do or as doing something that a reasonable and prudent person would not do.[2]

Malpractice. Malpractice is negligence committed by a professional. More specifically, *malpractice* is the failure of a physician or nurse to apply the degree of skill and learning in treating and nursing a patient that is customarily applied in the same community in treating and caring for those suffering similarly.[3] Recently, this community measurement has been expanded to more general national boundaries.

It is clear that professionals are not expected to perform above and beyond the standard of care. The nurse, for example, is not expected to be a "super nurse" or lay-attorney; yet the patient is protected. Professionals should strive to achieve the highest possible level of care for their patients.

RESPONSIBILITIES AND RELATIONSHIPS

Responsibility to the Patient

The nurse's responsibility to the patient supersedes, within reasonable limits, other relationships—namely, that between the hospital and the physician. If this principle is applied, the patient should receive good, safe care.

Responsibility for Oneself

An extension of the concept of responsibility to the patient is responsibility for oneself. Irrespective of other persons or agencies that may also be held liable for the actions of one professional, the professional is never exempted from responsibility for himself. A case in point is that of *Darling* v. *Charleston Memorial Hospital:*

> A young man of 18 broke his leg while playing football. He was taken to the emergency department where the physician applied a plaster cast. Not long after admission, the patient's toes became painful, swollen, and dark, eventually becoming cold and insensitive. On the next and subsequent two days, the cast was notched, trimmed, and split. In the course of cutting the cast, the patient's leg was cut. Blood and other drainage were observed by the nurse. After transfer to another facility several days later, the leg was amputated eight inches below the knee. Action was brought against the defendant hospital. On the basis of evidence, it was concluded that the nurses did not test for circulation as frequently as necessary and that skilled nurses would have promptly recognized the conditions that signalled a dangerous impairment of circulation in the patient's leg and known that the condition would become irreversible in a matter of hours. At that point, it becomes the nurse's duty to inform the attending physician, and if he fails to act, to advise the hospital authorities so that appropriate action may be taken.[4]

The Darling opinion posits a responsibility on the part of the hospital toward the patient, in addition to that on the part of the physician. However, hospital personnel should be considered agents of the hospital. Their actions, or lack of actions, reflect on the institution.

Respondeat Superior: Responsibility of the Employer

Failure to exercise the duty to bring appropriate matters before the proper authorities will lead to liability not only of professionals themselves, but also of the employing agency, under the legal doctrine of respondeat superior. This holds the employer responsible for the legal consequences of the acts of the employee while acting within the scope of employment, even though the employer's conduct is without fault. This doctrine does not absolve the employee. As a matter of fact, not only may the injured party sue the employee directly, but the employer may seek recovery from the employee as a result of being held liable for the employee's wrongful act.

SCOPE OF PRACTICE

Errors of commission constitute as serious a concern as errors of omission. It is possible that some emergency care activities infringe upon the area of medical practice. This question has been raised repeatedly in regard to nursing practice in special care units and in emergency departments. If a nurse engages in activities beyond the legally recognized scope of practice, she or he runs the risk of violating the state's medical and nursing practice acts. Paramedics who initiate medical treatments outside of established protocols or medical supervision incur the same risk. The critical issue related to scope of practice problems is determining the nature and range of judgment assigned to the professional. If a professional follows medically established guidelines or protocols applicable to specific situations that she or he, by virtue of specialized training or experience, is qualified to recognize, then she or he is not engaging in the illegal practice of medicine.

NURSE PRACTICE ACTS

Because of questions related to scope of practice, many states have revised their nurse practice acts to include a broader range of activity within the law and eliminate attempts to maintain an artificial division between nursing practice and medical practice. The trend is toward recognizing the individual's competence in light of education and experience to fulfill responsibilities without increasing risk to patients. For example, the California Nurse Practice Act allows the following:

> observation of signs and symptoms of illness, reactions to treatment, general behavior, or general physical condition, and (1) determination of whether such signs, symptoms, reactions, behavior, or general appearance exhibit abnormal characteristics; and (2) implementation, based on observed abnormalities, of appropriate reporting, or referral, or standardized procedures or changes in treatment regimen in accordance with standardized procedures, or the initiation of emergency procedures.[5]

Emergency Nursing Standards

The American Nurses' Association and the Emergency Department Nurses' Association have defined emergency nursing in this introduction to their Standards:

> Emergency nursing practice is the nursing care of individuals of all ages with perceived physical and/or emotional alterations which are undiagnosed and may require prompt intervention. Emergency nursing care is unscheduled and most commonly

occurs in a specific care setting, *i.e.,* an emergency department, a mobile unit, or a suicide prevention center. Thus, the nursing care is episodic, primary, and acute in nature.

> The scope of emergency nursing practice encompasses nursing activities which are directed toward health problems of various levels of complexity. A rapidly changing physiological and/or psychological status, which may be life-threatening, requires assessment of the severity of the health problem, definitive intervention, on-going reassessment, and supportive care to significant others. The level of physiological and/or psychological complexity may require life-support measures, appropriate health education, and referral. The scope of emergency nursing practice not only encompasses nursing activities which are directed toward the health problems presented by individuals, but also encompasses knowledge of and the observance of legal aspects, such as reporting an incident to appropriate governmental agencies, *i.e.,* police or public health departments, when a situation calls for such action. Emergency nursing practice is affected by the brevity of patient interaction with the nurse, the stressful climate created by lack of control over the numbers of individuals seeking emergency care, and the limited time frame in which to evaluate the effectiveness of intervention.[6]

Professional Liability Insurance

Rising levels of responsibility and the expanding scope of practice are becoming legally recognized and protected. Increasing responsibility entails an increase in accountability, which makes it necessary to consider the general issue of professional liability insurance.

There is no question that those who sue "go after the big money," and under respondeat superior, protection is usually provided by the employer. However, with the long overdue increase in the status of the nursing profession, we may see this trend changing. Emergency nurses should carefully investigate their agencies' policies, and even if covered, consider personal professional liability insurance. Emergency department nursing has been identified as one of the eight major problem areas related to malpractice loss.[7] It is becoming increasingly common in some areas of the United States to sue for the slightest cause. Careful, reasonable care of patients is the nurse's, as well as the patient's best protection, but it can be very costly to prove one's innocence.

LEGAL ASPECTS OF PREHOSPITAL PATIENT CARE

Good Samaritan Laws

Unavoidable circumstances sometimes call for the practice of emergency care outside of the hospital. Thus, many states have enacted Good Samaritan legislation which protects physicians, nurses, and others from liability in *ordinary* negligence when intervening in an emergency situation outside of the usual setting, for example, the roadway. These statutes do not eliminate liability for *gross* negligence but are applicable, provided that care was rendered in good faith, based on the judgment that the situation constituted an emergency. Defining an emergency, of course, is the difficult question, and considering it in retrospect may produce a different judgment.

Definition of an Emergency. A basic definition of an emergency, taken from instructions given to juries consid-

---

Chart 2-1

DEFINITION OF AN EMERGENCY

An emergency is an unforeseen combination of circumstances creating a condition which in the professional judgment of a physician and surgeon of good standing acting under the same or similar circumstances requires immediate care, treatment, or surgery in order to protect a person's life or health.[8]

(From instructions given to juries considering malpractice cases)

---

ering malpractice cases, is provided in Chart 2-1. The determination that a particular set of facts constitutes an emergency is legally correct only when it can be shown that reasonable and prudent persons would have reached the same decision under the same or similar circumstances.[9]

Mobile Intensive Care

In an effort to extend emergency care and provide previously unavailable medical care, many communities have instituted mobile intensive care programs. Accompanying these programs are new statutes that define roles, describe responsibility and reporting structure, regulate training, and delineate permitted treatment and liability. For example, in the California Health and Safety Code, the following is found:

> No physician or nurse who in good faith gives emergency instructions to a mobile intensive care paramedic at the scene of an emergency shall be liable for any civil damages as a result of issuing the instructions.[10]

Nurse Practitioner and Physician's Assistant

A relatively new and legally untested area of emergency care pertains to the nurse practitioner and physician's assistant. States are in the process of defining these roles and will determine standards of care and scope of practice. Those who practice in these roles and those who interact with practitioners and physician's assistants should have a clear understanding of the legal responsibilities and restrictions placed on them by their states, preceptors, and agencies.

LEGAL ASPECTS OF PATIENT CARE IN THE HOSPITAL SETTING

STANDARDS OF CARE FOR INSTITUTIONS

Just as nurses, physicians, and other professionals have standards of care with which they must comply, so do hospitals and other agencies. Among the applicable national regulations are the standards of the Joint Commission on Accreditation of Hospitals (JCAH) and the Medicare Conditions of Participation (see Chart 2-2).

Standards are also set by professional organizations such as the American College of Surgeons and the American College of Emergency Physicians and by individual states and local communities. Examples are individual states' Health and Safety Codes that affect staffing, equipment, and back-up services.

In addition to the more general standards, facilities maintain policies and procedures that constitute self-imposed standards. It is especially important that nurses play a large role in establishing policies and procedures in the emergency department. They should set a high standard of care for the protection of the patient, one that is not impossible to attain or maintain. Job descriptions should be included. Whatever the standard, whether recognized statewide or only within one's own facility, a deviation from this standard may lead to renewed negligence. Emergency department standards, policies, and management procedures are discussed in detail at the end of this chapter.

DUTY TO TREAT/RIGHT TO TREATMENT

Is there a duty to treat all who request emergency care? The law is not universally consistent on this issue, and each situation must be dealt with individually. However, the legal attitude that has evolved in recent years is that if a hospital maintains an emergency service, those in need may assume that emergency care will be available to them. The statutes of some states have specific references for this issue. Note the following example from the California Health and Safety Code:

> Emergency services and care shall be provided to any person requesting such service or care, or for whom such service or care is requested, for any condition in which the person is in

---

Chart 2-2

EXCERPTS FROM MEDICARE CONDITIONS OF PARTICIPATION: STANDARDS THAT APPLY TO PROFESSIONALS IN THE EMERGENCY DEPARTMENT[11]

Standard A. Factor 3. The emergency service is supervised by a qualified member of the medical staff and nursing functions are the responsibility of a registered professional nurse.

Standard C. Factor 1. The medical staff is responsible for insuring adequate medical coverage for emergency services.

Standard C. Factor 2. A physician sees all patients who arrive for treatment in the emergency service.

Standard C. Factor 4. Qualified nurses are available on duty at all times, and in sufficient numbers to deal with the number and extent of emergency services.

---

danger of loss of life, or serious injury or illness, at any health facility licensed under this chapter that maintains and operates an emergency department to provide emergency services to the public when such health facility has appropriate facilities and qualified personnel available to provide such services of care.

Neither the health facility, its employees, nor any physician, dentist, or podiatrist shall be held liable in any action arising out of a refusal to render emergency services or care if reasonable care is exercised in determining the condition of the person, or in determining the appropriateness of the facilities and the qualifications and availability of personnel to render such services.

Emergency services and care shall be rendered without first questioning the patient or any other person about his ability to pay therefor, provided that the patient or his legally responsible relative or guardian shall execute an agreement to pay therefor or otherwise supply insurance or credit information promptly after the services are rendered.

If a health facility subject to the provisions of this chapter does not maintain an emergency department, its employees shall nevertheless exercise reasonable care to determine whether an emergency exists and shall direct the patient to a nearby facility which can render the needed service including transportation services, in every way reasonable under the circumstances.[12]

The question is how to determine what an emergency situation is. The courts may hold that if a hospital maintains an emergency department, refusing care to a person in a true emergency may be cause for liability when such refusal causes injury. The following case is an important example of liability predicated on the refusal of services to a patient in an unmistakable emergency; two other examples are also cited.

An infant was taken to the emergency department with a history of temperature elevation and diarrhea. The nurse informed the parents that the hospital could not give treatment because the child was being medicated by a private physician and that medicine prescribed by the hospital might conflict with that of the physician. She did not examine the infant, but she did try, without success, to communicate with the private physician and instructed the parents to return to the pediatric clinic the next day. The parents took the child home, where, during the night, he died of bronchial pneumonia. The court refused to grant a summary judgment for the hospital and said the question was whether the nurse's decision to deny the infant an examination was within the reasonable limits of judgment of a nurse, or whether she did not discharge her duty in not recognizing an emergency when it was presented to her.[13]

In another case, a man who belonged to a prepaid hospital plan came to the emergency department of a hospital which had no relationship with the plan. He complained of severe chest pain radiating to his arms. The nurse on duty stated that the hospital did not take care of plan members, but did call a plan doctor, who told him to return when the plan clinic was open. After this exchange, the nurse refused to locate another doctor, whereupon the man went home and died before any further help could be summoned. An appeal court reversed the trial court's verdict for the hospital and said that there was a question as to whether the plan physician and the nurse who failed to obtain further help were negligent.[14]

Equality in availability of treatment for all is demonstrated in a judgment against a hospital who refused care to foreign parents who brought their burned children to the hospital for emergency treatment.[15]

It thus appears that for the legal health of the institution and, most importantly, for the health of the patient, hospitals that have emergency departments should maintain a policy of treatment for all. If there is a deviation from this philosophy, for the protection of the professionals staffing the emergency department, a clearly stated protocol should be drawn up by the hospital administration and reviewed by hospital's attorneys.

ADMISSION TO HOSPITAL

The issue of the emergency department's responsibility in the admission of patients into the hospital for further treatment also needs to be addressed. The following two cases are examples of how the courts considered refusal to admit from the emergency department:

After a car accident, a patient sustained an injury to his leg. He developed permanent footdrop after having been appropriately treated at one emergency department and transferred for admission to another hospital because he had no health insurance. He claimed that the cause of his disability had been the transferring hospital, but the court held for the hospital, stating that his injury had been irreversibly caused by the trauma, and not by the fact that he had been refused admission.[16]

In another case, a judgment was handed down in appeal against a hospital when the administrator refused admission to a patient with a diagnosis of frostbite of both feet. Apparently, the patient was unable to pay a $25 admission fee. The court held that the institution "was the only hospital in the immediate area, it maintained an emergency service, and plaintiff applied for emergency treatment and was refused, and that the members of the public had reason to rely on the hospital, and in this case, it could be found that plaintiff's condition was caused to be worsened by the delay resulting from the futile efforts to obtain treatment from the hospital."[17]

Consider also patients inappropriately transferred when their condition indicates an alternative course of action. A case in point:

A patient was brought to the emergency department with a gunshot wound of the thigh. No effort was made to control the bleeding by the nurses who examined him. After blood 30 inches in diameter formed around the wound, the patient was transferred at the order of the physician to another facility where he died from hypovolemic shock. The court ruled against the hospital, "holding that a hospital giving emergency treatment is obliged to do what is immediately necessary to preserve the life and health of the patient."[18]

The courts permit the transfer of patients to other facilities for admission, but only when the patient is medically stable and transported in a safe manner with appropriate personnel and equipment.

CONSENTS

There is a tendency to complicate the issue of consents. However, if considered reasonably, with the good of the patient in mind, consent need not be a problem. Generally speaking, treatment of the patient without consent is considered assault. People have the right to determine what is done with their own bodies. It is important, therefore, to obtain consent prior to treatment. It is not necessary to get a signature on the hospital's consent form, although it is preferable and the simplest form of documentation. Verbal consent and consent implied by the actions of the patient who knowingly accepts treatment should be documented on the chart.

Treatment Without Consent

Because of the nature of emergency care, some patients are unable to give consent before treatment. Consent in this setting is *implied,* that is, the professional can make the assumption that were the patient able, consent for treatment would be given in order to maintain health. To do otherwise might result in loss of life or a serious permanent disability and would not be considered reasonable.

Minors

The treatment of minors is regulated by individual states. Consent from a parent or legal guardian is required in treating a minor. The question of intervention in the absence of consent from a parent is always affected by judgment about the urgency of the patient's presenting problem. Only the physician should make this judgment, and in many cases, consultation is advised so that there is documentation of more than one medical opinion. It is also recommended that the efforts of the emergency department staff to locate the parent or guardian be noted on the chart. The age of 18 is usually considered the age of majority.

Some states allow minors who are emancipated to consent for their own treatment. Examples of emancipation may include the following:

- Minors on duty with the United States armed forces
- Minors receiving pregnancy care (excluding treatment not related to pregnancy)
- Minors requesting abortion
- Minors living apart from their parent or legal guardian and managing their own affairs
- Minors suffering from a reportable communicable disease (excluding treatment not related to the disease)
- Minors who have been married

Refusal of Consent

The situation in which medical intervention is required to preserve the life of a minor and the parent refuses is sensitive. The most desirable course of action is persuasion by medical personnel so that the parent will change his or her mind. However, in the event of failure, a court order allowing medical treatment may be necessary. Every emergency department should have vital information accessible for this purpose.

Similarly, a patient may refuse to consent to treatment or may rescind consent previously given. This presents difficulties for professionals who feel they know what is best for the patient. Adults who are conscious and mentally competent have the right to refuse any medical or surgical procedure. This refusal must be honored whether it is based on possible result, lack of confidence in the physician, religious beliefs, or no reason at all.[19]

When a patient refused a blood transfusion, the hospital requested authorization to perform the procedure in spite of the patient's refusal. The court held that a competent adult's wishes concerning his or her person must be honored. It was recognized that refusal of the transfusion might cause death, but the court would not authorize the treatment, saying that a competent individual has the right to make this decision, even though it may seem unreasonable to the medical experts.[20]

Some states differ from this opinion when there is concern for the welfare of the children of a critically ill patient or when the state recognizes a compelling interest in protecting the life of its citizens.[21,22]

The situation becomes even less clear when the patient's mental competence becomes questionable, especially under the influence of injury or illness. For example, a patient may refuse treatment because of hypoxia or alcohol and drug abuse. These cases should be considered individually, always with the well-being of the patient in mind, and when appropriate, the hospital's attorney should be consulted.

Another potential modifier of the ability to give consent is the administration of a narcotic for relief of pain. Because this might occur before a consent is secured, the professional should make every effort to ensure that the patient understands the proposed course of action and should document accordingly. Depending on the urgency of the emergency situation, staff members should make the effort to obtain consent before medication is administered.

When a patient refuses treatment contrary to the advice and recommendation of the physician, a form should be signed by the patient. If the patient will not sign a release of responsibility, the refusal of the treatment and the refusal to sign should be documented on the chart and preferably witnessed by two staff members.

The issue of informed consent in the emergency department is as yet untested. As part of the theory of reasonableness, there is a duty to disclose within reason any available therapeutic modalities that the patient may choose, if able, as well as inherent and potential dangers of the treatment. As was mentioned previously, circumstances may hamper the patient's ability to give informed consent (*i.e.,* unconsciousness).

Special Consents/Law Enforcement

In addition to consent for treatment, there is the question of consent for specific procedures requested by law enforcement agencies for evidence. If blood and urine are taken from a patient for legal purposes without consent, the patient can claim battery. In many states, possession of a driver's license implies consent on the part of the driver for analysis of blood, breath, and urine when he or she is taken into custody for alleged intoxication. However, this does not preclude the driver from withdrawing his consent. In other states, the driver may refuse consent for such tests, but refusal may result in revocation of the license.

In one case, when the defendant had not consented to the procedure, the court held that the results of a blood test were admissible as evidence and did not violate the defendant's right against self-incrimination. In addition, it was held that because the procedure was performed according to acceptable medical standards by a competent person, it met the test of reasonableness.[23]

The question of liability of emergency department staff, however, is not so clear. Although the court ruled that such evidence does not violate the driver's constitutional rights, the hospital itself might be liable for battery.[24]

Some states protect hospitals and their employees from liability resulting from obtaining a blood sample at the request of a police officer. The vehicle code of the State of California is an example:

> No physician, registered nurse, licensed vocational nurse, or duly licensed clinical laboratory technologist or clinical laboratory bioanalyst or hospital, laboratory or clinic employing or utilizing the services of such physician, registered nurse, licensed vocational nurse, or duly licensed laboratory technologist or clinical laboratory bioanalyst owning or leasing the premises on which such tests are performed, shall incur any civil or criminal liability as a result of the proper administering of a blood test when requested in writing by a peace officer to administer such a test.[25]

Emergency personnel are cautioned that whenever an action is taken without consent in this matter, battery may be claimed. There should be an emergency department policy and procedure written in conformity to state law.

REPORTING AND RELEASING INFORMATION

Confidentiality

Every patient who presents for treatment in the emergency department has the right to expect that information about his or her presenting complaint, course of treatment, diagnosis, and disposition is confidential. Information divulged without consent that results in injury to the patient may result in liability for damages against the person releasing the information.

Because of the nature of emergency care, there are circumstances in which confidentiality of information is affected by other factors, such as the position of the person in the community. A person whose activity is a matter of public record or whose livelihood depends on being kept in the public eye may forfeit, to an indefinable degree, the rights of privacy generally ascribed to a less prominent person. In these cases, general information such as name and condition may be released to the press. It is advisable, however, that the patient concur in the release of information. Similarly, information may be released when a disaster has occurred.

In order to maintain a set standard and to simplify the situation for the staff, it is recommended that no information be released from the emergency department itself. A designated person should be kept informed about the status of the patient, and all press inquiries should be referred to that person.

Many states have rules that require confidentiality about psychiatric patients, irrespective of other factors.[26]

Mandatory Reporting

The other issue involving the emergency patient's right to privacy is the mandatory reporting of specific disease entities and injuries and of death under certain circumstances. The usual tenets of confidentiality may be modified when the general good of the public requires the disclosure of confidential information. In this instance, the principle of the general good supersedes the patient's right to privacy. Agencies that may require information include the department of health, the local police authority, the department of motor vehicles, the welfare department, and the coroner. Examples

of diseases and other matters that may fall under the rules of reporting are the following:

- Communicable diseases
- Diseases characterized by lapse of consciousness
- Pesticide illness
- Abuse in nursing facilities
- Poisoning
- Drug abuse
- Attempted suicide
- Injuries inflicted by violence (including sexual assault, gunshot wounds, and stabbings)
- Illegal abortion
- Animal bites
- Motor vehicle accidents
- Deaths of a suspicious nature
- Radiation contamination
- Nonaccidental injuries to children

Child Abuse. Because of the seeming increase in the incidence of child abuse, or perhaps the increase in the reporting of it, amplification of this subject is justified. Emergency departments are the primary portals of entry for children who have been abused. It is probable that the emergency department personnel may represent the only chance for intervention that a child may have. For this reason, many states have enacted strict laws that protect not only the child but also the reporting individual. The following excerpt from the penal code of the state of California is an example:

> No person shall incur any civil or criminal liability as a result of making any report authorized by this section unless it can be proven that a false report was made and the person knew that the report was false.[27]

As a matter of fact, failure to report may result in a misdemeanor in addition to other legal liability.

The role of the physician, nurses, and hospital in child abuse reporting can be illustrated by the following case:

> After having been repeatedly beaten by her mother's common-law husband, 11-month-old G. L. was taken to a local emergency department. She was found to have a comminuted fracture of the right tibia and fibula, plus multiple bruises and abrasions on other parts of her body. The mother did not offer an explanation. There was no indication that the physician had considered a diagnosis of child abuse. No further x-rays were taken (which would have shown a linear skull fracture) and the incident was not reported to law authorities. The child was released into the same environment from which she came. Two months later, G. L. was taken to another hospital, suffering from traumatic blows to her right eye and back, puncture wounds on her left leg, and severe bites on her back. She also had third-degree burns on her left hand. This time, the child was correctly diagnosed as abused and taken into protective custody after appropriate reporting by the second hospital. The first hospital, for the action of the doctor as its agent, was held liable for failing to report child abuse, causing the child to be returned to her home, resulting in further injuries to the child due to lack of intervention.[28]

Although the nurse's responsibility when the physician does not report has never been tested, emergency nurses are reminded that they are responsible for their own actions and may be held liable, irrespective of the actions or responsibilities of others.

PROTECTION OF PATIENTS' PROPERTY

A practical as well as a legal problem in the emergency department is the disposition of the patient's possessions. This is a common cause of monetary claims against hospitals. Not only is the nurse responsible for any act of negligence involving a patient's property, but as an agent of the hospital she may subject her employer to liability as well. A procedure for the safekeeping of the patient's goods while he is in the department should be available. When a patient deposits personal property with another, a *bailment* is created. The description and disposition of the property should be carefully documented and signatures of receipt required. Only the owner of the property may decide its disposition. The nurse may be held liable if loss or injury results when property is given to another without permission.

Physical Evidence/Chain of Possession

Chain of evidence is important because many lawsuits hinge on the proper maintenance of evidence retrieved from patients seen in the emergency department. A most important consideration in evidence is the chain of possession. It is essential to maintain records that document the chain of possession of specimens recovered in order that they may constitute usable evidence. Attorneys must be able to trace back a particular object from the human source. For example, a retrieved weapon can be considered a specimen for the pathology laboratory or given directly to a police officer. In either case, careful documentation of the area of retrieval, the person who made the retrieval, and the individual who accepted the object must be noted. Receipts should be obtained for all items. All objects should be meticulously handled in order to avoid distortion or disturbance. (See Chap. 3, Forensic Aspects) Evidence in cases of sexual assault is extremely important. (See Chap. 7, Sexual Assault.)

SPECIAL CONSIDERATIONS IN EMERGENCY DEPARTMENT MANAGEMENT

STAFFING

The patient who presents to the emergency department for care expects that the professionals attending him will be skilled and that a sufficient number of them will be available. As was previously mentioned, Medicare regulations, the JCAH, and standards from professional organizations address the quality and quantity of nursing staff. In addition, the JCAH and state and local regulatory agencies may categorize hospitals according to their ability to respond to the needs of the patients on a primary, secondary, and tertiary care level. Requirements for staffing in the emergency department vary according to the determined category.

Job descriptions should delineate the qualifications and roles of emergency personnel: for example, the staff nurse must make rapid decisions, screen patients, be able to assist in all types of emergency cases, and have the ability to deal with people under stress.[29]

New staff members should be thoroughly oriented and should demonstrate knowledge by measurable objectives determined by the needs of the department. The JCAH offers a model orientation program and makes recommendations about continuing education.

Nurses with special functions above and beyond that of the staff nurse should also have appropriate training and be guided by specific job descriptions. The role of the triage nurse should be carefully defined. Physicians should participate in drafting such definitions because functions that are ordinarily their responsibility are often delegated to specially trained nurses in the emergency care setting.[30] The question of the physician's liability for the triage nurse's error has not been resolved, but no matter who else may be held responsible, the nurse is liable for her own actions. The following case illustrates the responsibility placed on nurses who make decisions in the absence of a physician.

> A 14-month-old child suffering from a rare form of croup-epiglottitis was sent to a hospital by his pediatrician. The nurse placed the child and mother in a bath room for steam treatment, where the child suffered cardiopulmonary arrest. He was resuscitated, but had brain damage, mental retardation, and quadriplegia. In a suit against the pediatrician, the nurse, and the hospital, the jury found the pediatrician not liable, and awarded damages against the hospital and nurse only.[31]

If the nurse, by virtue of specialized emergency training, had appreciated the severity of the illness, she might have summoned a physician and perhaps proper intervention would have been initiated.

Emergency personnel should be available in sufficient numbers. There is no easy answer to the question of proper staffing. Standards should be set by administration and nursing professionals. When staffing shortages occur, they should be documented. The courts are unsympathetic in their reaction to evidence of understaffing. When understaffing occurs, the nurse responsible should document the problem and make certain that administration is aware of it. Whoever is ultimately responsible should rectify the situation.[32]

EQUIPMENT

In addition to being appropriately staffed, the emergency department should be properly equipped. Some states have defined the necessary types of equipment for hospitals in specific categories. Nurses are required to notify their supervisors or other responsible persons whenever equipment is not functioning. If a nurse fails to notice defective equipment that he or she could have been reasonably expected to notice, or fails to report it, he or she is liable as a negligent employee and the employer is also at risk.[33]

In addition, professionals are expected to know how to use the special kinds of apparatus that are standard in emergency departments. The following example involves equipment commonly used in emergency departments and intensive care units.

A five-year-old boy suffered a cardiac arrest in the operating room and was quickly resuscitated. After recovery room care, transfer was made to the intensive care unit with orders for hypothermia. When he arrived, the resuscitator assigned to the unit was not working or was absent. Furthermore, there was no glass thermometer available that would register lower than 94°F, even though the nurses knew that the thermometer attached to the hypothermia machine was not always accurate. The boy's temperature started to rise and after many convulsions he became apneic. Mouth-to-mouth resuscitation was instituted until a resuscitator could be located. By change of shift, the boy had had two more seizures and the nurse noted improper ventilations: Ten minutes later, a kink in one of the respirator tubes was discovered and corrected. In a subsequent lawsuit, damages in excess of $294,000 were recovered by the plaintiff. It is obvious that the lack of proper equipment, as well as lack of understanding about use of the equipment, contributed to the patient's condition.[34]

NURSE-PHYSICIAN RELATIONSHIPS AND RESPONSIBILITIES

The nature of emergency services demands a team whose members work well together. The possibility exists that nurses and physicians working closely together may become legal adversaries. This need not occur if good medical and nursing care is provided and if roles are clearly defined and understood. Nurse practice acts are being revised to describe the roles and functions that nurses really perform. The questions of the nurse's expanded role and the physician's legal responsibility for the nurse are important ones, especially in emergency care, because many duties are delegated.

Captain of the Ship

The doctrine of Captain of the Ship addresses the physician's responsibility for the nurse. The legal principle behind it is *vicarious liability;* that is, one party is held responsible for the action or inaction of another. It is similar to the principle of *respondeat superior,* discussed previously. Fortunately, this concept is not adhered to as closely as it once was because more independent nursing functions have been defined. In addition, the question of liability is related to the amount of control exercised by the physician, for example, hiring or firing. The following case illustrates this point:

A physician ordered the administration of heparin subcutaneously every 6 hours for a patient with coronary disease. The nurse injected the medication directly into the femoral nerve, causing the patient permanent damage. The physician was not held liable, but personal liability was granted against the nurse as well as agency liability against the hospital. To hold the physician liable for routine hospital services performed by nurses would place an unbearable cloak of responsibility on him or her.

Can a nurse be held liable for negligent acts committed by a physician? Probably not, as long as he or she commits no negligent act of his or her own while caring for the patient. First and foremost is the responsibility to the patient. Ideally, such sensitive situations are handled among those involved.

What happens, then, when after exhausting every route, the nurse feels that he or she must intervene for the safety of the patient? The key here is a policy statement written with input from nurses, physicians, and administrators, wherein lines of communication are established to deal with the problem. Every institution is different, and such policies must meet the needs of the setting while protecting the patient. A word of caution: independent intervention by the nurse can result in disruption of relationships, division of the department, and even loss of the nurse's job. The nurse must be responsible and act appropriately, adhering to set procedures and keeping in mind the good of the patient.

Before leaving this subject, consider the setting in which no physicians are present in the department and the onus of responsibility is on the nurse. Treatment and disposition of a patient by means of telephone communication with the physician can be a delicate and potentially dangerous procedure. However, in some areas, this is the only practical way in which patients receive care. The following case is an example:

A patient was brought to the emergency department after a car accident, saying his back might be broken. The nurse telephoned the physician on call and told him that the patient could wiggle his toes and that she could find nothing wrong with him. In addition, she said that he and his friends had been drinking. Medication was given for pain, and the patient was released. The next day, after finding blood in his urine, he was seen in another emergency department, where he was diagnosed as having a fracture of the spine. The physician at the first hospital claimed he had instructed the nurse to have x-rays and other diagnostic studies done and to have the patient admitted. He denied that the nurse told him the patient was complaining of back injury and could not walk.[36]

One can see the difficulty that might arise if the intentions of the physician are misunderstood or incorrectly implemented. In addition, even if the physician did err, and the nurse was correct, it might be impossible to prove this point. A verdict was awarded against the hospital by virtue of the actions of the nurse as its employee.

Patient care in the absence of a physician is not advised. However, when there are no other alternatives, there should be careful communication. When there is any question about treatment, medication, or disposition, the nurse should request examination by the physician. Any dialogue between the nurse and the physician should be carefully documented.

SUPERVISORY RESPONSIBILITY

Every emergency department should have an identified nurse leader who is responsible for the smooth and safe functioning of the unit. Not only does this person set the tone and determine the style of the department, but he or she has legal liability as the supervisor. The extent of that liability is contingent upon the amount of control he or she exercises.

The issue of liability here is not specifically contingent upon the doctrine of respondeat superior such that the employer is responsible for the negligence of the employee. Rather, *supervisory liability* has its basis in what would be reasonably expected of the ordinary supervisor in the same or similar circumstances. For example, if the supervisor is aware that the department is dangerously understaffed and does nothing to alleviate this situation, he or she may be held liable if patient injury occurs because of it. Judgment will take into consideration the usual role and job description

---

Chart 2-3

CONTENT OF MEDICAL RECORD AND EMERGENCY LOG

1. Patient identification
2. Time and means of arrival
3. History and physical findings, allergies
4. Care given
5. Physician orders
6. Observations, including results of treatment
7. Reports of procedures, tests, and results
8. Impression (working diagnosis)
9. Conclusion, disposition, condition, instructions
10. AMA form where applicable.

(Requirements specified by the Joint Commission on Accreditation of Hospitals)

---

of that supervisor. If it is stated that the supervisor is responsible for safely staffing the unit, he or she will be held to that standard.

Delegation and Control

In addition, supervisory personnel may be held liable for the negligent act of another if there is inappropriate delegation or control. This holds true not only for identified leaders, but for every nurse who assigns another staff member to perform a task. If a nurse assigns another to carry out a treatment which by virtue of lack of education, experience, or licensure, he or she cannot perform, the nurse who makes the assignment may be held accountable for damages caused. The following case illustrates the concept:

> A patient died because of an infection caused by a sponge left in the abdomen. Judgment was entered against the supervisory nurse when evidence showed that the person responsible for the sponge count was not competent without immediate supervision, which was lacking.[40]

Nurses in emergency departments should exert care when assigning duties to other RNs, licensed vocational nurses (LVNs), nurse assistants, and prehospital care personnel. Not only may legal liability be involved, but state boards of nursing may intervene if the proper supervisory standard of care is not maintained. Consider the following opinion from the Attorney General of California:

> The Board of Registered Nursing may discipline registered nurses working in a supervisory capacity for authorizing untrained persons or licensed vocational nurses to perform tasks which such supervisory nurses knew or should have known they lacked the competency to perform.[41]

In addition to supervising staffing and assignments, the nurse manager should ensure a safe environment for staff and patients by acquiring and maintaining proper equipment and supplies. Communication of hospital policies and state regulations is another aspect of supervision that has legal overtones. There should be an effective mode of communication so that staff members will be kept aware of new procedures and statutes with specific application in the emergency department.

RECORDKEEPING

Standards and Regulations

The patient should have clear documentation of his course of treatment. The JCAH has specific requirements for the content of both the medical record and the emergency log.[37] These specifications are listed in Chart 2-3.

Even within the structure set by regulations, there are as many types of emergency department charts as there are emergency departments. Ordinarily, it is the responsibility of the physician to maintain the accuracy of the record, but the nurse also has an important role.

Record of Nursing Care. Nursing care, especially for the patient requiring a multitude of different procedures, should be noted on the patient's chart. This should include vital signs. If there is insufficient space on the record, add another sheet for documentation of nursing care.

Accurate recordkeeping can be of considerable help to the nurse who is asked for legal purposes to recall an event that may have occurred a year earlier. This is especially important when justifying an action, or lack of action, in observing a patient's status.

Freedom of Information

Occasionally a patient may want to see his medical record. Although the record is the property of the institution, the patient does have a right to the information contained in it. Some states require a legal action, such as a subpoena, for the individual's access to his record. Others do not. The most common procedure is referral to the medical records department where the patient's request can be attended to appropriately without disrupting hospital activities.

Incident Reports

Incident reports can be important in a legal action or defense. One should be familiar with the hospital's procedure for reporting unusual occurrences. The report should not be made in duplicate and does not become part of the patient's record. It should be given in a confidential manner to the designated administrative person. It is only when the report is intended exclusively for the hospital's attorney or insurance agent that it is privileged information and not available to the court.

DISPOSITION OF THE PATIENT

In most instances, patients are seen in the emergency department, evaluated, treated, and referred appropriately. It is only when the patient is not referred according to reasonable standards of care that legal liability may ensue.

Discharge Instructions

Every patient, or his agent or guardian, should be instructed about continued care or observation of his condition. Upon discharge from the emergency department, these instructions should be documented, either on a standard form or in writing, by the staff member giving the instructions. Generally speaking, it is the duty of the physician to inform the patient about his illness and instruct him in continued care. However, the nurse plays an important role in reinforcing the physician's instructions. The clerk or other staff member whose function it is to sign the patient out again reviews the directions while obtaining the patient's signature. The importance of providing discharge instructions is illustrated in the following example:

> An 11-year-old boy was brought into the emergency department after suffering a head injury in a fight. The intern who saw him felt that he should be admitted, but because he was not being treated by a private physician with privileges, he was discharged home after consultation with a staff pediatrician. The physician gave the father neither appropriate instructions nor a head injury instruction sheet. The boy's condition continued to deteriorate at home, and the father brought him back to the emergency department, where a diagnosis of epidural hematoma was made. After surgical intervention, the boy was mute and totally paralyzed from the neck down. The father was awarded $4 million.

It is difficult to predict what might have happened had proper discharge instructions been given, but the failure to provide them was felt to have adversely affected the boy's course.

Interhospital Transfer for Specialized Care

In many cases, patients require admission for further care. Legal aspects of referral and transfer were presented earlier in this chapter. Hospitals maintain secondary care at a level adequate to the needs of most patients requiring admission from the emergency department. However, in some communities, there are transfer protocols which provide guidelines for the transfer of patients to tertiary care centers for specialized care. Examples of such centers are burn units, spinal cord injury centers, and poison units.

Although these documents, signed by hospital administrators and chiefs of service, are not binding, there are indications that transfer for specialized services may become a standard of care. For example:

> Liability was imposed on a hospital that had treated a patient with third-degree burns for 53 days although not equipped to do so. The patient was ultimately transferred, but damages were awarded for the additional hospitalization and for permanent disability that resulted from delay of transfer.[39]

Psychiatric Detainment

Most hospitals do not maintain locked facilities for mentally disordered patients. This designation involves patients who are considered a danger to themselves or others, as a result of either a psychiatric disease or the use of drugs or alcohol. Each state has statutes that regulate the disposition of such patients, and procedures should be available to the emergency department staff.

REFERENCES

1. Cazalas MW: Nursing and the Law, 3rd ed. Germantown, Md, Aspen Systems, 1978
2. Prosser: Torts, 3rd ed. 1964, Sec 1, 2 Baudry-Lacantinerie: Précis de droit civil, 7th ed, par 1346–1347. Lee: Torts and Delicts. 27 Yale LJ 721 (1928) Salmond on the Law of Torts, 9th ed, Secs 3–5 (1936)
3. Valentin v la Societé Française de Bienfaisance Mutuelle de los Angeles, 76 Cal, App 2d l, 172, p 2d 359 (1956)
4. Darling v Charleston Memorial Hospital, 211 NE 2d 253 (West Virginia, 1965).
5. Nursing Practice Act, State of California, Business and Professions Code, Chap. 6, Art 2, Sec 272 5 d, p 9 (1974)
6. Standards of Emergency Nursing Practice. Kansas City, Mo, American Nurses' Association, 1975
7. Foster JT: What California is doing about it. Mod Hospital 112:84, February 1969
8. BAJI I, 6.15, p 5
9. Creighton H: Law Every Nurse Should Know, 3rd ed, p 81. Philadelphia, WB Saunders, 1975
10. Health and Safety Code, State of California, Sec 1483, p 130 (1976)
11. Social Security Administration, Document HI m-1, p 35 (1966)
12. State of California Health and Safety Code, Sec 1317, p 333
13. Wilmington General Hospital v Manlove, 54 Del 15, 174 A 2d 135 (1961)
14. O'Neill v Montefiore Hospital et al, 11 AD 2d 231, 202, NYS. 2d 436 (1960)
15. Guerrero v Copper Queen Hospital, 537 P, 2d 1329 (Arizona, 1975)
16. Harper v Baptist Medical Center, Princeton, 341 So 2d 133 (1976)
17. Stanhurf v Sipes 447 SW 2d 558, 562 (1969)
18. New Biloxi Hospital v Frazier, 146 So 2d 882 (Mississippi, 1962) and Creighton H: Law Every Nurse Should Know, 3rd ed, p 83. Philadelphia, WB Saunders, 1975
19. Cazalas M: Nursing and the Law, 3rd ed, p 43. Germantown, Md, Aspen Systems, 1978
20. Erickson v Dilgard, 44 misc 2d 27, 252 NYS 2d 705 (1962)
21. District of Columbia in re Osborne, 294 7 2d 372 (DC Ct App, 1972)
22. John F Kennedy Memorial Hospital v Heston 58 NJ 576, 279 A 2d 670 (1971)
23. Schmerker v State of California, 384 US 757 (1966)
24. Warren D: Problems in Hospital Law, 3rd ed, p 164. Germantown, Md, Aspen Systems, 1978
25. State of California Vehicle Code, Sec 13354 (d)
26. State of California Mental Health Act, Sec 5328
27. State of California Penal Code, Sec 11161-5
28. Landeros v Flood 551 D 2d 389 (Cal Sup Ct, 1976)
29. Creighton, H: Legal Responsibilities for the RN in the emergency room. Mississippi RN 30:35–40, October 1968
30. George, J: Emergency nurse triage: Beware. Emergency Nurse Legal Bulletin, October 1976
31. Hollinger v Childrens' Memorial Hospital (Ill Cir Ct, Cook Co, Docket No 70 L-10627, July 16, 1974)
32. Regan WA: Nurse understaffing: Legal liability. Regan Report on Nursing Law 14(12), May 1975
33. Creighton H: Liability for defective equipment. Supervisor Nurse 5:45–46, January 1974
34. Rose v Hakim, 335 F. Supp. 1221 (District of Columbia, 1971)
35. Muller v Likoff, 310 A 2d 303 (Pennsylvania, 1973)
36. Citizens Hospital Association v Schorlin, 262 So 2d 303 (Alabama, 1972)
37. Accreditation Standards: Emergency Services, 7th ed. Chicago, Joint Commission on Accreditation of Hospitals, 1979
38. Niles v City of San Rafael, 116 Cal. Rptr. 733 (Cal Ct of App, October 1974)
39. Carrascp v Bankoff, 33 Cal Rptr 673 (1963)
40. Piper v Epstein, 326 Ill App 400. 62 NE 2d 139 (1945)

APPENDIX A

A GLOSSARY OF LEGAL TERMS

Charitable immunity is the doctrine that a charitable hospital is not responsible for the negligence of its physicians and nurses in the treatment of patients. This doctrine has been overturned in some states.

Comparative doctrine of negligence is one in which the plaintiff is not necessarily barred from recovery, by his own negligence.

Contributory negligence is an act or omission on the part of a person, injured or ill, that contributes to that person's injury or death. It is an act or omission that a reasonably prudent person under like or similar circumstances would not allow.

A **defendant** is the person(s) the suit was filed against, *e.g.,* accused of neglect.

Derogate means contrary to or militate against. It may also mean partial repeal of a law or statute, as opposed to **abrogate** which means full repeal of a law or statute.

Distributees are a deceased's heirs.

Duty of care is the legal duty of the professional to the patient to have and use skills in care used by other prudent similarly trained professionals under similar circumstances.

Expert defines special training or special knowledge acquired from extensive experience.

False imprisonment is wrongful restraint of an individual against his will.

Gratuitous describes a service provided without recompense or compensation.

Guarantee against self-incrimination is the principle that one is not required to testify or give evidence against oneself.

Indemnification suit is one by which an employer (hospital) seeks to recover a loss by bringing action against its employee(s).

Injury in malpractice is the legal loss a patient suffers and claims was caused by the negligence of the professional. The loss can be physical, mental, or monetary.

A **judgment** is the court's determination, or the court's and jury's determination, that damages are or are not due, and if due, the amount payable.

Liability is the legal responsibility (that established by law) to account for any damages that may result from one's wrongful or negligent actions (as determined by law), by paying damages to the injured party.

Malpractice is the law of negligence when applied to a professional person's misconduct, lack of reasonable skill, or omission of a duty, when a person or his property is injured.

Mandatory means obligatory.

To commit **negligence** is to do something that a reasonable, prudent professional would not do, or to fail to do something that a reasonable, prudent professional would do in carrying out the care of a patient. (See also **compartive doctrine of negligence** and **contributory negligence**.)

Order of death is involved in a common disaster or multiple deaths (involving husband and wife, for example). It refers to the time sequence of each death and may be important in terms of property rights and testamentary (will) disposition.

A **plaintiff** is the person who files a suit.

The **proximate cause** of an event is that which, in a natural sequence unbroken by any new cause, produced that event and without which it would not have occurred.

Res ipsa loquitur is a rule of evidence in courts. In the case of certain injuries, "the thing (the injury) speaks for itself." The plaintiff does not then have the burden of proving the negligence.

Respondeat superior is the legal principle that the employer (the "superior") is liable for (responsible for) the negligence of his employee.

Sovereign immunity is the right of a governmental agency to be free from liability and suit unless it consents otherwise. (New York State, among others, has waived this immunity.)

A **statute** is a law enacted by a legislature.

Statute of limitations is the state law that sets forth a time limit within which a legal action must be started before the right to bring the action is lost.

A **suit** is the legal litigation between a plaintiff and a defendant. The court, with or without a jury, litigates or decides the respective rights of the parties. A **civil suit** is filed by a person for restitution (money) for an injury. A **criminal suit** is filed by the state for violation of a law.

Technical assault is touching another without his consent, express or implied.

Testamentary guardian is a person appointed by a will to act as guardian of a minor.

A **tort** is a legal wrong committed upon the person or property of another. A negligent act resulting in injury is a tort.

Uniform Anatomical Gifts Act is a law that provides that a person may, during life, request in writing that upon death one or more body organs may be used for transplantation or other medical purposes.

3

FORENSIC ASPECTS OF SUDDEN AND UNEXPECTED DEATH

BOYD G. STEPHENS

Death is no stranger in an active emergency department. In other settings, death most often follows a natural disease process and only reflects the frailty of mankind. Natural death that occurs as a result of known or diagnosed disease while a person is under the care of a physician is not of interest in this chapter. Rather, deaths that are sudden, unexpected, or unnatural or that result from the acts of another person are considered. Some natural deaths fall within this category—for instance, the unexpected death of a person who is apparently in good health and has not been under the care of a physician who can reasonably identify the cause of death. In some cases, the patient may be resuscitated long enough to allow a diagnosis, such as rupture of a berry aneurysm or acute myocardial infarction with classic ECG or enzyme changes. In many instances, there is no opportunity for diagnosis, such as when a 15 year old collapses while playing ball or a 25-year-old jogger collapses while running. Most frequently the patient is found collapsed, and a history cannot be obtained.

Forensic considerations are involved in most instances when death occurs suddenly or unexpectedly. Emergency care personnel should be aware of their responsibilities in these situations and familiar with recommended procedures. In emergency care, as in every other phase of health care, the well-being of the patient is the foremost consideration, and all necessary steps to diagnose and preserve life must be taken. But legal and moral responsibilities continue even when life cannot be maintained. These responsibilities include seeing that the body is not assaulted, protecting property and evidence, and reporting certain deaths to the medical examiner, coroner, or police. Health care personnel should also be alert for the possibility of death from defective hospital equipment, infectious disease, or human actions. These basic responsibilities are summarized in Chart 3-1. Procedures associated with forensic considerations, such as preservation of evidence and property, complete and accurate recording of data, and compliance with coroner's laws, are described in this chapter, and their application in specific situations is discussed.

Chart 3-1

SUDDEN AND UNEXPECTED DEATH: BASIC RESPONSIBILITIES OF EMERGENCY CARE PERSONNEL

- To see that the body is not assaulted
- To protect property
- To preserve evidence
- To report certain deaths to the medical examiner, coroner, or police
- To be alert to the possibility of death from defective hospital equipment, infectious disease, or human actions

---

DEFINITION OF DEATH

Death is still largely undefined from a legal standpoint. Although it may be possible to recognize death from simple inspection, there is still no basic universal legal definition or medical test to prove death accurately and rapidly. For many years, the law has avoided this issue by recognizing that death may be obvious in some instances, and that even a lay person can recognize certain signs of death. An accurate legal definition of death or the inability to return to an acceptable life form is a prerequisite for tissue donation and for determining when advanced life support can be removed without jeopardizing the patient's right of survival.

Every hospital should have a preestablished protocol for the minimum necessary examination to determine death. The protocol must be consistent with statutory regulations and must be reviewed periodically to ensure that it is in compliance with laws as they change. There must be some brief written documentation of why a person is dead, or why no life support is justified. The protocol may require another physician's review as a consultation. In making these decisions, one must be mindful of conditions that are known to mimic death and avoid hasty decisions. It is wise to check more than one modality and to record both the time when the decision is made and the basis for it. Be particularly cautious when it is technically difficult to hear or see the necessary findings; for example, when noise interferes with hearing heart or respiratory sounds.

EVIDENCE OF DEATH

Various groups of signs are important in determining death. These signs are listed in Chart 3-2. The designation *relative signs* essentially refers to the absence of vital signs. *Objective signs* involve the measurement of neurophysiologic function. *Observable signs* are, as the name implies, readily visible or obvious. Of the groups listed, relative signs are easily misleading and unreliable; they are most often the factor responsible for error in the diagnosis of death. Patients who meet all or most of these criteria have been known to survive in modern emergency and trauma facilities.

Conditions Known to Mimic Death

Profound shock, severe hypothermia, and barbiturate overdose are conditions that have been repeatedly associated with misdiagnosis of death in the past. All protocols must take these possibilities into account and should include requirements for a higher level of certainty before death is assumed. The conditions that are known to mimic death are listed in Chart 3-3.

Responsibility for Diagnosis of Death

It is generally advised that nonmedical personnel determine only whether the patient can benefit from medical therapy or resuscitation–not pronounce death. Because death is considered a diagnosis, only a person who is legally able to

---

Chart 3-2

EVIDENCE OF DEATH

Relative Signs (Physiologic aspects that can be seen or measured)

- Absent vital signs
   Blood pressure
   Pulse
   Respiration
- Loss of body temperature
   Core temperature 35°C (95°F) or lower
- Cyanosis, livor, and rigor mortis

Objective Signs (Measurements of neurophysiologic function)

- Deep coma—patient unresponsive to neurologic stimuli
- Flat ECG, EEG
- Loss of midbrain function
   No spontaneous respiration—patient fails apnea test (no mechanical assistance with O_2 at 6 L/min)
   Unresponsive, fixed, and dilated pupils
   No corneal or other neurologic response
   No motor activity
- For establishing brain death, requirements include 12 to 24 hours of observation without hypothermia and the absence of drugs known to produce deep coma, such as barbiturates, curare derivatives, etc.

Observable Signs

- Airway blocked with blood or other material for at least 5 minutes
- Body damage incompatible with life (decapitation, extensive burns)
- Changes due to decomposition

---

make a diagnosis can legally pronounce death. This may change in the future when laws are passed that define certain criteria and specify other persons who would be qualified to make such a pronouncement.

curred. The scene typically provides 60% to 80% of the evidence that allows an understanding of a death. This information is decreased or lost when the body is moved or transported to the hospital. It is important for emergency care personnel to be aware that the quality of the investi-

THE SCENE OF DEATH

For the investigator of the death, the scene is frequently the most important element in gaining an understanding of how, where, and why the person died. When death is obvious at the scene, the first obligation to protect the life of the patient ends, and the obligation to protect the scene begins.

The Need to Protect Evidence at the Scene

The position of the patient, blood, and other factors at the scene yield data about force, angle, movement, and sequence that are crucial in interpreting how and why the death oc-

---

Chart 3-3

CONDITIONS KNOWN TO MIMIC DEATH

- Profound, acute shock
- Severe hypothermia
- Drug overdose (*e.g.,* barbiturates, curare derivatives)

gation and the collection of evidence depends in part on how pure that evidence is at the scene. The loss, destruction, or damage of evidence can be costly to the taxpayer at a subsequent trial, or may lead to an improper court finding.

Responsibilities of Primary Responders

The chief responsibilities of primary or first responders at the scene of a sudden or unexpected death are care of the patient and protection of evidence.

Responsibility to the Patient.   The first responder has the initial responsibility of determining whether the patient can benefit from medical therapy. If death is not obvious, or there is reasonable doubt, most jurisdictions require that some action be taken to ensure that the patient receives the necessary medical care. When the patient is obviously dead at the scene, the primary responder is legally required to leave the scene undisturbed. Unless there is a previously established procedure or an order from an appropriate superior, the body should be left in the position in which it is found, and the person assessing the patient should back out of the scene in his or her own footsteps. Obviously, it is necessary that the determination be unquestionably accurate, and that others not be allowed to wander around the scene out of curiosity. Only authorized investigators should reenter the scene to document and collect evidence. This is especially true when there is a suspicion that the death is unnatural. If the death is natural, and the family is present, one should follow the protocol previously established.

Protection of Evidence.   When there is a question about whether the death occurred naturally, or when the death is obviously unnatural, there is almost always important evidence or information at the scene. A number of mistakes are easily—and all too commonly—made by first responders at the scene of an unnatural death. They include the following:
* Moving the body because it is in public view
* Changing the position of the body unnecessarily
* Walking through blood spatters
* Removing property to check for a name
* Using a telephone at the scene
* Destroying clothing because it is bloody
* Losing a piece of evidence, such as a bullet

As a result of carelessness in these matters, questions about the factors leading to death may remain unanswered. An unanswered question can become a legal loophole. It should be borne in mind that **there is rarely a scene of sudden and unexpected death that does not contain important information.** This is especially true when the death is due to violence or the act of another person.

Cooperation With Law Enforcement Agencies

The decision to transport a patient from the scene of death depends upon a tremendous number of variables, such as the presence of a trauma center, the training and capability of first responders, and the safety of others, to name only a few. These variables obviously differ from area to area, sometimes even within a large jurisdiction. Representatives of law enforcement agencies and medical facilities should cooperate in establishing guidelines for the necessary protocols and should maintain good working relationships to ensure that each party understands the legal requirements, needs, and limitations of the other.

Evaluation of the Scene of Death

In view of the serious responsibilities involved, it is essential for emergency care personnel to know the correct procedures to follow both in safeguarding the patient and in preserving evidence. A procedure for evaluating the scene of death is presented in Chart 3-4.

CORONER'S LAWS

In general, twenty-five to thirty percent of all deaths in a community have possible legal complications! This indicates that if the deaths are not skillfully investigated, the survivors may suffer serious consequences: including unjustified accusation of murder, failure to uphold a valid charge of murder, loss of insurance payments, loss of workmen's compensation benefits, loss of legal rights to bring suit or properly defend against such suit against a charge of wrongful death, failure to recognize contagious disease or the failure to recognize other dangers to society.

As early as September of 1194, and possibly before that time, an office identifiable as the coroner was described in England. Since that time, there have been many modifications of the role and purpose of the coroner, but English Law from the late 1700 to early 1800's established the legal purpose, principles and authority that is in common use through-out the world today.*

Most progressive states have laws that state specifically which deaths are reportable to the coroner, outline the authority of the office, and define its legal responsibility. Although laws can and do vary from state to state, generally they require the coroner to inquire into deaths that are sudden, unexpected, and unnatural. In most areas, a private physician cannot sign a death certificate if either the cause or manner of death is unnatural. Frequently, these laws require the coroner to investigate, take charge of the scene, give authority to perform an autopsy, carry out scientific testing, and hold an inquest (including the power of subpoena). The coroner's functions are summarized in Chart 3-5. Since there is variation from area to area, emergency care personnel should be familiar with the law and procedures that pertain in their area. When there is a question, it is always better to have a person who is fully familiar with the details about the care and death of the patient report the case to the coroner. This accurate reporting helps relieve other emergency personnel of legal responsibility, and allows the coroner, who is usually more knowledgeable about the current laws, to decide whether an investigation is required.

* Houts, Marshall JD: Cyclopedia of Sudden, Violent and Unexplained Death, vol I. Emerald Bay Publishers, 1969

Chart 3-4

SCENE EVALUATION PROCEDURE

Approaching the Scene

- Enter carefully.
- Avoid disturbing obvious evidence, for example: Gun or knife lying on the floor—avoid kicking Blood spots—avoid stepping in them if possible

Evaluating the Patient's Condition

- Do whatever is necessary to determine whether the patient can be treated or transported or whether he or she is obviously dead at the scene.
- If the patient cannot be considered alive, and there is no doubt (benefit of doubt is always in favor of the patient), carefully back out of the scene, avoiding blood or other evidence.

Documentation

- Record tersely in written form the minimum reason why this patient cannot benefit from medical treatment. (*Note:* Recall that only a person who is legally able to make a diagnosis can legally pronounce death.)

Actions to Avoid

- Do not search the body or the residence or wander around the scene out of idle curiosity.
- Do not use the telephone at the scene.
- Do not leave your fingerprints on doorknobs.
- Do not lean against the wall.

(These and other actions tend to destroy evidence such as fingerprints, which usually are not visible.)

Recommended Actions

- Leave the scene as soon as possible, keeping it intact for the responsible investigators.
- Initiate appropriate action in accordance with community regulations and as directed by the person with legal authority for the scene.
- Work with the other responsible authorities to help develop the best possible medical and forensic services for your community.

Chart 3-5

CORONER'S JURISDICTION: BASIC RESPONSIBILITIES AND AUTHORITY OF THE CORONER

In most states, the coroner has the following obligations and prerogatives:

- To inquire into deaths that are sudden, unexpected, and unnatural (In most areas, a private physician cannot sign a death certificate if either the cause or the manner of death is unnatural.)
- To investigate the death
- To take charge of the scene
- To grant permission to perform an autopsy and scientific testing
- To hold an inquest (including the power of subpoena)

DEATHS REPORTABLE TO THE CORONER

Deaths that must be reported to the coroner are described in Chart 3-6. Not all areas use each of these regulations; most have additional requirements. Emergency care personnel are legally responsible for knowing the reporting laws in their area. Most states have laws that require notification of the appropriate authority in a number of cases. Gunshot wounds, stabbings, child abuse, and contagious disease are typical examples. Some states require that sexual assault be reported when the victim is below a certain age; other states consider this child abuse and regard sexual assault as a matter of voluntary reporting.

Matters of policy and legal compliance must be discussed, established by protocol for the facility, and followed. If doubt exists, discuss it with your legal representative, or with the authority who has jurisdiction. It is always wise to report a case and to seek correct advice; failure to do so can lead to mistakes. The mandate to report a death does not necessarily require that the case be investigated further by the coroner. Once the report is reviewed, usually by telephone, the death certificate may be released for the physician's signature. However, some cases—such as homicide—can be handled only by the coroner.

Proximal Cause: Coroner's Cases

Legally, a condition or event that follows some other event may be related to the primary event through the doctrine of proximal cause if it cannot reasonably be supposed that the second event would have occurred at that time, or if the complication or illness is a natural and continuous ex-

tension of the primary event. For example, a person suffers a head injury that causes loss of consciousness resulting in pneumonia and death two weeks later from pulmonary complications. The death is directly related to the head injury, and whether the chain of events continues for 2 weeks or 2 years, would still be considered an accident or a homicide, depending on the cause of the original injury. Unless the chain of events is clearly broken, so that the causal relationship is disrupted, the probability that the doctrine of proximal cause would apply to any factor causing the medical death is very great. However, emergency personnel should not attempt to make this determination, since the decision involved is usually a legal one, not a medical one. Whenever death results directly from or as a consequence of a factor that places the case under the jurisdiction of the coroner, that case may be a coroner's case. Proximal cause may be involved in such cases. For example, a victim of an auto accident suffers injuries requiring surgery. Complications develop, requiring additional surgery at another facility. Further complications lead to sepsis and death six months later. If the death is directly related to injuries or complications from the initial injury, the death is an accident, and must be a coroner's case because only the coroner can sign the death certificate.

Proximal cause is not involved if the patient has reasonably recovered from the injuries and death is due to an unrelated cause. As an example of the latter, the patient just mentioned is recovering in a hospital. At about the time of planned discharge, the patient decides to undergo hair transplantation, which involves two additional exposures to an anesthetic associated with liver damage. The patient dies from the resulting liver necrosis. In this instance, the death is

---

Chart 3-6

DEATHS REPORTABLE TO THE CORONER

- All violent, sudden, or unusual deaths
- Unattended deaths—usually when a physician has not seen the patient for a specified period of time
- Deaths following or suspected of resulting from self-induced or criminal abortion
- Known or suspected homicide, suicide, or accident
- Deaths known to have resulted from or suspected of resulting from injury, recent or old.
- Sudden infant death syndrome (SIDS)—although technically a sudden death, SIDS is specifically mentioned in some states
- Deaths resulting from or related to sexual assault or crimes against nature
- Deaths from or suspected of resulting from contagious disease, constituting a public health hazard
- Deaths from occupational diseases or hazards
- Deaths of persons under sentence or in jail
- Deaths associated with any circumstance that affords reasonable grounds to suspect that the death resulted from the criminal act of another
- Death occurring within a specified time after a patient enters a hospital (in some areas)
- Death occurring while a patient is under anesthesia or its effects (in some areas)

(*Note:* Emergency care personnel are responsible for knowing the reporting laws in their area).

still accidental, but is not a result of the initial accident. Should the same patient, while in the hospital, die from cancer metastasis to the brain just before planned discharge, the death would be due to natural causes. It would be advisable to report any such case to the coroner, who would probably release the latter case for the physician's signature on the death certificate. Should a hospital autopsy be done that showed that the diagnosis of tumor was in error and that the death was really due to traumatic brain injuries, the coroner would again have jurisdiction.

CORONER'S JURISDICTION IN SPECIFIC SITUATIONS

Technically, the potential for coroner's jurisdiction never ends. To meet the criteria of the law and ensure the best treatment, protocols or written procedures must be established and implemented. Requirements and responsibilities associated with tissue donation, autopsy, gunshot wounds, stab wounds, blunt trauma, hospital deaths, and other situations are discussed in the sections that follow.

TISSUE DONATION

Confirmation of Death, Coroner's Consent

As a prerequisite for tissue donation, most states require the documentation or diagnosis of cessation of brain function in order to confirm death. This usually requires testing of midbrain function and satisfactory evidence of irreversible cessation of brain function. Since a coroner has jurisdiction from the second when death occurs, he must give clearance of the case before donation is made. Usually, autopsy or donation permits are not considered valid until the coroner has either released jurisdiction or consented to the procedure. Because of the time limits that apply to most types of tissue donation, there must be no unnecessary delays, and the procedure should be as routine and as foolproof as is humanly possible. Because most emergency departments have a fairly steady turnover of personnel, a checklist form

is suggested, to prevent mistakes or delays in obtaining consent and to ensure compliance. The form, which is recommended for all emergency department deaths, requires the physician to respond to a number of questions about the death. A sample checklist is shown in Chart 3-7. Many times the coroner reviews the case before death occurs, to determine if he will have jurisdiction and if he can agree to donation.

The checklist should be constructed so that a single negative response requires some specified action. In general, the treating physician should contact the coroner, since he is the person who knows his patient best. Finally, a supervising nurse or an experienced administrator should review the emergency department records to determine that the necessary treatment, procedures, and documents have been properly completed. A checklist ensures that the following requirements have been met:
- The relatives have been contacted by the appropriate person.
- The coroner or other law enforcement agency has been contacted as required.
- Tissue donor candidates have had the proper legal review, and contact with the required agencies has taken place.
- The required legal documents have been signed.
- The required chart entries have been made.

In some jurisdictions, it is required that in all sudden hospital deaths, all tubes and lines must be left in place and the patient closed off from the atmosphere. It is helpful to observe all IV solutions and life support equipment.

Cessation of Life Support. Special considerations are required for patients who are on life support and may become donors; protocol must be followed by emergency personnel. It is best to notify the coroner of this situation before discontinuing life support so that he can review the patient and the circumstances of the case. Timely notification of the coroner allows for a decision on the death as a coroner's case and, if so, for determination of whether donation can be authorized. It prevents delays in tissue harvesting when this is the wish of the patient or the family and prevents loss of evidence in cases for court presentation.

Chart 3-7

PHYSICIAN'S CHECKLIST FOR EMERGENCY DEPARTMENT DEATHS

- Is the death from apparent natural causes?
- Is there any suggestion of trauma, poison, or drugs?
- Is the patient under medical care for a condition that could reasonably cause death?
- Were you reasonably able to make a diagnosis of the cause of the patient's death?
- Is there a donor card, permit, or other legal document associated with the patient?
- Is there some other legal reason that requires reporting the death to an authority?

If the death is not natural, or if questions exist—report to the coroner.
(Telephone number _____)

Updating of Protocols. As new technology renders the diagnosis of death more accurate, mandatory periodic updating of transplant protocols will become necessary. New procedures for obtaining and storing tissue for long periods of time before transplantation will result in new laws. Emergency care personnel are responsible for knowing current laws and for being aware that the coroner has first authority.

Transplant and Autopsy Permits

Many legal and ethical considerations are associated with transplant and autopsy permits. Emergency care personnel should be aware of the following important points.

1. The next of kin should never be asked to sign a consent form until the patient is legally pronounced dead. Although it is correct to discuss donation or autopsy before death, a relative does not have the legal right to authorize such a procedure before the patient has died. In most states, the patient may authorize tissue donation or an autopsy prior to his death, as long as legal procedures are followed.
2. In the case of a predeath authorization by the patient, neither the procurement of tissue nor autopsy should be undertaken if the immediate family is protesting vigorously. Although most states clearly indicate that this would be within the legal rights of the emergency care nurse to do so, the risks to the transplant program probably outweigh the potential benefits, and the decision to proceed with the autopsy should be reviewed legally.
3. Be certain that the person signing the permit is the legal next of kin in accordance with state laws. It is helpful to have the law excerpted and summarized on the front or back of legal forms that are to be signed by next of kin. This helps to ensure informed consent and to prevent unauthorized signatures. Relatives and friends typically wish to make the "arrangements" rather than have the close family distressed; however, keep in mind that such signatures may not be legal.
4. The exact organ or tissue that is to be donated should be specified on the form. Do not accept statements such as "any useful organs" or "any necessary material"; such statements are not specific, may not be legal, and could invite trouble. The form should state specifically "both eyes," or "both kidneys," or "left humerus." Only the listed material can be taken. Because the family should not be approached again for additional tissue, there must be a coordinated program. Most important, the family should not be asked for too much from their loved one. Such an approach tends to arouse anger and hostility in the grieving family and may engender lawsuits.
5. No attempt should be made to add on to the form at a later time. Most families will respond to such an attempt by totally withdrawing permission, on the basis that they "aren't running a wrecking yard." Only one program or person should contact the family.
6. It is important to contact the coroner early and to have a good understanding of what he is likely to do. In general, most coroners want to be involved early so that evidence is not lost or damaged and so that they understand both the real injuries and the artifacts.
7. Currently, no coroner is authorized to donate tissue or materials from a patient; this is the legal right of the patient or the legal next of kin.

8. A case should be reported if there is any question about whether or not it should be reported.

These points are summarized in Chart 3-8.

SUDDEN INFANT DEATH SYNDROME (SIDS)

Sudden death due to natural causes is much more common in the young than most people realize. Death from natural cause can strike within seconds. The sudden infant death syndrome (SIDS) is a classic example of rapid, natural death in an apparently healthy child. This syndrome typically occurs during sleep. By definition, SIDS is usually considered to involve the death of a child between the age of 1 week and 1 year, in whom a complete investigation and autopsy have revealed no recognized cause of death. The peak incidence is between the second and third months of life. After the sixth month, the incidence is markedly reduced.

Assessment. Approximately 40% to 50% of SIDS children have a bloody, mucoid material in the upper airway or pharynx. There may be marked darkening and distortion of the soft tissue about the face. Livor mortis (settling of blood by gravity effect) may be misinterpreted by the inexperienced as ecchymosis from severe child beating. These signs are listed in Chart 3-9.

Effects on Parents. The sudden death of a child is a catastrophic blow to the parents, and guilt, remorse, and anger are common responses to the death. See Chapter 6, Death, Grief, and Sudden Loss, for insight into this problem.

Need for Investigation and Autopsy. Much information and reassurance for the parents can be gained from a properly conducted investigation and autopsy. Usually the coroner provides a letter or other material for the parents and the investigator talks with the family at the hospital or as soon as possible to ensure that the parents have the information on SIDS. The child should be autopsied by an experienced pathologist, preferably a forensic pathologist. Ignoring this is a serious mistake. Possibilities of infection, abuse, congenital or familial disease of significance to subsequent children, and knowledge of many other factors depend on a complete and careful autopsy. The coroner will want to ensure that the parents are aware of the disease and local support programs, and of how they can obtain the findings of the examination. The security of feeling reasonably certain that nothing preventable was present in the child that died is extremely important to the parents.

GUNSHOT WOUNDS

Assessment of the patient with gunshot wounds yields information that is important both in determining treatment (or confirming death) and in conducting the legal investigation of the injury. These two closely related aspects will be discussed together. It is helpful to be aware of some popular misconceptions about gunshot wounds and to understand some basic principles. Accurate observation and exact recording of data are crucial. However, interpretation

Chart 3-8

CONSIDERATIONS FOR TRANSPLANT AND AUTOPSY PERMITS

1. Show consideration in approaching patient's family.
2. Never request next of kin to sign consent form for tissue donation or autopsy until patient is legally pronounced dead.
   - Relative does not have legal right to so authorize prior to patient's death.
   - Patient may so authorize, in most states, if legal requirements are met.
3. In the case of predeath authorization by patient, do not proceed with procurement of tissue or autopsy if immediate family protests vigorously.
   - Have decision to proceed reviewed legally.
   - Do not jeopardize transplant program.
4. Be certain that person who signs permit is legal next of kin in accordance with state laws.
   - Provide summary of law on legal form signed by next of kin.
5. Be certain that form specifies exact organ or tissue to be donated (*e.g.*, both eyes, both kidneys, left humerus).
   - Only specified material can be taken.
6. Do not accept general statements on form (*e.g.*, any useful organ, any necessary material).
   - Such statements may not meet legal requirements.
   - Discussion of donor's intent may distress family.
7. Do not attempt to add anything to the form at a later time.
   - Family should not be approached more than once.
   - Only one person or program should contact family.
   - Requests for additional tissue may cause family to rescind permission entirely.
8. Contact coroner early so that he can secure evidence and evaluate injuries and artifacts.
9. Be aware that coroners are currently not authorized to donate tissue from a patient.
   - Only patient or next of kin has legal right.
10. If there is any question whether or not a case should be reported, **report it!**

Chart 3-9

SIGNS OF DEATH DUE TO SUDDEN INFANT DEATH SYNDROME (SIDS)

- Bloody mucoid material in upper airway or pharynx (40%–50% of cases)
- Marked darkening and distortion of soft tissue about the face
- Livor mortis (sometimes misinterpreted as ecchymosis due to severe child beating)
- Absence of recent significant illness

of technical data about the weapon, the missile, and the manner of injury must be left to experts.

Characteristics of Gunshot Wounds

Size and Shape. When a firearm discharges, the gas pressure produced by the burning powder can amount to thousands of pounds per square inch. If the muzzle of the gun is very close to the skin, especially if the skin is immediately over bone, this gas may be forced into the bullet entrance hole. The rapidly expanding gas may balloon the skin out into a large "blister" in a fraction of a second. When the "blister" pops, as the skin must do when the pressure becomes too great, it makes a characteristic cruciate or stellate wound. To the inexperienced, the larger wound appears to be the exit, whereas in fact the opposite is true. Obviously, in tight contact wounds, especially with large-caliber weapons, this gas pressure may actually blow part or all of the tissue away, especially in technically closed compartments, such as the head. Expansion injuries like this are quite uncommon in the chest or abdomen because there is an expansion compartment for the gas pressure. One must not base judgments on folklore, such as the notion that bullets always make small entry holes and large exit wounds.

Smoke or Soot Deposits.   The burning of gunpowder typically deposits smoke or soot in a near wound. This may be seen in the edge of the wound or its depths from a near or loose contact wound. If the wound is debrided, the resected material should always be saved in an approved fashion. Undermining at the entry wound may be extensive. Periosteum typically holds soot or gunpowder in close or contact wounds, where it appears as a black or black-grey layer on the bone. If the ballooning pressure is lower, then this "blister" of skin may expand rapidly enough to "slap" the muzzle of the gun, and an imprint of the front of the weapon may be left on the skin. In some instances, this image can be of great value in identifying the weapon, or at least the type of gun involved. If the muzzle is a short distance away, the gas pressure takes the path of least resistance, and there is no starburst injury. However, soot and gunpowder do strike the skin. This pattern constitutes the important information on the firing distance of the weapon. If possible, the pattern should be photographed, or at least the radius should be measured and the measurements placed in the chart with a diagram.

Expert Evaluation of Bullet.   The most likely place to find a bullet is under the skin opposite the point of entry. This is because the elastic fibers of the skin can stretch and trap the bullet. A velocity of 200 to 500 ft/sec is needed for the bullet to escape through the skin. Under certain circumstances, an exit wound can look almost like an entrance wound. Therefore, an expert should determine the actual direction of travel. If a hard, movable mass is palpated under the skin opposite a bullet wound, the path of the wounding and the organs most likely to be injured may be estimated.

It is important to know that bullets do not always travel in a straight line; the notion that they do so is quite misleading. A bullet may enter a large vessel and embolize, it may take other pathways, or it may be free within a cavity. It is also possible for a bullet to have just enough energy

to exit, making a slit-like opening that looks like a stab wound. This is most typical of a small-caliber, fully jacketed bullet like the .25 automatic, but it can happen with any bullet. In this instance, the bullet may fall back into the body, be trapped in the clothing, or fall out on the gurney. It is extremely important to realize that the caliber of a bullet cannot be determined by its size on x-ray, or by the size of the entry wound. It is also impossible to tell the position of a person at the moment of being shot with any accuracy. Only an expert *may* be able to do so after investigation and careful consideration of *all* the data.

Accurate Recording of Data

Hospital errors involving gunshot wounds frequently lead to problems in court. It is both unnecessary and incorrect to make chart notations about the caliber of the weapon or distance or direction of travel of the bullet. Unless there are legitimate reasons for being concerned about kinetic energy transfer, it makes no sense to make such uninformed statements. Hospital notes of this nature are incorrect more often than pure chance alone would explain. Many times, physicians have testified in court about the direction of travel or distance—and have been wrong. Obviously, it is important to know whether a bullet penetrated completely through a patient or whether there are two wounds on opposite sides (wounds of entry and wounds of exit). The wound path is important in determining what organs are likely to have been damaged. The only other necessity is a good description of the wounds. Guidelines for recording gunshot wound data are listed in Chart 3-10.

Preservation of Evidence

Emergency care personnel should know the procedures for saving clothing and other evidence for the forensic laboratory. Proper storage methods and precise documentation are essential. In general, the following information should appear on the label identifying the stored evidence: the patient's name and identification number; the place of re-

---

Chart 3-10

ACCURATE RECORDING OF GUNSHOT WOUNDS

Do record
- Exact number of wounds
- Exact location of wounds (indicate on diagram of patient)
- Exact appearance of wounds

Do not attempt to record
- Caliber of weapon
- Direction of travel of bullet
- Distance traveled by bullet

Chart 3-11

DOCUMENTATION/LABELING OF EVIDENCE

The following information is required:
- Patient's name and identification number
- Place of recovery of evidence (site)
- Date and time of recovery
- Name of person who made the recovery (both printed name and signature)*
- Name of a witness, if possible (both printed name and signature)*

* The printed name and signature are required to establish chain of possession.

---

covery (site); the date and time of recovery; the name of the person making the recovery; and, if possible, the name of a witness. These items are listed in Chart 3-11. Both the printed name and the signature are necessary to evaluate the chain of possession.

Chain of Possession. Chain of possession is a legal procedure that ensures that the specimen is always accounted for and always clearly under the control of a specific person. It is easy to carry out, yet cases are thrown out of court because someone neglected to do this vital thing. The evidence must be maintained in such a manner that its purity is documented and no person can have caused artifacts, switched, or in any way changed it in order to meet the necessary requirements for use in court. Some recent legal decisions strongly suggest that emergency personnel may have both a legal and a moral responsibility to collect and properly maintain evidence. A locked and secure place is required for storage until the evidence is signed out by the last person in possession to the police, who in turn sign for it in order to maintain the chain of possession (see Chart 3-12).

Clothing. The patient's clothing may be of critical importance because all of the firing distance information, as well as any other data pertaining to evidence from the scene, may be found on it. Even though it is bloody, it can be of considerable forensic importance. Clothing should be disposed of as follows:

- When cutting clothing away from wound, follow seam line if possible.
- Do not place clothing on floor.
- Do not shake clothing.
- Hang clothing up, handling it gently. Keep individual items separate.
- When blood is dry, store items of clothing in separate paper bags (not plastic).
- Label accurately.

Missile Collection and Storage. If a missile is recovered from within or about the patient, the recommended procedure is to place it in a preprinted envelope that specifies the information to be recorded (Fig. 3-1). It is crucial to establish chain of possession for a recovered missile. Bullets are stored in envelopes because although they look hard, they are easily damaged. The important information lies in the fine lines on the sides of the bullet that are produced by its forced passage through the barrel of the weapon. This area must not be damaged in the removal or storage of the evidence. Therefore, bullets are never picked up with instruments or stored in glass or plastic jars. Use fingers or rubber-shod tools for recovery.

As in other medical specialties, a complex body of special knowledge and procedures is involved in forensic medicine. Although it is not always possible to save the patient's life, it is vital to save clothing and other evidence for the police or the coroner. Nothing must be done or omitted that might jeopardize the proper adjudication of the case in court. The following are some important considerations about gunshot wounds:

- Accurately record only what you have seen.
- Do not make judgments about the following:
  Firing distance
  Direction of travel of the missile
  Caliber of the weapon
  Make or type of gun
- Do not make assumptions such as the following:
  That a big hole must be an exit wound
  That the path of a bullet is always a straight line
- Carefully store and document clothing and other evidence.
- Maintain the chain of possession.
- Do nothing that might jeopardize the proper adjudication of the case in court.

STAB WOUNDS AND INCISED WOUNDS

Technically, a stab wound is an injury produced by a cutting instrument; the wound is deeper than it is wide. The same instrument can easily make both stab and incised wounds. A cutting instrument is any item with a relatively sharp edge. This type of wound differs from a laceration in that it has a relatively well-defined, sharp skin edge, with the neurovascular bundles cut at the plane of the wall of tissue.

Chart 3-12

CHAIN OF POSSESSION: A LEGAL PROCEDURE FOR THE SAFEGUARDING OF EVIDENCE

Purposes
- To ensure that the specimen is always accounted for and under the control of a specific person
- To ensure the purity of evidence—protecting against artifacts, switching, or alteration

Requirements
- Complete, accurate documentation
- A locked and secure place for storage
- Control by a specified person
- Signed record of release and acquisition of specimen

Patient Assessment and Associated Risks

Assessment of the patient with stab wounds must be carried out with great care because of the numerous risks involved. It is also important to avoid damaging potentially crucial evidence.

Figure 3-1 Envelope used for storing a recovered bullet.

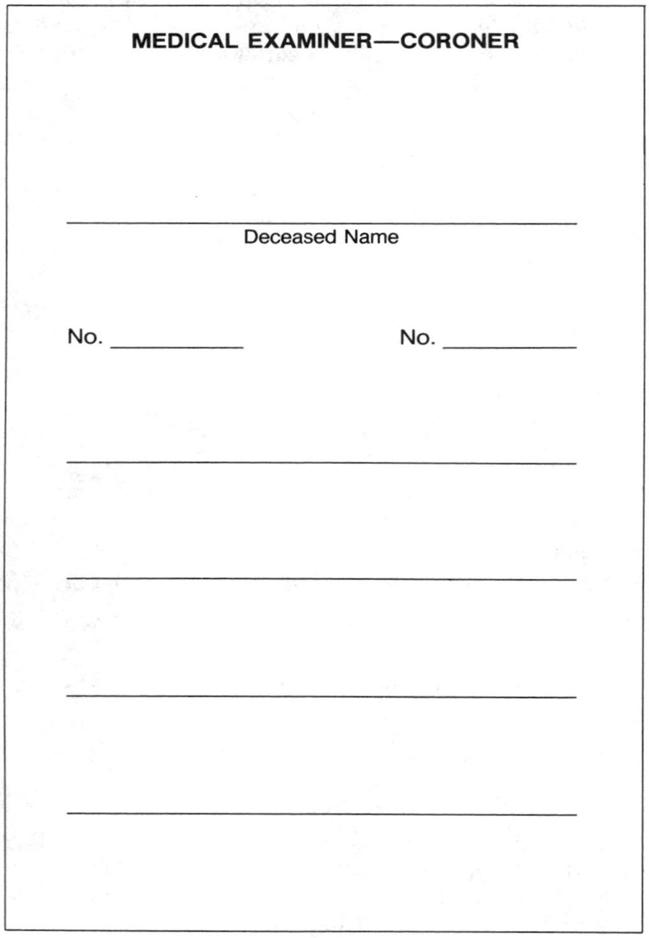

MEDICAL EXAMINER—CORONER

Deceased Name

No. _____   No. _____

Massive Bleeding. Not all stab wounds bleed to the surface. This is especially true of wounds to the chest because the blood can drain into the chest cavity as the lung collapses. Wounds into the head may not bleed because the brain may fall back and block the hole. In either case, *massive bleeding can occur when the patient is moved* or may have occurred internally.

Gas Embolism, Cardiac Arrest. Keep in mind that peripheral penetrating wounds of the lungs have a high potential for gas embolism. Embolism may occur immediately or when the lung is expanded, as with ventilation. Gas can enter the pulmonary circulation and pass directly into the left side of the heart. In the typical position for resuscitation, with the patient flat on his back, the coronary ostia is almost always directly at the highest point, so that even a small amount of gas—a few milliliters—may enter the coronary artery, act like a thrombus, and produce cardiac arrest. Since the volume may be small, the typical clinical features, including the "mill wheel" rumble, may not be present. Sudden cardiac arrest in a patient with a peripheral penetrating lung wound who was previously thought stabilized should put gas embolism high on the list of diagnoses. This may be one justification for an immediate emergency thoracotomy with blind aspiration of the coronary arteries and ventricle.

Neurologic Injuries. Be especially careful of wounds into or around major neurovascular bundles or the spinal cord. Hemorrhage into the closed space may not produce immediate symptoms yet may represent significant injury from nerve compression or infection. Infection can be a severe risk for the patient.

Missed Injuries. It is easy to become so involved with a visibly bleeding wound or with a cardiac arrest that one fails to look carefully at the other body surfaces. These wounds can easily be missed on casual examination. As soon as possible, look at all the body surfaces. Don't probe a stab wound that may enter a body cavity unless preparations are made for immediate surgery. Be alert for portions of the cutting instrument that may have broken off in the wound or bone. Although this is uncommon, it can be critical evidence or a source of infection. Either way, such a fragment should be recovered and saved if at all medically possible. If the patient is dead, *never probe the wound for any reason!*

Interpretation and Documentation of Stab Wounds

Stab wounds are frequently confused or misinterpreted by emergency personnel. The elastic fibers in the skin (the elastic lines of Langer) can pull incised wounds apart so that they appear round and may resemble bullet wounds. Additionally, a relatively small pocket knife can penetrate deeply into the body because of compression of the movable surfaces of the body, and can produce deep injuries to major structures. Stab wounds, like bullet wounds, may produce little external hemorrhage, especially in parts of the body associated with a potential cavity. A cutting instrument may be inserted to its full length, or only part way, and victim and assailant may move relative to one another, so that an L-shaped compound wound may result. The weapon may cut in the direction of pressure, or upon entering or leaving the body, so that the wound may have "tails" or other features. The weapon may cut an arc within the body, using the skin as the fulcrum. Because of the elastic fibers in the skin, the wound may be physically smaller or larger than the weapon that made it.

Be careful about assuming that you can tell the length or width of a knife by the surface injury size, or that you can judge the direction of travel within the body, the severity of the injury, the size of the swath internally, or the depth of penetration. No statement should be made about the relative height of the person with the knife, whether he or she is left-handed or right-handed, or what the victim was doing at time of the injury.

In some instances, the weapon may be introduced with such force that the hilt leaves an imprint. This can occasionally be of value in including or excluding a type of weapon or a specific weapon. Notice the recurring reference to "cutting instrument" rather than "knife." Many instruments may be used to produce sharp force injuries, and you must not limit your thinking to a knife alone.

Important considerations associated with stab wounds are listed in Chart 3-13.

BLUNT TRAUMA

Blunt trauma includes injuries due to jumps and falls, auto/pedestrian injuries, and endless other mechanisms of injury involving force from blows, impacts, and falls. Since a person may fall several times, or suffer multiple impacts from a single incident (*e.g.,* a fall down stairs), as well as suffer forces of varying energy (*e.g.,* a primary impact throwing a patient into another object), one has to be very careful in assuming exactly how the injury occurred. It may also be difficult to see several types of closed injuries.

Assessment

Transmitted Force. Force, in the form of kinetic energy, can be transmitted. This may occur along the length of the spinal cord, causing significant head injuries, or may produce shearing injuries of organs without any external signs of remote injury. When transmitted force results in injuries distant from the initial blow, these remote injuries can be lethal (*e.g.,* dissection or transection of the aorta from closed chest injury, rotational laceration of bridging vessels of the brain, laceration of solid organs). Transmitted force produces hydraulic pressure and other types of pressure that can cause fracturing of bone along the supraorbital plates. Compression forces may cause tearing or laceration of the brain. Sometimes the relative movement injuries to the brain are referred to

---

Chart 3-13

STAB WOUNDS: IMPORTANT CONSIDERATIONS

- Be aware that stab wounds, like bullet wounds, may produce little external bleeding or hemorrhage.
- Use great care when assessing and moving the patient because of risks of massive bleeding, gas embolism, cardiac arrest, spinal cord injury, etc.
- Carefully inspect all body surfaces for other wounds as soon as possible.
- Be alert for fragments of cutting instrument that may have broken off in the wound or bone and may cause infection.
- Be aware that the appearance of the surface injury may not indicate the following:
  Depth of penetration or extent of wound within the body
  Direction of travel of the instrument within the body
  Severity of the injury
- If patient is dead, *never probe the wound for any reason.*
  Evidence may be damaged or destroyed
- Do not attempt to make statements about the following:
  Relative height or left-handedness or right-handedness of assailant
  What victim was doing at the time of the injury

as coup and contrecoup (blow and counterblow) injuries to denote whether they are adjacent to the area of the force or distant from it. These important closed head injuries are of great significance because they explain why the major injury to the brain may be on the side opposite the point of injury. It is difficult to assess the extent of damage to an organ such as the liver by the size or shape of a patterned injury on the skin, since typically the visible injury does not reveal all the factors that could explain how the kinetic energy of the blow was dissipated by the tissue.

Lacerations.   Blunt trauma is frequently associated with lacerations. Blunt force lacerations have irregular skin edges and may leave intact neurovascular bundles, which are frequently visible at the base of the injury. Lacerations are typically produced by compression of the tissue between an object and an underlying structure and may undermine tissue, which helps identify the direction and sometimes the force.

Bruises.   Bruising can occur at or *near* the time of death and, to some extent, after death. Significant amounts of blood may collect within the fat layer or muscle without any initial evidence of a bruise. The *raccoon sign* (black eyes) following head trauma, gunshot wounds to the head, or acceleration/deceleration forces is a typical example. Bruising may form almost instantaneously with some injuries—for example, gunshot and blows to the head—and bruising about the eye may not indicate an earlier beating.

Interpretation of Blunt Trauma

Blunt trauma is the classic stuff that murder mysteries are made of. It is difficult for a nonexpert to tell whether the patient fell or was hit with an object. Sometimes, because of the pattern left on the skin of the patient, one can exclude, implicate, or include a particular object as the one that probably caused the injury. An additional factor is usually required before one can go to the next step and state that one specific object alone caused the injury. There may be an abrasion around the injury that can tell something about the object that produced it. Sometimes an object can be matched with the injury or eliminated as a possible cause of the wound by such examination.

For the expert, the position and nature of the injury can tell a great deal about how the injury was received, as well as how it could *not* have been received. A bite mark on the tongue or lips may suggest a seizure disorder, injuries on the anterior leg may suggest chronic alcoholism. This same experience and logic are used in the interpretation of blunt injury by the forensic scientist.

Documentation and Preservation of Evidence

Blunt trauma is probably seen more often than any other type of injury because there is an almost endless number of causes of these injuries. Important points about documenting and preserving evidence in blunt trauma are listed in Chart 3-14.

HOSPITAL DEATHS

With the increased use of sophisticated electronic equipment, better prehospital care, and advanced training in emergency care, most severely injured patients are being admitted to specialized care facilities. When one of these patients, or any patient, dies suddenly or unexpectedly, one should pause to consider the possibility that some medical problem, equipment failure, or other defect may have caused or contributed to the death. First, these are common charges in malpractice cases, and second, failure to correct the problem could expose another patient to the same danger. In some jurisdictions, regulations require that when any patient dies suddenly and unexpectedly in a hospital, *all* IV tubes and other apparatus must be left in place. The purpose is to facilitate documentation, determination of placement, and evaluation of complications such as gas embolism. It is important to recognize complications so that changes can be made to prevent recurrences. The following examples illustrate this principle.

Chart 3-14

BLUNT TRAUMA: DOCUMENTATION AND PRESERVATION OF EVIDENCE

- Don't include any statement in the chart without referring to its source (*e.g.*, "Ms. Jones stated that her husband beat her").
- Don't make statements that cannot be supported in court (*e.g.*, "the patient looks as though he was hit in the face with a fire ax, or a pint bottle").
- Be aware that the story heard in the emergency room is never the one heard in court, and hence no assumptions should be made.
- Clothing of a possible assault victim should always be saved—no matter how soiled it is. It must be stored in properly marked *paper* (not plastic) bags.
- Watch for foreign material in blunt trauma wounds. If there is reason to think that the injury was caused by another person, save any such material.

1. Following an auto accident leading to a flail chest and near drowning, a 21-year-old male was treated in a small hospital emergency room. His pulmonary compliance became progressively worse. There was a recurring problem of an air leak at the cuff of the endotracheal tube requiring increasing amounts of air in the cuff.

   Because of the difficulties in medical management, the patient was transferred to a major medical center. Within minutes of entering this facility, the patient suffered cardiac arrest, and death rapidly ensued. At autopsy, the cuffed endotracheal tube was still in place. The cuff was massively enlarged, and as a result, its normal symmetry was distorted so that it forced the lumen into the side of the trachea, causing complete blockage of the airway.

   The basic problem was that the tube initially selected for the patient was far too small for the airway. It had not been replaced by a larger size tube, and the problem of the recurrent leak had not been reported to the new hospital staff. This patient would have had a reasonable chance of recovery if proper respiratory assistance had been given.

2. In another instance, a patient developed prolonged hypotension during routine gallbladder surgery. To better monitor the patient's cardiac output, the anesthesiologist inserted a percutaneous central venous pressure (CVP) line. This prepackaged product was placed easily on the first attempt. In the recovery room, the patient developed arrhythmias that led to a series of arrests. A scheduled positional chest x-ray to check the CVP line was cancelled by a new staff member as being unnecessary. The patient died suddenly.

   At autopsy, it was seen that the plastic line had punctured the atrium, causing tamponade. The catheter was found to be damaged and had a sharp point. There were multiple lacerations of the interior of the heart where the point had been forced against the tissue adjacent to the conduction system. The failure to take positional x-rays and the subsequent withdrawal of the tube out of the heart led to the perforation and the patient's death. The line was thought to be defective when manufactured.

3. A patient with a 3-month-old mechanical heart valve was walking on a city sidewalk when she realized that she was once again in serious heart failure. She took a cab to the nearest emergency room and was seen immediately by a cardiologist. A chest x-ray was taken within 5 minutes of her arrival, at which point she suffered cardiac arrest. In spite of extensive resuscitation efforts, including placement of external pacing electrodes and multiple intracardiac injections, the patient was pronounced dead.

   At autopsy, it was observed that the disk that blocks the return of blood and therefore makes the valve work, was completely out of the heart valve because of a broken wire strut. Review of the initial x-ray proved that the strut was broken before resuscitation was attempted. The occluder was radiolucent and was found free in the aorta.

In the last two cases, the manufacturer was contacted, and changes were made in the production or quality control processes to prevent or improve diagnosis of complications. In the case of the heart valve, a radiopaque marker was inserted into the disk so that its function and position could be seen on x-ray, and the wire strut was strengthened, with the result that no deaths from this problem have occurred over the last 4 years. Removing the apparatus or failing to investigate would have obscured the real cause of death in each of these cases, would not have improved the quality of patient care, and would have unnecessarily endangered many lives.

Hospital Charting

Hospital charts are not used for documenting evidence—they are for patient care. But when a case has medicolegal implications, there is a good chance that part or all of the chart will appear in court. Medical personnel have a legal obligation regarding charting, and the law is tending toward enforcing that obligation. The following are some simple, logical steps that facilitate good charting:

- Always start every progress note or other entry with the date and time.
- Write all entries in legible form. Always write orders or notes carefully, and be certain that numbers and other data, such as units of measure, are always easy to read. **Print** if necessary.
- Avoid abbreviations at all times, especially for potentially critical portions of the chart. In physician's orders, the difference between a scrawled *mg* and *mEq* or similar term can cost a life.
- Be especially careful when writing orders for new, unusual, or unusually toxic drugs.
- The terms *accident, homicide,* and *suicide* are legal terms. They should not be used by emergency care personnel in describing the manner of death or injury or in making a definitive statement. "Possible suicide" and "possible homicide" are acceptable terms.
- Consent forms and operative permits are legal documents. Don't add to a form after the patient has signed it. Be certain that the patient or the legal next of kin has signed the appropriate form at the appropriate time.
- The language barrier is a common problem, and arrangements must be made to deal with patients who do not speak English. These may consist of a list of interpreters whom you can call on when necessary. Using a relative or another patient as an interpreter is not always the best way to get accurate information or to pass on important instructions.

These points are summarized in Chart 3-15.

Special Considerations

Securing and Keeping Blood and Urine Specimens. It often happens that a patient with serious head injuries dies after days of hospitalization, and lack of samples precludes a diagnosis of the cause or manner of death. In any case in which the initial diagnosis is not clear, and in which it is even remotely possible that a drug, industrial or agricultural poison, toxin, or virus may be involved, it is recommended that all blood and urine from the initial workup be saved for at least 1 or 2 weeks. In some instances, these specimens can make the diagnosis. They may have to be sent to another laboratory or to the coroner after death. In some areas, the hospital is required to draw and maintain a sample for ethyl alcohol analysis on all automobile drivers who enter with serious injuries. If the patient dies, the sample is sent to the coroner; if the patient lives, the sample is discarded.

Head Injuries. Be cautious about discharging a patient with a recent history of head injury, especially a child or an adult who has no one to look after him. In many instances, patients with minor or serious head injuries have been discharged before blood or urine was collected for testing, and have died at home. During an outbreak of some condition such as influenza, be sure to watch for head injuries, which

---

Chart 3-15

GUIDELINES FOR HOSPITAL CHARTING

- Start each progress note or other entry with the date and time.
- Write orders or notes carefully and **legibly**—Print if necessary.
- Take special care with numbers and units of measurement.
- Never use abbreviations. Confusion about an illegible *mg* or *mEq*, or a similar term, could cost a life.
- Do not use legal terms such as *accident, homicide,* or *suicide* in describing manner of death or injury or in making a definitive statement. "Possible homicide" and "possible suicide" are acceptable terms.
- Consent forms and operative permits are legal documents.
  Do not add to a form after the patient has signed it.
  Be certain that patient or legal next of kin has signed the appropriate form at the appropriate time.
- Provide for communication with patients who speak another language.
  Maintain a list of available interpreters.
  Avoid using relatives or other patients as interpreters.

---

can be overlooked. Do not assume that similar symptoms necessarily indicate the same condition.

Coroner's Cases. All deaths of persons under sentence or in jail become coroner's cases. These deaths should be investigated from the outset as homicides because when a case is opened at a higher level of investigation, the level can later be decreased, but it is almost impossible to increase the level of investigation without losing a great deal of evidence or information. Approximately 70% to 75% of prisoners who die are recent arrests, and most typically for problems associated with alcoholism. Jail suicides also typically occur within 1 or 2 days of arrest. Victims of sudden, unexpected, or violent death are likely to become matters of interest in civil or criminal court. A sizable number of these victims that do not die are equally likely to be involved in court proceedings. Emergency department personnel have a moral and legal obligation to help victims in a number of ways. Protection of evidence, patient rights, and documentation need not interfere with good patient care, nor does it necessarily add to time or effort needed for this care. Simple attention to detail and good charting, both prerequisites for patient care, plus some general forensic knowledge such as that above, will prepare you to work with almost any case you are likely to see in the emergency department.

BIBLIOGRAPHY

Adelson L: The Pathology of Homicide. Springfield, Ill, Charles C Thomas, 1974
Harris RI: Outline of Death Investigation. Springfield, Ill, Charles C Thomas, 1962
McNeese M, Hebeler JR: The Abused Child: Clinical Symposia. CIBA 29(5), 1977
Moritz AR, Morris RC: Handbook of Legal Medicine, 3rd ed. St. Louis, CV Mosby, 1970
Spitz WU, Fisher RS: Medicolegal Investigation of Death. Springfield, Ill, Charles C Thomas, 1973
Tedeschi CG, Eckert WG, Tedeschi LG: Forensic Medicine. Philadelphia, WB Saunders, 1977
Wecht CH (ed): Legal Medicine Annual. New York, Appleton-Century-Crofts, 1971

AGENCIES

National Foundation for Sudden Infant Death, 1501 Broadway, New York, NY 10036

4
ACQUISITION OF DONOR ORGANS

ALBERT D. MENNO

HISTORICAL CONSIDERATIONS

The use of tissues from one human being in the body of another is largely a 20th century development. Many slow, progressive steps were taken in the latter half of the 19th century. This early work by several skin transplant surgeons mainly involved various methods of transplanting skin. Thiersch, in 1874, described the microscopic details of how a graft "takes," that is, how it adheres in its new bed. A similar period of development occurred with corneal transplantation beginning in 1884.

It was not until 1943, however, that Gibson and Medawar first appreciated the significance of the *source* of tissue for transplantation and initiated research on the immunologic reactions that occurred in allografting and xenografting.* Organ transplantation, because of technical difficulties, was not attempted until the first decade of the 20th century, at a time when vascular surgery was just coming of age. Only short-term successes were recorded, however, until the classical work of Medawar, which described the standard rejection reaction and its variations occurring in transplantation of tissues.

The first successful transplantation with prolonged survival occurred in 1955, when a human kidney was taken from one identical twin and transplanted into the other. As of 1975, approximately 2500 kidneys had been transplanted in the United States, and at least five times that number had been transplanted worldwide. These figures have probably tripled since then. Other types of tissues that have been transplanted with varying degrees of success are blood vessels, bone, blood, skin, cornea, lung, heart, intestine, endocrine, glands, marrow, and liver.

IMPLICATIONS FOR EMERGENCY PERSONNEL

Although organ transplantation has only a brief history, it is now common in the practice of many medical specialties. Personnel in an emergency setting are not frequently involved in the care of patients during or following transplantation procedures. Skin grafting for a wound is probably the most notable exception. More often, emergency management centers on the care of a possible donor, the emotional support of his family, or the mechanisms for getting permission to obtain donor organs from the family of a dying patient. The emergency care professional may serve as a facilitator and liaison among those concerned with the acquisition, transport, and maintenance or storage of donor organs.

Thus, responsibilities may include the initial handling and storage of donor organs until they can be transported to the appropriate location. In other instances, for example, when the donor organ must be supported *in vivo,* the staff may become involved in life-support measures for the dying patient to provide adequate perfusion of the donor organ(s)

* See Terminology section.

until the necessary arrangements can be made. The specific responsibilities depend a great deal on where one practices and the types of transplants done in that area. Since these vary widely, one must become acquainted with the community and regional resources available for procuring, storing, and transplanting various donor organs.

TERMINOLOGY

Over the years, terms have evolved that express the relationship of the donor source to the recipient. An understanding of the following terminology is necessary to comprehend the variety of transplants that can be done.

The transplantation of any tissue or organ from one place in a given individual to another place in the same individual has been called an *isograft* in older literature and an *autograft* in more modern studies. The transplantation of any tissue or organ from one individual to another of the same species has been called a *homograft* in older literature and an *allograft* more recently. The transplantation of any tissue or organ from an individual of one species to an individual of another has been called a *heterograft* in the past and a *xenograft* in the more recent literature.

For example, a skin graft taken from a patient's thigh to be placed on the abdomen is an autograft. A kidney taken from patient A and placed in patient B is an allograft. Pigskin, which is used as a temporary dressing in burn patients, among others, is an example of a xenograft.

Immunologic Reactions

Under normal circumstances, autografts do not involve immunologic reactions. Success depends more on mechanical factors, such as the size of vessels, the characteristics of the donor organ, and the recipient space for the organ. Xenografts and allografts, on the other hand, involve clear-cut immunologic reactions, and success depends on both mechanical factors and the degree of similarity or difference between the donor and the recipient (see Tissue-Typing).

Host-Versus-Graft Reactions. These immunologic differences (between donor and recipient) are the stimulus for the generation in the recipient of antibodies against the "foreign" proteins in the donor tissue (antigens) and the inflow of lymphocytes into the donor tissue or organ. These are known as *host-versus-graft* reactions. To some degree, it is possible to modify these reactions by using combinations of steroids and cytotoxic agents, but this is successful only when the differences are not great.

Graft-Versus-Host Reactions. Recently it has been recognized that a reversed immunologic reaction can occur. In this *graft-versus-host* reaction, multiple organ damage can result from immunologic attack on a recipient whose own body defenses have been highly modified by the *immunosuppressive* agents mentioned above.

ORGAN TRANSPLANTATION

KIDNEY TRANSPLANTS

Kidney transplantation is a common type of organ transfer, and the matching of donor kidneys to potential recipients has been well organized. For these reasons, this type of transplantation and the network of cooperation that facilitates it is discussed in depth in this chapter. Similarities and differences that exist among the various types of organ transplants are outlined later in the chapter.

Selection of the Donor

Whenever siblings, parents, or children of patients are available, an attempt is usually made to use one of these family members as the source of the kidney for transplantation. These donations are usually completely elective and depend on a detailed study of the function of the donor organ, in addition to its tissue match to the recipient.

A problem arises when no relative is available or when a relative is not willing or physically healthy enough to donate an organ; in these circumstances, a cadaver becomes the only possible source for a kidney. Cadaver kidneys, however, are rarely used in children because of the difference in size, which may cause many technical problems.

Size and Age Factors. When a kidney from a child is to be used in an adult, the size of the organ is a more significant factor than the age of the donor. In the average-size child, the practical age limit falls at 7 to 8 years. The kidney at this age is almost always large enough to sustain a small to average-size adult; evidence shows that the organ enlarges rapidly within the first few weeks after transplantation.

Although kidneys from donors as old as 75 years of age have been transplanted, the common practical upper age limit for adult donors is approximately 50 to 55 years. Persons older than this commonly have sufficient sclerosis of the aorta or renal arteries to make the anastomosis of the artery technically very difficult. In addition, organs beyond this age are more likely to have undesirable vascular changes, glomerular changes, or pyelonephritic fibrosis. A rapid, complete evaluation of function on such donors would be necessary if they are to be seriously considered.

Cadaver Donors. The usual donor of cadaver kidneys is most likely to fall between the ages of 15 and 45 because of the prevalence of automobile accidents, a principal cause of death in this age group. The most appropriate cadaver donor for organs is one with an almost pure, severe cerebral injury; however, most severely injured patients have multiple injuries.

Screening of Donors. It is essential to have some reasonable knowledge of the donor's injuries, hospital course, and surgery, and if available, past medical history. Dying patients whose additional injuries affect the extremities present no problems. However, when actual or potential contamination of the abdomen (as from previous surgery involving colon leakage of intestinal content or obvious peritonitis) is a factor, the dying patient should be carefully screened. Since one of the most common causes of post-transplant complications seen in immunosuppressed patients is infection, the presence of any type of organism (even some low-grade pathogens and some organisms that are usually nonpathogenic) in the transplanted organ should be scrupulously avoided. For the same reason, when pyelonephritis is a cause of the recipient's renal failure, special preparation is required—such as bilateral nephrectomy or conduit construction for urologic obstruction, or antituberculosis prophylactic antibiotics.

Whenever there is suspicion of renal injury such as gross or microscopic hematuria, an intravenous pyelogram (IVP) should be done to prove renal integrity. Many contused but not otherwise damaged kidneys can be salvaged in this manner.

Legal Considerations. Most transplant surgeons currently avoid cadaver donors whose injuries have resulted from criminal assault or when a criminal charge is pending against a party of the associated accident. The cadaver of a suicide victim may be used, depending on the attitude of the medical examiner in the locality and on whether the suicide is clear-cut and unquestioned.

A good working relationship with the coroner or medical examiner is absolutely essential. Whenever a potential donor becomes available, it should be the custom to call the coroner or medical examiner to ascertain that he sees no medicolegal impediment to salvaging the kidneys. (See Chap. 3, Forensic Aspects of Sudden and Unexpected Death).

Recovery of the Donor Organ

It is necessary to transplant only one healthy kidney to maintain a person who is otherwise without kidney function. Therefore, when a cadaver donor becomes available and both kidneys can be salvaged, two different recipients may each receive a kidney simultaneously, often in two separate hospitals, each with its own transplant team. Obviously, a closely knit communications network is necessary to coordinate all these activities. Since 4 to 6 hours are necessary for tissue typing (discussed below), the person who is dead on arrival (DOA) or dies shortly after arrival at the hospital is usually not considered a donor candidate unless an organ perfusion apparatus is available. Local practice governs what can be done. A few transplant centers are willing to salvage kidneys from a recent DOA donor, place them in supportive perfusion and assess their function for possible use. Kidneys from patients who die a short time after arrival are used more often. Such kidneys are placed on a perfuser before transplantation.

Organ Perfusion. Belzer initially developed a perfusion apparatus that circulates a cold nutrient perfusate through a donor kidney. Although clinically capable of sustaining the kidney for 72 hours, organ perfusers are more commonly used for periods of 10 to 18 hours. Several similar machines, most of them portable, are now available. The perfusates are variable, but are similar in composition to Ringer's lactate solution, with some additives. The use of an organ perfuser is desirable for a number of reasons:

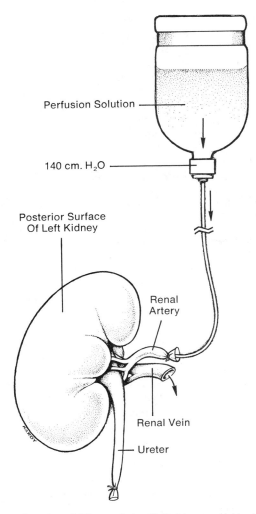

Perfusion Solution

140 cm. H$_2$O

Posterior Surface
Of Left Kidney

Renal
Artery

Renal Vein

Ureter

Figure 4-1 *Technique of kidney perfusion. Sterile intravenous tubing is inserted into the main renal artery and held in place by a suture tied around the exterior of the artery. The perfusion solution (4°C lactated Ringer's, with 50 mg heparin and 1 gm procaine per liter) is raised to a height of 140 cm of water above the donor kidney and allowed to run through the kidney by force of gravity. The cut end of the renal vein is open to allow the fluid to flow from the kidney.*

- Sustaining the organ while tissue typing is being completed
- Obtaining more time for recipient preparation
- Providing a means of testing the functional viability of the organ after salvage and before recipient implantation
- Transporting the organ over long distances

Ischemia Time. In the past few years, salvage of kidneys from cadavers has become a highly organized procedure. This is necessary because circulation through the kidney ceases with death and the termination of cardiac action. The absence of renal blood flow from the time of death until vascular anastomosis is completed in the recipient is called the *ischemia time*. The total ischemia time is the sum of the warm and cold ischemia times, which may be described as follows:

1. *Warm ischemia time.* It is generally accepted that no more than 45 minutes should elapse from the time of death to the time when the kidney is cooled to near-freezing temperatures. This is the warm ischemia time.

2. *Cold ischemia time.* A period of 3½ to 4 hours is allowed to place the donor kidney in the recipient, anastomose the renal artery and vein to the recipient vessels, and reestablish blood flow. This is the cold ischemia time.

Generally, the shorter the warm ischemia time, the longer the donor kidney can tolerate the total time of ischemia. When the warm ischemia time is as short as 10 minutes, the surgeon can work with approximately 10 hours of tolerance to total ischemia.

Organ Salvage Procedure. The donor kidneys are removed by surgeons in an operating suite under sterile conditions. Once the blood vessels are divided, arterial perfusion is initiated, using a solution that has been cooled to 4°C (39.2°F) (see Fig. 4-1). This perfusion is effected by gravity only; it flushes out the renal arteries and veins, rinsing out all the blood and cooling the kidney from within. The fluid most commonly used is a 5% glucose/Ringer's lactate solution with 50 mg of heparin and 1.0 gm of procaine added. A similar solution, but with additional magnesium and dibenzyline, is preferred. It can be prepared by the hospital pharmacy.

After 500 ml to 1000 ml are flushed through each kidney, the kidneys are placed in sterile plastic bags which are then put in a 1- to 2-liter nalgene jar and transported in styrofoam-insulated cartons (Polyfoam Packers) to the recipient hospital. Each kidney should be labeled *left* or *right* because, for technical reasons, it is desirable to place a right kidney in a left iliac fossa and vice versa.

Tissue Typing

The success of autotransplantation depends in part on matching compatible donors and recipients by tissue typing. This is a most delicate procedure, requiring 4 to 6 hours for completion. It involves the collection of 20 ml to 25 ml of blood, which is defibrinated and passed through a column of resin material to separate out the lymphocytes. The lymphocytes are then tested with antisera, and the positive reactions are noted. In this manner, the HL-A human lymphocyte antigen (HL-A) type of the donor is identified and compared with the HL-A types of all possible recipients until a match is found.

At one time, as many as 200 antisera might be used in a single typing. However, the antisera used in typing have been classified by Terasaki and others.[9] This made it possible to define human lymphocyte antigens reacting against groups of antisera. At present, 13 groups of transplantation antigens are accepted and used internationally in tissue typing. Many more are being used by various immunologists throughout the world who are engaged in various stages of analysis of those antigens. Undoubtedly, some of these may later become accepted. Those that are fully accepted bear the designation HL-A plus a number.

It is now accepted that four HL-A antigens usually define a *tissue type*. One pair of antigens occurs at one locus on a chromosome and presumably is derived from one parent; the second pair occurs at a second locus on the chromosome and is presumably derived from the second parent. In the present state of the art, results may not always be precise; occasionally, one or two of the antigens are not defined by the testing.

Only the antigens within the HL-A system are significant for the purposes of transplantation. They are present on all somatic body cells, but the lymphocyte, being a readily available "circulating cell," is used as typical for testing purposes. The lymphocyte is also a mediator in the immunologic response of rejection and thus is a logical choice as the model cell. From the technical standpoint, difficulties sometimes arise because of the inability to separate the lymphocytes from other white blood cells, particularly after trauma, when an excessive number of polymorphonuclear leukocytes may be present.

The red cell ABO antigens, so well known in blood crossmatching for compatibility, are also most important to match in transplants. These are very strong antigens that can evoke massive, rapid, and acute responses in the recipient within minutes of exposure to them. This phenomenon is called *hyperacute rejection.* Mismatching in the ABO system of red blood cell classification dooms the transplant to failure.

On the other hand, the red cell Rh antigen is very weak and of little significance. It is usually completely ignored when matching donors to recipients, and no transplant rejections are known to have resulted from ignoring this antigen.

OTHER TRANSPLANTABLE ORGANS

Cornea

The next most publicized transplantable tissue is the cornea, though this tissue was actually transplanted long before the kidney. Indeed, the organization of the renal "organ recovery" programs follows patterns developed by eye banks in many areas of the country.

Corneal transplant has several unique advantages. First, time is less pressing, since several hours are available from the moment of death to the time when the cornea must be salvaged, treated with antibiotic and saline solutions, and cooled. This allows time for obtaining consent from relatives and preparing the recipient. Second, there are no agonal physiologic changes in the cornea that limit its capabilities after transplantation. Thus, the corneas from a person who is DOA may be salvaged. Third, no tissue typing is necessary, since the cornea acquires no vascularization after transplantation. Indeed, its function requires that it not become vascularized; thus, there is no way for tissue antibodies to reach it.

The most important action to be taken when cornea salvage is a possibility is that of taping the lids to the donor closed to prevent drying. All remaining steps should be taken by a representative of the local eye bank, who should be called immediately. He has about 3 hours in which to complete the salvage.

Skin and Bone

Skin and bone are the tissues that can currently be "banked" in the strict sense of the word. Well-organized skin and bone banks exist in many metropolitan areas. Storage of these tissues involves cleansing and rinsing in saline solutions, treatment with antibiotics, and freezing. Both skin and bone are removed as soon after death as is convenient. At present

there is no set time limit, although 12 to 24 hours is a practical limit. Only diseased tissues or tissues containing tumors need be excluded from salvage.

Of all the organs or tissues used, bone creates the fewest problems in transplantation because eventually it is completely replaced by the recipient's own tissues. It merely acts as a strut and a source for calcium. No attempt is ever made to tissue type the donor or the recipient for this type of transfer.

Skin is handled similarly and is currently most useful for transplantation in burned patients. For this purpose, it acts mainly as an organic dressing to prevent the problems that occur with infiltration of bacteria into the burn wound. When skin is used solely in this fashion, there is usually no attempt at tissue typing because it is expected that it eventually will slough and disappear. Organic dressings allow the burned patient to recover more completely and to regenerate sites on his own body where skin may be obtained for an autograft. (See Chap. 28, Burns.)

When the allografted skin is intended to be permanently attached, tissue typing is necessary. A relative is usually a good donor for skin transfer.

Blood Vessels

Salvage of blood vessels has become unimportant in recent years because of the availability of prosthetic vessels. However, whenever natural vessels are desirable, the saphenous vein is usually chosen, and an autograft is done.

Aortic valves or aortic valve cusps are currently being used as allografts in open heart surgery. These are salvaged and stored by the individual surgeons who use them, usually from cadavers within their own institutions. They are rinsed in saline solutions, treated with antibiotics, and frozen, much as bone and skin are handled. No tissue typing is necessary, since they merely act as struts in the formation of new cusps within the aorta.

Other Organs

At present, transplants of endocrine glands, marrow, and spleen are being done only in isolated institutions, and for the most part are still highly experimental. Success rate data and details have not been widely publicized. The difficulties thus far appear to be mainly in the immunologic area; infection and other radiation-related problems may occur as a result of the large amounts of radiation and immunosuppressive agents that are required to control the rejection process.

Lung, heart, and liver transplantation are currently widely publicized but are always extremely difficult to perform. Each of these organs can be sustained outside the body for only short periods of time and only with the use of pump oxygenators during the transfer between the cadaver and the recipient. Therefore, salvage from patients who die within the institution where the transplantation will occur is most practical. Portable perfusion techniques are being perfected, however, to overcome this limitation.

At present, lung, heart, and liver transplants are performed in very few centers in any one country, and tissue typing is always necessary. The current success rate with these organs

UNIFORM DONOR CARD

OF_____

Print or type name of donor

In the hope that I may help others, I hereby make this anatomical gift, if medically acceptable, to take effect upon my death. The words and marks below indicate my desires.

I give: (a) _____ any needed organs or parts

(b) _____ only the following organs or parts

_____

Specify the organ(s) or part(s)

for the purposes of transplantation, therapy, medical research or education;

(c) _____ my body for anatomical study if needed.

Limitations or
special wishes, if any :_____

Signed by the donor and the following two witnesses in the presence of each other:

_____   _____
Signature of Donor   Date of Birth of Donor

_____   _____
Date Signed   City & State

_____   _____
Witness   Witness

This is a legal document under the Uniform Anatomical Gift Act or similar laws.

Figure 4-2 *Legal consent for donation of an organ or body part. This form is a legal document, when properly completed, under the Uniform Anatomical Gift Act and similar laws.*

is only mediocre because of inability to control immunologic reactions.

MEDICOLEGAL CONSIDERATIONS

Uniform Anatomical Gift Act

Almost all states have now adopted a *Uniform Anatomical Gift Act,* with the following provisions:

1. An individual of age 18 or older can, prior to his death, consent to the removal of any or all organs from his own body after death and can carry a signed, witnessed card to this effect.

2. Only the most available ranking legal next of kin* need sign a consent for removal of organs from a dead relative for transplantation (whereas all of the ranking next of kin must sign for postmortem examinations).

3. A state of cerebral death acceptable to both medical and legal communities can be determined when five criteria are met.

_____
* Legal next of kin refers to a specific listing of order of kinship and is usually defined in the state probate code.

Criteria for Cerebral Death

The five criteria for cerebral death are:
1. The absence of spontaneous respirations
2. The absence of all reflexes
3. Dilated fixed pupils
4. A completely flat electroencephalogram, taken on two occasions 24 hours apart
5. An unstable blood pressure

All five criteria must be present for cerebral death to be declared (obviously with the consent of the family) in hopeless situations so that salvage of the kidneys can be accomplished and the respirator turned off in an acceptable legal manner. The importance of early notification of the coroner or medical examiner cannot be overemphasized.

Consent Forms

For consent to be signed by the legal next of kin, a standard consent form, specifying the operative procedure as "removal of (specified organs) after death for transplantation purposes" is all that is required. For the person over 18 who wishes to sign his own consent, a card is currently available from headquarter offices of the National Kidney Foundation, which can be carried in the wallet (Figure 4-2). It must be signed by two witnesses. This card then represents the complete legal consent form in itself and can be used even when relatives cannot be contacted. Such cards are now acceptable in all 50 states. It specifies whether certain organs, all available and desired organs, or the entire body may be used for scientific purposes. This consent card is legally binding. The law holds health professionals blameless for acting solely on the basis of the consent card.

ESTABLISHING A SYSTEM TO FACILITATE TRANSPLANTS

A community-wide communication system is essential for matching donor kidneys to needed recipients. This system must possess at least two capabilities: (1) the ability to inform appropriate sources rapidly that donor kidneys have been obtained and (2) the ability to provide a continuously updated list of needed recipients and related information. While system differences exist, the model discussed is common to many areas. The reader is advised to become familiar with the procedure in his or her own locale by contacting any of the following:
1. The nearest hospital known to be involved in transplanting organs of any type
2. The regional chapter of the National Kidney Foundation
3. The chairman of the department of surgery of the nearest medical school.

The Operation of One System

In upstate New York and southern Ontario, lines of communication have been developed, as shown in the accom-

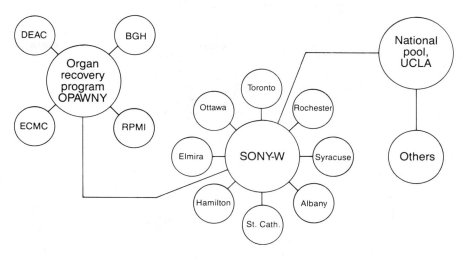

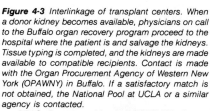

Figure 4-3 *Interlinkage of transplant centers. When a donor kidney becomes available, physicians on call to the Buffalo organ recovery program proceed to the hospital where the patient is and salvage the kidneys. Tissue typing is completed, and the kidneys are made available to compatible recipients. Contact is made with the Organ Procurement Agency of Western New York (OPAWNY) in Buffalo. If a satisfactory match is not obtained, the National Pool at UCLA or a similar agency is contacted.*

DEAC, Deaconess Hospital; ECMC Erie County Medical Center; RPMI, Roswell Park Memorial Institute; BGH, Buffalo General Hospital; SONY-W represents a city: Buffalo, Rochester, Syracuse, Albany, Elmira in New York State and St. Catherines, Hamilton, Ottawa, and Toronto in Ontario, Canada.

panying diagram (Fig. 4-3). The hospitals involved supply representatives on rotation to receive calls from hospitals with potential donors, arrange for tissue typing, select appropriate recipients, and salvage kidneys in hospitals anywhere in the region. In addition, a continually updated list is circulated to participating hospitals, containing names of potential recipients who have previously been tissue typed, their ABO types, and the names of their attending physicians. The salvaged kidneys are sent to the best-matched recipients, preferably in two different hospitals. When many equally matched recipients are found, the patients who have been waiting the longest are given preference.

The Organ Procurement Agency of Western New York functions as the local recovery program. If no satisfactory match is found locally, contact is made with other agencies, such as the SONY-West listing in Rochester, or others. This organization has been formed by representatives from hospitals in Buffalo, Rochester, Albany and Syracuse, New York, in addition to Hamilton, Toronto, St. Catherines, and Burlington, Ontario. SONY-West supplies a listing of the recipients in this larger area. To avoid problems at the border, customs officials are notified by telephone and transportation is provided by state and provincial police.

If no suitable recipient match is found within this larger area, contact may be made in a similar manner with a more distant regional listing such as that in Los Angeles. This listing contains a large number of patients in California and other western states, in addition to some in foreign countries.

SUMMARY

The transplantation of human tissues occurs every day in the United States. The tissues most commonly used are skin, cornea, and kidneys. While some tissues may be preserved and stored for long periods of time, others, such as the kidneys, must be implanted in the recipient within a matter of hours.

Transplant centers have been established in many areas of the United States. Many of these centers are linked across the country to allow for complete use of donor organs as they become available. Emergency personnel should be familiar with the transplantation services available in or near their regions; they should help establish procedures for obtaining suitable organs for human transplantation and should facilitate their use.

A Uniform Anatomical Gift Act has been enacted in most states. Many persons carry uniform donor cards. When properly completed and witnessed, such a card constitutes a legal document. Consideration must be given, however, to whether a particular individual is or is not suitable as an organ donor.

The primary limiting factor in transplantation is the availability of donor organs. Emergency personnel can play an important role by being aware of a seriously injured patient as a potential organ donor after death. When such a patient is seen in the emergency department, measures aimed at facilitating the acquisition of usable organs should be taken.

REFERENCES

1. Alexander JW, Good RA: Immunobiology for Surgeons. Philadelphia, WB Saunders, 1970
2. Brooks JR: Endocrine Tissue Transplantation. Springfield, Ill, Charles C Thomas, 1962
3. Juul-Jensen P: Criteria of Brain Death. Copenhagen, Munksgaard, 1970
4. Menno AD, Giordano ML: The operation of the kidney bank of Buffalo. Cryobiology 7:179, September–October 1970
5. Moore FD: Give and Take. Philadelphia, WB Saunders, 1964
6. Rappaport FT, Dausset J: Human Transplantation. New York, Grune & Stratton, 1968
7. Starzl T: Experience in Renal Transplantation. Philadelphia, WB Saunders, 1964
8. Starzl TE, Porter KA, Husberg BS, Ishikawa M, Putnam CW: Renal homotransplantation. Curr Probl Surg, 1974
9. Terasaki P: Histocompatibility Testing. Baltimore, Williams & Wilkins, 1970
10. Norman JC: Organ Perfusion and Preservation. New York, Appleton-Century-Crofts, 1968

UNIT TWO

PSYCHOSOCIAL ASPECTS OF EMERGENCY CARE

5

PSYCHIATRIC EMERGENCIES

M. KATHLEEN ROSE-GRIPPA

The intrusive behaviors associated with anxiety can and do hinder emergency department personnel in fulfilling their primary responsibility of saving lives. The result of these intrusions can be fatal. The patient, the family (or others accompanying the patient), the emergency department staff, or any combination of these persons may be the source of intrusive anxiety and its demanding behaviors.

The emergency department staff, by role and by definition, has the responsibility of handling and at least initially, treating these psychiatric emergencies. These tasks require the staff to

- Keep calm in order not to add to the anxiety
- Recognize and assess behaviors provoked by anxiety
- Successfully intervene in these behaviors
- Learn from each situation how to deal more effectively with the next psychiatric emergency

DEFINITION OF A PSYCHIATRIC EMERGENCY

Attempting to find an exact definition of a psychiatric emergency is like trying to find an exact definition of love. Each definer uses his own theoretical and experiential background to choose the words that best describe his experience with the phenomenon. Some common threads appear among the available definitions, one being the *suddenness* of the event—often described as "a sudden serious disturbance"[5] or "an urgent condition."[30] Another commonality involves references to the *overwhelming nature* of the event—"an obstacle seen as unsurmountable,"[8] "unable to cope with life forces;"[28] it "exceeds an individual's adaptive capacity."[30]

The implied but seldom stated third thread is that the person needs *psychological assistance* during this time of high stress. These three threads unite in a simple and pragmatic definition: a psychiatric emergency exists whenever "some person's anxiety has increased to the point that immediate aid is requested."[20] This definition, with its focus on the patient and on the present level of anxiety, provides guidelines for sound intervention.

Anxiety is highly contagious; at any moment the emergency department staff may be faced with anxiety—in themselves or in a patient. Staff members must be able to understand, accept, and handle their own levels of anxiety in a tense situation and be able to intervene successfully in the patient's anxious behavior. This is crucial because the most powerful intervention strategy the emergency department staff has is competent self-assurance. As Rogerson states:

> The composure of the emergency room staff in knowing how to handle psychiatric emergencies is an extremely valuable asset in dealing with such emergencies—especially when it is coupled with an accepting attitude and prompt decisive action.[30]

Long experience has shown that the insecurities of a staff in handling psychiatric emergencies decrease markedly with practice at well tested, specific interventions. Self-confidence and composure increase with each instance of successful intervention. This chapter, therefore, is designed to provide specific strategies and tactics for handling psychiatric emer-

gencies and to explain some of the reasons behind them so that even the novice can intervene successfully.

The Concept of Anxiety

A conceptualization of anxiety and its behaviors is basic to the understanding of people, whether these people be the patients or the staff of an emergency department. The behaviors associated with anxiety can be conceptualized in many ways. In this chapter, the concept of anxiety is presented as a horseshoe-shaped spectrum, with too little anxiety at one end and too much anxiety at the other.[4] The person is viewed as having the ability to react to stress in a variety of ways, depending on personality characteristics, experience, and the immediate environment. One person may exhibit the behaviors associated with panic, another those associated with severe depression. Either reaction may involve approximately the same amount of subjective anxiety (known only to the person). The horseshoe of anxiety is shown schematically in Figure 5-1.

This discussion is organized around four identifiable levels of *visible* anxiety:
1. Little or no visible anxiety
2. Mild to moderate anxiety
3. Severe anxiety
4. Panic

In addition to these levels of *visible* anxiety there is yet another level, referred to as *undefined anxiety*, which falls between the first and second categories. No one of these levels exists completely by itself, since the behaviors more frequently associated with one level can slide in and out of various other levels. Because it is difficult to discuss the staff's response to clinical situations without concrete examples, the patient is the primary focus in this discussion, and suggestions are provided for the staff's implementation of the ideas presented. The last few paragraphs of the chapter are directed exclusively to the emergency department staff.

THE PATIENT WITH LITTLE OR NO VISIBLE ANXIETY

Some level of anxiety is necessary for normal functioning. Experience with our own feelings teaches us to recognize when levels of anxiety in others are too low to be functional. The most reliable clue is that the seriousness of a situation and the person's response do not match. Thus, when a person shrugs off a 30-pound weight loss or responds, "Oh, yeah," to having come very close to a successful suicide, health care professionals should pay close attention. This incongruous lack of anxiety is seen most often in depressed persons or in those being treated following an attempt to commit suicide.

THE PERSON WHO ATTEMPTS SUICIDE

Most distressing to health care professionals is the patient who has attempted suicide. Emergency department person-

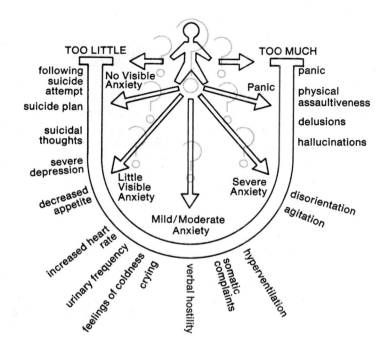

Figure 5-1 *The horseshoe of anxiety. This model illustrates: (1) that a person exhibiting little or no anxiety is not the complete opposite of the person exhibiting panic, and (2) that any person can respond to stress in a variety of ways.*

nel frequently interpret the attitude of a suicidal person as that of despondence. He seems to be saying, in effect, "What you value so highly isn't worth much." Sometimes it is difficult to remember that the primary consideration is to save the patient's life.

Life-saving procedures depend upon the type and severity of the means used to attempt suicide; since these procedures are outlined in other chapters, they will not be developed here. Procedures must be carried out with an accepting, nonpunishing attitude. Health professionals have long known that people are more inclined to talk when they believe they will be listened to and that more information can be collected from a verbal than from a nonverbal person. It follows logically that if the professional staff adopts behaviors that indicate an ability and desire to listen, the patient will be encouraged to talk more freely, more information will be collected, the nurse will be more likely to make an appropriate referral, and the probability that this person will return to the emergency department after another attempt at suicide will decrease.

While following procedures for gastric lavage, suturing, or other trauma-related measures, the nurse should speak in a modulated tone of voice and avoid being shrill or sharp or moving suddenly. She should not cram the lavage tube into the patient's throat, but rather should take the time to talk reassuringly while working, explaining the procedure. She must also watch what she says: punishing comments such as "This will teach you a lesson" or "Do a better job next time" should never be made. The patient feels bad enough without having someone add to his feelings of guilt and worthlessness.

Emergency department staff members are *the* health care profession as far as the patient is concerned. If he gets the message that he is not being heard, that it really does not matter what happens to him, that he should not be taking the staff's time away from someone who really needs it, it

is highly unlikely that he will seek help from another health care professional, *i.e.,* a psychotherapist. If psychotherapy is mandated and follows punishing treatment in the emergency room, it will take longer for a trusting relationship to be established between patient and therapist. This deprives the troubled person of support and help during the three dangerous months following a suicidal crisis[13] and increases the chances that he will make a second attempt. An accepting attitude lets the patient know that the staff members care about the person, no matter how they may feel about suicidal behavior.

Too frequently, after the hectic atmosphere of the initial life-saving procedures, the patient is left alone. On the surface, there appears to be little need to spend any additional time with him, since he is apparently no longer in danger of dying, and there is no behavior indicating that anxiety is present. The suicidal act seems to have drained all of the anxiety out of him.[7] But now is the time for the emergency care nurse to ask "What specifically happened right before you took the pills?" While talking and listening, the staff should ask the following questions:

- Did the staff member have to be insistent to get an answer from the patient?
- Does the patient respond slowly?. (If the staff member waits quietly, the patient will eventually answer the question.)
- Is the patient highly verbal? (If so, he needs only to be given a few open-ended questions—"How did this evening start?"—or statements—"Tell me how this happened"—and the whole story will unfold.)
- How does the patient respond to touch? By holding out his hand to the staff member? By accepting an offered hand? By withdrawing from touch?
- Is it easier for this patient to talk with a particular staff member?

This information can be jotted on a card and kept in a

specified place, available only to those who are fully aware of their responsibility in patient confidentiality. Then, if the patient is seen following another suicide attempt, the available information can be built upon and the same questions need not be repeated.

The actions discussed above serve three purposes. They say plainly to the patient, "I care enough about you to take this extra time." They provide the staff with something other than a "here we go again" focus for a patient who attempts suicide more than once. And they provide human contact for someone who desperately needs it.

Among possible difficulties involved in taking extra time with a depressed patient is that the staff member is vulnerable and may risk painful rejection by the patient. Another is that the staff's attention may be misused by patients who use suicide attempts as a means of controlling those around them. However painful the rejection or the feelings of being "used," it is helpful to remember that pure suicidal manipulators are few; it is better for the staff member, as well as for the patient, to provide attention than to withold it; and even though the patient shows rejection, the presence is reassuring.

Assessment and Prevention

Saving lives is the primary consideration of the emergency department staff. With persons who have attempted suicide, the life-saving role is rather well defined; but in *preventing* suicides, another aspect of saving lives, the role is less well defined. One reason for this is the common feeling among emergency department personnel that they never see a suicidal patient *before* he tries to take his life.

Certain facts and concepts about suicide are now known.
- 65% of all persons who commit suicide have had some contact with a health care facility or professional within the 3- to 6-month period before the suicide attempt.[40]
- No research study on suicide has demonstrated a positive relationship between good health and suicide.[18]
- The second most frequent warning about suicide (after direct expressions of suicidal intent) is a discussion of depressed feelings.[28]
- These depressive feelings are frequently masked by a variety of physical complaints.[20,28]
- Suicide-prone persons are likely to respond to any stress as a crisis.[18]

It is reasonable to expect that an emergency department staff will see a higher percentage of persons who are suicide risks than do other health care professionals. The persons in this anxiety category may come to the emergency department because of explicit or implicit depression, which may be viewed as either the cause or the result of physical symptoms. A number of patient characteristics that indicate suicidal risk have been identified and can be applied in assessing these persons. These factors are listed in Chart 5-1. Keep in mind that suicidal risk increases in proportion to the number of these characteristics that apply to the patient.

The person who is severely depressed (referring to a feeling, not a diagnosis) is usually brought to the emergency department by family or friends. Obviously, he will be sad. He will move slowly, be apathetic and unable to initiate any activity, and show the effects of decreased appetite, lack of sleep, and poor grooming.

Questons That Must Be Asked. Exploring the patient's thoughts about suicide is critical. Few people commit suicide while feeling and acting severely depressed. Suicide is more apt to occur as the patient starts to feel better. The staff cannot know where this person is on the depression scale, though, until someone asks. A direct inquiry in a matter-of-fact voice is necessary: "Have you thought of taking your own life?" "Have you felt that you wanted to kill yourself?"

Chart 5-1

PATIENT CHARACTERISTICS ASSOCIATED WITH SUICIDAL RISK*

- White male over the age of 45 years
- Nonwhite male between the ages of 20 and 35 years
- Female between the ages of 20 and 30 years
- Married and under the age of 20 years
- Single, divorced, or widowed
- Has made a previous suicide attempt
- Has been treated within the past 6 months for any psychological problem
- Has suffered a recent loss (in the past 6 months to 1 year) of anything *regarded by him* as important (*e.g.,* home, job, a person, a pet, or health)
- Firearms or hanging is the method of suicide being considered

Risk increases in proportion to the number of these characteristics present.

* For a more complete rating scale, see the Suicide Prevention Center Assessment of Suicidal Potentiality from the Los Angeles Suicide Prevention Center and the Institute for Studies of Self-Destructive Behaviors, 1041 S. Menlo Ave., Los Angeles, Calif. 90006.

or "Have you wished to be dead?" If the answer is no, the staff member has shown enough compassion to ask and that it is acceptable to talk about suicidal thoughts, thus leaving the door open should they occur later.

Emergency personnel often find it hard to do this, for fear of putting ideas into the patient's head. But it is extremely unlikely that a depressed person has not considered suicide. The thought of suicide has usually been entertained at least long enough to reject it. Staff members should assume that they will not be mentioning a subject that the person has not thought about.

If the patient expresses any positive response to the question (*e.g.,* "I've thought about ending it all" or "They'd be better off without me" or "I can't stand any more of this"), the next question to be answered is: "How do you think you might kill yourself?" or "Have you thought about how you might do it?" The staff should then find out if the person has the necessary items for carrying out the proposed plan. The more specific and detailed the plan, the more easily available the means for carrying it out, or the more violent the chosen method, the greater the risk of success. Thoughts of shooting and jumping are considered more lethal than thoughts of cutting oneself or swallowing pills.[31]

Interventions. When the data point to a high suicide risk, any one or all of the following are appropriate actions, depending upon the situation:
1. Inform family or friends of your concerns and suggest further immediate evaluation. If there are no family or friends to notify, the risk of suicide increases.
2. Notify an available crisis counselor (*e.g.,* a member of an on-call crisis team connected with your emergency department, the suicide/crisis telephone team, or the psychiatric outpatient clinic). Explain your concerns and request that someone come to the emergency department to do further evaluation.

3. If the community does not have a crisis team or a mental health/psychiatric worker available and the risk of suicide is too high to let the person leave, try any of the following until it is possible to reach the patient's personal physician:
   - If the patient can move and perform some tasks, put him to work under direct supervision. (How long has it been since there has been time to sort out the cupboard where the record forms are kept?) Keep in mind the patient's proposed method of suicide, and avoid allowing him access to the instruments associated with it. A person who has talked about cutting his wrists should not be asked to sort and wrap suture sets.
   - If the patient cannot muster the motivation for such tasks, find a place for him to sit where he can be readily seen. Explain to him the concern for his safety.
   - Make a point of frequent contact with the patient, about every 15 minutes. Offer him a magazine, coffee, a clean ash tray—and a little of your time. Let him know that he is not alone.
   - Get a physician, preferably his personal physician, to the emergency department as quickly as possible. These points are summarized in Chart 5-2.

The big "don't" is *don't* make promises that are impossible to keep, such as "I won't let you kill yourself." This is false reassurance. It immediately sets up a power struggle between the staff and the patient, one that the staff can never win.

Try to remember that the emergency department is probably the only place open. There is nowhere else for the depressed person to go. He is undecided whether suicide is the answer, or he would not have sought help. No matter how ridiculous it may seem, considering suicide is often a way of getting feedback about oneself: "Am I worthy enough as a person to even consider continuing to live?" Another's concern can swing the patient's feelings toward life.

Table 5-1 summarizes the characteristics of mild to moderate anxiety and presents appropriate staff behaviors.

Chart 5-2

HIGH SUICIDAL RISK: APPROPRIATE INTERVENTIONS

1. Inform patient's family or friends about this concern and suggest immediate further evaluation.
2. Notify available crisis counseling agency (on-call emergency department crisis team, suicide/crisis telephone team, psychiatric outpatient clinic) and request that a representative come to the emergency department to do further evaluation.
3. If crisis team or mental health/psychiatric worker is not available and risk of suicide is very high, keep the patient in the emergency department and try to reach his personal physician.
4. Meanwhile, try any of the following:
   - If the patient can move and perform a task, put him to work at an appropriate task. Prevent access to potentially harmful objects.
   - If the patient is unable to perform a task, seat him where he can be readily seen and explain that this is done for his safety.
   - Check with the patient frequently—about every 15 minutes; offer reading material, coffee, an ash tray. Spend time with him. Let him know that he is not alone.
   - Get a physician (preferably the patient's personal physician) to the emergency department as quickly as possible.

THE VICTIM OF SEXUAL ASSAULT

A second group of emergency room patients who may exhibit minimal anxiety are victims of sexual assault.

Emergency room personnel usually encounter the sexually assaulted victim shortly after the attack. Though these victims may display a wide range of behaviors, the behaviors associated with shock are common. The victim may act as though nothing traumatic has happened. She may be withdrawn and unable to talk about the attack; or she may be agitated and incoherent and exhibit the behaviors of a severely anxious person (see Table 5-3, p. 63).

Again, the staff's most basic intervention is acceptance. Acceptance and support can serve as the first step to full recovery for the victim of sexual assault.

Other interventions include providing the following:
1. Prompt and competent physical care
2. Empathetic listening
3. An opportunity for the victim to express her feelings
4. Information about and rationale for any necessary procedures

One should listen closely for the victim's wishes and decisions in coping with the trauma of sexual assault.[33] (See Chap. 7.)

THE PATIENT WITH UNDEFINED ANXIETY

The next group for consideration falls into a shadowy area between "little or no visible anxiety" (see Table 5-1) and "mild to moderate anxiety" (see Table 5-2, p. 62)—the group of patients who come to the emergency department for any of a wide range of physical complaints. This is not to say that everyone who comes in with a headache or an ingrown toenail is contemplating suicide. The nurse can develop the skills to differentiate between the headache that requires an aspirin and the one that needs further exploration.

Again, the first question to be asked is "Why now?" It can be phrased as "What made you decide to come to the hospital?" or "What happened right before the pain started?" or "What went on today that led up to this?" This can be asked while the preliminary procedures for assessing the physical complaint (*e.g.,* measuring vital signs, having the patient undress, or collecting blood or urine specimens) are being done. Then listen closely while the patient relates what happened, especially for any statements that hint at sadness, indicate a grim future, mention being better off dead, or indicate any thought of suicide or dying. If he makes any such statement, follow it with, "Something you said concerned me. [Repeat the statement of concern.] Can you tell me more about that?" The answer may be "Oh, I didn't mean that," or it may be a sudden outburst of feelings or tears, at which time an ear and a tissue are needed. It is also necessary to get answers to the questions mentioned in the section "Questions That Must Be Asked" and to bear in mind the factors listed in Chart 5-1, Patient Characteristics Associated With Suicidal Risk.

PATIENTS WITH MILD TO MODERATE ANXIETY

This is probably the most common of all levels of anxiety. Everyone has experienced that flush of exhilaration when faced with an exciting, challenging task. It provides the extra "oomph" to get over an obstacle or the fortitude to stay with a task until it is done—like the parent who is reassuring and calm until all of the stitches are in his child's scalp. And at least once, everyone has been gripped by that sudden tight feeling inside that would not let go—sweaty palms, heart pounding in the throat, labored breath, knees like not-quite-set aspic, and an urgent need to get to the bathroom. Such intense anxiety creates obstacles such as hyperventilation and respiratory alkalosis or verbal hostility, anger, and retaliation.

It is highly unlikely that an 8-hour shift in the emergency department can pass without the presence of at least one of these characteristics of moderate anxiety. The manifestations of mild to moderate anxiety are visible in nine out of every ten people who come to the emergency department and are easy to handle if recognized and responded to quickly.

Time does not allow a personality assessment of everyone who comes to the emergency department, although this would help one predict who will move from mild anxiety to more severe and less adaptive anxious behaviors. Therefore, a few precautionary measures, such as those in the following list, should be applied to everyone.

TABLE 5-1. LITTLE OR NO VISIBLE ANXIETY

Behaviors Observed	Common Interpretations	Expected Staff Behaviors
Complaints of a wide variety of physical problems, ranging from an ingrown toenail through pneumonia to cancer	Neurosis, depression	Listen and take patient seriously
	Involutional melancholia	Do an assessment of suicidal potential or intent to harm others
Somatic complaints: difficulty falling asleep; early morning awakening; fatigue; loss of appetite; constipation/diarrhea; decrease in sexual functioning or desire; aches and pains; strange taste or burning sensation in mouth	Schizoaffective, depression	
	Hypochondria	Make no derogatory remarks
		Show calm, reassuring acceptance of the *patient,* not necessarily acceptance of his behavior.
		Support and show acceptance of the victim of sexual assault

1. Provide a waiting room away from the mainflow of emergency traffic. Anxiety breeds anxiety. If a mildly anxious person is continuously reminded of the trauma and fear associated with the emergency department, his own anxiety will be reinforced, and he will spend much of his energy controlling this escalation of anxiety, leaving no reserve strength for coping with developments such as changes in the condition of a family member being treated.

2. Make sure that the person (clerk, nurses' aide, attendant/ orderly, nurse, or physician) who first sees the patient or family is friendly and warm, listens well, and respects people. These qualities are demonstrated by paying attention to people when they talk, looking at them, calling them by name and title, trying to pronounce names properly, and graciously accepting corrections when a name is mispronounced.

3. Take the following general preventive measures:
   - Offer a hot drink or food. This can be done by actually handing the person a cup of coffee, tea, or cocoa or by having a vending machine in the waiting room.
   - Have restrooms close to the waiting room, clearly marked and well maintained.
   - Have blankets available for use and waiting room seating out of drafts.
   - Have facial tissues or washcloths available, and offer them when someone is crying.
   - Make sure that people know that the staff is available. This can be accomplished by having the staff circulate in the waiting room and the treatment rooms.

The consistent application of any or all of these measures will reduce the anxiety of everyone involved. These measures support the current coping behaviors of the family or patient and make the emergency department staff's job easier.

Hyperventilation: Assessment and Intervention

The front-line staff member should be able to assess dizziness, complaints of being "lightheaded," sweating, and shallow breathing as signs of less-adaptive anxiety and should be able to take action or summon help. These symptoms indicate hyperventilation and respiratory alkalosis and may be the presenting complaint of a patient or may develop in anyone in the waiting room. The appropriate interventions include doing a physical examination, establishing normal respirations, and teaching the patient.

The physical examination serves to reassure the patient that he is being taken seriously and that his heart and lungs are functioning properly. Rebreathing his own exhaled air increases the carbon dioxide content of the lungs and increases the effectiveness of the person's breathing. This is done by providing the patient with a paper bag (or using a synthetic bag and mask especially designed for this purpose) and instructing him to place the bag over his nose and mouth and to breathe with the bag in place. The patient may be more comfortable lying down. A staff member must stay with the patient until regular breathing has returned.

The next step is to spend a few minutes teaching the patient how to hyperventilate. Instruct the patient to breathe rapidly for approximately 2 minutes, which reestablishes respiratory alkalosis, and then have him use the rebreathing bag again.[3] This demonstrates to the patient that he can control the situation if or when it occurs again.

Coping With Anger and Hostility

When anger and verbal hostility are the result of building anxiety, the emergency department staff needs all the patience and objectivity it can muster. There is nothing comfortable about being yelled at, sworn at, or constantly criticized for the care being given. This anxiety turned to anger may stem from the patient's feelings of frustration (*e.g.*, the staff's apparent preoccupation with filling out forms) or from the patient's unmet expectations of the staff (*e.g.*, the direct and immediate resolution of his problem). The anger is a substitute for anxiety and is being used to exert some control in a situation in which the patient feels powerless. The words may connote hostility, but the nonverbal message is fear: "I'm afraid something will happen to me. Are you doing everything you can to help me?"[8]

Staff members must respond to the nonverbal message in a reassuring and nonretaliatory manner. Returning a patient's angry comment with sarcasm, withdrawal, or placating statements only adds to the feelings of powerlessness and makes the situation more tense. Openly recognizing the feelings of anger and their relationship to anxiety and conveying the idea that there is nothing wrong with these feelings helps the patient. Here is an example of a commonly encountered exchange:

> *Patient's Wife:* You never do any work. You just sit there and write. . . . It seems you could find something better to do with your time.
>
> *Emergency Nurse:* Yes, I'm writing. It must be hard to sit and wait without knowing exactly what is happening to your husband. Is there anything I can do?

The staff must look beyond the surface hostility and respond in ways that will decrease the person's anger and anxiety rather than in words that will be regretted later. It is useful to remember that the anger is not directed at anyone personally; it just needs to be discharged.

Table 5-2 summarizes the features of mild to moderate anxiety and some useful coping behaviors for the staff.

THE PATIENT WITH SEVERE ANXIETY

The manifestations of severe anxiety may be primary or secondary. Consequently, the behaviors of severe anxiety may be the primary reason for a person's coming to the emergency department or may follow the onset of some other problem, such as diabetes, hepatic dysfunction, renal failure, degenerative disease, or the effects of drug use or withdrawal from drugs, including alcohol. Whatever the reason behind the occurrence, the behaviors are the same.

The patient suffering severe anxiety is confused. He is not able to attend to his surroundings and thus is disoriented to time, place, and person. He is incoherent and agitated, his behavior marked by restless and aimless movements, mumbling to himself, slamming doors, and swearing or physically striking out. The severely anxious person is incapable of doing any abstract thinking, including problem-solving; thus, if he feels the need to urinate, he may simply

TABLE 5-2. MILD TO MODERATE ANXIETY

Behaviors Observed	Common Interpretations	Expected Staff Behaviors
Hyperventilation, peripheral paresthesia, "pins and needles" in extremities, breathlessness	Anxiety	Rule out organic basis.
	Hypochondria	Reestablish normal respirations.
Sweating	Anxiety reaction	Make sure restrooms are clearly marked.
Urinary frequency and/or diarrhea	Neurosis: hysteria	Friendly, noncoercive *attention*
"Butterflies" in stomach	Adjustment reaction of adult life	Good listening skills
Nausea		Offer hot drink or food.
Increased heart rate		Separate from other anxious persons.
Silence or talking all of the time.		Do not take verbal hostility personally; answer the content (the words being said), and do not respond to the feeling tone (anger); recognize the feeling, but do not respond in kind.
Feelings of cold		
Verbal hostility		
Pacing in the waiting room		
Finger tapping		

do so in a corner of the treatment room instead of following the thought process of the less anxious person, who solves the problem by asking directions and going to the bathroom. He may exhibit a variety of emotions and move quickly from one to another; for example, he may be angry for 5 minutes, cry for 5 minutes, laugh for 5 minutes, and be soberly seductive for the next 5 minutes.

The severely anxious patient's internal controls are functioning minimally. The cerebral cortex is responding to a variety of stimuli that is wider than usual, with the result that he loses touch with or distorts reality. A person at this level of anxiety can move easily either to calmness or to panic. And since he has very little control left, persons in his environment have the greatest influence on which direction he takes.

Strategies

The task is to eliminate the source of the loss of control while providing the control that is lacking until the patient can reestablish self-control. This usually consists of preventing him from hurting himself or others while treatment for the specific etiology is begun.

Reorienting the Patient. The patient needs to be reoriented to time, place, and person frequently, perhaps as often as every 5 minutes. The emergency staff should use simple language with wide applicability, such as "I am a nurse," instead of "I am Mrs. Jones, the evening supervisor," and "You are in a hospital," instead of "You are in Metropolitan General Hospital on 76th Avenue East," and "Your name is _____."[28] Keep irritability out of your voice; it can be heard even when cognitive functions are minimal. If the temper fuse starts getting short, it is wise to go out into the hall and take a few deep breaths.

Providing a Calming Environment. The room should be well lighted. A balance should be found between soft light and glaring light. The former creates unwanted shadows, adds to illusion, and makes reality testing difficult. The latter is harsh and uncomfortable and is not conducive to relax-

ation. Well-balanced lighting helps the patient reassure himself—"I am seeing things; they'll go away," or "they (the staff) can see me, so they won't forget me." Similarly, the environment should be kept as simple as possible.

Communicating With the Patient. The staff member must explain each procedural step before touching him and should face him while talking. Seeing the staff member's lips move leaves very little room for doubt about the origin of the voice. A calm, reassuring voice and simple language should be used. If the patient demonstrates increased anxiety (pulling away, folding his arms around himself, looking desperately around the room) one should ask, "Is this procedure absolutely essential to this patient's well-being?" If the answer is no, then ask, "Why am I running the risk of pushing this person into a panic?" If the answer is "Yes, this procedure is essential," then ask, "Must I do it right now, or can I take some more time to explain and help decrease his anxiety?" If it must be done immediately and the confusion has increased, get assistance. This will decrease the probability of the patient's hurting himself or someone else—either of which creates in the patient loss of self-respect, increase in guilt, and fear of retaliation.

Staying With the Patient. A staff member should stay with a patient or have another responsible staff member or family member stay with him. If he *must* be left alone, leave the door of the treatment room open at least halfway, to decrease or eliminate any feelings of being trapped. Someone should check *with*—not check *on*—the patient every 15 minutes. This means recognizing his presence, announcing one's own presence, and orienting him to time, place, and person; it does not mean peering through the window in the door.

Helping the Family. It is also wise to remember that family members or friends may be in the throes of mild or moderate anxiety; using a few of the aforementioned intervention strategies can help them to stay calm in the presence of their confused relative or friend. In turn, this will decrease the patient's anxiety and reduce pressures on staff members.

TABLE 5-3. SEVERE ANXIETY

Behaviors Observed	Common Interpretations	Expected Staff Behaviors
Incoherence	Acute brain syndrome	Remove the source (through gastric lavage, hemodialysis, medications).
Disorientation to time, place, and person	Delirious intoxications: metabolic toxins, direct trauma to the brain, alcohol, drugs, infections	Reality orientation: identify yourself; use simple words; tell patient he is in a hospital; tell simply, repeatedly, and reassuringly who, what, and where.
Memory loss	Organic brain syndrome: arteriosclerotic, psychotic, or nonpsychotic.	
Loss of judgment		
Decreased ability to attend to surroundings	Drug dependency	Simplify the environment: use well-lighted room; move slowly; explain procedures; keep door of treatment room open; use one staff member consistently.
Hallucinations	Alcoholism	
Emotional lability, sadness, apprehension, euphoria		
Agitation: pacing, muttering, swearing, random striking out, picking at things		Avoid extra medications and physical or mechanical restraints.

Medication

Medication is sometimes necessary for a confused patient. The inherent risk is that most sedatives increase the degree of confusion and disorientation, either by their direct action or by creating within the patient a sensation of losing the little control he has left. Remember that elderly patients require less medication than do younger patients. If medications are given to an elderly patient, especially intramuscularly, he should be kept lying down for at least 30 minutes to decrease the danger of hypotension.[6] The constant presence of another person is the best restraint possible and usually makes the use of any restraints, either physical (cloth or leather wrist restraints or a Posey belt) or chemical, unnecessary.

The Intoxicated Patient

The person who is most frequently in need of all the preceding interventions and is often difficult to treat is the "drunk." Each emergency department has its own group of returning alcoholics with problems ranging from simple disorientation that sleep will cure to delirium tremens (DTs) or Korsakoff's syndrome.

Little else is as discouraging to emergency department staff as spending time and effort to get a person on his feet and then seeing him come back the next night, week, or month. The anger (Why doesn't he shape up?), the pity (How can he live that way?), the fear (I wonder exactly what started the drinking?), and the professional sense of injustice (This money and skill could be used to help someone who is really sick and who'll get well.) all combine to make the staff want never to see or treat another person with acute alcohol intoxication. But treatment must be started, for without treatment, three out of five alcoholics who suffer delirium tremens will die, thus defeating the purpose of the emergency department.

Alcoholics fit no one personality pattern, belong to no one particular occupational group, and come from no one socioeconomic background. They do share a low tolerance for tension and low self-esteem. Therefore, while administering the necessary intravenous fluids, vitamins, and/or medications, the emergency staff should try to focus on the patient's current acute distress and should not dwell on thoughts of how and why this distress came about. They should offer acceptance and reassurance by carefully attending to his physical needs and comfort and should avoid reinforcing his feelings of worthlessness with thoughtless remarks. A sense of humor is valuable, both for the staff's well-being and as a tool for encouraging a patient to stay in bed or not to knock over the intravenous fluids. Be patient.

Table 5-3 summarizes how the emergency department staff should cope with severe anxiety.

PANIC

The fourth level of anxiety, panic, is the most awesome. Panic is marked by lack of coordination in behavior and the disappearance of rational thought. The self is completely out of control. Fear is overwhelming, and the emergency department staff must expect the unexpected. Panic creates fear in the staff—whether because it touches off their own aggressive feelings or reveals their uncertainties about being able to handle the situation is unimportant for this chapter. What is important is to answer the question, "How do We provide control where there is none?"

A panicked person may be brought to the emergency room by the police, family, friends, companions, or strangers. The reason given for bringing him in may be, "He drank too much," or "He took too much and is on a bummer,*" or "He just flipped out." The panicked patient might also be the drunk in Treatment Room 3 whose delirium tremens' butterflies just turned into giant scorpions, or the kid in Treatment Room 1 who dropped street acid (LSD_{25}) and is alternating between deep, meaningful insights and intense sensations of his body dissolving; or it could be the person in the admitting room who starts yelling that everyone is part of a plot to make sure he dies and that this is the reason he is being refused treatment by a doctor.

Whatever the circumstances, the staff must stay calm and remember that the patient is afraid and wants help, that

---

* Bummer: a term used to describe unpleasant and very frightening experiences following the ingestion of psychedelic drugs.

people are more important than property, that it is their responsibility to act *before* someone is hurt, and that panic episodes are transient. They will end.

The panicked patient has two choices—to strike out at others or to attack himself. His fear and pain may be so acute that his only thought is to escape or end his life. He may jump out of a window, run through a plate-glass door or break a medicine jar and start slicing himself. In striking out at others, the patient may put his fist through a wall, destroy furniture, or hit people. He may be acting in a delusional system, obeying auditory hallucinations, trying to stop threatening visual hallucinations, or struggling for *any* definitive action that will end this horrendous fear and powerlessness. Table 5-4 summarizes how the emergency department staff should cope with panic.

STRATEGIES

Talking to the Patient

A staff member should start talking to the patient. A good rule of thumb is that if the person is talking, he will probably be able to listen. If he is being treated in the emergency department and thus is in contact with a staff member, that person should do the talking. A familiar face, no matter how recently familiar, can do wonders to decrease fear and confusion.

Other patients and all other persons not directly involved with the panicked person, including the family, should leave the room. A person with homicidal tendencies is more likely to attack members of his family than strangers.[30]

The person in contact with the patient should keep talking in a voice that is calm and low. Whispering is not called for, and there is no need to yell. Using simple language, the person should offer the patient the option of giving up a weapon, piece of furniture, or anything else he has that may be used as a weapon. This same person should *constantly* reassure the patient of the staff's awareness of how frightened he is and that everything possible is going to be done to *help* him. Be convincing with the statement, "I don't want you to hurt anyone."

It is important to keep talking and to listen to anything the patient says. It may be possible to find a clue to what started the "fight" behavior, and information or reassurance may then be realistically offered about it. Very few incidents of aggressive behavior start for absolutely no reason at all. The reason may seem insignificant to an outside observer, but it is a reason. In talking with the patient, do not worry about being repetitious. Making contact with the patient is what is important, not being a good conversationalist. Do not censure or reprimand; this is not the time to teach more appropriate behavior.

Obtaining Assistance. While the talking is going on, someone should go for assistance. A minimum of three persons and a maximum of six are needed to physically restrain one panicked person. Someone should also see that these extra persons do not burst upon the scene like a cavalry charge. They should wait immediately close by until they receive directions on how to proceed. Too big and too sudden a show of power will only increase the person's feelings of helplessness and anxiety and breed more assaultive behavior. *A single staff member should never try to restrain an adult patient.*

Physical Restraint

If talking is unsuccessful, then physical restraint must be used. The staff member who has the best rapport with the patient should direct all activity involved in physically restraining him. This is not the time to haggle over strategies and rationales; save these for a staff evaluation conference. Anything gained in discussing a more therapeutic approach will be lost if the patient perceives that the staff is not working together for him, and the disagreement will only add to the chaos.

Helpless inconsistency ("Here, let me do this" or "No, you do that, not this" or "No, that won't work") gives the patient the message that he is in control of the situation by creating so much anxiety in everyone else. The panicked person cannot cope with this extra burden. In addition, the

TABLE 5-4. PANIC

Behaviors Observed	Common Interpretations	Expected Staff Behaviors
Physical aggression: homicidal or suicidal	Schizophrenia, paranoid type	Stay calm.
Delusions: sees and hears things as others do but interprets them differently; fears others will harm him	Manic-depression, manic type	Act with confidence and assurance.
	Schizophrenic reaction, undifferentiated	Remember that the behavior is not directed toward anyone personally.
	Organic brain syndrome, acute or chronic	
Hallucinations: eyes move as though watching something; is preoccupied, does not hear you; tilts head in a listening manner; talks to himself; lips move with no sound	Acute alcohol intoxication	Use assistance (persons, drugs, mechanical restraints) *only to protect the patient* from harming himself or others.
	Fatigue	
	Psychotic reaction, undiagnosed	Never try to physically restrain an adult alone.
	Drug dependence	Talk; be repetitious and soothing. Give directions ("Do not bite") without anger.
		Medicate.
		Reinforce reality, don't insist on it.

staff then feels helpless and intimidated and may retaliate in anger to regain its status, self-control, and power. The patient responds to anger with anger, and the entire situation is out of control.

Panicked males tend to strike with an arm, a leg, or an object. Females do not exhibit such a pattern. Each team member should be assigned a specific appendage—arms, legs, or head. The team should approach the patient from the sides and/or rear; a direct frontal approach is a nonverbal invitation to fight. They should move calmly and quickly, then stay as close to the patient as possible; the less space between a staff member and the patient, the less momentum can be put into a swing or a kick. *Never* grab the patient by the throat, mouth, or nose. This is threatening to anyone and can only add to panic. If the patient's head must be restrained to prevent biting or self-inflicted wounds, the staff member should put one hand under his chin and one hand at the back of his neck and support his head against her body (Fig. 5-2). If the patient's arm must be restrained, it should be held with one hand over his elbow and the other over his wrist in such a way that the staff member's arms naturally move in the same direction as the patient's (Fig. 5-3).

The staff member should keep talking in a reassuring voice, explaining what she is doing and why. By standing to the side and the back of the patient, a single person can place one hand on his far elbow and the other on his wrist, for control and safety. Figure 5-4 illustrates this hold. If two staff members are available for restraint of the patient's arms, each can take one arm, using the hold shown in Figure 5-5. Then they should try to get the patient against a wall or on the floor. Getting him to sit on the floor with his back

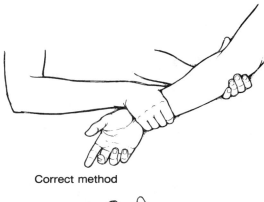

Correct method

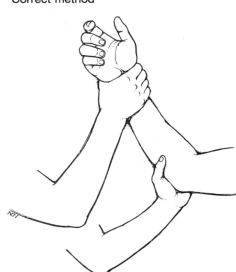

Incorrect method

Figure 5-3 *Correct and incorrect methods of restraining the arm of a person out of control. In the correct method (top), one hand is placed over the elbow and the other over the wrist in such a way that the staff person's arms flux in the same direction as the patient's arm. With incorrect placement (bottom), the patient cannot be controlled.*

Figure 5-2 *Supporting the head. The staff member places one hand under the patient's chin and the other hand at the back of his neck and supports the patient's head against her body.*

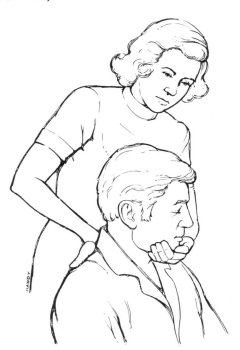

against the wall is most effective because the support of a solid structure poses the least physical threat. This position allows for direct eye contact and ease in administering oral or intramuscular medications and requires fewer staff members for restraint.

Gentle but firm pressure is required when restraining a patient. Staff should practice with each other, to get an idea of what this means. Slowly squeeze another staff member's arm, and determine how each degree of pressure feels, and especially when it causes pain.

Pressure that can be gradually released while still maintaining the position of restraint is desirable. The staff member then has the options of either allowing the patient to control his own behavior or quickly providing necessary control. It is imperative that the person be allowed as much control as is safely possible.

One must *never* strike a patient unless it is the only action that can determine life or death. Striking a patient only reinforces assaultive behavior as a means of coping with stress. A staff member who has a sense of losing control should get away from the patient. It is much more valuable

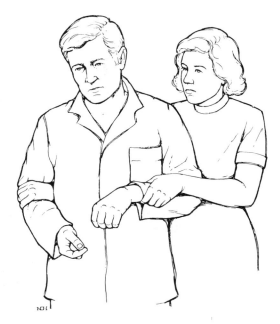

Figure 5-4 *Restraining a panicked patient. The staff member grasps the patient's near wrist and far elbow as shown for maximum control.*

for the staff member's self-esteem and the patient's well-being to recognize one's own limitations and leave than to stay and add to the patient's tension.

Sedation

Sedation will most likely be required. Someone who is not a member of the team physically restraining the patient should be available to prepare the medication. Choice of medication depends on the known or inferred basis for the

behavior. Phenothiazines are used when the patient is delusional or hallucinating, except when the hallucinations are induced by drugs. Then the drug of choice is diazepam (Valium); phenothiazines tend to bring a person down too quickly and increase the likelihood of flashbacks.*

When acute alcohol intoxication appears to underlie the behavior, chlordiazepoxide (Librium), chloral hydrate, or paraldehyde may be used; chlordiazepoxide is preferred. There are times when amobarbital (Amytal) can be used. It makes sense to have all available and ready for use.

It is easier to keep other people away from the patient until the sedating medication has started working than to try to move the patient away from others. If he must be moved, Figure 5-6 illustrates the safest way. The team restraining the patient should stay with him until the desired effect of the medication is evident. Someone should expect to spend time with the patient; he needs human contact.

HALLUCINATIONS AND DELUSIONS

All of us hear our own thoughts, but we do not answer. A hallucination† is really a thought becoming so loud and so persistent that it has to be answered, verbally or nonverbally. Indications that a person is hallucinating include the following:

1. Head tilted as though listening to someone
2. Lips forming words or moving with no sound
3. Talking aloud, apparently to oneself
4. Ears stuffed with cotton in an attempt to keep the voices out

---

* Flashback: the reliving of a previous drug-induced experience, frequently a bad one, without the ingestion of additional drugs.
† Hallucination: a perceptual disorder wherein "an inner experience is expressed as though an outer event."[13]

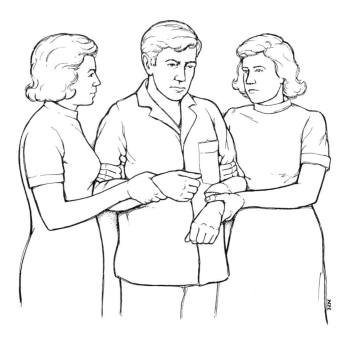

Figure 5-5 *Patient restraint by 2 staff members. When greater patient control is needed, 2 persons may become involved, each using on one arm the hold illustrated in Fig. 5-4.*

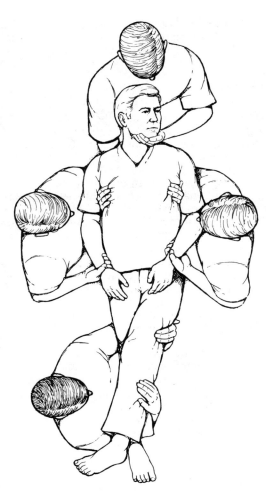

Figure 5-6 *Safe method of moving an agitated patient by a four-person lift. One staff member supports the patient's head, neck and upper back. The trunk is supported by two staff members, crossing their arms beneath the patient's trunk and grasping his arms. The fourth staff member clutches the patient's legs in adduction.*

what interested, and friendly. Do not waste time arguing; arguing shows the patient the discrepancies in his delusional system, which he will then proceed to correct, with the effect of strengthening it. If the patient asks directly whether you believe him, tell him, "I believe that your feelings are true and that you are telling me the truth as you see it." Listen without agreement or disagreement.

Avoid any behavior that could be construed as suspicious by the patient:

1. Do not talk to the patient's family or friends outside of his presence or where he might overhear.

2. Do not get into a power struggle with the patient over who is wrong or right.

3. Do not be overly sweet, solicitous, and supportive. Since the patient is aware that the staff member does not know him well enough to know the whole story, too much support only increases his suspicion that someone is trying to get something from him.

4. Do not use the pronoun "we"; use "I." "We" could be interpreted as an indication of a conspiracy. *Gentle* honesty goes a long way.

If the hallucinations and/or delusions plus the panic state are caused by psychedelic drugs, the staff should continually remind the patient that he has taken a drug, that what is going on is due to the drug, and that the effects of the drug will eventually wear off. Repeat what you say often. Little will be heard the first time.

"Talking the patient down" is contraindicated if he has taken phencyclidine (PCP, or "angel dust"). Such a patient is hypersensitive to auditory and visual stimulation. Any external stimulation, including verbal reassurance, can trigger agitation and violence. Earplugs may even be used to decrease the auditory stimuli received by these patients.[25,29,38] A quiet, controlled environment is necessary.

Patients are open to change when they are in the middle of a crisis. If the crisis is handled well by the emergency department staff, it can give the patient a strong start on a rapid recovery.

5. Describing an object or person that is not seen by anyone else

If the patient is actively hallucinating, the staff member should state her view of reality to him in simple, nonderogatory terms; for example, "No, I don't hear voices (or see snakes)." But the patient's perception of reality in seeing the objects or in hearing the voices should never be denied; they are very real to him. It is possible to state one's own perception of reality without telling the patient his is wrong.

At the same time, it is not wise to pretend that one is seeing or hearing something just to placate a patient. This increases the patient's fear and offers him no reassurance, but instead suggests to him that the hallucinations will never go away and the rest of his life will be as horrible as it is right now. If the hallucinations are not particularly frightening and do not urge destructive behaviors, it is best to state one's perception of reality and then ignore them.

As for delusions,* the best approach is to be calm, some-

---

* Delusion: a false, fixed belief about something that has no basis in fact and requires certain behaviors from the person who holds it.

WHEN THE PATIENT IS A CHILD[36]

A child's anxiety in the emergency room is usually associated with intrusive and painful procedures that are necessary for either diagnosis or treatment. The child's anxiety tends to range from moderate to severe for the following reasons:

1. Children have little or no control over the environment or what is happening to them.

2. They lack well-developed mechanisms for coping with stress.

3. They lack the language skills for expressing themselves.

4. They have very active imaginations, difficulty in separating fantasy from reality, and a keen fear of bodily injury and mutilation.

Strategies for Minimizing Anxiety

The emergency staff can intervene to minimize the child's anxiety by means of some simple but effective strategies.

Providing Security. Security can be provided through the consistent use of the same emergency personnel and other supportive adults. Parents or guardians are ideal. Provide security items if available—for example, a special blanket or a toy. Parents should be encouraged to stay with the child and comfort him. However, they should not be forced to stay when painful procedures are being done if they feel they will be unable to support and comfort the child. Parents should not be asked to help restrain a child or to assist in a painful procedure. The staff can do the restraining and let the parent do the comforting.

Explaining Procedures Truthfully. The emergency room staff can give the child simple, truthful explanations of the procedures. Say the procedure will hurt when it will. Tell the child that the procedure is being done to help him to get well and that it is not being done because he has been bad. Explain strange noises and smells. Provide children with an opportunity to handle equipment. Use toys and puppets to involve the child in the procedure. Through the use of a puppet and one's own imagination it is possible to discover what questions need to be answered and what the child is fantasizing.

Applying Restraints Gently. If restraint is required it should be done gently and with no more force than is necessary to prevent injury during the procedure. The person who is providing the restraint should do so in a caring manner so that the child does not detect hostility and interpret it as punishment for misdeeds. One good communication technique is to say, "I am going to help you lie still so the hurt will be over faster." Another is, "It is all right to cry when something hurts."

Allowing the Child to Maintain Control. The child should be allowed to control the situation as much as possible, for example, selecting an injection site or helping to apply an adhesive bandage after an injection. If it is feasible for a child to make a decision about any part of a procedure, give him the opportunity to do so.

STAFF CONSIDERATIONS

The many difficult aspects of anxiety described in this chapter may seem to suggest that one must be a model of patience, calmness, clear thinking, and nonirritability. How can anyone achieve all this? No *one* person can. Despite great effort, a given nurse may not be able to work with alcoholics. Another may be incapable of working with someone who has a long list of physical complaints without viewing this person as a hypochondriac. Still another may freeze if a patient yells and threatens. These shortcomings will not harm the quality of emergency care if staff members work together and support each other. Such support can be developed in several ways.

1. *Take care of yourself.* Emergencies are filled with the pain and problems of other people. It is not uncommon for emergency care staff to become emotionally burned out. By taking care of yourself, you can help to prevent burnout. Shubin recommends a "decompression rou-

tine,"[31] or a period of relaxing activity between leaving work and arriving home. The chosen activity can vary from a quiet, reflective time to a walk or strenuous physical activity. The activity should be enjoyable and result in reducing tension.

Learn to recognize the early signs of burnout, and take quick action. Indications of burnout include the following:

- Working extra hours frequently
- Feeling tired when thinking about work
- Becoming increasingly involved with the technical aspects of patient care
- Developing a cynical attitude
- Becoming disgusted with everybody

Be alert to changes in your behavior. When any one of these indications appears, start looking for the source. Once it has been identified, take appropriate action to remedy the situation.[31]

2. *Support each other.* Pat each other on the back when something is done well. Listen to each other, and when an emergency has been especially traumatic for one staff member (a battered child, a baby dead on arrival due to sudden infant death syndrome, or an injured neighbor or friend), the support can be genuine and instantaneous.

Compile a flip-card file of names and phone numbers of agencies (*e.g.,* Acoholics Anonymous, Sudden Infant Death Syndrome Foundation, Suicide/Crisis Center, Poison Control Center, Women Against Rape) and people who can provide on-call assistance or immediate referrals.

3. *Learn from each other.* Plan regular staff in-service seminars—a minimum of once a month, but preferably more often. Vary responsibilities and format. A nurses' aide may be responsible for one seminar and decide that the focus should be on the incident with Mr. Z last week and the reasons behind specific staff interventions. A resident may need help with some paperwork; the ward secretary can help him and everyone else learn just what happens to all of those pieces of paper. Some seminars could be lectures given by staff members or guest speakers. The hospital in-service educator should be available for consultation and assistance.

Help each other practice physical restraint holds. The first person you try these holds on should not be the panicked patient. Work so that each staff member knows what "firm and gentle holding pressure" means in relation to his own strength.

Consider the possibility of having a camera with a videotape recorder available. A flick of a switch could start the camera in a difficult emergency. The tape could later be played back and evaluated; suggestions could be made for similar situations in the future, and the tape would then be erased.

4. *Develop and use a sense of humor.* Laugh with and at yourselves. Joke about things. It is well known that the gallows humor associated with moments of personal stress, such as occur in the operating room or during autopsies, serves as a welcome alternative to screaming. Screaming may relieve a one's anxiety temporarily, but it will yield an unwanted harvest of anxiety in others.

Emergency department personnel are important people who work in an anxiety-laden environment. Recognition and management of this anxiety, whether it occurs in patients or in staff members and whether it is mild or severe, are necessary components of emergency care. It has been the intent of this chapter to outline some strategies for coping with the ever-present anxiety of an emergency department.

BIBLIOGRAPHY

1. Aguilera DC, Messick JM: Crisis Intervention: Theory and Methodology, 3rd ed. St. Louis, CV Mosby, 1978
2. Allison C, Bale R: A hospital policy for the care of patients who exhibit violent behavior. Nursing Times 169:375, March 22, 1973
3. Bartolucci G: An overview of crisis intervention in the emergency rooms of general hospitals. Am J Psychiatry 130:953–960, September, 1973
4. Bower FL, Pendleton MK (eds): Theoretical Foundations of Nursing 1. San Jose, Nursing Faculty Publications, San Jose State University, 1972
5. Brunner LS et al: The Lippincott Manual of Nursing Practice, 2nd ed. Philadelphia, JB Lippincott, 1978
6. Busse EW, Pfeiffer E: Behavior and Adaptation in Late Life. Boston, Little, Brown & Co, 1977
7. Choron J: Suicide. New York, Scribner's, 1972
8. Davis JW: Opportunity and techniques in crisis therapy. unpublished manuscript
9. Dorpat T, Anderson WF, Ripley HS: The relationship of physical illness to suicide. In Resnik HLP (ed): Suicidal Behaviors: Diagnosis and Management Boston, Little, Brown & Co, 1968
10. Enelow AJ, Wexler M: Psychiatry in the Practice of Medicine. New York, Oxford University Press, 1966
11. Farberow NL: Personality patterns of suicidal mental hospital patients. Genetic Psychology Monographs 42(1):3–79
12. Frost M: Violence in psychiatric patients. Nursing Times 68:748, June 15, 1972
13. Gravenkemper, KH: Hallucinations. In Burd SF, Marshall MA (eds): Some Clinical Approaches to Psychiatric Nursing New York, Macmillan, 1963
14. Hendin H: Black Suicide New York, Harper & Row, 1971
15. Johnson RN: Aggression in Man and Animals Philadelphia, WB Saunders, 1972
16. Kavalier F: The violent patient: HMC publishes new guidelines. Nursing Times 69:656, May 24, 1973
17. King JM: The initial interveiw: Basis for assessment in crisis intervention. Perspect Psychiatr Care 9:247–256, 1971
18. Lester G, Lester D: Suicide: The Gamble With Death. Englewood Cliffs, Prentice-Hall, 1971
19. Leib J, Lipsitch II, Slaby AE: The Crisis Team: A Handbook for the Mental Health Professional. New York, Harper & Row, 1973
20. MacKinnon RA, Michels R: The Psychiatric Interview in Clinical Practice. Philadelphia, WB Saunders, 1971
21. MacMahon B, Pugh T: Suicide in the widowed. Am J Epidemiol 81:23–31
22. Meerlo JAM: Patterns of Panic New York, International Universities Press, 1950
23. Menninger, K: Man Against Himself. New York, Harcourt, Brace & Co, 1938
24. Parkes CM: Bereavement: Studies of Grief in Adult Life. New York, International Universities Press, 1972
25. Petersen RC, Stillman RC (eds): Phencyclidine (PCP) Abuse: An Appraisal. Rockville, Maryland, Department of HEW, National Institute on Drug Abuse, August 1978
26. Pokorny AD: Myths about suicide. In Resnik HLP (ed): Suicidal Behaviors: Diagnosis and Management. Boston, Little, Brown & Co, 1968
27. Reid JA: Controlling the fight/flight patient. Canad Nurse 69:30, October 1973
28. Robinson, L: Coping with psychiatric emergencies. Nursing '73, 3:42–44, July, 1973
29. Rodman MJ, Smith DW: Pharmacology and Drug Therapy in Nursing, 2nd ed. Philadelphia, JB Lippincott, 1979
30. Rogerson KE: Psychiatric emergencies. Nurs Clin North Am 8:457–466, September 1973
31. Shneidman ES, Farberow NL (eds): The Cry for Help. New York, McGraw-Hill, 1965
32. Shubin S: Burnout: The professional hazard you face in nursing. Nursing '78 8:22–27, July 1978
33. Stuart GW, Sundeen SJ: Principles and Practice of Psychiatric Nursing. St Louis, CV Mosby, 1979
34. Sullivan HS: Conceptions of Modern Psychiatry New York, WW Norton, 1953
35. Susser M: Community Psychiatry, Epidemiologic and Social Theories. New York, Random House, 1968
36. Thompson M: Personal Communication, July 30, 1979
37. U.S. Public Health Service. Vital Statistics of the United States, 1979. II. Mortality, Part A. Rockville, Maryland, U.S. Department of HEW, Public Health Service, 1974
38. Vourakis C, Bennett G: Angel dust: Not heaven sent. Am J Nurs 79:649–653, April 1979
39. Webster WE: Uniform Crime Reports: 1979 Preliminary Annual Release. Washington, DC, U.S. Department of Justice, April 1979
40. Yolles SF: Suicide: A public health problem. In Resnik HLP (ed): Suicidal Behaviors: Diagnosis and Management Boston, Little, Brown & Co, 1968

6
DEATH, GRIEF, AND SUDDEN LOSS

RITA E. CAUGHILL

Death is an unwelcome topic at any time, but it is an event that all of us will experience. The feelings aroused by thoughts of death are intangible and frightening; they make us feel lost and uneasy. It is far easier to deny the fact that death is an inevitable part of life. Especially if one is young and full of life, it is preferable to view death as something that happens to other people but never to oneself.

CURRENT ATTITUDES: THE DENIAL OF DEATH

Western society has developed in such a way that it is difficult for its members to face death or relate to dying people in a meaningful way. Urbanization has been a major factor in removing people from contact with death. In simpler societies, children grow up close to nature, experiencing the cycle of life and death in the changing of the seasons and the shorter survival spans of plant and animal life. Urban living not only separates people from the basic laws of nature but actually fosters feelings of independence from nature and the inevitability of death. The increased longevity resulting from rapid advances in science in the last few decades also promotes the notion that man has mastered death.

Fifty years ago, American family life was built around a large, close-knit structure which included aunts and uncles as well as grandparents. Typically, close relatives lived within a few miles of each other, if not in the same household. If the mother of young children died, loving aunts or grandmothers were available and willing to step in as parent-substitutes. The nuclear family units of today, however, are likely to consist only of father, mother and children. This tends to increase family members' emotional investments in each other, so that the death of any one member causes a far greater sense of loss in the others, and there is no one to fill the void. The threat of such an overwhelming disaster is too terrible to think about: the average person finds denial of the possibility of death his best defense.

The removal of old people from the family home, where they were loved and respected by children and grandchildren, has contributed to the Western denial of death. Many older people freely choose to move to retirement communities. Others, physically or financially unable to make it on their own, are shunted off to nursing homes. Out of sight and all but forgotten, their deaths hardly create a ripple in the hurried flow of life.

As a result of all these factors, there is less need to develop a philosophy of life that takes both life and death into consideration. Very often, neither a concept of death nor a means of dealing with it is established. Death is viewed merely as the opposite of life, the complete end of everything, the extinction of self—a frightening phenomenon, indeed, with no significance but catastrophic annihilation.

Because of this typical attitude, it is hardly surprising that in Western society, when death must be dealt with, the goal is to remove its sting. Literautre, drama, television, and movies portray death frequently, but it is usually depicted as heroic or tragic, accidental or violent, rarely due to old age or chronic illness. Death is portrayed as an external power, a catastrophic force that happens to people against their will.

Denial of death also occurs quite naturally in the hospital and negatively influences the behavior of professionals caring for the dying. The fact that nurses and physicians are uncomfortable in the face of death is not surprising, since they are members and products of a society that fears death and taboos open and frank discussion of it. It is easier to avoid the situation than meet it, to spend as little time as possible with the dying person, to avoid talking about it.

RESPONSES TO LOSS AND GRIEF

Emotional problems also arise when emergency personnel are confronted by grief. The fact that grief invariably follows the event of death only adds to the discomfort experienced by staff members, who must interact in some way with the grieving survivors while still trying to deal with their own uneasy feelings.

Grief is an experience so common to human beings that hardly anyone can move into adulthood without experiencing it. Parkes[18] defines grief quite simply as "a reaction, emotional and behavioral," which is set in motion "when a love tie is severed." Since many of the familiar people and things in our lives are objects of our love—e.g., parents, spouses, pets, homes, jobs—the loss of any of these interrupts our sense of security and continuity and constitutes a threat to our psychological well-being.

Werner-Beland's definition of grief is a very broad one: "Grief is a state that occurs after the experience of a significant loss."[32] Though not very descriptive, this definition suggests the important point that grief occurs following *any* significant loss, varying in degree according to the nature and strength of the attachment. Even the familiar phenomenon of homesickness is a grief reaction, a response to separation from one's familiar surroundings.

Loss, in fact, is an inevitable accompaniment to the everyday activities of living. It could be said that the experience of loss begins with birth and the concomitant loss of the warm, safe environment of intrauterine life. Throughout a child's early development, he discovers new objects in his environment, develops attachments to some, and subsequently experiences loss if these objects are removed from him. Examples might include weaning from the bottle, the move from crib to bed, and so forth.

As he matures, each person experiences separation from, or loss of, familiar and loved persons and objects as a normal course of events. The process of learning and maturing, however, helps the individual to take these losses in stride, and he gradually develops adaptive responses and effective mechanisms of coping with deprivation and loss.

When a loss is traumatic, however, normal coping mechanisms may not be sufficient to deal with the ensuing crisis. The grief reaction that results is a disruption of normal emotional and behavioral patterns.

THE GRIEVING PROCESS

Since most of the early research on grief was done in relation to death, it is discussed in this context here, rather than as a response to loss in general. All of the descriptions of grief and grieving that follow, however, are equally applicable to any significant loss.

In the early 1940s, psychiatrist Erich Lindemann began his investigations into the grieving process with the study of large numbers of survivors of a disastrous nightclub fire.[16] His observations have been substantiated and augmented through the years by numerous others.[1,11,25]

The simplest and clearest delineation of the progressive steps through which the bereaved person moves was outlined by George Engel in 1964. Engel compares the grieving process with wound healing. He compares the experience of grief to a wound and subsequent psychological responses to the tissue healing process. Successful grieving, like successful tissue healing, follows a foreseeable pattern, by which one can judge if healing is taking place normally. But like physical healing, the grieving process takes times and cannot be hurried.[6]

Stages of Grieving

The series of reactions characterizing grief, as described by Engel, should be helpful in understanding what constitutes a *normal* response to grief. The first reaction to knowledge of death is usually shock and denial. The person cries out, "No! It can't be. I can't believe it!" He may try to disavow the fact in other ways, by throwing himself on the body, for example, as though this will somehow restore life, or as though he believes life is still there.

This initial reaction is frequently followed by a numb state of mind that permits the person to shut out conscious acknowledgment that the death has indeed occurred. He acts as though he is in a daze. He may force himself to carry out automatic activities as though nothing happened, or he may actually sit motionless, turned in upon himself, so that it is difficult to get through to him.

Some people, however, may be able to carry on in a seemingly normal way, after the initial shock response. They immediately begin to make the necessary arrangements, comfort and support other members of the family, and seem in general to be able to accept the death as a reality. It is important to realize that while this person may have accepted the loss intellectually, he has also suppressed its emotional impact and is still in a state of partial denial. "The mind knows, but the heart cannot accept."[6] Very often this state persists through the funeral preparations and rituals. These people are described as "taking it well" or "holding up well" and are generally admired for what is seen as a stoic reaction. It must be admitted, too, that staff members are pleased to see such a reaction in the hospital, since it relieves them of the stress of having to cope with overt grief.

This first stage, then, is characterized by the bereaved person's attempts to protect himself from overwhelming grief. He does this by denial, blocking out either the *reality* of the event or the painful emotions aroused by it. The stage of shock and denial is most intense when the death is sudden and unexpected, and therefore is of special importance to emergency personnel.

The grief-stricken survivor may move into the second stage within a matter of minutes after learning of the death, or it may take as long as 14 days or more.[18] But since it frequently develops very quickly, emergency personnel are quite likely to see this stage of grieving.

A conscious awareness of the death begins to develop, and an acute feeling of anguish ensues as the true meaning of the loss sinks in.

It is during this phase, in fact, that the greatest depths of anguish and despair are reached. In addition to emotional distress, the grieving person may feel intense pain in the chest or epigastrium, a painful lump in his throat, choking sensations, feelings of weakness or faintness or sighing respirations.

Crying is a typical response in this stage and should be encouraged, as it plays an important role in the grieving process. Cultural patterns determine to some extent the amount of public crying and lamentation that people will indulge in; some ethnic groups are very open in their expressions of emotion, while others tend to be more restrained. At a time of acute grief, cultural practices are extremely important and should never be discouraged, criticized, or belittled in any way.

Regardless of race, ethnic background *or sex,* crying is a legitimate release in the presence of death. We not only accept crying, we expect it; and we are not—or should not be—shocked at the sight of a man's tears under these circumstances. Crying may be a form of regression to the helpless days of childhood, and it does serve to evoke sympathy and support. The grieving person can cry and still retain his self-respect while acknowledging that he wants and needs the help and support of others.

Another very important emotion that may be openly displayed in this second stage of grieving is anger. Anger may be directed at the physician, the nurse, the hospital, or someone the grieving person feels must have "botched the job" and allowed his loved one to die. Personnel should be aware that this anger is rarely directed at anyone personally although it may appear to be: it is more a manifestation of the person's feelings of frustration and helplessness, his inability to *do* anything about it. Anger may also be felt toward another family member who somehow failed in an obligation toward the deceased. Or it may be directed against the self if the person feels himself to be at fault. Parents, especially, tend to feel guilt over the death of a child and may berate themselves or each other; they may even injure themselves in an impulsive gesture of aggression or self-destruction. Guilt, in fact, is probably felt to some degree by all bereaved persons as they search their minds for ways in which they may have failed the loved one, when it is now too late to make amends.

Engel's third stage of grieving is the "work of mourning." It may begin during the funeral rites or shortly after; therefore, it is rarely seen in the emergency setting. During this final stage, which may go on for a year or more, the bereaved person works through his feelings toward his loss in a series of halting steps, until he is finally able to resume a normal life that revolves around new interests.

The grieving process has been described in various ways by other psychiatrists, but similarities are readily apparent. Bowlby for example, describes the first phase of mourning as one in which the individual, just deprived of the lost object of his love, makes strenuous efforts to recover it but experiences repeated disappointment when he cannot. The second phase is one of disorganization, accompanied by pain and despair. Lastly he describes a prolonged phase during which reorganization of personality takes place, in connection with both the image of the lost object and a new object or objects.[1]

Stages of Dying

Kübler-Ross's familiar stages of dying are, of course, stages of grieving as well, in which the individual mourns the impending loss of self. As described by Kübler-Ross, shock and denial constitute the first phase, followed by an anger stage. The anger arises from feelings of frustration, injustice and resentment over one's situation. These first two stages parallel Engel's exactly.

Kübler-Ross's third stage of bargaining (with God or with some person who is perceived as being able to grant a temporary reprieve) is an emotional respite, an attempt to postpone the inevitable. The fourth stage, depression, is a time of mourning past losses or failures, a time to grieve and cry. Finally, Kübler-Ross describes the stage of acceptance as a time of peace and contentment but also of sadness.[15]

It is important to keep in mind that the stages of grieving, however described, are not clear-cut; rather, one merges into the other, and regression into an earlier phase may occur at times throughout the grieving process. Nevertheless, a *process* is worked through by the grieving person, and the process is much the same for each individual, whatever the loss he has sustained.

MAJOR LOSSES OTHER THAN DEATH

Divorce

Obviously, the strongest grief reactions follow the most severe, unexpected, and irrevocable losses. Death of a loved one is a clear example, but just as severe a reaction can occur in separation and divorce. Indeed, in some ways, divorce can be more traumatic than loss through death, since the added burdens of rejection and abandonment are prominent factors. A typical grieving process follows, with strong feelings of anguish and guilt, anger and frustration. Just as in death, resolution of the loss follows a long and painful course of at least 1 year, and frequently more.

Effects on Health and Longevity. An important point that is seldom considered when death or divorce causes the loss of a spouse is the increased incidence of morbidity and mortality in the grievers. Several studies in the 1960s clearly indicated an increased death rate in the first year of bereavement as compared to matched groups of nonbereaved persons.[19,23,34] As Parkes points out, however, this does not prove that grief causes death, but it may well aggravate a physical problem that would have occurred in any case.[18] Nevertheless, there is a great enough increase in physical

illness, as well as in symptoms that may be ascribed to stress and anxiety (*i.e.*, headache, digestive disturbances, asthma, arthritis) to warrant inquiry about recent stressful events in the patient's life as a part of the history. Often a sympathetic listener can do as much to relieve such symptoms as medication or other treatment can.

Disabling Illness or Injury

Acute grief responses are also evoked by severe threats to the self-system, such as disabling illness or injury, or the loss of a body part. These alterations in body image are mourned as is any other complete and irrevocable loss because they actually represent the death of a part of oneself.

Body Image. Body image is the mental picture that each person has of his or her own body—the way in which the physical self is perceived. The importance of body image to physical and psychological well-being cannot be overemphasized. It is an essential part of the individual's self-concept, his sense of integrity and intactness. Any disruption of the body image, even in a psychologically well-adjusted person, can result in a severe grief reaction with marked anxiety and feelings of deep depression. This fact must be recognized in order to help the patient cope with his initial reactions and to recognize when psychological intervention may be indicated or when follow-up care may be necessary.

Loss of an external body part is an example of change in body image. Such traumatic disfigurements as severed limbs, severe burns, and extensive lacerations of the face or other body parts are perceived by the individual as the death of that part of the body or of its appearance, and he reacts with acute grief.

Debilitating illness such as stroke is an enormous assault on the body image. Not only is the patient coping with severe physiological stress, but his loss of function creates great psychological stress as well. This is an aspect of stroke that emergency personnel may recognize themselves but do not always acknowledge to the patient. However, the stroke patient has an intense need for information and reassurance about the effects of stroke.

In all of these instances, it is the *suddenness* of the change that precipitates a crisis. Just as in the sudden death of a loved one, the person has had no warning, no time to adapt, no opportunity to incorporate the change into a new body image. And as in any grieving process, time is the necessary ingredient for recovery.

Sexual Assault

Some less obvious grievers are victims of sexual assault. Care of the sexually assaulted victim usually follows well-established protocols designed to protect the victim and provide for the collection of evidence. While many hospitals include a rape counselor as part of the emergency department team, this is not always the case, and the nurse may be the only person available to fill this important role. Keep in mind that these patients, too, are grieving and in crisis. Most victims of sexual assault see their experience as a life-threatening event, and they present in the same state of shock and bewilderment as any griever, often unable to believe it has happened to them. The victim suffers loss of self-esteem, feels guilty, and may say she feels dirty and untouchable. Calm, compassionate, and warm support are most important at this time. Above all, the victim needs to feel that she is safe and has an empathetic person to listen to her. Encourage—but do not push—her to talk about her feelings. At times, touching her is important, both to convey your warmth and caring and to reassure her that she is not repulsive to others. See Chapter 7 for a comprehensive discussion of care of the sexually assaulted victim.

The Recovery Process. Over a period of time, the sexual assault victim goes through a recovery pattern very similar to the grieving process as outlined by both Engel and Bowlby. Evans identifies three phases, as follows:
1. Numbness and disbelief.
2. Acute disorganization, with disturbed sleep patterns, weight loss, and inability to make decisions.
3. Reorganization, in which the victim develops a new self-image, self-confidence, and trust in others, although still subject to regression when threatened in any way with loss of control. Evans emphasizes that complete recovery may take years to accomplish.

SUPPORTIVE CARE OF THE PERSON COPING WITH LOSS AND GRIEF

Although grief is a syndrome with a predictable course and consistent symptoms, emergency personnel must also be aware that each individual's *expression* of grief will be a little different, depending on such variables as age, sex, ethnic background, past experience with grief, and usual coping patterns. Severe grief does cause a breakdown in normal coping patterns, yet some semblance of habitual response is usually retained. For example, the person who meets all of his life crises with denial will inevitably use denial when faced with sudden loss. Those who are openly emotional in every phase of their lives will be highly emotional in grieving.

Some responses to loss and grief may not conform to our expectations. The person who does not cry, for example, is sometimes perceived as not being very much affected by his loss. The person who jokes with the staff even when faced with severe loss, is felt to be behaving inappropriately, and the staff's reaction may be disapproving. Such judgments must not be made, however. Each person is coping in the best way he can, and any intervention should always be accepting and supportive. At the same time, one should not reinforce inappropriate behavior but should gently present the reality of the situation to the person.

Men may lose their customary control of their emotions and, when unable to regain their composure, may feel ashamed because of their "unmanly" behavior. It is important to accept their behavior without any hint of disapproval or scorn. It *is* all right for men to be frightened, to be emotional, and to cry when facing acute trauma.

Communication

It is a mistake, in fact, to assume anything from the facade that the patient presents. The person who *appears* to be calm and in control may be just as frightened and unable to cope with his anxieties as the person who overtly expresses his feelings. Communication is the key to handling all of these modes of grief; it involves conveying a warm, receptive attitude; meeting the person's eyes with concern; offering a touch, a gesture. Supportive measures in themselves are not necessarily helpful or comforting; it is the way in which they are administered that makes a difference.

In fact, if one had to choose the single word that best sums up a compassionate, supportive approach to the person coping with loss, it might well be communication—both verbal and nonverbal. Skillful use of communication techniques is desirable, but even if one is unskilled, communication can be effective if it is honest and sincere. Listening is one of the more important communication techniques. Help can also be offered in tangible ways: by physical presence, by calm acceptance of varying moods, by encouragement and reassurance when appropriate.

Patients faced with significant loss begin to grieve as soon as they are aware of the actual *threat* of loss. If they are alert and oriented, they need realistic support at all times. However, it is often difficult to determine what this means. If the person views his situation as precarious, he deserves to know as much about his prospects as he really wants to know. Encourage him to express his concerns. Answer his questions as honestly as possible, always maintaining as much hope as is reasonable. Patients usually fear the worst, and emergency personnel may, by their honest answers, be able to alleviate their worst fears.

The Patient Who Cannot Talk. The patient who is not able to talk but who is conscious or semiconscious should be assured that the emergency care team is aware of his concerns, and should then be given *realistic* assurance about his progress and prognosis. This patient has a basic need to know that those caring for him are aware that he has anxieties he cannot express.

Dealing With Anxiety. The person who seems to be overwhelmed by anxiety may be helped to come to grips with his situation if someone can show him how to separate some parts from the whole and deal with them individually. Is he, for example, more concerned about his own welfare, or that of a family member or of someone involved in the mishap with him? Help him sort out the smaller worries; if some of them can be alleviated, the whole situation may not be so overwhelming.

Dealing With Guilt Feelings. Persons mourning a loss should be allowed to express their guilt feelings. These expressions frequently begin with the phrase "If only . . .": "If only I had done this (or had not done that), this whole thing might not have happened." Such expressions are a normal component of the grief response, and need to be verbalized. Do not judge or indicate in any way that anyone is guilty. Do not reassure the person too quickly, even though this may be a natural impulse, since your response may in effect tell him to stop talking about it. Rather, let him express his guilt feelings freely, listen sympathetically, and after he has had the chance to express his feeling you can offer plausible comments and suggestions to relieve his guilt, if this is valid. Another nonjudgemental response might be: "I understand how you feel. It's natural for you to feel this way right now." You might want to add: "You may feel differently about it later."

Dealing With Anger. The anger that is a part of the grieving process may be difficult to deal with too. For some reason, it is easier to tolerate crying than anger. Try to understand where the anger is coming from; be aware that it is an expression of frustration and helplessness. Refrain from responding with anger or acting hurt at the injustice of accusations the person might make, but rather remain calm and sympathetic until the anger subsides.

Dealing With the Fear of Insanity. Grievers who express fear of going insane should be reassured promptly that there is no reason to be afraid. Tell them that the feelings they are having are a part of grief, that it is normal to have these feelings under the circumstances, and that they will go away in time.

Sedation

The question of whether or not to sedate persons in acute grief is hard to answer. Certainly it is easy for emergency department personnel to choose sedation. Sedation does quiet the sobbing and appears to help the person get hold of himself. Many physicians feel that a mild sedative is in order in the early stages of grief, to blunt the sharp edge of reality and enable the griever to make the kinds of pragmatic decisions that have to be made. On the other hand, Twerski states: "There is altogether too much emphasis in our culture on escaping from all types of discomfort through alcohol or some type of drug," and notes that giving a sedative to relieve acute grief reinforces the assumption that drugs are a necessary part of coping with some of the harsh realities of life.[31]

In any case, sedation only delays the grief reaction. It seems preferable to allow the person to cry and express his rage and frustration right there where there is a shoulder to cry on and he can vent his anger without injuring himself. If the person giving care can be patient and understanding and perhaps agree that he or she would probably feel the same way, the bereaved person may be able to recover to the point where it would be safe for him to be sent home.

Sending the Survivor Home

A survivor should never go home alone. The person who is utterly alone in the world, with no relative, no friend, no minister, not even a neighbor who can stay with him, presents a very real problem. Many people in acute states of anguish are suicidal for a time. It would be better to admit the person overnight, in the care of others who are warm and compassionate, with the hope and expectation that he will be able to cope tomorrow.

Important points in the care of the grieving person are summarized in Chart 6-1.

Chart 6-1

SUPPORTIVE CARE OF THE GRIEVING PERSON

- Accept any grieving behavior without judgment—anger, crying, passivity, laughing, etc. The person will cope in ways that are most comfortable for *him*.
- Convey a warm, receptive, supportive attitude through touch, helpful gestures, and listening; convey concern and a sincere desire to help
- Encourage expression of concerns and feelings.
- Discuss misunderstandings about what occurred during the emergency; answer questions honestly.
- Listen empathetically to expressions of guilt; offer nonjudgmental responses after the griever has had an opportunity to express his feelings.
- Recognize that anger is an expression of frustration and helplessness and is not to be taken personally.
- Avoid reinforcing griever's denials.
- Convey permission to view the body; show acceptance of the body.
- Assist griever in contacting a friend, family member, clergyman, crisis volunteer, or counselor.
- Never send griever home alone or leave him alone at home; many people become suicidal after profound loss.
- Give news of death in person, not over the phone. Calmly inform bereaved person of the injury; suggest bringing a friend or family member; and state that there is no need to rush.

SUPPORTIVE CARE OF THE DYING PATIENT

Death in the emergency department differs from death in most other areas of the hospital, and so do the problems it creates and the ways in which the staff tries to cope with them. In the emergency area, death usually *is* a sudden, catastrophic event caused by an outside force. Whether that causative force is a traumatic accident or a coronary occlusion, it is sudden, unexpected, and overwhelming.

According to seasoned emergency personnel, the victim who is dead on arrival (DOA) is never a real shock *per se* because this experience occurs so often that the care team is psychologically prepared to handle it. The reaction to the DOA victim comes rather from the severity of the injuries, the type and degree of mutilation, and the like.

However, the patient who is admitted alive but in imminent danger of death presents a different problem. His critical condition requires the total involvement of emergency department personnel. The skilled efforts, the teamwork, the very "busy-ness" of the task help the staff to maintain composure in tense situations. Saving lives is the primary function of the unit. The physical needs of the patient are so urgent and demanding that there is little time to think about his psychological needs.

Communication

If the patient is unconscious or semiconscious, the need to interact with him is less urgent. He may be in a state of physical and emotional shock and not really aware of what is happening to him. However, because there is a chance that the patient does know what is going on, emergency department personnel should avoid making any negative comments about his condition and prognosis. If the patient is conscious but seems confused, he should be oriented in a calm way and in simple language that he can readily understand. Explain what has happened to him causing him to be brought to the hospital, tell him who you are, and assure him that you and everyone else there is giving him the best possible care. This can be done without lengthy explanation or false reassurance; your tone of voice and manner of speaking should provide assurance that you care about him and will try to help him. Empty phrases such as, "You'll be OK, don't worry," should be avoided. They may make *you* feel better, but they do nothing for the anxious patient.

The patient who is aware of and concerned about his prognosis creates another kind of problem. He may not say anything, only plead with his eyes for some answer, for reassurance. Even if he asks directly whether he is going to die, he may not really want the answer. What he does want to know for certain is, first, that he is getting the best possible care and, then, that you are not going to leave him alone.

Dealing With the Fear of Dying Alone. One of the greatest fears of a dying person, or a person who suspects he may be dying, is the fear of dying alone. Stay with him, and if you must leave the room, see that someone else remains there with him. Do more than just be there—share yourself;

meet the patient's eyes, smile, touch him, hold his hand, make him feel that you care about *him,* not just his intravenous lines or the myriad other gadgets that one tends to become absorbed in to avoid the human contact that means so much to the dying patient.

Dealing With Questions About Impending Death. It is unfair to try to fool the patient who suspects the truth. But it is also cruel to answer "Yes" to the question, "Am I dying?" More than cruel, it is devastating, because it takes away hope, and the patient who has been stripped of hope never does as well as the one who has a degree of hope held out to him. It is much better to respond to the effect that you are all there fighting for him, and you need to have him fight too. If he then persists in the assertion that he is dying, you can agree that that is a possibility, but that you are doing everything you can to prevent it.

Kübler-Ross maintains that a patient should never be told he is dying. Only when the patient himself offers the information that he is fatally ill should one talk openly to him about his dying.[15] In the emergency department, of course, patients are less likely to *tell* the personnel they are dying than they are to *ask* them, and their questions may be prompted by fear, pain, or suspicion, or by self-conviction when they get no sensible response to their anxious queries. Try to assess what is behind the patient's questions. Knowledge of what is actually happening to him pathologically will also influence the reply. Be very alert and sensitive to each individual when assessing his need. Is he aware of what is happening to him? How much does he want to know? How much is he able to hear? Be honest in your reply, yet keep in mind that the whole truth may destroy him.

Spiritual Support

An important source of help and comfort for many patients is spiritual support. A priest should always be called for the Roman Catholic patients who are in danger of death. Patients of other faiths may or may not wish to have a clergyman attend them, but they should be given the choice. An appropriate time to suggest this might be when the patient is expressing concern about his possible death. For the patient who does not verbalize such fears, use judgment about when to offer him this option. Some nurses are reluctant to suggest a clergyman to patients who do not mention it themselves, fearing that the suggestion will alarm the patient and thus do more harm than good. It is largely a question of weighing advantages against disadvantages. It would seem unfair to deprive the patient of spiritual support if he would gain great comfort and strength from it but might be reluctant to request it of professional people who are obviously busy with physical care. The patient of opposite convictions, who has no interest in spiritual affairs, might be alerted to his precarious status if offered this option, but the staff can then reassure him in keeping with his emotional response.

While religion may or may not be important to a patient, it cannot be known unless he tells someone. For the patient who does have strong religious convictions, it becomes far more important to him when his life is in danger. If the patient dies, the knowledge that spiritual guidance and support were provided will be a source of comfort to the family.

THE FAMILY

While the patient is still living and the emergency personnel are absorbed in the many tasks necessary to try to save his life, contact with the family in minimal. Although this is not necessarily desirable, it is more important at that time that all energies be directed to the patient himself. Afterward, the care team may be exhausted and emotionally drained, wishing only to withdraw and pull their thoughts together, perhaps even cry—but there is the family to cope with. For it is then that the real emergency occurs for the survivors. It is urgent that they be given all the help necessary to face this crisis.

This is not an easy task. The death has come as a terrible shock to the family. One can be empathetic, but it may be hard to accept their reactions, especially if they are highly emotional and noisy, or angry and unreasonable. You may just wish they would sign the necessary papers and leave, to do their grieving at home.

In order to understand the family and assist them more effectively at this critical time, recall the symptomatology of the grief syndrome and all of the supportive measures previously discussed in relation to loss in general. Reactions to death, the ultimate, irrevocable loss, are usually more profound, more anguished, and more agonizing than reactions to other losses. In the emergency department, reactions are even more intense because of the sudden and unexpected nature of the event.

SUDDEN INFANT DEATH SYNDROME

As recognition of sudden infant death syndrome (SIDS) becomes more widespread, we are becoming more aware of the devastating problems faced by the parents of infants who die because of it. SIDS babies, discovered dead in their cribs without any previous hint of illness, are sometimes rushed to the emergency department in the arms of the distraught parents. The parents' experience there, unfortunately, has not been a source of comfort to them but rather has added to their misery.

Attitudes of Emergency Department Personnel

The concomitant increase in child abuse cases has made hospital staffs suspicious in the face of the sudden, unexplained death of a child. SIDS babies frequently exhibit areas of ecchymosis on the head and body (due to pooling of blood in dependent areas at the time of death) which resemble the bruises of a battered child. The staff's natural feelings of revulsion and dismay when confronted with the appearances of child abuse seem to outweigh rational thought, and they react to the parents with hostility and suspicion.

The following excerpts from an interview with a mother of a SIDS baby bring out some of the feelings and reactions emergency department personnel should be aware of.

Q: What was your first reaction when you discovered your baby dead in his crib?
A: Panic. At first I told myself he was just sound asleep, even though I could tell right away that something was terribly wrong. I picked him up, and I kept saying, "No! No! He can't be dead, he can't be!" I remember I kept hoping it was all a bad dream, that he would wake up in a minute and start to cry.
     Then my husband phoned the rescue squad. We knew nothing could be done, really, but we couldn't just give up. I kept hugging the baby, patting his back, rocking him with my body.
Q: What did the rescue squad do?
A: They gave the baby oxygen with a mask on his face. I think they knew it was hopeless, but they kept giving him the oxygen. They wouldn't say he was dead. I guess they can't do that. Anyway, they took us to the hospital, my husband and me and the baby, and they kept giving him the oxygen.
Q: How did they treat you? What was their reaction to the situation?
A: They were all right. They were concerned about the baby, and they really tried. They didn't say much to us, but they were polite, and I got the feeling they really felt bad when they couldn't bring the baby around with the oxygen.
Q: What happened when you got to the hospital?
A: Well, they took us up to the emergency entrance, and of course, we were taken care of right away. By that time, I was practically in a state of shock, but I remember that the police arrived about the same time we did. One of the policemen whispered to the doctor something about the baby being dead, or was he going to pronounce him dead, or something like that. Then they began to ask us all kinds of questions, like what had we done to the baby? Had he fallen recently? Had he been sick? Had either of us ever hit him? I was shocked when I realized what they were driving at. It had never occurred to me that anyone would think we had tried to hurt our baby. We loved him! We had wanted him for such a long time. My husband had doted on him—his little son! And I had waited for what seemed like ages to have a baby, because I had to work a few years after we were married. I just couldn't believe that everybody didn't *know* we adored our baby.
     It was then that I really began to go back over things and wonder if I had done anything wrong, if maybe I hadn't burped him enough after his last bottle before I put him to bed. He had had a little cold the week before, but he seemed to be all over that. Then I began to wonder if my husband was suspicious of me too, if *he* thought I had neglected the baby somehow.
Q: Did anyone support you at this time?
A: No. No one. I really felt that they were all just suspicious of us, that they thought we were some kind of abnormal parents, child-beaters or something. A nurse came in and told us we would have to sign for an autopsy, and I couldn't. I didn't want my baby cut up. She said if we didn't sign, the coroner would do the autopsy anyway, so then my husband signed the paper. I was crying by then, and my husband was shaking all over, and we just clung to each other because there was nothing else we could do.

Supportive Care of Parents

In a situation like this, what should be done to help the distraught couple? The principles that apply to the support of grieving relatives also apply here.

Nonjudgmental Attitude.   First, it is imperative that the staff not attempt to judge the parents in this situation. No one can possibly know how or why this infant died. No one can know whether the parents are guilty of neglect or abuse or whether they are completely innocent. Even if it is found later that kindness and support have gone to parents who did abuse their child, nothing has been lost by the effort. In fact, such parents may be genuinely remorseful by that time, their grief augmented by their guilt.

Providing Reassurance. Parents of SIDS victims need repeated reassurances that neither anything they have done nor anything they failed to do has caused the death of their child. It is helpful for the emergency care team to be informed about the characteristics of SIDS, its incidence, and some of the theories on etiology, so that they can use some factual information in reassuring parents. While the cause of the syndrome is not yet known, much information is available about it, and a national lay organization* provides professional counseling for parents, among other services.

The initial stages of grief are coped with in the emergency department, and staff members can help best by understanding the parents' ordeal, accepting their behavior, assuring them that they are in no way to blame for the death, and comforting, supporting, and showing willingness to help in any way possible. Keep in mind that these parents are acutely sensitive to the critical atmosphere they encounter at almost every turn. It is one of the cruelest aspects of their ordeal, and it compounds their grief and guilt.

HELPING CHILDREN COPE WITH DEATH

Although children may not be the direct recipients of emergency care following the death of a family member, emergency department personnel can nevertheless do much to help them indirectly. Most adults find it difficult to talk to children about death, yet when they leave the emergency department as survivors, they frequently have to go home and explain to a child what has happened to his parent or a sibling. Most are grateful for a chance to talk about this with a staff member, if only to help clarify their own feelings.

A staff member might broach the subject with the simple question, "Have you thought how you're going to tell the children?" Together they can explore the issue, guided by the client's religious and philosophic beliefs. The most important points to convey are that (1) children cannot be protected from the knowledge and pain of death, and (2) children grieve just as adults do and should therefore be included in the family's grieving so that they, too, can work through their feelings.

Children's Perceptions of Death

The child's perception of death depends on his age and on previous exposure to loss. Theories differ regarding death perceptions at various developmental levels, but generally speaking, the child under the age of three years has little if any comprehension of death. He does, however, under-

stand separation and suffers severely from maternal deprivation—or paternal deprivation if the father has been the primary source of love and attention. The young child who loses a parent has an intense need to be reassured that some one person will still be there to take care of him and give him the love and security he needs. His questions should be answered honestly but simply, in terms he can understand.

It is a mistake to tell a young child that mother has gone to sleep or gone on a trip. The former may make him afraid to go to bed, and the latter will be seen as abandonment. He can deal with the truth, simply stated as "he (or she) was so sick, or so badly hurt, that the doctors couldn't save him and so he died." Such statements, of course, must be made to the child by another loved person, and assurances of continued love and security be given.

Child psychologists note that television viewing may lead to confused perceptions about death—for example, when a character who has "died" in a TV drama seemingly comes back to life in a drama that the child sees later. Confusion about the nature of death—whether it is permanent or only temporary—may result.

School-age children have a more developed concept of death, especially after the age of nine, when they view death much as adults do, as a real event that can happen to them too.

Needs of Bereaved Children

It must be kept in mind, however, that children of any age, when faced with the death of a loved one, have the following needs:

- Assurance of the continuing love and protection of other family members
- Inclusion in the family's mourning rituals so that they, too, can work through their grief
- Assurance that they were not responsible for the death.

This last concern is an antecedent of the guilt feelings that always accompany grief. The child in anger has probably wished the loved one dead on occasion, and the actual death may be perceived as a fulfillment of this secret wish. Whether or not the child verbalizes this concern, he should be reassured that such a thing could never happen.

Attendance at the Funeral. Should children go to the funeral? School-age children should certainly be *allowed,* although never *forced,* to go. Very young children probably should not attend the funeral, although they might be taken to the funeral home to view the body. The decision should rest with the adults responsible for the child who are closest to him, know him best, and know his level of maturity and emotional status. In turn, however, these adults need to be made aware that it is *not* a social taboo to take the child, that in fact if it is done in an atmosphere of love and mutual family support, it can be a positive experience for the child.

STAFF RESPONSIBILITIES WHEN DEATH OCCURS

In the event of death, who announces the death to the family, and how should this be done? If at all possible, it is helpful

* The National Foundation for Sudden Infant Death, Inc., 1501 Broadway, New York, NY 10036. Local chapters exist in many cities throughout the country.

to give the family some advance warning that things are not going well, that death seems imminent and inevitable. This kind of advance "bad news" is often difficult to impart and staff members are reluctant to do it, but it actually softens the blow for the family by giving them a little time to prepare themselves for the unexpected bad turn of events. This is referred to as preparatory grief, or anticipatory grief, and it is helpful because it allows the survivors to work through some of their feelings before the final blow, death, actually arrives.

When a patient dies a lingering death, family members have time to go through a good deal of their grief work beforehand, so that when the patient finally dies, they may already be into the third stage, the restorative stage. When death is sudden and unexpected, however, there is little or no time for preparatory grieving, and the shock is then much greater. Emergency department staff can help, if there is time, by periodically reporting progressively bad news. This is preferable to holding out too much hope in an attempt to be kind. Sudden death is a fact that must be accepted; avoiding the family or offering false hope is not helpful.

Informing the Family.   It is almost always better if the physician tells the family of the death. He is the person that the relatives see as the primary authority. They have the opportunity to ask him questions if they wish and to ask his advice about immediate problems that they may have. Even if the physician has never had any previous contact with the family, which is often the case, he can still establish a meaningful relationship with the survivors in a very short interval. Varying experiences are reported by relatives informed of a loved one's death by a physician. Comments range from, "He used such technical language that we couldn't understand what he was talking about," to the opposite extreme, "The doctor was so kind. He had bad news to tell us, but he tried to be helpful. He made us feel that he really cared about us."

Emergency department nurses often maintain that they are better equipped to inform families than physicians are, that their "nurturing" role enables them to show their concern and sympathy more effectively, and that they are more supportive of the grief-stricken kin. This may be true, and if the task does fall to the nurse and she is comfortable in the role, the family surely benefits from her touch. Nevertheless, it is still important that the family have contact with a physician who has been in attendance with the deceased patient. If no physician is in evidence, they will be left to speculate whether there was actually one present, and the thought that their loved one might have been saved if a competent physician had been available may torment them later. The physical presence of a physician with whom they can talk and ask questions will reassure them that everything possible was done. The nurse can certainly accompany the physician if she wishes, can temper his remarks if she feels it is necessary, and can stay with the family after he leaves, to explain, amplify, and reinforce his information.

Informing by Telephone.   When the family is not present and must be summoned by telephone, the problem is somewhat different. Most authorities maintain, and personal experience verifies, that if the death has been sudden and completely unexpected, the family should never be notified

by telephone—or only as a last resort. It is impossible to estimate, on one end of the line, the situation on the other end. Heart attacks have been precipitated and acts of self-injury or even self-destruction have been attempted by distraught survivors who are alone when the devastating news comes. In addition, the harried relatives, in their haste to reach the hospital, may themselves become the victims of an automobile accident en route.

The all-important factor, if the family must be informed by telephone, is to keep calm. The caller sets the stage for the way in which the family reacts. If it can be quietly conveyed that there has been an accident and that they should come to the hospital as soon as they can, with no urgency in the voice, chances are they will be able to avoid panic. They will, of course, be alarmed and may immediately suspect the worst; but even if they ask if it is "serious" or if he is dead, one can still avoid the truth without denying, by saying, perhaps, "He has been badly injured, but he is receiving excellent care and everything possible is being done. There is no need for you to rush." When they arrive, and there is face-to-face contact, try to control the situation by being very composed and calm in approach. Explain what has happened clearly and in terms the family can understand, emphasizing the quality of care given. Again, the physician should speak with the family, even if he has to wait there for their arrival.

Providing for Emotional Needs.   It is always better if more than one family member is present or if a close friend is there. They provide support for each other, and grief that is shared is somehow easier to bear. In any case, the bereaved person should not be left alone. If it is the nurse who breaks the news to the family, and she is *really* too busy to remain long with them (not simply looking for an excuse to escape from this uncomfortable situation), another appropriate person must be found, a chaplain or spiritual advisor, perhaps. Or, an aide who is a warm, concerned individual can fill this role with a little training and a lot of support.

Many authorities recognize the pressing need in the emergency department for some sort of psychological consultation service for families. Quint and others see this as possibly a social worker's role, but they ask, realistically, who would pay for the 24-hours-a-day services of such a person? Is the public ready to assume the cost?[22] While in some instances a chaplain may fill the role of comforter to the bereaved, it is important to realize that the mere fact of being a clergyman does not necessarily equip one to meet the needs of people in the acute stages of grief. He, too, needs adequate preparation, often not provided in his training. Kübler-Ross suggests that specially trained volunteers might be used effectively.[14] They would have the advantage of being uninvolved in the efforts to save the patient, which is so emotionally draining, and could therefore devote all of their energies to comforting the family. Volunteers who have experienced grief in their own lives are ideal and can readily be trained in basic psychological and communication techniques. They could be available on a round-the-clock basis, with no added cost to the hospital.

Providing Privacy.   Another essential element, too often lacking in hospitals, is a room where grieving relatives can be provided privacy. Every area of the hospital should be able to provide such a room, but certainly in high-risk areas it is indispensable. To give the family this shocking news in a corridor or in a waiting room filled with curious and perhaps anxious observers is heartless and inexcusable. If no space can be found in the emergency department itself, a nearby chapel or any small empty room can be used. Emergency departments now in the planning stages would be improved by the inclusion of one or more such "crying rooms."

Supportive Approach.   Survivors must be allowed, indeed encouraged, to express their acute grief in whatever way it comes out. Accept their tears and anger, whether they are noisy or subdued, without comment. Touch is extremely effective in conveying sympathy and concern, an arm around the shoulders, a handclasp. A simple offer of services is comforting: "Can I get you a glass of water?" "How about a cup of hot coffee?" "Can I phone your sister to come and be with you?" What you say is not as significant as how you say it. What you do is not as important as being there.

The following case presentation illustrates how thoughtlessness and a judgmental attitude can result in a harsh and insensitive approach to the bereaved person and leave lasting aftereffects of pain and guilt.

> Mr. H., age 49, was admitted to the emergency department at 11 P.M. and was immediately pronounced dead. He had been discharged from the same hospital only 2 weeks before, following a lengthy hospitalization with a myocardial infarction. Earlier that evening, he had encouraged his wife to go to a party at the home of friends, since he was feeling fine and could manage quite well alone.
> Later in the evening, he developed chest pain, telephoned a neighbor for help, said a few words, and collapsed. The neighbor immediately came to the house and found him lying on the floor. An ambulance was summoned, and Mr. H. was rushed to the hospital, but was dead on arrival.
> Mrs. H. arrived at the hospital soon afterward, obviously dressed in party attire, concerned about her husband but with no thought of death on her mind. She immediately approached a nurse with a multitude of questions: "How is he? Is he able to talk? How sick is he? Can he sit up?" The nurse detected alcohol on Mrs. H.'s breath and responded coldly: "Your husband is dead. There are papers here that have to be signed right away. We would also like to know what undertaker to call."

This nurse may not have meant to be cruel, but she did not feel that undue kindness was in order, either. She judged Mrs. H. on the basis of her party attire, the fact that she had been drinking and, worst of all, the fact that she had gone off to a party and left her husband to die alone. Without doubt, Mrs. H. would be tormented by feelings of guilt for the very same reasons, even though her motives were innocent. The nurse reinforced her guilt, added to the hurt, and delayed a healthy resolution of the grieving process.

VIEWING THE BODY

Should the family be allowed to see the body? Staff members often feel that if there is severe mutilation, especially of the head or face, it is too shocking a sight for the family to endure. Difficult as it is, it is necessary if the family is to accept the death as a reality. Studies have shown that survivors who have the most difficulty resolving their grief are those who have never seen the body because the cause of death was drowning, an airplane crash, or some other tragedy in which the body was never recovered. In the emergency department, the body can be cleansed and made as presentable as possible. At least some identifiable part should be made visible for the relatives, to confirm the loss. Prepare the family ahead of time so that they will have some idea of what to expect, but always give them the option of seeing the corpse. It is a form of reality orientation that the numbed survivor needs.

The experiences of two young practicing nurses clearly illustrate the difficulties of working through the grieving process for the survivor when he has not viewed the dead body. One nurse lost a much-loved brother in a car accident. His body was sent immediately across the country to the city where their parents lived, and he was buried there. This young woman never saw his body and has never seen his grave. Although many years have passed, she still resents her mother for "taking Donny away from me." She feels that he should have been buried "here," but when asked if she has thought of going to the other city to visit his grave, she resists the idea and still irrationally blames her mother for the loss.

The other young nurse says her father died when she was about 12 years old and was cremated. She did not even see him while he was sick and hospitalized. His death is unreal to her, despite the fact that his ashes sit in an urn on the home mantelpiece. The family plans to sprinkle the ashes from a plane (which was his wish), and then there will not even be ashes to confirm the fact of his death. This young woman is in a state of partial denial of her father's death. She knows that he died, yet she has never had any proof of the fact and cannot wholly accept it.

OBTAINING PERMISSION FOR AUTOPSIES

The task of obtaining permission for an autopsy cannot be ignored. Reponsibility for this duty may be delegated to various staff members, depending on the institution, the time of day or night when death occurs, and probably many other factors. The situation is a sensitive one, and many approaches are possible. Two are illustrated in the following case history:

> Hours earlier, the grief-stricken woman had been happily married, enjoying a quiet evening at home with her husband and two small children. Now she was in the waiting area outside the hospital's emergency rooms, recently informed that her 42-year-old husband had died of acute myocardial infarction. The family physician was called but arrived after the patient had died. As he entered the room he found the wife sobbing uncontrollably while a resident she had never seen before asked her for permission to perform an autopsy. She immediately refused and when he started to pursue his request further, she became extremely angry and refused to discuss the subject.
> The family physician discovered that the wife had not yet been given a sedative, so he offered this and other practical assistance soon after he arrived. He shared her grief and gave her the solace and encouragement she needed at this tragic moment. Before long, after the initial impact of sudden death

had started to wear off, the physician brought up the subject of autopsy once again. After he told her the reasons behind the request and the benefits to be gained by the autopsy, she gave the physician her permission without hesitation.

Why did the family physician succeed where the resident failed? Two of the most obvious reasons are that, unlike the resident, he knew the family and had a satisfactory doctor-family relationship. Also, he waited until the shock had started to wear off before making the request. But perhaps the most important reason behind his success was the way in which he made the autopsy request.[30]

There are a number of techniques that any staff member can use to make the task a bit easier and success more likely. The physician in the case history used a method recommended by a panel of thanatologists, who describe the following steps in requesting an autopsy.

1. Wait for the proper moment. This means waiting until the initial shock has worn off, offering meanwhile sympathetic support and some practical assistance (coffee, phone calls).

2. Make the request in a positive manner, rather than in the form of a question. Instead of asking directly, you might say, "I'm sure you'll want us to perform a postmortem examination. There are many reasons why it should be done." Terms such as "postmortem examination" or "examination after death" are much more acceptable to the lay person than the word "autopsy."

3. Give the relative some valid reasons why the examination should be done. For example, it is the last chance to learn all the facts about the accident or illness that caused the death; it is easier to accept death when we know it was inevitable; the exact cause of death is often necessary for settling insurance or legal matters. Families are more receptive to the idea that *people* will be benefited by the findings in an autopsy. They are not too concerned about advancing the cause of science.

4. If the family members still resist, they should not be bullied or badgered into giving permission. Their voiced objections should be answered, and to do this without seeming to pressure is tricky and requires tact. As an example, a frequent objection is this: "No, my husband has suffered enough already." Of course, the autopsy will not cause him any more suffering, and the family knows this, but they need to be told. It might also be added that, in the long run, autopsies actually reduce human suffering.

If the relative has strong guilt feelings about the deceased, he is less likely to grant permission. Psychologists have found that relatives who had abandoned the patient during the dying process or who had rejected him were the least likely to grant autopsy permission.[30]

An attitude of conviction about the need for the autopsy is a positive factor in obtaining permission. Above all, the staff member's manner will strongly influence the decision. A warm and understanding approach—even the admission that it is hard for emergency personnel to discuss the matter—can do much to gain the family's cooperation.

STAFF SELF-SUPPORT

In the emergency department, which is geared to saving the lives of the critically ill and the critically injured, the death of a patient despite all efforts is like a defeat. Even when the staff is convinced that the death was inevitable, there is still the lingering doubt, the thought that maybe it was their fault, that there must have been something else that could have been done.

Reactions to Loss

Feelings are more acute when the victims are young: the child killed in a fall, the teenager caught in the shattered wreck of a collision, the young father with a fatal coronary. We are a youth-oriented culture, and we place a high value on the young. In earlier days, death of children was common; parents were lucky to raise even 3 out of 7 children to adulthood. Now we have conquered most of the childhood diseases, and the death of a young person is seen as a terrible, senseless waste.

In much the same way, we attach a greater social value to success, beauty, education, responsibility. We are far more devastated when the young mother with a toddler dies, than we are, for example, if the victim is old. People who become health professionals bring with them the set of social values they grew up with and have lived with all their lives. The fact that they view other people, including their patients, in the light of these values is nothing to be ashamed of. But it *is* something to be aware of and to guard against, lest it influence the kind of care given. Awareness of one's personal response to social loss can also increase one's courage and composure in the face of tragedy.

The following case history demonstrates the way in which an overwhelming social loss factor can influence the staff to act in direct opposition to their objective professional judgment:

It was a quiet Sunday afternoon when Wendy W., age 12, was rushed to the emergency room of a small suburban hospital. Struck by a speeding car, she had been thrown 500 feet in the air.

The staff was shaken at the sight of her. Every bone in her body appeared to be broken. Her bloodied limbs sprawled at grotesque angles; jagged pieces of bone protruded at several sites on her legs and arms. Her skull and neck were fractured, the head twisted at an odd, unnatural angle. There was no pulse, no blood pressure. But there was still a weak heartbeat.

Everyone knew she didn't have a chance, that it would be kindest to let her die. But everyone knew, too, that this child's younger brother had lost his life in the very same way in the very same emergency room less than 2 years ago. Everything in them rebelled against this horror, and they reacted accordingly. When the cardiologist said, "It's no use. Let her go," one of the nurses cried out in anguish: "Do something! Can't you do *something?* Anything." Who could refuse? They all went to work with one accord, and the next 2 hours were filled with feverish activity. Yet in the end, the child died, just as they had all known she would. When at last the staff gave up their efforts, there was not a dry eye in the room. No one said anything to anyone else. There was nothing to say.

It is very hard not to attempt to resuscitate a young person. In this situation, the physician made a very difficult decision. Yet he was easily swayed by the more emotional and less rational reaction of a young nurse. Staff members need help in overcoming their own fears of death and finding satisfactory ways of coping with their hang-ups. This would help to prevent some of the desperate efforts which are clearly doomed to failure and are so emotionally exhausting for the staff.

Emergency personnel are exposed to other kinds of emotional trauma, too. Often they identify closely with the patient or with a member of the family. A woman who is the same age as the staff member, a child who is as young as her own child, an older person who reminds her of her father—these are the ones who bring the tragedy closer to her own life and heighten the impact of death upon her.

Many patients are warm and magnetic and involve the staff in a deeper emotional attachment than is ordinarily developed. For example, an attractive, middle-aged woman was admitted to an emergency department with severe chest pain which was subsequently determined to be a coronary occlusion. She remained there for 3 hours before a bed was available on a unit, and in this time became much more comfortable. She was very friendly and likeable, and since the staff members were not busy, they spent a lot of time with her. When she was finally transferred to another unit, they discussed her chances of recovery and all hoped she would get along well, "since she was such a lovely person." About an hour later, a "code 5" was sounded. The emergency staff sensed that it could be "their patient" and waited anxiously to find out. When they learned it was indeed this lovely lady and that she had died, the staff was overcome with gloom. For the remainder of the shift, staff members went about their own duties in silence, deep in private thoughts.

Sometimes family members upset the staff as much as the patient. They may be excessively demanding, hysterical, and noisy in their lamentations. Possibly the hardest to tolerate is the family that accuses the staff of negligence or even of causing their loved one's death. Adding to the problem is the staff members' difficulty in coping with their own feelings after a death. They are tired, frustrated, and drained by their unsuccessful efforts. What they really need is a chance to vent their own feelings, but instead they must maintain their composure and attempt to calm the family.

Need for Support

Members of the staff who have recently suffered bereavement may have great difficulty coping with dying patients and their families. They need help in handling their own problems and the opportunity to discuss their own recent crises, as well as the emergency department experiences that have upset them.

Team Conferences. Staff members need to support and aid each other in the crises that develop so that each can grow in his ability to cope with his own feelings and to provide thoughtful care. Sociologists Glaser and Strauss suggest that members of *every* hospital unit, but especially the high-risk units, should sit down and examine closely the typical dying trajectory in their unit and the reaction patterns of various staff members when a death occurs: who does what, who should do what, where the problems are, how they might be solved. Who is the strongest member of the team and the weakest? How can they help each other improve not only the care but the emotional climate of the unit?[9]

In fact, all staff members should sit down together and express their feelings and emotions, support each other, help each other. This means physicians, nurses, aides, EMTs—everyone who is part of the emergency scene. All need to talk together as human beings, forgetting the hierarchy that for years has prevented physicians from sharing their feelings with nurses and has made nurses feel they must maintain an air of cool, professional detachment. All experience grief, anger, shock, frustration in emergency care. All need support. And all will be surprised at how much it helps to admit it openly and share feelings with each other. In every group in which discussions of death and dying are initiated, the reaction expressed after only a few sessions is usually, "I thought I was the only one who felt this way! I never knew other people had the same feelings I had." And all feel better just knowing it.

Role Play. In addition to team conferences, role play has been found to be a very useful tool in improving communication with the dying and the bereaved. The emergency staff may need assistance in getting started, but the continuing education department should be able to help. It is difficult initiating any of this activity, and the first attempts will be painful and may appear futile. One particular situation may require some psychiatric counseling, or one may benefit from pastoral counseling. Help is always available, but ultimately the greatest strength will come from each other.

After a time, as staff members gain insight into their feelings about death, they can look at more effective ways of helping dying patients and their surviving relatives. Only by working together in this way can they come to grips with their anxieties about death, integrate death into the process of living, and help those who truly need help at a time of great personal crisis.

REFERENCES

1. Bowlby J: Processes of mourning. Int J Psychoanal 42:317–338, 1961
2. Cain AC: The impact of SIDS on families. In Weinstein SE (ed): Mental Health Issues in Grief Counseling. Washington, DC, Dept. HEW, 1979
3. Caughill RE (ed): The Dying Patient: A Supportive Approach. Boston, Little, Brown & Co, 1976
4. Cleveland AP: Sudden infant death syndrome (SIDS): A burgeoning medicolegal problem. Am J Law Med 1:55–69, March 1975
5. Engel GL: An approach to teaching and learning about grief. In Weinstein SE (ed): Mental Health Issues in Grief Counseling. Washington, DC, Dept. HEW, 1979
6. Engel GL: Grief and grieving. Am J Nurs 64:93–98, September 1964
7. Evans HI: Psychotherapy for the rape victim: Some treatment models. Hospital and Community Psychiatry 29:309–312, May 1978
8. Gaffney KF: Helping grieving parents. J Emerg Nurs 2:42–43, July/August 1976
9. Glaser BG, Strauss AL: Time for Dying. Chicago, Aldine, 1968
10. Goldberg SB: Family tasks and reactions in the crisis of death.

In Moos RH (ed): Coping With Physical Illness. New York, Plenum, 1977
11. Jackson EN: Understanding Grief. New York, Abingdon Press, 1957
12. Kastenbaum RJ: Death, Society, and Human Experience. St. Louis, CV Mosby, 1977
13. Kavanaugh R: Dealing naturally with the dying. Nursing 6:24–29, October 1976
14. Kubler-Ross E: Taped lecture series: Lessons From the Dying Patient. Flossmor, Ross Medical Association, 1973
15. Kubler-Ross E: On Death and Dying. New York, Macmillan, 1969
16. Lindemann E: Symptomatology and management of acute grief. Am J Psychiatry, 101:141–148, September 1944
17. McCawley A: Help patients cope with grief. Consultant, pp 64–67, November 1977
18. Parkes CM: Bereavement. New York, International Universities Press, 1972
19. Parkes CM: Broken hearts: A statistical study of increased mortality among widowers. Br Med J 1:740, 1969
20. Patterson K, Pomeroy MR: Sudden infant death syndrome. Nursing 4:85–88, May 1974
21. Pepitone-Rockwell F: Patterns of rape and approaches to care. J Fam Pract 6:521–529, 1978
22. Quint JC: Symposium: Managing the Dying Process. Patient Care, May 31, 1970.
23. Rees W, Lutkins S: Mortality of bereavement. Br Med J 4:13, 1967
24. Robinson GE: Management of the rape victim. Can Med Assoc J 115:520–522, September 18, 1976
25. Schmale AH: Giving up as a final common pathway to changes in health. Adv Psychosom Med 8:20–40, 1972
26. Schoenberg B et al (eds): Anticipatory Grief. New York, Columbia University Press, 1974
27. Schultz C: Grieving children. J Emerg Nurs pp 30–36, January/February 1980
28. Schulz R: The Psychology of Death, Dying, and Bereavement. Reading, Mass: Addison-Wesley, 1978
29. Sleep studies and sudden infant death. Med World News, pp 55–60, October 5, 1973
30. Symposium: Managing the dying process. Patient Care, May 31, 1970
31. Twerski AJ: Over the edge. Emerg Med 27–34, 43ff, November 1976
32. Werner-Beland JA (ed): Grief Responses to Long-Term Illness and Disability. Reston, Va: Reston, 1980
33. Wilcox SG, Sutton M: Understanding Death and Dying. Port Washington, Alfred, 1977
34. Young M, Benjamin B, Wallis C: The mortality of widowers. Lancet 2:454, 1963

7

SEXUAL ASSAULT

JUDITH STONER HALPERN

Statistics show that the number of violent crimes in the United States has increased annually, sexual assault representing one of the more frequently committed offenses. Not only is there a higher incidence of this crime than ever before, but more and more people have become willing to report it. Invariably, emergency personnel will have to deal with victims who have been subjected to some form of sexual assault.

Emergency personnel who encounter such a victim can be either a help or a hindrance, depending upon their awareness of the victim's needs, their perceptions of how best to meet these needs, and their insights into their own personal feelings about sexual assault.

This chapter highlights the care of sexual assault victims—both children and adults—and sensitizes the health care professional to the issues that confront these victims. Although it is recognized that men are also victims of sexual assault, for the purposes of this chapter, the victims are presumed to be female.*

LEGAL ASPECTS OF SEXUAL ASSAULT

To understand the scope of the problem and the elements involved in caring for victims of sexual assault, it is important to understand what constitutes rape and how the legal and medical systems can play a significant role in helping victims to recover from this emotional trauma.

Each state has established a legal interpretation of sexual assault as a broad category, in which rape is usually defined in narrower terms. Generally, sexual assault refers to sexual contact, whether genital, oral, or manual. Rape, on the other hand, is defined as penile penetration of the genitalia (however slight) without the consent of the victim. Some states restrict the designation of rape even further by excluding husbands or blood relatives as possible assailants.

Since rape is a felony, criminal prosecution must be based on proof that a crime has taken place. Therefore, the minute the victim enters the emergency medical system, steps must be taken to preserve any evidence. Initially the victim should be instructed not to urinate, defecate, douche, bathe, or in any way remove evidence from the part of the body that was subjected to sexual contact. Only after the medical examination is complete and specimens have been obtained should the victim clean herself. Supportive evidence, such as torn clothing or debris in the hair or on the body, should be left undisturbed because they too will be collected. The victim should be informed of this procedure and advised to bring along a change of clothing that can be worn home from the examining facility. However, although the evidence must be preserved as is, care should be taken to cover the victim to avoid unnecessary exposure while en route to the medical or police facility. Chart 7-1 summarizes the steps

to take in collecting valid evidence from the victim of sexual assault.

To aid in protecting the victim from further injury, including emotional trauma, the police should be notified as soon as possible with the understanding that the victim has the right not to press charges. If time and circumstances permit, an advance call to the hospital can alert personnel to the arrival of the victim, thereby expediting the delivery of medical care and facilitating legal procedures as well.

The medical examination is usually carried out in the hospital and is done for the purpose of collecting evidence essential in providing care to the victim and in prosecuting the case. Various persons may be designated to carry out the examination, ranging from specially trained nurses to gynecologists. Since local police jurisdictions and state legislatures have designated who can examine victims of sexual assault, it is important to see that only authorized persons do so.

Whoever performs the examination must be aware of the state's definition of rape, because subjective errors in judgment can hamper the legal prosecution of a case. Misunderstandings can be reflected in the medical record, such as can occur if the examiner thinks that sperm or semen must be present or that an intact hymen precludes rape. An erroneous emphasis in looking for a particular physical finding has led some physicians to ignore bruises, tears, and other injuries, prompting them to write "negative findings" on the record. The use of standardized reporting forms such as are provided by the United States Department of Justice (Fig. 7-1) helps ensure that consistent procedures will be followed in carrying out the examination and in collecting evidence.

Personnel who are responsible for charting should be objective and nonjudgmental. The use of direct quotations and specific descriptions of behavior instead of subjective impressions such as "angry," "nervous," or "dull" helps prevent errors in interpreting the behavior of person who is in a crisis.

After the examination has been completed, the samples collected for the police should be handled by as few people as possible. This information, referred to as *chain of evidence,* pertains to the acquisition and transfer of evidence from the victim until it has been safely locked up. As the number of people who handle the material increases, so does the chance of reducing the validity of the proof. This could cause a case to be dismissed in court on technicalities. Although local standards vary, careful documentation of everyone who handles the evidence should be kept. In order to minimize the chance of loss, mix-up with other specimens, or ultimately, the inability to prove its source, evidence should not be left unattended or unlabeled.

CHARACTERISTICS OF SEXUAL ASSAULT

Anyone can be a victim of sexual assault. There are no guarantees that will protect people from being victimized. Victims have ranged in age from 9 months to 90 years; they represent both sexes (although fewer cases of male sexual assault are

---

* This presumption does not discriminate against either sex, but serves to facilitate the use of the language. Data about male sexual assault is lacking because of infrequent reporting of such incidences. Male victims of sexual assault as well as of domestic violence (see Chap. 8) probably constitute a much larger number than estimated.

Chart 7-1

COLLECTION OF VALID EVIDENCE FROM THE VICTIM OF SEXUAL ASSAULT

- Remind victim not to urinate, defecate, douche, bathe, or remove evidence until after medical examination.
- Be sure that evidence collection protocol has prior approval of law enforcement and judicial agencies, the hospital laboratory, and the medical examiner.
- When possible, notify police and receiving hospital to facilitate legal procedures and medical care.
- Be familiar with legal definition of rape in your own state and be aware of protocol for collecting evidence.
- Evidence collection must be done by experienced personnel who are familiar with proper procedures for collection and for maintaining continuity of possession.
- Prepare sexual assault kits beforehand, including a simple checklist to follow in collecting evidence (see Chart 7-2).
- Place clothing, dried, in separate paper bags and label. (Have someone bring a change of clothing to examination facility.)
- Note bruises, scratches, and other injuries and have them photographed if necessary.
- Collect all external samples before any internal examination or collection to prevent contamination and introduction of semen from the outside of the body into vaginal canal.
- Maintain chain of evidence.
- Clearly and legibly label all specimens immediately with patient's name and number, *exact* anatomic site of collection, date, and name of collector; *seal* specimen containers.
- Use labels that adhere, and will not lift off cleanly.
- Keep handlers of evidence to a minimum.
- Place all materials in a large, sealed envelope or container, store in an approved, secure place, and convey to an approved laboratory as soon as possible.
- Samples must be properly collected and stored.
- To ensure collection of intact sperm, the sample should be collected with a saline-moistened swab and smeared on a slide premoistened with a drop of saline.
- Slides must be air-dried or coated with a special spray according to protocol.
- Moist samples should be frozen as soon as possible to halt enzyme loss, protein decomposition, and bacterial growth.
- Chart all positive and negative findings clearly and objectively. An example of a form for recording this information is shown in Fig. 7-1.

reported); they have come from all socioeconomic levels and from all occupations. It can happen to anyone, anywhere.

Social biases have led the uninformed to believe that the victim somehow invited the attack. However, it should be clearly stated that victims do not instigate sexual assault. Housewives have been assaulted in their homes while their husbands were present, women have been abducted from their jobs and assaulted; students have been accosted and molested in libraries.

Frequently the assailant knows the victim, her daily habits, her personal friends, and her time schedules. It is estimated that approximately 71% of all sexual assaults are planned and that 85% are carried out under some type of physical force or other intimidating coercion.[1] Physical violence may have been used even if the victim shows no signs of injury. This is an important fact to keep in mind in order to avoid making snap judgments such as ". . . she doesn't look as if she's been raped." A victim who submits out of fear should not be considered a willing accomplice.

How the victim responds to a violent, threatening situation will be determined by her previous experiences and her manner of coping with a crisis. Because not everyone is conditioned to respond in the same manner, any number of possible behaviors may be exhibited. Medical personnel who have preconceived notions of how people should behave are often suspicious of the patient's complaint when she responds in an unexpected manner. The staff needs to be aware that it is their own perceptions that underlie their doubts and that, by expressing disbelief, they themselves can convey a negative message to a person who may be acutely sensitive as a result of what has happened to her. Suspicion, doubt, or worse yet, open disapproval is never therapeutic. On the other hand, a compassionate response by staff members who are treating a victim with a questionable complaint will do no harm. Permanent injury can be inflicted on a patient who is subjected to callous, condescending, or aloof treatment. A basic tenet to follow is to learn to expect and accept any emotional response or be-

MEDICAL REPORT - SUSPECTED SEXUAL ASSAULT

PRINT OR TYPE   FORM 923   HOSPITAL

INSTRUCTIONS: Each physician and surgeon in a county hospital or in any other general acute care hospital who conducts a medical examination for evidence of sexual assault is required by law to complete this form where the patient has consented to be so examined. Each part of the form must be completed unless inapplicable. If the patient consents only to treatment complete only 1 A&B and IV B&C to the extent they are relevant to treatment and mail to police or sheriff after reporting the same information by phone to law enforcement. In filling out this form no civil or criminal liability attaches. Additionally, no confidentiality is breached in releasing this form to local law enforcement. Prior to commencement of the examination local law enforcement shall be notified by telephone.

I. GENERAL INFORMATION

A. PATIENT'S NAME   HOSPITAL ID NO.

B. ADDRESS	CITY	COUNTY	STATE	PHONE

C.	AGE	BIRTHDATE	RACE (USE CODED SUB-GROUPS)	SEX	DATE AND TIME OF ARRIVAL	MODE OF TRANSPORTATION

D. ACCOMPANIED BY: NAME	ADDRESS	CITY	COUNTY	STATE	PHONE	RELATIONSHIP

E. OFFICER NO. 1	ID NO.	DEPARTMENT	PHONE
OFFICER NO.	ID NO.	DEPARTMENT	PHONE

II. PATIENT'S or PARENT'S or GUARDIAN'S CONSENT (Sign where indicated)

I UNDERSTAND THAT HOSPITALS AND PHYSICIANS ARE REQUIRED BY PENAL CODE SECTION 11160-11161.5 TO REPORT TO LAW ENFORCEMENT AUTHORITIES THE NAME AND WHEREABOUTS OF ANY PERSONS WHO ARE VICTIMS OF SEXUAL ASSAULT OR WHO HAVE SUFFERED INJURIES INFLICTED BY A DEADLY WEAPON OR IN VIOLATION OF A PENAL LAW AND THE TYPE AND EXTENT OF THOSE INJURIES. KNOWING THIS, I CONSENT TO INDICATED TREATMENT.

_____
PATIENT OR PARENT OR GUARDIAN

I FURTHER UNDERSTAND THAT A SEPARATE MEDICAL EXAMINATION FOR EVIDENCE OF SEXUAL ASSAULT AT PUBLIC EXPENSE CAN, WITH MY CONSENT, BE CONDUCTED BY THE TREATING PHYSICIAN TO DISCOVER AND PRESERVE EVIDENCE OF THE ASSAULT. IF SO CONDUCTED, THE REPORT OF THE EXAMINATION AND ANY EVIDENCE OBTAINED WILL BE RELEASED TO LAW ENFORCEMENT. KNOWING THIS, I CONSENT TO A MEDICAL EXAMINATION FOR EVIDENCE OF SEXUAL ASSAULT.

_____
PATIENT OR PARENT OR GUARDIAN

III. FINANCIAL RESPONSIBILITY OF LOCAL GOVERNMENT (Government Code Section 13961.5)

I HEREBY REQUEST A MEDICAL EXAMINATION & COLLECTION OF EVIDENCE FOR SUSPECTED SEXUAL ASSAULT OF THE ABOVE PATIENT AT PUBLIC EXPENSE.

OFFICER	ID NO.	DATE

IV. MEDICAL EXAMINATION

A. HISTORY	ANSWER LINES 4-6 YES OR NO, OR EXPLAIN FOR EACH CATEGORY.	1. DATE AND TIME OF EXAM	DATE AND TIME OF ASSAULT

2. PHYSICAL SURROUNDINGS (BED, FIELD, CAR, ETC.)   IF PHYSICALLY RESTRAINED, HOW

3. PATIENT'S DESCRIPTION OF ASSAULT AND ASSOCIATED PAIN (PARAPHRASE)

NAME(S) AND NUMBER OR ASSAILANT(S)

WEAPON USED (GUN, KNIFE, ETC.)   IF FOREIGN OBJECT USED, WHAT AND WHERE

4. ACTS COMMITTED	COITUS	FELLATIO	CUNNILINGUS	SODOMY

5. DURING ASSAULT   □ VAGINAL PENETRATION (HOW)   EJACULATION: □ VAGINAL □ ORAL □ ANAL □   OTHER:

□ ANAL PENETRATION (HOW)   □ CONDOM USED   □ VOMITED   □ LOSS OF CONSCIOUSNESS   □ OTHER:

6. AFTER ASSAULT   □ WIPED/WASHED   □ BATHED   □ DOUCHED   □ VOMITED   □ CHANGED CLOTHES   □ BRUSHED TEETH   □ DEFECATED

□ OTHER:

7. MENSTRUAL HISTORY:

8. BP	PULSE	TEMP.	RESP.	KNOWN ALLERGIES

CURRENT MEDICATION   LAST TETANUS

B. GENERAL PHYSICAL	1. PATIENT'S GENERAL PHYSICAL APPEARANCE	HEIGHT	WEIGHT	

61926-552 6-78 100M OSP

Figure 7-1 *Standardized reporting forms ensure uniformity of examination procedures and collection of evidence.*

PATIENT'S NAME	HOSPITAL ID NO.	HOSPITAL

B. GENERAL PHYSICAL (Cont.)   2. LOCATE & DESCRIBE IN DETAIL ANY INJURIES OR FINDINGS (SPECULUM & BIMANUAL EXAM): TRAUMA, BRUISES, ERYTHEMA, EXCORIATIONS, LACERATIONS, WOUNDS, STAINS/FOREIGN MATERIALS ON BODY-MUCOID OR LIQUID MATERIAL, LOOSE HAIR, BLOOD, GRASS, DIRT, ETC.

TRACE OUTLINE USED & INDICATE LOCATION OF WOUNDS/LACERATIONS, USING 'X' FOR SUPERFICIAL, 'O' FOR DEEP; SHADE FOR BRUISES. WRITE OVER UNUSED OUTLINES. DESCRIBE IN DETAIL SHAPE OF BRUISES (ON ARMS OR OTHER EXTREMITIES) WHICH MAY INDICATE FORCE.

C. PELVIC   IF A CHILD, PERFORM ONLY IF NECESSARY. (SAME INSTRUCTIONS AS GENERAL PHYSICAL; IN ADDITION, NOTE PUBIC HAIR COMBINGS, DRIED SECRETIONS AND RECENT INJURIES TO HYMEN WHERE INDICATED.) TRACE AND MARK OUTLINE AS ABOVE.

V. DIAGNOSTIC IMPRESSION OF TRAUMA AND INJURIES

VI. TREATMENT/DISPOSITION OF PATIENT

A. ☐ G C CULTURE   ☐ VDRL   ☐ PREGNANCY TEST   ☐ POST COITAL ESTROGEN   ☐ V.D. PRO-PHYLAXIS   ☐ OTHER:

B. ORDERS:

C. DISPOSITION: ☐ ADMIT   TRANSFERRED TO

D. FOLLOW-UP WITHIN: ☐ MEDICAL   ☐ SOCIAL SERVICES   ☐ PRIVATE MD   ☐ OTHER

HOURS DAYS   HOURS DAYS   HOURS DAYS   HOURS DAYS

☐ RELEASED   ACCOMPANIED BY: NAME   ADDRESS   RELATIONSHIP

I HAVE RECEIVED THE INDICATED ITEMS AS EVIDENCE AND A COPY OF THIS REPORT.

OFFICER: ID NO.:   DATE:

NURSE   SIGNATURE OF EXAMINING PHYSICIAN

VII. SPECIMENS

STAINS/FOREIGN MATERIALS (WHEN INDICATED)

LOOSE HAIR ___	FINGERNAIL SCRAPINGS ___
BLOOD ___	DIRT OR GRAVEL ___
THREADS ___	VEGETATION ___
GRASS ___	CLOTHING ___

DRIED SECRETIONS

MOTILE SPERM: ☐ PRESENCE ☐ ABSENCE ☐ NOT TAKEN

	SLIDES	SWABS
VAGINAL	___	___
RECTAL	___	___
ORAL	___	___
ASPIRATES/WASHINGS	___	___
BITE MARKS	___	___
OTHER:	___	___

PATIENT'S SAMPLES. TIME OF COLLECTION AT MD DISCRETION.

BLOOD	___
HAIR FROM HEAD	___
SALIVA	___
HAIR FROM PUBIC AREA	___

61926-552 6-78 100M OSP

havior. (See Chap. 6 for further discussion of related grieving behaviors.)

Among the most unsettling feelings a victim experiences immediately after sexual assault is the realization of just how vulnerable she is. She had thought that she could control her life, or at least deal with most situations. Now she realizes how easily she can be caught off-guard and victimized. The recent threat of death and physical harm, as well as the actual assault, can stir a wide range of feelings—from fear, guilt, and shame to humiliation. These feelings can be of particular importance to a woman whose cultural and social upbringing have placed high value on chastity, virginity, or faithfulness to one lover. Such feelings can account for a victim hysterically crying, "No one will want me now. I'm dirty."

The victim may fear that significant others might not believe her or might question her complete innocence. Unfortunately, health care personnel frequently intensify this feeling by following investigative techniques that suggest that their first concern is collecting evidence to substantiate the fact that a rape has occurred rather than the needs of the victim. A woman may recall stories of antagonistic defense lawyers, judgmental medical personnel, and suspicious friends or acquaintances. If fear of this sort immobilizes her enough she may hesitate to report the assault immediately. She may then have to justify having second thoughts and reporting the crime at a later date when evidence has been removed or destroyed. In such instances, credibility is lost. Because sexual assault is a crime that often has only one witness—the victim—an increased burden is placed on her to prove the incident.

PSYCHOSOCIAL ASPECTS OF CARE

Medical personnel frequently react to a rape victim in an aloof and distant manner, preferring to concentrate on the physical and technical tasks to be done rather than to take an empathetic approach. Such behavior can be offensive and painful to a person who needs personalized attention as a result of the trauma she has experienced.

"I don't know what to say to a rape victim. I've never been raped." Comments like this, common among emergency care personnel, show a lack of understanding of what the assault signifies. Rape or any other type of sexual assault can overwhelm the victim with a sense of loss and crisis, similar to the feelings experienced by grieving people. (see Chap. 6.) Interacting with victims of sexual assault is very much like dealing with other grieving people.

INTERACTION WITH THE VICTIM

Initial Contact. As soon as the victim enters the emergency care system, some type of supportive care should be made available. The person filling this role need not be a trained crisis worker. A peace officer, concerned citizen, EMT, or hospital clerk, will do. Victims have said that the person they remember best is the one who said, "You are safe here" or "I'm really sorry you were hurt, but we'll try to help you." Empathetic, sensitive comments such as these, accompanied by friendly gestures such as offering a cup of coffee or a warm blanket are reassurances that a caring person is near.

The initial contact is considered a main factor in determining how the victim will progress through the medicolegal system. Every effort should be made to expedite her care, although it may not always be possible to do so, especially in a large urban hospital where the emergency department is busy and forced to handle life-and-death cases first. At such times, if a caring, supportive person approaches the victim, greets her and her family or friends, and explains the medical process, including the need for long waits in a busy department, the victim is likely to feel that she is in a compassionate environment.

A trained support person should be contacted early in the process to provide a source of support that the victim can turn to in a time of need. This can be especially helpful in the postcrisis period when the victim would have difficulty establishing such a contact, especially if it involved retelling the story from the beginning. If the victim has an opportunity early in the process to establish a bond with a resource person who can act as a confidant, it is more likely that she will make use of this person during the readjustment period. Women who have not found such a support will often try to "just get over it" and only succeed in internalizing their problems. Rape crisis centers generally have volunteers who serve as counselors and are willing to meet with the victims and help them with their medical, legal, and personal problems.

Acceptance of Behavior. Since each woman will respond to sexual assault in her own manner, the emotional behavior displayed by the victim may not always be what the staff expects. Some victims may respond by crying or expressing intense fear, while others may be quite angry and aggressive. The reactions may cover a wide range of behavior, from composure one moment to tears and even laughter the next. Such emotional lability, though inappropriate at other times, can be expected in a person facing a crisis.

Anger is especially difficult for most to accept, especially if it is directed toward them personally. Comments such as "You have a right to be angry and to feel the way you do" will assure the victim that she has a right to express her feelings and allow her the freedom to use this approach as one means of establishing control over her environment—an important need for someone who has been assaulted.

If at all possible, the victim should not be asked questions about her reasons for acting as she does in order to avoid undermining her position or challenging her behavior. Such questions often provoke a defensive reaction and increase her sense that others think she is culpable.

Privacy. A victim of sexual assault like anyone else who is suddenly thrust into the public eye, wants to be as inconspicuous as possible to avoid any further exposure or embarrassment. If emergency personnel are aware of this normal reaction, they can help to prevent unnecessary anxiety on the victim's part.

Most victims are evaluated in the field and escorted to the hospital by a uniformed officer, an EMT, or a paramedic. Since people tend to stop and look whenever they see uniformed personnel attending to a problem, the victim should be protected from curious onlookers to minimize further embarrassment or publicity. This is especially true if she is distraught, disheveled, or disfigured.

The visit to the hospital involves further exposure in the form of more questioning by personnel seeking pertinent and personal information. This can be especially distressing to young girls in a modest stage of development, who may recoil at the thought that personal information of this sort must be shared with others. Additional stress may result when victims are placed in rooms marked "Police GYN" or that contain equipment with easy to read labels such as "Rape Kit." Hospital personnel may further exacerbate the problem by asking embarrassing questions in a loud voice, or by reaching for data forms in folders with the word *rape* written prominently across the cover.

As a means of providing privacy, the victim should not be placed in the general waiting area or in a room with other patients who may overhear the details of the questioning. If an inconspicuous entrance is available, it should be used by police officers and other personnel escorting the victim so that they can enter and leave without being scrutinized by others.

Frequently the press follows the victim to the emergency department. In such instances, reporters and photographers should be directed to the spokesperson for the hospital's administration. No one else should take it upon himself to discuss the details of the event with the press in order not to betray the patient's right to privacy.

Returning Control. It is crucial that a victim be helped to regain as much control of her life as possible. Following an assault, many women are so frightened by their vulnerability that they tend to surrender responsibility for what happens to them. The fact that they were forced to submit to the demands of another robs them of a sense of independence and promotes a feeling of helplessness.

One way to help the victim regain some sense of control is to offer an opportunity to make simple decisions. These may be prompted by open-ended questions such as: "You look tired. Would you like to sit in this chair?" "There will be about a half-hour wait; whom may I call for you?" (Not, "Would you like me to call someone?" This type of question can be answered with a yes or no.) Making simple decisions such as these can serve as the first step toward a return to a normal life and the resolution of the crisis.

Actions that can be taken by emergency personnel to reduce the emotional trauma experienced by the victim of sexual assault are summarized in Chart 7-2.

THE PHYSICAL EXAMINATION

A victim of sexual assault should be considered a priority case in view of the need to assess for further injury and to collect evidence for legal purposes. However, the emotional trauma must be dealt with first because many women after being sexually assaulted view the physical examination as another invasion of their privacy. Further psychological damage can be avoided if the examiner takes time to be supportive and to enhance the victim's comfort and confidence. If such steps are not taken, the victim may associate

---

Chart 7-2

ACTIONS TO REDUCE EMOTIONAL TRAUMA OF SEXUAL ASSAULT

- Recognize that victim's behavior reflects the grieving response. Accept any and all behavior. (See Chap. 6).
- Provide sensitive, kind, supportive care initially and throughout victim's care. Assist in contacting a friend, family member, or volunteer from advocate group.
- Avoid *why* questions that cast doubt on victim's judgment.
- Provide privacy at scene and in emergency department
- Use the term, *sexual assault* in all verbal and written communications. *Rape* is a legal term defined and determined by a court of law.
- Return control to victim when possible by offering her choices and opportunities to make decisions.
- Prepare for physical examination by explaining, in terms patient can understand, what is to be done and why.
- Encourage patient to express feelings about examination and care.
- Provide prophylactic treatment for pregnancy prevention, venereal disease, and infection secondary to trauma
- Arrange for continuing care for physical and emotional needs
  - Follow-up appointments with private physician or in clinic (continuity with same persons is important)
  - Early and continuing support from an advocate group crisis worker or professional counselor.

Chart 7-3

SEXUAL ASSAULT EVIDENCE KIT

Contents	Purpose
Clean comb	To comb the pubic hair
Large envelope (3″ × 6″)	To collect pubic combings
Small envelope	To hold "plucked" pubic hair from victim for comparison with pubic combings
Sterile wooden stick cotton swab	To swab vaginal area for sperm or semen
Screw top airtight container	To hold swab of vaginal area
Labels	To adhere to various items for identification
Red top vacutainer	Serology testing
Culture mechanism for gonorrhea	For as many specimens as indicated (i.e., vagina, anus, mouth)
Glass slides	To observe if sperm is motile
Sterile gauze	To collect saliva for "secretor" test for blood type
Sterile container	To hold gauze after saliva test is obtained
Nail file	Optional—to scrape fingernails if victim scratched the assailant

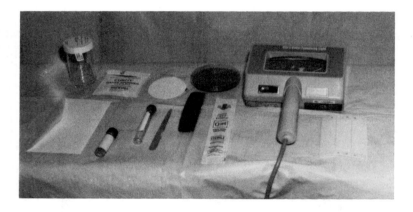

Materials for collection of evidence. Clockwise from top left: sterile container and 2 × 2 gauze for oral swab; two slides for motile sperm; chocolate agar plate for gonococcus; ultraviolet light for visualizing semen; labels; cotton-tip applicator for vaginal, rectal, or throat swab; comb for pubic hair combing; file for fingernail scraping; tube for blood sample; VDRL; tube for pregnancy test sample; small envelope for plucked pubic hair; large envelope for pubic combings.

the horror of the assault with this type of physical exam and tend to shy away from future health care.

Preparing for the Pelvic Examination. The internal pelvic examination is done on women (and little girls) who have experienced penile penetration as part of the sexual assault. Sodomized victims may require anoscopy and rectal examination. Since vaginal and rectal inspections are invasive, the victim may well come to associate this procedure with the sexual assault itself, especially since it is being carried out by a stranger and may be physically and emotionally discomforting. It should also be noted that instructing the victim to lie still and not move is similar to the orders given by the rapist.

In order to prevent the patient from making these negative associations, it is best to prepare her for the examination by explaining what will be done and why. Emergency personnel often forget that many people have limited experience with hospitals and may be intimidated, bewildered, or unnerved by the strange environment and the visions it conjures up of painful procedures and queasy sights and smells. It is natural to be unable to relax when there are so many unknowns.

Because this is a sensitive examination, it should be explained in terms that the patient can understand. "Pelvic" is not a familiar word to some people, especially the foreign born and the very young. It is best to find a reference point the patient can recognize (*i.e.,* Pap smear, childbirth) and then build the explanation from there. Younger patients

Chart 7-4

PROCEDURE FOR EXAMINATION OF SEXUAL ASSAULT VICTIM

The protocol to be followed *must* have the *prior* approval of the police, district attorney, public defender, courts, medical examiner, hospital, and laboratory. It should be reviewed before the evidence is collected in order to prevent invalidating specimens by inappropriate handling. *Only experienced, designated persons should perform the examination and collect evidence for legal purposes.* The following is a suggested procedure.

1. Prepare the patient for the examination by explaining what will be done.
2. Assist in history taking by either directing questions or by explaining what information will be necessary. In order to get a more accurate history, be sure to use terms that the patient will understand. Give the patient the opportunity to answer questions without friends or family present in order to avoid compromising confidential information.
3. Assist with the photographing of injuries and appearance.
4. Help the patient to undress. It is recommended to have the victim undress while standing on a white sheet. This allows the collection of debris that may have fallen from clothing or the body. Fold clothing carefully to avoid dislodging or removing evidence. Place clothing that is retained for evidence in individual bags of a type preferred by local police authorities.
5. Assist with physical examination. Notations should be made on the chart of any bruises, marks, bites, lacerations, abrasions, and debris that are found on the victim. Bite marks or patterned injuries may require special documentation, photography, and testing.
6. Cultures of the oropharynx and saliva specimens may be collected at this time. The saliva is used for blood typing by secretor tests. It is collected with a saliva swab from bite mark areas or from areas such as the nipples, according to protocol.
7. Assist with the pelvic examination. An explanation of each step should be given before it is done.
   - The perineal and thigh areas should be visibly inspected for semen. An ultraviolet light may be used to illuminate seminal fluid; if present, it will glow with a bright bluish-white fluorescent color. Swab the skin with saliva swabs and clip hair on which suspected semen is present.
   - Comb the pubic hair and collect all loose hairs in an evelope.
   - Pluck designated number of pubic hairs and place them in a separate evelope. Be sure the samples have the white follicle present on the tip.
   - If secretions are present in the vagina, a saline-lubricated pipette may be used to aspirate contents. Place in a test tube.
   - Swab the posterior fornix of the vagina with a cotton-tipped wooden applicator. Depending on local medical or crime laboratory methods, the swabs will either be used to make slides or be submitted for analysis. Prepare and handle as directed.
   - Saline swabs of all suspected areas of sexual contact should be collected to identify presence of sperm.
   - Swab areas of sexual contact (*e.g.,* rectum, cervix) for gonorrhea cultures.
     Note: to prevent mechanical disruption of evidence such as intact sperm, all swabs should be moistened with physiologic saline prior to collecting sample. In addition, a drop of saline should be placed on the receiving slide before it is smeared with swab content. The slide is then air dried or coated according to local protocol.
   - Complete the bimanual and rectal examinations to rule out injury or other pathology. Encourage the patient to keep her back on the table, breathe through her mouth, and concentrate on not tightening her lower abdomen during the internal inspection. Caution her that she may feel pressure.
8. Draw blood for serology testing. Some agencies also draw blood for typing or for specific studies such as blood alcohol or toxicology screens.
9. Present options for pregnancy control and venereal disease prophylaxis to the patient.
   a. If the patient chooses to be treated for pregnancy control:
      - Obtain a pregnancy test and await the results.
      - Obtain an informed consent regarding the use of postcoital estrogens. If a method other than medication is preferred, arrangements should be made for its completion.
   b. If the patient chooses prophylaxis for venereal disease:
      - Determine allergies, whether pregnant (so as to avoid tetracycline), and willingness to cooperate with treatment. A number of patients will refuse injections but will accept oral therapy.
      - Administer the antibiotic of choice.
      - Observe for at least 20 minutes after injection for possible allergic reaction.
10. Arrange follow-up care.
    - If the patient did not receive penicillin therapy, she should receive repeated testing. Gonorrhea retests should be done within 2 weeks; syphilis retesting is done at 6 weeks.
    - A follow-up appointment with an attending physician at 2 weeks is recommended for determining effectiveness of treatment and for identifying additional problems.
    - Assist the victim with counseling services for the emotional component of her care and encourage contacts with advocate groups. Know the services available in your community.

may need an explanation of basic anatomy before they can understand what will be done. Asking the child or his parent for familiar terms will help to provide information about what the child knows and how she will handle the examination. An apprehensive child who has been told that it is "dirty" to touch the perineal area may not understand that it is acceptable for a physician to do so.

All patients should be encouraged to consider the pelvic examination as a *normal procedure*—one that is being done in this instance under unusual circumstances. This will help to avoid the long-term stigmas attached to an intimate and important procedure. It is also appropriate to encourage the patient to express her feelings about the pelvic exam and to reassure her that it is quite natural for her to feel as she does. Verbalizing these feelings can help the patient to relax and regain control.

If evidence is to be collected during the exam, the pubic hair will be combed for loose hairs. Several strands of the hair will be plucked for comparison with the loose hairs. The vaginal vault (as well as any other area of sexual contact during the assault) will be aspirated and swabbed for semen and for gonorrhea cultures.* A sexual assault evidence kit, as described in Chart 7-3, is used.

Examination Procedure. The usual procedure followed for a pelvic exam of a victim of sexual assault is outlined in Chart 7-4.

TREATMENT

Pregnancy Prevention. A major concern of the sexual assault victim is fear of pregnancy—a fear that persists until the onset of the next menstrual period. The probability of conception from a single, random unprotected intercourse is estimated to be between 1 in 25 to 1 in 50 exposures, unless it occurs during midcycle (days 11–18 of a 28-day cycle); then the chances are 1 in 10 or 1 in 2 if it occurs on the day of ovulation.[14] The chance that a woman is already pregnant at the time of the assault are 2% to 3%.

If pregnancy prevention is considered necessary, then the patient's gynecologic history, the probability of her conceiving, and her religious convictions and personal desires must all be taken into account. *A pregnancy test and an informed consent are musts before any method is instituted.* See Table 7-1 for types of pregnancy prevention or termination.

Venereal Disease Treatment. Unprotected sexual activity with an unknown assailant carries the risk of venereal disease. Victims often are concerned not only about being infected, but also about the possibility of becoming carriers. To deal with these risks, cultures and serology tests should be obtained at the time of examination. Treatment may be given initially as a prophylactic measure or after the laboratory

---

* Local police and medical procedures may vary. The examiner and emergency staff should be aware of what is accepted procedure in their community and hospital and should be able to explain the procedure to the patient.

TABLE 7-1.   RECOMMENDED TREATMENT FOR PREVENTION OF PREGNANCY DUE TO SEXUAL ASSAULT

Regime	Comments
Ethinyl estradiol: 5 mg po/day for 5 days	Side-effects of nausea and vomiting can be prevented if the patient is given an antiemetic drug, such as triomethobenzamide (Tigan) or prochlorperazine (Compazine).
Norgestrel (Ovral): 2 tablets immediately and 2 tablets in 12 hr	

data confirm the diagnosis. However, it is preferable to give prophylactic treatment, since many victims do not return for follow-up care and are at risk of going untreated.

Evidence suggests that only about 3% of the victims will contract venereal disease as a result of the assault and that an additional 3% will prove to have unrecognized, established venereal disease.[14] Recommended antibiotic therapy for venereal disease prophylaxis is outlined in Chart 7-5.

Follow-up Care. No emergency visit is complete without arrangements for appropriate follow-up care because the victim's physical and psychological needs are usually of a long-term nature. In addition, complications of medical therapy can occur, such as failure to prevent pregnancy and superinfection secondary to antibiotic therapy. Somatic complaints are common, especially in areas that relate to sexual contact (*i.e.,* difficulty in swallowing, abdominal pain, dyspareunia).

Women may notice new difficulties with their interpersonal relationships with men. There may be a loss of self-respect or sense of independence, or even evidence of suicidal impulses or nightmares.[12] Much has been written about the aftereffects of sexual assault on daily living patterns. The patient should be informed that she may tend to relive the assault, awaken during the night, or become timid in certain situations. Forewarning the woman of such possible reactions will assure her that these feelings are part of the normal pattern of recovering from a frightening experience.

The quality of the initial care often determines whether the victim returns to the original hospital or facility for follow-up care. Every effort should be made to assure continuity of care, so that there is an opportunity for one facility to follow the patient's recovery. It can also help in identifying more unusual circumstances, as occurred in one instance in which the victim showed up at the emergency department with the complaint of being assaulted, only to have the record show that she was actually hallucinating and reliving an earlier assault, which had occurred several months before. The fact that a record or chart existed for the first visit revealed the real problem.

The victim may be scheduled for a follow-up visit to either her own private physician or a clinic to be sure that she is progressing without complications. In either instance, continuity of care should be assured to determine physical and emotional recovery. Follow-up of this type requires that assistance be arranged from an advocate group, a support

---

Chart 7-5

RECOMMENDED TREATMENT FOR PREVENTION OF GONORRHEA AND SYPHYLIS: Adults*

Regimen	Comments
Procaine penicillin G: 4.8 million units IM (given in 2 sites) with Probenecid: 1 gm po, preferably 30 min prior to penicillin injections	Therapy of choice Allows for single dose therapy in patients with low compliance to multidose drugs.
or	
Amoxicillin: 3.0 gm po or Ampicillin: 3.5 gm po with probenecid: 1 gm po, preferably 30 min prior to oral medications	Tolerated better by patients who refuse injections. Not as effective for anorectal or pharyngeal gonorrhea.
or	
Tetracycline HCl: 0.5 gm po, 4 times a day for 7 days (total dose 14.0 gm)	For patients allergic to penicillin. Effective for treating chlamydial infection if also present or suspected.
or	
Doxycycline hyclate: 100 mg po, 2 times a day for 7 days	May be used as a substitute for tetracycline.
or	
Spectinomycin HCl: 2.0 gm IM	For patients allergic to penicillin or who cannot tolerate tetracyclines. Ineffective for incubating syphilis.

Although it is difficult to determine the risk of a sexually assaulted person contracting a sexually transmitted infection, other infections are possible. If suspected, specific therapy should be used for chlamydial infections, genital herpes, cytomegalovirus, trichomoniasis, and hepatitis B.

* Defined as 100 lb (45 kg) or more in body weight.
(Sexually transmitted disease treatment guidelines, 1982. Morbid Mortal Week Rep (Suppl) 31:37S–60S, August 20, 1982)

---

person, or a professional counselor before the victim is discharged. Although the patient's preference in this regard should be respected, the staff can be especially helpful by suggesting the type of resource person they feel would be most appropriate.

THE CHILD VICTIM

Children who are sexually assaulted are usually victimized by an assailant who has frequent contact with them. In many cases, the offender is a trusted person in the home or neighborhood—often someone who can be viewed as a father figure.* Usually the assailant is male and the victim female. It is speculated that male victims involved in heterosexual

* A study conducted at the University of Washington on women who had been sexually molested as youngsters revealed that 26.5% were molested by their fathers; 15.2% by stepfathers, 10.2% by grandfathers, and 16% by brothers; strangers accounted for only 6.8%.[15] Another study found that almost half of the offenders of child sexual assault were family members. Of 20 men, 10 acted as the father in the home; 6 were uncles, and 3 grandfathers. According to Burgess[2] and to Holstrom,[9] "four of the offenders were involved with 10 of the victims, which emphasizes the frequency with which one family member is able to gain access to more than one female or male child in the family."

relationships are unlikely to report the incident because in all likelihood they regard the situation as an initiation into sexual activity rather than a violation of self.[15]

The type of sexual activity involved can vary. Many children are fondled or physically explored without intercourse, while others may experience penile penetration.

Various factors contribute to a child submitting to sexual assault over a period of time. Some studies indicate that such children tend to be affection seekers,[3] but other pressures play a role, such as pressures to obey one's elders, threats, misrepresentations of moral standards, and enticements such as candy or money. The children are often pressured into secrecy after the incident and as a result develop additional stress from this burden.

Often, the child conceals the sexual activity out of fear—fear of punishment from parents, of rejection by friends or family, of not being believed, or of being harmed by the offender.

TREATMENT OF A CHILD VICTIM

Assessment. In instances when the child does not readily admit to the sexual assault, health professionals must be aware of signs and symptoms that indicate sexual activity. Symptoms may include behavioral or physical manifestations such as nightmares, restlessness, withdrawal tendencies, hostility, phobias related to the offender, regression (*i.e.,* bedwetting) or truancy. Long-term effects may include guilt, a negative self-image (sometimes associated with self-destructive or suicidal intent) and difficulties in interrelationships with men (*i.e.,* mistrust, inadequate social skills, and sexual dysfunction).

In order to ascertain that sexual assault has occurred, the child should be encouraged to talk about the reasons emergency care has been sought, with emphasis on particular incidents when necessary. Encouraging the young child to draw pictures of the events can yield valuable information.

Emotional Impact. Children will perceive the importance and ramifications of sexual assault through the behavior of the adults around them. The reaction of adults will create an impression on the child— in some instances this impression has a greater impact than the actual incident. Children need to learn that although this type of sexual activity is not appropriate, it should not affect their entire outlook on sex. Rather than indicate to the child that some kind of irreversible damage has occurred, it is better to emphasize that "sex is simply a way in which people relate to each other, and it has the potential for being either good or bad."[15]

Physical Examination. A complete physical examination is done, including inspection of the genitalia. If evidence of penetration is found (bruises, red raised areas, marks) or if vaginal bleeding is present, only then is an internal examination indicated. An appropriately small-sized vaginal speculum or nasal speculum should be used. It may be necessary to use anesthesia if the child is especially apprehensive or if there is a likelihood that further trauma will result or that injuries need to be repaired. Depending upon the age and preference of the child, the parent(s) may remain in the room and participate in the examination. The small child may even be held on the patient's lap during inspection.

Collection of evidence includes obtaining loose hairs from the child's underclothing and perineal area, along with a sample of the child's pubic hair if it is present; wiping the thighs, buttocks, and genitalia for semen; collecting saliva for secretor tests to determine blood type; and procuring samples and cultures for venereal disease.

Management. Antibiotic therapy varies from that of the adult and is listed in Chart 7-6. Other treatment measures may include tetanus antitoxin when open wounds exist and sitz baths for discomfort.

Legal Responsibilities. If sexual assault is confirmed or suspected, any law that applies must be followed. In some

---

Chart 7-6

RECOMMENDED TREATMENT FOR PREVENTION OF GONORRHEA AND SYPHYLIS: Children*

Regimen	Comments
Amoxicillin: 50 mg/kg po plus probenecid: 25 mg/kg (max 1 gm), preferably 30 min prior to oral medications	
or	
Aqueous procaine penicillin G: 100,000 units/kg IM plus probenecid: 25 mg/kg (max 1 gm), preferably 30 min prior to injection	Recommended for patients with pharyngitis and/or proctitis.
or	
Spectinomycin: 40 mg/kg, IM	For patients allergic to penicillin. Ineffective for incubating syphylis.
or	
Spectinomycin: 40 mg/kg/day, po, in 4 divided doses for 5 days	For patients allergic to penicillin. Ineffective for incubating syphylis.
or	
Tetracycline: 40 mg/kg, po, in 4 divided doses for 5 days	Child should be over 8 years of age to prevent adverse effects in skeletal and tooth development.

Children with a sexually transmitted infection should be considered a vicitim of sexual abuse until proven otherwise. The risk of sexually transmitted disease appears to be lower in children than in adult victims.

* Defined as less than 100 lb (45 kg) in body weight

states minors may seek and be treated for sexual assault and venereal disease without parental consent. If sexual abuse of a child is identified, other authorities must also be notified according to regulations and policies followed by the reporting agency.

SUMMARY

The victims of sexual assault vary according to what has been done to them, how it was accomplished, and by whom. Even so, there are some similarities that generally hold true.

The adult is usually the victim of an attack that was planned and carried out with force and the threat of violence or death. The emotional trauma involved strips the victim of self-assurance and a sense of control over her life. The result may be long lasting after-effects. It also places her in the position of being subject to guilt feelings and possible repercussions from friends and family. The victim enters the medical system because of the legal requirements to gather evidence and because her physical condition needs to be assessed and attended to. Fear of possible pregnancy and of venereal disease will also direct her to seek medical assistance. How she is received by the staff members in terms of their sensitivity and awareness and the manner in which they react to her and interact with her can affect her for the rest of her life.

In the case of children, the sexual exploitation is accompanied by emotional overtones of betrayal and confusion. Often, the offender is a trusted close acquaintance. Revealing the sexual activity could generate a great deal of guilt or apprehension on the part of the child. Thus it is necessary for the adults in the child's life to be sure that their reactions do not complicate the resolution of the crisis and are such that the child can mature as normally as possible.

REFERENCES

1. Amir M: Patterns in Forcible Rape. Chicago, University of Chicago Press, 1971
2. Burgess A, Holstrom L: Sexual trauma of children and adolescents. Nurs Clin North Am 10(3), September 1975
3. Burton L: Vulnerable Children. New York, Schocken Books, 1968
4. California Medical Association Council: Guidelines for the interview and examination of alleged rape victims. West J Med November 1975
5. Division of Law Enforcement Investigative Services Branch, Dept. of Justice: Guidelines of physical evidence in sexual assault investigations. Physical Evidence Bulletin July 1977
6. Goldstein FL, Schaefer JL, Sullivan R: Special problems: Practice caring for the victim of rape. Patient Care October 30, 1978
7. Gorline L, Ray M: Examining and caring for the child who has been sexually assaulted. Matern Child Nurs J, 4(2)
8. Grossman M: Sexually transmitted diseases. In Pascoe DJ, Grossman M: Quick Reference to Pediatric Emergencies, 2nd ed. Philadelphia, JB Lippincott, 1978
9. Holstrom L, Burgess A: The Victim of Rape: Institutional Reactions. New York, John Wiley & Sons, 1978
10. Leaman K: The sexually abused child. Nursing 77, May 1977
11. Loebl S, Spratto G, Wit A: The Nurse's Drug Handbook. New York, John Wiley & Sons, 1977
12. Medea A, Thompson K: Against Rape. New York, Farrar, Straus & Giraux, 1974
13. Nadelson C, Notman M: Emotional repercussions of rape. Medical Aspects of Human Sexuality, March 1977
14. State of California Department of Health Services: Guidelines for Treatment of Victims of Sexual Assault. 1979
15. Tsai M, Wagner N: Incest and molestation: Problems of childhood sexuality. Resident and Staff Physician, March 1979

8

DOMESTIC VIOLENCE: ABUSE AND BATTERING

DIANN ANDERSON and JAMES H. COSGRIFF, JR.

ASPECTS OF DOMESTIC VIOLENCE

The term *domestic violence* includes all forms of violent behavior involving people who live together—a husband who beats his wife; a wife who beats her husband; one partner who beats the other in an unmarried, living-together relationship; a parent, guardian, or other family member who physically abuses or sexually assaults his or her child.[3] The abuse of elderly persons by their caretakers is also currently receiving widespread attention. Sexual assault, although related to domestic violence, is discussed in Chapter 7.

The incidence of abuse of spouses, elderly relatives, and children is greater than the most pessimistic estimates. Data are difficult to obtain because beatings usually occur in the privacy of the home, without witnesses. Incidents of abuse are buried in the records of domestic disturbance calls to police departments, in hospital emergency department records, and in the records of social service agencies and private psychologists and counselors. Only an estimated 10% of women report battering incidents.[18] Over 1 million American children suffer abuse and neglect,[7] and though data are lacking, it is estimated that abuse of elders is as prevalent as child abuse.

The abuse of spouses, children, or elders is a manifestation of domestic violence. More than one person within the same family unit—spouse, child, elder—may be subjected to abuse. Violence within the family affects all of the members—emotionally, physically, and developmentally.

Relationships Between Spouse Abuse and Child Abuse. Men or women who beat one another also beat their children.

> When violence becomes a pattern in the household it can take many forms. In her desperation, the battered wife may strike out at the children, scapegoating them as she has been scapegoated by a violent husband. And the man who beats his wife may also beat his children.[10]

Children who witness physical violence between their parents without being beaten themselves suffer emotional trauma—shock, fear, and guilt—as well as confusion about role expectation and how feelings should be expressed. They have seen one parent shower the other with expressions of love and affection, and then later break into uncontrollable rage and batter the spouse on the slightest provocation. If adult behavior is shaped by childhood learning, it is not surprising that these children grow up to be abusive adults. Emerging data strongly suggest that children who survive an abusive, unloving home are more likely to become spouse or child batterers and, later, abusers of their elderly parents; or they may become rapists or commit other violent crimes.[17] The incidence of violent crime increases yearly. Domestic violence and its eventual direct effect upon society provide food for some serious thought.

A form of prenatal child abuse can be identified in the battering of a pregnant woman when the physical assault is directed toward the unborn fetus. Some believe such acts to be a husband's attempt to terminate pregnancy and relieve him of the impending stress of another child. In fact, some beatings have reportedly resulted in miscarriages.[16]

Society not only permits but indeed condones discipline by force. Physical control of the wife is well documented in history, the Bible, literature, and modern media. Furthermore, the philosophy expressed by the axiom "spare the rod and spoil the child" is held by many and practiced to varying degrees. How the family conducts its affairs and how its members are disciplined are held to be the business of that family—and of no one else. This concept is reinforced by society's values as reflected in the enforcement, or lack of enforcement, of its laws. It is not surprising that victims of domestic violence are not recognized or cared for until the pattern of violence is well established and its deleterious effects on family members are all too obvious.

THE BATTERED SPOUSE

A battered spouse is any person who is subjected to physical abuse by his or her mate, whether married or unmarried and living together. Although victims and batterers can be of either sex, for the purposes of this chapter, the victims are generally presumed to be female and the attackers male.*

Spouse battering is not a new social phenomenon. The act itself can be traced back to some of the earliest historical accounts of the relationships between men and women. It has been and continues to be an expected and accepted part of many cultures. Spouse beating in our country, though not considered an acceptable form of the American way of life, is tacitly accepted by thoughtless tolerance and arbitrary application of the law.

Battered Women

The battered woman generally reports a battering incident only as a last resort, when she decides to leave her husband or male partner out of fear for her life or her children's. The instances reported represent only a small proportion of the total incidence. Reasons cited by battered women for not reporting and for staying with their partners include the following:

- Profound fear of what the man would do to her and her children if she tried to leave
- Belief that the man would change his behavior and stop beating her
- Lack of resources—no money, no one to turn to, and no knowledge of where to go for help
- Belief that she was the cause of her husband's violent behavior
- Belief that this is part of marriage and must be endured in order to keep the family together

Even when the woman has decided to leave her partner, some of the reasons just noted may eventually lead her to return. In spite of the beatings, there may have been times when he was very loving. Her ambivalent feelings and resulting loneliness become strong motives for returning.

---

* This presumption does not discriminate against either sex but serves merely to facilitate the use of language. Battered men are discussed on p. 102.

Characteristics of Wife-Battering. As battered women have sought protection and communicated their problems, some patterns and commonalities in their experiences have emerged:

- The beatings do not stop, even though the man may apologize and promise not to beat the woman again.
- The beatings often become more severe and more frequent.
- The beatings may occur without any provocation whatsoever.
- The man who has beaten the woman but not the children will at some point turn his violence toward the children and beat them.

Battered Men

Spouse battering is not limited to women. Men also are battered, but this is rarely reported. Society's concept of masculinity discourages disclosure; the humiliation suffered by a woman in the same situation is multiplied enormously for the man who reports battering.

Many men in violent domestic relationships feel as trapped as women do, and they suffer many of the same psychological and emotional effects—guilt, loss of self-esteem, and loss of control. But society is less empathetic toward the man who is beaten because it is generally accepted that he *could control* the situation—physically, financially, etc.—if he wanted to. Even fewer resources exist for men; many men, when seeking help, find assistance from organizations that support battered women.

Homosexual Relationships

Spouse battering can occur in homosexual relationships as well as in heterosexual ones. Homosexuals are conditioned by the same things in society as heterosexuals. They come from the same homes and culture and have the same responses to the human emotions of frustration, anger, jealousy, and insecurity.

Whether the beating has been sustained by a man, woman, or child, a homosexual or a heterosexual, there should be no difference in the quality of care given by emergency personnel. Care must be thorough, sensitive, empathetic, and free from judgmental comments and innuendo.

ASSESSMENT AND MANAGEMENT

Peace officers are often the first to be summoned to the scene of a domestic disturbance, and this poses a particularly dangerous problem for law enforcement intervention. Often, one or both partners are hostile to the officer and may attack him, often with a weapon. Because of the volatile atmosphere surrounding domestic quarrels, emergency care responders must be especially cautious when entering such a situation until they are certain that their own safety is not threatened. This may be particularly difficult when it is known that a severely injured victim lies within.

Assessment of the battered victim must proceed according to the principles observed when assessing any victim of traumatic injury.

- Determine the patient's status and maintain her life support systems (airway, breathing, circulation) as necessary.
- Complete a thorough secondary survey.
- Do a complete physical examination in the hospital. (Injuries are often inflicted on areas that are covered by clothing.)

Identifying the Battered Victim

Identifying the patient as a victim of battering may be difficult because the description of the injuries that is given may be incorrect, inaccurate, and protective of the attacker. Commonly, a woman will not seek medical treatment for bruises, lacerations, etc., out of embarrassment or fear of retaliation from her partner. When responding to questions, the woman may avoid eye contact and be hesitant or evasive about the details of her injuries. She may offer clues about her situation, however, in remarks such as, "Things haven't been going well lately," or, "There have been problems at home."

Approaching the Battered Victim

Directly questioning the woman is the best approach. Asking whether the difficulties ever led to physical harm, or whether the injuries were caused by her spouse or partner conveys your awareness and concern about her and her problem. She will feel a sense of relief that someone is aware and understands without her having to muster the will to introduce this forbidden subject. Once the subject has been introduced and the woman has shown a willingness to discuss it, it is important to remember the following key points:

Nonjudgmental Attitude. Avoid judgmental statements. Comments such as, "Oh, how awful. How could you let him do that?" imply that the woman who is battered is viewed as inferior, at a time when she is already struggling with the feelings of inferiority forced on her by the experience. Instead, be empathetic, trying to feel and understand what she has experienced; be aware that any woman who lives through batterings is a strong person and deserves respect and support.

Avoid "why" questions. These questions challenge the woman's judgment and threaten her. It is better to ask, "What sort of things would cause you to leave him?" than "Why don't you leave him?"

Supportive Attitude. Listen attentively. Support and encourage the woman in discussing what happened and her feelings about it. Battered victims commonly feel guilt and shame. Many believe that the battering evolved from their own failures to make their marriages work. Our culture reinforces the concept that the failure of a marriage represents failure as a woman, since it is a woman's responsibility to provide the home life conducive to a good marriage. Helping the victim to express her feelings is the first step in dealing with them. Helping her to become aware that she is not to blame for her battering will help reduce her feelings of guilt.

Return of Control. Help her to regain control over her life. Loss of self-esteem and self-respect follows battering with its subsequent guilt and shame. Much like the sexually assaulted victim (Chap. 7), the battered woman has suffered a loss—of her sense of self-worth, of control over her life. Often she feels that she has no choices or opportunities to leave the situation. She is trapped.

The first step is to have her identify what she wants for herself as a person and for her children, and to compare this with what she is getting from the relationship. If she determines that she is better off *without* the relationship, offer alternatives from which she can choose. Do not tell her what she *should* do, but support her ability to think and make her own decisions.

For the abuse victim, regaining a sense of control over her life may take some time and much encouragement and support from others. Encourage her to share her problem with someone that she can trust and run to in time of need. She must plan ahead for her safety and her children's.

Aids for Reestablishing Control. Discuss and provide information about available resources. Enrolling in a physical fitness program, especially one designed for self-defense, may help the victim physically as well as attitudinally. Though street-fighting techniques and tactics have limited applicability in the home, such training provides knowledge and skills that can be very useful in a crisis. Self-perceptions of helplessness can be replaced with feelings of control when the mind and body become practiced in self-defense skills.

The woman who feels trapped may benefit from a consciousness-raising group, one-to-one psychotherapy, or an assertiveness-training class. Any or all of these can help her regain a sense of her own identity and worth as a person and give her the support she needs in changing the direction of her life.

Community Resources. Discuss resources available to the victim and encourage her to use them. Community resources vary widely. Rural areas are typically woefully lacking in helping resources for the battered victim. Emergency personnel may become influential in organizing a group to help battered women. Be knowledgeable about the resources in your community, and be sure that this information is communicated to the battered victim.

Whether or not the victim leaves her partner is clearly a decision that she must make. Many communities have shelters for battered women where the woman and her children can be housed and protected* until she becomes self-sufficient, or until counseling or psychiatric treatment results in reconciliation with her partner.

Safety Precautions. Encourage the victim to take safety precautions as needed. If the woman's decision is to remain with her partner rather than seek protection elsewhere, encourage her to plan ahead. What is the quickest, most accessible escape route? Where can she go? Whom can she call? As a minimum, provide information and encourage her to contact some resource that may be of help in the future.

---

* Most emergency shelters for battered women keep their addresses confidential so that an attacker cannot find the woman who goes there. Usually a person from the shelter meets the victim in a neutral place to take her to the shelter. Victims are asked to maintain the confidentiality of the shelter's location.

This could be a psychiatric social service agency affiliated with the emergency department, a crisis hotline, or a self-help group active in the community. No woman identified as battered should leave the emergency department without resources for follow-up.

LEGAL ASPECTS

It is a crime for one person to beat another.[3] The crime of assault and battery is punishable as either a misdemeanor or a felony, depending on the amount of injury inflicted and the instrument used. To initiate legal action, the victim must contact the police or sheriff's department. In most jurisdictions, the attacker can be arrested by two means—police arrest or citizen's arrest. In both instances, the police must take the arrested person into custody.

If the attacker is arrested, he may be released within a few hours on his own recognizance (*i.e.,* his promise to return for a formal hearing) or upon posting bail. The victim must be prepared for this event and, anticipating the attacker's probable response, make appropriate arrangements for her children's and her own safety. Knowing that protective services are accessible to her may encourage her to follow through with prosecution.

For future protection, the victim should insist on a police report, whether or not she wishes to press charges and even if no arrest is made. A police report is required if the victim wishes to prosecute. If she decides against prosecution, the report will subsequently provide a record of threats or violence supportive of her case should she later decide to press charges or obtain custody of her children.

Many women who initially decide to prosecute withdraw their charges before trial and refuse to testify. For this reason, many prosecutors are reluctant to begin the prosecution process unless satisfied that the victim will not withdraw her complaint and refuse to testify.

Victim-Witness Assistance Programs. State and federally funded programs are available in some communities to provide a variety of direct services to victims of violent crime. Such services may include transportation, household assistance, notification of friends and relatives, arrangement for verification of medical benefits, referral to other agencies or community groups, assistance in applying for state victim compensation benefits, child care, and other related personal services as appropriate.

These programs also provide legal assistance. Participants in the program notify and inform witnesses prior to their being subpoenaed in criminal cases, assist them in reaching the hall of justice, provide reception and guidance at court, and explain unfamiliar procedures.

Important points in the psychosocial support of the battered spouse are summarized in Chart 8-1.

THE ABUSED ELDER

Abuse of elderly persons is a prevalent medical and social problem that has recently been widely recognized. Although

---

Chart 8-1

PSYCHOSOCIAL ASPECTS OF CARE OF THE BATTERED SPOUSE

Provide support, empathy, and respect.

- Avoid judgmental comments.
- Avoid "why" questions that discount her judgment.
- Encourage her to express her feelings, and listen attentively.
- Recognize her as a strong person, a survivor who is struggling with feelings of inferiority, ambivalence, and guilt.

Help her to regain control of her life.

- Encourage her to identify personal goals and alternatives.
- Do not attempt to make decisions for her.
- Support her ability to think and make her own decisions.
- Encourage her to share her problem with a trusted person.

Suggest aids to rebuild confidence and overcome feelings of helplessness.

- Self-defense training, consciousness-raising groups, psychotherapy, assertiveness training

Encourage her to take precautions for her safety and her children's.

- If she decides to stay with her partner:
  Plan ahead—someone to call, a place to go, the best and quickest escape route.
  Community resources—shelter for battered women, psychiatric social service agency, self-help groups, crisis hotline.
- If she takes legal action against her attacker:
  Sources of protection when he is released from custody
  Police report as documentation
  Victim-witness assistance programs

---

it has probably existed for some time, a number of factors may contribute to the current prevalence of the problem: increased life expectancy; physical and mental impairment, decreased productivity, and increased dependence associated with greater longevity; limited resources for care of the elderly; economic factors, including inflation, that create financial hardships for elderly persons and the family unit; and stress of middle-aged caretakers who must shoulder responsibility for two generations.

Characteristics of Elder Abuse

Emerging information suggests that certain patterns can be identified in the abuse of elders.
- Abused elders are more likely to be suffering from physical or mental impairment that necessitates greater dependence on their caretakers.
- Abusers are most often the children of the abused person, although spouses, grandchildren, and other relatives abuse elders almost as often.
- Like other abused dependents, elders are most often repeatedly abused by family members who are suffering from stress.

- Unlike other abused dependents, abused elders do seek help, but they are often unsuccessful in finding it.

Forms of Abuse

Abuse may take a variety of forms. An awareness of these common forms may prompt casefinding and reporting.
- *Physical abuse or neglect* may be manifested by obvious injuries and trauma, malnutrition, and poor personal hygiene.
- *Psychological abuse* is most often recognized by the victim's expressions of depression and loss of his sense of self-worth.
- *Violation of individual rights* may be revealed by the social history:
  - Has the elder been the victim of theft—of his money? personal property?
  - Has he lost his freedom of choice? Has he been removed from his home against his will?
  - How does he view his caretakers?

The cruel dilemma faced by many elderly persons is illustrated in the following example:

The man who lived with her since her husband's death drank too much. She said, he called her names. He pushed her around. He stole her social security checks. He mortgaged her home to buy himself a car. He left her alone for days with only canned goods in the cupboard and, being infirm, she could not cook for herself. So she went hungry. But no, said the woman, there was nothing she would do to stop the man. After all, she explained, "He is my son."[4]

MANAGEMENT

Once it is determined that an abusive situation exists, discuss with the patient the need for intervention and the possibilities that exist within his family structure and the community. It may be advisable to arrange for referral and follow-up with an appropriate social service agency or counselor. Provide the phone number or necessary information for contacting a helping resource in case further problems arise after the patient leaves the hospital. Be aware of advocate groups for the elderly and the local programs they sponsor (see Chart 8-5).

THE ABUSED CHILD

The various forms of child abuse and neglect and the physical or emotional impairment resulting from them come under the general heading of domestic violence. Child abuse involves the maltreatment of children (from infancy to 18 years of age in most jurisdictions) by their caretakers—parents, foster parents, stepparents, or babysitters. Violence against children is implied in the term; similar acts of violence inflicted on adults would be classified as assault and battery.

Neglect includes failure to provide physical care adequate to maintain health (nutrition, shelter, clothing) and sufficient human emotional interaction and stimulation for normal psychological development. Such failures are the result of indifference, disregard, or avoidable ineptitude on the part of the caretaker rather than inescapable environmental factors. Abuse and neglect involve nonaccidental injuries to children and the wide variety of failures to provide adequately for them. Both abuse and neglect demand early intervention to prevent further injury and to provide help for the abusive adult.

The importance of identifying the abused child lies in the fact that child abuse tends to be repetitive, each attack more savage than the one before. Many children who die or require hospitalization because of battering injuries have been treated previously, sometimes repeatedly, in an emergency department or a physician's office, for minor to moderate soft tissue injuries or fractures that were assumed to have resulted from accidents.[11] Had the true nature of the injury been recognized at an early stage, the cycle might have been interrupted before more serious, perhaps lethal, injury occurred.

Characteristics of Abusers

Child abuse is not related to social class, income, or level of education. Abusive persons have other common traits: history of a lack of early mothering, feelings of worthlessness about themselves or the child, resentment or rejection of the child, expectations that the child will satisfy personal or parental needs through behavior that is not attainable at the child's age and stage of development, and a need to discipline sternly and authoritatively.

The need to enforce rigorous discipline accounts for the cyclical nature of abuse, according to many authorities. The use of corporal punishment for corrective and educational purposes is well documented in history, and physical punishment is an accepted form of discipline in many cultures. A key element in the use of severe physical punishment is the repetition of patterns learned in childhood. Frequently the abuser was beaten as a child, and his way of disciplining his own child grows out of his early experience of harsh

---

Chart 8-2

BEHAVIORS OF THE CHILD ABUSER

- Evidences immature behavior and is preoccupied with himself.
- Has little perception of how a child could feel, physically or emotionally.
- Is critical of the child and has unrealistic expectations of him.
- Seldom touches or looks at the child or becomes involved in his care.
- Is unconcerned about the child's injury, treatment, and prognosis.
- Gives no indication of feeling guilt or remorse about the child's condition; rather, may blame the child or be angry with him for being injured.
- Is more concerned about what will happen to himself and others involved in the child's injury than about the child's welfare. Often disappears from the hospital during the examination or shortly after the child's admission.
- Asks to have the child return to the home only when interrogation has frightened him.

punishment. Even though he would prefer to use other forms of discipline, under stress the abuser tends to regress to the earliest patterns—that is, he will repeat with his children the treatment he himself received as a child.[14]

It is important to recognize that like all parents, most abusers love their children. However, their love is linked to the child's ability to satisfy their demands and expectations. The abusive parent fails to perceive that these expectations are often inappropriate for the child's age and stage of development. In an effort to make the "uncooperative" child live up to his expectations, the abusive parent uses physical punishment. If the abuser is under stress, he may lose self-control while administering punishment and inflict injuries on the child. Because repeated battering episodes tend to weaken self-control, breaking this cycle is crucial. Learning to recognize certain characteristic behaviors in the abuser and the abused may promote early identification and intervention. Behaviors characteristic of the abusive adult are described in Chart 8-2.

Signs of a Preabuse State. Occasionally, the potentially abusive adult (usually a parent) will actively seek help, fearful that he is losing self-control and may hurt his child. Emergency department personnel should be aware of the following patterns:

- Several emergency department visits within a 24-hour period. This behavior may indicate a plea for help.
- The parent who brings his or her child to the emergency department frequently for inconsequential symptoms. Whether or not the reason for the visit is apparent, one does exist. This behavior suggests that the parent is becoming unable to handle an impending crisis and is asking, albeit covertly, for help.

Characteristics of the Abused Child

The child's behavior offers important clues. This behavior is age-related. Typically, the child under 6 years of age is excessively passive; the child over 6 is aggressive. Rarely, at any age, will the child object to the parent's leaving the room.[5] Behaviors to look for in children are summarized in Chart 8-3. Any child over 3 years of age should be interviewed

privately. If the child says his injuries were caused by an adult, it is probably true.[12]

ASSESSMENT

History

The approach to the abused child and the abusive adult must be carefully considered. The sympathetic feelings that one has towards the abused child, or the hostile feelings aroused by the abusive adult often put the child in an adversary position relative to the parents. Yet, the child's primary resource for protection and security is a healthy family environment.

Any verbal or nonverbal communication that places the parents on the defensive will not serve the child's interest. It is important that the parent as well as the child be brought to sources of care that can correct the underlying problems and restore the family unit to a healthy state. When communicating with the parents, be objective and nonthreatening:

- Avoid statements that sound accusatory or judgmental.
- Remember that care of the child involves care of the family. If the parents are not alienated in the early phases of care, the first steps in breaking the child-abuse cycle have been successful.

The interview should be conducted with an attitude of concern and attentive listening. The information sought should include the complete details of the accident, who saw it, and whether a similar accident has happened before to this child or other children in the family. Determine, without raising suspicion, whether the history as given by parents and other observers is consistent, or whether it changes. Interview the child and each parent separately and compare the histories. Could the event, as described, cause the observed injuries in a child of that age? Was there a delay in seeking medical care? Delay of 1 to 4 days is common in nonaccidental abuse.[13] Do the parents and child exhibit any of the characteristic behaviors mentioned above?

Accidental vs. Intentional Injury. It must be remembered that accidental injuries are very common in children, and

---

Chart 8-3

BEHAVIORS OF THE ABUSED CHILD

- Cries hopelessly during treatment or examination without any real expectation of being comforted, or cries very little, in general.
- Does not look to parent (if abuser) for assurance, or may actively avoid parent.
- Is wary of physical contact initiated by abusive parent or others.
- Is apprehensive when other children cry and watches them with curiosity, especially when they are approached by another adult.
- Appears constantly on the alert for danger.
- May constantly seek favors, food, things, services.

health professionals lose much of their value if they become cynical and overly suspicious in dealing with parents, most of whom are struggling to deal with their own feelings of guilt over having allowed the injury to occur. When an accident is the cause of injury, the description of the incident is usually volunteered as a forthright and consistent story that accounts in a reasonable manner for the injury that has resulted.

If, in a private interview, the child is old enough to contribute his version of the way in which he was injured, he has lived through the age range when abuse is most frequent, but he is by no means immune. If his story is volunteered without hesitation and matches that given by a parent, child abuse is very unlikely. If he is hesitant and evasive or remains silent and terrified, the examiner may be justly suspicious.

Not all children in this latter category have been abused, however. Many simply feel guilty in the belief that wrongdoing on their part caused the accident. The older child who has been abused is particularly fearful that the parent will blame him for allowing the abuse to come to light and retaliate with further brutality. For this reason, great sympathy and tact are required to induce a child to reveal the true nature of the circumstances leading to his injury.

Distinguishing between an intentional injury and an authentic accident is a challenging problem that calls for intuitive questioning and careful examination.

Physical Examination

The physical examination is best done with another colleague. One person can examine for and describe the physical findings while the other validates and records the findings.[5] The recording must be scrupulously objective. Observations must be clearly described. Assumptions and personal perceptions must not be included because they may disqualify the medical record from being entered as evidence should the case be brought to trial. These notes must be terse and legible; they must include the date and time of observation or entry, and be signed, not initialed.

The examination of the child should be carried out kindly and gently, to prevent further pain, fear, and distrust of adults. All body surfaces and parts, including the genitals, must be examined by inspection and palpation.

Scrupulous adherence to collection and preservation of evidence is imperative. Saliva, hair, seminal fluid, blood, and broken fingernails are a few of the materials unique enough to eliminate or include an alleged abuser and can be the most critical evidence in the court presentation of the case. As detailed in Chapter 7, physiologic saline, not water, is used for collecting biological materials so that cell integrity is maintained.

The most common sites of physical trauma are the soft tissues, bones, head, and abdomen.

Soft Tissue Injuries. Soft tissue injuries are the injuries found most frequently in early abuse and may present in a variety of forms.*

* The material on soft tissue injuries was contributed by Boyd G. Stephens, M.T., M.D., Assistant Clinical Professor of Pathology, University of San Francisco, and Chief Medical Examiner/Coroner, City and County of San Francisco.

1. *Multiple bruises and ecchymoses* usually present in various stages of healing, from the black and blue of recent trauma to the greenish yellow of healing tissue. Suspicious bruises are those in areas where the child is unlikely to strike himself during activities normal for his growth and development.
   - Look for the presence of defense wounds—injuries commonly found on the ulnar aspect of the forearms, inflicted when the child is trying to protect himself from a blow.
   - Observe also whether the injuries are present on more than one plane of the body. If injuries are found on the face and back, for example, or on both sides of the body, chances are the injuries were inflicted intentionally by someone.

2. *Patterned injuries* are typically soft tissue injuries that reflect the shape or contour of the object that made them, suggesting the type of instrument that produced the injury and the manner in which it was used. A blow by a solid object tends to force blood through the microvessels by hydraulic force to the edge of the pressure area, producing a hemorrhagic outline of the shape of the striking face of the object. For example, a spanking with twin lead electrical cord leaves a characteristic mark consisting of three parallel lines, as shown in Figure 8-1. Similar markings may occur with other objects, such as a rope, a belt, or a hand.

   Patterned injuries can take many forms, and some, like bites, may have great significance. Delay cleansing suspicious wounds until evidence, such as saliva, can be collected according to established protocol. Crusting, swelling, and hematoma formation may distort or preclude the understanding or documentation of a patterned injury soon after it is incurred. Documentation with clear, balanced color photographs should be done as soon as the patient is medically stabilized.

3. *Scalds* are a common form of injury and abuse in persons of all ages, but the young and old are particularly susceptible. The initial pain is followed by a temporary anesthesia while the hot liquid literally "cooks" the tissue. Thus, a second-degree scald behaves medically as a third-degree burn. The period of time for this to occur is proportional to the temperature of the water, as shown in Table 8-1.

To prevent accidental scalds, tap water temperatures should not exceed 51.7°C to 54.5°C (125°F–130°F).

In some cultures hot water is used to punish or toilet train children. The latter may involve forcing the child's buttocks into hot water for soiling his pants. Often, one can duplicate the child's position in the water from examination of the burn pattern. A key feature suggesting this form of abuse is a sharp line of demarcation between burned and normal tissue (Fig. 8-2). At higher water temperatures, this exposure may be so brief that trapped air in hair or clothing may protect the skin from the burn.

Fractures. The second most commonly inflicted injuries are fractures, and x-rays make these the easiest to document. Their presence should be suspected when there is unexplained soft tissue swelling; the child may not be aware of any problem. It is surprising how little discomfort healing fractures seem to produce in young children. The examiner should be aware of the following:

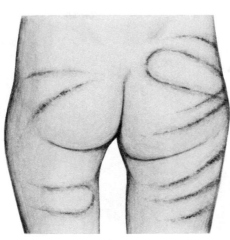

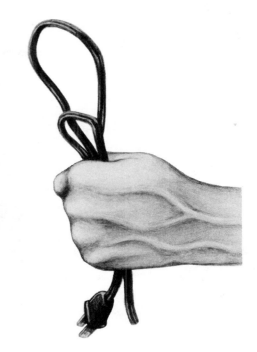

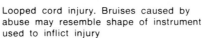

Figure 8-1 *Patterned injury inflicted with a twin-lead electrical cord. (© Copyright 1977, CIBA Pharmaceutical Company, Division of CIBA-GEIGY Corporation. Reprinted with permission from Clinical Symposia illustrated by John A. Craig, M.D. All rights reserved.)*

Looped cord injury. Bruises caused by abuse may resemble shape of instrument used to inflict injury

- *Twisting injuries* result in spiral fractures of the humerus or femur or in the elevation of the periosteum by a subperiosteal hematoma, which heals with more than normal callus formation.
- *Jerking injuries* result in epiphyseal separation, with callus formation at the junction of the shaft and growth center of the bone.
- *Rib fractures* result from forceful blows or from crushing injuries.
- Often, the fractures are multiple, some recent and some partially or completely healed, suggesting repetition of abuse. In the absence of metabolic bone disease, x-ray findings of multiple fractures of the long bones or ribs in varying stages of healing is pathognomonic for child abuse.

Head Injuries. Head injuries produce the highest mortality and result in the greatest amount of permanent disability.[1] Head injuries include scalp wounds, skull fractures, subdural or subgaleal hematomas, and repeated concussions.

The progression of abuse appears to be from the trunk and extremities toward the head as the major target of injury.

TABLE 8-1. RELATIONSHIP OF WATER TEMPERATURE TO TIME REQUIRED FOR SECOND-DEGREE SCALD TO OCCUR

Water Temperature		Time (Sec)
°C	°F	
68.9	156	1
65.0	149	2
60.0	140	5
56.1	133	15
52.8	127	60
51.1	124	180

Most children with severe head injuries show evidence of earlier peripheral injuries.

Abdominal Injuries. Abdominal injuries constitute a small but serious part of the abuse syndrome. Rupture of the liver and blunt injuries to the intestine and mesentery are potentially lethal, especially if there is delay in diagnosis of an abdominal injury.

Children who show evidence of neglect, multiple bruises, or other soft tissue injuries and who complain of abdominal distress should be carefully evaluated with the possibility of abdominal injury in mind.

MANAGEMENT

Treatment begins with the recognition that a child may have been abused. A sample protocol for dealing with suspected child abuse is shown in Chart 8-4. Following a complete assessment and documentation of all assessment data, a decision must be made whether the child has been abused. A suggested form on which data may be summarized is provided in Fig. 8-3. If there is any doubt, the child should be hospitalized immediately (not sent home first) and fully evaluated medically.

Protocols. Most emergency departments have protocols that guide their personnel in handling suspected child abuse cases. Further, every state and territory provides a mechanism for the reporting and investigating of real and suspected child abuse cases. It is suggested that emergency personnel become familiar with the hospital protocol and state reporting laws for suspected abuse.

Counseling. In addition to careful evaluation and protection of the child, the long-term treatment plan includes

Scalding Injuries

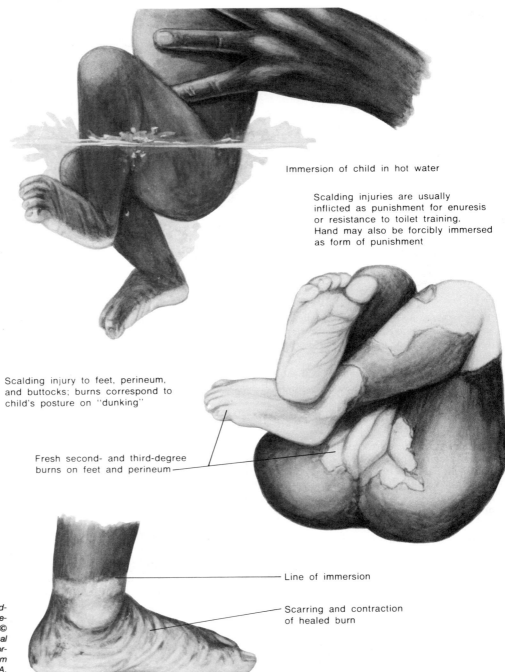

Immersion of child in hot water

Scalding injuries are usually inflicted as punishment for enuresis or resistance to toilet training. Hand may also be forcibly immersed as form of punishment

Scalding injury to feet, perineum, and buttocks; burns correspond to child's posture on "dunking"

Fresh second- and third-degree burns on feet and perineum

Line of immersion

Scarring and contraction of healed burn

Figure 8-2 *Signs of immersion in scalding injury. Note line of demarcation between burned and normal tissue. (© Copyright 1977, CIBA Pharmaceutical Company, Division of CIBA-GEIGY Corporation. Reprinted with permission from Clinical Symposia illustrated by John A. Craig, M.D. All rights reserved.)*

counseling of the abusive parent with the ultimate goal of providing a safe environment at home for the child. The abusive adult must be helped to realize that frustration and resentment of infants and children are natural and universal and that these feelings can and must be dealt with in an appropriate manner.

If such feelings are feared, repressed, and unrelieved, they are bound to surface again sooner or later, and may result in more vicious child abuse or other socially unacceptable behavior.

Protection of the Child. Usually the child need not be permanently removed from the home, though often a separation is needed. The child needs protection; the parent or adult needs help and counseling.

An interdisciplinary team approach to treatment is de-

Chart 8-4

PROTOCOL FOR SUSPECTED CHILD ABUSE

1. Every case in which a minor is brought to the emergency department and it appears to the physician or nurse from observation that the minor has physical injury or injuries that appear to have been inflicted upon him by other than accidental means, report of such fact must be made by *telephone* and *in writing* to:
   a. The local police authority having jurisdiction (where the injury occurred)
   b. The Juvenile Probation Department
   The ''Suspected Child Abuse Report'' form *must* be completed in every case (see Fig. 8-3).
2. Cases of suspected child abuse may require pediatric consultation. The attending physician may consider ordering a battered child series, pro-time, platelet count, urinalysis and other tests as he deems appropriate.
3. If the attending physician or a consultant feels additional studies including x-rays are required to make a proper evaluation, the legal consent for the evaluation should be obtained from the responsible adult, parent, or guardian. If the responsible party refuses consent, the physician's legal obligation to make such evaluation and reports should be explained. If the responsible party continues to refuse consent, the physician's recommendation for medical evaluation should be reported to the Juvenile Probation Department. An informal hearing may then be arranged at the hospital and the court order evaluation made. The local police authority should be notified if the party attending the minor otherwise impedes evaluation.
4. Contact Police Department for attending physician/pediatrician.
5. Contact the Juvenile Probation Department for the attending physician/pediatrician as follows:
   Monday–Friday 8:00 a.m.–5:00 p.m.
      Officer of the day: 299-3176 or
      Dependent Intake Unit: 299-3176
   Evenings and weekends:
      Juvenile Probation Department—evening office: 299-2250
      If no answer at any of the above, contact Children's Shelter
6. Note time of phone calls, name of officer and badge number on emergency department record for both police *and* probation.
7. State Penal Code (11161.5) protects the physician from any civil or criminal liability as a result of making this report. From Penal Code, Section 11161.5 ''. . . no physician and surgeon . . . shall incur any civil or criminal liability as a result of making any report authorized by this section. . . .''
8. In cases in which the registered nurse feels the injuries suffered by a minor appear to have been inflicted by other than accidental means and the attending physician disagrees, she will:
   a. State to the attending physician that she feels the case is suspect and discuss further that possibility with him. If physician and nurse cannot find agreement following discussion, she will then:
   b. Ask that he request consultation to obtain a second opinion. If the consultant feels the injuries appear to have been inflicted by other than accidental means, he will have the obligation to report as outlined above.
   c. If the attending physician refuses to request consultation, the nurse will immediately report the problem to the Chairman of the Department of Emergency Medicine (DEM), a member of the Executive Committee of the Department or the Assistant Hospital Nursing Director.
   d. Written reports of any such disagreement shall be prepared for the Director, DEM, by the nurse and physician within 24 hours of the event.

---

sirable, with the recognition that many factors contribute to child abuse and must be resolved. Treatment must be ongoing and comprehensive, and the child must be protected until his safety in the home is assured.

PREVENTION

Child abuse is a special form of pediatric emergency. Although much of emergency department practice involves the care and treatment of patients, in child abuse a third aspect of care is most important—that of prevention. As-

sessing injuries and behaviors that point to abuse and identifying and reporting them can activate the mechanism for protecting the child and rehabilitating the abusive adult.

SUMMARY

Child, elder, and spouse abuse—all forms of domestic violence—are democratic phenomena: they can happen to persons of any sex, race, religion, or socioeconomic or ed-

SANTA CLARA VALLEY MEDICAL CENTER
SUSPECTED CHILD ABUSE REPORT

Name: _____

Chart #: _____

Address of _____

parent: _____

_____

Date seen:

Area OPD _____

    Ward _____

    ER _____

    Other _____

Reason for
Report

a) Trauma _____

b) Failure to thrive _____

c) Neglect _____

d) Sexual abuse _____

e) Other _____

_____

Medical findings including history: _____

_____

_____

_____

_____

_____

_____

_____

_____

Physician signature _____

Lab:

_____

_____

X-ray:

_____

_____

Disposition of patient: _____
Reported to:
Juvenile Probation Dept. _____

Police Agency _____

DIAGRAM OF INJURIES OR CONTUSIONS

(Estimate times of injuries)

Section 11161.5 of the California Penal Code requires specified persons, including social workers and medical personnel, to report to the police and probation *or* health *or* welfare any physical injuries to minors which appear to have been inflicted by other than accidental means.

All forms to be sent to the Pediatric
Department for distribution.

    Copy 1-JPD   Copy 2-Police Dept.   Copy 3-Pt. Chart   Copy 4-Pedi. Dept.

Figure 8-3 *Example of a form for reporting data on suspected child abuse.*

Chart 8-5

RESOURCES FOR ABUSED PERSONS

- *American Association of Retired Persons,* 1909 K Street NW, Washington, DC 20049. (202) 872-4700. Advocate group to assist in preretirement planning and in providing educational, consumer, and community service programs for persons aged 55 and over. Publishes monthly newsletter, bimonthly journal, and informational material.

- *American Humane Association,* 5351 South Roslyn Street, Englewood, CO 80111. (303) 779-1400. A national center for promoting and developing child protective services in each community. Provides program planning, consultation, and education for persons working in field of child abuse.

- *Education Commission of the States,* 1860 Lincoln Street, Suite 300, Denver CO 80295. (303) 861-4917. A membership compact of 46 states and three territories organized to foster relationships among governors, legislators, and educators for the improvement of education. Has child abuse project. Does annual analysis of state reporting laws; has developed model state legislation; publishes materials on child abuse and on education.

- *Gray Panthers,* 3700 Chestnut Street, Philadelphia, PA 19104. (215) 382-6644. Promotes consciousness-raising and activism to combat age discrimination and to improve quality of life among the aging. Publishes bimonthly newspaper.

- *Golden Ring Council of Senior Citizens Clubs,* 1710 Broadway, New York, NY 10019. (212) 265-7000. Promotes social action to improve living conditions, social activities and legislation for the elderly.

- *Law Enforcement Assistance Administration,* United States Dept. of Justice, Washington, DC 20049. Publishes a national directory, *Programs Providing Services to Battered Women,* which provide information on victim witness assistance programs. These programs provide services to victims such as crisis intervention, transportation, emergency shelter, temporary child care, food and clothing, property return, information about the criminal justice system, resource and referral counseling, assistance in filing for financial reimbursement from Victim of Violent Crime fund.

- *Legal Research and Services for the Elderly,* 1511 K Street NW, Washington, DC 20005. (202) 638-4351. Association for persons and agencies working with the elderly in crime prevention. Conducts research, develops programs, provides technical assistance in program operations, publishes quarterly newsletter and resource materials.

- *National Center for the Prevention and Treatment of Child Abuse and Neglect,* Department of Pediatrics, University of Colorado Medical Center, 1205 Oneida Street, Denver, CO 80220. (303) 321-3963. Provides education, consultation, technical assistance, demonstration programs for treatment, evaluation, research to professionals working in the field of child abuse.

- *National Center on Child Abuse and Neglect,* United States Children's Bureau/DHEW, PO Box 1182, Washington, DC 20013. (202) 755-0587. Administers HEW funds for prevention and treatment of child abuse; funds ten regional centers that provide training and technical assistance to states; has clearinghouse for literature and statistical information.

- *National Committee for Prevention of Child Abuse,* 322 South Michigan Avenue, Suite 1250, Chicago, IL 60604. (312) 663-3520. Promotes public awareness and education, national volunteer network, technical and consultive services, primary prevention projects and advocacy. Membership association ($15.00 per year). Publishes quarterly newsletter.

- *National Council on Senior Citizens,* 1511 K Street NW, Washington, DC 20005. (202) 347-8800. Social/political action organization to foster health, education, recreation, and service programs and legislation for the elderly. Publishes monthly newsletter.

---

ucational level. The one common denominator is that abusive behavior perpetuates itself, and its expression, initially limited to the home, eventually expands into the community and society as a whole. The rising incidence of violent crime in American society has its roots in the home, in the family.[17] If a cure is ever to be found, it will have to be there.

Community and government resources available to abused persons are listed in Chart 8-5.

REFERENCES

1. Baron M, Bejar R, Sheaff P: Neurological manifestations of the battered child syndrome. Pediatrics 45:1003, 1970
2. Block, MR, Sinott JD: The Battered Elder Syndrome: An Exploratory Study. Paper presented at the 32nd Annual Meeting of Gerontological Society, Washington, DC, November 25–29 1979

3. California Dept. of Justice, Office of the Attorney General: Handbook on Domestic Violence, 3rd ed. Sacramento, California Dept. of Justice, Office of the Attorney General, Crime Prevention Unit, April 1979

4. Elderly Abuse. Tenth Anniversary Education Program. Emergency Department Nurses Association, July, 1980

5. Hansen MM: Accident or Child Abuse? Challenge to Emergency Nurses. J Emerg Nurs 2:13–20, 1976

6. Hendrix MJ, LaGodna GE, Bohen CA: The battered wife. Am J Nurs 650–653, 1978

7. Kempe CH: Eyewitness News. CBS, December 1, 1975

8. Langley R, Levy RC: Wife Beating: The Silent Crisis. New York, Pocket Books, 1977

9. Lieberkerknecht K: Helping the Battered Wife. Am J Nurs, 654–6, 1978

10. Martin D: Battered Wives. San Francisco, Glide Publications, 1976

11. O'Neill J, Jr, Meacham W, Griffin P, Sawyers J: Patterns of injury in the battered child syndrome. J Trauma 13:332, 1973

12. Schmitt B, Kempe CH: The pediatrician's role in child abuse and neglect. Curr Probl Pediatr 5:2–47, 1975

13. Silverman RN: Unrecognized trauma in infants, the battered child syndrome and the syndrome of Ambrose Tardieu. Radiology 104:337–353, 1972

14. Steele BF: The child abuser. In Kutash IL et al: Violence: Perspectives on Murder and Aggression. San Francisco: Jossey-Bass, 1978

15. Tintinalli JE: Child Abuse. J Am Coll Emerg Phys 7:110–113, 1978

16. Van Stolk M: Beaten women, battered children. Children Today 5:8–12, 1976

17. Violence in America. National Broadcasting Company, 1977

18. Walker LE: The Battered Woman. New York, Harper & Row, 1979

UNIT THREE

EMERGENCY PROCEDURES AND MANAGEMENT

9

CLINICAL ASSESSMENT *

JAMES H. COSGRIFF, JR. and DIANN ANDERSON

* Includes material by Barbara Bates, M.D., and Joan E. Lynaugh, R.N., M.S.N., in *The Practice of Emergency Nursing*, JB Lippincott, 1975

The assessment of a patient is not an isolated event but a dynamic ongoing process. In emergency situations, it involves the collection of historical data from the patient, family, friends, onlookers, emergency responders, and others; a detailed physical examination and appropriate adjunct studies; and the evaluation of the combined data. From this data base a plan of therapy is developed and implemented. Assessment requires the ability to ask relevant questions, identify life-threatening situations, establish priorities of care, and initiate resuscitative measures as indicated. All of one's senses should be used in the process of evaluating a patient, and one's manner of performing the examination should be calm, unhurried, and reassuring.

Assessment is begun at the scene of the incident by emergency personnel and continues during the entire out-of-hospital phase of care. The availability of highly skilled emergency medical technicians and paramedics on ambulances and rescue vehicles has resulted in better care at the scene because assessment and resuscitation can be carried out immediately to stabilize the patient. The extent to which on-site care should be given is controversial. Many advocate the "load and go" philosophy to expedite prompt transfer of the critically ill or injured patient to the hospital. The Committee on Trauma of the American College of Surgeons has developed a scheme for field categorization of the trauma patient using various parameters to determine the severity of injury. This concept may have important consequences because it allows the ambulance crew to match the severity of the injury with the level of treatment facility that can best serve the patient's needs.

Once the patient is in the hospital, an important aspect of assessment is the determination of the gradation of injury or illness and the capability of the hospital and its staff to deal with the problem. It is most important that emergency department personnel recognize their institution's limitations and provide for transfer of a critically ill or injured patient to a higher level facility when necessary.

With the advent of better trained and more highly skilled allied health professionals, including certified emergency department nurses, specialty nurse practitioners, and physician's assistants, protocols are used in many hospitals to allow such personnel to perform patient assessment and to engage in decision making to varying degrees.

OBSTACLES TO ASSESSMENT

In the emergency department, adequate assessment of the patient may be hindered by any of a number of factors, which may be related to the patient, the institution, or the health professional. Being aware of these challenges may help in overcoming them.

The Patient. Ordinarily, the patient presenting to the emergency department is assessed and treated promptly and leaves satisfied with his care. However, various difficulties in the encounter between the patient and emergency personnel may arise. Several examples follow:

- Impaired communication because of differences in language, custom, ethnic group, or social class. The patient may have difficulty expressing himself or understanding the questions asked of him. He may be too quiet or too verbose. To promote understanding, emergency personnel should be familiar with local customs and with colloquialisms used in the community. If emergency personnel feel the patient is not ill enough to receive treatment they may have difficulty establishing rapport.
- Mental aberration resulting from alcohol or drug intoxication, senility, delirium, fatigue, or apprehension
- Abnormal behavior such as drunkenness, aggression, hypochondriasis, or nudity

The Institution. Obstacles associated with institutions include the following:
- Disparity between patient load and number of available personnel
- Poor organization of an adequate staff
- Inadequate staff resources: interpreters, social services, patient advocates, laboratory and radiologic services

The Health Professional. A number of negative factors may hamper assessment:
- Professional inadequacy, incompetence, or lack of motivation
- Lack of the knowledge needed to deal with a particular problem
- Lack of interest in the assessment process
- Failure to identify one's role—the emergency department should have a written policy that clarifies the functions of the various staff members.

Knowledge, skills, attitudes, and the availability of adequate resources all come into play in surmounting the various obstacles to effective assessment.

METHODOLOGY: ORDER OF ASSESSMENT

Assessment should proceed in an orderly fashion. The essential steps in assessment and their proper sequence in the process should be kept in mind throughout. However, though the methodology does not change, the extent of assessment varies according to the severity and complexity of the patient's illness or injury and the gravity of his condition. Good judgment is called for. Clearly, a patient with a fractured finger does not require the in-depth evaluation needed by the patient with an acute myocardial infarction, arrhythmia, and hypotension.

In the emergency setting particularly, the examiner must be able to focus directly on the presenting condition. A critically ill or injured patient requires urgent assessment. Urgency calls for efficiency and may limit the scope of diagnosis and management. It rarely justifies the omission of any of the steps in assessment, however.

The steps in assessment are generally done in the following order. However, according to the requirements of the situation, the examiner may proceed with more than one step at a time.

1. Immediate survey
2. Resuscitation
3. History
4. Physical examination
5. Data analysis and problem definition
6. Reevaluation
7. Development of a plan of management

IMMEDIATE SURVEY

The first step in assessment is a quick overview of the patient, to determine his complaints and his reason for coming to the hospital and to identify any life-threatening conditions. It is essential to check the following immediately: airway patency, circulatory status, external bleeding, shock, evidence of fracture, and level of consciousness.

Airway Patency. Observe the patient's respiratory activity. Is the airway patent? If not, clear it by sweeping the mouth and pharynx with a finger to remove debris; aspirate mucus. Use the chin-lift or jaw-thrust maneuver if necessary to establish an open airway. If the patient is unconscious or a cervical spine injury is suspected, do not hyperextend the neck until the cervical-spine is determined to be intact.

Breathing Status. Observe the patient's chest for equal expansion and the rate, depth, and regularity of respirations. Note the presence of sounds accompanying respiration (*i.e.,* stridor, wheezing, rales, rhonchi), and whether retractions of accessory breathing muscles are present. Assist respirations and provide supplemental oxygen as appropriate.

Circulatory Status. Evaluate the patient's circulation by assessing his blood pressure and pulse. Pulse volume, rate, and rhythm are valuable indicators of circulatory status. It is generally believed that if the radial pulse is palpable, the systolic blood pressure is at least 80 mm Hg. If the patient is hypotensive, place two large bore veinways and initiate volume replacement with Ringer's lactate. In acute cardiac conditions, another fluid may be chosen to maintain the circulation. At the time of placing the IV lines, draw blood samples for basic laboratory tests and type and crossmatch if needed.

External Bleeding. Look carefully for evidence of external bleeding. If any is found, control the hemorrhage by direct pressure.

Evidence of Fracture. Disrobe the patient completely and examine for any obvious deformity or other evidence of fracture.

Level of Consciousness. Perform a rapid neurologic assessment to determine the level of consciousness and pupillary reflexes.

RESUSCITATION PHASE

- Give oxygen to all critically ill or injured patients.
- If the vital signs are unstable or the person is a known or suspected cardiac patient, electrocardiographic (ECG) monitoring is indicated. Note any arrhythmias.
- If the patient is in shock, the pneumatic antishock garment should be applied. Recall, however, that this is contraindicated in pulmonary edema. An intravenous line is placed to initiate volume replacement.
- Consider whether an indwelling bladder catheter or nasogastric tube is needed.

HISTORY

The history is an essential step in assessment. The examiner should introduce himself to the patient initially and explain what is to be done. If the patient is unable to communicate well, a member of the family or a friend accompanying him may be a good source of information. (The record should show whether the patient or another person is the source of information.) The examiner's questions should cover the following essential points:

1. *Exact location of the symptom(s).* Ask the patient to indicate a specific body region.
2. *Character or quality of the symptom(s).* Ask the patient to describe how it feels. This may be done by comparing the sensation to something else. For example, the chest pain of severe angina or myocardial infarction is often compared to "being squeezed around the chest" or having "someone sitting on my chest." Women may liken abdominal pain to labor pain.
3. *Time-related aspects of the symptom(s).*
   - Sequence of development. Ask when the symptom(s) *began,* and develop a *chronologic sequence* of the chain of events.
   - Relationship to other dates or events. Determine whether the occurrence of the symptom(s) is associated with specific dates or occasions, such as holidays or anniversaries. Such links are common.
   - Duration. Ask how long it lasts and if there are any symptom-free intervals.
   - Periodicity. Ask whether the symptom(s) recur at regular intervals. Determine whether they are related to any activity such as exercise, eating, change of position, sleeping, working, or social activity.
   - Progression. Ask whether the symptom is following a natural course—getting better or worse over a period of time.
4. *Effects of the symptom(s) on the patient's ability to function.* Ascertain whether the patient's *everyday functions,* both occupational and leisure activities, have been affected or limited in any way.
5. *Other associated symptoms or instances of dysfunction.* For example, it may be helpful to know whether the chest pain is accompanied by nausea, and if loss of weight, change in bowel or urinary habits, or disturbance of menstrual function has occurred.
6. *Environmental and stress factors.* Determine the *setting* in which the symptom occurs. Ask whether it is experienced at work or at home; while sleeping, eating, or reading; or during periods of physical or emotional

stress. Ask about the work and leisure environments in order to determine whether there is exposure to drafts, severe changes in temperature, or noxious fumes or substances.

7. *Factors that make the symptom(s) better or worse.* Establish whether the patient is aware of what makes the symptom better and what makes it worse, such as food, activity, or rest.

8. *Allergies and medications.* Determine whether the patient has any allergies. Ask about his use of medications currently and in the past.

9. *Family history.* Ask about the state of health of all members of the patient's immediate family.

10. *History of past illness(es).* Information relevant to the patient's present status may be obtained.

As experience in assessment grows, it becomes possible to develop the symptom complex fairly rapidly. Allow the patient to describe the complaint in his own words, being very careful not to lead him or put words in his mouth. Maintaining a calm outward appearance helps to reduce anxiety and apprehension on the part of the patient. Sensitivity to the patient's feelings and to his nonverbal cues is also helpful in putting him at ease and gaining information. When it would not obscure diagnosis, giving appropriate medication for pain relief may allow the patient to feel more comfortable and thus more cooperative. Privacy is also important, especially if the symptoms require personal questions.

Interviewing techniques in the emergency setting are necessarily modified and compressed, to allow for greater efficiency and to expedite care. Even so, each step of the history-taking process must be taken to avoid a serious omission.

PHYSICAL EXAMINATION

Like the history, the physical examination does not always follow the same steps but necessarily must vary with the needs of the patient. The assessment required by a patient with a simple laceration is entirely different from that needed by the patient with an acute myocardial infarction or with fever or coma of unknown cause. The examination outlined herein is not intended as a routine tool for emergency personnel. It is too detailed for some purposes and much less than adequate for others. Chapters on specific injuries include detailed assessment information. In performing physical assessment, the examiner should develop a systematic approach using the appropriate sequence.

General Survey

The first step of the physical examination is a general inspection of the patient; this completes the observation begun in the immediate survey and continued throughout the history-taking process. The following should be observed and noted:

- The patient's dress, grooming, and personal hygiene
- Any signs of distress
    wheezing, cough, and labored breathing (cardiopulmonary distress)
    cool palms and trembling fidgety movements (anxiety)

- Skin, nails, and earlobes
    clammy pallor or mottling (shock)
    cyanosis
    rashes
    bruises
- Position, gait, and motor activity
    Writhing, restlessness (renal colic)
    Quiet, guarded position (peritoneal irritation)
    Tremor of alcohol withdrawal
    Paralysis of an extremity
    Slurred speech
- Odors of alcohol, acetone, uremia, melena
- Facial expression—signs of anxiety, depression, pain, or panic
- Manner, mood, relationships to persons and things around him
- Speech—clarity, speed of response
- State of awareness, orientation, and rationality

Detailed Examination

Vital Signs. Take the temperature, pulse, respiratory rate, and blood pressure.

Head. Inspect and palpate for tenderness, masses, lacerations, changes in the contour of the skull, bleeding.

Eyes. Note position and alignment. Observe the conjunctivae for redness (*e.g.,* due to inflammation, marihuana use) or pallor (due to anemia), and the sclerae for jaundice. Note the size and shape of the pupils and their reaction to light and accommodation. Observe the range of extraocular movements. If indicated (*e.g.,* because of neurologic disease, trauma, or severe hypertension), examine the fundi with an ophthalmoscope, looking for papilledema, hemorrhage, and exudates.

Ears. Observe the earlobes for cyanosis. Inspect the ear canals and drums for inflammation or bleeding.

Nose. Inspect and palpate the external nose for deformity and tenderness. Inspect the nasal mucous membranes for swelling. Note the color (*e.g.,* redness denotes inflammation, grayness allergy), and the presence of any discharge or bleeding. Press and percuss the frontal and maxillary sinuses to detect tenderness (as in sinusitis).

Facial Bones. Inspect and palpate the facial bones, frontal area, zygomatic processes (cheek bones), maxilla (upper jaw), and mandible.

Mouth. Inspect the tongue and buccal mucosa for color and signs of dehydration. Inspect the teeth and note their state of repair; check the gums for inflammation, bleeding. If dentures are in place, have the patient remove them and carefully inspect the underlying area. Look at the throat and pharynx for swelling, inflammation, and exudate.

Neck. Palpate the neck for the position of the trachea. Tracheal deviation may indicate severe atelectasis or pneumothorax or neck mass. Palpate the thyroid and the neck for enlarged or tender lymph nodes.

Lungs and Thorax. Inspect the chest wall, noting the rate and rhythm of breathing, the excursion and symmetry of the chest wall. Note any signs of paradoxic movement of the chest wall. Palpate the chest wall for any masses or tenderness. Percuss the chest for any abnormal dullness (which may be due to pleural effusions or pneumonia). Auscultate the lungs for the quality and symmetry of breath sounds and for the presence of adventitious sounds such as rales, wheezes, rhonchi, and pleural friction rubs.

Breasts. Inspect for masses, inflammation, any change in the skin, *e.g.,* peau-d'orange (orange peel) or dimpling of cancer. Look for nipple discharge, palpate for masses or tenderness.

Axillae. Palpate for enlarged or tender lymph nodes.

Heart. Inspect the precordium for the apical impulse and abnormal pulsations. Identify by palpation the location of the apical impulse. Percuss the borders of the heart for enlargement. Auscultate the heart, identifying the two heart sounds at the apex and the base. Count the rate. Note the rhythm: Is it fast, slow, regular, irregular, affected by respiration? Note and describe any abnormal heart sounds and murmurs.

Abdomen. Inspect the abdomen, whether flat or distended. Note the presence of peristaltic loops or waves on the anterior abdominal wall that may be seen in intestinal obstruction. *Before palpation,* auscultate the abdomen with a stethoscope, noting the frequency and character of bowel sounds. Note any diminution or absence of peristalsis. Note any increase in peristalsis, high-pitched sounds, borborygmi. Palpate the abdomen in all four quadrants. If the patient has abdominal pain, begin the palpation away from the painful area, examining it last. Note any areas of tenderness, spasm, or guarding. Identify any masses or enlargement of the liver, spleen, or kidneys.

Genitalia. *Male Patient.* Inspect the penis, noting any lesions, urethral discharge. Inspect and palpate the scrotal contents, noting any swelling, masses, tenderness, or hernias. With the patient standing, check the inguinal rings for reducible hernias.

Female Patient. Inspect the external genitalia and the labia, noting any swelling, inflammation, or discharge. With a speculum, inspect the vagina and cervix, noting discharge, inflammation, or tenderness. Palpate the uterus for tenderness or enlargement. Move the cervix to check for adnexal pain. Palpate the adnexae for tenderness or masses.

Anus and Rectum. Inspect the anus, noting any lesions or bleeding. Palpate the anus, noting the tone of the anal sphincter. Note the character of the stool in the rectum if any and obtain a sample for visual examination and occult blood. Note any masses, tenderness, or blood. In males, inspect the membranous urethra and note the size and consistency of the prostate gland.

Extremities. Compare the extremity on one side with its opposite. Inspect the limbs for signs of peripheral vascular disorders (*e.g.,* pallor, cyanosis, hair loss, nail thickening, ulcers), musculoskeletal problems (*e.g.,* bony deformity of arthritis, fractures), neurological conditions (*e.g.,* atrophy, abnormal position or movement), clubbing of the fingers (pulmonary osteoarthropathy). Palpate the legs and feet for temperature difference, edema. Check the dorsalis pedis and posterior tibial pulses.

Neurologic Status. If indicated by evidence of neurologic disease, check motor function by inspection; test muscle tone, strength, and coordination, comparing one side with the other. Check sensation: light touch, pain, position, vibration, and discrimination. Test all superficial and deep tendon reflexes. Observe for meningeal signs.

Mental Status. Throughout the interview and examination, observe the patient's appearance and behavior, mood, thought processes and perceptions, and cognitive functions (*i.e.,* orientation, attention, concentration, memory, and judgment).

DATA ANALYSIS AND PROBLEM DEFINITION

The history and physical examination, the basic tools of clinical assessment, provide the data on which management will be based. The next step in assessment is to analyze the raw data and define the problem. This is a logical process that requires concentration, care, and thoroughness. A haphazard approach and hasty judgments can lead to error. The analytic process can be separated into six steps:

1. *Identify abnormal findings.* Review the history, physical examination, and laboratory work and identify symptoms, signs, and abnormal laboratory results that must be explained.
2. *Localize these findings anatomically.* Make an effort to determine what structures are involved and try to localize the problem to a body region (*e.g.,* abdomen, chest), more specifically to an organ system (*e.g.,* gastrointestinal tract, pulmonary tree), or to an organ (*e.g.,* stomach, gall bladder). When the abnormal findings are nonspecific, such as fever or fatigue, it may be difficult initially to ascertain what structures are involved.
3. *Interpret the findings in terms of the most likely underlying process.* This may be a pathologic process (*e.g.,* inflammatory, neoplastic, metabolic, traumatic, or toxic), a physiopathologic process (*e.g.,* increased gastrointestinal motility), or a psychopathologic process (*e.g.,* a depressive reaction).
4. *Make a hypothesis about the specific nature of the patient's problem.* This requires a wide range of clinical knowledge and has four components.
   - *Choose the most specific and significant problem(s) presented by the patient.*
   - Using the inferences you have made about the anatomic sites involved and the process going on, *match these problems* against conditions known to produce them. Obviously, the list will depend on the examiner's knowledge. Some may have sufficient knowledge to continue unaided through the analytic process. Others

may have to stop at this point and decide on referral, transfer, or consultation with another professional.

- *Eliminate diagnostic possibilities that fail to explain the patient's most significant findings* or are incompatible with the data. For example, a patient's chest pain may be matched against myocardial infarction but eliminated because it does not explain the associated pleurisy and purulent sputum. Here once again, and in subsequent steps of problem definition and management, a number of emergency personnel may participate and one take primary responsibility.
  - *Select the diagnosis most likely to explain the collected findings.* For this purpose, use the matching process described in the preceding paragraph and consider the statistical likelihood of the selected diagnosis in a person of the patients age, sex, race, geographic location, and so on.

5. *Test your hypothesis by further data collection.* More history, further physical examination, or additional laboratory studies may be called for. The process of formulating and testing a hypothesis guides the skilled examiner throughout the initial patient encounter.

6. *Establish a working definition (diagnosis) of the problem.* This definition should be made at whatever level of precision and certainty can be attained with the data available. For example, one might be limited to "abdominal pain, etiology undetermined" or be able to state quite precisely "acute retrocecal appendicitis with perforation." Any definition one makes is subject to further modification as the patient's course progresses and ongoing reevaluation is performed.

REEVALUATION

The patient must be assessed repeatedly while he is in the emergency department. This is done to identify any new symptoms and signs. As the initial problem is managed, other equally serious problems may develop. For example, a patient with an acute myocardial infarction whose blood pressure and chest pain are finally stabilized may suddenly develop a tachyarrhythmia of potentially life-threatening severity. Similarly, a patient with severe multiple trauma must be carefully observed and reevaluated for further unrecognized injuries. The accident or acute medical condition may have aggravated another underlying medical condition.

During this phase, the patient's vital signs should be monitored carefully and documented thoroughly. Hourly urine output is monitored in the shock patient and attempts made to maintain it at approximately 1 ml/kg/hour. Serial determinations of arterial blood gases, central venous pressure, and neurologic status are employed in critically ill or injured patients as indicated.

Repeated assessments should be performed at appropriate intervals. It is preferable that the continuing evaluation be performed by the person who made the initial assessment. If there is a change of personnel, the person leaving should review the patient's findings and status with the incoming person who will be responsible for the patient.

PLAN OF MANAGEMENT

Once the problem has been correctly identified and resuscitation accomplished as required, the goal is to outline and initiate definitive care. A plan of management should be developed that includes triage, further diagnostic procedures, referral, consultation, counseling, and support for the patient and family. They should be informed, to the fullest extent possible, about the nature of the problem and the requirements of future care. Detailed information on the management of specific clinical entities is provided throughout this book.

The steps in assessment are summarized in Chart 9-1.

CLINICAL EXAMPLE: STEPS IN ASSESSMENT

Clinical Situation

A 19-year-old female college student comes to the health service complaining of a sore throat and "feeling bad." She wants relief of symptoms so that she can take her examinations next week.

Immediate Survey

The patient's problem and her reason for coming to the emergency department are identified as described above. She is breathing freely, is not overtly hemorrhaging, is not in shock, is conscious and able to communicate, and does not appear to be seriously injured. Though she does not seem to be a "real emergency," assessment proceeds, according to the policy of the institution.

Resuscitation Phase

Not applicable.

History

The patient's illness began 1 week ago, when she first noted fatigue and malaise. These increased gradually, and 3 days ago she developed soreness in her throat. It occurs on both sides, is moderately severe, increases with swallowing, and is partially relieved by aspirin. The pain is getting worse. For 3 days she has also felt feverish but has had no chills. She has not taken her temperature. She has been anorexic, without nausea or vomiting, and has had no change in the color of her urine or stool. She recalls no exposure to similar illnesses. She has no other symptoms.

Physical Examination

On examination, the patient is thin, looks tired, and is somewhat flushed. Her skin is warm and moist, her hair straight; she wears no makeup. Although coherent in her history, she is somewhat impatient and irritable and prefers to lie down.

Pulse 110, respirations 20, blood pressure 120/75, temperature, taken orally, 102.4°F. Head and scalp are normal. Sclerae and conjunctivae are clear. Pupils are round, regular and equal, reactive to light and accommodation. Extraocular movements are intact. Fundi are normal. The nose is clear and the sinuses nontender. Ear canals and drums are normal. The tonsils are red and moderately enlarged and show a small amount of white exudate. The pharynx is moderately reddened. The tonsillar, superficial cervical, and posterior cervical lymph nodes are enlarged to about 2 cm to 2.5 cm in diameter; they are slightly tender, mobile, discrete, and firm. The lungs are clear. Bronchovesicular breath sounds are present in the right interscapular area. The heart is normal. The abdomen is negative, except that the area of splenic dullness is enlarged, and a spleen tip is just palpable below the left costal margin on deep inspiration. The remainder of the examination produces no abnormal findings.

Data Analysis and Problem Definition

- *Identifying abnormal findings*
  Symptoms: fatigue, malaise, sore throat, feverishness, anorexia.
  Signs: tachycardia; fever; red throat with exudate; enlarged tonsils; enlarged, slightly tender tonsillar, superficial, and posterior cervical nodes; splenomegaly.

Chart 9-1

SUMMARY OF STEPS IN ASSESSMENT

Immediate Survey

- Airway patency
- Breathing status
- Circulatory status
- External bleeding
- Shock
- Level of consciousness
- Fracture

Resuscitation Phase

- Oxygen administration
- ECG monitoring
- Antishock measures

History

- Description of symptom(s)
- Associated dysfunctions
- Environmental and stress factors
- Allergies and medications
- Family history
- History of past illness(es)

Physical Examination

- General Survey
    Appearance, grooming, personal hygiene
    Signs of distress
    Skin, nails, earlobes
    Position, gait, motor activity
    Odors
    Facial expression—anxiety, depression,
      pain, panic
    Speech
    State of awareness
- Detailed Examination
    Vital signs
    Head
    Eyes
    Ears
    Nose
    Facial bones
    Mouth

Neck
Lungs and thorax
Breasts
Axillae
Heart
Abdomen
Genitalia
Anus and rectum
Extremities
Neurologic status
Mental status

Data Analysis and Problem Definition

- Identify abnormal findings
- Localize findings anatomically
- Interpret findings to determine most likely underlying
    process
- Make specific hypothesis
- Test hypothesis by further data collection
- Establish working definition (diagnosis) of problem

Reevaluation

- Ongoing assessment to identify any new symptoms
    Monitor and record vital signs
    Serial determination of arterial blood gases, central venous pressure (CVP), neurologic status
    Monitor urine output

Plan of Management

- Definitive plan of care
- Further diagnostic procedures
- Patient education
- Referral, consultation, counseling, support of patient
    and family

- *Localizing abnormal findings*

Obviously it is impossible to localize some of these findings anatomically—for example, the fatigue, malaise, and fever. Nevertheless, there is good reason to believe that the patient's problem involves her pharynx, tonsils, lymph nodes, and spleen. The rationale includes the fact that although normal lymph nodes may be palpable in the neck, they are not usually so large or tender. A palpable spleen in an adult indicates splenic enlargement. Bronchovesicular breath sounds may normally be heard in the right interscapular space; therefore, there is no reason to include the lungs in the list of abnormal findings.

- *Interpreting findings—most likely underlying process*

The first thing to be considered is that the patient has had an acute febrile course. There are three classic manifestations

of inflammation present: redness, swelling, and pain. An acute infectious process is, therefore, most likely.

- *Formulating a specific hypothesis*

The first step in making a specific hypothesis on the cause and nature of the patient's disease is a review of all the conditions that can cause this clinical picture. Since pharyngeal exudate narrows the possibilities considerably and therefore is a central finding, the examiner might first list the causes of pharyngeal exudate with which one is familiar: monilia infection (thrush), adenovirus infection, streptococcal pharyngitis, infectious mononucleosis and diphtheria.

Then the examiner matches the patient's abnormal findings against the patterns of these diseases. Monilial infections of the mouth do not usually cause acute febrile illnesses and are, therefore, discarded. The only one of these diagnoses that readily explains the posterior cervical adenopathy as well as the splenomegaly is infectious mononucleosis. Diphtheria is unlikely on clinical grounds and is also statistically very rare (but not impossible) in the community. The tentative hypothesis is thus infectious mononucleosis.

- *Testing the hypothesis by collecting further data*

    The examiner will probably choose to test this hypothesis by laboratory work, including a white blood count, a differential white count and heterophil (or related) test. Since streptococcal pharyngitis can sometimes cause serious complications, such as rheumatic fever, the examiner may wish to take extra caution in ruling out this diagnosis by culturing the patient's throat.

- *Establishing a working definition (diagnosis) of the problem*

    If the test results support the hypothesis, the assessor has a working definition of the patient's problem, which in this situation is a definitive diagnosis of infectious mononucleosis.

Reevaluation

Reassessment has been going on during the process of testing the hypothesis.

Plan of Management

The patient will need information about the course, treatment, and prognosis of infectious mononucleosis. She may also need permission to adopt "the sick role" for the time being. It will probably be useful to help her talk through and evaluate her school situation and necessary life adaptations during her illness. Perhaps she will need written confirmation of her illness if she does not recover sufficiently by examination time. Reasonable self-care measures should be suggested, and follow-up should be planned. Specific instructions for subsequent care should be provided.

BIBLIOGRAPHY

DeGowin EL, DeGowin RL: Diagnostic Examination, 3rd ed. New York, Macmillan, 1976

Delp MH, Manning RT: Major's Physical Diagnosis, 8th ed. Philadelphia, WB Saunders, 1975

Krupp MA, Chatton MJ: Current Medical Diagnosis and Treatment. Los Altos, Lange Medical Publications, 1983

Petersdorf RG et al: Harrison's Principles of Internal Medicine, 10th ed. New York, McGraw-Hill, 1983

Sabiston DC, ed: Davis-Christopher Textbook of Surgery, 12th ed. Philadelphia, WB Saunders, 1981

Silen W: Cope's Early Diagnosis of the Acute Abdomen, 15th ed. New York, Oxford University Press, 1979

10
TRIAGE: ESTABLISHING PRIORITIES OF CARE

DIANN ANDERSON and JAMES H. COSGRIFF, JR.

Triage is a method designed to provide the greatest benefit to patients when treatment facilities are limited. Care is given to those who may survive with proper therapy rather than to those who have no chance of survival or who will live without treatment. The system was first devised in wartime as a method of managing large numbers of battlefield casualties. Today, it is applicable to the treatment of multiple victims of illness or injury outside and within the hospital setting.

PREHOSPITAL TRIAGE

In sorting the ill or injured outside of the hospital, the basic principles of clinical assessment are applied to determine the nature and severity of patient problems. The goal in group situations is to establish which patients should receive primary attention, stabilization, and transportation to a hospital emergency department. With the development of emergency medical service (EMS) systems, the concept of triage has expanded to include matching the patient's illness or injury to an appropriate facility for treatment. Advances in technology, the development of specialty services in medicine, and the recognition of special areas of health care expertise make it possible to provide a high level of care. Intensive coronary care, acute alcoholic detoxification, burn treatment, spinal cord injury care, and multiple trauma management are a few examples of specialty care; in some areas, specialized treatment centers are available. Categorization of hospital facilities helps to ensure the placement of the patient in the appropriate facility (see Chap. 1). In addition, local ordinances or EMS system directives may specify the hospital(s) to which acutely ill or injured patients should be transported.

Multiple Patient Triage

Triage of numbers of victims may be necessary in simple situations like two-car collisions, as well as in massive disasters, such as earthquakes, floods, and explosions. The principles of triage in either extreme vary little, though the methods used to communicate triage information and to match victims with available resources may vary.

Triage at the scene is done by the first qualified person to arrive (*i.e.,* the one with the most medical training). It is his responsibility to perform immediate primary surveys on all victims and to determine and communicate the numbers and types of resources needed to provide initial care and transport.

In disasters, three or four triage categories may be used, depending on local protocol. These categories are outlined in Chart 10-1. In some communities, triage categories are indicated by nonmedical terms such as *now, later,* and *dead.* Examples of injuries included in the *now* and *later* categories are shown in Chart 10-2. Using either triage system, victims are tagged (Figs. 10-1 and 10-2) or marked in some other obvious manner (*e.g.,* grease pencil on forehead) to communicate the extent of injuries and urgency of need for care

to other rescue workers and emergency responders. All first responders should be knowledgeable about the disaster plans in their communities and the triage classifications used. Participation in disaster simulations facilitates practice and learning in disaster scene triage and patient management.

In incidents involving multiple victims, especially disasters with dozens of casualties, proper triage requires life-and-death decisions for the injured. In order to provide the best level of care to ensure the highest number of survivors, those who are mortally injured but alive are necessarily given a low treatment priority, though this will almost ensure their death. These decisions are best made by an experienced physician. Therefore, in any situation with a large number of casualties, one or more physicians should be present at the site to lead the triage effort. Furthermore, it is not within the province of nonphysician emergency personnel to pronounce a patient dead; however, properly trained ambulance or rescue personnel can and should recognize the signs of death for the purpose of triage until physicians become available.

HOSPITAL TRIAGE

Triage in the hospital must involve decisions to ensure that prompt attention is afforded to the patients who most urgently need care. In a hospital with a large, active emergency department, a continuing annoyance to patients, relatives, and attendants is the long wait that patients with minor complaints must endure as they are bypassed in favor of more acutely ill patients. If facilities are available or can be established, a separate "walk-in" or convenience clinic should be set up for patients with minor or less urgent problems. This arrangement proves beneficial to patients and personnel alike by keeping the less acutely ill patients away from the excitement and bustle accompanying the more severely ill or injured patients.

The design of the emergency department can facilitate this goal, especially if several small, adequately equipped examining rooms are available to allow the staff to care for a large number of patients.

The triage area should be close to the patient entrance area but should allow the patient and examiner a quiet location for examination. The triage room should be properly furnished and include adequate lighting, an examining table, thermometers, sphygmomanometer, stethoscope, otoscope, ophthalmoscope, flashlight and other diagnostic equipment.

The Triage Officer

An important component in such a system is the designation of a member of the emergency department staff, usually an experienced emergency department nurse, to function as the triage officer. This person must have the professional maturity to tolerate the stresses inherent in the wide variety of acute problems seen on a day-to-day basis. The position involves the need to assess the patient's problem rapidly

Chart 10-1

TRIAGE CATEGORIES

Triage Category	Description
I	Injured patients who probably can survive with available appropriate care
II	Seriously injured patients who *may* survive with adequate care
III	Injured patients who can survive with little or no care
IV	Injured patients who exhibit evident signs of death, or who have little possibility for survival given available resources

Chart 10-2

TRIAGE CATEGORY GUIDELINES: Priorities for Triage and Care

In planning and organizing for the care of mass casualties, especially under circumstances in which local medical personnel, hospital facilities, and supplies are scarce, it is necessary to establish a list of priorities for triage and care.

Now (Priority I)

Asphyxia
Respiratory obstruction from mechanical causes
Sucking chest wounds
Tension pneumothorax
Maxillofacial wounds in which asphyxia exists or is likely to develop
Shock caused by major external hemorrhage
Major internal hemorrhage
Visceral injuries or evisceration
Cardiopericardial injuries
Massive muscle damage
Severe burns *over* 25% or burns with respiratory involvement
Dislocations
Major fractures
Major medical problems that are readily correctible
Closed cerebral injuries with increasing loss of consciousness

Later (Priority II)

Vascular injuries requiring repair
Wounds of the genitourinary tract
Thoracic wounds without asphyxia
Severe burns under 25%
Spinal cord injuries requiring decompression
Suspected spinal cord injuries without neurologic signs
Lesser fractures
Injuries of the eye
Maxillofacial injuries without asphyxia
Minor medical problems
Victims with little hope of survival under the best of circumstances of medical care

(Council of Santa Clara Valley Medical Society, Medical Catastrophic Disaster Plan for Santa Clara County, April 1980)

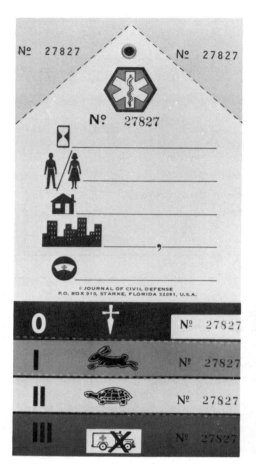
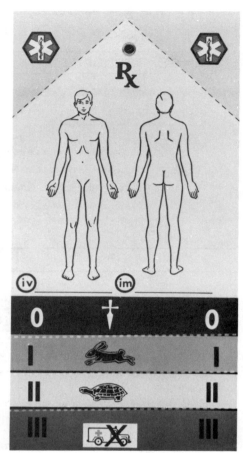

Figure 10-1 *Example of triage tag for sorting victims into one of four categories. This commercially available tag is color coded and perforated and provides information about the victim's injuries and destination. Color code: Triage category 0 is indicated by black, I by red, II by yellow, and III by green. (METTAG [Medical emergency triage tag], Starke, Florida)*

and make informed judgments on priorities of care. In addition, the triage officer must maintain a calm composure that serves to reassure and settle excited patients and relatives. Triage training includes didactic and practical experience in history taking, physical assessment, and interpretation of the collected data. In addition, the triage officer must know how to handle patients who are hostile, intoxicated, belligerent, frightened, anxious, or in pain and how to work against odds to establish rapport with the patient and relatives. The learning experience is an ongoing process that continues during the working period as one gains experience with patients, their families, and their friends.

The triage officer, as the first person in the emergency department to interview the patient, must gather and document as many facts as possible from prehospital emergency personnel, law enforcement officers, or family and friends of the patient. She or he also coordinates activities outside the emergency department, such as dealing with the press and facilitating the patient's acquisition of other services (social service, clinic appointments, resources for continuing care).

The triage officer must be organized, clear thinking, and able to communicate with many different people on a variety of levels. She or he must be an expert clinician with a broad knowledge and experience base and astute assessment skills.

Emergency Department Triage

The triage officer receives and records as much pertinent information as possible about the patient's reason for seeking care. This begins with a clear statement of the chief complaint in the patient's own words, followed by historical data and related relevant information, such as time of onset, duration of symptom(s), what aggravates or relieves the symptom(s), and so on. A brief physical assessment is done; an overall evaluation is made of the acuteness and severity of the condition, and vital signs are checked. From these data, the triage officer can judge the gravity of the problem and determine the need for immediate or delayed care.

Patients with acute conditions that threaten life or limb should receive the highest priority; those with chronic disease or minor illness or injury are assigned a lower priority. It is not possible to categorize the patient correctly in all instances, but it is better to err on the side of more serious illness. Priorities of care related to specific presenting signs and symptoms are discussed later in this chapter.

The triage officer may initiate diagnostic tests, such as x-rays and laboratory work, to facilitate treatment. All data are recorded on the emergency department patient care record or on a triage record. The triage record may be a checklist or flow sheet that allows for optimal collection of

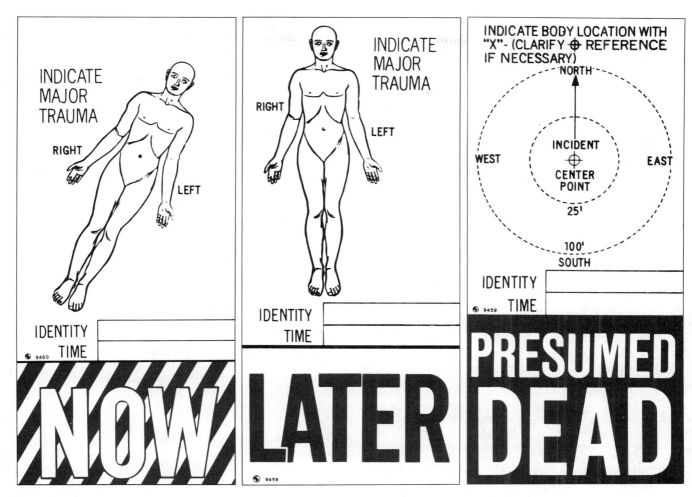

Figure 10-2 *Examples of triage tags for sorting victims into one of three categories. (Council of the Santa Clara County Medical Society, Medical Catastrophic Disaster Plan for Santa Clara County, April, 1980)*

information in a manner that is easily read and understood by those who give definitive care to the patient. The triage sheet should become a permanent part of the hospital record.

STEPS IN TRIAGE

HISTORY AND GENERAL SURVEY

History

Initially note the general appearance of the patient and obtain a more detailed history about the chief complaint and principal symptoms that brought the patient to the hospital. When inquiring about the problem, its time of onset, and its duration, seek the patient's own opinion on the severity and acuteness of his symptoms. Often the patient may provide some information that alerts the listener to a serious condition that is not immediately apparent. An apprehensive patient whose fears cause him to magnify a minor problem should be encouraged to voice his concerns; an explanation of his condition may be all that is needed to allay his anxiety. Other important information to be elicited and recorded includes:

- Previously diagnosed chronic diseases such as diabetes, heart, kidney, or lung disease, or cancer
- Abnormal bleeding tendencies (try to have the patient quantitate his loss as accurately as possible)
- History of allergies or drug sensitivities
- Medications formerly or currently used by the patient, especially cardiac drugs, antihypertensives, diuretics, tranquilizers or other sedatives, narcotics, steroids, hormones, anti-inflammatory drugs, aspirin, analgesics, anticoagulants, and antibiotics
- Prior hospitalizations or surgical procedures

General Survey

This phase of the assessment is performed to some extent during the history taking.

1. Note the *general appearance* of the patient and his awareness of his surroundings. His *state of consciousness* can be graded between the extremes of alertness and orientation to coma. Note the level of consciousness *and* any change in this state during the period of observation (see Chap. 18, The Comatose Patient).

2. Observe for *restlessness* or unusual activity. Restlessness is often due to low blood oxygen (hypoxemia) and may indicate that the patient with blood loss or a pulmonary or cardiac problem is on the verge of decompensation.

3. *Abnormalities of color,* such as jaundice or cyanosis, are best observed in the mucous membranes, nail beds, or lines of the palms of the hands in dark-skinned people. Record any abnormalities.

4. *Abnormalities of speech* (slurring, hesitation) may be the earliest or most obvious sign of neurologic damage. If the observer is not certain of the color or speech patterns of the patient, confirm through consultation with a relative or friend whether either are normal. This applies to other possible aberrations in behavior or appearance as well.

5. *Vital signs* must be considered in the light of circumstances at the time.

   - *Pulse.* Normal resting pulse rate in the adult is generally 65 to 80. Because of the nervous tension felt by many patients in the emergency department, rates of 80 to 90 or higher may reflect nothing more than excitement or apprehension. Conversely, some patients, especially well-conditioned athletes, have a normal pulse of 60 or lower per minute. Even after trauma, they may have little increase in pulse rate. Rates of 50 to 60 do not necessarily indicate a pathologic condition. However, slowing of the pulse frequently accompanies spinal cord injury, and when found in a comatose patient, may be a sign of serious brain damage. A pulse rate below 40 almost always indicates heart block, which is clearly abnormal and demands further study. Although the pulse rate characteristically rises in traumatic shock, this is not always the case, and occasionally patients with all other signs of profound shock will exhibit pulse rates of 75 to 80 per minute.

     While palpating the pulse, note its rhythm. Determine whether it is regular, or marked by skipped or extra beats, or grossly irregular. Alterations in the rhythm may indicate cardiac abnormality.

   - *Blood pressure* values normally range from 110 to 140 mm Hg systolic to 70 to 90 mm Hg diastolic, with some exceptions. Blood pressure normally varies with the position of the patient (lower when recumbent and higher when standing). Also, it must be evaluated in light of the patient's past history. For example, a blood pressure of 120/70, normal in most people, may represent shock level in a patient who usually has a pressure of 190/120. The patient or a relative may be able to give the patient's "normal," or usual, values.

   - *Respiration.* The character and rate of respiration may be significant. Dyspnea may indicate chronic lung disease, pneumothorax, cardiac decompensation, or pulmonary thromboembolus, or it may mean that a simple upper respiratory infection has become complicated by pneumonia. The patient with a healthy pink color who exhibits a deep respiratory effort at rest (Kussmaul breathing) may be a diabetic in ketoacidosis. Slow, shallow breathing may indicate a drug overdose.

ESTABLISHING PRIORITIES OF CARE

To provide guidelines for triage, certain clinical symptoms or conditons are grouped in order of importance. Highest priority conditions demand immediate medical attention.

Highest Priority

Acute Respiratory Difficulty. Acute respiratory difficulty with cyanosis or respiratory stridor in the undiagnosed patient may rapidly lead to death. A patient with acute respiratory infection or acute laryngitis may breathe noisily and have frequent coughing episodes that may further embarrass his respiration. When such a patient is working hard at breathing and exhibits a high-pitched inspiratory crow, his functional respiratory balance may decompensate rapidly, with coma and death following in minutes. Note respiratory rate *and* ventilation. Acute respiratory distress, especially when accompanied by cyanosis or stridor, is a high-priority emergency. (See Chap. 15, Respiratory Emergencies.)

Seizure. A person in seizure requires immediate attention and protection from hurting himself, even though he may be a known epileptic. The patient in seizure with no prior history or diagnosis requires urgent care and diligent investigation to identify the etiology of the seizure, whether cerebral injury, anoxia, drug withdrawal, or other cause. This patient must be watched closely for any sign of deterioration.

Coma. The patient in coma needs prompt initiation of diagnostic and therapeutic measures to forestall brain injury or imminent death. (See Chap. 18, The Comatose Patient, and Chap. 20, Injuries to the Head, Neck, and Spine.)

Shock. Both the shock state and its underlying cause(s) demand a high priority of care. Shock is a dynamic, unstable condition that may worsen rapidly. If untreated, it may result in damage to the brain, kidney, liver, and heart and can lead to death quite suddenly, even when the patient's general condition appears fairly good up to the point of cardiac arrest. Sudden decompensation is unpredictable.

Chest Pain, Dyspnea, Cyanosis. The patient with chest pain, acute dyspnea, or cyanosis may have an acute life-threatening condition such as a tension pneumothorax or severe acute myocardial infarction. This is especially true if the patient's blood pressure is below its normal baseline level.

Severe Hemorrhage. Severe hemorrhage from whatever cause is a high-priority condition, especially when accompanied by pallor and restlessness such as are found in oxygen hunger. A patient in this condition may progress rapidly to shock without prompt intervention.

Multiple Injuries. The patient with multiple injuries must be examined promptly to detect evidence of impending shock and initiate measures to treat it. Potentially life-threatening injuries must be identified and treatment initiated as outlined under *The Trauma Patient,* below.

High Fever. The patient with fever over 40.5°C (105°F) may soon experience seizures or delirium and requires prompt attention.

Secondary Priority

The following conditions are less urgent than those described above, but nonetheless require treatment promptly or as soon as possible.

Decrease in Level of Consciousness. The patient in whom the state of consciousness is dulled or obtunded requires observation. If this patient shows evidence that his condition is deteriorating, he requires a higher priority of care.

Chest Pain. Chest pain must be considered a sign of a potentially urgent condition, especially if it suggests myocardial ischemia (squeezing, crushing, vise-like substernal pain with radiation to the neck, shoulder, arm, or hand). Any undiagnosed chest pain is similarly urgent.

Dyspnea, Cyanosis. Dyspnea or cyanosis is a sign of respiratory or ventilatory decompensation. Although the patient's condition may otherwise appear to be good, the underlying cause should be recognized and treated as soon as possible, since in many situations deterioration may progress rapidly.

Bleeding. Active bleeding, unless readily and promptly controlled, should receive prompt attention, even if there are no signs of shock. This includes active gastrointestinal bleeding, the precise amount of which is always difficult to estimate, and severe bleeding from incomplete abortions. Bleeding patients may seem relatively stable when first seen, and then rapidly develop shock.

Prolonged Emesis, Diarrhea. Continuous or repeated bouts of emesis or diarrhea demand care without delay to make the patient comfortable and to correct fluid and electrolyte imbalance. The condition may progress to shock if untreated.

Severe Pain. Patients with severe pain of any type need prompt attention because of the potential threat of the underlying cause, *e.g.,* perforated ulcer, pancreatitis, dissecting aneurysm. Though analgesia can obscure findings necessary to make an accurate diagnosis, humane treatment demands relief of the pain *as soon as possible* after adequate steps have been taken to establish a diagnosis.

Fever. Persons with fevers of 38.8°C to 40.5°C (102°F–105°F) deserve attention as soon as possible. Although some of these patients will have readily treatable low-mortality conditions, others may be dangerously ill.

Caution Indicators

Some presenting symptoms should alert the triage officer to the possibility of impending danger for the patient. When a patient presents with the following symptoms, close observation is required until medical attention is available.

Disorientation. Any alteration in orientation, mentation, or consciousness or sudden onset of severe headache in a previously well patient falls into this category.

Chest Pain and Abdominal Pain. Chest pain and abdominal pain can be symptomatic of many conditions, ranging from mild disorders to mortal illnesses. The most dangerous disease can have an insidious onset, so that when care is first sought, the pain may be mild and may be the only symptom, the others not having surfaced. The patient's condition can worsen in a relatively short time. For example, the patient with a spontaneous pneumothorax may at onset have mild pain with no interference with respiratory efficiency. This may convert to a tension pneumothorax, leading to extreme hypoxia and death in a short time if untreated.

Tachycardia. A heart rate of 120 beats per minute or more at rest, without apparent reason, demands careful consideration. It may be due to obscure hemorrhage, incipient cardiac failure, "silent" myocardial infarction, hyperthyroidism, or other serious but obscure conditions.

Injury in the Alcoholic. The injured alcoholic or drug-dependent patient often presents a problem in diagnosis because the effects of alcohol may obscure or confuse the diagnosis of all types of injuries. Of particular concern is the presence of a concomitant head injury.

Comatose Patient With Injuries. The injured patient in coma requires special consideration. Since he is unable to give a history, it is most important that the first staff member who comes in contact with the patient obtain as much information as possible from those who accompanied the patient to the hospital. Cervical spine injury *must* be suspected in all such patients. Therefore, measures must be taken to protect the cervical spine until fracture or dislocation is ruled out by appropriate x-rays that demonstrate *all seven cervical vertebrae.*

Special precautions must be taken in evaluating and treating comatose patients who may be, or are known to have been, taking drugs, such as alcohol, or patients who have diabetes. Finding the cause of the coma in such a patient may be difficult but can be accomplished with appropriate diagnostic studies. (See Chap. 18, The Comatose Patient.)

THE TRAUMA PATIENT

PREHOSPITAL ASSESSMENT

To assist prehospital emergency personnel in identifying high-risk trauma victims, the American College of Surgeons

Committee on Trauma has developed a scheme of field categorization of trauma patients on the basis of anatomic injuries and physiologic derangement (Chart 10-3). The purpose of this approach is to grade the severity of the injury in order to ensure transport of the patient to the proper facility.

Theoretically, the application of this plan would mean that the most severely injured patient category is transported to a Level I or Level II hospital, depending on available resources. However, rigid matching of patients to appropriate levels of care may be impractical depending on the size of the community and the availability of resources. The field categorization schemes are intended as guidelines for health professionals and may require modification to suit community need.

PREHOSPITAL CARE

The patient with serious or potentially serious multiple injuries due to trauma is unique. The infinite variety of combinations of injuries of varying relative importance makes

---

Chart 10-3

FIELD CATEGORIZATION OF TRAUMA PATIENTS

System	Category 1	Category 2	Category 3
Soft tissue	Avulsion type injuries, severe uncontrolled bleeding	Soft-tissue injuries with stabilized bleeding	Soft-tissue injuries of moderate degree
Fractures	Open fractures, pelvic fractures, severe maxillofacial injuries	Single open or closed fractures	Uncomplicated fractures
Abdomen	Blunt or penetrating abdominal injuries especially when associated with hypotension	Blunt abdominal or penetrating trauma not producing hypotension	No abdominal injuries
Chest	Unstable chest injuries, respiratory rate > 30 or < 10	Multiple rib fractures without flailed segments, respiratory rate > 20 or < 10	No respiratory distress, respiratory rate 10–20
Head and neck, upper respiratory	Severe maxillofacial injuries, open penetrating and blunt trauma to face, neck, and cervical spine, multiple facial fractures, and injuries affecting vision	Facial trauma with single facial fractures, (without airway or major cervical vascular or cervical spine involvement)	Simple contusions of the head and neck, nasal fractures
Neurologic	Prolonged loss of consciousness, posturing, lateralizing signs, open cranial injuries, paralysis	Transient loss of consciousness, oriented to time, place, and person	No neurologic injuries
Vital signs	BP < 90 systolic P > 100 or < 60 Skin—cool, ashen, pale	BP > 90 systolic P—60–100 Skin—warm to slightly cool	BP > 100 systolic P—60–100 Skin—dry, warm

(American College of Surgeons Committee on Trauma: Field Categorization of Trauma Patients and Hospital Trauma Index, Bulletin of American College of Surgeons, Appendix E, p 29. February, 1980)

it impossible to follow a single pattern of assessment and treatment. Generally, priorities of care can be established so that the most urgent conditions are dealt with first. Priorities of care for trauma patients occur in the following order of decreasing urgency:

A—airway patency with control of the cervical spine
B—breathing to ensure adequate ventilation
C—circulation support, including assessment of the circulation (heart rate and quality, skin color and moisture, level of consciousness), and control of hemorrhage
D—wound care
E—fracture immobilization

1. *Airway patency and adequate ventilatory exchange* must be assured early on. The most common conditions that seriously affect airway patency and ventilatory exchange include maxillofacial fractures, open or sucking wounds of the chest, tension pneumothorax, and multiple segmental rib fractures with flail chest. Each demands recognition and stabilization.

2. *Cervical spine fracture* must be suspected in any trauma victim who is unconscious, has a maxillofacial injury, severe multiple trauma, or any injury above the clavicle. In the conscious trauma patient consider such an injury when there is evidence of paralysis or sensory deficit, by history or physical assessment. (See Chap. 20, Injuries to the Head, Neck, and Spine.)

3. Treatment of *shock* and *external hemorrhage* by the application of pressure dressings combined with restoration of circulating blood volume by intravenous fluid replacement is the next priority of care. This should be done by appropriately trained personnel. The application of a pneumatic antishock garment (PASG) is beneficial in the management of patients with major blood loss and fractures of the lower extremities.

   How long an injured patient in uncontrolled shock can survive is unpredictable. It is common for a patient in hemorrhagic shock to maintain a blood pressure barely adequate to preserve consciousness and some urine output and then collapse suddenly and die within a few minutes.

4. In the field, *open wounds* are carefully examined and covered with dry, sterile dressings. No attempt is made to cleanse the wound. Objects with which the patient is impaled should not be removed. Active bleeding is controlled with pressure dressings on the site and elevation of the part when possible. If the patient has suffered an amputation, the amputated part should be found and placed in a sterile wrapping, preferably cooled, to be taken to the hospital with the patient.

5. *Fractures,* when present or suspected, are immobilized in the position in which they were found in order to alleviate pain and minimize the possibility of further injury during transport. When a grossly displaced fracture or dislocation produces circulatory or neurologic deficit(s) in the distal limb, repositioning may restore function. Wounds involving bones and joints are more susceptible to infection than other wounds of the extremities are. Dry, sterile dressings are placed on wounds that occur with open fractures. (See Chap. 32 for detailed discussion of musculoskeletal injuries).

   Generally, *head injury* is less urgent than the three top-priority conditions (airway, breathing, and circulation). However, an open fracture of the skull demands prompt

cleansing and debridement. Urgent action is also required by the patient suspected of having an epidural hemorrhage. Prompt decompression with control of intracranial bleeding may lead to a successful result. The patient must be transported promptly and supportive care administered en route.

HOSPITAL ASSESSMENT AND CARE

Some clinical conditions that are commonly encountered in trauma patients are discussed in the section that follows. However, no such list can be considered complete, and although the relative urgency of each condition is indicated, the word *relative* is significant. Keeping this relativity in mind, some problems in the care of the trauma victim can be considered in the context of the general order of priorities discussed above. Hemorrhage means abnormal bleeding. Bleeding from a cut finger, while occasionally frightening to the patient, is rarely significant to his health; yet in the hemophiliac the same injury assumes much greater importance. Furthermore, bleeding from a severed femoral artery poses an immediate threat to life until it is controlled.

Highest Priority

1. *Progressively increasing dyspnea* requires immediate attention. Acute cessation of respiration or total obstruction of the airway is incompatible with more than a few minutes of life. However, many patients exhibit some degree of difficulty in breathing after injury, ranging from mild limitation because of pain from one or two fractured ribs to more acute problems related to other serious chest wall, oral, or cervical injuries. These more obvious injuries usually get the prompt attention they demand. However, the patient who comes to the emergency department with little or no respiratory difficulty and then experiences it with increasing severity may be developing a tension pneumothorax or compression of the trachea from hematoma.

2. *Shock unresponsive to adequate fluid replacement therapy* (rapid infusion through two or three large intravenous needles or catheters) requires urgent intervention. The patient with this condition most often has massive bleeding, usually concealed, and a decision about an immediate operation must be made at once.

3. *Progressively declining pulse pressure and rising venous pressure,* the latter often obvious from distended neck veins, indicate probable cardiac tamponade. Here, too, speed in making a diagnosis and instituting treatment is life-saving, and the time available may be short.

Secondary Priority

The following are situations of a slightly lower order of urgency but still calling for very careful observation and prompt attention:

1. *Airway or chest wall problems producing dyspnea or cyanosis of a minor degree* may not appear to be serious when first seen, but coupled with continued blood loss and fatigue from the effects of bleeding and other injuries, may result in rapid decompensation and deterioration. The basic mechanical problem must be evaluated promptly. In the meantime, the patient needs support

HOSPITAL TRAUMA INDEX

	initial impression	Name _____ Hosp. # _____ Date Adm. _____ Discharge _____	final impression		
SYSTEM		**INJURY**		**CLASS**	**INDEX**
RESPIRATORY		NO INJURY		no injury	0
		chest discomfort—minimal findings		minor	1
		simple rib or sternal fracture (fx), chest wall contusion with pleuritic pain		moderate	2
		1st or multi-rib fx, hemothorax, pneumothorax		major	3
		open chest wounds, flail chest, tension pneumothorax normal (nl) blood pressure (bp), simple lac diaphragm		severe	4
		acute resp. failure (cyanosis), aspiration, tension pneumo. c̄ ↓ bp, bilateral flail, lac(s) diaphragm		critical	5
CARDIOVASCULAR		NO INJURY		no injury	0
		<10% (<500 cc) blood volume (bv) loss. no change in skin perfusion		minor	1
		10–20% bv loss (500–1000 cc). ↓ skin perfusion, urine normal (+30 cc/hr). myocard. cont. bp normal		moderate	2
		20–30% bv loss (1000–1500 cc). ↓ skin perfusion, urine (>30 cc). tamponade, bp 80.		major	3
		30–40% bv loss (1500–2000 cc). ↓ skin perfusion, urine (<10 cc). tamponade, conscious, bp < 80.		severe	4
		40–50% bv loss. restless, agitated, coma, cardiac contusion or arrhythmia, bp not obtainable.		critical	5
		50% + bv loss. Coma. Cardiac arrest. No vital signs		fatal	6
NERVOUS SYSTEM		NO INJURY		no injury	0
		head trauma c̄ or s̄ scalp lactns. no loss consciousness (coma). no fracture (fx).		minor	1
		head trauma c̄ brief coma (<15′), skull fx, cervical pain c̄ minimal fndgs, one facial fx.		moderate	2
		cerebral injury c̄ coma (+15′). depressed skull fx. cervical fx c̄ neuro fndgs. multi facial fxs.		major	3
		cerebral injury c̄ coma (+60′) or neuro findings. cervical fx c̄ major neuro findings, i.e., paraplegia		severe	4
		cerebral injury c̄ coma c̄ no response to stimuli up to 24 hrs. Cervical fx c̄ *quadriplegia*		critical	5
		cerebral injury c̄ no response to stimuli & c̄ dilated fixed pupil(s).		fatal	6

Figure 10-3 *Example of a hospital trauma index. (American College of Surgeons Committee on Trauma: Field categorization of trauma patients and index, Bulletin of American College of Surgeons, Appendix E, pp. 32–33. February 1980)*

SYSTEM	initial impression	HOSPITAL TRAUMA INDEX INJURY	final impression	CLASS	INDEX
ABDOMINAL		NO INJURY		no injury	0
		mild abdominal wall, flank or back pain & tenderness s̄ peritoneal signs.		minor	1
		acute flank, back or abdominal discomfort and tenderness. fx of a rib 7–12.		moderate	2
		one of: minor liver, sm bowel, spleen, kidney, body pancr. mesentery, ureter, urethra. fxs 7–12 rib		major	3
		2 major: rupture liver, bladder, head pancr, duodenum, colon, mesentery (large).		severe	4
		2 severe: crush liver. Major vascular including: thor & abdom aorta, cavae, iliacs, hepatic veins		critical	5
EXTREMITIES		NO INJURY		no injury	0
		minor sprains & fx(s)—no long bones		minor	1
		simple fx(s): humerus, clavicle, radius, ulna, tibia, fibula. single nerve		moderate	2
		fx(s) multiple moderate, cpd moderate, femur (simple), pelvic (stable), dislocation major, major nerve		major	3
		fx(s) two major, cpd femur, limb crush or amputation, unstable pelvic fx.		severe	4
		fx(s) two severe, multiple major		critical	5
SKIN & SUBCUTANEOUS		NO INJURY		no injury	0
		<5% burn. abrasions, contusions, lacerations		minor	1
		5–15% burn. extensive contusions, avulsions 3–6″ extensive lacerations (total 12″2).		moderate	2
		15–30% burn. avulsions 12″2+.		major	3
		30–45% burn. avulsions entire leg, thigh or arm		severe	4
		45–60% burn (3rd degree)		critical	5
		60%+ burn (3rd degree)		fatal	6
		COMPLICATIONS			
		NO SIGNIFICANT COMPLICATIONS		none	0
		subq. wound infection, atelectasis, cystitis. superficial thrombophlebitis. temp < 38.5° (101 °F).		minor	1
		major wound infection, atelectasis, pyelonephritis septic or deep thrombophlebitis. temp > 38.5°.		moderate	2

SYSTEM	initial impression	HOSPITAL TRAUMA INDEX COMPLICATIONS	final impression	CLASS	INDEX
		i.p. abscess, pneumonia, anuria or oliguria c̄ ↑ BUN (no dialysis). jaundice. <6 u gi bleed. rds < 1 day		major	3
		septicemia, empyema, peritonitis, pulm embolis (nl bp). renal failure (dialysis < 1 wk) > 6 u bleed < 3 d rds.		severe	4
		septicemia c̄ ↓ bp. pulm emb c̄ ↓ bp. renal failure 7–40 d. gi bleed > 12 u. resp arrest. > 3 d rds c̄ vent.		critical	5
		pulm emb c̄ card arrest. cardiac arrest. renal fail > 6 wks. coma > 6 wks. > 30 d rds c̄ vent or > 80% O_2 > 7 d.		fatal	6

DEFINITIONS:

minor = trivial injury

moderate = minimal injury, short hospitalization anticipated

major = major injury, not immediately life-threatening

severe = life-threatening but survival probable

critical = survival uncertain

fatal = survival unlikely

ABBREVIATIONS:

bp—blood pressure

bv—blood volume

cpd—compound

c̄—with

d—days

fndgs—findings

fx—fracture

i.p.—intraperitoneal

lac-lactns—lacerations

mult—multiple

nl—normal

rds—resp. distress synd.

s̄—without

sgns—signs

u—units

vent—ventilator

wnd—wound

↑—increased

↓—decreased

>—greater than

<—less than

Brief History: _____

_____

_____

for his overloaded respiratory function. When available, blood gas studies are invaluable in following the progress of treatment of such problems.

2. *Neck injuries producing stridor and dyspnea* need immediate care. Increasing edema around an injury of the larynx or trachea may produce rapid changes in the patient's ability to breathe.

3. *Hypotension with no obvious hemorrhage* should lead to a prompt search for sites of potential occult bleeding. These may include abdominal injury producing splenic or hepatic damage or fractures of the pelvis, femur, or other long bones. A myocardial contusion that is interfering with cardiac function may produce hypotension, often with few other symptoms of heart injury. Brain injury does not produce hypotension until the final stage of decompensation, just before death. Hence, the patient with an altered level of consciousness who develops hypotension must be considered to have some injury in addition to his head injury.

4. The patient whose shock responds at first to replacement therapy only to develop *hypotension without apparent cause* almost certainly has undiscovered bleeding. Further diagnosis and treatment become an urgent need.

5. Evidence of *continued intrathoracic bleeding* (physical findings, x-ray evidence, or thoracostomy tube drainage) call for very close observation of patients. If profuse or obviously from arterial sources, such continued bleeding demands open operation.

6. *Gunshot wounds in the vicinity of large vessels* should be treated with the greatest caution. Even though distal pulses are apparently normal, serious damage may have occurred, and such patients should be watched carefully for changes in color, temperature and pulse, as well as for external bleeding or hematoma formation at the site of injury.

7. *Progressive or unusual swelling* in the presence of already apparent or obscure injury should be noted. Its presence will give a clue to massive bleeding. This can occur with few other symptoms in intra-abdominal injury. It can also be seen as a result of fractures of the pelvis or femur, when massive swelling of hips or thighs reveals extensive hemorrhage. Appropriate blood replacement may consist of many units of blood, and immediate surgical intervention is frequently needed.

Caution Indicators

These are situations in which the observer must be doubly cautious in examining, reexamining, and carefully observing the patient.

1. *The person who has been subjected to a great force* needs close watching; for example, the pedestrian who is struck

by a car, the person who has fallen from a considerable height (15 feet or more), or one who was in a car that crashed at high speed and who initially appears to have no injuries. Such patients must be assumed to have all manner of injuries and must be examined carefully and repeatedly over a period of hours. It is fortunate for the patient that in such circumstances he is often rushed to the hospital within minutes after his accident. But the nurse or physician who first sees the patient may have too little time to observe for symptoms of shock, respiratory distress, or coma to develop, and the temptation is great to do a quick examination and discharge the patient. If this is done, occasionally a serious injury may be overlooked, and eventual definitive treatment undertaken too late.

2. Any person with a history of *loss of consciousness* must be treated seriously. This situation may require a long period of observation, 12 to 24 hours or more.

3. The "frightened boy" who may have been injured while doing something he should not have been doing may tend to *minimize his symptoms and thereby obscure a serious injury*. Indeed, the young boy of 8 to 10 years is often trying to preserve his machismo by denying pain or other symptoms that could help the examiner find obscure and often serious injuries.

4. The *injured alcoholic* is often a problem in diagnosis, because the effects of alcohol may obscure or confuse the diagnosis of all types of injuries. There frequently is no way to rule out serious injury (especially head injury) in the intoxicated patient except by a period of observation long enough for the acute stupor and analgesia of the alcohol to wear off.

5. Special consideration is essential for *the injured patient in coma*. First, since the patient can give no history, it is of paramount importance that the first emergency department staff member who sees the injured person obtain as much information as possible from those who accompanied the patient to the hospital.

Second, until ruled out by appropriate means, the comatose patient should be assumed to have injuries that could be aggravated by injudicious handling. This means that the patient must be moved as if he had cervical or other spinal injuries until they are ruled out by x-ray. Fractures of the extremities must be ruled out by careful examination, and by x-ray if indicated. Appropriate splinting or support must be used in moving such patients until the exact nature and extent of the injuries are known. (See Chap. 20, Injuries to the Head, Neck, and Spine.)

Physical findings such as tenderness may be altered by coma, but only in the most deeply comatose patient is tenderness completely obliterated. Moreover, muscle spasm created by adjacent injury is not obliterated by head injury and is revealed by careful examination.

Special caution should be exercised in comatose patients who may be or are known to have been taking various drugs, including alcohol, or who have diabetes. Discovering the precise cause of the coma in these patients may be difficult but can be done if all possibilities are considered and appropriate studies carried out.

One means of standardizing and quantitating degrees of injury is the use of the Hospital Trauma Index (Fig. 10-3). Injuries to systems are evaluated and given a numerical value from 0 to 6, according to severity. These guidelines for grading patient injury facilitate comparison of mortality and morbidity in patient groups and may promote improvement in emergency postoperative and rehabilitative care within a community or region.

BIBLIOGRAPHY

Albin SL, Wassertheil-Smoller S et al: Evaluation of emergency room triage performed by nurses. Am J Public Health 65:1063–1068, 1975

Estrada EG: Advanced triage by a RN. Journal of Emergency Nursing 5:15–18, November–December 1979

Gross PL, Schmiedel S: Emergency ward triage. In Wilkins EW Jr (ed): MGH Textbook of Emergency Medicine. Baltimore, Williams & Wilkins, 1978

Mills J et al: Effectiveness of nurse triage in the emergency department of an urban county hospital. JACEP 5:877–882, 1976

Nyberg J: Perceptions of patient problems in the emergency department. Journal of Emergency Nursing 4:15–19, January–February 1978

Willis DT: A study of nursing triage. Journal of Emergency Nursing 5:8–11, November–December 1979

11
LABORATORY STUDIES

JAMES H. COSGRIFF, JR. and PAULA BAUDA

The hospital clinical laboratory plays an important role in providing emergency personnel with data for use in the diagnosis and treatment of the acutely ill or injured patient. The relevance of the information depends in part on its ready availability and accuracy. The results of laboratory tests on emergency patients may aid in the early diagnosis of disease, in differentiating one disease process from another, and in determining the activity of the disease and the effect of therapy.

The services provided usually include hematology, biochemistry, urinalysis, blood banking, bacteriology, and pathology. The range of services in a given hospital depends on its size, the nature of its patient load, and the activity of its emergency department. A large urban hospital center must have a full range of services available on a 24-hour, 7-day-a-week basis, whereas a small community or rural hospital may have a narrower range of services available for a limited number of hours per day. Many small hospitals contract with larger hospitals or independent laboratories to supplement their own capabilities with a broader range of services, especially less commonly used tests.

Test and Measurement Systems

With the advent of automation, a battery of biochemical and hematologic tests has become available. The instruments used may be capable of performing as many as 12 tests at a time, and test results are presented in a computer printout sheet that records both daily and cumulative results (Fig. 11-1). These tests are referred to collectively as sequential multiple analysis (SMA). One or more of several available computerized analysis systems may be used. The battery of tests performed includes biochemical and electrolyte determinations in addition to routine hematologic analyses (a complete blood count).

Test results are reported in a variety of terms, depending on the nature of the element or compound being evaluated. The metric system is used most commonly (Table 11-1), although test results may also be expressed as volumes, partial pressures, units, or dilutions.

Milligrams percent (mg%) and milligrams per deciliter (mg/dl) are used interchangeably. Blood gases are reported in millimeters of mercury (mm Hg) or Torr (international unit of reference).

Emergency personnel should be familiar with the tests available to them and should know the method of reporting and the normal range of values for each in order to interpret the results properly in light of the patient's clinical status.

Although certain factors such as age, chronic disease states, and some medications may cause alterations in data, these data may be considered within normal limits for a specific patient at a given time. For example, the oxygen content (pO_2) of arterial blood ranges from 60 to 70 mm Hg in the newborn, 75 to 85 mm Hg in patients over age 65, and 80 to 90 mm Hg in a normal adult. The patient with chronic obstructive pulmonary disease normally has an elevated pCO_2 and lowered pO_2 in arterial blood. Similarly, the time of day may also influence the test data. Plasma cortisol values are normally highest in the morning (7 to 25 μg/dl) and lower in the evening (2 to 9 μg/dl).

Collection and Disposition of Specimen(s)

Proper collection and disposition of the specimen(s) involves several important considerations, as follows:
- The patient must be correctly identified as the source of the specimen.
- The specimen must be labeled correctly.
- The correct type of container must be used.
- When indicated, an appropriate anticoagulant or preservative should be added to the specimen and mixed properly with it. For example, blood should be mixed gently with anticoagulant or preservative in order to prevent hemolysis.
- Sampling in a limb in which an intravenous line is in place should be avoided.
- Incorrect or prolonged application of a tourniquet combined with fist exercise should be avoided because erroneous laboratory findings may result from this practice.
- *All samples should be taken to the laboratory without delay.*

Specific Laboratory Studies

The number of tests commonly used on emergency patients represents but a fraction of those available in a hospital clinical laboratory. The specific laboratory studies discussed on the following pages are those most often requested in the emergency department. They include methods of evaluating blood, urine, cerebrospinal fluid, abdominal fluid, thoracic fluid, wound fluid, and body discharges.

BLOOD STUDIES

Blood is sampled and tested more than any other body fluid. The main categories of blood tests include the following:
- Hematology
  Complete blood count
  Differential count
  Platelet count
  Sedimentation rate
- Coagulation
  Prothrombin time
  Partial thromboplastin time
  Bleeding time
  Fibrinogen
- Biochemistry
  SMA-6
  SMA-12
- Other
  Serum amylase
  Serum lipase
  Ammonia
  Creatine phosphokinase (CPK)
  Blood gases
  Culture

```
                              CUMULATIVE REPORT

                *** FOR PEDIATRIC REFERENCE VALUES SEE SEPARATE SHEET IN CHART ***

                                      09/21
        Jane Doe                AGE  68                      4 WEST
        595743                  SEX  F                       ROOM NO.  45
                                                             DR. COSGRIFF
```

CHEMISTRY		NA	K	CL	CO2	BUN	GLUC	2 HR GLUC
REF VALUES		(135-145)	(3.5-5.0)	(95-105)	(24-32)	(10-20)	(65-110)	(65-110)
9/06	0815AM	134*	5.0	98	26	5*	206*	
9/07	0700AM	132*	5.0	97	23*	17	214*	
9/09	0805AM	130*	5.3*	98	20*	23*	153*	
9/11	0700AM	131*	5.5*	99	21*	27*	265*	
9/13	0700AM	130*	5.2*	97	24	25*	198*	
9/15	0700AM	132*	4.7	99	26	14	310*	
9/17	0700AM	125*	4.8	94*	14	16	185*	
9/18	0700AM	126*	5.0	96	21*	16	166*	
9/19	0700AM	129*	5.2*	95	23*	17	150*	
9/21	0700AM	132*	4.8	98	27	12	102	

CHEMISTRY--SMA		T. PROT.	ALB	CA	P	CHOL	T. BILI
REF VALUES		(6.0-8.0)	(3.5-5.0)	(8.5-10.5)	(2.5-4.5)	(150-300)	(0.15-1.0)
9/06	0815AM	6.8	3.9	10.0	2.7	343*	10.0*
9/07	0700AM	6.7	3.7	9.5	3.5	342*	11.5*
9/09	0805AM	6.8	3.4*	9.8	3.5	351*	15.5*
9/11	0700AM	6.7	3.7	9.6	3.6	380*	6.4*
9/13	0700AM	7.3	4.0	10.3	4.2	352*	4.8*
9/15	0700AM	5.9*	3.2*	9.1	2.8	252	3.6*
9/17	0700AM	5.7*	3.1*	8.7	3.2	225	3.1*
9/18	0700AM	5.8*	3.2*	8.9	3.6	223	2.8*
9/19	0700AM	7.0	3.5	9.3	3.9	229	2.6*
9/21	0700AM	6.4	3.3*	9.3	4.1	219	2.6*

CHEMISTRY--SMA		CREAT	ALK. PHOS	LDH	SGPT	SGOT	URIC ACID
REF VALUES		(0.7-1.4)	(30-105)	(100-225)	(7-40)	(7-40)	(M 3.9-8.5, F 2.2-7.5)
9/06	0815AM	0.8	295*	250*	530*	320*	4.1
9/07	0700AM	0.8	308*	240*	350*	257*	3.7
9/09	0805AM	0.8	334*	207	276*	237*	3.9
9/11	0700AM	0.8	321*	174	146*	128*	3.0
9/13	0700AM	0.7	291*	201	171*	174*	3.1
9/15	0700AM	0.7	254*	186	237*	220*	3.3
9/17	0700AM	0.6*	223*	184	120*	105*	1.9*
9/18	0700AM	0.6*	233*	202	123*	118*	2.7
9/19	0700AM	0.7	249*	268*	187*	189*	2.8
9/21	0700AM	0.8	276*	273*	395*	335*	4.3

CHEM-DISCRETE		T. BILI	D. BILI	CK	LDH	SGOT
REF VALUES		(0.2-1.1)	(0.1-0.4)	(M 0-160, F 0-130)	(109-193)	(10-30)
9/05	0700AM		6.3*			
9/09	0804AM		11.3*			

STAT LAB		SER AMYLASE	LIPASE	U AMYLASE	U AMYLASE--TIMED
REF VALUES		(15-200)	(0-1.5)	(0-500)	(35-275)
9/07	0230PM				62

Figure 11-1 *Example of an SMA printout.*

Type and crossmatch

Toxicology

Collection of Blood

The blood may be drawn from a vein or capillary (finger prick, earlobe prick). If multiple tests are requested, the venous approach is used. All blood necessary for the entire gamut of tests should be drawn at one time in order to lessen the number of venipunctures the patient must endure. The blood is best taken from a vein in which there is no infusion running, because the infusion fluid may cause erroneous results. A proper container appropriately labeled with the patient's name is required. Since the sight of the needle

TABLE 11-1. METRIC SYSTEM MEASUREMENTS

Unit	Abbreviation	Metric Equivalent
Length		
meter	m	
centimeter	cm	1/100 m
millimeter	mm	1/1000 m
micrometer	μm	10^{-6} m (1/1000 mm)
nanometer	nm	10^{-9} m
Weight		
kilogram	kg	
gram	gm	1/1000 kg
milligram	mg	1/1000 gm
microgram	μg	10^{-6} gm (1/1000 mg)
nanogram	ng	10^{-9} gm
picogram	pg	10^{-12} gm
femtogram	fg	10^{-15} gm
Volume		
liter	L	
deciliter	dl	1/100 L
milliliter	ml	1/1000 L
microliter	μl	10^{-6} L (1/1000 ml)

may cause undue apprehension on the part of the patient, calm reassurance by emergency personnel is helpful. Patients tend to imagine that large amounts of blood are being withdrawn, though at the most 30 ml to 50 ml may be taken. Reducing this to its equivalent in teaspoonsful (six to ten) may have a quieting effect on the patient.

HEMATOLOGICAL TESTS

Complete Blood Count

The complete blood count (CBC) consists of a series of tests to determine the numbers and proportions of various entities in the blood. The tests most commonly required in emergency practice are the following: hemoglobin, red blood cell count, hematocrit, reticulocyte count, platelet count, white blood cell count, and differential count. Normal values and test interpretations are summarized in Table 11-2.

Erythrocyte Sedimentation Rate

The erythrocyte sedimentation rate (sed rate or ESR) is the rate at which the red blood cells settle out of unclotted blood in 1 hour. It is measured in millimeters per hour. Depending on the method used, the rate may vary from 0 to 15 mm/hr in men and 0 to 20 mm/hr in women. The ESR is nonspecific and viewed by some as unreliable. It increases in acute disease processes.

BLOOD COAGULATION TESTS

The blood platelets, fibrinogen, and several enzymes make up the coagulation system. Although there are many laboratory tests to evaluate the clotting function of the blood, those used most frequently in the emergency department are the following: platelet count, fibrinogen, prothrombin time, partial thromboplastin time, and bleeding time.

Platelet Count

Platelets play a major role in the clotting process. Causes of aberration in the platelet count are listed in Table 11-2. A low platelet count causes an increase in bleeding time but does not affect the other clotting tests mentioned. The normal platelet count varies from 140,000 to 350,000/mm^3 of blood.

Fibrinogen

Fibrinogen is a protein substance found in the plasma in amounts of 200 to 400 mg/dl. It is essential to the coagulation process. The protein is synthesized in the liver and may be deficient in severe liver disease. Hypofibrinogenemia may be found in disseminated intravascular coagulation, severe bleeding of pregnancy, especially abruptio placentae, and septic abortion and eclampsia. It may be found in snakebite, septicemia, and chronic liver disease, among other conditions.

Prothrombin Time

The prothrombin time (PRO time or PT) is a measure of five different coagulation factors: prothrombin, fibrinogen, and factors V, VII, and X. It is used mainly in evaluating the coagulation process and in maintaining anticoagulant therapy. The PT is measured against a laboratory control and normally should equal the control, which is usually in a range of 10 to 16 seconds. It is unduly prolonged when any of the coagulation factors mentioned above are deficient or when the patient is receiving anticoagulants. This test is important in the initial evaluation of any patient with acute hemorrhage, to identify any preexistent or concurrent coagulation defect or as a baseline for further care. Values in excess of 2½ times the control indicate anticoagulant excess.

Partial Thromboplastin Time

The partial thromboplastin time (PTT) gives a measure of deficiencies in coagulation factors other than VII and XIII. It is not affected by platelet deficiencies. It is also used to evaluate maintenance of anticoagulant therapy with heparin. Values greater than two times the control indicate heparin overdosage. The normal range is less than 1½ to 2 times the control. PTT is an important screening test in patients with acute blood loss, to assist in identifying coagulation defects.

Bleeding Time

The bleeding time is used to measure deficiencies of certain clotting factors, especially platelets. The Ivy method is recommended. The normal range by this method is 3 to 6 minutes. Prolonged bleeding time is found in patients with thrombocytopenia and vascular abnormalities.

TABLE 11-2.   COMPLETE BLOOD COUNT

Test	Abbreviation	Normal Range	Cause of Abnormal Increase	Cause of Abnormal Decrease
Hemoglobin	Hgb or Hb	Men: 14.5–16.5 gm/dl Women: 13.0–15.5 gm/dl	Polycythemia vera Cardiac decompensation Dehydration High altitude	Acute or chronic blood loss Chronic infection Pernicious anemia
Red blood cell count	RBC	Men: 4.8–5.5 million/mm³ Women: 4.4–5.0 million/mm³	Same as above	Same as above
Hematocrit	Hct	Men: 43–50 vol/dl Women: 40–45 vol/dl	Same as above	Same as above
Reticulocytes	Retic	0.5%–1.5% of RBC	Acute blood loss After iron therapy After B_{12} therapy	Decreased RBC formation Hemolytic disease
Platelets		140,000–350,000/mm³	Iron deficiency anemia Malignancy, advanced Postsplenectomy Polycythemia vera Cirrhosis	Thrombocytopenic purpura Hypersplenism
White blood cell count	WBC	6000–9000/mm³	Infections, acute Intoxications, metabolic Acute blood loss Tissue necrosis Leukemia Acute myocardial infarction	Infections, chronic Drugs and chemicals Radiation Hematopoietic disease
Differential count	Diff	Neutrophils: 60%–70% of WBC	Acute infections Acute blood loss Myeloproliferative disease	Chronic infections Drugs Hematopoietic disease
		Lymphocytes: 30%–40% of WBC	Normally higher in children Viral infections Infectious mononucleosis Lymphatic leukemia Mesenteric lymphadenitis	Acute infections
		Basophils: 0%–3% of WBC	Myelogenous leukemia Polycythemia Hodgkin's disease Viral infections	Hyperthyroidism
		Eosinophils: 0%–5% of WBC	Allergic disease Granulomatous bowel disease Parasitic infestation	
		Monocytes: 0%–5% of WBC	Lymphoma Granulomatous bowel disease	

BIOCHEMICAL TESTS

For practical purposes, the vast majority of biochemical tests for emergency patients are those that can be performed with automatic equipment. The names applied to these tests vary from one hospital to another depending on the laboratory equipment used. New micromethods are not available in all hospitals and the volume of the specimen required must be checked with the laboratory. The tests are divided into electrolyte and biochemical determinations, as noted in Table 11-3.

BLOOD CULTURE

Blood is normally sterile. Blood specimens for culture are taken if bacterial invasion is suspected. Infection of the bloodstream tends to be episodic, hence repeated cultures are taken over a 24- to 48-hour period. It is preferable that samples be drawn before antibiotics are started. Specimens must be drawn using sterile technique to minimize the possibility of contamination. They are usually placed in a broth medium and may be subcultured in the laboratory onto both aerobic and anaerobic media. Sensitivity studies should be performed routinely on any organism that grows, to determine proper selection of antibiotic(s) for therapy.

TYPE AND CROSSMATCH

Before a patient is given blood, this ABO group and Rh type (blood type) must be determined. The patient's blood must also be tested for red cell antibodies. The main blood groups are A, B, AB, and O. The Rh type is either positive or negative. The frequency of the various types in the general population is listed in Table 11-4.

TABLE 11-3. SIGNIFICANCE OF ABNORMAL FINDINGS IN BIOCHEMICAL TESTS

Test	Abbreviation	Normal Range	*Cause of Abnormal Finding
Electrolyte Group			
Glucose		65–110 mg/dl	↑in diabetes, in insulin reaction, and other types of hypoglycemia
Blood urea nitrogen	BUN	10–20 mg/dl	↑in renal failure, dehydration, circulatory failure, gastrointestinal bleeding ↓in advanced liver disease, malnutrition
Sodium	Na$^+$	135–145 mEq/L	↑in dehydration, hyperosmolar coma ↓in diarrhea, vomiting, pyloric obstruction, Addison's disease, diabetic acidosis, prolonged tube drainage, prolonged diuretic use
Potassium	K$^+$	3.5–5.0 mEq/L	↑in renal failure, ketoacidosis, Addison's disease ↓in pyloric obstruction, vomiting, diarrhea, prolonged use of K$^+$-losing diuretics, alkalosis
Chloride	Cl$^-$	95–105 mEq/L	↑in renal or metabolic disease ↓in pyloric obstruction, vomiting, diarrhea
Carbon dioxide combining power	CO_2	24–30 mEq/L	↑in metabolic alkalosis, respiratory alkalosis ↓in metabolic acidosis
Biochemical Group			
Glutamic-oxalacetic transaminase	SGOT	5–40 U/L	↑in liver disease, biliary tract disease, disease of smooth muscle, and myocardial necrosis
Glutamic-pyruvic transaminase	SGPT	5–40 U/L	↑in liver disease (more than SGOT), biliary tract disease
Lactic dehydrogenase	LDH	100–225 U/L	↑in myocardial infarction, liver and biliary tract disease, pulmonary infarct, muscle damage
Alkaline phosphatase*	Alk phos	30–105 U/L	↑in children and adolescents, liver disease, bone disease, biliary tract disease
Total protein	TP	6.0–8.0 gm/dl	↓in liver disease, malnutrition, albuminuria
Albumin	Alb	3.5–5.0 gm/dl	↓in liver disease, albuminuria, nephrosis, malnutrition
Bilirubin		0.2–1.2 mg/dl	↑in liver disease with jaundice, hepatitis, cirrhosis, hemolytic anemia, biliary tract disease
Creatinine		0.7–1.5 mg/dl	↑in renal disease
Calcium	Ca	8.5–10.5 mg/dl	↑in hyperparathyroidism, some forms of malignancy ↓in hypoparathyroidism, rickets, intestinal malabsorption, some renal disease
Total cholesterol	Chol.	150–300 mg/dl	↓in children, hyperthyroidism ↑in primary or secondary hypercholesterolemia
Phosphorus	PO_4	2.5–4.5 mg/dl	↑in children, in renal failure, hypoparathyroidism ↓in hyperparathyroidism
Uric acid		Men: 3.9–8.5 mg/dl Women: 2.2–7.5 mg/dl	↑in gout, leukemia, renal failure, use of antihypertensive medication, glycogen storage disease
Other Tests			
Amylase		6–150 Somogyi Units	↑in pancreatitis, perforated ulcer, parotitis, pancreatic trauma, morphinism; greatest rise occurs with acute pancreatitis but returns to normal rapidly
Lipase		1.0–2.0 U/ml 1.0–2.0 U/ml	↑in acute pancreatitis, pancreatic trauma; returns to normal levels more slowly than amylase

TABLE 11-3. SIGNIFICANCE OF ABNORMAL FINDINGS IN BIOCHEMICAL TESTS (*CONTINUED*)

Test	Abbreviation	Normal Range	*Cause of Abnormal Finding
Ammonia		15–110 µg/dl	↑in advanced liver disease, gastrointestinal bleeding, some inborn errors of metabolism, hepatic coma
Creatine phosphokinase contains four enzymes	CPK	Male: 5–55 µg/L Female: 5–35 µg/L	↑in muscle disease, after surgery, in myocardial disease, in infarction (Isoenzymes are fractionated to establish the tissue of origin [skeletal or cardiac muscle].)
Arterial blood gases pH	ABG	7.35–7.45	↑in alkalosis, vomiting ↓in acidosis, chronic pulmonary disease, impaired perfusion
O_2 tension	pO_2	Adult: 80 mm–90 mm Hg* Over 65 yr: 75–85 mm Hg Newborn: 60–70 mm Hg	↓in chronic pulmonary disease, hypoventilation, hypoperfusion, pulmonary arteriovenous shunt
O_2 saturation	O_2 Sat	96%–97%	↓in chronic pulmonary disease, hypoventilation
CO_2 tension	pCO_2	35–45 mm Hg*	↑in chronic pulmonary disease, hypoventilation ↓in metabolic acidosis
Bicarbonate		20–30 mEq/L	↓in metabolic acidosis, respirator alkalosis ↑in metabolic alkalosis, respiratory acidosis
Base excess		0 ± 2.0 mEq/L	↑in alkalosis ↓in acidosis

* These values are often significantly different in pediatric patients.

The vast majority of the population (85%) is Rh positive. Rh typing is significant because patients with Rh-negative blood may form antibodies if given Rh-positive blood in a transfusion.

The dangers of blood transfusion include a number of untoward reactions, for example, ABO incompatibility that results from typing error or other causes. (See Chap. 13, Parenteral Fluid Therapy.)

Recent studies on emergency patients have demonstrated the feasibility of using type-specific noncrossmatched blood when rapid replacement is required to treat posthemorrhage hypovolemia. A full type and crossmatch takes up to 60 minutes to complete, while typing alone may require only 10 to 15 minutes. The incidence of untoward reaction is small.

URINE STUDIES

Urine is one of the most important fluids of the body. The excretion of urine is a necessary element in maintaining homeostasis. Urine is a valuable source of information about

TABLE 11-4. FREQUENCY OF BLOOD TYPES

Blood Type	Percentage of Population
A	38
B	12
AB	5
O	45

many of the body's biological processes. Both gross studies and microscopic studies are ordinarily performed on urine samples. Gross studies include appearance, pH, specific gravity, sugar, protein, occult blood, ketones, bilirubin, and urobilinogen (Table 11-5). Microscopic studies include epithelial cells, white blood cells, red blood cells, casts, bacteria, and formed elements (Table 11-6).

Collection of Urine

Of the utmost importance is the manner in which the specimen is collected and submitted for study. Urine deteriorates very rapidly; bacteria may grow and the pH may change. Therefore, the sample should be analyzed as soon as possible after collection.

In the emergency department, routine urine samples are usually collected at random, by voluntary voiding. Clean wide-mouthed containers are best suited for collection. Special methods of collection are needed for culture studies and are discussed later.

URINE OSMOLALITY

This is an index of renal function that is more sensitive than the test for specific gravity. Osmolality reflects the number of solute particles in the urine. The normal range is between 50 to 1400 mOsm/kg. Urea is a major contributor to osmolality. Some substances that affect specific gravity, such as glucose, x-ray contrast media, or abnormal proteins, do not affect osmolality. Urine osmolality is increased in dehydration, hemoconcentration, shock, acidosis, hyperglycemia, and inappropriate ADH secretion. It is reduced in induced or osmotic diuresis.

TABLE 11-5. URINE STUDIES

Test	Abbreviation	Normal Range	Cause of Abnormal Findings
Appearance, color	—	Pale straw to dark amber	*Colorless:* large output, granular kidney *Orange:* excreted drugs such as santonin, pyridine *Milky:* chyluria, purulent infections of the urinary tract *Pink to Red:* bleeding, trauma, hemoglobinuria *Greenish yellow:* jaundice
pH		6.0–7.0	*Above 6* (alkaline urine): certain infections, alkalosis, K⁺ depletion, large doses of alkali *Below 6* (acid urine): metabolic or respiratory acidosis, high fever, some metabolic disorders
Specific gravity	SG	1.003–1.030	↑in glycosuria, proteinuria, dehydration ↓in chronic renal disease, renal failure overhydration
Glucose		Negative	Present in diabetes mellitus, following infusion of glucose
Protein		Negative to a trace	↑in proteinuria, chronic renal disease, nephritis inflammatory processes of the kidney, prostate
Occult blood	OB	Negative	Present in some renal disease states, myoglobinuria
Ketones		Negative	Present in diabetic acidosis, dehydration, starvation
Bilirubin		Negative	Absent in hemolytic jaundice Present in jaundice, usually of the extrahepatic obstructive type, hepatitis, chemical intoxication
Urobilinogen		0.3–2.0 Ehrlich Units	↑in hepatitis, hemolytic jaundice, cirrhosis ↓biliary obstruction

TABLE 11-6. MICROSCOPIC EXAMINATION OF THE URINE

Test	Abbreviation	Normal Range	Cause of Abnormal Findings
Epithelial cells	Epith cells	None–2	Present with renal disease, abnormal conditions of the urinary tract, bladder
White blood cells	WBC	None–2	↑in urinary tract infections, tuberculosis, pyelonephritis, nephrosis
Red blood cells	RBC	None to occasional	↑in nephritis, tumors of the urinary tract, trauma
Casts		None to occasional	↑in renal disease, shock, fever, heart failure, renal failure
Bacteria		None	Urinary tract infection
Formed elements		None	Occasional spermatozoa, *Trichomonas* in some vaginal infections

URINE CULTURE

Normally, urine is sterile. Bacteria may be present at the urethral orifice, but they do not invade the urinary tract epithelium. In urinary tract infection, however, bacteria are present and may be cultured. The method of collecting the sample for culture is extremely important. Disposable sterile collection kits are available in most hospital emergency departments. Urine for culture may be collected by the clean-catch method, or a catheterized specimen may be obtained.

Obtaining a Clean-Catch Specimen

A clean-catch specimen is obtained from the female patient by holding the labia apart and cleansing the vulvar area from front to back with benzalkonium chloride (Zephiran) or povidone-iodine (Betadine) solution. While the labia are held apart, the patient voids and the midstream portion is collected in a sterile container, care being taken to ensure that the container does not touch the clothing or skin. The specimen is taken immediately to the laboratory.

In the male patient, the glans penis and the surrounding area are cleansed with sponges soaked in benzalkonium or povidone-iodine solution. The midstream voiding is collected in a sterile container, using the same precautions as those used for the female patient, and is taken to the laboratory immediately.

Obtaining a Catheterized Specimen

If a fresh catheterized specimen is taken, the catheter is inserted using sterile technique and the urine collected as it drains into a sterile container. If an indwelling catheter is already in place, proceed as follows: using a sterile needle and 10-ml syringe, cleanse the catheter drainage apparatus thoroughly with benzalkonium or povidone iodine, withdraw a syringeful of urine from the sampling port of the tubing, and place it in a sterile container.

CEREBROSPINAL FLUID STUDIES

The cerebrospinal fluid (CSF) originates from the choroid plexus of the ventricles; it fills the ventricles and the subarachnoid space that surrounds the surface of the brain and spinal cord. CSF contains a number of electrolytes, usually in concentrations that are different from those in plasma. (See Chap. 18, The Comatose Patient.) CSF samples are obtained using sterile technique.

Lumbar Puncture

In the emergency setting, CSF is usually obtained by lumbar puncture (LP). The indications for lumbar puncture are numerous. In general it is used as a diagnostic measure in suspected disease of the central nervous system. Extreme caution must be taken when considering LP in the presence of increased intracranial pressure. A drop in CSF pressure as a result of removing even a small amount of fluid may cause herniation of the brain stem through the foramen magnum and possibly death.

Examination of CSF includes the following: appearance, pressure, cell count, chlorides, colloidal gold, glucose, protein, and bacteria. These tests are summarized in Table 11-7.

TABLE 11-7.   CEREBROSPINAL FLUID

Test	Normal Range	Causes of Abnormal Findings
Appearance	Clear, colorless	Abnormally varies from opalescent → bloody → xanthochromic → purulent in infections of the meninges or brain, hemorrhage
Pressure	75–200 cm H_2O	↑in meningitis, some brain tumors, cerebral hemorrhage ↓in some spinal cord tumors
Cell count	0–10 WBC/mm³ (all lymphocytes)	↑in infections of CNS, meningitis, encephalitis RBCs found in cerebral hemorrhage Blood found in traumatic tap
Chlorides	110–125 mEq/L	↓in meningitis Chloride levels may be invalidated if an intravenous infusion of electrolyte solution is running
Colloidal gold	Not more than one in any tube	Abnormal curve in CNS syphilis, multiple sclerosis Not always diagnostic
Glucose	45–80 mg/dl (60%–80% of blood glucose level)	↓in meningitis ↑in diabetic acidosis
Protein	15–45 mg/dl	↑in meningitis, cerebral thrombosis or hemorrhage, CNS tumor
Bacteria	None	Present in bacterial meningitis

ABDOMINAL FLUID STUDIES

Abdominal or peritoneal fluid may be found in a variety of diseases, including trauma. Intra-abdominal fluid is often referred to as ascites. It frequently accompanies chronic liver disease (cirrhosis), congestive heart failure, and metastatic malignancy and sometimes occurs in malnutrition. Fluid in the peritoneal cavity may be associated with acute inflammatory diseases of the gastrointestinal tract, including perforated ulcer, pancreatitis, and mesenteric vascular occlusion. Blunt or penetrating abdominal trauma can result in free fluid in the peritoneal cavity.

Collection of Abdominal Fluid

Abdominal fluid is recovered by abdominal paracentesis, peritoneal tap, or peritoneal lavage. Fluid recovered in this manner should be analyzed for blood cells (WBCs and RBCs), specific gravity, appearance, amylase content, bacteria, and tumor cells. Cultures should be performed routinely on any recovered fluid.

In the emergency department, the examination of peritoneal fluid is most important in the patient with abdominal trauma. (See Chap. 21, Thoracic and Abdominal Trauma.)

THORACIC FLUID STUDIES

Fluid in the pleural cavity may result from thoracic trauma, pneumonia, pulmonary infarct, congestive heart failure, and primary or metastatic tumors of the lung or pleura. Diagnosis may be suspected by physical examination and confirmed by chest x-ray.

The fluid may be removed by thoracentesis. Complete examination of the fluid includes appearance, cell count, tumor cells, bacteria, and culture for organisms.

WOUND FLUID STUDIES

Fluid may be collected from seromas, hematomas, and abscesses. Fluid removed from a surgical or traumatic wound by aspiration or by incision and drainage should be taken under sterile conditions and a specimen sent to the laboratory for aerobic and anaerobic culture and sensitivity studies. A gram stain should be performed on the fluid to identify any pathogenic organisms before culture.

CULTURES OF BODY FLUIDS

Bacterial contamination may occur in various fluids of the body causing a variety of clinical problems. Sampling of these fluids for bacteriologic study to isolate and identify the pathogens is of great value in initiating a plan of therapy including appropriate selection of antibiotic(s). This sampling technique is referred to as a culture, and it consists basically of obtaining a specimen of the body fluid and inoculating it in a suitable culture medium. Certain organisms require special media for growth. These are discussed in specific chapters where applicable. If there is any doubt about which media should be used, the hospital bacteriologist should be consulted to ascertain the appropriate culture medium.

Generally, prepackaged containers are available commercially to receive specimens of body fluids for culture. These containers are sterile when unopened and contain an applicator and culture medium into which the specimen is inoculated before transport to the laboratory. This is done to keep the specimen moist. The fresh specimen should be taken to the bacteriology laboratory as soon as possible. A culture may be taken from any body orifice. All personnel should be aware of the need to handle bacteriology specimens with great care in order to avoid contamination of the specimen (and thus alter the results) and to prevent exposing themselves and others to a potentially serious infectious agent. Hospital procedures should be followed. Cracked or broken containers should not be used. The specimen should not be spilled on the outside of the container(s). The container and accompanying laboratory slip should be properly labeled to identify the patient and the source of the specimen correctly. If the patient is on antibiotic therapy, the laboratory should be informed.

The sites and fluids commonly cultured are described below.

Nasal Culture. A culture of the nasal passage is taken by gently inserting the swab into the nares to contact the mucous membrane. Rotate the swab to obtain the specimen and immediately place it in the culture medium.

Throat Culture. Inspect the involved area looking for an exudate; remove some exudate with the swab and inoculate the medium. If a membrane is present, scrape off a portion of it and take a specimen from the underlying tissue. This technique is likely to be more productive in recovering the offending bacteria.

Vaginal Culture. This procedure is usually performed by a physician, although this restriction may be modified by hospital policy. The patient is placed in the lithotomy position and a sterile unlubricated speculum placed in the vagina. Samples are taken from the vagina and cervix individually and placed in the medium for immediate transport to the laboratory.

Stool Culture. To obtain stool for culture, have the patient defecate into a bedpan and take a representative sample of stool from the pan and place it in a clean cardboard receptacle. The specimen should be taken to the laboratory without delay.

Sputum Culture. Sputum for culture may be taken from a patient in the emergency department before the initiation of antibiotic therapy. The patient should be asked to cough and expectorate into a sputum bottle. He should be told that he must *cough* to obtain material from the pulmonary tree. In acute pulmonary infections, in addition to plating the sputum for culture, a gram stain may be indicated to identify an offending organism.

To obtain sputum from a patient who is too weak to raise the pulmonary secretions, nasotracheal suction is used. Sterile technique is employed by emergency personnel using a sterile suction catheter and sterile glove. The sputum is collected in a bronchial trap (Luki tube) and taken promptly to the laboratory.

TOXICOLOGY

The detection of abnormal or noxious substances in the body fluids, particularly blood and urine, is important in evaluating patients suspected of having been exposed to or injesting a noxious agent. It may be particularly helpful in the diagnosis of the comatose patient.

The two body fluids most commonly used for study are blood and urine. Information should be sought from the hospital laboratory about directions for collecting specimens for analysis. Substances commonly tested in body fluids are listed in Table 11-8.

TABLE 11-8. SUBSTANCES COMMONLY TESTED IN BODY FLUIDS

Agent	Acceptable Levels	Toxic Levels (4 hr postingestion)
Acetaminophen	5–2.5 µg/ml	300 µg/ml
Acetone		>200 mg/dl
Amitryptyline		1.0 µg/ml
Alcohol		
(serum)		400 µg/ml
(urine)	Qualitative	
Amobarbital	2.0–10 µg/ml	>30 mg/ml
Amphetamine		
(serum)		1 µg/ml
(urine)	Qualitative	
Butabarbital	2.0–10 µg/ml	>30 µg/ml
Carbon monoxide	1%–2% saturation (Nonsmokers)	>20% saturation
Chlordiazepoxide	1.0–3.0 µg/ml	20 µg/ml
Chlorpromazide		1.0 µg/ml
Diazepam	0.1–1.5 µg/ml	2.0–20 µg/ml
Diphenylhydantoin	10–20 µg/ml	60 µg/ml
Disopyramide (Norpace)	2.0–5.0 µg/ml	>7.0 µg/ml
Ethchlorvynol (Placidyl)	3.0–5.0 µg/ml	40 µg/ml
Flurazepam (Dalmane)		1 µg/ml
Glutethimide (Doriden)	2.0–5.0 µg/ml	>20 µg/ml
Meperidine (Demerol)		20 µg/ml
Methadone (Urine)		6.0 µg/ml
Methyprylon (Noludar)	5.0–10.0 µg/ml	30–60 µg/ml
Pentazocine (talwin)		2.0 µg/ml
Pentobarbital (Nembutal)	1.5 µg/ml	20 µg/ml
Propoxyphene (Darvon)		1.0 µg/ml
Salicylate	6–30 mg/dl	>30 mg/dl
Secobarbital (Seconal)	2.0–5 µg/ml	20 µg/ml
Thioridazine (Mellaril)		1.0 µg/ml

Blood Toxicology Screen. This multianalysis study tests levels of: alcohol, salicylates, barbiturates, diazepam, glutethimide and methyprylon.

Urine Toxicology Screen. This includes studies for: amphetamine, cocaine, codeine, meperidine, methadone, heroin, pentazocine, phencycline, propoxyphene, quinine, methaqualone, and alcohol.

BIBLIOGRAPHY

1. Bormanis J, Shepherd FA, Hynie I: Your guide to clinical laboratory procedures. Can Nurse 25, 1979
2. Blumberg N, Bove JR: Uncrossmatched blood for emergency transfusion. JAMA 240:2057, 1978
3. Free AL, Free H: Urinalysis in Clinical Laboratory Practice. Cleveland, CRC Press, 1975
4. French RM: Guide to Diagnostic Procedures. New York, McGraw-Hill, 1980
5. Goldfinger D: Uncrossmatched blood for emergency transfusion. JAMA 237:1826, 1977
6. Metheny NA, Snively WD: Perioperative fluid and electrolytes. Am J Nurs 78:840, 1978
7. Raphael SR: Lynch's Medical Laboratory Technology. Philadelphia, WB Saunders, 1976
8. Sirridge MS: Laboratory Evaluation of Hemostasis. Philadelphia, Lea & Febiger, 1974
9. Widmann FK: Clinical Interpretation of Laboratory Tests. Philadelphia, FA Davis, 1979

12
SHOCK

JAMES S. WILLIAMS

Even today, many still think of shock as a clinical state manifested by rapid pulse and low blood pressure. In reality, the simple term *shock* denotes a complex series of alterations of physiologic processes associated with reduced blood flow and resulting in a syndrome manifested by a variety of clinical findings. For years, shock was a well-recognized but poorly understood chain of events which, if allowed to proceed unaltered, became irreversible and terminated fatally. Today, a certain percentage of shock patients die; however, the therapeutic modalities available allow for a significant salvage rate. Much of this progress is due to the persistent and innovative work of a large number of dedicated medical scientists applying the sophisticated methods made possible by modern technology.[2,3,8,9,11,12,13]

In the *emergency* setting, the patient in shock should be assigned the highest priority of care. Early, thorough evaluation should be done to make the proper diagnosis and determine the etiology of the shock state. Appropriate treatment is instituted to stabilize vital signs and functions, ideally within a 30-minute time period. In some patients, particularly those with massive bleeding, stabilization may not be possible without operative intervention, and a rapid and shorter workup should be done, with early institution of therapeutic measures and transfer to the operating theater. In other patients in shock, stabilization may require many hours of intensive care, with close observation and use of a variety of laboratory aids and monitoring techniques, in addition to numerous therapeutic modalities.

It has been shown that shock is a dynamic state, with a stress-response pattern. This invariably is associated with a deficiency of peripheral blood flow combined with lowered tissue perfusion, which if prolonged or untreated produces alterations in cellular metabolism that may eventually impair physiologic processes.[7] To properly manage the patient in shock one must have knowledge of these processes; appropriate intervention techniques can then be applied to interrupt and reverse the abnormal chain of events.

Because the shock state is dynamic and because of the nature of the therapy, more than one mechanism may be involved. For example, an elderly patient in oligemic shock may, as a result of fluid replacement, develop cardiogenic shock. Thus, those caring for the shock patient must be familiar with the parameters used in assessing his response to therapy in order to detect any deviation from the desired or anticipated course.

It is important to avoid making premature judgments about the shock patient's prognosis because this tends to limit the therapeutic approach and can adversely affect the eventual outcome. One must guard against this kind of thinking and outline a plan of management designed for survival until it is apparent that death is imminent or cerebral death has occurred. While it is important to prolong useful life, it is also important not to prolong death. This judgment may be the most difficult one that has to be made in caring for the shock victim. The definitive decision is made by the physician.

The complexity of the shock state challenges and may tax the expertise and judgment of emergency personnel; a multitude of factors are involved. The material covered in this chapter alludes to many of these factors. An effort is made to elucidate the basic changes in the homeostatic mechanism that occur in the shock state as the result of lower tissue perfusion and alterations in cellular metabolism. The newer concepts of human shock are discussed in order to give the reader an appreciation of the stress-response pattern that occurs in the patient in shock. The management of specific causes of shock is discussed in the appropriate chapters.

DEFINITION OF SHOCK

Shock is present when there is reduced perfusion of body tissues leading to cellular hypoxia and damage of vital organs. If it is uncorrected and allowed to continue, eventually a critical number of cells will be injured beyond repair, resulting in cessation of vital organ function and progressive, unrelenting death of the remaining cells in spite of treatment. This is *irreversible shock*.

CLASSIFICATION OF SHOCK

The circulatory system can be divided into five parts: arteries, capillaries, veins, heart, and blood. Using these divisions, with the exception of arteries, shock can be classified according to etiology into oligemic (blood loss) shock, capillary shock, venous "pooling" shock, and cardiogenic (myocardial, pump failure) shock. (See Fig. 12-1.)

- *Oligemic shock (blood loss or hypovolemia)*. Oligemic shock results from loss of whole blood or its parts from the circulatory system at a rate sufficient to produce reduced effective circulating blood volume and inadequate tissue perfusion.
- *Capillary shock*. Capillary shock occurs when circulating blood volume is sequestered in the capillary bed. This results in an inadequate tissue perfusion.
- *Venous pooling shock*. Venous pooling shock results when circulating blood volume is sequestered on the venous side of the heart.
- *Cardiogenic shock (pump failure)*. Cardiogenic shock results when cardiac action is unable to deliver a circulating volume at a rate sufficient to produce adequate tissue perfusion.

PATHOPHYSIOLOGY

OLIGEMIC SHOCK

Acute loss of blood volume stimulates the volume baroreceptors in the aortic arch and carotid arteries, resulting in vasoconstriction through increased sympathetic nervous system tone. In addition, adrenalin is released from the adrenal cortex, aiding the vasoconstriction and causing tachycardia by direct action on the heart. If loss if rapid enough, the oxygen-carrying capacity of the blood decreases.

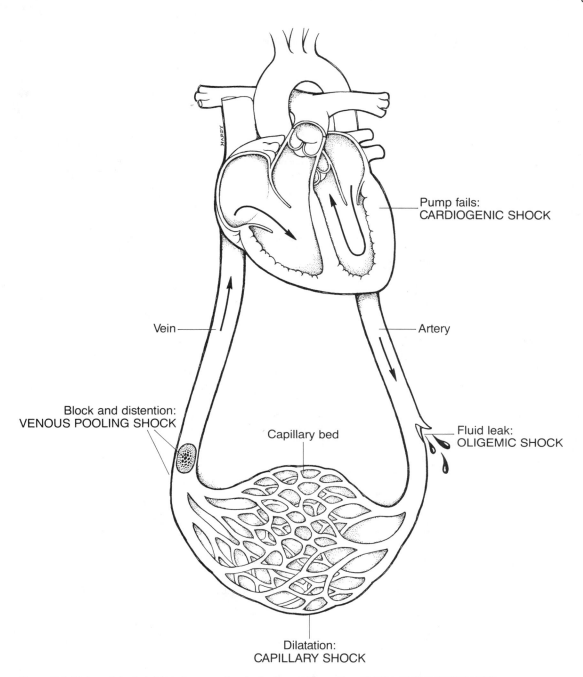

Figure 12-1 *Etiology of shock. A fluid leak causes oligemic shock; excessive capillary dilatation results in capillary shock; blood trapped in the venous system causes venous-pooling shock; and when the heart pump fails, cardiogenic shock ensues. (After material of the Photography Unit of the University of Rochester Medical Center, Rochester, New York)*

This is marked by shortness of breath (air hunger) and is frequently associated with cerebral symptoms. There may not be enough circulating blood volume for the patient to manifest cyanosis.

Depletion of circulating volume may involve either whole blood or merely the fluid portion (plasma). Examples of whole blood loss are major vessel damage associated with internal or external bleeding. Examples of loss of parts of whole blood are the decrease in plasma fluid as a result of

protracted vomiting or diarrhea and fluid loss from burns or peritonitis. (See Table 12-1, for other secondary causes.)

The following clinical signs and symptoms are associated with oligemic shock:

- Pallor
- Clammy extremities
- Hypotension
- Tachycardia

TABLE 12-1. PRIMARY AND SECONDARY CAUSES OF SHOCK BY ETIOLOGY

Etiology	Primary Cause	Secondary Cause
Oligemic	(1) Loss of whole blood (2) Loss of plasma (3) Loss of fluid	(1) Internal or external bleeding (2) Burn or peritonitis (3) Crush injury (4) Dehydration, vomiting (5) Diarrhea (6) Bowel obstruction
Capillary	(1) Dilatation of the capillary bed, with sequestration of whole blood	(1) Vasodilator damage (2) Spinal cord ''shock'' (cord transection) (3) Septicemia (4) Addisonian crisis (5) Anesthetic agents (6) Drug overdose
Venous pooling	(1) Entrapment of whole blood on the venous side of the heart	(1) Massive pulmonary embolus (2) Air embolism (3) Cardiac tamponade (4) Tension pneumothorax
Cardiogenic (myocardial)	(1) Failure of the heart muscle to pump adequate blood	(1) Myocardial infarction (2) Myocarditis (3) Extensive arteriovenous shunt (4) Pericarditis

- Apprehension
- As time progresses, cold, pale, or cyanotic extremities and lips are noted, and the victim eventually succumbs.

CAPILLARY SHOCK

There are some 70 miles of capillaries in a normal adult, and only 10% of these are open at one time. If a major percentage of the capillary beds were to open up, a large quantity of circulating volume would be easily sequestered.

Causes of capillary shock are numerous. Examples include septic shock, spinal cord shock, neurogenic shock, types of anesthetic shock, anaphylactic shock, drug shock (antihypertensives and tranquilizers) and adrenal insufficiency. (See also Table 12-1.)

The following clinical signs and symptoms are associated with capillary shock:
- Initially, the extremities are warm, and the patient is hypotensive, usually without tachycardia.
- As time passes, the sustained inadequate circulating volume stimulates the sympathetic nervous system through baroreceptor mechanisms, and vasoconstriction becomes a prominent feature.
- The cardinal symptoms and signs of shock ensue (see *Assessment*).

VENOUS POOLING SHOCK

The veins are normally very distensible; they have a considerable reservoir capacity and thus can harbor large quantities of blood. Anything that mechanically prevents blood from entering the heart chamber will cause blood to accumulate in the vast area of the venous reservoir. Effective circulating volume will drop sharply, and inadequate tissue perfusion will ensue.

The following are examples of venous pooling shock:
- Shock associated with a pulmonary embolus that is obstructing the pulmonary arteries
- A tension pneumothorax with mediastinal shift, causing obstruction of the vena cava due to kinking as it enters the thorax through the diaphragm
- An air embolus, whereby blood is churned into froth in the right heart chambers, preventing normal flow of blood through the heart
- Pericardial tamponade, whereby pressure in the pericardial sac collapses the atria, preventing filling

The following *clinical signs and symptoms* are associated with venous pooling shock:
- Increased venous pressure
- Rapid pulse
- Marked drop in blood pressure
- Cyanosis
- Rapid onset of the other cardinal signs and symptoms of shock (see *Assessment*)

CARDIOGENIC SHOCK

In pump failure shock, the heart is not strong enough to pump blood into the arterial tree with sufficient force to maintain adequate perfusion pressure, and therefore it backs up into the pulmonary circulation and subsequently into the systemic venous and capillary circulation. The victim experiences shortness of breath because of venous distention in the atrium, pulmonary circulation, and vena cava. Fluid accumulates outside the capillary beds and in the alveoli of the lungs and other extravascular tissues. Examples of this type of shock include acute or chronic myocardial infarction and any cause of acute or chronic myocardial degeneration. (See Table 12-1.)

The clinical signs and symptoms of cardiogenic shock are related to the rate of onset as well as the degree and locale of the myocardial damage. The usual cardinal symptoms are the following:

- Pain
- Dyspnea
- Restlessness
- Venous distention, edema, and finally the classic signs of shock (see *Assessment*).

Table 12-1 summarizes the pathophysiology of the four types of shock described above.

DISSEMINATED INTRAVASCULAR COAGULATION

Any discussion of the pathophysiology of the shock state would not be complete without mention of this entity. Disseminated intravascular coagulation (DIC) has also been known by a number of other terms: consumption coagulopathy, defibrination syndrome, and intravascular coagulation fibrinolysis syndrome. Basically, it involves alterations in the blood clotting mechanism; initial hypercoagulability is followed by hypocoagulability. It occurs in a variety of clinical situations,[1,4,6,10,15] but of particular interest to emergency personnel is its association with shock in patients with multiple injuries, and in those with bleeding in the last trimester of pregnancy.

Experimental studies have shown that DIC occurs particularly in shock due to hemorrhage or sepsis.[14] It is described as a functional state with intravascular clotting caused by activation of the normal coagulation system. The fibrinogen-fibrin reaction is accelerated, with the result that fibrinogen elements in the blood are reduced. Other factors, especially the blood platelets, are depleted. The results are:
1. Clot formation in the microcirculation, with subsequent impairment in flow
2. A hemorrhagic diathesis

Thus, in the same patient, the result can be abnormal hemorrhage and/or thrombosis.

The most dramatic result of DIC is the acute generalized hemorrhagic state. Diagnosis is difficult and depends on the clinical picture combined with adjunct studies, a number of laboratory tests (including a partial thromboplastin time, fibrinogen level and fibrin degradation products (FDP), peripheral blood smear for study of red cells, platelet count, and evaluation of various clotting elements in the blood). An excellent review of the subject was prepared by Damus and Salzman.[10] The reader is referred to this article for in-depth study of this problem.

EFFECTS OF SHOCK ON CELL METABOLISM (ENERGY PRODUCTION)

Cells must have oxygen in sufficient quantity to produce energy for maintaining normal cell function. Since shock, by definition, results in inadequate tissue perfusion and cellular hypoxia, it follows that cellular energy production is impaired during shock.

Normally, cell energy is supplied by adenosine triphosphate (ATP) molecules. Every time the alpha phosphate bond is split, 7000 calories of energy are released for cell use. The ATP molecules are manufactured primarily by the use of glucose (see Fig. 12-2). Glucose, either from ingestion or split from glycogen stores in muscle or liver, is converted into high-energy phosphate by way of the Krebs–tricarboxylic acid (TCA) cycle. During this process, hydrogen ions accumulate and must be carried away. Normally, in the presence of oxygen, they are transported through the cytochrome system. With hypoxia, however, they accumulate and are stored as lactate. As long as there is oxygen deficiency (debt), manufactured pyruvate is converted into lactate in order to store the ions. Energy production is drastically reduced and lactate accumulates in excess as lactic acid.

The major source of lactate is the muscle mass. It is normally metabolized in the liver and heart. In shock, more lactate is produced than can be utilized by these organs. The excessive accumulation of lactate as lactic acid, as well as other acid metabolites, results in acidosis, which has an unstabilizing effect on cell membranes.

Normally, the cell membranes, which are made up of lipoprotein, are maintained by ATP (see Fig. 12-3). It is evident that if ATP production is faulty, membrane stability will be in jeopardy. Indeed, as shock progresses, membrane function is impaired. Normal transfer of sodium and potassium in and out of the cell (the so-called sodium pump) is impaired, and water accumulates within the cell. The hydrolytic enzymes normally contained within the lipoprotein lysosomal membrane leak into the cell cytoplasm and begin to digest the cell components. Eventually they enter the general circulation and act on distant cells. If treated in time, cell membrane damage is reversible. If not, death occurs.

If shock progresses untreated, tissue levels of ATP decrease progressively as stores are used up. The PO_4 ion released during ATP breakdown accumulates in the serum. Likewise, glycogen stores, in the liver particularly and in the body in general, are depleted. In severe experimental shock models, after 2 hours glycogen was virtually absent and ATP was reduced as much as 75%, depending on the organ.

EFFECTS OF SHOCK ON SPECIFIC SYSTEMS

The effect of shock stress on specific body systems varies and is related to several factors. The following must be considered:
- General health of the victim prior to shock
- Age of the victim
- Duration and degree of shock
- Preexisting specific organ system disease
- Coexisting illness or injury
- Drugs or medications

Central Nervous System

Since blood flow to the brain and spinal cord is regulated by metabolic needs and not by the sympathetic nervous

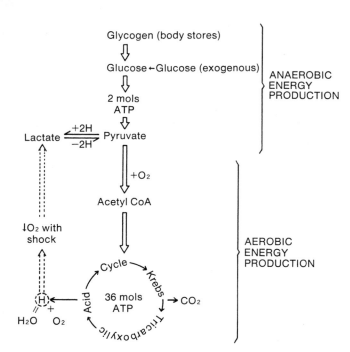

Figure 12-2 *Anaerobic and aerobic energy production. Glycogen and exogenous glucose are converted to pyruvate. Two mols of ATP are formed and (without oxygen) represent the sole source of high energy phosphate to sustain cell function. Excess hydrogen ions generated in this process convert pyruvate to lactate. In the presence of oxygen, lactate can be converted back to pyruvate, which in turn is changed to a 3-carbon molecule, acetyl CoA. This material enters the Krebs cycle and results in the formation of CO_2, H_2O and 36 mols of high energy ATP. If insufficient O_2 is present, excess hydrogen ions are stored as lactate. (After material of the Photography Unit of the University of Rochester Medical Center, Rochester, New York)*

system, blood flow is maintained to these areas in shock in preference to all other organs. The one exception is the heart, which shares equal-flow priority. An elevation in pCO_2 or a drop in blood *p*H will increase cerebral flow. If the patient has been hyperventilating, respiratory alkalosis may be present and the pCO_2 reduced. In this case, blood flow to the brain may decrease and oxygen disassociation from oxyhemoglobin be reduced, with a resultant degree of anoxia. Anoxia may also result from intracranial or extracranial vascular disease or perfusion pressure of less than 50 mm Hg.

Peripheral Nervous System

Although peripheral vasoconstriction is a prominent element of shock in most instances, peripheral nerves, as organ structures, are extremely resistant to shock.

Circulatory System and Myocardium

Adaptation of the heart muscle to changes in pressure and volume is regulated by Starling's law and mediated through the sympathetic and myocardial catecholamines. Regulation can occur in two ways:

1. *Homeometric adaptation,* by which the heart puts out an increased volume, but the end diastolic blood volume in the ventricle remains unchanged.

2. *Heterometric adaptation,* by which the end-diastolic volume increases to accommodate the increased volume.

The second method is quicker but less efficient, since the heart muscle is more dilated and contraction requires more work.

In cardiogenic pump failure shock, the heart muscle is unable to handle the increased blood volume, and heterometric adaptation quickly occurs. This may be followed by homeometric adaptation through increased sympathetic stimulation of myocardial catecholamines and result in a temporary decrease in the end-diastolic volume. Extra cardiac catecholamines may help during this phase.

However, hypoxia and depletion of myocardial catecholamines soon result in unresponsiveness of the myocardium to sympathetic activity, and adaptation reverts back to heterometric, resulting in an increasing end-diastolic volume heralding myocardial decompensation. Energy for maintenance of myocardial function is gradually reduced. The myocardial fibers become disarranged, the heart wall dilates, and irreversible arrhythmias occur. Subendocardial hemorrhagic necrotic areas have been observed, due to either anoxia or circulating lysosomal hydrolytic enzymes. One fraction of these enzymes from the gut and pancreas has been labeled *myocardial depressant factor* (MDF), but its clinical significance is uncertain.

Arterial System

With blood volume depletion, the elastic arterial wall constricts in an attempt to accommodate. Aided by arterial constriction, particularly in the periphery (extremities), blood pressure is maintained. As volume continues to decrease, arteriovenous shunts open, and blood bypasses peripheral capillary beds. Eventually, the same process occurs in the splanchnic and renal beds. The blood in these beds moves more and more slowly, finally sludging. Anoxia results in increased capillary permeability and in interstitial and intracellular edema. When arteriolar constriction can no longer be maintained, dilatation occurs, with additional fluid loss. A pressure sufficient to reestablish venular flow cannot be generated. Stagnant anoxia persists, and cell death progresses.

If restoration of volume is attempted at this point, the tissue edema will be picked up in the lymphatics, along with acid metabolites. This lymph volume added to the circulation is generally inadequate to reverse shock.

In capillary shock there is an early hyperdynamic state due to a low peripheral resistance and high cardiac output. This gives way to a hypodynamic state as fluid leaks out of the capillaries, hypovolemia ensues, and cardiac output drops. Sympathetic tone increases and the path described above is followed.

Respiratory System

Of all systems, the respiratory system is most vulnerable to the subtle changes of shock and its treatment. Multiple external and internal stresses are brought to bear on the lungs.

Early in shock, because of pain or apprehension, the victim splints the chest or breathes rapidly and shallowly. Deep

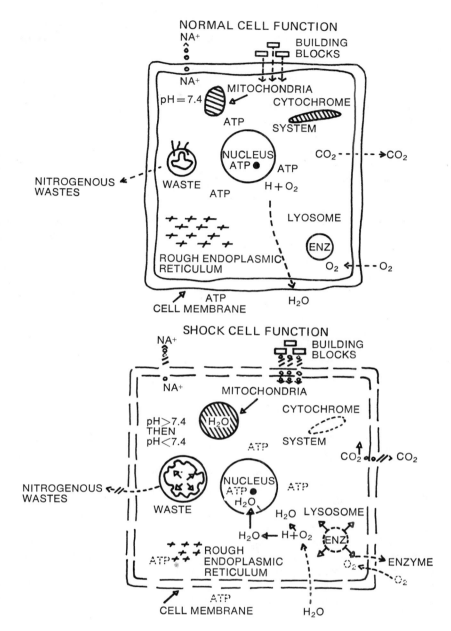

Figure 12-3 *Normal and shock cell function. Normally, ATP maintains the cell. Excess Na⁺ is pumped out and building blocks are brought in. The endoplasmic reticulum uses this material to produce integral cellular parts. CO₂, excess water, and wastes are expelled. O₂ enters the cell. In shock, ATP stores are depleted and not replaced. H⁺ ions, Na⁺ ions, CO₂, H₂O, and wastes accumulate. Cell membranes deteriorate. Hydrolytic enzymes escape from the lysosomes. Important intracellular systems disintegrate. pH rises early and then drops to severely acidotic levels. Eventually, the cell digests itself and dies. (After material of the Photography Unit of the University of Rochester Medical Center, Rochester, New York)*

breathing does not occur, and atelectasis results. With an increased respiratory rate, the effective alveolar ventilation decreases. Arteriovenous shunting occurs through the non-ventilated atelectatic lung. Arterial oxygen saturation falls. The problem is compounded by an increased pulmonary vascular resistance, in response to local pulmonary vascular compression, acidosis, hypoxia, and humoral and neural factors.

As time passes, vasodilatory substances such as arachidonic acid (from damaged polymorphonuclear leukocytes, platelets, and endothelial cells), complement components (particularly C3, C5, and C5A), lysomal enzymes, and the endorphin precursor β-lipotropin may cause the capillaries to leak. As a result, increased albumin-rich fluid accumulates in the interstitial spaces of the lungs. (This capillary leak syndrome is commonly seen in septic shock.)

Progressive respiratory deterioration during and after shock is enhanced by the following factors that contribute to adult respiratory distress syndrome (ARDS).

1. *Preexisting pulmonary disease,* such as chronic bronchitis, congestive heart failure, emphysema, or pneumoconiosis, leave the shock victim little pulmonary reserve.

2. *Pulmonary trauma* or injury to the chest wall results in early alteration in pulmonary function.

3. *Aspiration of gastric contents* or blood may result in extensive damage to cilia activity and bronchial mucosa.

4. *Overzealous fluid replacement* with blood, colloid, or crystalloid can produce pulmonary edema more readily in the shock-stressed lung than in the normal lung.

5. *Embolization of fat particles* after long-bone fractures or soft-tissue trauma results in conversion of the neutral fat to fatty acids that are toxic to pulmonary tissue.

6. *Microemboli* are common; they may be in the form of platelet aggregates secondary to sludging, thrombi from traumatized veins or intravascular coagulation, or particulate matter from transfusion.

7. *Oxygen toxicity,* characterized by intra-alveolar transudation and hyalinization, results from prolonged exposure to high concentrations of O_2.

8. *Supervening pulmonary infection* severely compounds the already stressed respiratory system.

9. *Cardiac failure* superimposed on shock results in pulmonary congestion and elevated pulmonary vascular pressure.

10. *Vasoactive substances* released during shock, such as serotonin, catecholamine, bradykinin, and histamine, cause pulmonary venous constriction and vascular congestion.

11. *Surfactant activity* is markedly reduced owing to inadequate phospholipid production secondary to ischemia and thus contributes to atelectasis.

12. *Massive head injury* has been associated with progressive pulmonary insufficiency, perhaps secondary to respiratory neuroregulatory dysfunction.

13. *Iatrogenic causes,* such as intravenous air, incompatible medication (allergens, depressants, vasoactives), anesthesia, and the like, must be included as contributing causes for progressive pulmonary insufficiency.

Digestive System

During shock, there appears to be a redistribution of blood flow away from the gastrointestinal tract secondary to sympathetic activity causing splanchnic vasoconstriction. The anoxia that ensues results in reduced energy, producing oxidative phosphorylation, injury to the intestinal mucosal cells, release of hydrolytic enzymes from the lysosomal membrane, and sequestration of fluid in the gut (from increased capillary permeability due to local acidosis and hypercarbia). The vasoconstriction affects the liver as well, but is well tolerated unless there is preexisting liver disease.

Excretory System

With decreased perfusion pressure, renal blood flow decreases. Glomerular filtration drops, and although renal venous oxygen saturation decreases only slightly, urine oxygen tension falls drastically, indicating that oxygen dissolved in urine may be an important source of oxygen supply to the renal parenchyma. The excretory regulatory function of the kidney is impaired. If the decreased perfusion is sufficient in degree or duration, *i.e.,* if the ischemic injury affects a sufficient number of nephrons to produce acute tubular necrosis, the kidney ceases to function.

Endocrine System

With stress there is an increased output of adrenocorticotropic hormone (ACTH) from the anterior pituitary gland.

This results in release of glucocorticoids from the zona fasciculata cells of the adrenal gland. They have glucogenic effects, increasing the release and manufacture of glucose. They keep vascular smooth muscle reactive to catecholamines. In addition, they are necessary for the conversion of norepinephrine to epinephrine in the adrenal medulla.

From the zona glomerulosa of the adrenal cortex, aldosterone is released. This salt-retaining hormone is released in response to renal hypotension. (The proteolytic enzyme renin, coming from the juxtaglomerular apparatus in the glomerulus of the kidney, causes the formation of angiotensin I in the plasma. This, in turn, is changed to angiotensin II, which initiates the release of aldosterone.) Aldosterone then acts on the proximal tubule of the nephron to increase sodium retention.

Catecholamines are released from the adrenal medulla in response to increased sympathetic nervous system tone. Epinephrine predominantly is released, as well as some norepinephrine. They increase vasocirculation tone and result in the conversion of glycogen to glucose.

ASSESSMENT

The clinical signs and symptoms of shock depend on the etiology and the physiological compensatory mechanisms the body employs to counter the shock. The classic clinical picture of shock is related to the increased sympathetic activity that eventually predominates irrespective of the cause of shock. The symptoms of shock that the patient relates are the cornerstones not only of the etiology of the shock but also of the diagnosis.

Appropriate treatment is based on an accurate diagnosis. Historical data will establish a diagnosis in over 80% of all cases. Physical examination will increase the percentage to about 90%. Laboratory data (including x-ray), monitoring, and observation will reveal the diagnosis in the remaining cases.

HISTORY

Depending on the type and phase of shock, historical data are gathered from the patient when possible and from family, friends, and emergency personnel as necessary. The following considerations are important:
- Develop a time sequence from the moment when the patient was last stable to the present.
- Note previous illness, infirmity, or disease.
- Record any drugs the patient takes; record allergies.
- Record data about the accident and characteristics of the pain.

PHYSICAL EXAMINATION

The first concern of the examiner is to assess the level of consciousness and record the patient's vital signs. Regional examination is done as rapidly as the situation warrants.

Level of Consciousness

- Early in shock, the victim may be lucid, restless, and anxious, in response to the increased circulating catecholamines.
- As anoxia sets in, the patient becomes restless, agitated, and irrational.
- As deterioration continues, the patient becomes obtunded, depressed, and stuporous.
- It must be kept in mind that age is a factor; thus it is not uncommon to find a lucid youngster in profound shock without obtainable blood pressure, or an elderly person who is restless and obtunded in mild shock.

Skin Temperature and Appearance

- Sympathetic hyperactivity causes vasoconstriction of the skin vessels, stimulation of the sweat glands, and contraction of the erector pilae muscles; the observable results are:
  - Pale, cool, clammy skin
  - Hair standing on end
- When the insult is severe, the skin may be cyanotic or exhibit patchy cyanosis (*livor*).
- Early in capillary (*e.g.,* septic) shock, skin may be warm, pink, and dry because of capillary dilatation. As time passes, sympathetic tone increases, and this situation is reversed.

Mucous Membranes

- The mucous membranes become pale as they undergo vasoconstriction and thus are a good index of carboxyhemoglobin level.

Nail Beds

- Vasoconstriction affects the nail beds. Therefore, their color and capillary refill times provide a reasonably good index of the degree of peripheral vascular "clamping."
- The time of capillary refill of the nail beds is prolonged in shock. Refill is considered prolonged if it does not occur within the time it takes the examiner to say "capillary refill" (about 2 seconds).

Peripheral Veins

- Peripheral veins collapse with volume depletion and sympathetic venoconstriction; they are valuable in evaluating the degree of shock.
- Distended veins signify obstruction of the venous return, as in venous pooling shock or heart failure.

Pulse

- Increased pulse rate is produced by the effects of catecholamine activity on the heart.
- The quality of the pulse weakens and becomes thready as intravascular volume decreases and vasoconstriction increases.
- An irregular pulse signifies a diseased or severely stressed myocardium.

Respiration

- Fear response and hyperventilation are caused by release of epinephrine.
- Gasping respiration (air hunger) occurs with a decrease in effective circulating blood volume or a marked reduction in oxygen-carrying capacity.
- Labored or tugging respiration indicates obstructed airway due to bronchospasm, lung collapse, or foreign material.

Blood Pressure

- Blood pressure is maintained by peripheral vasoconstriction and by increased cardiac output produced by the inotropic action of epinephrine on the heart until circulatory collapse is imminent.
- In some instances, peripheral blood pressure cannot be obtained because of such severe sympathetic "squeezing," although the central pressure is near normal.

As assessment continues and care is instituted, the following should be monitored:
- Vital signs
- Urine output
- Central venous pressure
- Electrocardiogram
- Blood gases
- Laboratory studies

The patient's clinical course should be documented in the chart as it evolves.

ADJUNCT STUDIES

A number of laboratory studies are used in assessing the patient in shock. Blood studies, radiographic studies, electrocardiograms, and pertinent cultures are done.

1. *Blood Studies*
   - Blood samples are drawn at the time of the intravenous catheter placement. Important blood studies include:
     Electrolytes
     Hematocrit
     White blood count and differential
     Arterial blood gas determinations
     Other studies as indicated
   - A blood type and crossmatch should be obtained.

2. *X-ray Studies*
   - Important roentgenograms should be taken, including a chest film to establish a baseline cardiopulmonary status.
   Note: During this period, the care of the patient must not be relegated to the x-ray technician, who is not trained in patient care.

3. *Electrocardiogram* (ECG)
   - An early heart conduction tracing is useful in evaluating the myocardial status and should be repeated when indicated.

4. *Cultures*
   - Blood and pertinent cultures should be obtained early.
   - Pus or sputum smear should be stained and examined under a microscope for early tentative diagnosis.

MANAGEMENT

Most cases of shock, when treated early, will respond and be successfully reversed. When the insult producing the shock has been massive or prolonged, reestablishment of a normal physiologic state is much more difficult and less successful. The therapeutic goal in the treatment of shock is to reverse the inadequate tissue perfusion. In order to accomplish this goal, the defects in the oxygen delivery cycle must be recognized and corrected.

VOLUME REPLACEMENT

Hypovolemia occurs in all types of shock. Anoxia is followed by capillary dilatation and tissue edema. Therefore, early fluid replacement in the form of lactated Ringer's solution or normal saline has therapeutic merit. One liter administered within a 30-minute period often stabilizes vital signs.

When whole blood or plasma is lost, it should be replaced volume for volume, with the realization that additional fluid is still necessary. Administration is monitored by central venous pressure (CVP) and urine output. A CVP of 15 mm H_2O indicates incipient pulmonary edema.

If the shock problem is complex, a pulmonary artery pressure (PAP, or Swan-Ganz) catheter should be placed in a small branch of the pulmonary artery to measure the wedge pressure and thereby monitor left heart competency. Dextran, albumin, or plasma, because of their osmotic qualities, may be used to hold fluid in the intravascular space until whole blood or packed red cells are available.

Dextran given as a 10% solution is a polymer of glucose with a molecular weight of 75,000 that helps to restore normal osmotic pressure. Excessive use, however, may promote bleeding.

Plasma protein fraction, a 5% solution of stabilized human plasma protein in normal saline, is an excellent temporary substitute for whole blood. Formulas are available for determining the rate of fluid administration, particularly in burns (Brooke Army and Evans formulas). Volume replacement may result in pulmonary congestion or edema because of sequestered extravascular fluid being drawn into the intravascular space by the increased osmotic pressure. If so, it should not be allowed to progress without continuous supervision.

OXYGENATION

The availability of oxygen to the tissue depends on airway patency and lung function. An obstructed airway or damaged lung will result in inadequate oxygenation. To maintain a clear airway, an endotracheal tube or tracheostomy may be required. If pulmonary congestion, trauma, or edema is present, constant positive pressure breathing (CPPB) may be necessary to drive the fluid back into the circulatory system and keep it out of the gas exchange area of the lung.

Restlessness and hyperventilation are the first clinical signs of poor oxygenation, but these are late in comparison to arterial oxygen pressure (pO_2).

Therefore, all shock patients should be given 40% oxygen by mask at a flow of 8.0 L/min. Assisted ventilation using a volume ventilator should be started early if the patient is dyspneic or has a low pO_2. Failure of arterial pO_2 to rise above 60 mm Hg with 100% oxygen ventilation indicates physiologic shunting through unaerated atelectatic segments of lung tissue and means that the patient has ARDS. The shunt may account for 15% to 30% of the cardiac output and aggravate cardiac compensation.

If improvement in cardiac function is not associated with improvement in arterial pO_2, the insult to the lung may be so great that progressive pulmonary insufficiency has developed. Eventually, oxygen can no longer enter the circulatory system, and carbon dioxide cannot escape. The arterial pO_2 falls, and the pCO_2 rises. Metabolic acidosis and lactic acidemia herald a terminal illness.

DRUG THERAPY

Cardiotonics

The cornerstone of adequate tissue perfusion is a smoothly functioning myocardium. During shock, the heart muscle adjusts to the stress with its own intrinsic mechanisms. Eventually, these mechanisms may fail. If there is clinical evidence that this is indeed occurring, medication can be given to improve cardiac function.

Digitalis Glycosides. Digitalis acts to slow ventricular rate by decreasing conduction through the atrioventricular node, decreasing myocardial irritability and thus preventing attacks of supraventricular tachycardia. In addition, it has a positive inotropic action on the heart, strengthening cardiac contractions.

Steroids. Massive doses of steroid preparations, given as a "slow push," have a direct inotropic effect on the heart and increase coronary artery flow. In addition, steroids counteract the effects of bacterial endotoxin, promote peripheral vasodilatation, stabilize the lipoprotein membranes of the cell and increase the flow of lymph back into the circulation. Methylprednisolone sodium succinate, 30 mg/kg, or dexamethasone sodium phosphate, 3 mg/kg, is recommended and may be repeated in 4 hours.

Lidocaine. Lidocaine, a potent smooth muscle relaxant with vagal blocking action on the atrioventricular node also reduces myocardial irritability. It increases refractoriness of the myocardium without affecting the conducting system and is therefore useful in the treatment of ventricular arrhythmias.

Diuretics

Maintenance of renal function during shock is important for regulation of fluid and electrolyte balance. Diuretics are used in this effort.

Mannitol. This osmotic diuretic is of great value in shock because it produces an obligatory urine flow by interfering with the nephron transport mechanism. It is postulated that the dissolved oxygen in the urine prevents anoxic tubular cell damage and acute tubular necrosis. The usual dose is 12.5 gm to 25.0 gm by slow push.

Furosemide. This powerful diuretic inhibits the active reabsorption of sodium in the proximal tubule and should be used after blood volume has been restored. It acts rapidly and is effective in treating pulmonary edema. The usual dose is 40 mg to 100 mg IV every 4 hours as necessary.

Vasoactive Medications

It is generally accepted that vasoconstrictor drugs such as norepinephrine and metaraminol have no place in the treatment of established shock. In certain situations, however, the blood pressure fails to respond in spite of volume restoration and other therapeutic measures. In these patients, vasoactive medications are indicated to ensure tissue perfusion.

Phenylephrine Hydrochloride. This medication is a powerful alpha receptor stimulant with little effect on the heart beta receptors. It is a vasoconstrictor but dilates the coronary arteries. It is administered intravenously (2 μm/ml) at a rate sufficient to keep systolic blood pressure between 80 and 100 mm Hg and is frequently useful in capillary shock states.

Isoproterenol. This medication is a beta adrenergic blocking agent that increases myocardial contractility and heart rate but produces peripheral vasodilation. The usual dose is 0.25–1.0 mcg/min. With large doses (4.0 mcg/min), tachycardia and subendocardial ischemia may result.

Dopamine Hydrochloride. This medication has an inotropic effect on the heart through release of norepinephrine from the nerve endings and a chronotropic effect from the molecule itself. It is given intravenously in a dosage of 5.0 mcg/Kg/min according to response. Prolonged use leads to production of norepinephrine, which may require the vasodilator phentolamine.

Dobutamine Hydrochloride. This medication is a cardiotonic because of its direct inotropic effect on the adrenergic receptors in the heart. It is useful in pump failure and capillary shock states because it does not increase peripheral resistance in moderate doses. It is given intravenously in a dosage of 1.0 to 40.0 mcg/Kg/min, according to response.

PNEUMATIC ANTISHOCK GARMENT

The pneumatic antishock garment (PASG), shown in Fig. 12-4, is a compartmentalized device that can be inflated after being applied to the lower extremities and torso. The device is thought to effect a redistribution of blood from the lower extremities. Its action may also be mediated by a humoral mechanism that is not yet fully understood. The PASG is of

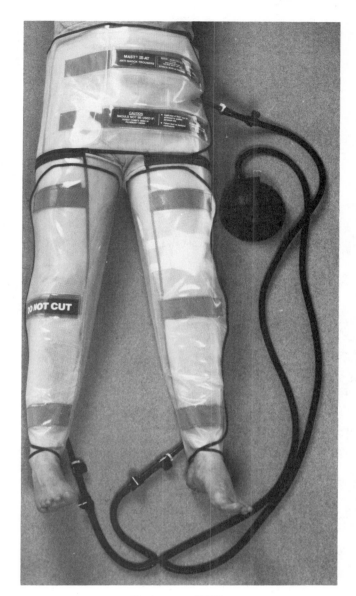

Figure 12-4 *Pneumatic antishock garment (PASG).*

use primarily in hypovolemic shock of almost any etiology. It is particularly useful in stabilizing long bone fractures of the lower extremities and controlling hemorrhage from such fractures and fractures of the pelvis. It can also be used in patients with hemorrhagic shock from any cause, including ruptured abdominal aortic aneurysm and massive gastrointestinal bleeding. It is being used more widely in the prehospital phase of care but has application in the emergency department setting also. The garment is used in conjunction with vigorous fluid volume replacement. It has been used successfully for as long as 48 hours. Emergency personnel should be cautious when deflating the garment making sure to constantly monitor the patient's blood pressure while deflating the abdominal compartment first. If the systolic blood pressure falls 5 mm Hg, immediate reinflation is indicated.

REFERENCES

1. Attar S, Kirby WH Jr, Masaitis C, Mansberger AR, Conley RA: Coagulation changes in clinical shock. Ann Surg 164:34, 1966
2. Baxter CR, Canizaro PC, Carrico CJ, Shires GT: Fluid resuscitation in hemorrhagic shock. Postgrad Med 48:95, 1970
3. Border JR: Advances and new concepts in the management of shock: Kidney. In Cooper P (ed): Surgery Annal, pp 108–109. New York, Appleton-Century-Crofts, 1969
4. Bounous G, Sutherland NG, McArdle AH, Gurd FN: The prophylactic use of an elemental diet in hemorrhagic shock and intestinal ischemia. Ann Surg 166:312, 1967
5. Clermont HG, Adams JT, Williams JS: Effect of cross-circulation in hemorrhagic shock. Surg Gynecol Obstet 135:593, 1972
6. Clermont HG, Adams JT, Williams JS: Source of a lysosomal enzymes acid phosphatase in hemorrhagic shock. Ann Surg 175:19–25, January 1972
7. Clermont HG, Williams JS: Lymph lysosomal enzyme acid phosphatase in hemorrhagic shock. Ann Surg 176:90–96, July 1972
8. Clermont HG, Williams JS, Adams JT: Liver acid phosphatase as a measure of heptocyto resistance to Hemorrhagic Shock. Surgery 71:868–875, June 1972
9. Crowell JW, Read WL: *In vivo* coagulation: A probable cause of irreversible shocks. Am J Physiol 183:565, 1955
10. Damus PS, Salzman EW: Disseminated intravascular coagulation. Arch Surg 104:262, 1972
11. deDuve C: Lysosomes: A New Group of Cytoplasmic Subcellular Particles. New York, Ronald Press, 1959
12. Deykin D: The challenge of disseminated intravascular coagulation. N Engl J Med 283:642, 1970
13. Fitts CT: Vasoactive drugs in treatment of shock. Postgrad Med 48:105, 1970
14. Glenn TM et al: Circulatory responses to splanchnic lysosomal hydrolases in the dog. Ann Surg 176:120–127, July 1972
15. Guenter CA, Hinshaw LB: Comparison of septic shock due to gram-negative and gram-positive organisms. Proceedings of the Society of Experimental Biology and Medicine, 134:780, 1970
16. Hardaway RM: The role of intravascular clotting in the etiology of shock. Ann Surg 155:325, 1962
17. Hinshaw LB, Archer LT, Black MR, Greenfield LJ, Guenter CA: Prevention and reversal of myocardial failures in endotoxin shock. Surg Gynecol Obstet 136:1, 1973
18. Hinshaw LB, Shanbour LL, Greenfield LJ, Coalson JJ: Mechanism of dumased venous return: Subhuman primate-administered endotoxin." Arch Surg 100:600, 1970
19. Hopkins RW: Septic shock: Hemodynamic cast of inflammation. Arch Surg 101:298, 1970
20. Horwitz DL, Moquin RB, Herman CM: Coagulation changes of septic shock in the subhuman primate and their relationship to hemodynamic changes. Ann Surg 175:417, 1972
21. Knisley MH: Intravascular erythrocyte aggregation (blood sludge). In Handbook of Physiology, sec 2, vol III, p. 2257. Washington, DC, American Physiological Society, 1965
22. Mayer GG: Disseminated intravascular coagulation. Am J Nurs 73:2067, 1973
23. Sarnoff SJ, Mitchell JH: The control of the function of the heart. In Hamilton WF, Don P (eds): Handbook of Physiology: Circulation, vol 1, pp 489–532. (American Physiological Society). Baltimore, Williams & Wilkins, 1962
24. Schumer W: Septic shock. JAMA 242:1906–1907, 1979
25. Schumer W: Hypovolemic Shock. JAMA, 241:615–616, 1979
26. Shine KI, Kuhn M, Young LS, Tikisch JH: Aspects of the management of shock. Am Int Med 93:723–34, 1980
27. Shires GT et al: Alterations in cellular membrane function during hemorrhagic shock in primates. Ann Surg 176, September 1972
28. Shires GT, Canico J, Canizaro PC: Pulmonary responses: Shock. In Dunphy JE (ed): Major Problems in Clinical Surgery, pp 62–64. Philadelphia, WB Saunders, 1973
29. Somenschien RR: Physiology of the Central Circulation Blood Vessels and Lymphatics, pp 241–245. New York, Academic Press, 1962
30. Sugerman HJ, Peyton JWR, Greenfield LJ: Grams-Negative Sepsis. Curr Probl Surg, 1981

13
PARENTERAL FLUID THERAPY

JAMES H. COSGRIFF, JR. and PAULA BAUDA

Parenteral fluids are perhaps the most common pharmacologic substances used in the management of the critically ill or injured patient. Appropriate use of them is a hallmark of good emergency care.

Parenteral fluids are used for the following purposes:
- To restore circulating blood volume in a hypovolemic patient
- To replace lost blood cells and other components
- To replace electrolytes in metabolic derangements
- As vehicles for administering medications such as antibiotics and cardiac drugs

Improvements in manufacture, particularly packaging, and the availability of plastic containers and presterilized infusion sets have made it feasible to use parenteral fluid therapy at all levels of emergency care. Proper use of parenteral fluid therapy requires a thorough knowledge of the physiology of the circulation and the physiologic derangements that may result from illness or injury. The principles to be followed when using parenteral fluids and in dealing with complications of parenteral fluid therapy are presented in this chapter.

PHYSIOLOGY OF CIRCULATION

The circulatory system is a continuous circuit that consists of three components: (Fig. 13-1)
- The heart, which serves as a pump
- The systemic circulation, which supplies blood to all the tissues of the body. It is also called the greater or peripheral circulation.
- The pulmonary circulation, which carries blood from the right heart through the lungs to the left heart. It is also called the lesser circulation.

Systemic Circulation

The systemic circulation consists of a series of blood vessels that include arteries and veins of varying sizes and capillaries. The functions of the systemic circulation are to transport oxygenated blood to the various organs and structures of the body, exchange nutrients with the cells, and return deoxygenated blood to the heart for passage into the pulmonary circulation.

Pulmonary Circulation

This component of the circulation consists of a series of blood vessels that include the pulmonary arteries, veins, and capillaries. The functions of the pulmonary circulation are to transport deoxygenated (venous) blood from the right side of the heart to the lungs for gas exchange of oxygen and carbon dioxide and to return oxygenated blood to the left heart for passage to the systemic circulation.

The functional integrity of the circulatory system is evaluated by a number of parameters, including the following:
- Pulse rate
- Arterial blood pressure
- Central venous pressure
- Pulmonary artery and wedge pressures
- Cardiac output
- Urine output

Blood Volume

The integrity of the circulation (the cardiovascular system) depends on an effective blood volume. A functionally effective blood volume exists when the amount of blood and the tone of the vascular compartment result in an adequate filling pressure of the heart. Alterations in either factor may produce significant changes in the function of the cardiovascular system.

The circulating blood volume (BV) accounts for 5% to 9% of body weight. Fat tissue is lower in blood volume than is muscle. The average male has a volume of 7% and the average female 6.5% of body weight. BV may be calculated as follows:

1. In the average 70-kg (150 lb) male:
   7% BV = 70 ml/kg
   70 ml × 70 kg = 4900 ml BV

2. In a 60-kg (130 lb) female:
   6.5% BV = 65 ml/kg
   65 ml × 60 kg = 3900 ml BV

A muscular man has a slightly higher volume of blood (75 ml/kg), and a fat woman a slightly lower volume (55 to 60 ml/kg).

Blood volume may also be estimated from body surface area, which is derived by a nomogram. The average blood volume calculated by this method is 2700 ml/M². Most of the circulating blood volume, nearly 80%, is in the systemic circulation. The nomograms for estimating body surface area are shown in Figure 13-2.

The blood flow varies from one organ to another, depending on the size and physiologic importance of the structure. The liver receives about 27% of the circulating blood, the kidneys 22%, and the brain 14%. The muscles, which form the bulk of the soft tissue, receive about 15% of the blood flow in the resting state. This figure increases significantly during exercise.

Distribution of Blood. At any given time, under normal conditions, the distribution of blood in the vascular tree is as shown in Fig. 13-3.

Components of Circulating Blood

The essential components of circulating blood are:
- Red blood cells—2% to 4% of body weight (BW)
  ∴ 70 kg × 20 or 40 ml = 1400 to 2800 ml of RBCs. Avg = 2100 ml
- Plasma—3% to 5% of BW
  ∴ 70 kg × 30 or 50 ml = 2100 to 3500 ml of plasma. Avg = 2800 ml

Other cellular factors in the blood are:
- White blood cells (about 1% of all blood cells)
- Platelets

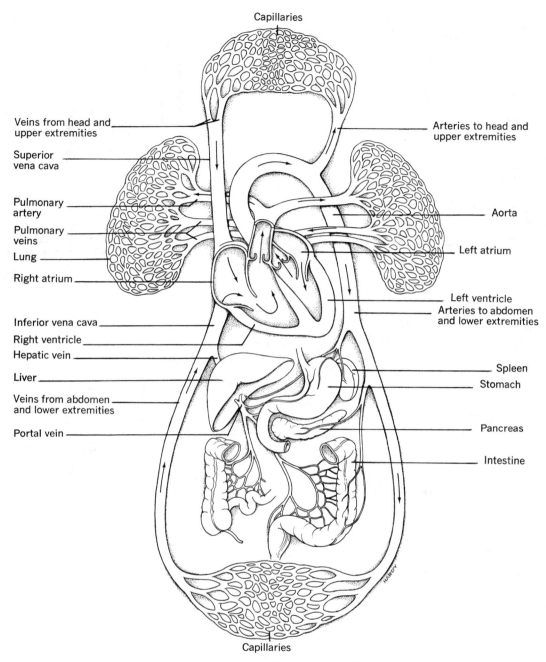

Figure 13-1 *Diagram of the pulmonary and systemic circulations. The pulmonary circulation includes the pulmonary arteries, capillaries, and veins. The systemic circulation includes all the other arteries, capillaries, and veins of the body. (Chaffee EE, Greisheimer EM: Basic Physiology and Anatomy, 4th ed. Philadelphia, JB Lippincott, 1980)*

BODY FLUIDS

The main component of body mass is water. In an adult, water accounts for about 50% to 60% of body weight; in a newborn, 70% to 80% of body weight is water.

Intracellular and Extracellular Fluid. Body water is divided into two major compartments:

- Intracellular, which amounts to 40% of body weight
- Extracellular, which amounts to 20% of body weight

Intracellular fluid is found in the cells of:

Skeletal muscle

Intestine

Viscera

Bone marrow

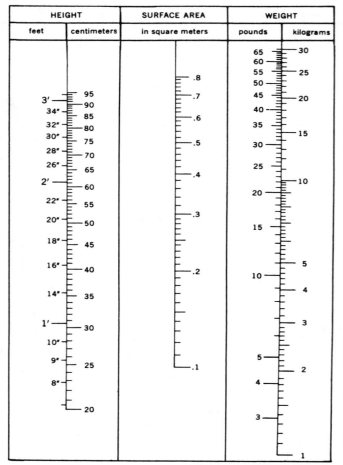

Figure 13-2 Nomograms for estimating body surface area. To determine the surface area of the patient draw a straight line between the point representing his height on the left vertical scale to the point representing his weight on the right vertical scale. The point at which this line intersects the middle vertical scale represents the patient's surface area in square meters. Surface area in square centimeters: $Wt.^{0.425} \times Ht.^{0.725} \times 71.84$. (Courtesy Abbott Laboratories.)

(Courtesy, Abbott Laboratories.)

Glands

Red blood cells

Extracellular fluid includes the water in:

Plasma

Lymph

Interstitial fluid

Bone, tendon, fascial elements

The *interstitial fluid* consists of the extracellular water between the tissue cells *outside of the vascular bed*. It accounts for 15% to 16% of body weight.

Fluid Balance. Body fluids move back and forth between the intracellular and extracellular spaces and between the blood vessels and the tissues outside the vessels. This movement is the result of the balance or differences between the net filtration (hydrostatic) pressure and the colloid osmotic pressure of the blood. In the arterial end of the capillary, the filtration pressure is high, pushing water out of the blood vessels. In the venous end of the capillary, the osmotic pressure is high and draws the water back into the blood vessels.

Conditions that cause a fall in filtration pressure, such as shock or dehydration, allow fluid to move back into the capillary bed in an effort to correct hypovolemia.

Third-Space Fluid. In certain clinical states the extracellular fluid is lost or sequestered in a portion of the body where it cannot be used to fill the fluid needs of the patient. This compartment of sequestered, unusable fluid is referred to as the *third space*.

Examples of third-space fluid are:
- Fluid trapped in the lumen of the bowel in instances of intestinal obstruction or ileus
- Fluid that pours into the peritoneal cavity in peritonitis
- Fluid in soft tissues due to burn injury (burn edema) or cardiac failure.

Third-space fluid can amount to several liters in critically ill or injured patients.

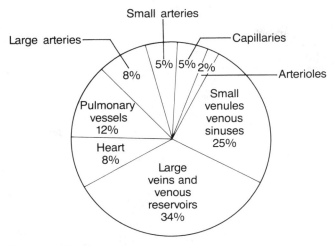

Figure 13-3 *Distribution of blood in the vascular tree under normal conditions.*

Electrolytes. The fluids of the body contain a variety of cations (positively charged ions) and anions (negatively charged ions). The sum of the cations equals that of the anions, to maintain electrical neutrality (Fig. 13-4).

1. The predominant cations are:
   Intracellular
   Potassium (K^+)
   Magnesium (Mg^{++})
   Extracellular
   Sodium (Na^+)
2. The anions are:
   Intracellular
   Phosphate (PO_4^-)
   Protein
   Extracellular
   Chloride (Cl^-)
   Bicarbonate (HCO_3^-)

Protein is present in both intracellular and extracellular fluid.

FLUID REPLACEMENT: DAILY REQUIREMENTS

Fluid replacement is based on an evaluation of the gains or losses of water daily. Assuming no oral intake, the daily basic fluid needs are calculated by adding the sensible and insensible losses.

1. *Sensible loss/24 hr*
Urine output	800 ml–1500 ml
Stool water	125
2. *Insensible loss/24 hr*
Skin and lung (as water vapor, not sweat)	600 ml–850 ml
Total/day	1525–2475 ml

These calculations indicate *basic* fluid needs in a stable patient. Larger or smaller amounts of fluid replacement are required by those who have sustained greater losses, such as occur in dehydration or shock, and by patients with intestinal fistulas or peritonitis. Smaller amounts are required by patients with cardiac or renal disease with limited output (oliguria).

The daily requirements of fluid replacement should be given over a 24-hour period. For ease of care, calculate the fluid dosage on an hourly rate, as follows:

Total fluid needs—3000 ml/24 hr

$$3000 \text{ ml} \div 24 = 125 \text{ ml/hr}$$

When parenteral fluid intake is restricted, the fluid dosage can be regulated by the drop. The infusion sets in current use are calibrated for this purpose and are so marked on the package. Infusion sets used for adults are calibrated at 10 drops/ml and pediatric minidrip sets are calibrated at 50 drops/ml. The sets used in a specific hospital should be checked for calibration.

EMERGENCY FLUID REQUIREMENTS

In the emergency setting, the most common indication for fluid replacement is a body deficit. Indications for fluid replacement are presented in Chart 13-1.

TYPES OF FLUID ADMINISTERED

The type of fluid given depends on the cause(s) of the deficit, for example:
- Major hemorrhage requires blood replacement.
- Intestinal obstruction requires water to which electrolytes have been added.

The makeup of replacement fluid, when other than blood, is determined from an assessment of laboratory data including the following:
- Hemoglobin and hematocrit
- Serum electrolytes Na^+, K^+, Cl^-; CO_2 combining power
- Arterial blood gases

RATE OF ADMINISTRATION

The rate of administration is determined by the patient's underlying condition and response. In major blood loss, fluid and blood replacement can be given at rates of 1 liter of fluid through one veinway in 15 to 20 minutes, if necessary. Urine output is monitored in any patient requiring large amounts of parenteral fluid and should be maintained at a rate of 0.5 to 1.0 ml/kg/hr.

Figure 13-4 *The electrical neutrality of the electrolyte components of the blood is shown above.*

Cations (+) 154		Anions (−) 154	
Na	142 mEq	Cl	105 mEq
K	5	HCO_3	24
Ca	5	Protein	18
Mg	2	Organic acids	4
		HPO_4	2
		SO_4	1

Chart 13-1

INDICATIONS FOR EMERGENCY FLUID REPLACEMENT

Causes of Fluid Deficits

- Insufficient intake
- Excessive losses
- Combination of the above

Clinical Conditions That Require Major Fluid Replacement

- Massive gastrointestinal hemorrhage
- Ruptured abdominal aortic aneurysm/major vessel
- Long-bone or pelvic fractures
- Severe crushing injury
- Second- and third-degree burns
- Gastrointestinal perforation with peritonitis
- Gastrointestinal obstruction
- Dehydration due to major fluid loss

Symptoms and Signs of Dehydration

- Thirst
- Decreased skin turgor
- Decreased eyeball tension
- Reduced urine output
- Lowered blood pressure
- Collapsed veins
- Low venous pressure

ROUTES OF ADMINISTRATION

The route of choice for fluid replacement is the intravenous route, through an extremity vein. In patients who have sustained abdominal trauma with possible major vein injury, the lower limbs should not be used. In major injury to the neck or upper thorax, the upper-extremity veins should be avoided. In conditions in which site selection is not influenced by the location of an injury, upper-limb sites are preferred.

When rapid replacement is necessary, two or three lines may be placed. Insertion of an indwelling venous catheter into a central vein such as the superior vena cava is a popular and well-chosen method of fluid replacement. This vessel is approached percutaneously through the subclavian or internal jugular veins. In infants, the external jugular route is used.

These procedures are invasive and should be performed using strict aseptic technique to minimize the possibility of infection.

MANAGEMENT OF FLUID THERAPY

Chief parameters monitored during fluid therapy are the following:

- *Vital signs*—pulse, blood pressure, respiration
- *Central venous pressure (CVP)* assesses the filling pressure of the right heart. It is not a reliable measure of cardiac function. Do not rely on individual pressure measurements, but instead evaluate *changes* in the CVP as an index of the patient's response. Accurate charting of serial CVP measurements is vital. The normal CVP may vary from −2 to +10 cm of water in children and adults.
- *Urine output*—maintain between 0.5 to 1.0 ml/kg/hr.
- *Pulmonary artery pressure (PAP)* and *pulmonary wedge pressure (PWP)* are excellent guides to cardiac function in critically ill or injured patients. Placement of a balloon flotation (Swan-Ganz) catheter in the pulmonary artery is required. This device is used in some emergency departments, but more often it is placed in the critical care unit.

- *Cardiac output determinations* are not generally used in the emergency setting. This parameter is easily measured by the thermodilution technique with a multilumen Swan-Ganz catheter.

COMPLICATIONS OF FLUID THERAPY

Complications Due to the Replacement Fluid(s)

- Transfusion reaction (see p 173)
- Fluid overload causing overhydration (see Chart 13-2)
  - Hypervolemia
  - Acute pulmonary edema
- Metabolic or electrolyte disturbance
- Adverse reaction because of drug incompatibilities (see p 174)
- Septicemia from contaminated fluid
- Vein thrombosis
- Tissue necrosis

Complications Due to Venipuncture

- Phlebitis at the puncture site
- Cellulitis, local sepsis
- Septicemia
- Air embolism
- Local edema

Complications Due to Hyperalimentation

- Hyperosomotic hyperglycemia
- Hyperchloremic acidosis
- Hyperammonemia

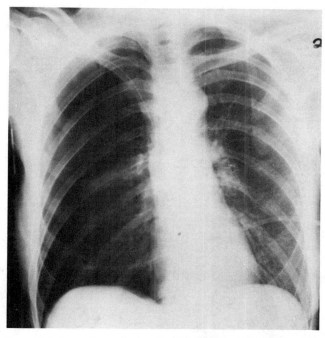

Figure 13-5 *Pneumothorax after insertion of central vein catheter. Note catheter in vein on right.*

- Azotemia
- Hypovitaminosis and trace metal deficiency
- Hypophosphatemic hemolytic anemia

Complications Due to Central Vein Catheters

These depend on the approach used, but are as follows:
- Local sepsis
- Thrombosis at puncture site
- Damage to subclavian artery with arteriovenous fistula
- Pneumothorax (Fig. 13-5)
- Hemothorax or hydrothorax
- Brachial plexus injury
- Subcutaneous emphysema
- Air embolism
- Thoracic duct injury
- Inadvertent injection of fluid into mediastinum or pleural cavity
- Catheter embolus (Fig. 13-6)
- Misdirection of catheter (Fig. 13-7)

TECHNIQUE OF VENIPUNCTURE

Sites of Administration (Fig. 13-8)

A vein large enough to accommodate the selected needle or catheter is chosen. The locations most commonly used are:

Chart 13-2

SIGNS AND SYMPTOMS OF FLUID OVERLOAD

- Dyspnea
- Pitting edema in dependent portions of the body
- Elevated blood pressure
- Tachycardia
- High venous pressure
- Basilar rales in the lungs
- Ascites and/or pleural effusion
- High urine output
- Acute weight gain, usually in excess of 0.25 to 0.5 kg/day

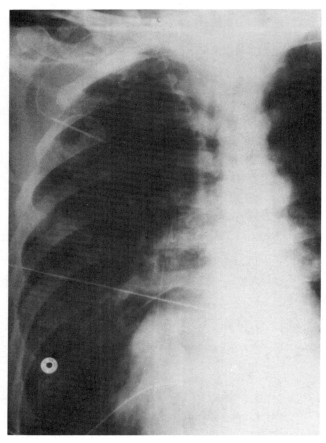

Figure 13-6 Catheter embolus. Note catheter in right heart with snare to retrieve it.

1. Upper extremity
   • Hand and wrist—dorsal vein
   • Forearm—volar or dorsal aspect of forearm
   • Elbow—volar (antecubital) aspect of elbow, basilic or cephalic vein

2. Lower extremity
   • Foot—dorsal vein
   • Ankle—greater saphenous vein just anterior to medial malleolus
3. Scalp
   • Used in infants
4. Central vein
   • Superior vena cava—The indwelling catheter is usually passed percutaneously through the subclavian, antebrachial, or jugular routes.

The choice of a site is affected by the following factors:
• If the needle is not to be left indwelling in the vein, a vessel in the antecubital space is chosen.
• If the needle or cannula is to be used for prolonged periods, select a vein on the dorsum of the hand, wrist, or forearm—in other words, the most remote peripheral vein large enough to accept the indwelling device.

Equipment

Needles—18 to 25 gauge needles (23 and 25 gauge are scalp vein needles)

Indwelling vein catheter—this consists of a 14 to 20 gauge cannula-needle assembly

Povidone-iodine scrub pad (alcohol if the patient is sensitive to iodine)

Tourniquet

Arm board

2-in × 2-in gauze pad

Adhesive tape

Procedure

1. Apply a tourniquet to the limb between the site of venipuncture and the heart. The tourniquet should be applied tightly enough to occlude outflow from the su-

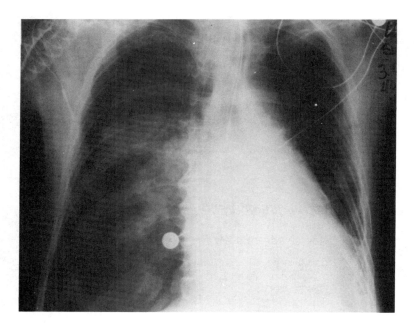

Figure 13-7 Misdirection of central vein catheter from right subclavian artery to left internal jugular vein.

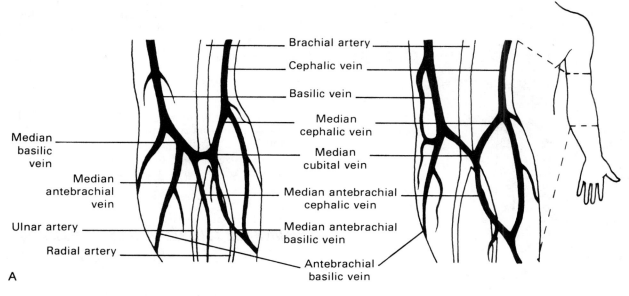

A

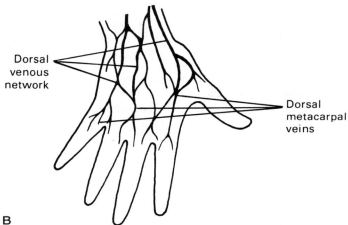

B

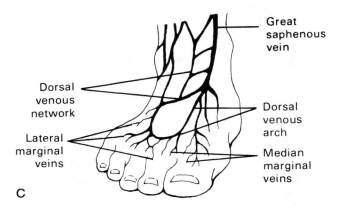

C

Figure 13-8 *Common sites for intravenous infusion in the upper and lower limbs. The preferred site is in the periphery of an upper extremity, remote from a joint (wrist, elbow), in order to maintain joint mobility and patient comfort. A. Two common configurations of the superficial veins of the inner aspect of the forearm. B. The dorsal venous system of the hand. C. Superficial veins of the foot and leg. (Sager DP, Bomar SK: Intravenous Medications. Philadelphia, JB Lippincott, 1980)*

perficial veins of the limb without occluding arterial inflow. If the skin is delicate, apply tourniquet over the patient's gown.

2. Prepare the skin with povidone-iodine (or alcohol). Apply with friction, working from the center out toward the periphery in an area 5 cm to 8 cm (2 in to 3 in) in diameter.

3. Introduce the needle or cannula-needle device, bevel up, at the selected site into the subcutaneous tissue to one side of the vein or in the crotch of a bifurcation, 1.5 cm to 2.0 cm (0.5 in to 0.8 in) below or distal to the main vein.

4. Pass the needle parallel to the vein for a distance of 1 cm to 1.5 cm (0.4 in to 0.6 in). See Figure 13-9.

11. Check the patency of the system and the position of the device by lowering the infusion bottle below the level of the vein, and observe the return of blood into the flash chamber or adapter.

12. Place the infusion solution approximately 30 inches above chest level.

13. Set the crimping device to regulate the rate of flow as ordered.

14. Tape the extremity to an arm board to minimize the chance of dislodging the indwelling device if it lies near a joint.

15. Record the size of the cannula and the date and time of insertion on the outer dressing (Fig. 13-10).

TECHNIQUE FOR CENTRAL-VEIN CATHETERIZATION

Sites of Administration

* The central vein is usually entered through a peripheral vein. In infants and small children, a venous cutdown may be necessary to insert the catheter; in adults, percutaneous puncture is usually accomplished without difficulty.

* The peripheral veins most commonly used are the brachial vein at the antecubital fossa, the internal jugular vein, and the subclavian vein.

* The subclavian vein is most favored, and its approach by the infraclavicular route is described below.

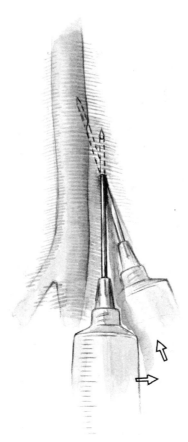

Figure 13-9 *Technique of venipuncture: preferred method for inserting needle.*
* *Introduce the needle, bevel up, at the site selected for venipuncture, through the skin into the subcutaneous tissue to one side of the vein.*
* *Pass the needle parallel to the vein for a distance of 1 to 1.5 cm.*
* *With the thumb of the free hand, apply pressure to the vein distal to the skin puncture to fix the vein in position and prevent it from rolling away from the needle.*
* *Once the vein is fixed, maneuver the needle to enter the side wall of the vessel at an angle of 20 to 35 degrees and firmly pass the point of the needle into the vein.*
(Cosgriff JH Jr: Atlas of Diagnostic and Therapeutic Procedures for Emergency Personnel. Philadelphia, JB Lippincott, 1978)

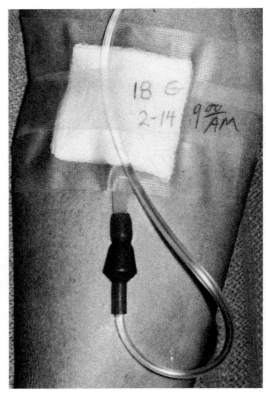

Figure 13-10 *Size of cannula and date and time of insertion recorded on outer dressing.*

5. With the thumb of the free hand, apply pressure to the vein distal to the skin puncture site to fix the vein in position and prevent it from rolling away from the needle.

6. Do not enter the vein by direct puncture through the overlying skin, lest the posterior wall of the vein be penetrated inadvertently. Once the vein is fixed, the preferred technique is to maneuver the needle to enter the side wall of the vessel at an angle of 20 to 35 degrees (Fig. 13-9).

7. Penetrate the vein. After entry, aspirate the syringe gently or observe blood entering the flash chamber of the cannula.

8. Remove the tourniquet.

9. If the needle is to be removed, place an antiseptic swab over the puncture site to minimize hematoma formation.

10. If an indwelling device is used, place an antiseptic 2-in × 2-in gauze pad with povidone-iodine over the puncture site and secure the catheter in place with adhesive tape.

Equipment

- The equipment is prepackaged and sterilized by the manufacturer.
- Either a catheter-over-needle or a catheter-through-needle device is used.

Procedure

1. Since this is an invasive procedure, strict aseptic technique is used.
   - The operator and assistant(s) should be properly gowned, gloved, and masked. In urgent situations, the gown may be eliminated.
   - The operative site should be shaved and widely prepped with povidone-iodine (or alcohol if the patient is sensitive to iodine).
2. Place the patient flat or in a slight Trendelenburg position to increase the pressure in the subclavian vein and minimize the chance of air embolism.
3. Rotate the patient's head 90 degrees to the side opposite the point of entry.
4. Raise a skin wheal with a local anesthetic agent, one fingerbreadth below the inferior border of the midpoint of the clavicle.
5. Introduce the needle and syringe assembly into the wheal.
6. Place the index or middle finger of the opposite hand in the suprasternal notch as a target and slowly advance the needle-syringe assembly toward it, keeping the syringe parallel to the line of the lateral half of the clavicle and the skin. (Fig. 13-11)
7. Advance the needle deep to the clavicle but *above* the first rib.
8. Once past the rib, aspirate gently. A free return of venous blood indicates that the needle is in the subclavian vein.
9. Carefully detach the syringe and cover the needle hub with the gloved finger.
10. Insert the catheter the desired distance through the needle.
11. Hold the catheter in position and withdraw the needle over the catheter.
12. Place the blunt needle into the catheter and secure it to the skin.
13. Apply povidone-iodine ointment at the site where the catheter penetrates the skin.
14. Cover with an outer sterile dressing.
15. At the completion of the procedure, check the position of the catheter in the superior vena cava by chest x-ray. The lower end of the vena cava is at the level of the interspace between the 7th and 8th thoracic vertebrae (Fig. 13-12).

Care of Indwelling Vein Catheters

- After application of an outer sterile dressing, record the date, time of insertion, and size of the catheter on the outer layer of the dressing.
- Avoid placing clamps on the IV tubing, which can be damaged by this maneuver.
- Change the infusion tubing every 24 hours.
- Check the infusion site for any evidence of sepsis. If any is present, remove the catheter to another site.
- Ideally, replace the catheter every 72 hours.
- In the elderly patient, check for any leak or fluid from the puncture site.

In Infants

1. A central vein line is usually placed through the external jugular vein and the catheter brought out through a subcutaneous tunnel in the neck or scalp.
2. Initiate measures to secure the line in place.
   - Cover the site with a plastic or paper cup (Fig. 13-13) when a peripheral line is used.
   - Restrain the limbs.
   - Keep restraints loose enough to allow for slight motion.
   - Cover the infant's hands with a cotton stockinette to prevent him from grasping the IV line.

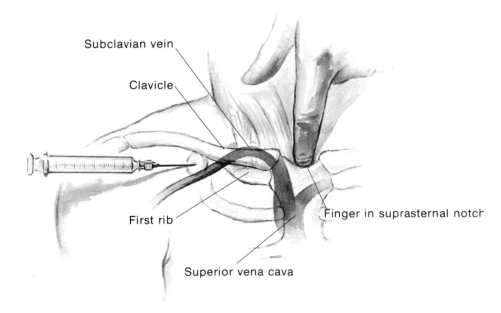

Figure 13-11 *Insertion of central venous catheter, subclavian approach. (Cosgriff JH Jr: Atlas of Diagnostic and Therapeutic Procedures for Emergency Personnel, Philadelphia, JB Lippincott, 1978)*

Subclavian vein

Clavicle

First rib

Finger in suprasternal notch

Superior vena cava

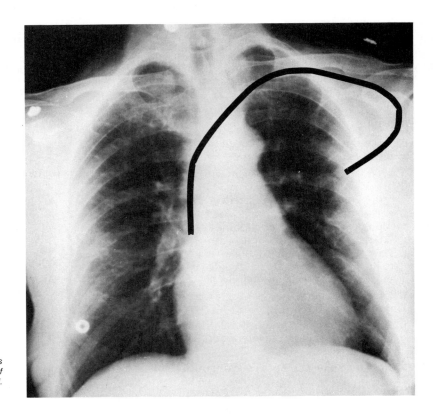

Figure 13-12 *Chest x-ray film showing position of central venous catheter in the superior vena cava. (Cosgriff JH Jr: Atlas of Diagnostic and Therapeutic Procedures for Emergency Personnel. Philadelphia JB Lippincott, 1978)*

3. Keep all lines out of the child's reach.
4. Tape all tubing connections.
5. Maintain an accurate record of time and amount of fluid infused.
6. Use an infusion pump for accurate delivery of the fluid.
7. Assess fluid needs by measuring weight daily.

BLOOD REPLACEMENT

Transfusion of blood is a common practice in the United States. Blood replacement therapy has changed in recent years in that whole blood is rarely used and blood components are usually given. Approximately 6 million units of blood are given annually. It is estimated that 2% of this amount is associated with unfavorable reactions, the most common of which is hepatitis. The use of blood components has reduced the incidence of untoward reactions. Adverse reactions to blood administration, their cause, signs and symptoms, and management are listed in Table 13-1.

Figure 13-13 *Paper cup taped over venipuncture site for protection. (Brunner LS, Suddarth DS: The Lippincott Manual of Nursing Practice, 3rd ed. Philadelphia, JB Lippincott, 1982)*

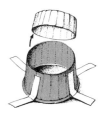

TYPES OF BLOOD PRODUCTS

The types of blood products available for replacement are:
- Whole blood
- Red blood cell concentrate (RBCC)
- Platelet concentrate
- Fresh frozen plasma
- Stored plasma
- Cryoprecipitate
- Factor IX complex
- Albumin
- Immune serum globulin

Whole Blood and Red Cell Concentrate

In the emergency setting, the two most commonly used products are whole blood and RBCC. Replacement with whole blood should be limited to situations in which there

TABLE 13-1. CHARACTERISTICS OF WHOLE BLOOD AND RED CELL CONCENTRATES

Characteristics	Whole Blood	Red Cell Concentrate
Volume, ml	500 ± 25	300 ± 25
Hematocrit, %	40 ±	70 ± 5
Red cell volume, ml	200 ±	200 ± 25
Plasma volume, ml	300 ±	100 ± 25
Albumin content, gm	10–12	4–5

(Blajcham, MA et al: Clinical use of blood, blood components and blood products. Can Med Assoc J 121:33–42, 1979)

is acute blood loss requiring more than 3 units. If hemorrhage is controlled, red cell concentrates are preferred. For more detailed discussion of this point, see Chap. 12, Shock. Characteristics of whole blood and RBCCs are listed in Table 13-2.

The advantages of red blood cell concentrates are as follows:

- The per-unit volume of hemoglobin is almost twice that of whole blood
- Circulatory overload is less likely

TABLE 13-2.   ADVERSE REACTIONS TO BLOOD ADMINISTRATION

Type	Cause	Signs/Symptoms	Treatment
Hemolytic reaction	ABO incompatibility	Onset during or shortly after transfusion Chills, fever Chest pain Headache Burning sensation along the vein Shock Hemoglobinuria, may produce renal tubular necrosis, a potentially fatal complication	Stop the transfusion immediately. Obtain sample of the patient's blood and urine for hemoglobin indicating intravascular hemolysis Monitor hourly urine output Return the unused blood to blood bank for recrossmatching
Hemolytic reaction	Allergy to blood products	Urticaria Pruritus Facial edema Anaphylaxis	Give antihistamines parenterally Give epinephrine if reaction is severe or associated with respiratory distress
Febrile reaction	Leukocyte antibodies	Chills, fever Headache Flushing Tachycardia Nausea, vomiting	Stop the transfusion immediately Give aspirin or acetoaminophen to reduce fever Check temperature at close intervals Substitute another unit of blood
Circulatory overload	Too-rapid infusion Excessive transfusions	Tachycardia Chest tightness Labored breathing Pulmonary edema	Stop transfusion Have patient sit up Use rotating tourniquets or phlebotomy Consider digitalizing patient
Bacterial contamination	Contamination of blood or infusion equipment	Chills, fever Hypotension Abdominal pain Vomiting Bloody diarrhea	Stop transfusion Obtain blood cultures Treat shock Administer broad-spectrum antibiotics Return unused blood to blood bank for bacteriology study
Hypothermia	Infusion of cold blood	Lowered body temperature Chills Cardiac arrhythmia leading to arrest	Perform external warming of patient Warm blood with warming coil may be heated to 40°C without significant hemolysis
Air embolism	Introduction of air into the infusion system Possibly, infusion of blood under pressure	Dyspnea Cyanosis Shock Cardiac arrest	Remove pressure infusor Turn patient on left side to collect air in the right atrium and divert it from the pulmonary tree Lower head Treat symptoms
Hyperkalemia	Transfusion of old blood that is partially hemolyzed Stored blood that contains increased amounts of potassium	Nausea, colic Diarrhea Apprehension Elevated serum K^+ Cardiac arrhythmias with high, spiking T waves	Obtain serum K^+ level K exalate Hydrate Insulin K^+ losing diuretic
Hypocalcemia	Massive transfusions. Ionized calcium is removed by the anticoagulant in donor blood	Muscle cramps Chvostek's sign* Trousseau's sign† Hyperactive reflexes Convulsions Low serum Ca^H	Obtain serum Ca^H level Give intravenous calcium chloride or calcium gluconate

* Chvostek's sign is pathognomonic of tetany due to low serum calcium. It is elicited by tapping sharply with the finger just anterior to the external auditory meatus over the course of the facial nerve. It produces a contraction of the muscles on the same side of the face due to hyperirritability of the nerve.
† Trousseau's sign is elicited by inflating a blood pressure cuff on the arm, causing a tetanic contraction of the wrist and fingertips. It indicates hypocalcemia.

- Transfusion reactions occur less often
- Transfusion hepatitis is less common
  The indications for blood replacement are as follows:
- To maintain or increase blood volume
- To maintain or increase the oxygen carrying capacity of the blood.

Each unit of blood will increase hemoglobin by 1.0 gm–1.5 gm.

Generally, blood replacement is made with type-specific, crossmatched blood. Depending on the hospital laboratory and the availability of blood, a crossmatch may take 30 to 60 minutes to complete. In clinical emergencies, type-specific, uncrossmatched blood may be used with a high degree of safety. Untoward reactions occur less than 0.5% of the time. Even so, it may take 10 to 15 minutes to perform a blood typing. Type O Rh-negative universal donor blood may also be used in emergencies.

Until blood is available, volume replacement may be initiated using Ringer's lactate solution or a plasma expander such as dextran 70, dextran 40, albumin, or hydroxyethyl starch (Hespan).

Other Blood Components

Because RBCCs replace only red cells, other blood components must be given in a timely manner. The following protocol may serve as a guideline.
- *Fresh frozen plasma*—used to supply coagulation factors. Give 1 unit for every 5 units of RBCC.
- *Platelet concentrate*—used to supply platelets, contain 10 to 12 units of platelets. Give one pack after replacement of 1 blood volume (10 units RBCC) or if platelet count is less than 55,000.

- *Cryoprecipitate (Factor VIII)*—give if partial thromboplastin time (PTT) is greater than 45 seconds.
- *Factor IX complex*—give if prothrombin time (PT) is greater than 18 seconds.

Other products to be used:
- Calcium chloride ($CaCl_2$)—give 1.0 gm/4 units RBCC. Do not exceed 3.0 gm total.
- Sodium bicarbonate ($NaHCO_3$)—give 1 ampule (55 mEq) for every 4 to 5 units RBCC; evaluate response by checking blood gases
- *Fresh* whole blood—give 1 unit after replacement of 1 blood volume (10 units RBCC)

BLOOD TRANSFUSION PRECAUTIONS

Precautions to be observed when transfusing blood are reviewed in Chart 13-3.

DRUG INCOMPATIBILITY

Drug incompatibility is an undesired reaction between a drug and its container, a primary solution, or another drug. It may adversely affect the therapeutic efficacy of the drug or result in unwanted side effects. Incompatibility may result from inadequate solubility or from chemical antagonism by which one drug may deactivate another. The factors that influence compatibility are many. For this reason, many hospitals allow only registered pharmacists to prepare drug ad-

---

Chart 13-3

BLOOD TRANSFUSION PRECAUTIONS

- Check vital signs, hemoglobin, and hematocrit for baseline information. Repeat at intervals during administration. If rapid infusion is necessary, monitor CVP.
- Check donor blood for correct type, patient's name and type, and expiration date.
- Warm blood to room temperature. If rapid replacement is needed, a warming coil may be used.
- Use a Y-type infusion set. Flush the tubing with normal saline or Ringer's lactate solution before and after administration. Do *not* use 5% dextrose in water because hemolysis of the donor cells can result.
- If the RBCCs are too viscous for easy flow, add 50 ml to 100 ml saline to the red-cell pack.
- Use a macropore filter in the infusion line to minimize the chance of cell aggregates' entering the circulation.
- Do not add medications to the blood; use a separate IV line for these.
- Observe the patient closely for adverse reactions to blood administration (Table 13-2).
- Administer blood within 20 minutes of removing it from the blood bank refrigerator.
- Administer blood at a rate compatible with the patient's needs.
- Generally, if an adverse reaction occurs, the transfusion should be discontinued immediately. The intravenous line is kept open with saline or Ringer's lactate solution and measures are taken to identify the type of reaction. Specific countermeasures are then initiated.

mixtures. If emergency personnel are required to mix or add medications to an intravenous fluid, they must be thoroughly familiar with any possible incompatibilities. The hospital pharmacist should be consulted if one is uncertain about the compatibility of drugs to be mixed.

BIBLIOGRAPHY

Blajchman MA, Shepherd FA, Perrault RA: Clinical use of blood, blood components and blood products. CMAJ 121:33, 1979

Blumberg N, Bove JR: Uncross-matched blood for emergency transfusion. JAMA 240:2057, 1978

Boral LI, Henry JB: The type and screen. Transfusion 17:163, 1977

Buickus BA: Administering blood components. Am J Nurs 79:937, 1979

Chaplin H: Packed red blood cells. N Engl J Med 281:364, 1969

Collins JA: Problems associated with the massive transfusion of stored blood. Surgery 75:274, 1974

Cullins LC: Preventing and treating transfusion reactions. Am J Nurs 79:935, 1979

Cosgriff JH Jr: Central vein catheterization. In Atlas of Diagnostic and Therapeutic Procedures for Emergency Personnel, p 133. Philadelphia, JB Lippincott, 1978

Ehrlich A: Avoiding the cross-match mismatch. Emerg Med 9:101, 1977

Fisher RE: Measuring Central Venous Pressure. Nursing 79 79:74, 1979

Goldfinger D: Uncrossmatched blood for emergency transfusion. JAMA 237:1826, 1977

Hogman CF, Hedlund K, Zetierstrom H: Clinical usefulness of red cells preserved in protein-poor mediums. N Engl J Med 299:1377, 1978

Isbister JP, Scurrm RD: Blood transfusion therapy: Components, indications, complications and controversies. Anesth Intensive Care 6:197, 1978

Johnston DG: Blood transfusion: Use and abuse of blood components. West J Med 128:390, 1978

Manzi CC, Masourli S: Troubles with IVS? Nursing 78 78:78, 1978

McCurcy PR: Blood component therapy. Postgrad Med 62:143, 1977

Millam DA: How to insert an IV. Am J Nurs 79:1268, 1979

Myrhe BA: Fatalities from blood transfusion. JAMA 244:1333, 1980

Silberman S: Less waste—and fewer complications—in blood component therapy. Consultant 16:97, 1978

Smith RN: Invasive pressure monitoring. Am J Nurs 78:1514–1521, 1978

Valeri CR: Blood components in the treatment of acute blood loss. Anesth Analg 54:1, 1975

14
RESUSCITATION: PRINCIPLES AND TECHNIQUES

BARBARA SECORD-PLETZ

Resuscitation is defined as "restoration to life after apparent death."[1] "Apparent death" is generally characterized by unresponsiveness, absence of spontaneous breathing, and pulselessness (cardiopulmonary arrest). Current resuscitation techniques include airway management, ventilatory and circulatory support, and use of electricity and drugs to restore an effective heart rhythm. The potential for success depends upon several factors; these include etiology of arrest, the speed with which basic life support (BLS) and advanced life support (ALS) are provided, and the expertise of the providers.

Resuscitative techniques have been evolving since ancient times. Successful resuscitation was recorded as long ago as 300 B.C., when the Prophet Elisha revived a child.[2] In 1744 Tossach documented success using mouth-to-mouth ventilation in humans. (This technique was replaced by the less effective arm-lift method, which remained in common usage until the mid-1960s.) Use of electrical shock to restore heart rhythm was reported in 1775 by Squires. Experimentation in resuscitation escalated in the mid-1800s and proliferated during the 20th century with the development of cardiac massage (open and closed chest techniques), AC and DC defibrillation, and advances in airway management and ventilation techniques. In 1960, Kouwenhoven, Jude, and Knickerbocker reported sucessful resuscitation in eight patients using closed chest massage, mouth-to-mouth ventilation, and defibrillation.[3]

During the 1960s, hospitals established coronary care units, staffed by specially trained nurses, where myocardial infarction (MI) patients were continuously observed and their heart rhythms monitored. These units demonstrated that many cardiac arrest victims could be successfully resuscitated with immediate cardiopulmonary resuscitation, defibrillation, and drug therapy. Despite the success of these units, high mortality rates continued for victims of cardiac arrest that occurred outside the hospital.

The largest group of patients who suffer prehospital cardiac arrest are victims of sudden cardiac death. It is estimated that in the United States there are 640,000 deaths annually from coronary heart disease and 350,000 of these occur before the patient reaches the hospital. Most deaths (60%) occur within 1 hour of symptoms, and in many instances, cardiac arrest happens without warning.[4]

STANDARDS

In 1973, the National Conference on Standards for Cardiopulmonary Resuscitation (CPR) and Emergency Cardiac Care made some important recommendations, including the following:
1. CPR training must be extended to the public.
2. Training in CPR and emergency cardiac care (ECC) must be in accordance with the standards of the American Heart Association, using a nationally standardized curriculum.
3. Basic life support (BLS) and advanced life support (ALS) delivery must be required for all life-support units and hospitals on a stratified and integrated community-wide basis.
4. Recognition of early warning signs should be stressed.
5. Emphasis on access to the emergency medical service (EMS) system should be included in emergency cardiac care.[5]

Definitions of BLS and ALS appear in Chart 14-1.

The American Heart Association has largely accomplished these goals. Training programs in BLS and ALS are becoming readily available. Prehospital care systems have been generally upgraded; prehospital BLS is almost universally available and many systems offer prehospital ALS as well. Prehospital ALS is often directed by physicians or emergency department nurses by radio communication to paramedical personnel. Large numbers of citizens have been trained in CPR. (Comparative studies have shown that survival rates for out-of-hospital arrest are significantly improved when bystander CPR has been initiated.[6])

The impact of BLS and ALS in conjunction with improved EMS-system access and citizen CPR training is becoming increasingly evident. The best survival rates for patients suffering out-of-hospital arrest have been in EMS systems in which BLS is often provided within 4 minutes and ALS within 8 minutes. Additionally, there is evidence that stabilization of myocardial infarction patients before transport, using BLS and ALS, decreases the incidence of cardiac arrest en route.[7]

CARDIOPULMONARY ARREST

Cardiopulmonary arrest may occur suddenly, without warning, or it may be the final event of a progressively life-threatening disorder. Although organic heart disease is by far the most prevalent cause of cardiac arrest, many other conditions may produce it. Broad categories for underlying causes of cardiac arrest include hypoxia and anoxia, neurologic dysfunction, and metabolic and chemical dysfunction.[8] Any condition that results in hypoxia or acidosis or otherwise interrupts vital cellular functions can cause cardiac arrest.

A large number of cardiac arrests fall into the category of sudden cardiac death. Patients in this category most often suffer arrest outside of the hospital or shortly after admission to the emergency department. The American Heart Association currently defines sudden cardiac death as cardiac death that occurs within 1 hour of symptoms. Although the majority of these patients are found to have underlying heart disease such as severe diffuse coronary atherosclerosis, many do not show evidence of acute myocardial infarction.[9] See Chapter 16, Cardiac Emergencies.

THE PREARREST PHASE

The primary goals in caring for patients in the prearrest phase of acute myocardial infarction are preventing cardiac arrest and limiting the extent of myocardial infarction. Medical interventions to achieve these goals are aimed toward:

Chart 14-1

BASIC AND ADVANCED LIFE SUPPORT

Basic Life Support

Basic life support (BLS) includes recognition of unconsciousness and maintenance of the airway, breathing, and circulation without the use of adjunctive equipment.

Advanced Life Support

Advanced life support (ALS), as defined by the American Heart Association, includes the following:
* Basic life support
* Use of adjunctive equipment for ventilation and circulation
* Cardiac monitoring for dysrhythmia recognition and control
* Defibrillation
* Establishment and maintenance of an intravenous infusion line
* Definitive therapy, including drug administration, to correct acidosis and maintain an effective heart rhythm and circulation
* Stabilization of the patient's condition
* Transportation with continuous monitoring

---

1. Providing sufficient oxygen to the myocardium
2. Decreasing myocardial oxygen consumption by decreasing the heart's work load
3. Preventing life-threatening dysrhythmias
4. Controlling dysrhythmias that increase myocardial oxygen consumption or decrease the blood supply to the coronary arteries.

Treatment

Early medical intervention may prevent cardiac arrest. When the presentation suggests myocardial ischemia, cardiac monitoring should be instituted immediately and a specific treatment plan initiated. This plan should include:

1. *Administration of supplemental oxygen.* Oxygen is administered at 6 L/min with a nasal cannula. This method achieves an oxygen concentration of 25%–40% and is well tolerated by patients. In patients with a history of chronic obstructive pulmonary disease (COPD) and carbon dioxide retention, an oxygen mask equipped with a Venturi-type metering device should be used with the initial oxygen concentration at 24%.[10]

2. *Establishment of an intravenous route.* An intravenous line of 5% dextrose in water (D_5W) should be established as a route for administering medications. The line should be kept open for a full flow.

3. *Pain relief.* Relief of pain by the administration of nitroglycerin or morphine sulfate should receive a high priority in the treatment plan. Pain increases anxiety, which in turn stimulates catecholamine release. High blood levels of catecholamine increase the myocardial work load and hence myocardial oxygen consumption, and predispose to irritable heart rhythms. Besides pain relief, nitroglyc-

erin and morphine sulfate have additional hemodynamic benefits. They decrease myocardial oxygen consumption because they lessen the heart's work load by reducing both preload and afterload.[11]

4. *Treatment of dysrhythmias.* Dysrhythmias can be divided into two general groups: active (irritable, tachycardic) and passive (bradycardic). Both types pose a threat to the patient.

* Does the dysrhythmia have the potential to progress to a more life-threatening one? (*e.g.,* multifocal premature ventricular contractions → ventricular fibrillation)
* Does the dysrhythmia substantially increase myocardial oxygen demand (*e.g.,* atrial fibrillation with a rapid, uncontrolled ventricular response)?
* Is the cardiac output generated by the rhythm inadequate (*e.g.,* sinus bradycardia associated with hypotension or ventricular ectopy)?

Even when dysrhythmias are not present, antiarrhythmic therapy may be indicated. Lidocaine is currently recommended in the early course of acute myocardial infarction because primary ventricular fibrillation frequently occurs without any warning dysrhythmia.[12]

Management of the patient in the prearrest phase of cardiac arrest is summarized in Chart 14-2.

ARREST PHASE

The term *cardiopulmonary arrest* means the absence of both pulse and spontaneous breathing. Its hallmarks are apnea, pulselessness, and unresponsiveness. At least initially, arrest is not always cardiopulmonary. When patients suddenly

---

Chart 14-2

MANAGEMENT OF THE PATIENT IN THE PREARREST PHASE OF CARDIAC ARREST

Primary Objectives

- Prevent cardiac arrest.
- Limit the size of myocardial infarction.

Objectives of Medical Intervention

- Provide sufficient oxygen to the myocardium.
- Decrease myocardial oxygen consumption by decreasing cardiac work load.
- Prevent life-threatening dysrhythmias.
- Control dysrhythmias that increase myocardial oxygen consumption or increase blood supply to coronary arteries.

Treatment Plan

1. Institute cardiac monitoring.
2. Administer supplemental oxygen.
   - Nasal cannula, 6 L/min, for oxygen concentration 25%–40%
   - Oxygen mask with Venturi-type metering device—initial oxygen concentration 24% (for patient with COPD and carbon dioxide retention)
3. Relieve pain.
   - Administer nitroglycerin or morphine sulfate to relieve pain and anxiety, hence reduce cardiac work load, myocardial oxygen consumption, predisposition to irritable heart rhythms.
4. Treat dysrhythmias.
   - Institute drug therapy as indicated

General Management

- Convey attitude of calm, competence, and confidence.
- Recognize anxiety and emotional needs of patient and family.
- Reduce all physical stresses on patient

---

develop ventricular fibrillation, spontaneous respirations often continue briefly. Respiratory arrest may precede cardiac arrest, as in patients with narcotic overdose. Unresponsiveness may not be immediate in cardiac arrest. Monitored patients sometimes remain awake briefly after the cardiac monitor displays ventricular fibrillation.

Cessation of cardiac function and breathing leads quickly to anoxia and acidosis. Intervention must be swift to prevent irreversible cell damage. These interventions include CPR, oxygen administration, drug therapy, and the use of electricity to reestablish an effective heart rhythm.

Anoxia. Anoxia occurs because respirations have ceased and oxygen is no longer available for transport to tissues. Hypoxia is also present because tissues are no longer being perfused. Some of the effects of anoxia and hypoxia include:[13]
- Increased release of catecholamines (which decrease the fibrillation threshold of the heart)
- Vagal stimulation (which can propagate conduction disturbances and slow heart rates

- Cerebral vascular dilatation and structural cell damage. Additionally, because oxygen is not available, cells convert to anaerobic metabolism, which produces metabolic acidosis.

Acidosis. In cardiopulmonary arrest both respiratory and metabolic acidosis are present. Respiratory acid (carbonic acid derived from carbon dioxide and water) is not being excreted by the lungs. Metabolic acidosis occurs because anaerobic metabolism produces lactic and pyruvic acids, which cannot be metabolized without adequate tissue perfusion. The adverse effects of acidosis on the myocardium include increased irritability, decreased fibrillation threshold, decreased response to catecholamines, and decreased contractility.[14]

Cell Damage. Cells become damaged as a result of anoxia and acidosis. In the heart, myocardial cells, coronary microvasculature, and the conduction system are affected. The brain is particularly sensitive to oxygen deprivation. At normal temperatures, irreversible cerebral ischemia occurs within 8 to 10 minutes after cardiac arrest.[15]

It is important to note that cold temperatures produce hypothermia (*e.g.*, submersion in cold water). In hypothermia cell damage is delayed. Successful resuscitation is possible without neurologic sequelae after prolonged anoxia in hypothermic patients.

OBJECTIVES AND METHODS OF RESUSCITATION

Ideally, the primary goal of resuscitation is to restore the patient to his prearrest state of health without sequelae. The overall objective is to reestablish an effective heart rhythm and spontaneous breathing while preventing irreversible cell damage. The specific therapeutic objectives involved in resuscitation and the methods of achieving them are as follows:

1. *Provide sufficient oxygen to tissues.* Tissues must receive adequate oxygen to prevent permanent cell damage and so that other medical interventions will be successful. Methods to provide adequate oxygenation include:
   - Airway maintenance
   - Ventilation with high concentrations of oxygen
   - Chest compressions to circulate oxygenated blood
2. *Correct acidosis.* Acidosis must be corrected to enable the heart to respond well to drug therapy and electrical countershock. Acidosis decreases myocardial contractility. There are two methods of treating acidosis; both methods must be used in cardiopulmonary resuscitation.
   - *Ventilate.* Respiratory acidosis is caused by retention of carbon dioxide. Carbonic acid is volatile and is excreted by the lungs during ventilation. Therefore, respiratory acidosis is treated by ventilating the patient so that gas exchange can be accomplished.
   - *Administration of sodium bicarbonate.* Metabolic acidosis during cardiopulmonary arrest is the result of anaerobic metabolism and insufficient tissue perfusion. It is treated by administering sodium bicarbonate.
3. *Maintain adequate tissue perfusion.*
   - Chest compressions
   - Maintenance of an adequate circulating volume. This is a major concern when cardiopulmonary arrest is secondary to hypovolemia.
   - Drug therapy. Sometimes drugs that improve cardiac contractility and blood flow are necessary (*e.g.*, Dopamine).
4. *Restore an effective heart rhythm.* Restoration of an effective heart rhythm is a primary objective in resuscitation. Methods of achieving this may include:
   - Maintenance of optimal oxygenation of tissues
   - Correction of acidosis
   - Use of electricity
     Defibrillation
     Synchronized cardioversion
     Artificial pacing
   - Drug therapy
     Drugs that suppress irritable heart rhythms (*e.g.*, lidocaine)
     Drugs that increase the heart's ability to respond favorably to electrical countershock (*e.g.*, epinephrine)
     Drugs that increase heart rate (*e.g.*, atropine)

INITIAL ASSESSMENT AND TREATMENT

An organized, rapid, and appropriate patient assessment is performed while resuscitation efforts are being instituted. Assessment is important because the treatment plan will be based on this information. The assessment incorporates both physical findings and, if possible, historical data. Critical patient care is provided simultaneously with the assessment steps as they are performed. The basic sequence is described in Chart 14-3.

PRIORITIES IN RESUSCITATION

It is essential to adhere carefully to priorities in conducting resuscitation. These priorities follow a logical and easily remembered sequence:
1. Airway
2. Breathing
3. Circulation

After the initial ABCs are accomplished, it is important to consider the probable etiology of arrest in the light of physical findings and historical data. For instance, if bleeding is a likely etiology, volume replacement (through inflation of antishock trousers and administration of intravenous fluids) will receive a high priority in the treatment plan.

RESUSCITATION TECHNIQUES

The resuscitation techniques described in the sections that follow include basic and advanced life-support measures for airway management and ventilation, maintenance of adequate tissue perfusion, and restoration of an effective cardiac rhythm.

AIRWAY MANAGEMENT AND VENTILATION

Establishing and securing a patent airway and providing adequate oxygenation are of primary importance in resuscitation. Airway patency and adequacy of ventilation must be continually reevaluated throughout the resuscitation process.

ESTABLISHING PATENCY

The first step in establishing a patent airway is to attempt repositioning the patient. The airway is often occluded by the tongue lying against the posterior pharyngeal wall. Effective airway positioning may restore spontaneous breathing. Positioning should always be attempted before airway adjuncts are used.

Head-Tilt Maneuver. The head-tilt maneuver is performed by placing one hand under the victim's neck and gently lifting upward while placing the other hand on the victim's forehead and pressing downward. This maneuver is effective in opening the airway and places the rescuer in an ideal position for performing rescue breathing (Fig. 14-1*A*). This technique cannot be used if cervical spine injury is suspected; in this instance, the modified jaw-thrust maneuver should be used.

Chart 14-3

INITIAL MANAGEMENT OF THE PATIENT IN CARDIOPULMONARY ARREST

Primary Objectives

- Reestablish effective heart rhythm and spontaneous breathing.
- Prevent irreversible cellular damage.

Initial Assessment and Care

1. Evaluate responsiveness—shake and shout.
2. Airway
   - Assess airway patency.
   - If patient is not breathing, open the airway.
3. Breathing
   - Determine whether patient is breathing spontaneously after airway is established—look, listen, and feel.
   - If breathing is absent, begin rescue breathing.
4. Circulation
   - Feel for a carotid or a femoral pulse.
   - If no pulse can be felt, begin chest compressions.
5. Evaluate heart rhythm.
   - Institute cardiac monitoring and evaluate heart rhythm.
   - Proceed with treatment as appropriate.
6. Establish an intravenous line.
   - For administration of medications
   - For maintenance of circulating volume
7. Secure the airway.
   - Endotracheal intubation is the preferred method.

Ongoing Assessment

- How much does the patient weigh?
- Are there any signs of trauma?
- Is the skin color bluish or pale?
- Are the head and neck grossly cyanotic in comparison with the trunk and periphery?
- Are the neck veins flat or grossly distended?
- Are the breath sounds equal bilaterally during ventilations, and is chest expansion equal?
- Are the lung sounds moist?
- Is the abdomen distended?
- Are there recent surgical scars?
- Are there signs of chronic illness?

History

If possible, elicit pertinent historical data:
- How long has the patient been in cardiopulmonary arrest?
- Where was the patient found and what was he doing when cardiopulmonary arrest occurred? (*e.g.,* eating at a restaurant, riding in a motor vehicle)
- Did the patient complain of feeling ill prior to cardiopulmonary arrest, and if so what were his complaints?
- Is the patient wearing any medical-alert tags?
- Is the patient under a physician's care? Does he have any known medical problem?

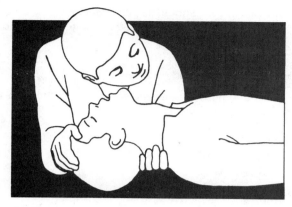

A. Airway

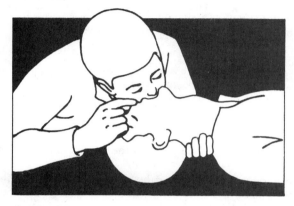

B. Breathing

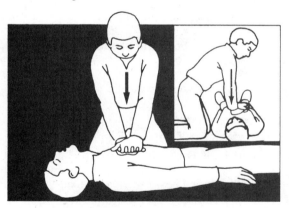

C. Circulation

Figure 14-1 *The ABCs of cardiopulmonary resuscitation include (A) opening the airway, (B) restoring breathing, and (C) restoring circulation with external cardiac compressions. (American Red Cross poster No. 321064, March 1981)*

Modified Jaw-Thrust Maneuver. The modified jaw thrust maneuver is effective in opening the airway while keeping the cervical spine in alignment. The rescuer's hands are placed behind the angle of the victim's jaw and the jaw lifted forward. This brings the tongue forward and away from the posterior pharyngeal wall. The jaw-thrust maneuver is probably more effective than the head tilt and it can be safely performed when cervical spine injury is suspected. It is more awkward for the rescuer and requires more skill. Once the

airway is positioned, the rescuer looks, listens, and feels for spontaneous breathing. This is done by placing your cheek next to the victim's mouth to feel air movement while looking at the victim's chest for chest rise. Good airway position, with the jaw lifted forward, is mandatory during ventilation until the airway is secured by an endotracheal tube.

RESCUE BREATHING

If the victim does not resume breathing spontaneously, rescue breathing must be started (Fig. 14-1*B*). To perform rescue breathing, you must seal the patient's airway. This is usually done by pinching the victim's nostrils with one of your hands, while maintaining good airway position, and placing your mouth over the victim's.

Give four full, quick breaths in rapid succession without allowing the victim's lungs to deflate fully between breaths. The four breaths should fully inflate the victim's lungs. Small air sacs often collapse when breathing ceases. While delivering these four quick breaths, watch to see the chest rise. Also note whether you feel resistance as you ventilate. If the chest does not rise, proceed with treatment for airway obstruction.

If the victim's chest rises with ventilation, continue rescue breathing until spontaneous breathing is restored or another means of ventilating the patient is established. If chest compressions are not required (as when the patient has palpable pulses), ventilate the patient at 5-second intervals.

Chest Compressions. If cardiac arrest is present, chest compressions are begun. For one-rescuer CPR, 15 compressions followed by 2 ventilations are given (Fig. 14-1*C*), except in pediatric patients, for whom the ratio is always 5:1. If two rescuers are present, 5 compressions are performed and then 1 ventilation is interposed on the fifth compression upstroke.

Special Situations. The method for sealing the airway can be adapted for special situations. The nose and mouth are sealed by the rescuer's mouth and ventilated in infants and small children. For a patient with a permanent laryngectomy, the stoma is sealed and ventilated by the rescuer's mouth. A patient who has a tracheostomy tube in place is ventilated through the tube while the rescuer seals the victim's nose and mouth manually.

Gastric Distention. Rescue breathing often causes gastric distention. Gastric distention can cause vomiting with subsequent aspiration, limit lung volumes, and produce increased vagal tone. If vomiting occurs, immediately turn the victim to his side and wipe out or suction the mouth before resuming CPR. Eventually the stomach can be decompressed with nasogastric intubation.

RELIEVING AIRWAY OBSTRUCTION: BASIC LIFE-SUPPORT TECHNIQUES

Airway obstruction can have a variety of causes. Aspiration of foreign bodies or material, laryngeal edema, laryngospasm, and obstructing tumors are examples. Prompt recognition and treatment of these conditions is a first priority.

Airway obstruction can be partial or complete. Partial obstruction is characterized by crowing respirations, wheezing, and coughing. When choking occurs, as with a bolus of food, the victim commonly clutches his hand to his throat. Efforts to relieve partial airway obstruction can result in just enough movement of the foreign body to cause complete airway obstruction. If the victim remains awake and can speak, it is best to encourage forcible coughing. If the victim cannot speak, is not moving air, and is becoming cyanotic, prompt action is necessary.

Conscious Victim (Chart 14-4)

The basic life-support techniques are back blows, abdominal thrusts, and chest thrusts. These will be successful only in airway obstruction due to a foreign body. Obstruction from other causes must be treated by other techniques.

Back Blows. The first maneuver for relieving obstruction in a conscious victim is to deliver a series of four back blows with the victim standing. These are delivered with the heel of one hand over the spine between the shoulder blades while the free arm supports the victim's chest.

Abdominal Thrust. If back blows are unsuccessful in dislodging the foreign body, the abdominal thrust maneuver is attempted. This technique is performed with the rescuer positioned behind the victim and with both of the rescuer's arms wrapped around the victim's waist. The rescuer forms a fist with one hand and positions the thumb side between the victim's waist and rib cage. The rescuer grasps the fist with one hand, and then performs four rapid thrusts directed inward and upward.

Chest Thrust. A modification of the abdominal thrust is the chest thrust. For this maneuver the rescuer is positioned similarly but the fist is placed over the midsternum. The thrusts are then delivered posteriorly. The chest thrust is preferred in pediatric patients, in advanced pregnancy, and in very obese patients.

Unconscious Victim (Chart 14-4)

When the victim is unconscious, these maneuvers are performed with the victim lying and the rescuer kneeling beside him. For the abdominal thrust, one of the rescuer's hands is placed on top of the other. The heel of the bottom hand is positioned between the victim's waist and rib cage and the thrusts are directed upward (toward the head) and downward (toward the back). For the chest thrust, the hand is positioned as it is during chest compressions and the thrusts are delivered in a downward direction.

The sequences currently recommended by the American Heart Association are described in Chart 14-5.

RELIEVING AIRWAY OBSTRUCTION: ADVANCED TECHNIQUES

If the airway remains occluded despite repeated attempts to relieve obstruction by basic life-support techniques, more advanced techniques are required. These techniques demand skill and practice and should be performed only by qualified persons. If performed improperly, they can result in serious complications.

Removal of Foreign Body

The safest and least invasive technique is to attempt to visualize the foreign body and remove it.

Equipment
Laryngoscope handle and blade
Magill forceps

Positioning
- Place victim's head and neck in "sniffing" position. (This allows for good visualization of the glottic opening when laryngoscope is correctly positioned; foreign bodies are most often located just above the glottic opening.)

Procedure
1. Grasp laryngoscope handle (with blade snapped in place) with your left hand, with the blade inferior to the handle.
2. Hold the Magill forceps in your right hand.
3. Gently insert the blade into the victim's mouth, to the right of the midline.
4. As you advance the blade, lift the tongue to the left and move the blade to the midline.
5. Advance the blade, lifting the handle upward and slightly toward the victim's feet, until the glottic opening (or the foreign body) comes into view.
6. If a foreign body is visualized, maintain laryngoscope position and reach into the pharynx with the Magill forceps.
7. Grasp the foreign body with the forceps and remove it. Use great care not to push the foreign body deeper into the airway.
8. Attempt to ventilate the patient.

Cricothyroid Puncture and Transtracheal Catheter Ventilation

If no foreign body is visualized, or if the body cannot be removed by the procedure described above, cricothyroid puncture and transtracheal catheter ventilation can be attempted.

Equipment
Antiseptic agent and cotton swabs
14-gauge plastic intravenous catheter-over-needle assembly attached to a syringe or 14-gauge short-bevel intravenous needle
Intravenous plastic extension tubing
Hand-operated release valve
Oxygen tank or wall oxygen with a pressure adjustment valve

Procedure
1. Locate cricothyroid membrane (Fig. 14-2).
   - It is located between the thyroid cartilage (Adam's apple) and the cricoid cartilage. The cricoid cartilage is found below the thyroid cartilage.

Chart 14-4

RELIEVING AIRWAY OBSTRUCTION: BASIC LIFE-SUPPORT TECHNIQUES

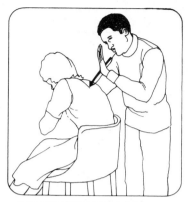

Conscious Victim

BACK BLOWS

Back blows are delivered between the scapulae with the heel of an open hand. The victim is supported with one hand on his upper chest and is positioned forward so that gravity can aid expulsion of the obstructing material.

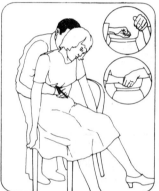

ABDOMINAL THRUSTS

The rescuer stands behind the victim, makes a fist, and places the thumb side of the fist in the midline beneath the victim's rib cage and above his waist. Grasping the fist with his other hand, the rescuer administers four quick thrusts directed inward and upward. (Chest thrusts are administered posteriorly with the fist at the midsternum. Chest thrusts are preferred for pediatric victims and those who are very obese or in advanced stages of pregnancy.)

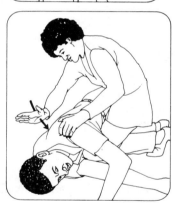

Unconscious Victim

BACK BLOWS

The victim is rolled toward the rescuer and is supported by the rescuer's legs. Four quick back blows are delivered between the scapulae.

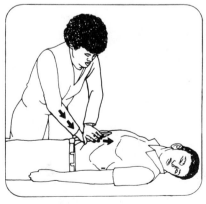

ABDOMINAL THRUSTS

The victim is then rolled onto his back and four abdominal thrusts are delivered. One hand is placed on top of the other, with the heel of the lower hand positioned in the mid-line below the victim's rib cage and above his waist and the fingers pointing toward the sternum. The thrusts are delivered with a quick, upward motion. (Chest thrusts are administered in the same manner as chest compressions, except quickly and in a series of four.)

(Illustrations from American Red Cross poster)

Chart 14-5

ACTION SEQUENCES FOR RELIEVING AIRWAY OBSTRUCTION*

Conscious Choking Victim Who Is Unable to Speak

1. Support victim with your body.
2. Deliver four back blows.
3. Deliver four abdominal or chest thrusts.
4. Repeat sequence until obstruction is relieved.

Complete Airway Obstruction in an Unconscious Victim

1. Attempt to ventilate patient.
2. Reposition airway and attempt to ventilate patient again.
3. Deliver four back blows
4. Deliver four abdominal or chest thrusts
5. Sweep the *adult* victim's mouth with a finger. In *pediatric* patients, maneuvers to remove the foreign body are done only when foreign material is seen.
6. Position airway and attempt to ventilate patient.
7. Repeat sequence until obstruction is relieved.

* Sequences recommended by the American Heart Association

- The cricothyroid membrane is the indentation between the two cartilages.
2. Prepare site with antiseptic agent.
3. Stabilize the trachea between the thumb and the index and middle fingers of one hand.
4. With catheter-over-needle, puncture cricothyroid membrane in the midline.
5. Advance the catheter-over-needle assembly at a 45-degree angle downward and toward the victim's feet while applying negative pressure with the syringe (Fig. 14-3). When the trachea is entered, air should enter the syringe.
6. Advance the catheter over the needle; remove the syringe and needle.
7. To ventilate, attach intravenous tubing to the catheter, connect the tubing to the oxygen source, and press the toggle valve.

8. Observe for chest rise with ventilation. When the lungs are inflated, release the valve so that exhalation can occur.
9. Oxygen pressure is adjusted to the minimum necessary to inflate the lungs.

Complications
Hemorrhage

Esophageal perforation

Subcutaneous and mediastinal emphysema

Overinflation of the lungs (can occur if there is a tight obstruction above the vocal cords)[16]

Surgical Cricothyroidostomy

Surgical cricothyroidostomy is an incision through the cricothyroid membrane with insertion of a permanent airway

Figure 14-2 *The cricothyroid membrane is located between the thyroid cartilage (Adam's apple) and the cricoid cartilage. An indentation is felt between these two structures. (Cosgriff JH Jr: Atlas of Diagnostic and Therapeutic Procedures for Emergency Personnel. Philadelphia, JB Lippincott, 1978)*

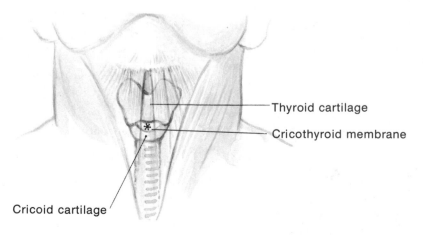

Thyroid cartilage

Cricothyroid membrane

Cricoid cartilage

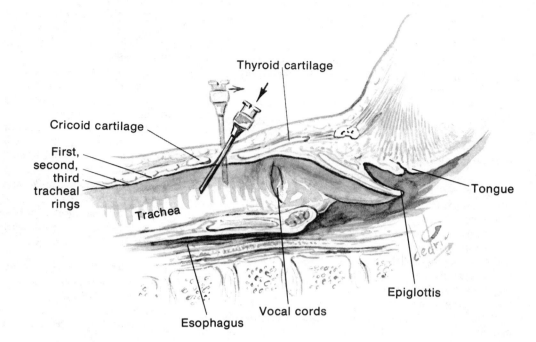

Figure 14-3 Inserting needle for cricothyroid puncture. Stabilize the trachea and firmly insert the needle perpendicularly into the cricothyroid membrane. Once air passes through the needle, indicating that the trachea has been entered, the needle is advanced at a 45° angle then stabilized with adhesive tape. A plastic catheter-over-needle device may be used (see text). (Cosgriff JH Jr: Atlas of Diagnostic and Therapeutic Procedures for Emergency Personnel. Philadelphia, JB Lippincott, 1978)

Labels on figure: Thyroid cartilage · Cricoid cartilage · First, second, third tracheal rings · Trachea · Esophagus · Vocal cords · Epiglottis · Tongue

device. It provides more rapid and easier access to the airway than the standard tracheostomy and in fact may be converted to a tracheostomy if desired. The anatomic considerations are the same as for cricothyroid puncture.

Equipment

Six small curved hemostats

Two #3 scalpel handles

#15 scalpel blade

#11 scalpel blade

10 ml syringe

25-gauge ⅝-inch needle

22-gauge 1½-inch needle

Tracheostomy tube #4 or #6 with low-pressure inflatable cuff

Two tissue forceps with teeth

Two tissue forceps without teeth

Two skin hooks

Two small rake retractors

One tracheal spreader

Small needle holder (Webster)

Small dissecting scissors

Suture scissors

Four towels

Twenty 4-inch × 4-inch gauze sponges

3-0 absorbable suture on a needle

4-0 nonabsorbable suture on a needle

Prep cup

Local anesthetic agent

Antiseptic prep solution

Procedure

1. Locate the cricothyroid membrane with patient in supine position.
2. Prepare the anterior neck with an antiseptic agent.
3. Stabilize the thyroid cartilage with the thumb and index finger of the left hand.
4. Make a transverse skin incision 2.5 cm to 3.0 cm in length over the cricothyroid membrane, through the subcutaneous tissue.
5. Control bleeding by clamping and tying blood vessels.
6. Identify the cricothyroid membrane and incise it carefully. Avoid injury to the cricoid cartilage.
7. Spread the incision by inserting the scalpel handle into it and rotating the handle 90 degrees to open the airway. A tracheal spreader may be used if available.
8. Insert an appropriate-sized cuffed tracheostomy tube (size 4 or 6) into the opening, directing the tube toward the lower trachea.
9. Inflate the cuff and ventilate the patient.
10. Place one or two nonabsorbable sutures in the skin incision.
11. Apply a sterile dressing over the operative site.

Complications

Bleeding, hematoma formation

Subglottic stenosis or edema

Laryngeal stenosis

Injury to the cricoid cartilage

Cellulitis, infection

Laceration of the esophagus or trachea

Mediastinal emphysema

Vocal-cord paralysis

AIRWAY ADJUNCTS

Oropharyngeal Airway

The oropharyngeal airway is often helpful in keeping the victim's tongue forward. It is useful in maintaining airway patency in unconscious patients who are breathing spontaneously. It cannot be used in patients with an intact gag reflex. It is often used to assist in maintaining a patent airway for nonbreathing patients who are being ventilated with rescue breathing or mechanical devices. This airway is semicircular and is made of plastic, rubber, or metal. Size must be selected for the individual patient; the oropharyngeal airway is available in many sizes to accommodate people of any size, from tiny infants to large adults. When the airway has been positioned correctly, its tip lies in the lower posterior pharynx, over the back of the tongue, and the entrance of the tube is anterior to the patient's mouth. If not inserted and positioned properly, the oropharyngeal airway may push the tongue backward into the posterior pharynx, causing airway obstruction. For best results, insert the tube into the victim's mouth with the curvature in the direction of the roof of the mouth, and advance it until it approaches the posterior pharynx. At that point rotate the airway 180 degrees so that it is positioned correctly.

Nasopharyngeal Airway

The nasopharyngeal airway is made of soft rubber. It is useful when the patient is breathing spontaneously but having difficulty maintaining a patent airway. It is tolerated quite well by the patient with an intact gag reflex. The tip should be well lubricated, preferably with a local anesthetic lubricant, and then gently inserted into a nostril near the midline. It is advanced gently along the floor of the nasal passage into the posterior pharynx. It must be inserted gently, since exerting force can cause epistaxis.

Esophageal Obturator Airway

The esophageal obturator airway (EOA) and its newer model, the esophageal gastric tube airway (EGTA) is used primarily in an unconscious patient in the prehospital setting to ensure ventilation. Its primary action is to occlude the esophagus to prevent vomiting and aspiration. It is a hollow plastic tube with a blind (closed) tip and vents at the level of the patient's pharynx. The tube fits into a specially designed face mask. When properly positioned, the tip of the tube is in the victim's esophagus. A balloon near the tip is inflated to occlude the esophagus. The balloon must lie below the level of the tracheal bifurcation (carina), to prevent airway obstruction. The mask is firmly seated on the victim's face; the rescuer carries out the jaw-thrust maneuver and breathes through the port on the mask. Air enters the patient's airway through the vents. No air should escape if the victim's mouth and nose are well sealed with the face mask (Fig. 14-4). The EGTA is essentially the same device with a central channel for passage of a nasogastric tube into the stomach for nasogastric decompression.

Procedure for Esophageal Intubation. To perform esophageal intubation, the following procedure is used:

1. Snap the face mask onto the obturator.
2. Lubricate the tip.
3. Approach the patient from his head.
4. Position the patient's head and neck in a neutral position or flex the neck slightly forward (if cervical spine injury is excluded).
5. Grasp the patient's jaw by placing your thumb inside his lower jaw and lift the jaw forward.
6. Insert the tube with its curvature in line with the patient's airway.
7. Advance the tube until the mask is firmly seated on the victim's face.
8. If the EGTA is used, insert a nasogastric tube into the stomach.
9. Ventilate the patient by blowing into the mask's port while maintaining a jaw thrust.
10. Observe for chest rise with ventilation.

If the chest rises with ventilation and bilateral breath sounds are audible by auscultation, the tube is positioned correctly. The balloon can then be inflated with 35 ml of

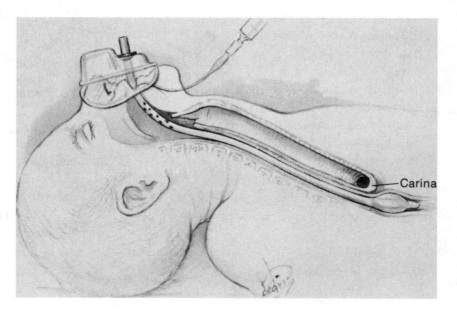

Figure 14-4 *The esophageal obturator airway (EOA). The tube has a closed end, which is inserted into the esophagus after adequate lubrication. The cuff at the lower end of the tube is inflated to occlude the esophagus, and the mask is applied tightly over the patient's mouth and nose to form a closed system. Air is then introduced into the open end of the tube either by a bag-valve device or mouth-to-tube insufflation. The air passes out of the perforations seen in the upper half of the tube and inflates the lungs. (Cosgriff JH Jr: Atlas of Diagnostic and Therapeutic Procedures for Emergency Personnel. Philadelphia, JB Lippincott, 1978)*

Carina

air to occlude the esophagus and the patient ventilated with a bag-valve or positive pressure system. If the chest does not rise or breath sounds are not heard on auscultation, immediately remove the tube and ventilate the patient by other means. *Note:* Observe frequently for signs of increased gastric distention when using the EOA. This condition often occurs when the EOA has been positioned in the trachea.

Good airway position is mandatory when using the EOA because it does not secure the airway as does an endotracheal tube. Endotracheal intubation can be done with the EOA in place. The EOA should not be removed until the airway has been secured by endotracheal intubation or until the patient becomes sufficiently responsive to maintain his own airway. The balloon must be deflated before the EOA is removed. Because vomiting frequently occurs when the EOA is removed, the patient should be positioned on his side and suction must be ready. This complication is unusual when the EGTA is used.

Use of the EOA is not without complications. These include tracheal intubation (*in which case the trachea is obstructed*) and esophageal rupture and laceration. The EOA is contraindicated in patients with known esophageal disease. Since no pediatric sizes are available, the EOA cannot be used in children younger than 17 years of age. Its use may be contraindicated in the presence of maxillofacial trauma with severe oral/nasal hemorrhage, since the blood may enter the tracheobronchial tree when the esophageal balloon is inflated.

Endotracheal Intubation

Endotracheal intubation secures the airway better than any other method. The tube is passed directly into the trachea to seal the airway and prevent aspiration. Endotracheal intubation requires more expertise and practice than esophageal intubation.

Equipment
- Laryngoscope with handle and lighted blade. The handle contains batteries. The blades are changeable and of varying sizes and shapes suitable for infants and adults.
- Endotracheal tubes. These are available in graduated sizes with an internal diameter of 3.5 mm to 9 mm to fit all patients. These devices are disposable. Each is fitted with a connector that is adaptable to standard resuscitation equipment. (Some tubes may cause tracheal irritation, particularly in infants and children. A tube should not be used unless it is implant tested and free of toxicity—these are marked IT and Z79.)

  To obtain an airtight fit in the airway, the distal end of the tube is fitted with an inflatable rubber cuff. Cuffs are usually not used on tubes with an internal diameter of less than 4 mm.
- Water-soluble lubricating jelly
- Topical antiseptic spray solution
- Stylet (optional)
- Suction machine—tonsil (rigid) suction tip
- 10 ml syringe

Anatomic Considerations. The tube may be passed into the trachea through the mouth (orotracheal route) or nose (nasotracheal route). The orotracheal method is most commonly used and performed under direct vision, whereas the nasotracheal route is essentially a blind technique.
- The trachea is in the midline of the neck, its superior entry being the glottis, which contains the vocal cords. In orotracheal intubation, the vocal cords must be visualized before the tube is passed into the trachea.
- The uvula, suspended from the midline of the soft palate, is used to guide the operator in placing the laryngoscope properly.
- The epiglottis is attached to the base of the tongue and should be visualized and elevated to expose the glottis and vocal cords. In thick-necked patients, the glottis may be more easily visualized by applying external pressure on the thyroid cartilage while the base of the tongue and the epiglottis are being elevated with the laryngoscope blade.
- The trachea extends to the level of the second intercostal space anteriorly and bifurcates into left and right bronchi. The right main bronchus comes off at a very slight angle to the trachea, while the left takes off at a 45-degree angle. This anatomic configuration allows the endotracheal tube to be passed easily into the right bronchus. This point is important because, if the tube is passed accidentally into the right bronchus, occluding the origin of the left main bronchus, atelectasis of the left lung occurs with aggravation of pulmonary insufficiency.

Procedure
1. Lubricate the endotracheal tube with water-soluble jelly.
2. Stand at the patient's head. It is preferable to have the patient in the supine position. Extend his neck by elevating the neck or jaw and applying pressure on the forehead. Use caution in patients suspected of having an injury to the cervical spine.
3. Retract the lips onto the teeth or gums to avoid pinching them in the blade.
4. Grasp the lower jaw with the right hand and draw it forward and upward. Remove any dentures.
5. With the laryngoscope in the left hand, insert the blade into the mouth over the tongue toward the right side, pushing the tongue to the left. Continue to advance the blade into the mouth and identify the uvula.
6. Keep the blade closer to the floor of the mouth. Then elevate the tongue until the epiglottis is seen (Fig. 14-5). Observe the mouth and oropharynx for any foreign bodies or secretions, and, if any are present, remove them for better visualization of anatomic landmarks and to prevent aspiration into the trachea.
7. Advance the laryngoscope blade over the epiglottis and elevate the tongue and epiglottis by firmly raising the handle of the laryngoscope. Do not push the laryngoscope blade against the upper teeth (to prevent injury or loss of a damaged or carious tooth). With the tongue and epiglottis raised, the glottis should be visualized.
8. If the patient gags or if the vocal cords are closed (adducted), spray the cords with the topical anesthetic solution. If the patient is breathing spontaneously, the cords may open during inspiration.
9. With the cords in full view, pass a tube of the appropriate size into the trachea (Fig. 14-6). In an adult, a 7-mm tube may be used. In infants a 4-mm to 5-mm tube is

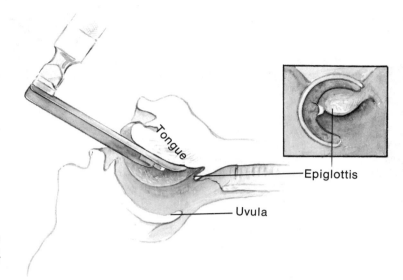

Figure 14-5 *The laryngoscope is used to visualize structures in the mouth and throat and to facilitate insertion of the endotracheal tube. (Cosgriff JH Jr: Atlas of Diagnostic and Therapeutic Procedures for Emergency Personnel. Philadelphia, JB Lippincott, 1978)*

preferable, whereas in a newborn a 3.5-mm tube should be used.

10. Check the position of the tube in the airway by placing the ear next to the end of the tube and compressing the chest. If the tube is properly placed, air will be expelled through it with this maneuver.

11. Inflate the cuff with 5 ml to 8 ml of air.

12. Attach tube to a mechanical ventilator or resuscitation bag device (Ambu bag) as indicated.

13. Once the patient is being ventilated, auscultate the chest to be certain that both lungs are being aerated. If the breath sounds are decreased or absent in the left lung, the tube may have been passed into the right mainstem bronchus and may have occluded the origin of the left main bronchus. If this is the case, deflate the cuff, withdraw the tube 1 cm to 2 cm, and auscultate again.

14. Withdraw the tube until both lungs aerate equally; continue as before.

15. Place an oropharyngeal airway in the mouth to prevent the patient from biting the endotracheal tube. Tape the endotracheal or oropharyngeal tubes to the side of the face to prevent expulsion.

Figure 14-6 *The endotracheal tube is inserted after the glottic opening is visualized. (Cosgriff JH Jr: Atlas of Diagnostic and Therapeutic Procedures for Emergency Personnel. Philadelphia, JB Lippincott, 1978)*

Complications
Esophageal intubation

Intubation of a mainstem bronchus

Tracheal rupture

Esophageal trauma

Intubation of the pyriform sinus.[18] The intubation procedure can produce increased vagal tone with resulting bradycardic rhythms.

VENTILATION DEVICES

Providing a high concentration of oxygen to the patient in cardiopulmonary arrest is a high priority. Rescue breathing provides an oxygen concentration of approximately 16% to 17%. As soon as possible, supplemental oxygen should be given. A concentration approaching 100% is ideal.

Pocket Mask

The pocket mask is an excellent tool for maintaining good airway position and ventilating the patient. It can be used with supplemental oxygen. It consists of a transparent vinyl

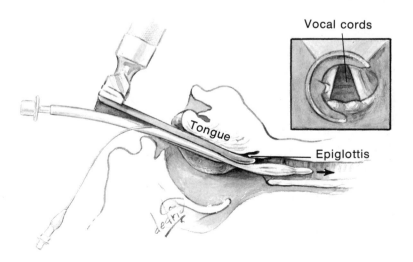

mask surrounded by an inflatable cuff (for face seal), a ventilation port, and a one-way valve for supplemental oxygen delivery. This mask is intended primarily for use with rescue breathing, but it can also be used with a bag-valve system or with positive pressure breathing devices.

To use the pocket mask with rescue breathing, the rescuer approaches the victim from the behind-head position and places the mask over the mouth and nose. The rescuer performs the jaw-thrust maneuver with both hands while holding the mask to achieve a tight face seal and ventilates the patient by blowing into the ventilation port.

The pocket mask has some real advantages over standard mouth-to-mouth rescue breathing and may be superior to the bag-valve-mask and positive pressure breathing device-mask techniques. It has the following advantages:

- It provides an excellent mask-to-face seal.
- Both hands of the rescuer are available to maintain optimal airway position.
- Supplemental oxygen can be provided.
- It is easy to use properly and can be performed well by persons with small hands.
- In addition to these features, a recent study indicates that even the unskilled can provide excellent tidal volumes by this method.[19]

Bag-Valve Systems

Bag-valve systems can be used with a face mask, EOA, EGTA, or endotracheal tube. The bag-valve is a self-inflating bag with an adaptor that can be attached to a mask or tube. The rescuer squeezes the bag so that air enters the patient's airway. The bag is then allowed to reinflate before the next ventilation. An oxygen reservoir can be used to allow for an oxygen concentration of 90% or greater to be delivered if the oxygen flow rate is adjusted to 10 L/m to 15 L/m. Bag-valve ventilation is ideal for use with an endotracheal tube. One can recognize decreases in lung compliance because increased resistance is felt when the bag is squeezed. However, it is difficult to adequately ventilate patients with a bag-valve mask (especially for rescuers with small hands), since it is difficult to maintain good airway position and squeeze the bag simultaneously.

Manually Triggered Oxygen-Powered Breathing Devices

These devices can be used with masks, endotracheal tubes, EOAs, EGTA, or tracheostomy tubes. The device connects to the oxygen source and has a valve that the rescuer presses to ventilate the patient. This valve functions on demand and can be triggered by spontaneous breathing. It inflates the lungs to a pressure of 40 mm Hg and delivers 100% oxygen. These devices are not recommended for children under the age of 12 years and should be used with caution in patients with a history of lung disease.

TECHNIQUES FOR MAINTAINING ADEQUATE TISSUE PERFUSION

Adequate perfusion of tissues with oxygenated blood is vital. In most situations, this is accomplished by manual chest compressions. The patient must be lying on a firm surface. The lower half of the sternum (but not the xyphoid) is compressed rhythmically at a rate of 60 per minute. These compressions will produce a cardiac output. Blood flow to the cerebral circulation is estimated to be one-fourth to one-third of normal during resuscitation with external chest compressions.

MANUAL CHEST COMPRESSION

One-Rescuer Method

1. *Position yourself* close to the victim's side. If the victim is on a stretcher, you may need to stand on a stool to obtain an optimal position. If the victim is on a soft surface, you will need to place him on the floor or put a board beneath him.
2. *Locate the correct compression point* (Fig. 14-7). The area to be compressed is the lower half of the sternum, excluding the xyphoid. To locate the compression point, locate the lower margin of the rib cage using the middle finger of the hand closest to the victim's feet. Run your finger along the rib border toward the midline until it is in the notch where the rib joins the sternum. With your middle finger in this notch, bring your index finger next to it. Then bring the heel of your other hand to the sternum in the midline and position it next to your index finger.
3. *Position your hands, arms, and body.* Place the hand that you used to locate the lower rib border on top of the hand that now rests on the lower half of the sternum. The fingers of both hands are extended or interlaced. The fingers must not be in contact with the chest when compressions are performed. Straighten both arms and lock your elbows. Position your shoulders directly over your hands.
4. *Begin compressions.* The sternum is depressed 1½ inches to 2 inches for adults. The direction of force should be straight down. In order to produce optimal cardiac output, the compression duration should be longer than the relaxation phase.[20] The compressions should be delivered rhythmically. Following compression, release pressure fully but do not allow your hand to lose contact with the victim's chest. For single-rescuer CPR the ratio is 15 compressions to 2 ventilations.

Two-Rescuer Method

When two rescuers are available, one performs compressions while the other ventilates the patient. The ratio is 5 compressions to 1 ventilation (which is performed on the fifth compression upstroke). In this situation the rate of compressions should equal 60 per minute. Performing chest compressions is tiring. If two rescuers are present they may periodically exchange roles, but must not interrupt the rhythm when they do so.

Complications

Complications associated with chest compressions include the following:[21]
- Rib fractures
- Sternal fracture
- Costochondral separation

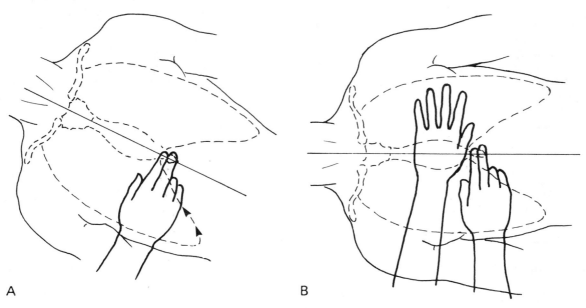

Figure 14-7 *Placement of hands for closed chest cardiac compression. A. With the middle and index fingers of the lower hand, follow the lower edge of the rib cage to the notch where the ribs meet the sternum. B. With the middle finger on the notch and the index finger placed next to it, place the heel of the other hand on the lower half of the sternum, next to the index finger. (After Manual for Instructors in Basic Cardiac Life Support, pp 48–49. Dallas, American Heart Association, 1977. Reproduced with permission. Copyright © 1977, American Heart Association)*

- Pneumothorax
- Hemothorax
- Lung contusions
- Liver lacerations
- Fat emboli

Performing the procedure correctly usually prevents these complications, but rib fracture may still occur.

OPEN-CHEST CARDIAC MASSAGE

Certain specific situations necessitate open-chest cardiac massage. This procedure should be performed only by a physician skilled in the procedure. Special surgical instruments are required and every emergency department should have a sterile emergency thoracotomy tray available at all times.

Indications. According to the American Heart Association, current indications for open chest cardiac massage are:

1. Cardiac arrest associated with penetrating chest trauma
2. Cardiac tamponade
3. Cardiac arrest occurring in the operating room
4. Crushed-chest injury
5. Certain anatomic deformities of the chest
6. Rarely, failure of appropriately applied closed-chest compressions to produce adequate cardiac output.[22]
7. Penetrating wounds suspected of involving the heart.

Another authority also recommends the procedure in tension pneumothorax with mediastinal shift and in certain cases of severe emphysema associated with extreme barrel chest.[23]

PNEUMATIC ANTISHOCK GARMENT

The important role of antishock trousers in the emergency management of severe hypovolemic shock has been widely recognized since the Vietnam war. Inflation of antishock trousers shunts approximately 2 units of blood into the central circulation from the venous beds of the lower extremities and pelvis. Recent studies suggest that this apparatus may be useful in increasing the effectiveness of chest compressions during CPR.[24] More data are needed before it can be clearly recommended for routine use in humans.

Indications. The trousers should unquestionably be used in the resuscitation of trauma victims and in cardiac arrest secondary to hypovolemia. There has been some experimentation and conjecture that inflation of antishock trousers may be beneficial in cardiogenic shock with "forward failure" in patients who do not exhibit signs of pulmonary congestion. This is considered experimental and is not currently recommended as standard therapy.[25] The fluid challenge provided by inflation of antishock trousers is totally reversible by deflation of the trousers.

Note: The trousers are contraindicated in the presence of pulmonary edema.

TECHNIQUES FOR RESTORING AN EFFECTIVE CARDIAC RHYTHM

Methods of restoring an effective cardiac rhythm include the use of electricity, precordial thump, and administration of drugs. Electricity is used to terminate irritable heart rhythms by simultaneously depolarizing all myocardial cells and to stimulate the heart to beat with artificial pacemakers. Drug therapy includes drugs that enhance the heart's electrical activity, alkalinizing agents, drugs that improve myocardial contractility, and drugs that suppress myocardial irritability.

Cardiac arrest is characterized by the absence of central (carotid and femoral) pulses. Any condition that results in a cardiac output insufficient to produce these pulses will cause cardiac arrest. Dysrhythmias that produce cardiac arrest are:

1. Ventricular fibrillation
2. Nonperfusing ventricular tachycardia
3. Ventricular asystole
4. Atrioventricular blocks that produce a very slow ventricular rate
5. Idioventricular rhythm

Electromechanical dissociation is not categorized as a dysrhythmia, but it does produce cardiac arrest. These rhythms often respond to electrical countershock and drug therapy by converting to other dysrhythmias. (For information on conversion dysrhythmias see Chap. 16, Cardiac Emergencies.)

DYSRHYTHMIAS OF CARDIAC ARREST: CHARACTERISTICS AND INITIAL TREATMENT

Life-threatening dysrhythmias are discussed in detail in Chapter 16, Cardiac Emergencies.

Ventricular Fibrillation

Mechanism: This is a disorganized dysrhythmia in which there is chaotic multifocal depolarization of the ventricles and uneven repolarization. The heart muscle quivers in response to the electrical activity but no contraction is produced.

ECG features: Electrical activity is demonstrated by irregular waveforms that are not at all uniform in shape. There are no identifiable P waves or QRS complexes. "Coarse" ventricular fibrillation has waveforms of high amplitude, and electrical activity is rapid with frequent, relatively narrow waveforms. It is often combined with waveforms that resemble ventricular tachycardia. "Fine" ventricular fibrillation is characterized by waveforms of low amplitude with complexes that are less frequent and wider in configuration.

Initial treatment: (In general, coarse ventricular fibrillation responds more favorably to electrical countershock than does fine ventricular fibrillation. Fine ventricular fibrillation usually needs to be coarsened with epinephrine prior to electrical countershock.)

Witnessed (and Monitored) Ventricular Fibrillation
1. Perform a precordial thump (see pp. 294–295).
2. If this treatment is not immediately effective in terminating the dysrhythmia, proceed with the treatment described below for unwitnessed ventricular fibrillation.

Unwitnessed Ventricular Fibrillation
1. Begin CPR immediately and continue until a perfusing rhythm is established.
2. Defibrillate as soon as equipment is available. (See Chart 14-6 and pp 246–247.) The energy setting is 200 to 300 joules of delivered energy for adults. Observe the monitor. If a rhythm has been established, palpate for central pulses and proceed with the indicated treatment.
3. If the patient remains in ventricular fibrillation, immediately repeat defibrillation at 200 to 300 joules. Observe the monitor and evaluate the rhythm.
4. If the patient remains in ventricular fibrillation, administer epinephrine and sodium bicarbonate.
5. Repeat defibrillation at a dose not to exceed 360 joules of delivered energy. Observe the monitor and evaluate the rhythm.
6. If the patient remains in ventricular fibrillation, reevaluate adequacy of ventilations, oxygen delivery, pulses with chest compressions. Failure of the heart to respond to appropriate therapy is often related to inadequate oxygenation.
7. Further therapy will include repeating sodium bicarbonate (based on arterial blood gas results when they are available), additional epinephrine, and repeating defibrillation. Additional drugs that are indicated for refractory ventricular fibrillation include lidocaine, procainamide, and bretylium.

Ventricular Tachycardia

Mechanism: Ventricular tachycardia is repetitive firing at a tachycardic rate on an ectopic focus (or multiple foci) in the ventricles. Atrioventricular dissociation (an unrelated atrial rhythm) may be present. The ventricles usually contract in response to the electrical activity but the cardiac output produced may be minimal. The cardiac output generated by ventricular tachycardia depends upon the amount of ventricular dysfunction present (*i.e.,* size of a noncontracting area of the myocardium), as well as the rate of the tachycardia. A general rule is that the faster the rate is, the poorer the cardiac output will be.

ECG features: Wide (greater than 0.12 sec), bizarrely shaped QRS complexes are seen at a rapid rate (100 to 220/min). The T waves have a polarity opposite to that of the QRS complexes. The rhythm is usually regular but may be slightly irregular. Independent P waves may be seen. Occasionally, a fusion beat (Dressler beat) may occur.

Initial treatment:

Perfusing Ventricular Tachycardia (with sufficient cardiac output to maintain consciousness and blood pressure)
1. Administer lidocaine. Other drugs that may be useful if lidocaine is not effective are procainamide and bretylium.

Nonperfusing Ventricular Tachycardia (creating unconsciousness or hemodynamic instability)
1. If the *onset* of ventricular tachycardia is witnessed on the cardiac monitor, perform the precordial

thump and observe whether a rhythm is restored. If so, check for pulses and administer lidocaine to prevent recurrence.

2. If the patient remains in ventricular tachycardia, or if the onset was not witnessed, immediately perform synchronized cardioversion at 20 to 200 joules of delivered energy. (See Chart 14-6 and p 246.)

3. If the patient remains in ventricular tachycardia, CPR is necessary. Drug therapy will include lidocaine and sodium bicarbonate. Procainamide and bretylium may also be used.

4. Occasionally, overdrive pacing of the ventricles is effective in overriding ventricular tachycardia that is refractory to other treatment.

Ventricular Asystole

Mechanism: There is no electrical activity in the ventricles and therefore no ventricular contraction.

ECG features: Ventricular asystole is recognized by a "flat-line" pattern with no discernable waveforms. P-wave activity may be seen. Extremely "fine" ventricular fibrillation with minute waveforms should be considered ventricular asystole.

Initial treatment:
1. Start and continue CPR until an effective heart rhythm is restored.
2. Administer epinephrine.
3. Administer sodium bicarbonate.
4. Administer high-dose atropine.
5. Administer calcium chloride.
6. If the patient remains in asystole, additional therapy may include repeating epinephrine, calcium chloride, and sodium bicarbonate. An isoproterenol infusion can be useful. Occasionally, a temporary pacemaker can restore an effective rhythm in persistent asystole.

AV Blocks That Produce Slow Ventricular Rhythms

Atrioventricular (AV) blocks that frequently produce slow ventricular rates and cause hemodynamic instability are second-degree AV (Mobitz II) block and third-degree AV block (complete heart block). These two rhythms do not always result in hemodynamic instability. The degree of instability depends on the amount of ventricular dysfunction present and the ventricular rate. A general rule is that the faster the ventricular rate is, the better the cardiac output will be.

Second-Degree AV (Mobitz II) Block

Mechanism: This conduction disturbance is below the AV-node level (most commonly across both bundle branches). It frequently progresses to third-degree AV block. The atria are depolarizing normally, but some of the impulses are not conducted to the ventricles. For those that are conducted, the AV conduction time is consistent. If a "high-grade" block is present (with many impulses blocked) the ventricular rate may be dangerously slow. The bases for this dysrhythmia's life-threatening status are its tendency to progress to complete heart block and the slow ventricular rates it may produce.

ECG features: P waves are present and are regular. Some P waves are not followed by a QRS complex. The PR interval for the conducted beats is constant. (Most often the QRS complexes have a bundle branch block pattern.)

Initial treatment:
1. A temporary pacemaker is inserted as soon as possible.
2. Administer atropine. This may or may not be effective in improving AV conduction.
3. If the patient is hemodynamically unstable and a pacemaker cannot yet be inserted, an isoproterenol infusion may be given *very cautiously.*

Third-Degree AV Block (Complete Heart Block)

Mechanism: This conduction disturbance may be located at the level of the AV node, the bundle of His, or the bundle branches. The atria fire normally but no impulses are conducted to the ventricles. An escape pacemaker will pace the ventricles below the level of the conduction defect. Two independent rhythms, one for the atria and one for the ventricles, result. The ventricular rhythm is regular and its rate is less than 60 per minute. If the conduction disturbance is below the bundle of His, a very slow rate is probable.

ECG features: The P-wave rhythm is regular and has a faster rate than the QRS complexes. The QRS complexes are regular and slow (less than 60/min). There is no relationship between the P waves and the QRS complexes. The QRS complexes may be normal in width or abnormally wide.

Initial treatment:
1. A temporary pacemaker is inserted as soon as possible.
2. Administer atropine. This may or may not be effective in improving AV conduction.
3. If the patient is hemodynamically unstable and a pacemaker cannot yet be inserted, an isoproterenol infusion may be given *very cautiously.*

Electromechanical Dissociation

Mechanism: Electromechanical dissociation (EMD) is not a rhythm diagnosis but rather a condition. The heart has orderly electrical activity but is not contracting. It is characterized by an absence of pulses in the presence of an electrical rhythm that would normally be sufficient to produce them. EMD is caused by disorders of calcium transport or by severe ventricular dysfunction. It can be mimicked by pericardial tamponade, tension pneumothorax, and exsanguination. Treatment for these conditions should be definitive for them.

ECG features: As above.

Initial treatment:
1. Begin and maintain CPR until pulses are palpable with heart rhythm.
2. Drugs that may be effective include calcium chloride, epinephrine, and sodium bicarbonate.

PRECORDIAL THUMP

A single precordial thump may convert ventricular fibrillation and ventricular tachycardia if it is performed immediately at the outset of the dysrhythmia. Its mechanism of action is similar to that of electrical countershock at a very low energy setting. Additionally, repeated precordial thumps ("fist pacing") can sometimes stimulate ventricular depolarization sufficient to produce muscle contraction in ventricular asystole.

The precordial thump is currently reserved for "witnessed arrest" situations in which the patient's cardiac rhythm is being observed at the onset of these dysrhythmias. The precordial thump must be delivered *immediately* in order to produce a favorable result.[26] The precordial thump is not performed on pediatric patients.

The precordial thump is a single, sharp blow to the midsternum delivered from a level of 8 inches to 12 inches above the chest. The blow is given by the fleshy portion of a clenched fist.

For ventricular tachycardia or ventricular fibrillation, deliver one precordial thump and observe the monitor to determine if it has been effective. If the dysrhythmia persists, institute CPR and proceed with standard therapy.

For ventricular asystole secondary to third-degree AV block, repeated precordial thumps are given at a rate of 60 per minute. Observe the oscilloscope to see if QRS complexes are produced. Palpate the carotid pulse to see if the QRS complexes are producing pulses. If none are produced, begin CPR and proceed with standard therapy.

ELECTRICAL COUNTERSHOCK

The goal of electrical countershock is to depolarize all myocardial cells simultaneously in order to terminate irritable heart rhythms so that an effective rhythm can be restored. A single direct current (DC) electrical shock is delivered to the myocardium.

Defibrillation and Synchronized Cardioversion

The defibrillator consists of a power source (portable battery-operated or line-powered), a dosage meter, discharge switch(es), and two chest paddles. It is usually connected to a cardiac monitor. Some defibrillators are equipped with "quick-look" paddles that can be used as ECG electrodes. The paddles are positioned on the victim's chest, and the machine discharged so that direct electrical current travels through the heart.

Rhythms that respond favorably to electrical countershock are "irritable" (tachycardic) in origin. They include ventricular fibrillation, ventricular tachycardia, and supraventricular tachycardias (*e.g.,* atrial flutter, atrial fibrillation). In countershock rhythms other than ventricular fibrillation, the synchronizing switch is activated. This procedure (synchronized cardioversion) synchronizes countershock to the patient's ECG and avoids countershock during the "vulnerable" period (the upstroke of the T wave on the ECG), which might produce ventricular fibrillation.

Skin Preparation. In order to reach the myocardium, electrical energy must penetrate the skin. Increased impedance (resistance to flow of electrical current) can prevent the entry of sufficient current. Skin, especially when dry,

has a high resistance to electrical current. Conductive material must be applied between the defibrillator paddles and the patient's skin. Conductive gel pads, electrode paste, or saline-soaked pads can be used. Successive countershocks decrease impedance. For this reason, a second countershock is delivered immediately if the first attempt is not successful.

Paddle Placement. Correct placement of the paddles is important because electrical energy must flow *through* the heart. Standard paddle placement consists in one paddle over the apex and the other below the right clavicle to the right of the sternum. This standard is utilized in most emergency situations. An alternative method is anteroposterior paddle position. For this method the anterior paddle is placed over the precordium and the posterior paddle on the patient's back, behind the heart. The posterior paddle is flat so that it can be positioned with the victim lying upon it. Consider anteroposterior paddle placement if the patient is very large, has a barrel-shaped chest, and has not responded to repeated countershocks in the standard paddle position. There is some evidence that anteroposterior paddle position increases current delivery to the myocardium by 2½ times.[27]

Paddle Size. The ideal size of defibrillator paddles has not been conclusively established. Paddle size of approximately 13 cm (5 inches) is recommended. Smaller paddles are less effective and can cause greater myocardial damage. Larger paddles are also less effective.[28] The recommended size for pediatric paddles is 4.5 cm (1⅞ inches) for infants and 8.0 cm (3¼ inches) for older children.[29]

Dosage. Currently, the recommended adult dosage of electricity for ventricular fibrillation is 200 to 300 joules of *delivered* energy. The initial dosage for children is 2 joules per kilogram (2.20 lb) of body weight, and the energy setting may be doubled for repeat attempts.

Ventricular tachycardia and supraventricular tachycardias usually respond to a lower electrical dosage than is necessary to convert ventricular fibrillation. The initial dosage in these situations is 20 to 200 joules.

Failure to Respond. If the dysrhythmia fails to respond to repeated countershocks despite appropriate drug therapy, the patient's acid-base and oxygenation statuses should be reevaluated. Other factors that may preclude conversion are hypothermia, digitalis toxicity, and the underlying etiology of arrest.

Ventricular fibrillation sometimes converts to ventricular asystole in response to electrical countershock. This occurs most often when the duration of arrest has been prolonged without effective CPR and when fine ventricular fibrillation is present. In these situations, it may be advantageous to perform good CPR and institute drug therapy before defibrillation.

Side-Effects. Myocardial damage and skin burns may result from electrical countershock. Significant myocardial damage is most often sustained when paddle size is too small, energy levels are excessive, and the number of countershocks is numerous. Skin burns may occur even when the correct procedure is used but are minimized by using enough paddle pressure, ensuring full contact of the paddle surface to skin, and using sufficient but not excessive conductive material. Electrical bridging, or arcing of electrical current between the paddles, causes skin burns and prevents the electrical current from reaching the myocardium. Electrical bridging often results from applying too much conductive material and from failure to maintain complete contact between paddle surface and skin.

Precautions. Defibrillation can be dangerous for medical personnel. The electrical current can be conducted to anyone who is in direct contact with the patient or with conductive material that is touching the patient when countershock is delivered. For this reason, make sure that all present are out of danger before discharging the defibrillator.

PHARMACOLOGIC INTERVENTION

Drug therapy is an important component of cardiopulmonary resuscitation. Drugs are used to improve myocardial contractility, correct metabolic acidosis, suppress myocardial irritability, increase heart rate, stimulate electrical activity, enhance the heart's responsiveness to electrical countershock, and improve perfusion.

MECHANISMS OF DRUG ACTION

In order to achieve these results, resuscitation drugs have a variety of mechanisms of action. Some drugs achieve their therapeutic effects by direct chemical action. An example of this is sodium bicarbonate, which directly combats metabolic acidosis by combining with a strong metabolic acid

---

Chart 14-6

PROCEDURE FOR DEFIBRILLATION

1. Turn on defibrillator.
2. Apply conductive gel to the paddles and spread it evenly, or put saline pads on the patient's chest (in position for paddle placement).
3. Set wattage.
4. Charge the paddles.
5. Position the paddles on the patient's chest, one under the right clavicle to the right of the sternum and the other over the apex.
6. Apply and maintain firm pressure on the paddles (to ensure good contact and decrease impedance).
7. Call "Stand clear" and look to see if anyone, including yourself, is in contact with the patient or with conductive material that is in contact with the patient.
8. Discharge the machine by pressing the discharge button(s).
9. Visualize the monitor to observe the rhythm. If rhythm is restored, palpate the carotid pulse.

Procedure for Synchronized Cardioversion

1. The patient must be attached to a cardiac monitor that is linked into the defibrillator.
2. Turn on the defibrillator and set the synchronization switch to "on" position.
3. Apply conductive gel to the paddles or put saline pads on the patient's chest.
4. Ascertain that the machine is sensing the patient's QRS complexes. This is usually demonstrated by a flashing light at the synchronization switch when a QRS is displayed. If the machine fails to sense properly, increase the gain until synchronization is accomplished. (*Note:* Be careful not to adjust the size too large because this can cause the machine to sense the T waves as well as the QRS complexes. Some equipment will not synchronize unless an upright QRS complex is produced.)
5. Set wattage.
6. Charge the paddles.
7. Place the paddles in proper position.
8. Apply and maintain firm pressure to the paddles.
9. Call "Stand clear" and look to see if anyone, including yourself, is in contact with the patient or with conductive material that is in contact with the patient.
10. Discharge the machine by pressing the discharge button(s). Expect a slight delay before the machine discharges.
11. Watch the monitor to observe the rhythm and palpate the carotid pulse.

to form a weak acid. Certain resuscitative drugs have a more indirect action, and many of these achieve their effects by chemically manipulating the body's autonomic nervous system.

AUTONOMIC NERVOUS SYSTEM

The autonomic nervous system exerts specific influences on the heart and vascular system. It has direct actions on heart rate, conductivity, and irritability. It increases and decreases force of contraction and dilates and constricts blood vessels. The autonomic nervous system also has effects on respiratory function, specifically bronchodilation and bronchoconstriction.

The autonomic nervous system consists of two branches: a *sympathetic* (also called *adrenergic*) *branch* and a *parasympathetic* (also called *cholinergic*) branch. The two branches have opposing actions on the body: the sympathetic branch increases heart rate, and the parasympathetic branch decreases it. Both are continually active, but certain biologic factors may cause one branch to be more active than the other. The sympathetic branch becomes most active when cellular metabolism is increased (*e.g.,* during exercise) or when the supply of oxygen and other nutrients is less available to cells (*e.g.,* when cardiac output is inadequate). The parasympathetic branch is most active during the body's more vegetative functions, such as digestion.

Parasympathetic Branch. The parasympathetic branch arises from the brain stem through the vagus nerve. The chemical mediator for impulse transmissions between parasympathetic nerves and an organ is *acetylcholine*. An increase in stimulation of the parasympathetic branch (increased vagal tone) has specific effects on the heart. These effects include
1. Decreased rate of sinus-node depolarization
2. Slower conduction of impulses through the AV node
3. Some decreases in contractility.
Therefore, anything that increases vagal tone can cause a slower heart rate and prolonged AV conduction. Certain actions produce vagal stimulation, for example, retching, the Valsalva maneuver, and carotid sinus massage. Atropine achieves its action by preventing uptake of acetylcholine at the parasympathetic nerve endings, thereby blocking parasympathetic effects. When parasympathetic actions are blocked, the sympathetic branch has a more pronounced effect. As a result, the sinus node rate increases and AV conduction occurs more rapidly.

Sympathetic Branch. The sympathetic nerves arise from the spinal cord. The chemical mediator for impulse transmissions between sympathetic nerves and an organ is *norepinephrine*. The body manufactures and secretes many chemicals that stimulate sympathetic activity. These substances, called *catecholamines,* include a few that are also used as resuscitation drugs (norepinephrine, epinephrine, and dopamine). Basically, increased sympathetic activity results in a faster heart rate and more forceful myocardial contraction.

The sympathetic nervous system also exerts effects on blood vessels. There are pharmacologic receptors at the cellular level that mediate sympathetic activity. These are called α and β receptors. When α receptors are stimulated they cause blood vessels to constrict. Beta$_1$-receptor stimulation produces:
1. An increased rate of depolarization of the sinus node
2. Increased pacemaker cell rate throughout the heart's conduction system (AV junction and ventricles)
3. Increased myocardial irritability
4. Increased force of contraction.
Beta receptors called β_2 are also present in the blood vessels and in the bronchioles. Beta$_2$ stimulation produces peripheral vasodilation and bronchodilation.

Certain drugs stimulate sympathetic activity. Some do so by activation through α receptors (causing vasoconstriction), some through β_1 receptors (causing increased rate, irritability, and force of contraction), and some through β_2 receptors (causing peripheral vasodilation and bronchodilation). Many drugs produce combined α and β activation.

The actions of the sympathetic branch can be blocked by drugs. For example, propranolol is a β-blocking agent. Its effects include decreases in irritability, rate, and force of contraction.

ROUTES OF ADMINISTRATION

The route of administration for drugs during resuscitation is usually intravenous. This route achieves rapid action because the drugs are administered directly into the circulation. However, during CPR, circulation is decreased compared to normal cardiac function, so that the time required for the drug to achieve its effect is delayed. Allow intravenous medications to circulate with CPR for 90 seconds before expecting maximal effect. Intravenous push medications should be given slowly to permit them to dilute in the circulation, and to prevent these potent medications from reaching the heart in a highly concentrated form.

Some medications can be given by endotracheal tube (*e.g.,* epinephrine). Intracardiac injection is rarely indicated and can cause serious complications, including pneumothorax, hemopericardium, pericardial tamponade, laceration of coronary arteries, and injection of medication into the cardiac muscle.[30]

PRINCIPAL DRUGS FOR CARDIAC ARREST

The drugs most commonly used in the treatment of cardiac arrest are described in Chart 14-7.

PEDIATRIC CONSIDERATIONS

Resuscitative techniques for infants and children differ from those for adults in that procedures, equipment, and drug dosages must be adapted for their smaller size and anatomic differences. The other major consideration is that the etiology

Chart 14-7

PRINCIPAL DRUGS FOR CARDIAC ARREST*

Atropine

Mechanism of action

    Blocks parasympathetic activity

    Increases sinus node rate

    Speeds AV conduction

Indications

    Sinus bradycardia—when accompanied by significant hypotension or frequent ventricular ectopic beats

    AV blocks—at the nodal level

    Ventricular asystole

Dosage

    Adult—0.5 mg IV, may be repeated at 5-minute intervals (total dose not to exceed 2.0 mg). In ventricular asystole, the initial dose is 0.5 mg to 1.0 mg; a repeat dose of 1.0 mg to 2.0 mg may be given.

    Pediatric—0.01 to 0.03 mg/kg

Special considerations:

    Should be given only if the patient is hemodynamically or electrically unstable. May cause ventricular tachycardia and ventricular fibrillation.

Bretylium Tosylate

Mechanism of action

    Actions are not well understood. Has some sympathetic blocking properties. Increases the ventricular fibrillation threshold. Improves myocardial contractility.

Indications

    Ventricular fibrillation, Ventricular tachycardia (when these dysrhythmias have not responded to lidocaine, procainamide, and repeated countershocks)

Dosage

    Adult—initial dose is 5 mg/kg undiluted and given rapidly IV push. After initial dose, repeat countershock. If not successful, the dose can be increased to 10 mg/kg, and repeat countershock.

    Pediatric—not established

Special considerations

    Not a first-line drug. It is given only when ventricular fibrillation and ventricular tachycardia are refractory to first-line treatment. Contraindicated in the presence of digitalis toxicity.

Calcium Chloride

Mechanism of action

    Increases force of contraction

    Increases automaticity

Indications

    Electromechanical dissociation

    Ventricular asystole

Dosage

    Adult—5 to 7 mg/kg of a 10% solution IV slowly. May be repeated at 10-minute intervals if necessary.

    Pediatric—0.3 ml/kg of 10% solution

Special considerations

    Can cause slowing of a beating heart. Use with caution in digitalized patients because it may potentiate digitalis toxicity. Precipitates in the presence of sodium bicarbonate.

Chart 14-7

PRINCIPAL DRUGS FOR CARDIAC ARREST (*CONTINUED*)

Dopamine

Mechanism of action

A naturally occurring catecholamine. Has both α- and β-stimulating properties; effect varies with amount given. Low-range midrange (2–10 μg/kg/min) effect is primarily β. At higher doses, α-effects are seen. At low doses dilates renal and mesenteric blood vessels. The desired therapeutic effects are increased myocardial contractility, improved perfusion, and maintenance of adequate renal and mesenteric blood supplies.

Indications

Cardiogenic shock and hemodynamically significant hypotension. It is not the treatment of choice for hypovolemic shock, but may need to be used in conjunction with definitive therapy for this condition.

Dosage

Adult—2 to 10 μg/kg/min by IV infusion. At higher doses, α-effects are seen. The correct dosage is the minimum necessary to produce desired effects.

Pediatric—as above

Special considerations

Can cause side-effects related to sympathetic actions, including myocardial irritability. Alpha side-effects include undesirable vasoconstriction. Can cause angina. Dosage must be decreased in patients taking monoamine oxidase (MAO) inhibitors. Inactivated by sodium bicarbonate. Must be given with an infusion pump. Extravasation can cause tissue sloughing.

Epinephrine

Mechanism of action

A naturally occurring catecholamine. Has both α- and β-stimulating properties. Primary actions include increased heart rate, increased force of contraction, increased automaticity, increased myocardial irritability, bronchodilation, and vasoconstriction. Makes the heart more susceptible to defibrillation in ventricular fibrillation. Elevates perfusion pressure.

Indications

Ventricular fibrillation not responsive to countershock.
To ''coarsen'' fine ventricular fibrillation.

Ventricular asystole.

Occasionally, for *pulseless idioventricular rhythm.*

Dosage

Adult—0.5 mg to 1.0 mg of 1:10,000 solution by IV push. May be repeated at 5-minute intervals. May be given through endotracheal tube. Rarely, may be given by intracardiac injection.

Pediatric—0.1 ml/kg of 1:10,000 solution.

Special considerations

May be partially deactivated by sodium bicarbonate.

Isoproterenol

Mechanism of action

Stimulates sympathetic β-receptor sites; therefore increases rate of all pacemaker cells, increases irritability, increases contractility, and vasodilates.

Indications

Atrioventricular blocks resulting in hemodynamic instability (when not improved by atropine). Also used for hemodynamically significant sinus bradycardia not responsive to atropine.

Ventricular asystole after first line drugs have been given.

Chart 14-7

PRINCIPAL DRUGS FOR CARDIAC ARREST (*CONTINUED*)

Isoproterenol (*continued*)

Dosage

Adult—administered by intravenous infusion at 2 to 20 μg/min titrated to heart rate (desirable heart rate of 60/min). If ventricular irritability is seen, immediately decrease or terminate the infusion.

Pediatric—initially by infusion at 0.1 μg/kg/min. Precautions as above.

Special considerations

Give only when absolutely necessary. It is a potent and dangerous drug when cardiac activity is present. Frequently produces serious ventricular irritability (including ventricular fibrillation). Increases myocardial oxygen consumption. Must be given with an infusion pump.

Lidocaine

Mechanism of action

Suppresses ventricular ectopy. Raises the ventricular fibrillation threshold.

Indications

Premature ventricular contractions that are frequent, fall close to the T wave, are multifocal, or occur in succession

Ventricular tachycardia

Ventricular fibrillation

Suspected myocardial ischemia—many authorities now recommend prophylactic lidocaine to prevent onset of primary ventricular fibrillation

Dosage

Adult—initial intravenous bolus of 50 to 100 mg, followed by an infusion of 1 to 4 mg/min. An additional 0.5 mg/kg may be given 10 minutes after the initial dose if necessary to control continued ventricular ectopy.

Pediatric—1 mg/kg as an initial bolus, followed by an infusion at 30 μg/kg/minute.

Special considerations

Signs of toxicity are primarily related to the central nervous system. They include drowsiness, confusion, parasthesias, and muscle twitching. Can cause seizures. Caution should be exercised in administering to patients with known conduction disturbances. Dosage must be decreased in patients with hepatic dysfunction.

Norepinephrine

Mechanism of action

A naturally occurring catecholamine. Actions include both α and β properties. Its most significant action is α-receptor related—causes profound vasoconstriction.

Indications

Hypotension, especially if total peripheral vascular resistance is low. Not indicated for shock secondary to hypovolemia.

Dosage

Adult—an intravenous infusion of a solution with a dilution of 16 μg/ml titrated to maintain a low normal blood pressure.

Pediatric—initial dosage by infusion at 0.1 μg/kg/min

Special considerations

Increases myocardial consumption. Contraindicated in hypovolemic shock. Can cause irritable heart rhythms. Must be infused with an infusion pump. Extravasation causes tissue sloughing.

Chart 14-7

PRINCIPAL DRUGS FOR CARDIAC ARREST (*CONTINUED*)

Procainamide

Mechanism of action

Suppresses ventricular irritability.

Indications

Ventricular irritability. Significant premature ventricular contractions, ventricular tachycardia, ventricular fibrillation when these dysrhythmias have been resistant to lidocaine.

Dosage

Adult—100 mg titrated intravenously every 5 minutes (20 mg/min) until the dysrhythmia stops or the patient becomes hypotensive, or until 1 gm has been given. After the initial dose, intravenous infusion at 1 to 4 mg/min.

Pediatric—not established

Special considerations

Can cause hypotension, conduction disturbances, cardiac arrest. Infusion pump should be used.

Propranolol

Mechanism of action

A β-blocking agent; therefore decreases heart rate, myocardial irritability, and force of contraction.

Indications

Recurrent ventricular tachycardia, ventricular fibrillation refractory to standard therapy. Can be especially useful when digitalis toxicity is responsible for dysrhythmias.

Dosage

Adult—1 to 3 mg very slowly intravenously. An initial test dose of 0.1 mg to 0.3 mg is recommended.

Pediatric—not established.

Special considerations

Should not be used in patients with atrioventricular block or bradycardia. *Use with extreme caution in patients with asthma or heart failure.* May precipitate bronchoconstriction and congestive heart failure.

Sodium Bicarbonate

Mechanism of action

Combats metabolic acidosis by combining with hydrogen ions to form a weak acid.

Indications

Metabolic acidosis

Dosage

Adult—1 mEq/kg IV push as an initial dose. Subsequent doses are based on arterial blood gas results. For out-of-hospital situations, half the initial dose may be repeated every 10 to 15 minutes while the patient remains in cardiac arrest.

Pediatric—Initial dosage 1–2 mEq/kg

Special considerations

If given in excess can cause metabolic alkalosis. Can cause overload of sodium and water. Do not administer with calcium chloride or catecholamines.

* (Dosages listed are those recommended in the Textbook of Advanced Life Support. American Heart Association, 1981.)

of arrest is much more likely to be respiratory in origin rather than cardiac. For this reason, pediatric resuscitation is especially focused on airway maintenance, ventilation, oxygenation, and acid-base balance. A detailed discussion of pediatric resuscitation is presented in Chapter 27, Pediatric Emergencies.

ANATOMIC CONSIDERATIONS

There are some significant anatomic differences between children and adults. These include:

- *Body size:* Drug dosages must be adjusted for body weight. Equipment must be modified.
- *Airway:* The diameter of the pediatric airway is smaller (and occludes more easily) and is more flexible (hyperextension of the neck can cause airway obstruction).
- *Heart:* Located higher in the chest
- *Chest:* More pliable
- *Temperature control:* Small body mass with a large surface area, along with immature temperature regulation, makes hypothermia a major concern (especially in infants).

VENTILATION AND OXYGENATION

Providing optimal ventilation and oxygenation is the key to pediatric resuscitation. The airway is best maintained by the head tilt–neck lift maneuver.

Airway Suctioning at Birth

- It is extremely important to remove mucus, blood, amniotic fluid, and meconium by suctioning the newborn's airway.
- Both the nose and the mouth must be suctioned, because infants are obligate nose breathers.[31]

Assessment Considerations

Aspiration of Foreign Bodies. Aspiration of foreign bodies is especially common in toddlers. Sudden respiratory distress or cardiopulmonary arrest in a previously healthy child is very likely because of foreign body aspiration.

Hypoxia. Bradycardic heart rhythms terminating in asystole are common as a result of hypoxia in children. In planning treatment, it is important to consider this factor before focusing on drug therapy.

Pediatric Modifications of Rescue Techniques

1. *Rescue breathing*
   - Technique depends on the age and size of the infant or child.
   - Rescuer must make a seal over the airway in order to ventilate the patient.
     Infant: Mouth and nose are sealed with the rescuer's mouth.
     Larger child: Airway may be sealed in standard fashion.

- The ventilating volume should be large enough to produce chest rise. Children's lungs, especially those of infants, have small volumes. Their smaller air passages provide a greater resistance to ventilation.
- The ventilation rate is more rapid for pediatric patients because they normally breathe faster than adults.
  Ventilation rate for infant: 20 per minute
  Ventilation rate for child: 15 per minute
- Rescue breathing alone is frequently successful in resuscitating pediatric patients.

2. *Ventilation*
   - It is difficult to ventilate infants and young children using a bag-valve system unless an endotracheal tube is in place.
   - Manually triggered oxygen-powered breathing devices should not be used for pediatric patients.
   - Methods of providing supplemental oxygen during rescue breathing:
     The rescuer wears a nasal cannula, with oxygen flowing, while performing rescue breathing.
     The pocket mask is used as an adjunct to rescue breathing, and supplemental oxygen is provided through the port.

3. *Endotracheal intubation*
   - The esophageal obturator airway cannot be used in children
   - Endotracheal intubation should be attempted only by personnel who are experienced in pediatric intubation.
   - Equipment:
     Pediatric laryngoscope blade
     Uncuffed endotracheal tubes for children under 8 years of age

Note: Guideline for selecting appropriate size of endotracheal tube—the size of the nail bed of the patient's little finger corresponds to the outside diameter of the endotracheal tube.[32]

4. *Relief of airway obstruction caused by a foreign body*
   - Back blows and chest thrusts are used.
   - Abdominal thrusts are not recommended.
   - If relief is not achieved, visualization with a laryngoscope and removal of the body with McGill forceps may be attempted.

Note: Use of laryngoscope and McGill forceps is contraindicated when epiglottitis is suspected. A cricothyroid puncture or cricothyrotomy may be required.

PERFUSION

Assessment of Pulses

- To assess pulses in an infant it is usually best to palpate the brachial pulse.
- Carotid pulses are difficult to palpate.
- It is often difficult to hear the heartbeat with a stethoscope.

Modified Technique for Chest Compression (Fig. 14-8)

- Compression point is higher because a child's heart lies higher in the chest.

  Compression point in infant: midsternum

  Compression point in child: slightly higher than for adult

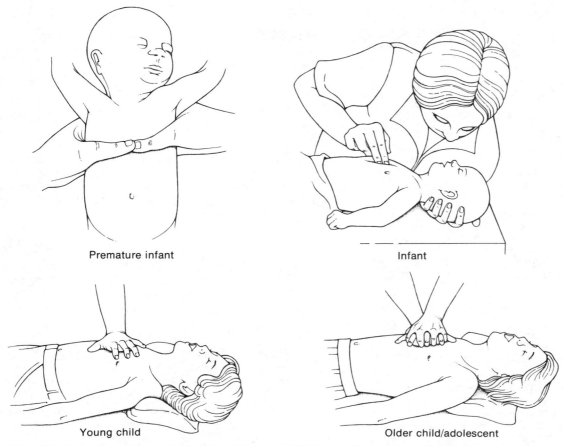

Premature infant

Infant

Young child

Older child/adolescent

Figure 14-8 *Cardiopulmonary resuscitation in children. In the young child, the heel of the hand is placed over the lower midsternum. In older children and adolescents, both hands are used. (Brunner LS, Suddarth DS: The Lippincott Manual of Nursing Practice, 3rd ed. Philadelphia, JB Lippincott, 1982)*

- Compression depth is more shallow because the chest is more pliable. Methods of compressing to the appropriate depth correspond to the age and size of the child.

    Infant and very young child:

    Compression depth: 1.3 cm to 2.5 cm (½ inch to 1 inch)

    Method 1: Rescuer uses two or three fingers of one hand to perform compression.

    Method 2: Rescuer encircles infant's chest with both hands and performs compressions with the thumbs. (Thumbs may have to be superimposed in small infants.)

    Larger child (large enough so that the sternum does not compress adequately with the three-finger technique)

    Compression depth: 2.5 cm to 3.8 cm (1 inch to 1½ inches)

    Method: Rescuer performs compression with the heel of one hand.

- Rate of compressions is faster for pediatric patients than for adults.

    Rate of compressions for infant: 100 per minute

    Rate of compressions for child: 80 per minute

- The compression-to-ventilation ratio is always 5:1, whether there are one or two rescuers performing CPR.

COORDINATING CARDIOPULMONARY RESUSCITATION IN THE EMERGENCY DEPARTMENT

Successful resuscitation is not possible without careful preparation, a well-organized plan, and competent team members. Being prepared is imperative. Actions must be swift and correct. In order to contribute fully, team members must have in-depth knowledge of resuscitation principles and be expert in resuscitative techniques. They must be able to communicate effectively and act decisively. Resuscitation situations are stressful, and good planning can minimize confusion, duplication of tasks, and errors of omission. Preparedness includes environmental considerations, equipment and supply availability, and a teamwork plan that ensures that all team members are aware of and able to perform in their assigned roles.

ENVIRONMENTAL CONSIDERATIONS

- The emergency department should be designed to permit efficient resuscitation.
- Traffic patterns must be considered and wasted motion minimized.
- The area must be well lighted.

- There must be enough space to permit personnel to perform effectively.
- All of the necessary equipment must be located in the immediate patient care area.

EQUIPMENT AND SUPPLIES

Equipment and supplies must be readily available and conveniently located. Equipment should be kept in good working order.

1. *Major equipment*
   - Cardiac monitor/defibrillator
   - Intubation equipment
   - Ventilating devices
   - Oxygen
   - Suction
   - Pacemakers
   - Infusion pumps
   - X-ray facilities must be accessible.
2. *Supplies*
   - Tracheostomy tray
   - Intravenous equipment for peripheral and central-vein cannulation
   - Pacemaker wires (transvenous and transthoracic)
   - Airway adjuncts
   - Nasogastric tubes
3. *Special needs*
   - A well-stocked crash cart containing all necessary medications, intravenous solutions, and tubings
   - Equipment for adult and pediatric patients
   - Special equipment and supplies for treatment of trauma-induced arrest, *e.g.,* antishock garment

TEAMWORK: ASSIGNED ROLES

The resuscitation team members must have assigned roles. There must be enough personnel to carry out the necessary tasks but not so many as to create additional confusion or cause congestion. Specific roles are described in Chart 14-8.

Communication

Good communication between team members is vital. The stressful atmosphere, numerous personnel present and the urgency of the situation demand careful and clear communication to prevent errors and maximize effectiveness.

Critique Sessions

A critique session immediately following the resuscitation is helpful. Team members are encouraged to evaluate the team effort and to offer suggestions for improvement in the future. In general, the sooner the critique session is conducted the more informative it will be.

The critique session has the additional benefit of allowing team members to detraumatize by expressing their feelings with their peers in a supportive atmosphere. Resuscitation is extremely stressful for emergency personnel, especially when it is not successful. Anger, frustration, and grief are common emotions at such times. Verbalizing and sharing with peers can help combat the stress and burnout syndromes.[34]

Chart 14-8

RESUSCITATION TEAM ROLES

Medical Director	Directs all medical care. It is best for the medical director to observe and direct care rather than to be a hands-on participant.
Coordinator	Coordinates team-member activities, facilitates equipment procurement, and serves as the primary communicator to other departments. The coordinator is responsible for "scene" control and should request persons who are not needed to leave.
Scribe	Records events and care rendered. (This should be done by one designated person).
Care Providers	Specific assignments include the following: • Airway management and ventilation responsibilities • Chest compressions • Establishing intravenous lines • Performing defibrillation • Administering medications
Procurement	At least one team member must be available to procure any additional equipment or supplies that are needed.

REFERENCES

1. Stedman's Medical Dictionary, p 1383. Baltimore, Williams & Wilkins, 1966
2. The Bible, King James Version, Kings II, 4:34–35
3. DeBard ML: The history of cardiopulmonary resuscitation. Ann Emerg Med 9(5):273–275
4. Textbook of Advanced Cardiac Life Support, p I-1. American Heart Association, 1981
5. Standards and guidelines for cardiopulmonary resuscitation and emergency cardiac care. JAMA 244(5):453–455
6. McElroy CR: Citizen CPR: The role of the lay person in prehospital care. Topics in Emergency Medicine 1(4):37–45, 1980
7. Textbook of Advanced Cardiac Life Support, p I-3. American Heart Association, 1981
8. Budassi SA, Bander JJ, Kimmerle L, Eie K: Cardiac Arrest and CPR, p 7. Rockville, Aspen Systems, 1980
9. Textbook of Advanced Cardiac Life Support, II-1. American Heart Association, 1981
10. Textbook of Advanced Cardiac Life Support, p IV-6. American Heart Association, 1981
11. Textbook of Advanced Cardiac Life Support, pp VIII-13, IX-7. American Heart Association, 1981
12. Textbook of Advanced Cardiac Life Support, pp III-2, 3. American Heart Association, 1981
13. Budassi SA, Bander JJ, Kimmerle L, Eie K: Cardiac Arrest and CPR, pp 8–9. Rockville, Aspen Systems, 1980
14. Textbook of Advanced Cardiac Life Support, p II-5. American Heart Association, 1981
15. Budassi SA, Bander JJ, Kimmerle L, Eie K: Cardiac Arrest and CPR, p 14. Rockville, Aspen Systems, 1980
16. Textbook of Advanced Cardiac Life Support, pp IV-9, 10. American Heart Association, 1981
17. Textbook of Advanced Cardiac Life Support, p IV-9. American Heart Association, 1981
18. Textbook of Advanced Cardiac Life Support, pp IV-5, 6. American Heart Association, 1981
19. Harrison R et al: Mouth-to-mask ventilation: A superior method of rescue breathing. Ann Emerg Med 2(1):39–41
20. Textbook of Advanced Cardiac Life Support, pp IV-5, 6. American Heart Association, 1981
21. Standards and guidelines for cardiopulmonary resuscitation and emergency cardiac care. JAMA 244(5):469
22. Textbook of Advanced Cardiac Life Support, p V-4. American Heart Association, 1981
23. Budassi SA, Bander JJ, Kimmerle L, Eie K: Cardiac Arrest and CPR, p 100. Rockville, Aspen Systems, 1980
24. Textbook of Advanced Cardiac Life Support, p V-2. American Heart Association, 1981
25. Wayne MA: The MAST suit in the treatment of cardiogenic shock. JACEP 7:107–109
26. Standards and guidelines for advanced cardiac life support and emergency cardiac care. JAMA 244(5):491
27. Budassi SA, Bander JJ, Kimmerle, Eie K: Cardiac Arrest and CPR, p 141. Rockville, Aspen Systems, 1980
28. Textbook of Advanced Cardiac Life Support, p VII-3. American Heart Association, 1981
29. Textbook of Advanced Cardiac Life Support, p VII-6. American Heart Association, 1981
30. Textbook of Advanced Cardiac Life Support, pp XIV-16, 17. American Heart Association, 1981
31. Textbook of Advanced Cardiac Life Support, pp XVI-2. American Heart Association, 1981
32. Textbook of Advanced Cardiac Life Support, pp IV-6. American Heart Association, 1981
33. Standards and guidelines for advanced cardiac life support and emergency cardiac care. JAMA 244(5):476
34. Graham N: How to avoid a short career, part 2. JEMS, pp 25–31, February 1981

15
RESPIRATORY EMERGENCIES

JAMES H. COSGRIFF, JR. and CAMILLE RATAJCZYK

Patients with acute respiratory problems are commonly seen in the emergency department and require the highest priority of care.

Compromise of respiration may result from infections, trauma, degenerative disease such as chronic obstructive lung disease, cardiac disease, neoplasms, aspiration of foreign bodies, and environmental factors.

A patient may seek assistance with a primary complaint of respiratory impairment or may develop airway difficulty while in the emergency department—for example, patients in coma or with thoracic injury.

There is perhaps nothing that can arouse more anxiety in emergency personnel than a patient with acute respiratory distress. Emergency personnel must be able to: properly assess a patient with respiratory distress, identify the causative factor(s), and initiate corrective measures. On occasion, the necessary intervention requires rapid, split-second decisions and actions to save the patient's life. To attain these skills, one must be familiar with respiratory physiology, the mechanics of respiration, the pathologic processes that alter normal respiratory function, and correct methods of respiratory assessment and emergency care. Resuscitation techniques and equipment are discussed in detail in Chapter 14, Resuscitation: Principles and Techniques.

ANATOMY AND PHYSIOLOGY

Respiration is broadly defined as the gaseous interchange that occurs between an organism and its environment. Humans depend on oxygen to maintain normal cellular activity.

The two phases of respiration are:
1. *External respiration*—in which oxygen (O_2) and carbon dioxide (CO_2) are transferred between the inspired air and the pulmonary capillaries
2. *Internal respiration*—in which O_2 and CO_2 are transferred between the peripheral blood capillaries and the tissue cells

The transfer of gases occurs by diffusion, which depends on the partial pressure of each of the gases in the air and the body tissues. Table 15-1 shows the partial pressures of O_2 and CO_2 in the atmosphere, alveoli, and venous and arterial blood. The pressure gradient of O_2 between atmospheric and alveolar air is 57 mm Hg (157 − 100). The gradient of O_2 between alveolar air and venous blood is 60 mm Hg (100 − 40).

The lungs are contained within the chest, or thorax. The chest wall is composed of the bony rib cage and supporting soft tissue structures, primarily the intercostal muscles. The lungs are paired organs lying within the lateral portions of the chest cavity. They consist of millions of tiny air-containing sacs called *alveoli,* in which external respiration takes place. Each lung is covered by a serous membrane that consists of two layers: (1) the *visceral pleura,* a thin cellular layer, that adheres closely to the lung, and (2) the *parietal pleura,* a parietal layer, which is reflected to form the lining of the chest wall and cover the upper surface of the diaphragm. Although it is only a potential space, the area between the visceral and the parietal pleurae is called the *pleural cavity* or the *pleural space.* Normally, a thin layer of serous fluid between the two pleural surfaces prevents friction and allows them to move smoothly over one another during breathing.

The lung compartments lie on either side of the *mediastinum,* the area in the central portion of the chest. The mediastinum contains several major structures: the esophagus, trachea, lymphatics, and heart and great vessels.

The borders of the lung compartments are described as follows:
Inferior—the diaphragm, which separates the thoracic and abdominal cavities

Superior—the apex of the pleura, which extends above the clavicles to the supraclavicular space

Lateral, anterior, posterior—the rib cage

Medial—the mediastinum

The entrance to the respiratory tract is the *upper airway,* which includes the mouth, nasal cavity, pharynx, larynx and glottis (vocal cords), and trachea. The trachea is a fibrocartilaginous tubular structure extending from the level of the thyroid cartilage, in the neck, to the sternomanubrial joint (the angle of Louis) at the 2nd intercostal space anteriorly. At the angle of Louis, it divides into the left and the right main bronchi, each of which leads into a lung and subsequently divides into smaller and smaller branches until the alveolar sacs are reached. The pulmonary capillaries are located within the walls of the alveoli. It is here that the pulmonary capillary blood is separated from the alveolar air by two very thin membranes through which the transfer of O_2 and CO_2 takes place.

As air enters the alveoli on inspiration, the difference in partial pressure of gases in the alveolar air in the pulmonary capillary (venous) blood results in a free diffusion of O_2 and CO_2 within the lungs. External respiration takes place within the alveoli. This blood, now oxygenated, returns to

TABLE 15-1. PARTIAL PRESSURES OF OXYGEN AND CARBON DIOXIDE IN ATMOSPHERE, ALVEOLAR AIR, AND BLOOD (AT SEA LEVEL, 760 MM HG)

Gas	Atmosphere (mm Hg)	Alveolar Air (mm Hg)	Venous Blood (mm Hg)	Arterial Blood (mm Hg)
Oxygen	157	100	40	93
Carbon dioxide	0.3	40	46	40
Percentage oxygen saturation of hemoglobin			75	97
Plasma pH			7.35	7.38

(After Best CH, Taylor NB. In Brobeck JR (ed): Physiological Basis of Medical Practice, 9th ed, pp 6-5, 6-6. Baltimore; Williams & Wilkins, 1973)

the left heart by way of the pulmonary veins and is then pumped into the systemic circulation. (Fig. 15-1) As this blood reaches the arterial capillaries in the body, there is diffusion of O_2 and CO_2 between the capillaries and adjacent tissue cells. This is called internal respiration. The venous capillary blood leaving these tissues contains a lower pressure of O_2 and a higher concentration of CO_2 and is returned to the right heart and the lungs for reoxygenation.

The pleural space (the space between the visceral pleura and the parietal pleura) is unique in that the intrapleural pressure is negative in relation to atmospheric air and the air in the alveoli.

The negative pressure varies with the stage of respiration. At rest, it is approximately −2.5 cm of water. This negative pressure assists in keeping the lungs expanded. Normal respiratory action occurs as follows: the intercostal muscles contract, raising the ribs and expanding the chest wall, while simultaneously the diaphragm descends, acting as a bellows. Air is thus drawn into the lungs (inspiration) until they are fully expanded. At the end of inspiration, the intrapleural pressure rises to −7 to −8 cm of water.

Expiration is essentially a passive action, since the elastic recoil of the lungs causes the air to be expelled. The amount of air taken in during an ordinary inspiration averages 500 ml in an adult; it is called *tidal air* or *tidal volume*. It can be measured easily by a respirometer and is one index of pulmonary function.

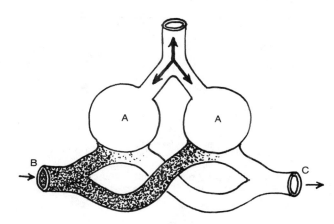

Figure 15-1 *Diagrammatic illustration of the normal process of respiration. Air enters the pulmonary alveoli (A). Pulmonary venous blood (B) is oxygenated through the alveolocapillary membrane, thus producing arterialized (oxygenated) blood (C), which is then returned to the left side of the heart.*

RESPIRATORY ASSESSMENT

The extent of assessment depends on the condition of the patient. In an urgent situation, assessment, diagnostic studies, and treatment may proceed concurrently. In the prehospital phase, a rapid assessment is made at the scene and immediate care is given as required. In the hospital, a thorough respiratory assessment and general physical examination are performed, adjunct studies are done, and definitive treatment is instituted. Important points in the assessment of the patient with respiratory distress are outlined in Chart 15-1.

PREHOSPITAL PHASE

The initial assessment and immediate care of the patient with respiratory distress or chest pain not related to trauma include the following:
- Assess airway patency.
- Check mouth and oropharynx for foreign body or excessive retained secretions; remove or bypass obstruction as indicated.
- Give oxygen by mask or nasal catheter as indicated.
- Provide assisted ventilation with bag-valve mask as indicated.
- Record vital signs
- Assess level of consciousness.
- Observe for cyanosis of lips, earlobes, nail beds.
- Observe rate, depth, rhythm, and ease or difficulty of respiration.

- Prepare patient for transport.

Patient should be assisted or carried to the litter and not allowed to walk. Transport patient in a sitting or semi-sitting position, whichever is more comfortable.

HOSPITAL PHASE

History

In the emergency setting, the history may be gathered while assessment and initial care are going on. The following information is needed:
- Was the onset of symptoms abrupt or was it insidious (occurring over a period of days or weeks)?
- Do the respiratory symptoms occur at rest or with exertion?
- Is there any associated chest pain?
- Ask the patient to describe any pain (*e.g.,* sharp, dull, constant, intermittent, related to respiratory activity). Does it radiate? If so, in what direction?
- Are there any cough, fever, chills?
- Is any sputum raised? If so, describe the color (white, yellow, green, bloody); consistency (thin, thick); quantity (teaspoonful, tablespoonful, cupful).
- Does the patient have any known associated disease, *e.g.,* heart disease, hypertension, emphysema, bronchitis, asthma, allergy?
- Is the patient a smoker? If so, identify type (cigarette, cigar, pipe); quantity; and duration of smoking.
- Was there any exposure to noxious fumes, chemicals, coal?

Physical Examination

In order to evaluate a patient with dyspnea or chest pain, the two most common symptoms of respiratory embarrassment, emergency personnel must have a clear understanding of normal physical findings in the chest. Familiarity with the topographic anatomy of the thorax is important in assessing the normal findings and localizing those that

Chart 15-1

ASSESSMENT OF THE PATIENT WITH RESPIRATORY DISTRESS

Prehospital Phase

INITIAL ASSESSMENT AND IMMEDIATE CARE

- Assess patient for airway patency and adequate ventilation.
  Remove or bypass mechanical obstruction as required.
  Give oxygen by mask or nasal catheter as indicated.
  Give assisted ventilation with bag-valve mask as indicated.
- Assess and record vital signs, skin color, and level of consciousness.
- Prepare patient for transport.
  Assist or carry; do not allow patient to walk.
  Transport in sitting or semisitting position.

Hospital Phase

HISTORY

- Onset of symptoms—abrupt or insidious?
- Effects of rest or exertion on symptoms
- Pain?
  Sharp, dull, constant, intermittent
  Relationship to respiratory activity
  Location, radiation
- Cough, fever, or chills?
- Sputum?
  Color—white, yellow, green, bloody
  Consistency—thin, thick
  Quantity—teaspoonful, tablespoonful, cupful
- Associated disease(s)
  Heart disease
  Hypertension
  Emphysema
  Bronchitis
  Asthma
  Allergy

---

are abnormal. Major thoracic landmarks are shown in Chart 15-2.

The patient's chest should be bared for examination. Privacy and good lighting should be provided; a comfortable room temperature, when available, prevents shivering and permits more accurate observation. The usual mode of physical assessment is followed: inspection, palpation, percussion, and auscultation.

Inspection.   Observe for the following signs and symptoms of respiratory embarrassment.
- Feeling of apprehension
- Supraclavicular tugging or retraction
- Intercostal retraction
- Flaring of the nares with inspiration
- Alterations in consciousness, disorientation, confusion
- Paleness to cyanosis
- Increased rate of breathing (tachypnea)
- Splinting of the chest (pleurisy, rib fracture)
- Audible wheezing (asthma)
- Frothy sputum at the mouth or nose (pulmonary edema)

In a good light, observe the chest wall for any deformity, alteration in shape, the rate, depth and rhythm of respiratory movement. Look for labored breathing, which may be manifested by retraction of the intercostal spaces or the supra-

---

Chart 15-1

ASSESSMENT OF THE PATIENT WITH RESPIRATORY DISTRESS (*CONTINUED*)

Hospital Phase

- Smoking habit?
    Type, quantity, duration
- Exposure to noxious fumes, chemicals, coal?

CHEST EXAMINATION

1. Inspection
   - Observe for signs and symptoms of respiratory embarrassment.
   - Observe chest wall for deformity, alteration in shape; rate, depth, and rhythm of respiratory movement.
2. Palpation
   - Identify any areas of tenderness.
   - Check range of motion during respiration.
   - Palpate for subcutaneous emphysema (crackling under the skin).
   - Test tactile fremitus.
3. Percussion
   - Percuss entire chest.
   - Compare one side with the other.
   - Identify any areas of dullness or flatness.
4. Auscultation
   - Examine entire area of lung with stethoscope.
   - Listen to one or two complete breaths in each area.
   - Compare one side with the other.
   - Identify any abnormal breath sounds.

GENERAL PHYSICAL EXAMINATION

- Complete the remainder of the physical assessment in the usual manner.

ADJUNCT STUDIES

- Routine blood studies
- Chest x-ray
- Arterial blood gas determinations
- Electrocardiogram (ECG)
- Sputum examination
- Pulmonary function tests (rarely done in emergency department)

---

clavicular or subxiphoid areas. Determine whether the chest wall moves equally on each side. Is the patient breathing at a normal rate (12–16/min), or rapidly (tachypnea); with deep breaths (hyperventilating), or slowly (bradypnea) or irregularly (Cheyne-Stokes)?

Palpation. Confirm the findings noted on inspection. Identify any areas of tenderness. Place the hands on the lower chest posteriorly and observe the excursion of the thumbs to detect the range of motion (Fig. 15-2). Palpate for subcutaneous emphysema (crackling under the skin). Place the palm of the hand on the chest wall posteriorly to test tactile fremitus and ask the patient to say "eeee."

Percussion. Percuss the entire chest. Normally the chest will give a hollow percussion note similar to that of a drum. Dullness or a flattened percussion note indicates the absence of air in the underlying lung and suggests the presence of fluid in the pleural space or inside the alveolar sacs. Compare one side with the other.

Auscultation. With a stethoscope, examine the entire area of the lung. The patient is asked to breathe through his mouth during auscultation. Listen to one or two complete breaths in each area and compare one side with the other. Normal and abnormal breath sounds are described and illustrated in Chart 15-3.

Chart 15-2

THORACIC LANDMARKS, AIDS TO ASSESSMENT

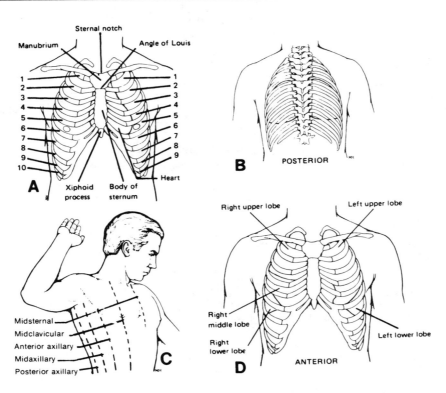

Anteriorly, the lungs extend from above the clavicles to the level of the 6th rib in the midclavicular line. Posteriorly, the lower margin of the lung is at the 10th thoracic vertebra. It may descend two additional vertebrae on deep inspiration. The trachea normally lies in the midline and is easily palpated just above the suprasternal notch. It enters the mediastinum and divides into the left and right bronchi at the level of the angle of Louis anteriorly and the 4th thoracic vertebra posteriorly. Here, the airway is close to the chest wall.

(Illustrations from Brunner LS, Suddarth DS: Lippincott Manual of Nursing Practice, 3rd ed. Philadelphia, JB Lippincott, 1982)

Differential Diagnosis

The two most common symptoms of respiratory embarrassment are dyspnea and chest pain. It is important to be aware of the many factors involved in evaluating each of these symptoms. These factors are described in Chart 15-4.

Adjunct Studies

Adjunct studies commonly ordered for the patient in respiratory distress include routine blood studies, chest x-ray, arterial blood gas determinations, electrocardiogram (ECG), and sputum examination. Pulmonary function tests are rarely done in the emergency department.

Routine Blood Studies. Routine blood studies include a complete blood count (CBC) and SMA-18. Leukocytosis of-

ten accompanies infectious processes; eosinophilia is found in many patients with asthma because of an underlying allergic condition. Anemia may be a causative factor in respiratory difficulty. The electrolytes, especially CO_2, may be deranged in respiratory acidosis.

Chest X-ray. X-ray of the chest is one of the most useful studies in a patient with respiratory distress. Some of the conditions that may be identified on a routine chest x-ray are mass lesions (tumors), infectious processes (chronic bronchitis, bronchiectasis, pneumonia), atelectasis, pulmonary edema, emphysema, pneumothorax, and pleural effusion.

Arterial Blood Gas Determinations. Arterial blood gas determinations are the single most important method of

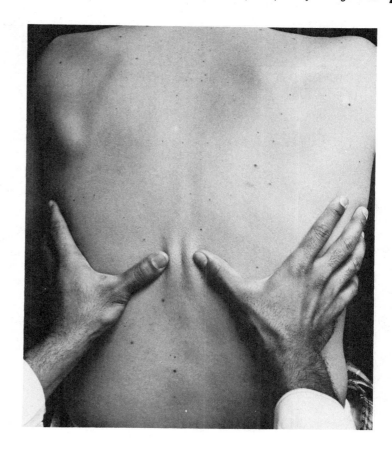

Figure 15-2 *Palpation of the lower posterior chest.*

assessing cardiopulmonary function in the emergency department. Normal values for arterial blood gases are listed in Table 15-2. Normal values vary with the age of the patient and are altered by any condition that affects the following:

1. The *diffusion of gases* across the alveolar-pulmonary capillary membrane (as in pneumonia, acute pulmonary edema) (Fig. 15-3)
2. The *perfusion of blood* through the pulmonary vessels due to changes in blood flow within the lungs (as in precapillary shunting, mass lesions [Fig. 15-4], or shock).

The blood gases reflect the quality of pulmonary function based primarily on the pH and O_2, CO_2, and bicarbonate content.

Electrocardiogram. ECGs may be helpful in identifying certain types of heart disease that can contribute to or cause pulmonary difficulties.

TABLE 15-2. NORMAL VALUES FOR ARTERIAL BLOOD GASES

Gas	Value
pH	7.4 ± 0.3
pCO_2	40 ± 4 mm Hg
pO_2	80–100 mm Hg
Standard bicarbonate	24 ± 2 mEq/L
Base excess	0 ± 2.5 mEq/L
Buffer base	46 ± 1 mEq/L
Oxygenation saturation	95–97%

Sputum Examination. *Sputum examination* is useful in patients with infectious disease of the lung. Sputum studies, including gram stain and acid-fast stain in addition to culture and sensitivity, may be obtained in the emergency department before initiation of antibiotic therapy.

Pulmonary Function Tests. *Pulmonary function tests* are used to evaluate lung function but are rarely used in the emergency setting.

Figure 15-3 *Impaired diffusion of gases. Thickening of the alveolopulmonary membrane (A) impairs diffusion of gases. Pulmonary venous blood (B) is incompletely oxygenated on return to the left side of the heart through the pulmonary veins (C).*

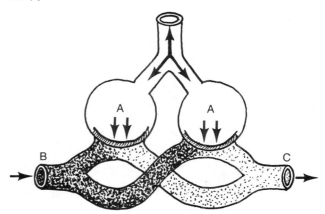

Chart 15-3

DiFFERENTIATION OF BREATH SOUNDS

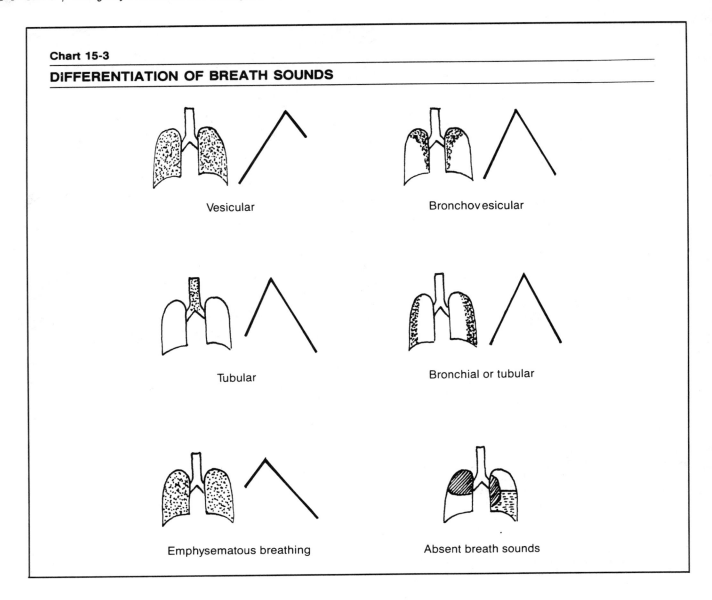

Vesicular

Bronchovesicular

Tubular

Bronchial or tubular

Emphysematous breathing

Absent breath sounds

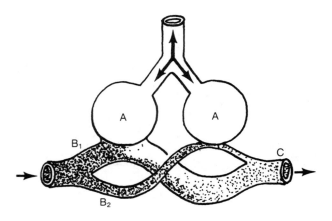

Figure 15-4 *Perfusion variations due to selective shunting. Diminished perfusion of alveoli by selective shunting within the lung causes incomplete oxygenation of the venous blood. The diagram above illustrates normal flow through one pulmonary vessel (B$_1$) and diminished flow through another (B$_2$). The end result is incomplete oxygenation of blood in the pulmonary vein.*

SPECIFIC CAUSES OF ACUTE RESPIRATORY DISTRESS

There are many types and causes of acute respiratory distress (ARD). The problems most commonly seen in the emergency department are inhalation injuries, acute pulmonary edema, spontaneous pneumothorax, pulmonary thromboembolism, chronic obstructive pulmonary diseases (COPD), and acute respiratory acidosis (respiratory failure).

INHALATION INJURY

Lung damage due to the inhalation of smoke or other noxious products of combustion is considered the leading cause of death among fire victims. It is estimated that 50% to 60% of fire-related deaths are due to inhalation injury. Functionally,

Chart 15-3

DIFFERENTIATION OF BREATH SOUNDS (*CONTINUED*)

Normal Breath Sounds

Type	Location (Where Heard)	Pitch	Amplitude (Loudness)	Relative Duration of Inspiration, Expiration
Vesicular	Over most of lung area, except close to midline over trachea and bronchi	Low	Moderate (soft)	Inspiration much greater than expiration
Broncho-vesicular	Over apices of lungs and larger airway passages near midline anteriorly and posteriorly	Medium	Greater than moderate	Equal
Tubular	Over trachea	High	Very great (loud)	Inspiration may be shorter than expiration

Abnormal Breath Sounds

Bronchial or tubular breathing	Over periphery of lung	High	Louder than vesicular sounds	Equal
Emphysematous breathing	Over most of lung area	Medium	Moderate (soft)	Expiration longer
Absence of breath sounds	Indicates lack of aeration of the underlying lung, as occurs in pneumothorax, large pleural effusion, and atelectasis			

Adventitious Sounds

Friction rub — Caused by irritation of the pleura by inflammation or tumor and rubbing of the visceral and parietal pleural surfaces during breathing. Heard as a grating sound, usually on both inspiration and expiration; not affected by coughing.

Wheezes, rales, rhonchi — Indicate narrowing of the air passages by spasm or mucus/fluid in the tracheobronchial tree, as in chronic bronchitis, asthma, and emphysema.

inhalation injury may affect the upper respiratory tract (mouth, pharynx, larynx, trachea) or the lower respiratory tract (lung), or both.

CAUSES

Carbon Monoxide

Carbon monoxide (CO) is a colorless, odorless, tasteless gas formed by the combustion of organic materials such as paper or wood. It causes damage by producing hypoxia. CO has an affinity for hemoglobin, which is 200 times greater than that of O_2. As a result, CO replaces O_2 on the hemoglobin molecule, forming carboxyhemoglobin, which interferes with O_2 transport.

Smoke Poisoning

Smoke injury results from the thermodegradation products of synthetic materials. The combustion of these substances produces noxious gases containing acids and nitrogen and sulfur oxides. These gases may cause corrosive damage to the air passages, primarily in the lower respiratory tract.

Chart 15-4

DIFFERENTIAL DIAGNOSIS OF DYSPNEA

The term *dyspnea* refers to any labored, difficult, or painful respiration. It may be observed either subjectively or objectively. Four types of dyspnea are described below:

Exertional Dyspnea

- Associated with physical exercise or exertion
- Persists for varying periods of time after exercise has ceased

Paroxysmal Dyspnea

- Usually occurs at night, when patient has been recumbent for a period of time (often referred to as paroxysmal nocturnal dyspnea)
- Associated wtih congestive heart failure
- Redistribution of edema fluid from lower portions of body to lungs occurs when patient is recumbent, because of gravitational effects of this position
- Symptoms may be relieved by getting out of bed and breathing at an open window.

Positional Dyspnea (Orthopnea)

- Occurs as soon as patient assumes recumbent position
- Associated with a number of cardiac abnormalities or diseases
- May be relieved by using several pillows to elevate head and chest

Continuous Dyspnea

- Present at all times, even at rest
- Aggravated by slight exertion
- Associated with chronic pulmonary disease and obesity

Possible Causes

Dyspnea may be associated with or secondary to the following:
- Primary pulmonary disease such as chronic bronchitis, emphysema, asthma
- Environmental pollutants
- Anemia
- Cardiac disease, especially rheumatic heart disease with mitral stenosis, aortic stenosis, coronary artery disease

DIFFERENTIAL DIAGNOSIS OF CHEST PAIN

Pain in the chest may be due to conditions arising in a number of sites, as follows:

Heart and Great Vessels

PAIN OF ANOXIA

- Chest pain due to myocardial anoxia is usually associated with coronary artery disease; it may also be found with pericarditis
- Associated with some form of physical exertion, often relieved by rest

Chart 15-4

DIFFERENTIAL DIAGNOSIS OF CHEST PAIN (*CONTINUED*)

- Often occurs after exertion or a meal and is interpreted by some patients as indigestion
- Commonly referred to as *angina*
- Described as a squeezing, tightness, pressure, or heaviness in the chest
- Location of pain
  Usually anterior chest or epigastrium
  May be in posterior interscapular region, in neck, or at the angles of the jaw
  Commonly radiates to the neck and shoulders and down one or both arms
- Pain of pericarditis is also located in anterior chest, but may mimic pleuritic pain because it can be aggravated by respiration.

  PAIN ARISING FROM THE GREAT VESSELS

- Usually associated with a dissecting thoracic aortic aneurysm
- Characteristically sudden in onset
- Pain moderate to severe and constant
- Located in anterior chest, but may be noted in the back, usually on the left side.

Lungs, Pleurae, Chest Wall, and Mediastinum

- Pain arising in the lungs and pleurae may be secondary to an acute infectious process, pleurisy, or pulmonary thromboembolism with infarct.
  Pain usually dull to sharp
  Aggravated by respiratory activity but rarely by body movement
- A *pulmonary embolus* is not painful unless infarction of the lung has occurred.
  Pain felt at site of lesion
  If lesion is near diaphragm, pain may be referred to shoulder.
- *Spontaneous pneumothorax*
  May cause sudden pain and dyspnea of varying degrees
  Pain usually continuous
- *Tension pneumothorax* that develops spontaneously
  May be marked by pain, severe dyspnea, and hypotension (see Chap. 21)
- *Mediastinal emphysema*
  May follow a pneumothorax or rupture
  Marked by rather constant retrosternal pain that is not aggravated by respiration
  Hammans' sign (mediastinal crunch synchronous with heart beat) is pathognomonic.

Esophagus

- Pain of esophageal origin may mimic cardiac pain.
- Usually due to reflex esophagitis, achalasia, peptic ulcer of the esophagus, or rupture
- The most common cause is reflux esophagitis
  Burning pain in anterior lower chest (heartburn)
  Often follows ingestion of a meal, lying down, or bending forward (as if to tie one's shoe)
  Relieved by taking an antacid
  Reflux often associated with a hiatal hernia

Cervical Spine

- Herniation of a lower cervical intervertebral disk may produce chest pain.
- May be aggravated by motion of neck, coughing, wheezing, or straining
- Pain usually located in anterior or posterior upper chest

Thermal Injury

The heat generated by a fire, especially in a closed space, may reach temperatures in the range of 1000°F. Soot and particulate matter may form as a result of incomplete combustion and cause direct damage to the air passages when inhaled. The inhalation of hot, dry air may cause damage primarily to the upper airway.

ASSESSMENT

History

Consider the possibility of smoke inhalation in any patient who was:

- Exposed to fire in a closed space
- Found unconscious or has a history of loss of consciousness

Physical Examination

The signs of possible inhalation injury are:
- Burns about the face and mouth
- Singeing of the nasal hairs
- Carbonaceous (soot-stained) sputum
- Hoarseness, cough
- Respiratory distress
- Rales, rhonchi, wheezes on auscultation of the chest

Adjunct Studies

- Arterial blood gases should be obtained early in the management of the patient. Typically, decreased O_2 and increased CO_2 are found.
- Increased carboxyhemoglobin level is one of the characteristics of inhalation injury. It is tested separately from routine blood gas determinations.
- Chest x-ray may reveal no abnormality during the early hours after injury but hours or days later may reveal infiltrates and increased hilar markings.
- Bronchoscopy is a simple and accurate method of identifying inhalation injury.
- Xenon-133 clearance has been used to diagnose inhalation injury but is not often performed during the emergency phase of care.

MANAGEMENT

Prehospital Care

- Remove the patient from the noxious environment, taking care to protect yourself from exposure.
- Clear the airway by suction, if available, or position the patient for drainage.
- Remove visible debris.
- Insert a nasopharyngeal or nasotracheal airway.
- Give 100% O_2 (humidified if possible) by mask or through the airway.

Hospital Care

- Establish and maintain an airway, preferably by endotracheal intubation in severe injury.
- Obtain baseline blood gases and carboxyhemoglobin levels
- Give 100% O_2. Assisted ventilation with positive end expiratory pressure (PEEP) is indicated in severe hypoxemia.
- Suction airway frequently, as indicated. Maintain sterile technique.
- Consider bronchodilators such as aminophylline or terbutaline.
- Obtain sputum samples for bacteriologic study.
- The prophylactic use of antibiotics is controversial; some clinicians wait until specific organisms are identified in the sputum.
- The use of steroids is also controversial but is advocated by some to diminish the inflammatory response.
- Observe closely for airway difficulty, since the onset of lower respiratory tract difficulty may have an insidious, delayed onset hours to days after exposure.

ACUTE PULMONARY EDEMA

Pulmonary edema is defined as an abnormal accumulation of liquid and solute in the extravascular tissues and spaces of the lung.[13] It results in widening of the alveolopulmonary capillary membrane.

1. Basic causative factors in pulmonary edema:
   - Increased pressure in the pulmonary capillaries due to cardiac disease, pulmonary venous disease, fluid overload
   - Altered permeability of the alveolopulmonary capillary membrane, as in pneumonia, uremia, drowning, aspiration, inhalation of noxious fumes
   - Decreased oncotic pressure associated with low albumin due to nutritional, kidney, or liver disorders
   - Other causes, such as high altitude, heroin overdose, pulmonary embolism, eclampsia
2. Common specific causes of pulmonary edema:
   - Cardiac disease with acute myocardial infarction, hypertension, or mitral stenosis. This is the most common cause.
   - Pulmonary embolism
   - Inhalation of noxious fumes
   - Pulmonary infection

PATHOPHYSIOLOGY

Although the mechanisms may vary, the underlying physiologic alterations are:
- Increased permeability of the alveolopulmonary capillary membrane with passage of fluid across the barrier from the capillaries into the interstitial space and the alveoli

- Diminished gas exchange with:

    Hypoxemia (decreased O_2 tension in the blood)

    Hypercarbia (increased CO_2 tension in the blood)

As the patient becomes dyspneic and tachypneic, the cardiac rate increases, causing the heart to function less efficiently and leading to further aggravation of the condition by the outpouring of more fluid into the alveoli. The mechanism of pulmonary edema in low-albumin states, high altitude, and heroin overdose is not as clearly understood as that associated with primary cardiac disease and congestive heart failure.

ASSESSMENT

History

The patient may give a history of cardiac disease, but in many instances the initial episode is the first evidence of cardiac abnormality. The nature of the heart problem may be related to arteriosclerosis, hypertension, dysrhythmia, or an earlier myocardial infarction. The onset of acute pulmonary edema may be sudden or may be heralded by gradually progressive paroxysmal nocturnal dyspnea.

In acute myocardial infarction, the patient may complain of substernal or precordial pain. With pulmonary emboli and infarction, pleuritic pain may be present.

In other patients, exposure to fumes, drugs, or high altitude may be causative factors.

Physical Examination

- The patient appears apprehensive and breathless, unable to lie flat.
- Cyanosis of the lips, earlobes, and nail beds is frequently present.
- Frothy white or pink-tinged sputum may be flowing from the mouth or nose.
- Blood pressure may be normotensive, hypertensive, or hypotensive depending on the underlying etiology.
- Tachycardia and tachypnea are usually present.
- With cardiac disease, dysrhythmias, especially auricular fibrillation, may be noted.
- The superficial neck veins are distended owing to an increase in venous pressure.
- Chest auscultation reveals generalized rales with impaired breath sounds
- Peripheral edema may be noted
- Hepatojugular reflex may be noted
- Ascites and the stigmata of liver disease may be seen.

Adjunct Studies

- Arterial blood gases reveal a decrease in O_2 tension and increased or lowered CO_2 tension

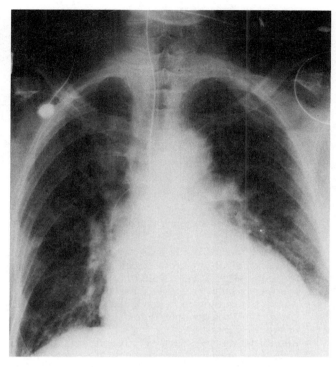

Figure 15-5 *Pulmonary edema marked by increased bronchovascular markings, increased heart size, and left pleural effusion; note central venous catheter in place.*

- Chest x-rays characteristically show (Fig. 15-5):

    Increased bronchovascular markings

    Increased heart size with widening of the diameter of the heart

    Pleural effusion (hydrothorax); commonly seen in noncardiac states. Heart size is normal or widened. Special x-ray studies may be needed to rule out pulmonary emboli (p 222).

- ECG may demonstrate:

    Findings of acute coronary artery disease (see Chap. 16, Cardiac Emergencies)

    Dysrhythmias, usually tachyarrhythmia

- CBC and SMA-18 are done. In infectious or allergic states, leukocytosis, or eosinophilia may be noted. Hypoalbuminemia or deranged liver function tests are seen in chronic liver disease or malnutrition.
- Cardiac isoenzyme studies
- Urinalysis may demonstrate hematuria, proteinuria, and casts in patients with chronic renal disease.

MANAGEMENT

Objectives of Treatment

- Improving ventilation
- Correcting the etiology of the problem

Prehospital Care

- Aspirate excessive oropharyngeal secretions.
- Give 100% O₂ by mask.
- Transport patient in a sitting or comfortable upright position.

Hospital Care

1. Insert a large-bore intravenous line to draw blood samples and give medication. All medication should be given intravenously, particularly in cardiac patients or those with hypotension.
2. Insert central-vein line to measure venous pressure.
3. For cardiac patients, morphine sulfate, 0.008 gm or 0.010 gm, may be given to allay apprehension and slow the respiratory rate.
   - Give 40% to 60% O₂ by mask or O₂ bubbled through 50% ethyl alcohol with intermittent positive pressure breathing (IPPB). The alcohol lowers the surface tension in the lungs and acts as a sedative.
   - Administer cardiotonic drugs to strengthen myocardial contractility, for example, digoxin, ouabain, inotropin, or other β₁ drugs.
   - Administer diuretics such as furosemide or ethacrynic acid; these are given intravenously to decrease blood volume and diminish preload on the heart.
   - Manage cardiac arrhythmias as indicated (see Chap. 16, Cardiac Emergencies).
   - If patient is severely hypertensive, trimethaphan camphorsulfonate (Arfonad) can be given by intravenous drip.
   - Keep patient on continuous cardiac monitor.
4. For patients with pulmonary thromboemboli, manage accordingly (p 222).
5. For patients with nutritional, renal, or hepatic disease
   - Give O₂ by mask as for cardiac patient, above.
   - Administer diuretics intravenously.
6. In poisoning, near-drowning, or exposure to noxious fumes
   - Give O₂ by mask.
   - Maintain pulmonary hygiene.
   - Give specific antidote if available in poisoning.

SPONTANEOUS PNEUMOTHORAX

Spontaneous pneumothorax is a rather common clinical condition characteristically found in apparently healthy young persons between 20 and 40 years of age. Eighty percent of these patients are men. Spontaneous pneumothorax is almost always caused by rupture of a subpleural bleb. In older patients, it is sometimes associated with emphysema. Spontaneous pneumothorax is recurrent in approximately one-third of patients.

ASSESSMENT

History

- Sudden onset of chest or shoulder pain, with or without antecedent exercise

- Pain may increase with respiratory activity.
- Dyspnea, especially with exertion, present in 70% of patients
- Nonproductive cough, present infrequently

Physical Examination

- Patient may be dyspneic at rest.
- Respiratory rate may be increased.
- Breath sounds diminished over affected lung.
- Trachea may be shifted to opposite side.

Adjunct Studies

- Chest x-ray is diagnostic and characterized by a lack of lung marking in the apex and periphery of the lung. Mediastinal shift to the contralateral side may be identified (Fig. 15-6).
- Films should be taken on inspiration and expiration.

MANAGEMENT

Except for minimal pneumothorax (5% to 10% collapse) a tube thoracostomy is recommended. The chest tube is inserted into the 2nd intercostal space anteriorly in the midclavicular line. (Some prefer to insert the tube in the 5th or 6th interspace in the midaxillary line.) The tube is directed toward the apex of the lung and connected to an underwater seal (PleurEvac). Have the patient cough a few times and repeat the chest x-ray, which often demonstrates complete reinflation of the lung. Usually, the patient is admitted, but in some hospitals, a one-way flutter valve (Heimlich valve)

Figure 15-6 Pneumothorax. Total collapse of right lung is shown. Note the mediastinal structures shifted to the left. Patient was treated by intercostal tube drainage (closed thoracostomy), with full reexpansion.

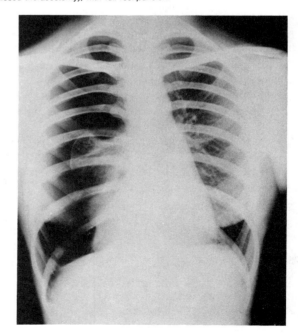

is attached to the intercostal tube and the patient is sent home.

The tube is left in place until the lung is completely reexpanded. It should be removed in 3 to 5 days. If expansion is slow to occur, the chest tube may be attached to a thoracic suction pump. In recurrent spontaneous pneumothorax, or in patients with a major lung leak, open thoracotomy may be needed to remove the blebs to promote reexpansion of the lung.

Note: Tension pneumothorax is a serious complication of spontaneous pneumothorax; it is life-threatening and requires emergency decompression of the pleural space. Needle decompression will suffice until an intercostal tube can be inserted. (See Chap. 21, Thoracic and Abdominal Trauma.)

PULMONARY THROMBOEMBOLISM

Pulmonary embolism is among the most common pulmonary problems requiring acute care. It is a serious disease accounting for 200,000 deaths annually. There are an estimated 630,000 symptomatic episodes in the United States each year.

PATHOPHYSIOLOGY

Pulmonary emboli most often result from thrombi in the peripheral venous system. Less frequently, emboli may consist of fat, bone marrow, amniotic fluid, or tumor masses.

Following the formation of a thrombus in a vein of the pelvis or lower extremities, a portion may fragment and pass upward in the vena cava to the right heart. It is then propelled through the right atrium and ventricle into the pulmonary circulation and lodges in a branch of the pulmonary artery.

The site of embolization depends on the size of the embolic fragment. Large emboli arising from a major vein in the thigh or pelvis may lodge in the main pulmonary artery or its first main branch in either lung. Small emboli pass into the smaller branches of the pulmonary artery in the periphery of the lung. A single embolus or showers of emboli can occur. Sudden occlusion of the main trunk of the pulmonary artery or one of its major branches may cause death in as short a time as a few minutes. Smaller emboli, either singly or in showers, may cause varying degrees of respiratory embarrassment.

Fat emboli commonly follow long-bone fractures. Amniotic fluid embolus occurs in complicated pregnancy or labor and can cause death. Embolization may be present with or without pulmonary infarction.

ASSESSMENT

A number of clinical studies have shown that there is no single symptom or sign that is specific for pulmonary embolism. Emergency personnel must perform an adequate history and physical assessment and maintain a high degree of suspicion in making the diagnosis.

Predisposing Factors

- Thrombophlebitis or phlebothrombosis of the pelvic or lower extremity veins
- Varicose veins
- Disseminated carcinoma
- General surgical procedures on the abdomen
- Operative procedures on pelvic organs
- Pregnancy
- Obesity
- Use of birth control pills
- Congestive heart failure
- Multiple fractures with damage to peripheral veins

History

Most instances of pulmonary embolus occur in the hospital, but others happen at home, either spontaneously or in postoperative patients. Question the patient carefully about the predisposing factors listed above.

Physical Examination

- The most common symptoms of pulmonary embolus, as described in a recent Urokinase Pulmonary Embolism Trial (UPET) study, are shown in Table 15-3. The more common signs are shown in Table 15-4.
- Dyspnea was designated as the chief symptom. Dyspnea, apprehension, sweats, and syncope are essentially nonspecific findings.
- Pleuritic pain is not found unless infarction of the lung has occurred.
- The physical findings may be deceptively insignificant and nonspecific.
- The following triad of symptoms has been described in conjunction with emboli:

  Dyspnea

  Hemoptysis

  Pleuritis

- Maintain a high degree of suspicion when evaluating a patient, because of the widely varied clinical picture. Bear in mind the predisposing factors, symptoms, and signs to determine which adjunct studies may be of use in making a correct diagnosis.

TABLE 15-3. SYMPTOMS OF PULMONARY EMBOLISM

Symptom	Percentage
Dyspnea	81
Pleuritic pain	72
Apprehension	59
Cough	54
Hemoptysis	34
Sweats	26
Syncope	14

(After the Urokinase Pulmonary Embolism Trial [UPET])

TABLE 15-4. SIGNS OF PULMONARY EMBOLISM

Sign	Percent
Tachypnea (16)	87
Rales	53
Increased P2	53
Tachycardia	44
Fever (> 37.8)	42
S_3, S_4 gallop	34
Diaphoresis	34
Phlebitis	33
Edema	23
Murmur	23
Cyanosis	18

(After the Urokinase Pulmonary Embolism Trial [UPET])

Adjunct Studies

- Routine blood and urine studies should be obtained but do not ordinarily contribute to the diagnosis.

- Arterial blood gases may reveal impaired oxygenation. It has been suggested that an arterial oxygen tension of less than 80 mm Hg supports the diagnosis of pulmonary emboli.[11] This too is nonspecific, but is important when considered in conjunction with other clinical findings.

- Chest x-ray findings of significance are

  Elevation of the diaphragm(s)

  Pleural effusion

  Pulmonary infiltrate or atelectasis

  These findings may be present singly or in combination

- Perfusion lung scan documents the interruption of pulmonary blood flow and is most useful in the diagnosis of pulmonary emboli. The most significant findings are multiple segmental or lobar defects throughout the lung fields (Fig. 15-7).

- Ventilation lung scan aids in distinguishing defects that may be seen on the perfusion scan in patients with COPD. Pulmonary emboli generally produce perfusion defects without related ventilation defects.

- ECG, although nonspecific, may reveal an acute right bundle branch block with sudden right-axis deviation. These findings are present in a high proportion of patients with underlying cardiopulmonary disease.

- Gallium scan is useful in distinguishing large pulmonary inflammatory infiltrates from infiltrates associated with pulmonary emboli, because gallium is taken up preferentially by leukocytes.

- Pulmonary angiography is a highly specialized study that is unfortunately not available in many hospital radiography departments. It is the most accurate study available for use in difficult diagnostic situations. The classic findings in emboli are:

  1. Sudden cut-off of the column of dye in a vessel
  2. Filling defects in the major vessels of the lungs

  Pulmonary angiography may be indicated if surgical intervention is anticipated in the presence of massive emboli.

MANAGEMENT

Prehospital Care

The patient should be rapidly assessed, given oxygen by nasal catheter or mask, and prepared for early transport to the hospital.

Hospital Care

1. Ensure a patent airway.
2. Obtain baseline blood studies, including arterial blood gases.
3. Give 100% oxygen by mask or nasal catheter.
4. Evaluate for underlying cardiac or pulmonary disease.
   - Obtain baseline blood coagulation studies, prothrombin time (PT), partial thromboplastin time (PTT), clotting time, platelet count.
5. If no contraindication exists, start anticoagulant therapy with intravenous heparin. A loading dose of 10 to 15

Figure 15-7 Top. Ventilation scan showing homogenous uptake of radionuclide in both lung fields, indicating normal ventilation. Bottom. Perfusion scan with multiple defects in both lung fields. Findings are consistent with multiple pulmonary emboli.

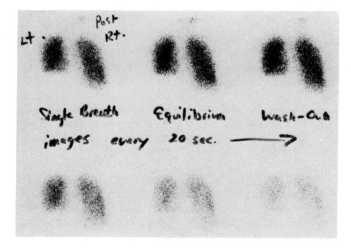

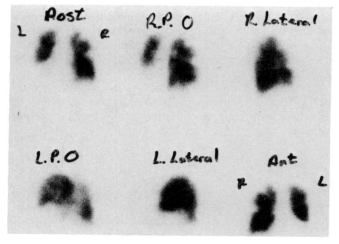

units/kg is given, followed by a continuous infusion using a continuous infusion pump. It is suggested that patients receive 25,000 to 30,000 units daily.

6. Obtain PTTs at 4- to 5-hour intervals during the first 24 hours of treatment and daily thereafter. Maintain PTT at 1½ to 2 times the control.

7. Chest x-ray and perfusion scans should be performed early in the course of treatment.

8. Oral anticoagulation medication with coumadin may be started on the first day or several days later. When therapeutic PTs are reached, at 2 to 2½ times the control, heparin may be discontinued.

9. Thrombolytic agents such as streptokinase and urokinase appear to be particularly useful when major embolization has occurred (>50% occlusion of the pulmonary vascular bed). These two drugs are not without serious complications, some fatal, and must be used with caution.

10. Emergency surgical treatment, pulmonary embolectomy, is indicated in a patient with a massive embolus. This requires cardiopulmonary bypass.

11. *Indications for pulmonary embolectomy:*
    - Persistent shock unresponsive to nonoperative therapy
    - Angiographic evidence of 50% or more occlusion of the pulmonary arterial circulation
    - Other surgical procedures, not used in an emergency setting, are insertion of a transvenous vena cava filter and vena cava interruption.

The mortality rate from untreated emboli is approximately 30%. In treated patients it is 8% to 9%. In acute *massive* pulmonary thromboembolism, the death rate is 60% to 80%.

CHRONIC OBSTRUCTIVE PULMONARY DISEASE

Chronic obstructive pulmonary disease (COPD) constitutes a spectrum of diseases of the lungs that result from long-standing, persistent inflammation of the air passages. Although there are a number of causative factors, cigarette smoking is perhaps the single most important. The following are common examples of COPD:
- Emphysema
- Chronic bronchitis
- Small airways disease
- Asthma
- Bronchiectasis

Emphysema, chronic bronchitis, and asthma are seen in the emergency setting. Emphysema and chronic bronchitis are characterized by chronic cough and obstruction of airflow. Distinguishing features of bronchitis and emphysema are listed in Table 15-5.

CHRONIC BRONCHITIS

Chronic bronchitis is characterized by:
- Chronic cough
- Expectoration for at least 3 months of the year for at least 2 years
- Higher incidence among persons under age 50

It is often found in conjunction with emphysema.

PATHOPHYSIOLOGY

Chronic bronchitis is a lingering disease of the airways associated with hypertrophy and hyperplasia of the mucus-producing glands in the submucosa of the large cartilaginous airways (those with cartilage in their walls).

Other changes include an increase in goblet-cells and inflammatory cells, edema, fibrosis, and mucosal plugs in the small airway. The smooth muscle in the walls of the air passages is also thickened. As the disease process continues, airflow obstruction occurs and eventually progresses to true emphysematous change. Changes develop in ventilation-perfusion with CO_2 retention and hypoxemia. With further progression, pulmonary hypertension and cor pulmonale are commonly seen. Factors that contribute to these changes include:
- *Smoking*—perhaps the single factor most commonly associated with chronic airway obstruction
- *Air pollution*—the disease is more common in highly industrialized areas.
- *Occupation*—bronchitis is more common in workers exposed to noxious fumes or organic dusts.

TABLE 15-5. DISTINGUISHING FEATURES OF BRONCHITIS AND EMPHYSEMA

	Emphysema	Bronchitis
Age at onset of Dx	±60	±50
Dyspnea	Severe	Mild
Cough	After dyspnea starts	Before dyspnea
Sputum	Scanty, mucoid	Copious, purulent
Bronchial infections	Less frequent	More frequent
Respiratory insufficiency episodes	Often terminal	Repeated
Chest x-ray	Hyperinflation, small heart	↑ Bronchovascular markings, large heart
Hematocrit	35–45	50–55
Chronic $PaCO_2$ mm Hg	35–40	45–60
Chronic PaO_2 mm Hg	65–75	45–60

(After Isselbacher KJ et al: Principles of Internal Medicine, 9th ed, p 1238. New York, McGraw-Hill, 1980)

- *Heredity*—The relative importance of this factor is yet unknown. The incidence of respiratory illness is higher in children of smoking parents. What part heredity plays as opposed to the exposure of the child to air pollutants in the household requires further study.

ASSESSMENT

History

The striking findings are:
- Cough for years
- Sputum production—copious amounts of mucopurulent material
- Dyspnea that is mild and may be more severe after coughing
- Frequently recurring bronchial infections that aggravate the underlying symptoms
- Prior episodes of respiratory failure

Physical Examination

- The patient is frequently overweight and cyanotic.
- Respiratory rate is normal or only slightly increased.
- Dyspnea at rest is uncommon.
- Chest is resonant to percussion.
- Auscultation reveals coarse rhonchi and wheezes, which may change with coughing.
- Abnormal cardiac sounds are common secondary to the pulmonary abnormality.

Adjunct Studies

- CBC may reveal secondary polycythemia. Leukocytosis is found with active respiratory infection.
- Arterial blood gases reveal an increase in CO_2 tension (45–60 mm Hg) with low O_2 tension (45–60 mm Hg).
- Chest x-ray demonstrates increased bronchovascular markings. Often, cardiomegaly is present with prominence of the pulmonary artery.

MANAGEMENT

- Bronchodilator drugs such as aminophylline are given intravenously or orally.
- Beta$_2$ receptor agonists such as isoproterenol or metaproterenol (Alupent, Metaprel) are given by aerosol inhalation.
- O_2 by nasal cannula or venti mask for hypoxemia in low concentration so as not to remove the respiratory CO_2 drive
- Postural drainage or pulmonary physical therapy
- Expectorants such as potassium iodide may assist in liquefying secretions.
- Smoking should be discontinued.
- Antibiotics are considered if evidence of infection is present.

- Late treatment of infection of the diseased tracheobronchial tree as seen in patients with chronic bronchitis may lead to acute respiratory failure.
- Arterial blood gases should be carefully monitored.
- Agitation, insomnia, and increasing dyspnea may herald impending respiratory failure.
- Sedatives and narcotics are withheld or used cautiously in such patients, lest they precipitate frank respiratory failure.

EMPHYSEMA

Emphysema is the most common chronic lung disease, progressing slowly over a period of 10 to 20 years. It may be defined as an irreversible disease of the lung with destruction of the parenchyma in the most distal portions of the airway. Emphysema is characterized by:
- A long history of smoking
- Exertional dyspnea
- Minimal cough
- Higher incidence in persons over age 60

It often follows long-standing lung disease such as chronic bronchitis and asthma.

PATHOPHYSIOLOGY

Chronic disease of the lungs marked by airway obstruction leads to increased pressure in the distal (peripheral) portions of the airway, particularly the alveoli. The walls of the individual alveoli rupture, causing a coalescence of these alveolar sacs. The pulmonary capillaries in the alveolar walls may tear or become fibrotic and thrombosed, reducing blood perfusion through the alveolar walls. The destroyed alveoli lose their elasticity, which reduces their effectiveness as functional air spaces, thereby reducing ventilation. With the airways' obstruction and alveolar disruption, the lungs lose their elasticity, and become overinflated, increasing the external anteroposterior diameter of the chest (barrel chest). Pulmonary ventilation-perfusion is seriously impaired, resulting in varying degrees of respiratory insufficiency.

The factors contributing to emphysema are essentially those contributing to chronic bronchitis.

ASSESSMENT

History

- Dyspnea, usually exertional initially
- A long history of cigarette smoking is usually obtained.
- Cough, not common, may occur late in the disease or with associated infection.
- Ease of fatiguability
- Loss of weight and appetite
- An acute episode may have been precipitated by an acute respiratory infection or by exposure to noxious fumes or air pollutants.

Physical Examination

- With acute respiratory embarrassment, the patient may be apprehensive and extremely dyspneic.
- Cyanosis may be present.
- Tachycardia is often noted.
- The patient uses accessory muscles of respiration and expires between pursed lips.
- Auscultation reveals prolonged expiration, wheezes, and rales. These findings are due to airway obstruction.
- Increase in anteroposterior diameter of the chest

Adjunct Studies

- CBC may be within normal limits
- Arterial blood gas evaluation reveals a low O_2 tension with a low-to-normal CO_2 tension.
- Chest x-ray reveals hyperinflation of the lungs. Bullae may or may not be seen in the apices. The heart may be normal sized or small. The diaphragms are low. The retrosternal air space is increased.

MANAGEMENT

- Bronchodilators such as aminophylline and theophylline are given orally or intravenously. Maintain theophylline levels at 10–20 mg/L.
- Isoproterenol or metaproterenol are given by aerosol.
- Antibiotics are indicated if an active pulmonary infection is present.
- Give O_2 by nasal catheter or ventilation mask at a rate of 2–3 L/min.
- IPPB with humidification is beneficial.
- All forms of smoking must be discontinued.
- Monitor ventilation and, therefore, therapy by periodic arterial blood gases.
- Ventilatory assistance with an endotracheal tube or tracheostomy may be needed in patients with advanced respiratory impairment.

ASTHMA

Asthma is defined as a reversible obstruction of the airways due to increased responsiveness of the tracheobronchial tree due to noxious stimuli.

It is characterized by:
- Spasm of the tracheobronchial musculature with narrowing of the airway
- Increased secretions
- Edema of the mucosa and submucosa of the bronchial passages

Normally, the air passages widen during inspiration and narrow somewhat in expiration. The three features mentioned above combine to cause narrowing of the airways, which functionally may close the lumen during *expiration*.

Thus, expiration is interfered with and pulmonary ventilation considerably altered (Fig. 15-8).

ETIOLOGY

The causes are related to many factors, including:
- Allergy—the cause of asthma can be established when due to an allergy. This etiology has received much attention because it provides a good basis for treatment.
- Infection—respiratory infection causes increased reactivity to bronchoconstrictors such as histamine, thus precipitating an asthmatic episode.
- Irritants—these include noxious gases, fumes, dusts, or powders in the home or work environment.
- Heredity—there is an inherited tendency toward asthma, but the exact role or importance of the genetic causes is difficult to assess.
- Psychosomatic effects—although disputed, these effects may contribute significantly to the etiology of asthma, especially in children.

PATHOPHYSIOLOGY

The autonomic nervous system controls the bronchi. Bronchoconstriction is produced by vagal or parasympathetic stimulation. The sympathetic innervation to the lung is not very rich; most of the sympathetic influence is humoral. Most of the bronchial sympathomimetic receptors are β receptors. Thus, bronchodilation is caused by both epinephrine and norepinephrine. Bronchoconstriction is due to an α-adrenergic effect.

In an acute asthmatic episode, patients respond to an antigen stimulus by the formation of immune globulin (IgE) antibodies, which attach to mast cells in the bronchial wall. As the antibody-antigen reaction continues, the mast cells secrete a number of biochemical substances including histamine, eosinophil chemotactic factor of antiphylaxis (ECF-A) and slow-reacting substance of anaphylaxis (SRS-A), which are partly responsible for the response. Other agents include prostaglandins and adrenergic and cholinergic agents. This

Figure 15-8 *Bronchial asthma. Spasm of the bronchial tree, combined with an increase in secretions (A), causes a decrease in airflow and, thus, inadequate oxygenation of pulmonary, arterial blood (C).*

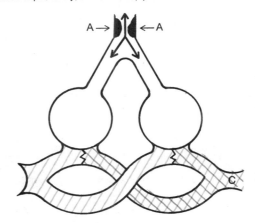

combination of factors leads to the pathologic changes that characterize the disease.

Of particular significance is the discovery of three types of adrenergic receptors, α, β_1, and β_2, which serve as a basis for pharmacotherapy. *Alpha receptor* stimulation causes contraction of the smooth muscles in the vessels and airways. *Beta$_2$ receptor* stimulation causes bronchodilatation without cardiac side-effects.

ASSESSMENT

History

The patient usually gives a history of previous asthma attacks. Often, the acute episode may follow a period of exercise or exposure to fumes, a noxious substance, or a known allergen. In some patients, the episode follows emotional stress.

The onset of the attack may be characterized by:
- Vague sensations in the neck or pharynx
- Tightness in the chest with breathlessness
- Loose but nonproductive cough; difficulty in raising sputum
- Labored respiration, particularly on expiration, as the episode continues
- Apprehension and tachypnea may follow as the patient becomes hypoxic.
- Audible wheezing

Physical Examination

1. In mild attacks, vital signs are stable. Auscultation of the chest reveals inspiratory and expiratory wheezes.
2. In a full-blown attack, the patient:
   - Appears anxious and agitated
   - Is unable to lie flat and is usually sitting, leaning forward, gasping for breath
   - Has an increased anteroposterior diameter of the chest
   - Has wheezes on inspiration and expiration
   - Has a prolonged expiratory phase of respiration
   - Has rhonchi and rales bilaterally
   - Has pulsus paradoxus (disappearance of a peripheral pulse on inspiration) in about 50% of cases
   - Has central cyanosis in severe attacks

Be alert to the high-risk patient, *i.e.,* one whose ability to ventilate is impaired. Such patient may be in a life-threatening condition. See Chart 15-5 for a profile of the high-risk patient.

Adjunct Studies

- CBC—look for leukocytosis or eosinophilia. An increase in eosinophiles may indicate an allergic etiology.
- Total eosinophil count—if elevated, this may indicate an allergic etiology. Repeat counts may be done to check the response to therapy.
- SMA-18—pay particular attention to the potassium (K^+) and chloride (Cl^-), which may be sharply reduced in patients with long-standing respiratory acidosis.
- Arterial blood gases—hypoxemia, hypercarbia, and respiratory acidosis are often encountered. Repeat arterial blood gases at intervals to assess ventilation. In mild cases, hypocarbia may be present.

Chart 15-5

HIGH-RISK PATIENT: ASTHMATIC ATTACK

The following findings indicate a high-risk patient:
- Grossly overinflated chest
- Central cyanosis
- Tachycardia
- Pulsus paradoxus
- Use of accessory muscles of respiration
- Silent chest on auscultation

- Sputum studies—wet-mount study of the sputum for eosinophils and polymorphonuclear leukocytes (polys). Presence of a large number of polys may indicate secondary infection.
- Chest x-ray may show hyperinflation of the lungs. Infiltrates may be seen in secondary infection.
- Laboratory studies to measure IgE antibodies.

MANAGEMENT

Prehospital Care

- Give O_2 by nasal catheter at a rate of 2–3 L/min or 24% to 35% by ventilation mask.
- Do not give a high concentration of O_2, which could lead to hypoventilation.
- Place patient in Fowler's position.
- Bring medications from home.
- Prepare for early transport.

Hospital Care

Treatment is based on the severity and chronicity of the illness.

1. *Simple Measures: Mild Attack*
   - Ask the patient about prior treatment. Patients who have responded to subcutaneous epinephrine previously most likely will do so again. On occasion, mild asthmatics are unpredictable.
   - Give epinephrine 1/1000 in a dose of 0.01 ml/kg to a maximum of 0.3 ml subcutaneously or give terbutaline sulfate (Brethine, Bricanyl), 0.25 mg subcutaneously. A response should be noted in 10 to 20 minutes. The initial dose of terbutaline may be repeated in 30 to 60 minutes and then every 4 to 6 hours.
   - As an alternative, isoetharine HCl (Bronkosol) or metaproterenol sulfate (Alupent, Metaprel) may be given by inhalation. Terbutaline and two aerosol compounds are β_2 agonists and effective bronchodilators without cardiac side-effects.

2. *Progressive measures: moderately severe attack, no response to simple measures, status asthmaticus*
   - Do not continue "simple measures" more than 3 to 4 hours if no response is noted.

- Give aminophylline intravenously.

  If the patient has been on this medication, give a maintenance infusion of aminophylline, 0.6 to 0.9 mg/kg/hr.

  If the patient is not taking aminophylline, give a loading dose of 5 mg/kg intravenously over a 20-minute period, then a constant infusion at a rate of 0.6 to 0.9 mg/kg/hr. The lower dose is given to patients with congestive heart failure or liver disease in whom the half-life of aminophylline is prolongted.

Note: The infusion is preferably given with an infusion pump, but *not in a central vein line.*

- A patient who responds well may be sent home with oral or aerosol bronchodilators.

- A patient who does not respond in 3 to 4 hours, or whose condition deteriorates, should be admitted.

- Obtain periodic arterial blood gases to assess ventilation.

- Obtain blood levels of aminophylline to maintain a therapeutic level between 10 to 20 mg/L. Levels above this are considered toxic.

- Observe for toxicity, manifested by:

  - Nervousness

  - Tremors

  - Gastrointestinal symptoms

- Obtain serum electrolytes to check for low K^+ and Cl^-, which are reduced in chronic respiratory acidosis

- Give fluid replacement intravenously, 5% glucose/dextrose in water (G/D_5W), to assist in clearing secretions by hydration. Use caution in cardiac patients.

- Give broad-spectrum antibiotics, especially if there is an underlying infection or a large number of polys on sputum smear.

- Steroids must be considered if the patient is to be admitted. Patients who are currently receiving steroids should be given methylprednisolone (Solu-Medrol) immediately, 0.1 to 0.2 gm, and repeat doses every 4 to 6 hours.

- Continue O_2 by nasal cannula or ventilation mask.

- Endotracheal intubation and assisted ventilation may be needed if the PCO_2 rises above normal, indicating respiratory failure.

- Avoid sedatives, which may suppress the respiratory drive.

- A number of promising drugs are now under study in the United States that may be helpful to the asthmatic patient. These include salbutamol, Sch 1000, carbuterol HCl, and fenoterol, which are primarily β_2 receptor stimulants.

The patient with an acute asthmatic episode requires complete assessment, early, well-chosen pharmacologic management, and continued monitoring to assess response, which is marked primarily by improved ventilation.

ACUTE RESPIRATORY ACIDOSIS (RESPIRATORY FAILURE)

Acute respiratory acidosis occurs whenever there is sudden failure of ventilation. Respiratory failure exists when the lungs do not provide sufficient gas exchange to meet the body's need for O_2 consumption, CO_2 elimination, or both. Acute respiratory failure may result from a number of causes.

PATHOPHYSIOLOGY

When alveolar ventilation decreases, the arterial O_2 tension falls, and the CO_2 rises. The rise in arterial CO_2 tension produces increased amounts of carbonic acid in the blood and the pH falls, resulting in respiratory acidosis.

If uncorrected, the lowered arterial O_2 tension combines with low cardiac output to produce diminished tissue perfusion and tissue hypoxia. This causes a shift to anaerobic tissue metabolism with formation of increased amounts of lactic acid, which aggravates the acidosis caused by CO_2 retention. In the process, a wide range of symptoms develop, involving the central nervous and cardiovascular systems. The single most significant finding is hypercapnia with the CO_2 tension above 45 mm Hg.

ASSESSMENT

History

Patients seen in the emergency setting are often frequent visitors for treatment of chronic pulmonary disease with superimposed infection. They are usually well-known to emergency personnel. The history is typically that of a patient with COPD.

Physical Examination

1. Findings of the underlying lung disease
2. Signs of hypercapnia (increased CO_2 tension) include:

   - Disturbances of consciousness, ranging to coma
   - Headache
   - Restlessness
   - Apnea with slow, gasping respiration
   - Tachycardia, bounding pulse, hypertension
   - In severe respiratory failure, the following occurs:

     Hypotension
     Generalized vasodilatation
     Diaphoresis
     Papilledema
     Flapping tremor of the hand

Adjunct Studies

- Arterial blood gas studies confirm the diagnosis.

  O_2 tension is low, usually less than 80 mm Hg (hypoxemia).

  CO_2 tension is elevated above 45 mm Hg (hypercarbia), which is diagnostic.

  pH is low.

- Sputum for smear, culture, and sensitivity studies are obtained to identify any unusual predominant organism

- CBC

- Urinalysis

- Chest x-ray to identify specific lung disease

- ECG

- A careful search should be made to identify any specific cause(s) of acute respiratory failure.

MANAGEMENT

Principles of Care

- Continuous treatment of hypoxemia
- Correction of hypercapnia
- Correction of acidosis
- Identification and correction of the specific cause

Patient Breathing Spontaneously

1. Give O_2 by ventilation mask (24%) or nasal cannula (1 L/min). Proper humidification is essential. Adjust oxygen therapy by following arterial blood gases at 15- to 20-minute intervals. An effort is made to achieve an O_2 tension of 85 to 90 mm Hg.
2. Give sodium bicarbonate, especially when the *p*H is 7.2 or lower. The first dose is 50 mEq $NaHCO_3$ given by intravenous push; 50 mEq should be given for each base deficit multiple of 3.
3. Perform tracheal suction for brief intervals to clear the airway of mucus plugs.
4. Bronchodilators by parenteral or aerosol routes
5. IPPB to improve alveolar ventilation
6. Monitor arterial blood gases closely to assess patient response

Patient Not Breathing Spontaneously

1. Initiate ventilatory assistance mouth-to-mouth or by endotracheal tube.
2. Once an endotracheal tube is in place, use a volume-cycled ventilator.
3. Humidify air properly.
4. Use other means as mentioned under *Patient Breathing Spontaneously,* above.
5. Try to identify the specific cause of the problem and initiate appropriate therapy.

PNEUMONIA

Pneumonia is an acute inflammatory condition of the lung parenchyma that may be caused by a variety of viral and bacterial organisms, fungi, and parasites.

The inflammation is usually caused by organisms that enter the air passages, causing an outpouring of inflammatory cells into the involved segment of lung tissue. It may occur in previously healthy persons, but more often it is associated with conditions that impair the body's defense mechanisms.

ASSESSMENT

History

The predominant symptoms are combinations of:
- Cough
- Chest pain, usually pleuritic
- Dyspnea
- Fever, with or without chills
- Sputum, which may be mucoid, purulent, or bloody
- Abrupt or gradual onset

Physical Examination

- Tachypnea
- Fever
- Tachycardia
- Cyanosis may be present.
- Diminished respiratory excursion due to pleuritic pain
- Auscultation may reveal end-respiratory crackles or rales. Tubular or bronchial breathing may be heard over areas of consolidation

Adjunct Studies

- CBC usually shows leukocytosis.
- Chest x-ray reveals varying types of infiltrates, interstitial, segmental, or lobar.
- Sputum smear, culture, and sensitivity usually reveal specific organisms. Examine the smear for leukocytes.
- Blood cultures, especially if the patient is febrile, often reveal bacteremia.
- Arterial blood gases may reveal hypoxemia and often hypocarbia.

Management

1. Broad-spectrum antibiotics are begun orally or parenterally. The sputum smear may assist in the selection of the antibiotic.
2. Provide adequate hydration.
3. Humidified O_2 by mask or nasal cannula.
4. Analgesics to diminish chest pain and improve respiratory activity. Codeine serves this purpose well.
5. Mechanical ventilation is not required unless there is some underlying cardiopulmonary disease.

REFERENCES

1. Alexander JK: Differential guide to chest pain. Hosp Med 11:38, 1975
2. Artz CP, Reiss E: The Treatment of Burns, pp 127–129. Philadelphia, WB Saunders, 1957
3. Ashbaugh DG, Petty TL et al: Continuous positive pressure breathing (CPPB) in adult respiratory distress syndrome. J Thorac Cardiovasc Surg 57:31, 1969
4. Ashbaugh DG, Petty TL: Sepsis complicating the acute respiratory distress syndrome. Surg Gynecol Obstet 135:865, 1972
5. Associated clinical and laboratory findings (chap XIII): Uro-

kinase Pulmonary Embolism Trial. Circulation 47(Suppl. II):81, 1973

6. Blaisdell W: Pathophysiology of the respiratory distress syndrome Arch Surg 108:44, 1974

7. Bone RC, Hiller C: Modern treatment of bronchial asthma. JACEP 7:269, 1978

8. Dailey RH: Asthmatic, acute—and adult. Emerg Med 5:127, 1973

9. Dalen JE, Alpert JS: Natural history of pulmonary embolism. Prog Cardiovasc Dis XVII(17):259, 1975

10. Fuhs M et al: Nursing in a respiratory intensive care unit. Chest 62:145, 1972

11. Greenberg MI, Walther J: Axioms on smoke inhalation. Hosp Med 14:100, 1978

12. Heimlich HJ: Pop goes the café coronary. Emerg Med 6:154, 1974

13. Israel HL, Goldstein F: The varied manifestations of pulmonary embolism. Ann Intern Med 47:202, 1957

14. Kettel LJ: Acute respiratory acidosis. Hosp Med 12:31, 1976

15. Lichstein E: Evaluation of chest pain. Hosp Med 11:8, 1975

16. Luisada AA: The differential diagnosis of dyspnea. Hosp Med 11:38, 1975

17. McGlynn IJ et al: Pulmonary embolism. JACEP 8:532, 1979

18. Motley HL: Pulmonary Emphysema. Hosp Med 9:8, 1973

19. Reichel J: Pulmonary emphysema. Hosp Med 16:8, 1980

20. Robin ED, Cross CE, Zelis R: Pulmonary edema. N Engl J Med 288:239, 1973

21. Rothfield A, Bromberg PA: Pneumothorax: Diagnosis and management. Hosp Med 14:66, 1978

22. Sloggin CH: Asthma: Changing concepts and therapies. Mod Med 48:26, 1980

23. Sokol WN, Beall GN: Asthma. Hosp Med 13:10, 1977

24. Sugarman HJ et al: Positive end-expiratory pressure (PEEP): Indications and physiologic considerations. Chest 62:86S, 1972

25. Szucs MM Jr et al: Diagnostic sensitivity of laboratory findings in acute pulmonary embolism. Ann Intern Med 74:161, 1971

26. Trunkey DD: Inhalation injury. Surg Clin North Am 58:1133, 1978

27. Webb-Johnson DC, Andrew JL: Bronchodilator therapy. N Engl J Med 297:758, 1977

16
CARDIAC EMERGENCIES

JILL D. HOLMES

Cardiovascular diseases affect 40 million people in the United States. Though there has been a decline in mortality from coronary heart disease since 1968, cardiovascular disease still accounts for 52% of all deaths in this country. Subjective effects of cardiovascular disease on persons who have significantly altered life-styles owing to their disease cannot be measured directly, but these effects are important in terms of productivity and individual well-being. Major cardiovascular diseases include hypertension, myocardial infarction, cardiovascular accident, congestive heart failure, rheumatic heart disease, and congenital defects. Because of the number of persons affected and the dollars and time given to their treatment and rehabilitation, cardiovascular emergencies are a concern of all emergency care professionals. The methods of assessment and treatment of the patient with a cardiovascular emergency can directly affect the outcome of his illness and ultimate recovery.

ANATOMY AND PHYSIOLOGY OF THE CARDIAC SYSTEM

As a working pump, the heart's capacity for long and usually trouble-free service to its owner surpasses that of any man-made pump. Essential to life, the heart propels blood around the body to bring nutrients, oxygen, and hormones to each cell. Within 5 seconds of cardiac arrest, there is loss of con-sciousness, and irreversible brain damage can commence within 4 to 6 minutes.

The heart beats 100,000 times a day. With each beat the heart pumps 2 oz (60 ml) of blood, or about 5 quarts per minute, 75 gallons an hour, and 70 barrels a day through 60,000 miles of blood vessels. All of this is done on a minimal amount of rest—the heart rests just three-tenths of a second per beat.

THE CORONARY CIRCULATION

Blood is supplied to the myocardium by the right and left coronary arteries, which arise from the base of the ascending aorta close to the leaflets of the aortic valve. (Fig. 16-1) The heart muscle extracts up to 75% to 80% of the oxygen from its coronary blood supply.

The left coronary artery is short and divides into two branches almost immediately after its origin. One branch, the left anterior descending (LAD) coronary artery, runs down a groove lying between the right and left ventricles to the apex of the heart; it supplies blood to the left ventricular wall and to the anterior portion of the ventricular septum. The second branch of the main left coronary artery, the circumflex, circles the heart to the left, lying in a groove located between the left atrium and the left ventricle, and descends down the posterior wall of the left ventricle. The circumflex supplies blood to the lateral portion of the left atrium and ventricle.

Figure 16-1 *The coronary circulation, showing the coronary arteries that arise from the aorta and some of the coronary veins. A. Anterior view. B. Posterior view. (Porth C: Pathophysiology: Concepts of Altered Health States. Philadelphia, JB Lippincott, 1982)*

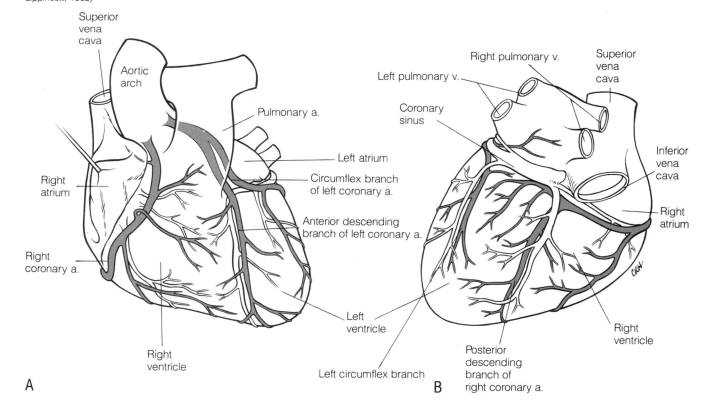

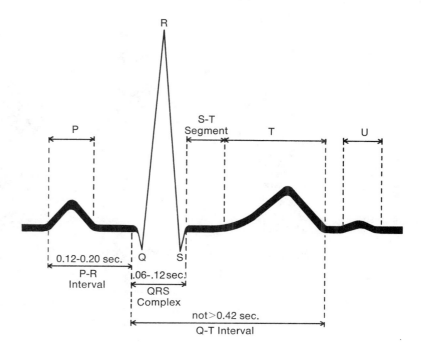

Figure 16-2 *Anatomy of a heart beat. P wave: represents atrial systole as a result of electrical excitation (depolarization) of the atrium arising from the sinoatrial (S-A) node. P—R interval (including the P-R segment): represents time span from S-A impulse origin, spread through atria, atrial systole, conduction of the impulse across the atrioventricular (A-V) junction, bundle of His, and bundle branches to the ventricular musculature. QRS complex: represents ventricular systole as a result of impulse conduction through ventricular muscle (depolarization). T wave: represents ventricular repolarization. S–T segment: represents time span from the end of the QRS complex to the beginning of the T wave. Q–T interval: represents complete depolarization and repolarization from the beginning of the QRS to the end of the T wave. U wave: cause not clear; some experts believe it is the result of residual repolarization of the ventricle while it is relaxing. (The T occurs during ventricular contraction.) It is any wave seen after the T wave but before the next P wave.*

The right coronary artery and its branches supply the right atrium and right ventricle, a small portion of the left ventricle (the inferoposterior wall), the sinoatrial (SA) node, the atrioventricular (AV) node, the bundle of His and the posterior portion of the ventricular septum.

From the epicardium, arteries branching from the main vessels penetrate the muscular walls of the heart, dividing into a fine network of capillaries. Once oxygen is extracted by the myocardium, a network of veins returns the deoxygenated blood through the coronary sinus to the right atrium, where it mixes with the deoxygenated blood from the peripheral (systemic) circulation.

Because it depends on just three arteries lying along the surface, the heart's blood supply is vulnerable. Disruption of blood flow in a major coronary artery without developed collateral circulation can be catastrophic. Portions of the heart supplied by this artery become ischemic, and if circulation remains diminished or blocked, these affected portions begin to die. Occlusion of the coronary arteries is most commonly due to coronary artery disease (CAD) and currently affects 4.2 million people in the United States.

Because the coronary artery and its branches lie on the surface of the myocardium, subjected to the forces and movements of contraction, most of the blood flow to the myocardium occurs during diastole, when the chambers of the heart are filling. (During systole, blood flow to the myocardium is minimal.) This arrangement works well enough in the normal heart even when, because of excitement or exercise, the heart rises to 180 beats per minute (bpm), reducing the resting phase of the heart. But in the damaged or aged heart, accelerated heart rates may significantly reduce the needed blood flow to the heart muscle, producing ischemia and pain. Thus, sustained tachycardia in patients with damaged hearts should be watched carefully and treated.

ELECTRICAL CONDUCTION OF THE HEART

The electrical impulse originates in the SA node (the pacemaker) located in the right atrium. The impulse leaves the node and speeds through the atrial myocardium through specialized pathways. Once the electrical impulse has depolarized (stimulated) both atria, mechanical activity follows and the right and left atrial musculature contracts, ejecting a small volume of blood into the resting and filling ventricles. The atrial depolarization produces a *P wave* on the ECG. (Fig. 16-2)

As the electrical impulse enters the AV node above the interventricular septum the speed of conduction slows, allowing the atria time to contract and to eject their blood volume. After the temporary slowing of conduction through the AV node, the electrical impulse then travels more rapidly down the bundle of His and splits into two main bundle branches, the right and left bundles. Like a tree, the two main branches separate into other branches, which end in a fine network of fibers called the Purkinje fibers. (Fig. 16-3) Here, the impulse rapidly conducts the electrical charge throughout the right and left ventricular endocardium. Mechanical contraction of the ventricular muscle fibers occurs. Ventricular depolarization is represented on the ECG by the *QRS complex*. Ventricular repolarization (recovery) becomes the *T wave*.

PRELOAD, AFTERLOAD, AND STARLING'S LAW

In general, the cardiac cycle runs smoothly. Minute-to-minute adjustments by the heart to the volume load it receives from the body and to the demand by body cells for appropriate cardiac output are made quickly and simply. As changes in volume occur, the heart can alter its force of contraction

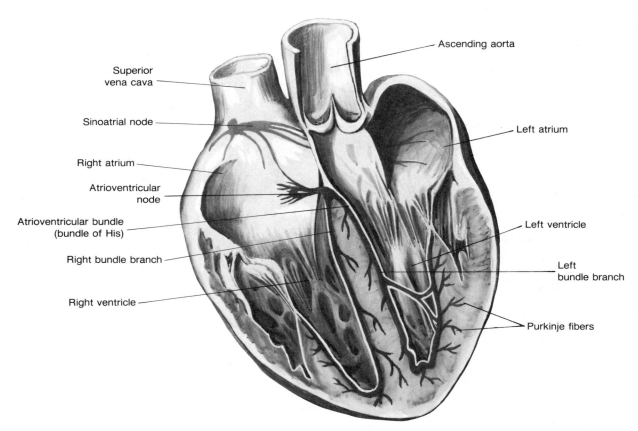

Figure 16-3 Conduction system of the heart. (Chaffee EE, Lytle IM: Basic Physiology and Anatomy, 4th ed. Philadelphia, JB Lippincott, 1980)

accordingly. For example, as more volume is returned to the ventricles, the ventricular fibers stretch to accommodate the greater volume. Because of the stretch, the fibers contract more vigorously and eject the volume more forcefully, emptying the heart's chambers. In this way, the heart prevents venous congestion and is able to maintain good arterial flow and cardiac output. This relationship of increased stretch to greater force of contraction is called Starling's law of the heart.

Because the heart obeys this law until physiologic limits are reached, the heart's cardiac output and response to stretch can be manipulated. Drugs such as isoproterenol and low-dose dopamine can increase the volume returning to the heart. This end-diastolic ventricular volume increases pressure and stretch inside the ventricles (preload), and can improve cardiac output.

Additional factors are the systemic blood pressure and vascular resistance against which the heart has to pump. Peripheral vascular resistance is called afterload and it too can be manipulated by drugs or mechanical devices to assist the heart.

Treatment of a patient with cardiac disease often concentrates on manipulating the preload, the afterload, and the individual Starling response of the heart. Monitoring techniques, using equipment such as arterial lines, central venous pressure (CVP) lines, Swan-Ganz catheters, transducers, and monitors, enable one to assess preload, afterload, and cardiac output values continually.

ASSESSMENT

INITIAL ASSESSMENT

Evaluation of the patient with a cardiovascular condition begins with assessment of his airway, breathing, and circulation—the ABCs. Once it is determined that these are adequately maintained, proceed with a general body survey, collect the data base, and identify and list patient problems.

HISTORY

Chief Complaint

The patient's chief complaint is of major importance. The patient or his family has sought medical aid because of the presence of some sign or symptom. Ask what signs, symptoms, or concerns brought the patient into the emergency medical service (EMS) system. The patient's chief complaint, when written in his record, should always be stated in his own words. Common chief complaints associated with cardiovascular disease include chest pressure, chest pain, sudden onset of weakness or dizziness, sudden onset of intense diaphoresis, acute onset of shortness of breath, noticeable heart palpitations, or a syncopal episode.

Chest Pain. The mnemonic PQRST provides a structure for assessing pain. This assessment tool is presented in Chart 16-1.

Associated Signs and Symptoms. Ask the patient about problems or symptoms accompanying the chief complaint, such as the presence of weakness, syncope, nausea, vomiting, dyspnea, orthopnea, dependent edema, and fatigue. Keep questions simple and direct, stating them so that the patient can respond with a yes or no or with short, descriptive answers.

Past Medical History. Consider preexisting factors known to increase a person's risk for developing cardiovascular disease—hypertension, diabetes, smoking, obesity, lipidemia, sedentary or stressful life-style, and heredity.

Ask about the patient's current medications in order to acquire information about the presence of acute or chronic disease. Also, determine whether the patient has been taking his medications as directed. Patient compliance with certain groups of medicines, such as antihypertensives, is less tenacious than for others. Because of untoward side-effects, the patient may avoid taking the medications for his "asymptomatic" hypertension. Finally, ask about allergies to any drugs taken in the past.

PHYSICAL EXAMINATION

Draw a general impression of the patient's state of health—healthy, acutely ill, chronically ill—and his level of nutrition—undernourished, well-nourished, obese, cachectic.

Look for signs of distress in facial expressions, body position and movements, and skin color and moisture.

1. Palpate the radial pulse. This establishes physical contact with the patient and allows you to assess skin temperature and moisture and pulse rate, quality, and regularity.
2. Determine the level of consciousness.
3. Note the patient's skin color.
   - Cyanosis seen at the lips, mouth, and fingertips indicates a central cyanosis that often accompanies heart or lung disease.
4. Assess pupils for size and response to light.
5. Observe for venous congestion in the jugular veins of the neck.
   - Normally, with the patient lying at an angle of 30 degrees or less, venous pulsations are barely visible.
   - If the neck veins are engorged and easily visible, suspect right-sided heart failure, valvular disease or cardiac tamponade.
6. Examine the patient's chest. Observe for rate and rhythm of respiration and for bilateral movement of the rib cage.
7. Inspect and palpate the chest for the presence of pulsations and thrills in the area overlying the heart.
8. Auscultate the chest in a planned sequence, working from the upper lung area to the lower.
   - Compare breath sounds between right and left lung segments and note the presence of rhonchi, rales, and wheezes.

Chart 16-1

ASSESSMENT OF CHEST PAIN: PQRST METHOD

P = provokes: What brought the pain on? Ask about the patient's activity at time of onset:
"What were you doing right before the pain began?"
"Have you noticed some chest discomfort and pressure in the past with increased activity?"
"Is there anything that you did that made the pain better? worse? go away?"

Q = quality: What is the pain like? Example: *"What does the pain feel like?"* If describing pain is difficult for the patient, provide descriptive adjectives such as *heaviness, tightness, pressure, squeezing, dull, sharp, constant, jabbing, burning.*

R = region: Where exactly is the pain? Cardiac pain can and does radiate away from the midsternum, down the left arm, down both arms, to the back, up the neck, in the jaw or in the throat. The patient may also experience tightness, pain, or pressure in the arms, neck, jaw, or throat without any midsternal or chest pain. Example:
"Please point or indicate where your chest pain is located."
"Does your pain go to any other region?"

S = severity: How severe is the pain? Pain is a subjective experience, but the professional needs to know how the patient feels he is tolerating pain and how the patient looks in relation to his pain. Example:
"How comfortable are you with this chest pain?"
"How bad does the pain feel right now?"
"When the pain first occurred, how severe was it?"

T = time: What is the duration of the pain? Example:
"How long ago did this chest pain begin?"
(with disclosure of other episodes of chest pain):
"How long ago did those other episodes last?"
"How often have these chest pain episodes occurred?"
"In the past, what was done for those chest pains?"

9. Palpate the point of maximum impulse (PMI), located near the 5th intercostal space just medial to the mid-clavicular line, to determine the location of the apex.
   - A lateral shift may indicate an enlarged left ventricle.
   - In barrel-chested, obese, or very muscular patients, the PMI is difficult to find.
10. Assess the peripheral pulses bilaterally.
    - Evaluate for strength, rhythm and rate (Table 16-1).
    - An irregular pulse may not transmit all beats to the peripheral vessels being palpated. Therefore, with irregular pulses, an apical rate is taken and compared to determine the pulse deficit.
11. Assess the blood pressure.
    - Take a *palpated* pressure in patients suspected of being hypertensive before taking the auscultated reading. Thus, the true systolic pressure will be obtained in the presence of an auscultatory gap, a common phenomenon in hypertensive patients with wide pulse pressures.
12. Determine whether edema is present. Press firmly in edematous areas to evaluate the presence and degree of pitting edema.
13. Assess heart sounds.
    - Use the stethoscope *bell,* pressed *lightly* to hear low-pitched sounds.
    - Use the *diaphragm,* pressed *firmly,* for high-pitched sounds.
    - The diaphragm picks up the normal "lub-dub" of the heartbeat (the first and second heart sounds) and the bell picks up murmurs, clicks, rubs and low-pitched third and fourth heart sounds.

Heart Sounds

There are four areas on the chest wall where sounds and blood flow through the valves can be heard: the aortic, pulmonic, mitral (apex) and tricuspid areas (Chart 16-2). These areas are named for the valve sounds best transmitted to that area and do not overlie the valves anatomically.

First Heart Sound. The first heart sound (S_1) is produced by the closure of the mitral and tricuspid valves just as ventricular contraction begins. The sound is heard best at the mitral (apex) area. The mitral valve closes slightly before the tricuspid valve owing to different pressures in the ventricle. Normally, this splitting of the first sound is difficult to hear and usually presents as one sound.

Second Heart Sound. During ventricular contraction, the aortic and pulmonic valves open as the pressures within both lower heart chambers rise above pressures in the pulmonary and aortic arteries. After the blood is ejected, pressures in the ventricles drop, causing the aortic and pulmonic valves to shut. The closure produces the second heart sound (S_2). Though heard throughout the precordium, it is loudest in the aortic area.

Aortic and pulmonic valve closure is not simultaneous. During inspiration, atmospheric pressure in the chest cavity permits a larger venous return to the right side of the heart. With this larger volume to eject, right ventricular systole is prolonged and the pulmonic valve closes slightly later than the aortic valve. This creates a physiologic splitting of the

TABLE 16-1. SIGNIFICANCE OF PULSE VARIATIONS

Palpated Pulse Variation	Description	Clinical Significance
Strong, bounding pulse	Very full, strong, high pressure pulses.	Pain, fear, anxiety, hyperthyroidism, anemia, patent ductus arteriosus, aortic regurgitation, complete heart block, extensive arteriosclerosis in older people ("pipe-stem" arteries), exercise.
Weak pulse	Small cardiac output that doesn't generate strong pressure at the peripheral arteries; difficult to palpate or feel easily.	Severe failure of the left ventricle for any intrinsic or extrinsic reason; aortic stenosis.
Irregular pulse	A pulse in which beats come early or late, these often differ in strength. The irregularity may appear consistently with a regular pattern or may be completely unpredictable.	With suspected MI, PVCs are most probable. In patients with known rheumatic heart disease, coronary heart disease or hyperthyroidism, atrial fibrillation is likely.
Pulsus alternans	The pulse, though regular, differs in strength or pressure in an alternate manner—strong–less strong–strong–less strong. If not perceptible from palpation of the pulse, it can usually be detected by auscultating the BP.	Left ventricular failure
Pulsus paradoxus	In some normal persons, the pulse diminishes in pressure during inspiration. This is demonstrated by auscultating the BP at the systolic level and having the patient breathe normally. The difference between hearing the beats only during expiration and hearing all the beats throughout the respiratory cycle should be no greater than 10–12 mm Hg.	Severe CHF, severe pulmonary disease, cardiac tamponade.

Chart 16-2

RELATION OF HEART SOUNDS TO CHEST WALL

Chest Area	Location	Sounds Best Heard
Aortic (base)	2nd intercostal space just to the right of the sternum	Aortic valve murmurs, intense second heart sounds
Pulmonic	2nd intercostal space just to the left of the sternum	Split second heart sound, inspiration
Tricuspid	5th intercostal space at lower left sternal border	Split first heart sound, S_3 ventricular gallop
Mitral (apex)	5th intercostal space left of the sternum, medial to the midclavicular line	Intense first heart sound S_3—ventricular gallop S_4—atrial gallop

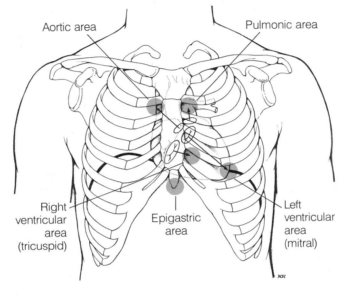

Aortic area

Pulmonic area

Right ventricular area (tricuspid)

Epigastric area

Left ventricular area (mitral)

(Illustration from Brunner LS, Suddarth DS: Textbook of Medical-Surgical Nursing, 4th ed. JB Lippincott, 1980)

second heart sound that can be heard best over the pulmonic area. During expiration, right and left systoles are nearly equal in length, so valve closure is almost simultaneous.

Third Heart Sound. The third heart sound (S_3) occurs early in diastole and is produced by the rapid flow of blood from the atria into ventricles. This low-frequency sound can be heard by placing the bell at the mitral area with the patient in a left lateral position. Of significance in the older patient with known cardiac disease, S_3, called a ventricular diastolic gallop, indicates congestive heart failure (CHF). It is normal in children and adolescents.

Fourth Heart Sound. A cardiac filling sound, the fourth heart sound (S_4) is not heard in normal hearts. It is believed to be caused by increased resistance of the ventricle to atrial filling. Occuring late in diastole, it is heard best with the

bell at the mitral area. Its presence is associated with hypertensive cardiovascular disease, CAD, aortic stenosis, and heart block. The patient who has had myocardial infarction may have a fourth heart sound.

Summation Gallop. Summation gallop, a combination of S_3 and S_4, may occur in rapidly beating diseased hearts.

Murmurs

Murmurs are sounds caused by increased turbulence of the blood. They can be produced by turbulent flow across a partial obstruction such as a stenosed valve, or by regurgitation through an incompetent valve or defect.

Murmurs heard between the S_1 and S_2 are designated systolic murmurs; those occurring after systole are diastolic murmurs. Murmurs vary in intensity and may be described as rumbling, blowing, harsh, musical, high-pitched, or low-pitched.

Murmurs do not always indicate valvular disease. They can occur in healthy young people and are called functional murmurs. Brief and quiet, these murmurs occur during systole because of the ejection force and rapid flow of blood. Functional murmurs become more evident during exercise, pregnancy, high fever, and anemia.

ADJUNCT STUDIES

Laboratory tests most often ordered are electrocardiograms, blood studies, cardiac enzymes and chest x-rays. Noninvasive tests such as phonocardiography and echocardiograms help extend the knowledge gained by the bedside examiner. Phonocardiography is useful in analyzing heart sounds and murmurs, and echocardiograms help to visualize the four cardiac valves and the dimensions of three of the four heart chambers.

Stress testing and invasive procedures such as cardiac catheterization and coronary arteriograms may be used in selective cases. Nuclear studies, using small amounts of radioactive substances, help to visualize the great vessels, heart, and pulmonary vessels. In patients with nonperfusing portions of the myocardium, radioactive isotopes are used to visualize the size and location of the infarcted area.

Electrocardiogram. The 12-lead electrocardiogram (ECG) permits observation of the electrical activity of the heart from 12 different views. Changes occurring in the conduction system or in the heart muscle itself may not be evident immediately after the acute emergency. Yet the initial ECG tracing provides a baseline for comparison of serial ECGs.

Chest X-Ray. The chest x-ray illustrates heart size and shape, and the lung vasculature. Though persons with known CAD may have no cardiac enlargement, serial x-rays over time can show significant change.

Heart size is categorized as normal, significantly abnormal, or borderline. A general rule is the transverse diameter of the heart should be less than one-half the transverse diameter of the bony thorax.

Lung vasculature may give important clues to the status of both the pulmonary and cardiac systems. For example, with left ventricular failure, pulmonary congestion shows as prominent and distended blood vessels in the upper lung fields. Pulmonary edema may present as cloudiness beginning in the central portion of the lung, spreading to the periphery as the edema worsens.

Serum Enzyme Studies. When the myocardium has irreversible damage to an area of muscle, the dying and dead cells release enzyme-rich cell contents into the blood. Blood serum levels of these enzymes are a diagnostic test for cardiac muscle necrosis and can be used as a general guide for patient prognosis.

The three enzymes elevated in blood serum following cardiac muscle damage are creatine phosphokinase (CPK), serum glutamic oxalacetic transaminase (SGOT), and lactic dehydrogenase (LDH). Each enzyme has its own individual release, elevation peak, and return-to-base profile as outlined in Table 16-2.

Elevated enzyme levels may occur with injury to other organs and muscles. If there is a disease process concurrent with suspected cardiac damage, the elevated enzyme levels may point incorrectly to myocardial infarction. Primary liver disease or liver congestion due to right-sided failure, pulmonary infarction, pericarditis, shock, cardioversion, or any surgical procedure may elevate the SGOT and LDH levels. In addition, hemolysis of red blood cells, leukemia, or CHF can cause LDH enzyme levels to rise. CPK levels may elevate with multiple intramuscular injections, muscle damage or disease, alcohol intoxications, and convulsions or other vigorous muscle activity.

The search for cardiac-specific enzymes led to the discovery of CPK and LDH isoenzymes, CPK-MB and LDH_1, respectively. CPK-MB is of greater diagnostic value if the patient is seen within 48 hours of experiencing chest pain. After 48 hours, the LDH_1 isoenzyme determination is more helpful.

Enzyme levels may have prognostic value. If the serum blood levels are four to eight times the normal values, the appearance of complications like ventricular arrhythmias, CHF, and shock are more likely.

TABLE 16-2. SERUM LEVELS OF ENZYMES FOLLOWING CARDIAC INJURY

Name	Activity			Values*
	Begins Elevation	**Peaks**	**Returns to Normal**	
Creatine phosphokinase (CPK) Isoenzyme MB Cardiac specific	6 hr	24 hr	72 hr	Male: 0–50 milliunits Female: 0–30 milliunits CPK-MB 15% of total
Lactic dehydrogenase (LDH) LDH_1 isoenzyme Cardiac specific	6–12 hr	3–4 days	10 days	150–450 units/ml (Wroblewski unit) 71–207 IU/L 80–120 (Wacker units)
Nonspecific serum glutamic-oxaloacetic transaminase (SGOT)	8–12 hr	24–48 hr	3–4 days	8–40 units/ml (Karmen unit) 6–8 IU/L

* Values may vary with individual laboratory procedures and test determinations.

ATHEROSCLEROSIS

Atherosclerosis, a form of arteriosclerosis, is the pathology that ultimately causes CAD and its resulting complications. Atherosclerosis is a slow, progressive disease in which plaque is deposited along the intimal lining of arteries, gradually restricting and occluding blood flow.

Risk Factors

The development of atherosclerosis depends on the inter-relationships of metabolic, chemical, physical, biologic, and mechanical factors. The following factors have been iden-tified as increasing the risk of developing atherosclerosis:

Elevated Blood Lipids Such As Cholesterol and Triglyc-erides. Diets high in animal fats, dairy products, and sat-urated fats have been implicated, though studies showing the relationship of diet to incidence of CAD are inconclusive. The ratio of low-density lipoprotein (LDL) to high-density lipoprotein (HDL) may be important; the HDL may remove excessive cholesterol or inhibit its role in plaque formation.

Cigarette Smoking. Smoking speeds the development of atherosclerosis. Though the pathophysiology is not identi-fied, it is known that substances in cigarettes increase heart rate, constrict peripheral blood vessels, and promote hypoxia by means of inhaled carbon monoxide.

Diabetes Mellitus. Diabetes mellitus seems to accelerate the process of atherosclerosis. The process is also more diffuse, involving smaller arteries in addition to the more common sites such as the middle-sized and larger arteries. Persons who develop diabetes mellitus have a higher in-cidence of stroke and CAD.

Hypertension. Hypertension appears to increase devel-opment of atherosclerosis. Complications of CAD such as CHF occur more frequently in the presence of preexisting hypertension.

Obesity. Overweight, a national health problem, contrib-utes to the development of adult-onset diabetes and hy-pertension. Heart work load is increased because blood must be pumped through increased body mass and a larger vas-cular network.

Age, Race, and Sex. Middle-aged and older white males are at greater risk. Before menopause, women have a sig-nificantly lower risk than men; after menopause, the inci-dence of atherosclerosis rises rapidly.

Positive Family History. Having immediate family mem-bers who have developed CAD before age 65 indicates a greater risk potential for the individual.

Sedentary Life-Style. High-level (aerobic), vigorous, and routine exercise is best for reducing risk when started early in life. Also, high-level exercise or high-energy work pro-motes the development of collateral coronary circulation.

Personality Traits. The competitive, aggressive, fast-moving executive, the "type A" personality, appears to be at greater risk. Further scientific study is needed to relate personality to development of atherosclerosis.

Combinations of risk factors may increase the process of atherosclerosis. Some risk factors, such as age, sex, or a positive family history, cannot be changed. Others can be altered if the person is aware of what they are and of their significance to his well-being.

CORONARY ARTERY DISEASE

Symptoms of atherosclerosis in the heart's coronary artery system appear when the blood flow is reduced by 75% or more. The artery most affected is the left anterior descending coronary artery, followed by the right coronary and the cir-cumflex arteries, respectively.

Even with total closure of one coronary artery by ath-erosclerosis, the patient may remain symptom-free because of the development of collateral circulation. This supportive network may be so extensive that myocardial tissue is still well perfused. Without collateral circulation and with sig-nificant narrowing, the patient remains symptom-free when not under stress; however, with exercise, or in situations demanding greater flow to the myocardium, the patient mo-mentarily has vascular insufficiency and chest pain.

Atherosclerosis involving the coronary arteries may present as angina pectoris, cardiac insufficiency, acute myo-cardial infarction, or sudden death. An individual may de-velop all three manifestations over time or may develop only one.

ANGINA PECTORIS

Angina pectoris is a clinical syndrome in which the cardiac muscles' need for oxygen momentarily exceeds the supply, resulting in myocardial ischemia. Most commonly, angina pectoris is due to incomplete blockage of one or more cor-onary arteries by atherosclerotic lesions. The episode is usu-ally triggered by some form of exertion: unusual physical exercise, emotional stress, ingestion of a large meal, sexual intercourse, or exposure to cold.

Assessment

- Angina pectoris is characterized by the sudden onset of chest pain, which may range from a mild pressure to crushing pain accompanied by dyspnea, diaphoresis, light-headedness, and palpitations. One cannot differentiate between angina pectoris or myocardial infarction based upon the pain intensity, radiation, or location.
- Angina is a temporary condition in which there is no damage to the myocardial cells and consequently, no rise in cardiac serum enzymes or permanent ECG charges. During an attack, changes occur in the ECG—ST segment depression or T-wave inversion; however, after the chest pain has disappeared, the ECG returns to normal.
- Frequency of angina attacks may range from many a day to infrequent episodes occurring once in a matter of weeks

or months. The duration, intensity, and factors producing the pain can remain stable or may disappear if the patient develops good collateral circulation or if he develops an infarct of the marginal area of the hypoxic myocardium.

- Certain worrisome patients appear to lie on the disease scale between stable angina pectoris and myocardial infarction. This clinical state may be called coronary insufficiency, preinfarction angina, or unstable angina pectoris. Chest pain occurs at rest and not as a result of unusual exertion or stress. The duration of pain is longer (up to 30 minutes) and the episodes occur more frequently. Such patients may be at high risk for developing a myocardial infarction and are often hospitalized for observation and treatment.

Treatment

The treatment goal is to reduce the discrepancy between myocardial demand for oxygen and the available supply of oxygen. Rest and nitroglycerin relieve the pain of angina pectoris, usually within 10 to 15 minutes.

Patient Education. Patients should appreciate the following about nitroglycerin:
1. Headache, tachycardia, a sensation of warmth, and a slight burning sensation under the tongue as the tablet dissolves are common side-effects.
2. In some, temporary hypotension may occur; these patients should remain sitting or lying while the drug is taking effect.
3. Nitroglycerin is light- and heat-sensitive. Even when the drug is kept in a cool, dark place, the patient should plan on replacing his supply every 3 to 6 months.
4. The patient cannot become addicted to the drug and he may take it as many times a day as needed for his chest pain attacks.
5. If, during an attack of chest pain, the patient has taken up to 3 nitroglycerin spaced 5 to 10 minutes apart without relief, he should seek medical help immediately.

Other drugs used in the treatment of angina pectoris are the long-acting drugs such as isosorbide dinitrate (Isordil), long-acting nitroglycerin ointment, and propranolol (Inderal).

MYOCARDIAL INFARCTION

Myocardial infarction (MI) is the death or necrosis of a segment of myocardial cells due to a disruption of coronary artery blood flow. Most commonly, obstructed coronary blood flow is the result of atherosclerosis in the coronary vessels. Less commonly, it is due to coronary artery spasm or to an embolism in the artery.

When the blood flow stops, cells beyond the blockage begin to die. The higher the location of the block in the coronary artery, the greater the area of myocardium that is deprived of oxygen. The loss of a percentage of the pumping myocardium is a major medical emergency, and prompt action is required of all who come into contact with the patient. Statistically, 50% to 60% of all acute myocardial infarction (AMI) victims die within 2 to 4 hours after onset and before being seen by any medical person.

If the patient reaches a hospital, however, his chance of survival improves. With the advent of coronary care units (CCUs), in-hospital mortality of all admitted patients has dropped from 30% to 12% to 15%. Most of the gains against the mortality percentages have been in the area of treatment of arrhythmias.

Assessment

- Associated signs and symptoms are dyspnea, diaphoresis, weakness, light-headedness, nausea, vomiting, and a feeling of impending doom.
- The patient appears pale, his skin is often cool and moist, and he is anxious.
- Often, his heart rate is elevated above 100 bpm and his blood pressure is variable.

As with angina, pain may vary in severity from minimal discomfort to crushing pain. The chest pain of AMI lasts longer than 30 minutes. Rest, nitroglycerin, and oxygen alone do not provide relief, and narcotics are needed to provide pain relief. With some patients, especially elderly diabetics, pain may be absent even if the associated signs and symptoms are present. The duration of pain may vary and cannot be used to differentiate between coronary insufficiency and MI. The severity of pain does *not* correlate with the extent of the infarct. A patient with moderate pain may have an infarct affecting 30% to 40% of his ventricle in contrast to another patient who has severe anginal pain with no residual damage.

Clinically, with the death of cardiac cells, AMI produces:
1. A rise in cardiac enzymes
2. Left ventricular dysfunction (the left ventricle is most often affected)
3. Onset of arrhythmias
4. Changes over time in the ECG such as ST elevation, significant Q waves, and T-wave inversion.

Management

General objectives of care:
- Prevent additional damage to myocardium
- Conserve ischemic areas of the myocardium that are salvageable
- Observe, anticipate, and treat cardiac dysrrhythmias
- Observe for development of complications, such as CHF, cardiogenic shock, and pulmonary edema
- Provide emotional support for the patient and his family.

Prehospital Care. Chest pain has numerous etiologies; however, all patients complaining of heavy substernal chest pain must be treated as heart attack victims until proven otherwise. There is no certain way to decide in the field whether the patient is suffering from acute anxiety or AMI. The treatment protocol and rationale for trained paramedic personnel are outlined in Chart 16-3.

Hospital Care. Upon arrival in the emergency department, care of the patient with AMI must be prompt. Equipment must be readily available for efficient assessment and treatment; it should include the following:
- Electrodes, patient wire for monitor system
- Functioning cardiac monitor
- Blood pressure cuff, stethoscope, suction, and O_2 equipment

---

Chart 16-3

PREHOSPITAL CARE OF PATIENT WITH ACUTE MYOCARDIAL INFARCTION

Management/Treatment	Rationale
Check airway, breathing, circulation	
Oxygen, 6 L/min by nasal cannula or 10 L/min by mask, in patient with no known chronic pulmonary disease	Myocardial ischemia produces chest pain. By enriching the air with oxygen, greater oxygen extraction can be achieved by the myocardium with some relief of the hypoxic state.
Rest, assurance, position of comfort	Patients with chest pain have an increased level of catecholamine release, which increases heart rate and exacerbates myocardial ischemia.
Monitor cardiac status and vital signs.	With myocardial ischemia, cardiac cells become electrically unstable and are capable of ectopic activity. Arrhythmias, particularly premature ventricular ectopic beats, must be monitored carefully. Other arrhythmias such as sinus tachycardias, AV conduction defects, or bradyarrhythmias need to be watched and, if need be, treated.
IV of 5% dextrose in water at keep-open rate	In the event of arrhythmias or total cardiovascular collapse, an IV line should be in place for IV drug administration.
Pain relief: Nitroglycerin (optional)	A smooth muscle relaxant and vasodilator, nitroglycerin can reduce afterload and dilate coronary arteries. Work load of the heart is lessened and blood flow increased. Monitor BP, watch for syncope.
Morphine sulfate	This opiate lessens severe chest pain and reduces patient anxiety, thus improving oxygen availability to myocardium. Monitor respiration rate and BP.
Transfer to the nearest hospital with CCU, code 2	Whenever possible, transport of the patient should be accomplished without lights and siren since these elements can contribute to patient anxiety and apprehension and ultimately increase cardiac work load and oxygen need.

- 12-lead ECG and technician on stand-by
- Resuscitation cart
- Intravenous (IV) solution of 5% dextrose in water (D_5W), microdrip tubing, IV tray
- Lab slips, blood tubes for cardiac enzymes, serum electrolytes, complete blood count (CBC), glucose, blood urea nitrogen (BUN), creatinine, and clotting studies

Management of the patient with suspected AMI is outlined in Chart 16-4. Chapter 14 discusses resuscitation of the patient in cardiopulmonary arrest.

Complications of Acute Myocardial Infarction

Following an MI, the patient is susceptible to complications that can accompany the heart crisis. Two major complications are the development of arrhythmias and cardiogenic shock.

ARRHYTHMIAS

With the advent of monitoring, less than 2 decades ago, cardiologists and the staffs of CCUs became aware of the high incidence of arrhythmias in the patient with an AMI within the first 24-hours. As many as 90% of all patients with AMI develop arrhythmias, the two most common being premature ventricular contraction (PVCs) and sinus tachycardia.

Arrhythmias play havoc with cardiac output, good coronary artery flow, and myocardial perfusion. Following an AMI, there is an ischemic zone of myocardial tissue that lies between the dead, infarcted myocardium and the perfused healthy tissue. This zone is an unstable, marginally perfused area, susceptible to blood flow disruptions. Decreases in blood flow to this area can occur with arrhythmias, which may convert the ischemic zone into part of the infarction. Extension of the infarcted area adds overall to the total amount of lost myocardium, which is inert, adynamic tissue. The net loss of functioning myocardium decides the ultimate outcome.

This ischemic zone also is the site generating arrhythmic disturbances. Chart 16-5 describes arrhythmias and ECG changes in relation to infarct location and indicates appropriate management. Other contributing factors are hypoxia, electrolyte imbalance (particularly potassium and calcium), acidosis, alkalosis, high levels of catecholamines, CHF, and drugs such as epinephrine, digitalis, and isoproterenol. Car-

---

Chart 16-4

HOSPITAL CARE OF PATIENT WITH ACUTE MYOCARDIAL INFARCTION

Management/Treatment	Rationale
1. Receive patient in the ED. Introduce yourself, visually assess patient.	A patient who is awake and responds verbally has demonstrated the ABCs: he has an airway, is breathing, and has circulation. An attempt to establish staff-patient relationship may aid in reducing emotional stress and decreasing the amount of circulating catecholamines.
2. Begin oxygen therapy; 6 L/min by nasal prongs 10 L/min by mask.	Oxygen is routinely administered to AMI patients to improve the PO_2 and to conserve ischemic areas of the myocardium. Extra care must be taken with patients who have known lung disease; increasing the oxygen percentage could be dangerous for these patients. Monitoring the blood gases and assessing the patient's level of consciousness and respiratory rate are essential.
3. Establish IV 500 D_5W at keep-open rate using a micro-drip (60 drops = 1 ml).	The IV route is immediately available for drug administration. Whenever possible, narcotics and antiarrhythmics should be given IV to better control drugs effects and patient responses and to eliminate skeletal muscle injury, which would raise the CPK serum level.
4. Monitor cardiac status and vital signs.	90%–95% of patients with AMI have arrhythmias. In addition to developing a life-threatening arrhythmia, the patient with untreated arrhythmias may develop an increased infarcted area, CHF, or cardiogenic shock.
5. Assess the patient for degree of chest pain and obtain order for medication.	Pain can cause coronary artery spasm and increase the secretion of catecholamines. High levels increase the heart rate, oxygen consumption, work of the heart, and potential for arrhythmias. Morphine sulfate is best given in 3-mg to 5-mg IV boluses. In patients with a potential for bradyarrhythmias or AV block, meperidine HCl may be ordered, since morphine is a vagomimetic agent and can potentiate slow rates and block. Monitor vitals following administration.

---

diac arrhythmias are classified as tachycardias, bradycardias, or irregular rhythms. The rhythms may occur along with either a normal or abnormal heart rate.

Tachycardias present a problem in interference with normal cardiac output due to decreased ventricular filling time. The arrhythmias included in this classification are sinus tachycardia, atrial fibrillation-flutter, paroxysmal atrial tachycardia, ventricular tachycardia, and ventricular fibrillation.

Bradycardias interfere with normal cardiac output because of a decreased rate of ventricular ejection. The arrhythmias included in this classification are sinus bradycardia, partial heart block and complete heart block.

Irregular heart rhythms may indicate myocardial irritability. They may not necessarily interfere with normal cardiac output, so they do not usually cause any immediate concern. They include the partial heart blocks, dissociation, and PVCs.

Of concern to emergency personnel are arrhythmias that require immediate intervention to prevent rapid death. They include ventricular tachycardia, ventricular fibrillation, third-degree (complete) heart block, and asystole.

VENTRICULAR ARRHYTHMIAS

Premature Ventricular Contractions

The most common ventricular arrhythmia is the premature ventricular contraction (PVC), also called ventricular premature contraction (VPC). It is a premature (early) occurrence of the QRS complex whose configuration is bizarre and wide, since it arises from the ventricles. The T wave is usually large and is opposite the main deflection of the QRS. No P wave precedes it, but occasionally a sinus P wave may be seen just before the premature ventricular beat. If the premature QRS has the same configuration each time it appears on the scope, the PVCs are said to be unifocal (originating from one site). If the configuration alters, the PVCs are considered multifocal, since they may be arising from more than one focus within the ventricle (Fig. 16-4).

The causes of PVCs are numerous. PVCs are particularly common in digitalis toxicity, but other drugs such as epinephrine, aminophylline and isoproterenol may enhance their appearance. In the patient with an AMI the appearance

Chart 16-4

HOSPITAL CARE OF PATIENT WITH ACUTE MYOCARDIAL INFARCTION (*CONTINUED*)

Management/Treatment	Rationale
6. Obtain 12-lead ECG, and blood samples—if possible, get blood during venipuncture for IV.	Diagnosis of AMI depends basically on three findings: cardiac enzymes, 12-lead EKG, and physical exam and history. Baseline data are gathered in order to compare developments over the next 12 to 36 hours. Common tests include CBC, serum electrolytes, glucose, BUN, creatinine, cardiac enzymes, clotting studies (PT, PTT, TT), and arterial blood gas studies.
7. If appropriate, do secondary survey and assess patient's response to initial treatment.	Now check for presence of edema, abnormal breath or heart sounds, distended neck veins, etc. Evaluate cardiac output by checking skin temperature and color, level of consciousness, blood pressure, and urine output.
8. Administer prophylactic loading dose of lidocaine according to protocol.	The most common cause of death during the prehospital phase of AMI is ventricular fibrillation. Lidocaine is most effective in abolishing ventricular ectopic activity.
9. Continue to monitor and obtain orders immediately for treatment of arrhythmias should they appear.	Hemodynamically, any arrhythmia can adversely affect cardiac output and coronary artery blood flow. Ischemic margins surrounding the infarcted area are potentially salvageable areas if they continue to receive oxygenated blood. Prompt treatment of arrhythmias prevents extending the infarction and prevents more unstable and lethal arrhythmias from developing.
10. Prepare the patient for transfer to the CCU. Inform family of the transfer; introduce staff of CCU to patient/family.	Explanations and common courtesy to both patient and family provide emotional support and demonstrate concern and caring. A nurse or physician should accompany patient with continuous monitoring and portable oxygen administration during transfer. A portable defibrillator, bag-valve-mask, and small cardiac emergency drug tray should also accompany patient.

of PVCs can be due to the electrical instability of the ischemic zone of myocardium surrounding the infarction, the presence of electrolyte imbalance, particularly hypokalemia, the coexistence of CHF, or hypoxia.

Treatment. PVCs indicate an electrically irritable heart that has the potential to produce lethal rhythms: ventricular tachycardia, and ventricular fibrillation. The usual criteria for treating PVCs are as follows:
1. PVCs appear near the vulnerable period during repolarization (R-on-T phenomenon).
2. They are multifocal.
3. They occur more than 5 to 6 times in one minute.
4. They appear in runs of three or more consecutively.
Any one of these criteria should prompt the emergency nurse to treat a patient for PVCs.

However, careful documentation has indicated that ventricular fibrillation can be precipitated by late-occurring PVCs and not just by R-on-T PVCs, and some emergency department personnel now treat PVCs promptly even if they do not meet any of these criteria.

The treatment for PVCs associated with suspected AMI is a lidocaine bolus of 1 mg/kg of body weight followed by an IV drip of 1 gm of lidocaine in 250 ml or 500 ml D_5W IV and administered at a 1 to 4 mg/min drip.

Administration of Lidocaine. The following precautions should be kept in mind:
- Lidocaine has a half-life of 20 minutes; the initial bolus should be followed by an IV drip or a second bolus to maintain a therapeutic plasma concentration.
- Total dosage should not exceed 300 mg in an hour.
- Monitor drug dosage, using a pediatric microdrip administration set (1 gt/ml).
- Consider concentrating the IV solution (1 gm in 250 ml) when the patient is elderly or unable to handle large amounts of IV fluids.
- Continue to monitor the patient after drug administration; note and document his response to treatment by counting

Chart 16-5

CLINICAL SIGNIFICANCE AND MANAGEMENT OF MYOCARDIAL INFARCTION ACCORDING TO LOCATION

Location of Infarction	Significance	Management
Anterior wall (extensive)	Involves main left coronary artery. ECG changes seen in leads V_{1-6}, depending on extent, and in leads I and aVL. Owing to extensive damage and loss of functioning muscle, pump failure is common. AV conduction disturbances, though not as common as with inferior-wall AMI, have an intrinsic heart rate of less than 45 bpm with a wide QRS and are associated with Mobitz II second-degree heart block and complete heart block. With complete heart block associated with pump failure, mortality is 75%.	Assess patient for signs of pump failure: 1. Listen to the chest for rales; observe for shortness of breath. 2. Watch monitor for the development of rhythms associated with heart failure: • Sinus tachycardia • Atrial arrhythmias such as PACs and rapid atrial arrhythmias such as PAT. Watch patient's monitor for the development of AV conduction disturbances: 1. Report promptly because onset of complete heart block can occur rapidly from the appearance of first rhythms. 2. Keep isoproterenol on hand to be added to an IV solution if necessary. 3. Have IV pacemaker on stand-by.
Limited areas Anteroseptal wall	Involves the left anterior descending branch of the left coronary artery. ECG changes seen in leads V_1 through V_4.	
Anterolateral wall	Involves the circumflex branch of the left coronary artery. ECG changes seen in leads V_{4-6}, and aVL and I.	
True posterior wall	Involves the circumflex branch of left coronary artery. ECG changes are seen in leads V_{1-2}, the R waves of V_{1-2} become abnormally tall. The normal infarct pattern is not seen on ECG.	
Inferior wall (diaphragmatic)	Involves right coronary artery. ECG changes seen in leads II, III, and aVF. Because the right coronary artery supplies blood to the SA and AV nodes, ischemia occurs, vagal tone increases, and bradyarrhythmias such as sinus bradycardia and AV blocks (first-degree and Mobitz I) are seen. With block, rates greater than 45 bpm with a narrow QRS occur temporarily. Associated with sinus bradycardia is AIVR. Rate ranges from 50–90 bpm. Rhythm is usually benign and self-limiting.	1. Be prepared for the appearance of first-degree heart block, Mobitz I (Wenckebach), or sinus bradycardia. 2. Unless the patient is affected hemodynamically and is unstable, he may simply be observed. 3. Keep atropine on hand if patient begins to deteriorate.

the frequency of PVCs per minute and their location in relation to the preceding T wave.

• Observe the patient carefully for onset of central nervous system (CNS) side effects such as dizziness, confusion, or seizures.

• Lidocaine is metabolized by the liver; consider dose reduction in patients with altered liver function.

• Do not treat only the arrhythmia. Look for other contributing causes such as hypoxia or hypokalemia, and treat them as well.

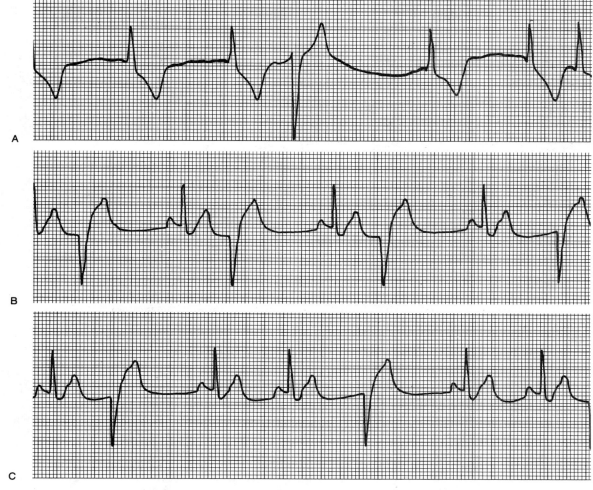

Figure 16-4 *Premature ventricular contractions (PVCs) A. Unifocal PVCs. B. Bigeminy PVCs. C. Trigeminy PVCs.*

Figure 16-5 *Ventricular tachycardia. A. Common ventricular tachycardia. B. Arrows indicate the occurrence of fusion beats. (B is from Constant J: Learning Electrocardiography, p 547. Boston, Little, Brown & Co, 1973. Copyright © 1973 by Little, Brown & Co)*

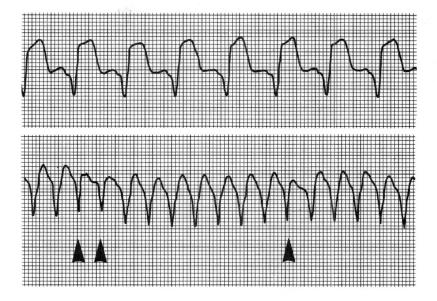

TABLE 16-3.   COMPARATIVE DIFFERENCES BETWEEN DEFIBRILLATION AND CARDIOVERSION

Defibrillation	Cardioversion
Life-saving first aid measure Patient is in a lethal arrhythmia or clinically dead.	Elective measure Patient is alive, sedated or anesthetized for the procedure; done in the hospital.
Unsynchronized shock; *defibrillator* will fire when triggers are pushed. In *adult* emergencies, a dead victim after CPR may be "shocked" with 400 watt-sec.	Synchronized shock; *cardiovertor* will fire *only* when switches are pushed and an R wave is sensed. The countershock energy administered by the physician is selected. It may vary with size of patient and knowledge of successful use of cardioversion therapy with this patient in the past.
It may save the life and probably will do no serious damage.	May or may not convert the undesirable rhythm. Patient will be managed on drug therapy. Life not in peril.
Paddles must be well lubricated with electrically conductive jelly. It is essential to avoid contact with other monitoring electrodes, wires, metals, etc., during defibrillation.	Paddles must be well lubricated with electrically conductive jelly. In cardioversion it is essential to avoid contact with monitoring electrodes, wires, etc. Metal neck chains should be removed.

PVCs appearing in patients without AMI may require other therapy such as avoiding coffee and tobacco or, in the digitalis-toxic patient, administration of phenytoin (Dilantin).

Ventricular Tachycardia

Ventricular tachycardia is a series of bizarre, wide QRS complexes of three or more in a sequence occurring at ventricular rates between 120 and 250 bpm (Fig. 16-5). This rhythm must be terminated immediately, since it can have serious hemodynamic effects on the patient and may deteriorate into ventricular fibrillation (see Fig. 16-7). Contributing factors are AMI, intrinsic slow rates (like sinus bradycardia), drug toxicity (quinidine, procainamide, and digitalis), hypoxia, electrolyte imbalance, and CHF.

Treatment.   If the patient is maintaining his level of consciousness and does not appear to be in severe distress, the rhythm can be treated with a bolus of lidocaine, 1 to 2 mg/kg of body weight (50 mg–100 mg). The dose may be repeated, or if the rhythm persists, the patient may be cardioverted by direct current (DC) shock.

However, when the patient deteriorates rapidly, DC cardioversion is the treatment of choice. Rapid deterioration may be seen as the onset of sudden, severe chest pain, the development of CHF, or a hypotensive state. Unlike DC shock for ventricular fibrillation, low watt-second settings synchronized to the QRS complexes are used. (See comparison of countershock therapies in Table 16-3).

Following conversion, begin an IV drip of lidocaine, 1 to 2 gm of lidocaine in 250 ml to 500 ml D5W, to prevent recurrence. If not given before cardioversion, an IV bolus should precede the IV drip to raise the plasma level. Maintain the lidocaine drip for 24 to 48 hours.

Resistant ventricular tachycardia may respond to bretylium tosylate (Bretylol), 5 mg/kg of body weight, given IV slowly over a 15-minute period. Procainamide HCl (Pronestyl) may also be used. It is given in a 50-mg to 100-mg IV bolus slowly over a 3-minute period. With both drugs, monitor the blood pressure for hypotension.

Accelerated Idioventricular Rhythm

Accelerated idioventricular rhythm (AIVR) may be misdiagnosed as a slow ventricular tachycardia because the rate of this rhythm is 60 to 100 bpm. The rhythm is ventricular in origin and is common in patients with inferior-wall AMIs who develop sinus bradycardia or who have digitalis toxicity. As the sinus rate falls, the pacemaking function is assumed by a faster-than-normal ventricular focus. (Fig. 16-6)

Treatment.   This rhythm is transient and usually does not require treatment. If the patient does appear to be in difficulty or if the rhythm becomes unstable, increasing the intrinsic rate of the sinus node with atropine, 0.5 mg IV push, may be tried. The dose may be repeated up to 2.0 mg. Have transvenous pacemaker equipment available.

Ventricular Fibrillation

Ventricular fibrillation appears to be totally chaotic with no clear-cut QRS complexes evident. Instead, the baseline un-

Figure 16-6 Accelerated idioventricular rhythm.

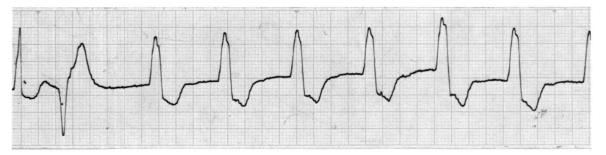

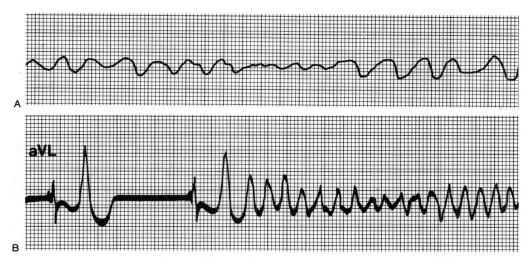

Figure 16-7 *Ventricular fibrillation. A. Common ventricular fibrillation. B. Shows the sudden onset of ventricular fibrillation by a ventricular ectopic beat. (B is from Constant J: Learning Electrocardiography, p 550. Boston, Little, Brown & Co, 1973. Copyright © 1973 by Little, Brown & Co)*

dulates, with up-and-down waveforms (Fig. 16-7). Waveforms of large amplitude ("coarse" ventricular fibrillation) suggest that onset of fibrillation occurred recently. If measures to combat the hypoxia and acidosis are not instituted, the amplitude diminishes to a fine, small baseline fluctuation and eventually, to asystole.

Ventricular fibrillation occurs in patients with AMI, CAD, AV block, drug toxicity (digitalis, quinidine, procainamide), hypothermia, and hypoxia. Hemodynamically, this arrhythmia is catastrophic for the patient. Cardiac output falls, coronary artery and cerebral perfusion cease; the patient loses consciousness and stops breathing. He may also have seizures. Treatment must be initiated immediately.

Treatment. Treatment is immediate DC countershock. No time should be wasted on intubating or other extra steps if a working DC defibrillator is available within 30 to 45 seconds of onset to deliver 300 to 400 watt-seconds. Artificial ventilation by means of a bag-valve-mask may be done by a second staff member while the paddles are being positioned and the machine charged. Delays necessitate the use of sodium bicarbonate and other measures to combat the inevitable metabolic acidosis. (See Chap. 14, Resuscitation.)

With successful termination of ventricular fibrillation, the patient's rhythm should be stabilized with a loading dose bolus of 50 to 100 mg. of lidocaine (1 mg/kg of body weight) followed by a lidocaine drip of 2 to 4 mg/min.

Electric Countershock. The term *electric countershock* includes cardioversion and defibrillation. The techniques use controlled high-energy electric current in order to interrupt unacceptable cardiac rhythms. The rationale for this approach is to stop chaotic, lethal arrhythmias and to convert both dangerous tachyarrhythmias and atrial problems which are difficult to manage and which compromise the cardiac output. These disorders of the heartbeat may include atrial fibrillation (especially when control by drugs has not been satisfactory), ventricular tachycardia in AMI, and ventricular flutter and fibrillation.

The major distinguishing element between the two countershock therapies is that defibrillation is employed as a life-

saving measure in cardiac arrest and cardioversion is employed as a therapeutic approach in controlling certain cardiac rhythm disturbances not being controlled adequately by drugs. Comparative differences of these two therapies are outlined in Table 16-3.

Defibrillation produces a simultaneous depolarization of the heart muscle. If the myocardium is oxygenated and not acidotic, the spontaneous heartbeat may resume. Defibrillation is used most often in patients with ventricular fibrillation. It has not been effective with the heart in ventricular asystole, but it is used when the heart is in ventricular tachycardia without a peripheral pulse.

When defibrillating a patient, one paddle should be to the right of the upper sternum below the clavicle and the other to the left of the cardiac apex (or left nipple line) (see Fig. 16-8). The paddles should be lubricated with electrically conductive gel to provide for good conduction. While the shock is administered, be sure no one else is near the bed.

In emergencies, it is customary to deliver a shock of 400 watt-seconds for adults with ventricular fibrillation. The amount of myocardial damage is proportionate to the amount of energy used; therefore, some physicians elect to initiate defibrillation at a lower setting and work up the scale until it is effective. This protocol is more applicable to slender patients with small frames. *Never start defibrillation at less than 200 watt-seconds* except for a child.

SINUS AND ATRIAL DISTURBANCES

Sinus Tachycardia

Sinus tachycardia is a sinus-initiated rapid, regular rhythm. The QRS complex is normal, indicating that the initiating impulse is supraventricular. The P wave may be hidden in the slope of the preceding T wave. Thus, the electrical conduction follows the normal pathway, but the rate is accelerated to 100 to 180 bpm.

Pain, anxiety, hypovolemia, fever, CHF, and AMI may provoke this rhythm disturbance. Unrelieved tachycardia may produce chest pain in the susceptible patient.

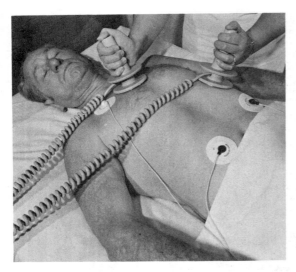

Figure 16-8 *Proper positioning of defibrillator paddles. Note that the patient also has fixed electrodes in place. (Courtesy Mennen-Greatbatch Electronics, Inc.)*

Treatment. Treating the underlying cause, such as relieving pain and anxiety, administering fluids, or drug therapy for CHF or infection may be indicated, depending on the clinical presentation and cause. If the rapid rate is dangerous to the patient, propranolol HCl (Inderal), 1 mg slow IV push every 5 to 10 minutes up to 5 mg, may be administered. Additional measures are as follows:

- Continue patient assessment to establish the underlying cause(s) for the rapid heart rate.
- Unless contraindicated, give supplemental oxygen.
- Reduce anxiety.
- Assess patient with prior AMI for signs and symptoms of CHF. This possibility is most common in patients with an extensive anterior-wall MI.
- If propranolol is given to the patient, watch monitor carefully and have atropine, 0.5 mg, on hand for a symptomatic bradycardia. Check blood pressure; watch for hypotension.

Sinus Bradycardia

Sinus bradycardia appears normal, except that the rate is below 60 bpm. P wave and QRS complex configuration are both normal and the PR interval of normal duration.

Etiologies include inferior-wall MI, increased vagal tone, hyperkalemia, and drug toxicity with antiarrhythmic drugs such as digitalis, quinidine, propranolol, and procainamide. It is also found in highly trained athletes. It may develop in the patient who inadvertently increases vagal tone by vomiting, straining at stool, or any other activity involving the Valsalva maneuver.

Treatment. Recent data suggest that in an AMI patient who has a heart rate greater than 50 bpm and is free from ventricular arrhythmias and signs of heart failure the arrhythmia should not be treated. Sinus bradycardia in such a patient may serve as a protective mechanism, reducing oxygen consumption and the work of the heart.

Atropine, used to block vagal (parasympathetic) tone, is used to increase the heart rate in carefully selected patients. Caution is advised because driving the heart of an asymptomatic patient with atropine can do greater harm by extending the infarction into the marginally perfused zone of the infarct.

For patients who show signs of decreased cardiac output, have a rate of less than 50 bpm, or develop ventricular escape beats, atropine, 0.5 mg IV push, may be given.

Premature Atrial Contractions

Premature atrial contractions (PACs) are premature beats originating in the atria with a normal-appearing QRS complex. (Fig. 16-9). The P wave may be altered and the P-R interval is normal or prolonged. Use of drugs, excessive intake of coffee or tobacco, and anxiety states can provoke their appearance. In a patient who has an AMI, PACs are early signs of impending heart failure and may forewarn of the onset of other, more serious atrial tachyarrhythmias such as atrial tachycardia, flutter, or fibrillation.

Treatment. If PACs appear with increasing frequency or in runs, or if the patient shows signs of CHF, treatment is initiated for the underlying cause. Drug therapies may include digitalis and quinidine or procainamide.

Paroxysmal Supraventricular Tachycardia

Paroxysmal supraventricular tachycardia includes paroxysmal atrial tachycardia (PAT) (Fig. 16-10), and atrioventricular

Figure 16-9 *Premature atrial contractions (PACs). Patterns like this warn of atrial fibrillation.*

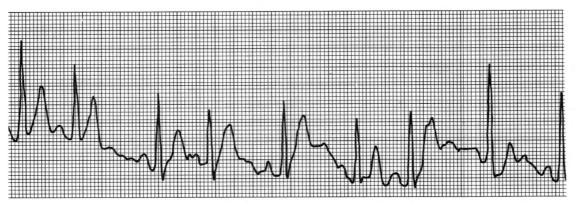

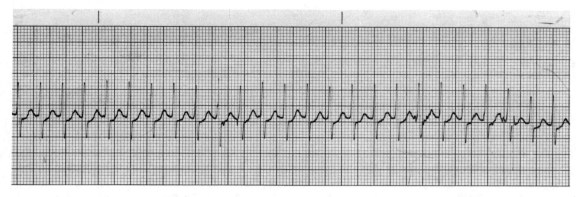

Figure 16-10 *Paroxysmal supraventricular tachycardia (PAT).*

junctional tachycardia. Identifying features include a rapid, regular rate of 120 to 220 bpm. The QRS complex and T wave appear normal. The adjective "paroxysmal" means that the rhythm begins and terminates abruptly. Clinically, with either rhythm, the patient may deteriorate quickly because of the rapid rate. With preexisting heart disease, the patient can develop chest pain or CHF.

Most commonly, PAT occurs in persons with normal hearts; the initiating factor can be alcohol, caffeine, tobacco, or emotional stress. For these patients, despite their obvious distress with the situation, the outlook is good.

Treatment.   Treatment depends on how well the patient tolerates the rhythm. In addition to reassurance and sedation, measures to increase vagal tone, such as carotid sinus massage, gagging, and Valsalva maneuvers, are often effective. If they are not effective, drug therapy may be tried. Cholinergic drugs like edrophonium chloride (Tensilon), pressor drugs like metaraminol (Aramine), and rapid-acting digitalis preparations such as ouabain, digoxin (Lanoxin), or deslanoside (Cedilanid-D) may be tried. Carotid sinus massage may be used 1 hour after the digitalis preparation is given if the arrhythmia is still present.

If the patient has not converted or is unable to tolerate the rapid rhythm and is decompensating, electrocardioversion synchronized to the ECG at low power may be used.

Atrial Flutter

Atrial flutter characteristically has a saw-tooth pattern on the baseline of the ECG (flutter waves) (Fig. 16-11). Atrial contractions occur at 250 to 350 bpm, producing these regular waves. Since the AV node is unable to conduct each atrial impulse through the ventricle at this rapid rate, it blocks every other beat at a ratio of 2:1. With an atrial rate of 300 bpm, the ventricular rate with a 2:1 block will be 150 bpm. Less commonly, the ratio may be 4:1 or 3:1 or may vary.

This rhythm rarely occurs in normal persons, it is usually associated with CAD, mitral stenosis, atrial septal defect, pulmonary embolization, and chronic obstructive pulmonary disease (COPD).

Treatment.   If necessary, prompt treatment with low-voltage DC cardioversion with synchronization can be tried. Pharmacologic treatment may include propranolol, 1 mg–3 mg IV bolus or 10 mg–40 mg po, in an attempt to slow the ventricular rate and possibly convert it to a sinus rhythm. The use of a fast-acting digitalis preparation may be used instead of propranolol to slow ventricular response.

Atrial Fibrillation

Atrial fibrillation produces no defined atrial contraction. No P waves are visible on the monitor; instead, the baseline appears undulating or "rough" in appearance (Fig. 16-12). The atrial rate is 350 to 600 bpm. Since the AV node conducts atrial impulses to the ventricles erratically, the ventricular rhythm becomes grossly irregular and usually rapid (100–160 bpm). The rapid, irregular ventricular rhythm alters cardiac output and adversely affects coronary artery blood flow.

Atrial fibrillation, when chronic, is associated with underlying heart disease. Other causes are enlarged heart, hypertension, thyroid disease, mitral stenosis, and pericarditis.

Figure 16-11 *Atrial flutter. Notice the "sawtoothed" appearance of the flutter (F) wave.*

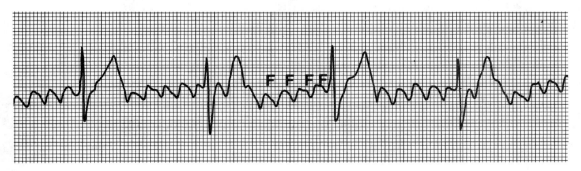

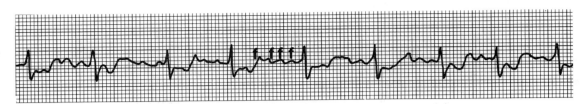

Figure 16-12 Atrial fibrillation. Notice the "wavy baseline" of fibrillatory (f) waves. P–R interval is irregular.

Treatment. The treatment of choice, aimed at reducing the rapid ventricular response and converting the rhythm to sinus rhythm, depends on the patient's clinical status. DC cardioversion with low watt-second settings may be necessary. Digitalis, administered alone or with propranolol or quinidine, is used to reduce the rapid ventricular rate and improve cardiac output.

AV CONDUCTION DISTURBANCES

AV conduction blocks produce difficulties in transmission of the electrical impulse between the atria and ventricles. Depending on location, severity, and extent of disruption to the normal cardiac cycle, these blocks range from benign to potentially lethal. AV blocks are classified into three types: first-degree, second-degree (including Mobitz I-Wenckebach and Mobitz II), and third-degree (complete) heart block.

First-Degree AV Block (Fig. 16-13)

A delay in conduction between the atria and the ventricles results in a PR interval longer than normal (>0.20 sec) on ECG. Every P wave is conducted through the AV node to the ventricle.

Second-Degree AV Block

Mobitz I (Wenckebach Phenomenon) (Fig. 16-14A). In this condition, a progressively longer PR interval occurs with each beat until the P wave is no longer conducted and a ventricular beat is dropped. The cycle is repeated every 3 to 6 beats. This rhythm is associated most commonly with inferior wall AMI due to ischemia of the AV node. It is generally reversible and less serious than Mobitz II.

Mobitz II (Fig. 16-14B). Periodically, a QRS complex does not follow a P wave and is dropped. The PR interval remains constant, and the ratio of P waves to QRS complexes may be constant (2:1, 3:1, or 4:1) or may vary. This rhythm, Mobitz II block, is seen with anterior-wall AMI and is associated with a more serious and permanent disruption in the conduction system than is Mobitz I. The conduction defect is located lower in the conduction system (below the bundle of His).

Third-Degree AV Block: Complete Heart Block (Fig. 16-15)

In third-degree AV block, the impulse from the SA node is not transmitted through the AV node to the ventricles. The atria beat at their own rate as determined by the sinus node, whereas the ventricles beat independently at whatever rate is intrinsic to the AV node or to the ventricular pacemaker. The higher the site of the block in the conduction system, the faster is the ventricular rate and the more narrow the appearance of the QRS complex. With the patient who has an anterior-wall AMI, onset of this rhythm is often sudden, without preliminary warning. The rate is lower than 45 bpm and the mortality is greater than 70%.

Significance of Acute Myocardial Infarction Location in Heart Block

Inferior-Wall Acute Myocardial Infarction. In patients with inferior-wall AMI, which indicates right coronary involvement, AV blocks are two to three times more common than in patients with anterior-wall AMI. Disruptions of the AV conduction system in inferior-wall AMIs are due to myocardial ischemia and edema of the AV node with an increase in vagal tone. They are regarded as usually reversible and temporary. Even in third-degree block, in which the block has occurred higher in the electrical conduction system, the QRS complex is narrow, the "take-over" pacemaker's intrinsic rate is greater than 45 bpm, and the patient may be asymptomatic. Mortality is 20% to 40%.

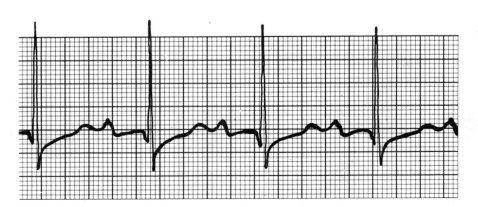

Figure 16-13 First degree A-V block. (Hudak C: Critical Care Nursing, 3rd ed, p 131. Philadelphia, JB Lippincott, 1982)

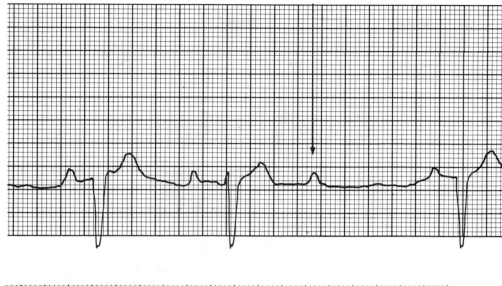

A

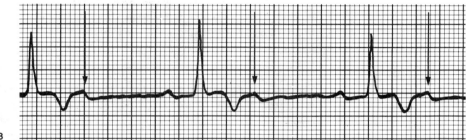

B

Figure 16-14 *Second degree block. A. Mobitz I (Wenckebach). The arrow indicates the nonconducted P wave in this sequence. B. Mobitz II. Arrows denote blocked P waves. (Hudak C: Critical Care Nursing, 3rd ed, p 132. Philadelphia, JB Lippincott, 1982)*

Anterior Wall AMI. In contrast, AV conduction disturbances with anterior-wall AMIs occur suddenly because of an actual area of infarction in the ventricular septum and involvement of the bundle branches of the conduction system. Mobitz II can be a preliminary rhythm, prior to complete heart block. In this case, the heart rate is set by a low-paced pacemaker in the ventricles, the QRS complex is wide, and the intrinsic pacemaker rate is below 45 bpm, producing degrees of circulatory failure. The mortality is high.

Treatment of Heart Block

Treatment of the various degrees of block depends on the clinical status of the patient and the potential for the patient's developing more severe forms of block.

First-degree AV block, with its concomitant PR prolongation, is not treated unless a new bundle branch block is associated with it. Mobitz I second-degree block normally is not treated either unless the patient develops significant

Figure 16-15 *Third degree block (complete A-V block). (Hudak C: Critical Care Nursing, 3rd ed, p 133. Philadelphia, JB Lippincott, 1982)*

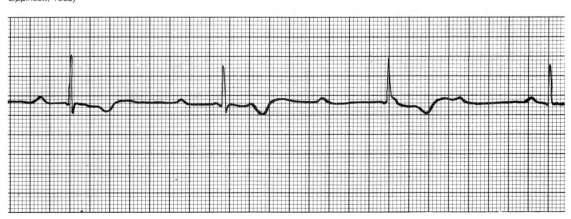

symptoms. However, Mobitz II second-degree block, associated with an anterior-wall AMI, should alert the emergency department staff that the patient could be in danger of developing complete heart block rather quickly. The treatment of choice for Mobitz II or complete heart block is a pacemaker. If not immediately available, an isproterenol (Isuprel) drip should be prepared for administration to increase the rate of ventricular contraction until the pacemaker and the cardiologist are ready.

Assess the patient to see how well he is tolerating the ventricular rate. Rates below 45 bpm significantly alter the hemodynamic status; expect the patient to show changes in level of consciousness, decreased blood pressure, cold, clammy skin, and lung rales. The ECG will show a slow, wide idioventricular rhythm.

Adams-Stokes (or Stokes-Adams) syndrome is a loss of consciousness with or without seizures, resulting from a sudden decrease in cerebral perfusion. The underlying pathology is cardiac arrhythmia, usually a sudden onset of transient complete heart block. Diagnosis of the underlying cause is assisted by the use of an ambulatory cardiac monitoring system.

CARDIOGENIC SHOCK

Cardiogenic shock is the one clinical problem that has remained resistant to treatment despite the tremendous advances in medicine. Mortality from "heart attack" for the hospitalized patient has remained at a 10% to 15% level for many years and is caused mostly by cardiogenic shock. The mortality for this complication is greater than 80%. Studies have suggested that there is a higher incidence of shock with documented anterior-wall infarcts. Typically, the patient is elderly and has a history of previous MI.

Cardiogenic shock is a severe impairment of pump function, producing inadequate perfusion to all body tissues, which is precipitated by an AMI. There is a direct relationship between the percentage of myocardium destroyed by the infarction and the degree of impairment of the pump function of the heart. If 40% or greater of the left ventricle is infarcted, the pumping action of the heart is critically hampered and severe left ventricular failure can be expected. Initially, a patient may have less than 40% of his left ventricle affected but the infarction may be extended by inadequate treatment of arrhythmias, hypotensive states, or less severe forms of heart failure. The theory of extension after initial infarct is supported by the fact that most patients develop cardiogenic shock some hours after the initial MI.

ASSESSMENT

In addition to the signs and symptoms of cardiac distress that may be present, the patient manifests:
- Cool, clammy, pale skin
- Systolic blood pressure less than 90 mm Hg in the normotensive individual

- Altered level of consciousness and behavior changes such as increased lethargy, restlessness, or agitation
- Urinary output less than 20 ml per hour
- Clinical findings suggesting metabolic acidosis

TREATMENT

Goals of treatment are to improve cardiac output and contractibility without increasing stress and oxygen consumption of the heart. No one therapeutic approach has been uniformly successful: several therapies may be tried until the patient's response becomes as close to optimal as possible. Treatment modalities, in general, aim at manipulating the patient's preload or afterload. (See pp 233–234)

The preload and afterload should not be lowered too drastically lest it decrease the coronary blood flow. Conversely, raising the blood pressure too high, to preinfarction levels, increases the work load of the failing heart and costs too much in terms of energy. Hemodynamic monitoring with a pulmonary artery catheter and transducer is essential. Treatment measures for cardiogenic shock are presented in Chart 16-6. Drug therapy is outlined in Table 16-4.

ACUTE PULMONARY EDEMA CAUSED BY CONGESTIVE HEART FAILURE

Acute pulmonary edema of cardiac origin is a common cardiovascular emergency. Congestive heart failure is the most severe manifestation of this underlying disease state.

Congestive heart failure (*CHF*) is a syndrome in which the heart's cardiac output is insufficient to meet the metabolic needs of the body's tissues. The disease state involves either the left or the right ventricle initially (termed *left ventricular failure* or *right ventricular failure,* respectively).

Most CHF involves the left side of the heart, because CAD and hypertension chiefly affect the left side. When right ventricular failure does occur, it is usually secondary to left ventricular failure with pulmonary involvement: the weaker, lower-pressured right side cannot eject blood into a pulmonary system made hypertensive by the increased fluid pressures from the failing left side. Similarly, patients with chronic lung disease, congenital heart defects, or rheumatic mitral valve disease can develop right-sided heart failure.

Less common heart failures involving a normal heart but excessive body demands include conditions such as hyperthyroidism and anemia. These are examples of *high output failure,* a term indicating that cardiac output is normal or even greater than normal, but still inadequate.

This discussion is limited to the "low-output failure" resulting from conditions such as CAD, MI, hypertension, valvular disease, and COPD.

PATHOPHYSIOLOGY OF CONGESTIVE HEART FAILURE

The weakened left ventricle has an impaired ventricular contractile force; cardiac function is diminished and output falls. With each ejection, the ventricle does not empty itself as completely and the pressure within the ventricle rises because of increased residual volume.

Sympathetic stimulation increases the heartbeat and the force of contraction. Sympathetic stimulation also increases peripheral vascular resistance and shifts blood flow to the vital organs, such as the heart and brain. This mechanism augments the volume load in the heart (preload), and the heart responds to a degree.

With increased peripheral vascular resistance, blood flow to the kidney is reduced; the kidney responds by activating a complex feedback mechanism to conserve water and sodium. This action raises the total volume of body water and sodium and increases blood volume. Augmented blood volume can be seen as the body's attempt to increase the volume load in the heart and therefore, again, encourage the Starling response of the myocardial fibers to contract more vigorously.

These mechanisms work well over time, but are limiting when the heart's ability to respond begins to diminish. Additional compensatory mechanisms may develop. The ventricular muscle hypertrophies and the heart dilates, but these are less effective measures to maintain cardiac output.

ASSESSMENT

Early Signs/Symptoms of Left Ventricular Failure

Signs and symptoms of left ventricular failure may begin slowly. The following are common early signs and symptoms.

Fatigue. One of the earliest symptoms is *fatigue,* which increases as the day wears on.

Nocturia. Another early finding is *nocturia;* body fluid is pooled in the periphery during the day and is not handled by the kidney because of poor cardiac output and poor kidney perfusion. The fluid rejoins the vascular compartment when the patient retires and lies down. Mobilized fluid can then be filtered through the kidneys owing to the improved renal blood flow and the patient begins voiding large amounts of urine after retiring.

Orthopnea. If the movement of the water from the periphery into the vascular compartment is large enough and if the left ventricle is unable to handle it, fluid "backs up" into the pulmonary capillary space, exceeding normal pulmonary capillary pressures. Movement of fluid (transudation) into the interstitial tissues of the lung occurs. The patient discovers he is more comfortable with his head elevated on two or more pillows at night (*orthopnea*).

Paroxysmal Nocturnal Dyspnea. If the fluid fills some lung alveoli, the patient awakens in a panic, feeling highly anxious and dyspneic. This is paroxysmal nocturnal dyspnea (PND).

Sinus Tachycardia. Persistent unexplained sinus tachycardia may be present—a compensatory mechanism to improve cardiac output.

Other Arrhythmias. Additional arrhythmias seen with CHF are PACs, atrial fibrillation, PAT, and PVCs.

Cardiac Asthma. With increased movement of fluid from the interstitial space of the pulmonary tree into the alveoli and bronchioles, a reflex spasm of the bronchioles produces a wheezing similar to asthma. Such wheezing, associated with heart failure, is referred to as "cardiac asthma." Fine "crackling" rales can be heard in the lower lobes of the lungs.

Abnormal Heart Sounds. Abnormal heart sounds, such as ventricular or atrial gallops (S_3, S_4) may be noted at the mitral (apical) area. The abnormal third heart sound closely follows the second and is an important sign of left ventricular failure.

Signs and Symptoms of Acute Pulmonary Edema

Acute pulmonary edema is a medical emergency in which the heart's ability to match output to body need fails dramatically.

Increasing Pressures. Pressures increase in the left ventricle, left atrium, and pulmonary vasculature. Increased pulmonary capillary pressure causes a rapid transudation of fluid into the interstitial spaces, alveoli, and bronchioles.

Extreme Dyspnea and Anxiety. Oxygen exchange is hampered. The pO_2 falls. Carbon dioxide exchange is adequate initially because carbon dioxide exchanges in a wet atmosphere better than oxygen does. As fluid fills the bronchioles, the patient begins to cough; small capillaries that have ruptured because of the increase in lung pressure tint the frothy sputum pink. The patient struggles to breathe. Breath sounds are audible; rales, rhonchi, and wheezing may be present, and the patient appears highly anxious.

Pale, Cold, Wet Skin. High levels of circulating catecholamines contribute to the pale, cold, and wet skin. They enhance cardiac irritability, producing arrhythmias.

Restlessness, Confusion. With poor oxygen exchange and cardiac output, the patient's cerebral function is affected and he becomes confused, irrational, or hostile.

Reduced Level of Consciousness. As the patient's condition worsens, his carbon dioxide level begins to rise because of his increasingly ineffectual respiratory movements. Simultaneously, anaerobic metabolism in the periphery contributes large amounts of lactic acid, producing a metabolic acidosis that further depresses cardiac muscle function and lowers the level of consciousness.

Falling Blood Pressure. As the cardiac output falls, so does the blood pressure; the initial increase in peripheral vascular resistance can no longer be maintained. Immediate treatment is mandatory to prevent death.

Chart 16-6

MANAGEMENT OF THE PATIENT IN CARDIOGENIC SHOCK

Management/Treatment	Rationale/Comment

Prehospital Care

1. Place patient in position of comfort, usually low to semi-Fowlers position.
2. Administer oxygen as soon as it becomes available.
3. Cover patient to maintain body heat.
4. Give nothing by mouth.
5. Monitor vital signs, level of consciousness, and skin color, paying particular attention to the blood pressure and pulse strength and regularity.

Rationale: Some head elevation will ease respiratory efforts yet maintain cerebral blood flow.

Advanced Prehospital and Hospital Care

1. Determine presence of other conditions that cause the hypotensive state—arrhythmias, pain, overuse of morphine, antiarrhythmic drugs, hypoxia, acidosis.
     If arrhythmias such as bradycardia or a tachycardia are present, treat promptly and check patient's response to treatment.
     Provide O_2, pain relief.

Rationale: In addition to pump failure, many factors can predispose to hypotensive state.

2. Assist the physician with the placement of hemodynamic monitoring catheters
   - CVP

   - Swan-Ganz catheter

   - Arterial pressure catheter

Rationale: The CVP catheter measures pressures in the right side of the heart; it indicates the general state of hydration in the body and is a reflection of right-side heart pressures. It does not reflect left ventricle pressures.
The Swan-Ganz catheter is a four-lumen catheter that can measure four different parameters: CVP, cardiac output, pulmonary artery pressure, and pulmonary artery wedge pressure. These last two pressures give important information about pressures in the left ventricle.
An arterial pressure catheter directly measures systolic/diastolic pressures and mean arterial pressure. Also, it makes arterial blood available for blood gas assessment.

3. Obtain arterial blood sample

MANAGEMENT

Management of the patient with acute pulmonary edema is detailed in Chart 16-7. Emergency personnel should consider this added precaution: Drugs such as morphine sulfate, furosemide (Lasix), and aminophylline can be provided by paramedic services in many communities. Starting this treatment may be life saving to the patient with acute pulmonary edema. However, the patient must be assessed carefully before administration of such potent drugs: giving morphine to a patient who is dyspneic because of an exacerbation of COPD would be a grave error.

CARDIAC TRAUMA

With the increase in high-speed automobile accidents and violent crimes, the number of victims of cardiac trauma has

---

Chart 16-6

MANAGEMENT OF THE PATIENT IN CARDIOGENIC SHOCK (*CONTINUED*)

Management/Treatment	Rationale/Comment

Advanced Prehospital and Hospital Care (*continued*)

4. If the patient's CVP and pulmonary artery pressures are low, begin a fluid challenge and monitor all parameters closely. Report changes promptly. Watch for rales, decrease in BP. Fluid challenge may be done with dextran, serum albumin, or D₅W. Fluid should infuse at 20–50 ml/min. Stop infusion if CVP > 20 mm Hg, if pulmonary wedge pressure is >20 mm Hg, or if CVP rises more than 3 mm Hg after 50 ml of infusion.

   Occasionally, owing to use of diuretics, excessive diaphoresis, vomiting, peripheral pooling after morphine, or hemorrhage, the patient may be volume depleted. Correction of this deficit may reverse the shock state.

5. If the patient's status or hemodynamic parameters do not indicate a fluid challenge, prepare for administration of drugs such as vasopressors, inotropic agents, steroids, and vasodilators (Table 16-8)

   Hypotension must be corrected to improve coronary blood flow and support ventricular function. The treatment goal is to maintain the systolic BP at 90–100 mm Hg.

6. If the patient's status remains unchanged or deteriorates, the intra-aortic balloon pump may be used as a temporary measure.

   To assist the failing heart, an inflating/deflating balloon is introduced through a large catheter that has been inserted through the patient's femoral artery and placed in the descending aorta. The balloon inflates during diastole, and blood is propelled forward through systemic arteries and backward (retrograde), thus improving flow into the coronary arteries. It deflates before systole and reduces pressure in the aorta against which the heart has to work (afterload).

Important Points to Remember

- Assess the patient frequently. Arrhythmias, pain, and hypovolemia are correctable and can alter the patient's status if treatment is begun early. Check on the possibility of excessive morphine use in the prehospital phase, which could account for the decrease in blood pressure.
- Monitor vital signs, level of consciousness, and hemodynamic parameters carefully and frequently. Observe ECG monitor closely. Urine output should be checked hourly.
- Administer drug therapy as ordered; understand the rationale for the treatment and the expected, desired effect. Use an IV infusion pump or controller.
- Supplement oxygen intake. Monitor arterial blood gases. Be alert for acidosis.
- Keep the family informed. The patient is seriously ill and family anxiety is high. Obtain the help of a social worker, priest, minister, or rabbi if it is in the best interests of the patient and family.

---

also increased. Gains achieved by advances in prehospital care and transportation have brought victims of potentially lethal trauma to emergency departments in time to be saved.

In many hospitals, a trauma room is set aside within the emergency department for trauma victims so that resuscitation may proceed without dangerous delays prior to transfer to the operating suite. Because surgical intervention will probably be required, the cardiac trauma patient is best transported to a hospital that has a ready surgical staff and equipment capable of handling extracorporeal circulation.

Cardiac trauma falls into two main categories:

1. *Nonpenetrating cardiac injury:* Blunt chest trauma associated with auto injuries in which the chest strikes an object or with falls, crushing injuries, explosions, and cave-ins

2. *Penetrating cardiac injury* involving a weapon such as a knife, icepick, shotgun, or handgun. According to one source, this type of injury is more rapidly fatal; over 50% of the patients die before reaching the hospital. The most deadly weapon of the four mentioned is the shotgun because of its ability to cause massive tissue injury.

TABLE 16-4. DRUG THERAPY IN CARDIOGENIC SHOCK

Class	Dosage	Expected Response
Vasopressors		
Norepinephrine (Levophed)	5–30 µg/min (8–16 mg/500 D_5W)	A powerful vasoconstrictor; raises BP and improves coronary blood flow when the patient is hypotensive. Caution: increases O_2 consumption of the myocardium. Systolic pressure of 90–100 mm Hg is adequate for perfusion yet will not increase the work of the heart excessively. A direct heart stimulant, but not to the degree of epinephrine or isoproterenol.
Metaraminol (Aramine)	0.5 mg–5.0 mg (100 mg/500 D_5W)	A vasoconstrictor and a moderate direct heart stimulant. Assists release of stored catecholamines from nerve endings; if body has been depleted by continued stress or if drug has been used for several days, it will not be effective.
Inotropic agents		
Dopamine (Intropin)	5–20 µg/kg/min 200 mg/250 D_5W IV drip	Both sympathomimetic agents boosts cardiac output. Dopamine at high doses vasoconstricts peripheral vessels and raises arterial pressure.
Dobutamine (Dobutrex)	2.5–10 µg/kg/min 250 mg/ 250–500 ml D_5W IV drip	
Isoproterenol (Isuprel)	2–4 µg/min (1–2 mg/500 D_5W)	A potent β-adrenergic drug that increases heart rate and cardiac output and dilates arteriole smooth muscle. Dobutamine does not increase the heart rate as much as dopamine and does not constrict the peripheral vessels. However, increases O_2 consumption of the myocardium and the work of the heart. May be dangerous in patient with AMI or cardiac disease.
Vasodilating agent		
Sodium nitroprusside (Nipride)	0.5–10 µg/kg/min (50 mg/500 D_5W)	This vasodilator helps reduce afterload and lessen the work load and O_2 consumption of the heart. Also by decreasing arterial resistance, more volume circulates to the periphery, reducing preload. This drug is used only on specific patients with high arterial pressure. Swan-Ganz monitoring for left heart pressures is necessary.

NONPENETRATING CARDIAC INJURY (See Chap. 21)

An automobile accident involving rapid deceleration is the most common cause of nonpenetrating cardiac injury. The heart, suspended in the pericardial sac within the chest cavity, moves forward and slams against the chest wall, which itself may have been thrown against the steering wheel. Because of the strong forces and speed involved, isolated injuries are not likely. Injuries to the pericardium, myocardium, cardiac valves, coronary arteries, great vessels, pulmonary structures, and abdominal organs are all possible. The most common injuries to the heart from blunt trauma are myocardial contusion and myocardial rupture.

Myocardial Contusion

Bruising of the heart muscle may range from mild edema of a small area to large-scale necrosis of the myocardium. Chest pain, ECG and serial cardiac enzyme profile findings are similar to those of a patient with an AMI. If the area of cardiac contusion involves the electrical conduction system, various degrees of heart block or other ventricular arrhythmias may result.

Treatment. Treatment is similar to that for AMI: bed rest, pain relief, monitoring, and antiarrhythmic medications as appropriate. Recovery without other complicating injuries is likely with less extensive contusions.

Cardiac Rupture

Cardiac rupture, when it involves the ventricle, has a high mortality rate; some patients have survived atrial rupture.

Occasionally, the ventricular septum may be the sole site of rupture as a result of a previously contused and necrosed segment.

Treatment. Surgical treatment is necessary to repair the ruptured site.

Blunt Trauma to the Aorta

Blunt trauma to the aorta may occur with deceleration injuries. With the forward movement of the heart, the aorta is stretched, resulting in hemorrhage on the intimal or medial surfaces—partial or complete laceration—or in formation of an aortic aneurysm. Physical findings that suggest injury to the aorta include severe chest pain radiating to the scapula region, dyspnea, pulse inequalities, hypertension of the upper extremities, widening of the mediastinum (on x-ray), and tracheal deviation.

Treatment. Treatment depends on the extent of the patient's injuries and his physical status. If it is desirable to delay surgery (because of coexisting injuries) the patient may be treated with antihypertensive drugs and monitored carefully. Otherwise, surgical intervention for aorta repair is done immediately.

PENETRATING CARDIAC INJURY (See Chap. 21)

Because of the anatomic position of the heart within the thoracic cavity, penetrating heart injury most often involves the ventricles (70%–77%). The right ventricle is more frequently injured because it lies in an anterior and more prominent position than does the left ventricle. Of all cardiac wounds, 10% to 11% involve the atria; 16% to 20% involve the great vessels and the pericardium.

Cardiac Tamponade

Cardiac tamponade is the common underlying pathologic event in penetrating cardiac injury. Bleeding into the pericardial sac producing tamponade is common with stab wounds. Between 80% and 90% of victims develop tamponade after penetrating injury because of self-sealing of the pericardium. The tamponade, in turn, may slow the bleeding from the initial wound in the myocardium and may contribute initially to the patient's survival. However, the tough, nonelastic pericardium can only accommodate 80 ml to 120 ml of fluid without seriously affecting cardiac muscle function and output. If the leak into the pericardial sac is slow enough, the sac can distend and stretch over time, accommodating large volumes of fluid without effect on the pumping activity of the heart. However, in sudden penetrating injuries, the volume of blood collects too rapidly.

In early tamponade, when the pericardial volume is less than 200 ml, the first observable signs are an increase in heart rate and a rise in central venous pressure (CVP). As the pericardial volume increases to about 200 ml, cardiac output and stroke volume decrease and the classic Beck's triad of signs appears:

1. Hypotension with a decrease in pulse pressure
2. Neck-vein distention
3. Muffled or distant heart sounds

With further volume increases within the pericardial sac, the CVP rises as high as 30 cm to 40 cm of water. Cardiac output and stroke volume drop to very low levels and the patient may be close to cardiac arrest. The time sequence for these events varies from minutes to hours.

Other signs suggesting tamponade include pulsus paradoxus, in which there is a greater-than-normal inspiratory decrease in systolic arterial pressure, and ECG changes such as electrical alternans and low-voltage QRS complexes.

Treatment. Treatment is aimed at making the diagnosis, relieving the tamponade, improving cardiac function, and stabilizing the patient for cardiac repair. Pericardiocentesis can aid in both establishing the diagnosis and relieving the tamponade, if only temporarily. Dramatic improvement is seen with the removal of only a small volume of blood from the sac; this buys time for the emergency department staff to stabilize and further assess the patient.

Thoracotomy for exploration and repair of the cardiac wound is the recommended treatment. Some studies suggest that patient mortality from stab wounds drops when patients are treated aggressively and reach the operating room for thoracotomy within 2 hours of the initial event. Treatment measures are summarized in Chart 16-8.

HYPERTENSION

An estimated 20% of adults in the United States have elevated blood pressures; of that total group, only 15% to 25% are under treatment and adequately controlled. Untreated hypertension increases the risks of developing the following cardiovascular problems: cardiomegaly, CHF, stroke, AMI, and renal insufficiency. However, with good control, patients with hypertensive disease can reduce such risks by 70% to 90%.

Parameters used to diagnose hypertension are not absolute, and such factors as age, sex, and race can alter blood pressure interpretation. In general, blood pressure equal to or greater than 140/90 may signify hypertension, but serial readings over time are required to establish the diagnosis.

In 80% to 90% of cases, the etiology of hypertension is unknown, and the terms *essential, primary,* or *idiopathic* hypertension are used.

As research continues, however, the role of the kidney in the development of hypertension becomes more suspect. Other factors contributing to the development of primary hypertension include sodium intake, obesity, high stress, smoking, elevated serum cholesterol, and heredity.

Hypertension is associated with accelerated atherosclerosis and all of its attendant complications; statistics show that untreated hypertension will shorten the life span by 10 to 20 years, most often because of the accelerated atherosclerosis process.

Secondary hypertension, in which the elevated blood pressure is secondary to some primary disease, accounts for less than 10% to 12% of all cases of hypertension. Endocrine diseases involving the adrenals (pheochromocytoma, aldosteronism, Cushing's syndrome), the pituitary gland (acromegaly), and the thyroid (hyperthyroidism) should be considered. Renal diseases, especially those involving the renal vasculature such as renal artery stenosis, can cause secondary hypertension.

Hypertensive diseases range from mild, labile blood pressure elevation to the hypertensive crisis, a medical emergency.

LABILE HYPERTENSION

Labile, or borderline, hypertension occurs in response to physical and psychological stress. As the stress disappears, the pressure returns to normal. Such patients should have regular blood pressure checks because persons with demonstrated labile hypertension can develop sustained blood pressure elevation.

CHRONIC HYPERTENSION

A patient who has sustained elevated blood pressures and other objective signs of the disease is said to have chronic hypertension. Since the patient with a mild to moderate elevation may be in the emergency department for reasons unrelated to hypertension, the goal is to assess the reason(s) for the blood pressure elevation and to institute a program of blood pressure control and for follow-up care.

Assessment

Assessment of a patient with chronic hypertension may include an ECG to observe signs of left ventricular hypertrophy and laboratory tests such as CBC, electrolytes, BUN, creat-

Chart 16-7

MANAGEMENT OF THE PATIENT WITH ACUTE PULMONARY EDEMA

Management/Treatment	Rationale/Comment
Prehospital Care	
Offer reassurance to patient and family.	Reducing stress decreases work load of the heart.
Place patient in position of comfort, usually upright. If able, he should dangle legs over the edge of stretcher.	Upright position makes use of surface area of the lung in the apex for gas exchange and decreases the work of breathing. If the patient were to lie flat, a greater lung area would be covered by lung water. Placing legs in a dependent position helps to pool some of the blood volume in the extremities and lessen preload (venous return) to the heart.
Begin oxygen therapy. Use IPPB if available.	O_2 given under pressure may encourage fluid to move from the alveoli into the capillaries and improve O_2 exchange, reducing hypoxemia.
Advanced Prehospital and Hospital Care	
Begin lifeline of D_5W; use microdrip drip chamber, monitor infusion rate carefully.	Drugs should be given IV for faster response and more accurate titration to patient status. Fluid monitoring is crucial to prevent further fluid overload.
Monitor cardiac rhythm; obtain baseline rhythm strip.	With the hypoxic state, low cardiac output, and high catecholamine levels, cardiac arrhythmias are common. Treatment of the underlying cause often eliminates arrhythmias without additional drug therapy.
Begin drug therapy Furosemide (Lasix) (40–120 mg IV push)	A powerful diuretic such as furosemide reduces circulating blood volume by means of rapid diuresis and lessens the high pulmonary capillary pressure. Furosemide also reduces blood volume returning to the right side of the heart by decreasing venous tone in the periphery, which helps to pool blood volume. Diuresis begins within 30 min.
Morphine sulfate (3 mg–5 mg IV push)	Morphine reduces venous return by venodilation (a "pharmacologic tourniquet"), reduces respiratory rate, and decreases anxiety and pain.
Rotating tourniquets	Tourniquets reduce blood return to the heart by pooling venous blood in the peripheral vessels. Tourniquets are not as effective as prompt drug therapy but may be a useful adjunct.

Chart 16-7

MANAGEMENT OF THE PATIENT WITH ACUTE PULMONARY EDEMA (*CONTINUED*)

Management/Treatment	Rationale/Comment

Advanced Prehospital and Hospital Care (*continued*)

Management/Treatment	Rationale/Comment
Aminophylline (250 mg in 20 ml–30 ml over 20–30 min)	Aminophylline relaxes smooth muscle; it relieves bronchospasm when present in pulmonary edema (reflex action brought on by fluid entering the bronchioles). It also increases heart rate, which may or may not be desired. In addition, there is a mild diuretic effect. Avoid this drug in patients with AMI because it increases ventricular irritability and work for the myocardium.
Continue or begin all measures noted in prehospital care protocol. Place patient in acute bed; have resuscitation equipment on standby.	
Continue to monitor patient's rhythm, vital signs, breath sounds, and level of consciousness. Administer O_2.	
Monitor results from blood gas studies and draw blood for lab work.	A falling PO_2 (<50 mm Hg) with a PCO_2 greater than 50 mm Hg indicates that the patient is facing acute respiratory failure and is unable to maintain adequate ventilation unassisted.
Note times all drugs are administered. Begin I & O sheet; insert Foley catheter if ordered. Obtain 12-lead ECG	
Begin drug therapy Digitalis (0.5 mg–0.75 mg IV push initially)	Digitalis increases myocardial contractibility but is not a first-line drug. It can be dangerous in a patient with AMI because of the unpredictability of patient response. Avoid unless CHF is severe enough to warrant its use. If so, use with caution.
Vasodilator therapy: Nitrates (sublingual, oral paste) Nitroprusside Phentolamine Trimethaphan Hexamethonium Hydralazine	These drugs may be used in patients whose clinical course is not responding to traditional pharmacologic agents. Depending on the drug, vasodilator therapy may reduce arterial resistance (afterload) and thereby lessen the work load on the left ventricle and improve cardiac output. Or, the drug(s) may reduce preload volume by reducing venous tone.
Assist with phlebotomy.	This therapy is a second-line measure used when other therapies seem ineffective and the patient remains overloaded with blood volume. Drawing off 100 ml to 500 ml of blood will reduce volume quickly.
Prepare for hospital admission.	

Chart 16-8

MANAGEMENT OF THE PATIENT WITH CARDIAC TRAUMA

Management/Treatment	Rationale/Comment

Prehospital Care

- Carefully evaluate airway, breathing circulation, vital signs, level of consciousness, skin color, and evidence of chest injury. Be prepared to initiate CPR in the critically injured patient.
- Begin high-flow oxygen as soon as possible.
- Control external bleeding, stabilize impaled objects or flail section, apply occlusive dressing to sucking chest wound.
- Obtain details of trauma, description of weapon or mechanism of injury.

Description of the patient at the scene and associated components of the trauma or accident facilitate assessment. For example, the presence of a collapsed steering wheel, the severity of explosion, the approximate distance of fall, the length of the knife, or the caliber of the gun can give clues to the possibility or severity of injury.

Advanced Prehospital and Hospital Care

- Assess pulses for rate, rhythm, quality, and character and attach patient to cardiac monitor. Have crash cart available.

Cardiac arrhythmias or arrest are likely.

- Begin IV therapy; insert large-bore catheters into peripheral veins. Infuse IV solution at prescribed rate. If CVP line is to be inserted, assist and take baseline reading.

Successful resuscitation depends on good body fluid replacement.

- Draw blood for baseline studies; request stat handling. Instruct lab to set up sufficient units of blood for surgery.

If necessary, type O-negative blood can be used in extreme emergencies.

Continue to monitor patient's vital signs.
- Anticipate the development of signs and symptoms of shock or tamponade.
Record.

Beck's Triad (suspect cardiac tamponade):
- Low BP with narrow pulse pressure
- Neck-vein distention
- Muffled heart sounds

- Prepare for chest tube insertion. Obtain thoracotomy tray, underwater seal drainage system.

An unrelieved pneumothorax or hemothorax can reduce lung tissue available for effective and necessary oxygenation.

- Assist. Note drainage obtained, patient's pre- and post-treatment status.
- If necessary, prepare for pericardiocentesis; obtain tray, dual-channel monitor-ECG machine, defibrillator, crash cart, and support personnel.

If procedure reveals blood in the pericardium, prepare patient for transport to OR, since cardiac repair will be needed.

- Assist. Note amount and quality of fluid obtained from pericardiocentesis and patient's response.
- If patient deteriorates rapidly or arrests, stand by to assist with CPR, thoracotomy. Ready suction tubing, switch defibrillation paddles to internal and reduce watt-seconds.

inine, calcium, uric acid, cholesterol, and triglycerides, blood glucose, and urinalysis.

Management and Treatment

Management and treatment of chronic hypertension may include the following:
- Reduce sodium intake
- Reduce body weight
- Decrease intake of saturated fats in the diet
- Reduce alcohol and coffee consumption
- Eliminate smoking
- Reduce stress factors by relaxation techniques or exercise, or by altering environmental factors.

Patient education is essential in order to promote understanding of the outlined regimen and compliance with it.

Drug therapy may be necessary. The three classes of drugs used either singly or in combination are (1) diuretics to decrease the peripheral vascular resistance, (2) sympatholytic agents to counteract the vasoconstrictive effects of the sympathetic nervous system, and (3) vasodilators to relax smooth muscle and reduce vascular tone.

Although it is unlikely that emergency department personnel would be involved in the long-term treatment of patients with diagnosed chronic hypertension, they can participate in case-finding and referral. Patient compliance can be aided by supportive professionals willing to emphasize and explain key points of management.

ACCELERATED OR MALIGNANT HYPERTENSION

Accelerated or malignant hypertension denotes a sudden, sustained rise in blood pressure leading to a diastolic pressure greater than 120 mm Hg. This complication occurs in 2% to 7% of patients with known hypertensive disease. These patients, between 40 and 60 years of age, give a history of having chronic hypertension, usually poorly controlled, for at least 2 years. Depending on the clinical picture and the degree of involvement or damage of other organ systems, a treatment plan aimed at blood pressure reduction may be spread over several days or may be more immediate. Malignant hypertension is regarded as one type of hypertensive crisis.

HYPERTENSIVE CRISIS

Prolonged elevation of blood pressure (greater than 120 mm Hg diastolic) can lead to a variety of clinical conditions indicating organ damage. Systems particularly at risk are the optical, cardiovascular, kidney, and CNS.

Assessment

- Changes in the eye, such as the presence of retinal hemorrhage and exudates and papilledema (choked disk), can occur.

- Kidney involvement may be manifested by elevated BUN, gross hematuria, and a decrease in urinary output.
- Cardiovascular system damage is observed with chest pain, acute left ventricular failure, pulmonary edema, AMI, or dissecting thoracic aneurysm.
- Acute hypertensive encephalopathy is suggested by the sudden onset of a severe elevated diastolic pressure (often greater than 150 mm Hg), severe headache, altered level of consciousness, and increased intracranial pressure with cerebral edema and retinal changes. Death may result if the condition is not treated.

Treatment and Management

The treatment plan for anyone presenting with an abnormally high diastolic blood pressure depends on the presence and degree of organ involvement. Rapid blood pressure reduction and control using parenteral drug therapy isn't always indicated for a hypertensive condition in which oral antihypertensive drugs, bed rest, and hospitalization will bring about the same results over time. Care should be taken to rule out other disease states that may present but are correctible through other treatment approaches, like a hypertensive crisis. Neurologic emergencies, pulmonary edema with left ventricular failure, and labile hypertension with acute anxiety fall into this category. Management of the patient in hypertensive crisis is outlined in Chart 16-9.

INFLAMMATION OF THE HEART

The onset of inflammatory problems can be sudden, severe, and life-threatening. Treatment for the specific condition may also include procedures involving other organ systems such as the pulmonary, central nervous, or genitourinary systems.

Infective endocarditis (acute or subacute bacterial endocarditis) is a microbial infection of the valves or endocardium. Pericarditis is an inflammatory process of the pericardium, including the pericardial space. Though it does not normally affect heart function, pericarditis can lead to complications such as cardiac tamponade. Pericarditis can be due to an infective process or can arise from other causes such as metastatic carcinoma, collagen diseases, acute rheumatic fever, or trauma.

Chart 16-10 outlines the etiology, significant patient data, presenting signs and symptoms, and complications associated with these inflammatory diseases of the heart.

Treatment

Patients with infectious endocarditis are treated with antibiotics selected according to the sensitivity of the organism to various antibiotic drugs available. The patient should un-

Chart 16-9

MANAGEMENT OF THE PATIENT IN HYPERTENSIVE CRISIS

Prehospital Care

- Prehospital emergency personnel cannot diagnose a true hypertensive crisis in the field because needed diagnostic tests are available only in the hospital. Drugs and monitoring systems used to treat hypertensive crisis are not commonly carried by field personnel.
- Initiate supportive treatment.
- Obtain an accurate history and list of current medications.
- Assess the patient and gather on-site information.

Hospital Care

Management/Treatment	Rationale/Comment
1. Assist with general assessment, history, physical exam, vital signs. Continue to assess BP, pulse rate, and respirations q 5–15 min as indicated by patient's clinical status or drug therapy. Record all data.	Most commonly, patient or family will affirm that patient has a hypertensive history.
2. Obtain a list of current medications; check whether patient has complied well with prescribed regimen.	
3. Elevate bed 30°. Reduce physical, emotional stress.	
4. Assist with specific exams to check for retinal or neurologic damage. Check level of consciousness, pupil response, motor-sensory parameters frequently.	Existence of positive retinal or neurologic findings along with elevated diastolic pressure supports the diagnosis of hypertensive crisis.
5. Obtain blood and urine for baseline lab data—CBC, BUN, creatinine, electrolytes, glucose, urinalysis, and culture.	The lab tests help determine functional renal status and blood serum changes, which could indicate an unknown underlying disease state. Electrolyte blood glucose alterations may accompany antihypertensive drug therapy.
6. Obtain 12-lead ECG for baseline. Place patient on monitor; obtain rhythm strip.	If underlying primary cardiac disease is suspected, serial ECGs are indicated.
7. Monitor airway and breathing. Begin O_2 therapy if indicated.	
8. Start IV in large vein with D_5W to keep open. Obtain infusion pump if treatment plan involves the use of parenteral drugs.	Antihypertensive drugs are potent and need to be infused carefully at the exact rate prescribed.
9. Assist with placement of a CVP line or pulmonary artery catheter and arterial line; attach to transducers and monitoring system. Obtain baseline pressures.	Monitoring devices may be inserted in a cardiopulmonary lab, a special procedure room, or the ICU after the patient is transferred; this is essential for close monitoring.
10. Place indwelling urinary catheter. Monitor I & O.	Accurate I & O is essential for deciding effectiveness of therapy.
11. Continue to monitor patient's neurologic status. Keep airway and bitestick at bedside. Keep suction equipment ready and crash cart nearby.	Altered level of consciousness is due to loss of autoregulation of cerebral perfusion. The end result is cerebral edema along with multiple small thrombi.
12. Transfer quickly to ICU or CCU. Accompany patient, continuing to monitor. Keep family members informed; introduce them to unit nurse.	Report baseline data and assessment information to ICU personnel. Don't forget the family. They're in crisis, too.

Chart 16-10

INFLAMMATORY HEART DISEASE

Disease	Etiology/Significant Patient Data	Presenting Signs/Symptoms	Complications
Acute infectious endocarditis	Onset: Sudden with rapid, fulminating course. Patient often has a normal heart. Responsible organism (bacterial or fungal) is highly pathogenic. Preexisting infection (*i.e.*, skin infection) often evident. Common among IV drug abusers. Can involve right side of heart, affecting the tricuspid valve. Aortic and mitral valve involvement occurs more often with drug addicts.	Fever (higher than in less acute form), malaise. Chills, petechiae common. Patient appears acutely ill with rapid deterioration. Other findings: Cardiac murmurs (most common), CHF, leukocytosis, anemia. Positive blood cultures, microscopic hematuria.	Septic infarction Rapid valvular destruction and rupture of the chordae tendineae may produce severe cardiac failure, pulmonary edema. Emboli to lung, kidney, coronary arteries, brain, or extremities. Metastatic abscesses to kidney, brain, liver. Conduction defects due to abscesses, heart block.
Subacute infectious endocarditis	Onset: Insidious, slowly progressive. May be related to dental work, urethral or vaginal procedures, tonsillectomy, URI. (Any structural irregularity in the heart may permit thrombi formation at the site, which in turn attracts bacteria implantation). Left side of heart most often involved (mitral and aortic valves). Responsible organism: Indigenous, of low pathogenicity.	Fever (most common), weakness, night sweats, loss of appetite, weight loss, joint aches. Physical exam: Patient pale, appears chronically ill; petechiae present in mucous membranes, conjunctiva, commonly on upper, anterior trunk. Painful nodules on fingers (Osler's nodes)—a classical sign but rare. Enlarged spleen. Cardiac valvular murmurs. Lab findings: Anemia, leukocytosis, elevated ESR, presence of rheumatoid factor in serum, alteration in serum protein ratio; positive blood culture.	Emboli to the lung, kidney, coronary arteries, brain, or extremities Heart failure/arrhythmias, TIA, encephalopathy, abscess, renal disease.
Acute pericarditis	Many etiologies; a good patient history will help differentiate. *Infective:* Bacterial, viral fungal, parasitic. *Posttraumatic* *Postmyocardial infarction* *Collagen Diseases:* Rheumatic fever, rheumatoid arthritis, lupus erythematosus *Metastatic disease* *Radiation*	Characteristic pain: Precordial, sharp and severe; worsens with inspiration or supine position, pain may radiate to neck, left arm/shoulder. Pericardial friction rub; may be intermittent. ECG changes (ST, T); supraventricular cardiac arrhythmias. Infective or inflammatory signs; chills and fever, sweats, headache. Ewart's sign (with pericardial effusion): bronchial breathing; percussive dullness, egophony posteriorly below angle of left scapula	Pericardial effusion: heart sounds distant Cardiac tamponade due to large effusion: above sign plus dyspnea, orthopnea, tachypnea, elevated venous pressure, hepatic engorgement, tachycardia, low pulse pressure, pulsus paradoxus >10 mm Hg

derstand the importance of taking the drug or drugs for the full prescribed course of treatment. For the patient who has developed heart failure, medical treatment with digitalis or diuretics or surgical treatment with valve replacement should be considered.

Pericarditis has many etiologies, and the treatment plan depends on the underlying cause. For patients whose in-flammatory process is caused by bacteria or fungi, antimicrobial therapy is used.

For viral inflammations, supportive therapy consisting of analgesics and anti-inflammatory agents is selected. Other treatment modalities include antiarrhythmics, antineoplastic agents, and, in the event of a cardiac tamponade or large pleural effusion, pericardiocentesis.

BIBLIOGRAPHY

BOOKS

Alpert JD, Rippe JM: Manual of Cardiovascular Diagnosis and Therapy, 1st ed. Boston, Little, Brown & Co, 1980

Andreoli KG et al: Comprehensive Cardiac Care: A text for Nurses, Physicians and other Health Practitioners, 4th ed. St Louis, CV Mosby, 1979

Baldwin L, Pierce R: Mobile Intensive Care: A Problem-Oriented Approach. St Louis, CV Mosby, 1978

Berkow R, Talbott JH (eds): The Merck Manual of Diagnosis and Therapy, 13th ed. Rahway, New Jersey, Merck Sharp & Dohme, 1977

Berndt TB, Schroeder JS, Harrison DC: Unstable angina pectoris. In Mason DT (ed): Cardiac Emergencies. Baltimore, Williams & Wilkins, 1978

Chung EK (ed): Cardiac Emergency Care. Philadelphia, Lea & Febiger, 1980

Chung EK: Principles of Cardiac Arrhythmias, 2nd ed. Baltimore, Williams & Wilkins, 1977

Coggins CH: Management of hypertensive emergencies. In Wilins EW (ed): MGH Textbook of Emergency Medicine. Baltimore, Williams & Wilkins, 1977

Combating Cardiovascular Diseases Skillfully. Horsham, Intermed Communications, 1978

Costrini NV, Thomson WM (eds): Manual of Therapeutics, 22nd ed. Boston, Little, Brown & Co, 1977

Ganong WF: Review of Medical Physiology, 8th ed. Los Altos, Lange Medical Publications, 1977

Goldman MJ: Principles of Clinical Electrocardiography, 10th ed. Los Altos, Lange Medical Publications, 1979

Isselbacher KJ, Adams RD (eds): Harrison's Principles of Internal Medicine, 9th ed. New York, McGraw-Hill, 1980

King OM: Care of the Cardiac Surgical Patient. St Louis, CV Mosby, 1975

Kones RJ: Cardiogenic Shock: Mechanism and Management. Mt Kisco, Futura, 1974

Mason DT (ed): Cardiac Emergencies. Baltimore, Williams & Wilkins, 1978

McGurn WC: The Heart: Principles of function, pathophysiology and goals of cardiac nursing care. In Kintzel KC (ed): Advanced Concepts in Clinical Nursing, 2nd ed. Philadelphia, JB Lippincott, 1977

Pepine CJ: Pericarditis. In Coo HF (ed): Current Therapy 1981. Philadelphia, WB Saunders, 1981

Rowe JW, Landsberg L: Hypertensive crisis. In Donoso E, Cohen SI (eds): Critical Cardiac Care. New York, Stratton Intercontinental, 1979

Spirak JL, Barnes HV: Manual of Clinical Problems in Internal Medicine. Boston, Little, Brown & Co, 1974

Vinsant MO, Spence MI, Hagen DC: A Commonsense Approach to Coronary Care, 2nd ed. St Louis, CV Mosby, 1975

JOURNALS

Allen RP, Liedtke AJ: The role of coronary artery injury and perfusion in the development of cardiac contusion secondary to nonpenetrating chest trauma. J Trauma 19:3, 1979

Barker LR et al: Hypertension: Spectrum of problems and guidelines for management. Ann Emerg Med 9:4, 1980

Breau EP et al: Cardiac tamponade following penetrating mediastinal injuries: Improved survival of early pericardiocentesis. J Trauma 19:6, 1979

Callaham M: Acute traumatic cardiac tamponade: Diagnosis and treatment. JACEP 7:8, 1978

Dawber TR: Annual discourse: Unproved hypothesis. N Engl J Med 299:9, 1978

DeManuelle MS et al: The recognition of infective endocarditis. JACEP 8:9, 1979

Dracup KA, Breu CS, Tillisch JH: The physiologic basis for combined nitroprusside-dopamine therapy in post-myocardial infarction heart failure. Heart Lung 10:1, 1981

Ellrodt GT, Singh BN: Adverse effects of disopyramide (Norpace): Toxic interactions with other antiarrhythmic agents. Heart Lung 9:3, 1980

Franciosa JA: Nitroglycerin and nitrates in CHF. Heart Lung 9:5, 1980

Gazes PC, Gaddy JE: Bedside management of acute myocardial infarction. Am Heart J 97:6, 1979

Harmovici H: Atherogenesis: Recent biological concepts and clinical implications: David M. Hume Memorial lecture. Am J Surg 134:2, 1977

Havlik RJ et al (eds): Proceedings of the Conference on the Decline in Coronary Heart Disease Mortality. Dept. HEW, Public Health Service, National Institute of Health, NIH 79-1610, May 1979

Heger JJ, Prystowsky EN, Zipes DP: New drugs for treatment of ventricular arrhythmias. Heart Lung 10:3, 1981

Huss P et al: The new inotropic drug dobutamine. Heart Lung 10:1, 1981

Krosgseng BA: Assessment of coronary risk factors. J Emerg Nurs, p 19, March/April 1979

Kuhn LA: Management of shock following AMI. I. Drug therapy. Am Heart J 95:4, 1978

Kuhn LA: Management of Shock following AMI. II. Mechanical circulatory assistance 95:6, 1978

Kumpuris AG, Raizner AE, Luchi RJ: The role of serum digitalis levels in clinical practice. Heart Lung 8:4, 1979

Markovchick VJ et al: Traumatic acute pericardial tamponade. JACEP 6:12, 1977

Trinket JK et al: Affairs of the wounded heart. J Trauma 19:6, 1979

APPENDIX B

EMERGENCY CARDIAC DRUGS

Drug	Dosage/Administration	Actions/Indications	Comments
Antiarrhythmics			
Bretylium tosylate (Bretylol)	IV for immediate use, 500 mg in 10-ml ampule to dilute in 50 ml D₅W Initial dose 5–10 mg/kg over 8 min. For life-threatening VF, give undiluted Bretylol, 5 mg/kg body wt by rapid IV push. May repeat and increase to 10 mg/kg body wt.	Prolongs action potential duration and effective refractory period. Increases or raises threshold for ventricular fibrillation. Indications: used for ventricular arrhythmias that have been unresponsive to first-line drugs such as lidocaine.	Can produce postural hypotension during IV administration. Keep patient flat and monitor BP. Nausea and vomiting can also occur. Keep patient on cardiac monitor.
Disopyramide phosphate (Norpace)	Oral, 400–800 mg/day total given q6h in divided doses	A cardiac depressant; depresses myocardial excitability and conduction velocity and prolongs action potential and effective refractory period. Action is similar to quinidine and procainamide. Indications: prophylactic agent for ventricular arrhythmias following AMI, such as unifocal or multifocal PVCs and for control of acute and chronic ventricular tachycardia. Side-effects: Anticholinergic signs and symptoms: dry mouth, urinary retention, visual disturbances. Has negative inotropic effects on the myocardium. Watch for ECG changes, QT prolongation.	Observe for signs of cardiac failure: decreased BP, dyspnea, skin signs, decreased urine output. Caution in patients with glaucoma, urinary
Lidocaine HCl (Xylocaine)	IV, 1–2 mg/kg body wt. as a loading dose. Following with an IV infusion of 1–4 mg/min. Solution: 1 gm in 250–500 ml D₅W. Not to exceed 300 mg/hr.	Decreases automaticity of ectopic fibers. Indications: Drug of choice to treat ventricular arrhythmias seen with AMI, digitalis toxicity. Side-effects: CNS depression ranging from disorientation to convulsions. Hypotension.	Has short half-life and can be titrated to effect. Patient must be monitored. In patients with hepatic disease or enlarged liver, decrease loading dose and IV infusion pump so as not to exceed 4 mg/min. Caution with all forms of heart block
Procainamide HCl (Pronestyl)	Oral or IM. In emergency may give IV: 50 mg–100 mg every 5 min slowly to max 1 gm (administration rate 25–50 mg/min). May give by infusion: dilute 500 mg in 250 D₅W and infuse at constant rate over 25 min.	A cardiac depressant—decreases excitability, conductivity, contractility, and automaticity; increases refractory period. Indications: Used for treatment of PVCs, tachyarrhythmias, following unsuccessful use of lidocaine. May also be used for atrial arrhythmias, such as AF. Side-effects: With IV administration of large dose, heart block, asystole, ventricular arrhythmias, severe hypotension.	Caution when patient's cardiovascular status is already compromised by conduction defects, digitalis toxicity, heart block, CHF. Patient must be monitored for ECG changes and BP drop. Keep patient flat; have vasopressors on hand.

APPENDIX B

EMERGENCY CARDIAC DRUGS (CONTINUED)

Drug	Dosage/Administration	Actions/Indications	Comments
Quinidine (different preparations)	Oral (preferred) or IM, IV Dose varies with clinical condition and quinidine preparation. Quinidine gluconate may be used parenterally. Oral: 200 mg q2–3h conversion of atrial fibrillation. 200 mg–300 mg tid or qid for treatment of PACs, PVCs. 400 mg–600 mg q2–3hr treatment of paroxysmal atrial/junctional tachycardias. IM: initial dose is 600 mg to be followed by 400 mg q2h IV: dilute 10 ml in 40 D_5W. inject slowly 1 ml/min.	Action: Cardiac depressant— decreases cardiac contractility; increases refractory period. Indications: Used to treat atrial fibrillation and flutter, premature atrial and ventricular contractions; paroxysmal atrial and ventricular tachycardias, fibrillation; maintenance after cardioversion. Side-effects: Hypotension, worsening CHF, varying degrees of block, cardiac asystole; widening of the QRS complex, prolonged QT interval. Toxicity: Nausea, vomiting, diarrhea, dizziness, visual problems, tinnitus.	If given parenterally, monitor ECG and BP. Watch for widening QRS, (>25%) and prolonged QT interval. IV administration may produce asystole, heart block, arrest. Have vasopressors, isoproterenol on hand. Undesired effects more likely in a previously damaged myocardium than in a normal heart.
Verapamil HCl (Isoptin, Calan)	IV administration 5-mg–10-mg bolus given over 2 min; may repeat 10 mg in 30 minutes. Slower rate for older patients.	Drug is a calcium antagonist that acts on the slow-current action potential (which is carried by calcium.) Actions on the heart include interruption of reentry at AV node, slowing of AV conduction, a decrease in myocardial contractility, and dilatation of peripheral and coronary arteries. Indications: Paroxysmal supraventricular tachycardia (with conversion to sinus rhythm), control of rapid ventricular rate in atrial fibrillation/flutter. Side-effects: hypotension, bradycardia, AV block, atrial systole.	Have on hand vasopressors and inotropic drugs such as norepinephrine, isoproterenol; patient should be monitored, ECG and BP taken frequently.
Investigational Antiarrhythmic Agents			
Amiodarone	Oral, IV	Indication: Resistant ventricular and supraventricular arrhythmias	
Aprindine	Oral	Indication: Treatment of acute and chronic ventricular and supraventricular arrhythmias	
Encainide	Oral, IV	Indication: Prevention and control of acute ventricular ectopy associated with WPW.	
Mexiletine	Oral, IV	Indication: Prevention and control of chronic ventricular arrhythmias similar to lidocaine	
Tocainide	Oral	Indication: Similar to lidocaine, for oral administration. Prevention and control of chronic ventricular ectopy.	
Adrenergic Agents			
Dobutamine HCl (Dobutrex)	IV administration by infusion: 250 mg in 500 ml D_5W; usual dose range: 2.5–10.0 μg/kg/min	Positive inotropic effect: Increases stroke volume, cardiac output. Less effect on heart rate and rhythmicity than	As with a dopamine infusion, ECG and BP monitoring is essential. If possible, wedge pressures and

APPENDIX B

EMERGENCY CARDIAC DRUGS (CONTINUED)

Drug	Dosage/Administration	Actions/Indications	Comments
		dopamine. Does not directly affect the mesenteric and renal arteries and blood flow to those areas as does dopamine. Indications: Low cardiac output states due to chronic CHF, organic heart disease, cardiac surgery. Side-effects: Angina, palpitations, ectopy (ventricular), nausea, headache.	cardiac outputs should be monitored. Watch for PVCs, increase in heart rate and BP.
Dopamine HCl (Intropin)	IV administration by infusion; 200 mg in 250 ml–500 ml D₅W. 2–10 μ/kg/min for β-receptor stimulation of the heart. 10–20 μ/kg/min for α and β effects. >20 μ/kg/min α-receptor stimulating activity produces vasoconstriction of renal and mesentery arteries.	Positive inotropic effect; increases cardiac output, ventricle contractility. Increases heart rate and BP. In low and medium dose range improves blood flow to kidney and gut; therefore improves (increases) urinary output. Indications: Cardiogenic, bacteremic, traumatic shock. May be used in patients with low cardiac output. May be used in hypovolvemic shock once fluid is replaced. Side-effects: Nausea, vomiting, headache, tachycardia, angina.	Physiologic effects of the drug are dose related. High-dose administration increases renal vasoconstriction and reduces kidney function. Monitor carefully. Watch for development of tachycardia, appearance of arrhythmias, or decrease in urine output. Monitor BP. Give in large vein.
Epinephrine (Adrenalin)	For cardiac arrest: IV administration 1:1000 (1 mg/ml): dilute with 9 ml of normal saline if no preload syringe available, or 10 ml 1:10,000 preload (1 mg/10 ml). Give 0.5-mg–1.0-mg IV bolus. May also give 1 mg–2 mg epinephrine in 10 ml sterile water through endotracheal tube directly into tracheobronchial tree.	Direct myocardial stimulant; increases cardiac automaticity irritability, increases force of ventricular contraction, heart rate. Most potent vasopressor; increases vasoconstriction in skin, mucosa, and kidney. Indications: Used in cardiac arrest (asystole) to restore cardiac rhythm; in VF to coarsen fine VF prior to DC shock. Also used for bronchospasm in allergic patients and in anaphylactic shock. Cardiac side-effects: tachycardia, arrhythmias, angina. Others: increased anxiety, headache, tremor, and weakness; pallor, clammy cool skin.	With a patient who has arrested, correct for acidosis before administering epinephrine. Patient's ECG and peripheral pulses need to be monitored.
Isoproterenol (Isuprel)	IV infusion: 1 mg–2 mg in 250 ml–500 ml D₅W to make a solution of 2-4-μg/ml. Infusion rate begun at 5 μg/min, titrate to effect or appearance of ectopy or tachycardia. Bolus: 1 ml–3 ml of 1:50,000 solution.	Action: Drug stimulates β-adrenergic receptors; relaxes smooth muscles in bronchial tree and arterioles. In the heart: increases heart rate and force of contraction; promotes an increase in cardiac output. Also promotes an increase in O₂ consumption of heart muscle. Enhances automaticity, especially in the ventricles. Indications: AV block (3rd°, or Mobitz II) until pacemaker is	Patient needs to be monitored continuously because of the possibility of ventricular ectopy (onset of PVCs, VT and VF). Watch for sinus tachycardia greater than 110 bpm or onset of angina. Decrease drip to keep rate at 90–100/bpm and rhythm free from ectopy. Use microdrip and infusion. Avoid using in patients with AMI.

APPENDIX B

EMERGENCY CARDIAC DRUGS (CONTINUED)

Drug	Dosage/Administration	Actions/Indications	Comments
		available. Can be used in shock when the myocardium is healthy, fluid replacement is adequate, and there is severe vasoconstriction. Side-effects: Tachycardia, ventricular arrhythmias, coronary ischemia, angina pectoris.	
Norepinephrine, levarterenol bitartrate (Levophed)	IV infusion: 1–2 ampules (8 mg–16 mg) in 500 ml– 1000 ml D$_5$W may add 2 ampules of phentolamine (Regitine) to IV solution to combat intense vasoconstriction. Administer at 8–12 μg/min or to desired effect.	Intense vasoconstrictor, affecting chiefly α receptors in blood vessels. Peripheral ventricular resistance (PVR) increases, cardiac output may stay the same, fall slightly, or increase. Decreased blood flow to renal, skin, and mesenteric vessels. Indications: Hypotensive states in which PVR is decreased, cardiogenic shock. Side-effects: Bradycardia, hypertension, chest pain, headache, vomiting, arrhythmias.	Infuse through large vein; inspect insertion site frequently— drug can cause tissue sloughing if extravasation occurs. Use microdrip and infusion pump. Monitor BP and ECG frequently; do not push BP to levels higher than necessary for desired effect. Intra-arterial pressure monitoring may be necessary.
Atropine	IV bolus adults: 0.5 mg–1 mg; may repeat every 5 min up to 2 mg. Child: 0.01 mg/kg dose up to 0.4 mg	Blocks vagal action on SA and AV nodes, therefore increases heart rate. Indications: Sinus junctional bradycardias, bradyarrhythmias such as escape rhythms. CPR: ventricular asystole. Side-effects: Urinary retention, especially in older males; flushing, agitation, dry mouth, mydriasis and blurred vision, fever.	With repeat doses, the incidence of severe side-effects increases. With the older patient, watch especially for confusion and agitation. In the elderly male, check for inability to void. In patients with AMI, atropine should be used only in situations in which bradycardia is accompanied by serious hypotension or frequent ventricular escape beats.
Propranolol HCl (Inderal)	Oral (usually) but may be given IV in emergencies. 1 mg IV slowly, (over 2 min), not to exceed 0.2 mg/kg.	Blocks effects of catecholamines on the heart: decreases heart rate, cardiac output, ventricular contractility, myocardial O$_2$ consumption; suppresses atrial, ventricular ectopy. Prolongs AV conduction. Indications: Atrial and ventricular tachyarrhythmias associated with digitalis toxicity. Also angina pectoris attacks, hypertensive crisis, and, when patient sustains a heart rate greater than 100 bpm with a normal or elevated BP, AMI. Prophylactic use following AMI to prevent recurrence, sudden death. Side-effects: Can increase airway spasm in susceptible patients (asthmatics).	When given IV, patient's ECG and arterial BP must be monitored continuously. Watch for hypotension, acute left ventricular failure or collapse, bradycardia, heart block. Have vasopressor, atropine, pacemaker at hand. Incompatible with any other percutaneous drug. Sudden withdrawal of oral propranolol for treatment of angina may worsen degree or frequency of angina, increasing ischemia and leading to possible AMI and appearance of ventricular ectopy.
Beta-adrenergic blocker Nadolol (Corgard)	Oral administration	Drug blocks effects of cateholamines on the heart. Indications: Hypertension, angina pectoris.	Has a longer half-life than propranolol

APPENDIX B

EMERGENCY CARDIAC DRUGS (CONTINUED)

Drug	Dosage/Administration	Actions/Indications	Comments
Metoprolol (Lopressor)	Oral administration	Indications: Hypertension	
Timolol		Indications: Hypertension	
Pindolol		Indications: Hypertension	
Antihypertensive Agents			
Diazoxide (Hyperstat)	IV bolus: 300 mg or 5 mg/kg IV push rapidly (less than 30 sec) May repeat after 30 min if BP decrease is inadequate.	Potent, fast-acting drug: acts by a direct vasodilation effect on the arterioles that decreases the peripheral vascular resistance, systolic and diastolic pressure. Indirect effect is an increase in cardiac output and left ventricular ejection velocity due to catecholamine release. Indications: Hypertensive crisis associated with acute hypertensive encephalopathy. Also used with toxemias of pregnancy. Side-effects: Na$^+$ retention, reflex tachycardia, chest pain, hyperglycemia, GI upset.	Keep patient flat; monitor BP every 5 min × 30 min. Rapid IV injection is necessary since this drug quickly binds with serum albumin: there must be enough unbound drug available in circulation to interact at receptor sites. Insulin-dependent diabetics may need an increase in insulin. Because of the risk of reflex tachycardia, drug is not used with patients who have coronary artery disease or dissecting aortic aneurysm. Important: Due to Na$^+$ retention with this drug, diuretics must be given before or during administration.
Hydralazine HCl (Apresoline)	When urgent, may be given IM or IV 20 mg–40 mg. Transfer to oral medication within 24–48 hr.	Relaxes arteriolar smooth muscle. Causes a reflex increase in cardiac output and heart rate. Indications: Severe preeclampsia or eclampsia; malignant hypertension. Side-effects: Na$^+$ and H$_2$O retention, tachycardia, headache.	Slower onset (15 min) with longer duration (3–4 hrs) than nitroprusside and diazoxide. Monitor patient's ECG for arrhythmias. Should not be used in patients with coronary artery disease or dissection of aortic aneurysm.
Sodium nitroprusside (Nipride)	IV infusion 50 mg in 250 ml–500 ml D$_5$W 0.5–10 µg/kg/min (average dose 3 µ/kg/min)	Dilates arterioles and veins (resistance and capacitance vessels). Also causes reflex tachycardia. Indications: Most potent and consistently effective drug for hypertensive emergencies, especially those associated with acute left ventricular failure or with cerebral hemorrhage. Can be used with dissecting aortic aneurysm with prior propranolol administration. Side-effects: Nausea, vomiting, headache, restlessness, sweating due to rapid hypotension produced by drug.	Given by slow IV infusion with continuous monitoring. Infusion pump must be used with microdrip. Has very rapid onset, short duration. Light sensitive—bottle must be covered. Solution is stable for 24 hr. Note: Check patient's thiocyanate serum levels if on Nipride longer than 24 hr. A buildup of this metabolic by-product can be toxic.
Trimethaphan camsylate (Arfonad)	IV infusion: 500 mg in 500 ml D$_5$W 3–4 mg/min.	A short-acting ganglionic blocker. Decreases cardiac contractility and cardiac output. Indications: Dissecting aortic aneurysm; cerebral or subarachnoid hemorrhage.	Patients should have head of bed slightly elevated to improve effect of drug. Constant monitoring of BP necessary. Use with infusion pump and microdrip. Be aware of

APPENDIX B

EMERGENCY CARDIAC DRUGS (CONTINUED)

Drug	Dosage/Administration	Actions/Indications	Comments
		Side-effects: Postural hypotension, urinary retention, decreased GI motility, dry mouth, mydriasis.	pupillary effects during neurologic exam.
Nitroglycerin	0.2 mg–0.6 mg sub ling IV infusion: 50 mg in 500 *glass* bottle D$_5$W or NaCl. Initial dose 5 μg/min. Increase by 5 μg q3–5 min	Relaxes vascular smooth muscle, decreases peripheral vascular resistance, which drops systolic BP; dilates the venous system, which reduces preload. Also dilates coronary arteries. Indications: angina pectoris. AMI complicated by heart failure. Side-effects: headache, hypotension, syncope.	After administration of drug, monitor BP every 3 min $\times$ 3; watch for moderate drop in systolic reading. If no response and pain is unrelieved, may repeat $\times$ 3. Record patient response, degree of pain relief. With IV infusion, use special plastic administration set to decrease absorption of drug. Use glass IV bottle.
Diuretic Agents Furosemide	40 mg–80 mg IV bolus, given slowly, over 1–2 min	Drug acts at the ascending loop of Henle in the kidney nephron, preventing Na$^+$ absorption. H$_2$O and Na$^+$ are lost in the urine. Also, induces K$^+$ and H$^+$ loss. Indications: Patients who are unresponsive to other diuretics, or who have poor kidney function; congestive heart failure; pulmonary edema, hypertensive crisis. Also, given concurrently with Na$^+$-retaining antihypertensives such as diazoxide. Side-effects: K$^+$ loss and associated symptoms, hyperuricemia, hyperglycemia, deafness (less common with furosemide).	Watch for hypovolemia, and electrolyte changes which could prove dangerous. Monitor BP, cardiac rhythm; keep accurate I and O.
Ethacrynate sodium (Edecrin)	50 mg in 50 ml D$_5$W IV Bolus 0.5–1.0 mg/kg body wt	Same actions. Same indications.	Same considerations.
Cardiac Glycosides Digitalis (many preparations) Digoxin (Lanoxin)	Oral or IV Loading dose 1.0 mg–2.5 mg oral 0.5 mg–2.0 mg IV IV effect in 5 to 30 min Therapeutic serum levels: 0.5–2.0 mg/ml	Increases the force of myocardial contraction (a positive inotropic effect), slows ventricular rate by prolonging period of AV node. Slows heart rate by effect on SA node. Indications: Congestive heart failure; used to treat supraventricular rhythms; atrial fibrillation, flutter, PAT, junctional tachycardia. Cardiac side-effects: Sinus bradycardia, SA block, atrial arrhythmias, PVCs, VT, heart failure. Others: Anorexia, nausea, vomiting, diarrhea, visual disturbances, headache, lassitude.	Needs a loading dose to reach plasma concentration and to maintain therapeutic levels. If digoxin is ordered IV, it is to be diluted in 10 ml normal saline (because it is an irritant) and administered slowly over 5–10 min. Digoxin and related preparations have a narrow therapeutic window; toxicity occurs often. Most common cause is concurrent use of diuretics, which promotes K$^+$ loss and increases susceptibility of the heart to digitalis effects.

17
VASCULAR EMERGENCIES

JAMES H. COSGRIFF, JR. and CAMILLE RATAJCZYK

Patients with urgent vascular problems are being seen with increasing frequency in hospital emergency departments. A number of causative factors for this can be identified. Increased mechanization, high-speed travel, and acts of violence account for many vascular emergencies. The extension of the average American's life span into the eighth decade, with related degenerative disease of the cardiovascular system; the increasing use of birth control pills; exposure to weather elements, especially cold; and iatrogenic factors also contribute significantly to these statistics.

The prognosis for many patients with vascular disease or injury has improved dramatically in the past two to three decades. Advances in diagnostic and therapeutic techniques have resulted in superior methods of evaluating patients with vascular problems, higher rates of limb salvage, and lower morbidity and mortality. Particularly noteworthy is the development of noninvasive studies to assess vascular integrity or compromise. Acute vascular problems involving the extremities, though often serious, are usually more of a threat to limb than to life. Early, appropriate, effective assessment and management of the patient with such a problem is essential to forestall an often fatal outcome. In trauma, one is concerned with the cause and extent of the injury, whereas in occlusive disease, the concern is whether the condition is acute or chronic. Vascular emergencies may be:

- Secondary to trauma
- Associated with degenerative disease of the vessels
- Venous in origin
- Associated with exposure to cold; lower temperatures cause a decrease in circulation, leading to tissue damage and actual cell injury.

VASCULAR EMERGENCIES SECONDARY TO TRAUMA

Patients with traumatic vascular damage may have associated multiple organ injury. As when caring for other such patients, one must be familiar with the basic principles of assessment, and able to identify damaged organ systems and establish priorities of care.

The causes of vascular injury include stabbings, gunshot wounds, vehicular accidents, falls, and iatrogenic factors.

An artery or a vein, or both, may be damaged. The arterial tree is a high-pressure system; when it is damaged, significant blood loss can result. In the majority of patients, such injury is obvious, but in a small percentage of cases, vascular damage may not be immediately apparent or recognized. These occult injuries are often associated with long-bone fractures or major joint dislocation, in which instance bleeding into a closed compartment of the limb occurs as a result of partial or incomplete disruption of the vessel.

The mechanism of injury can be an important factor in determining the extent of blood loss and the degree of vascular damage. Iatrogenic injuries to blood vessels are being seen with increasing frequency owing to the common use of cardiac catheters, central vein lines, and intra-arterial lines.

Types of Vascular Injuries

The types of vascular injuries commonly seen in emergency practice are simple laceration, complete transection, false aneurysm, contusion, and arteriovenous fistula.

- A sharp, incised *laceration* of an artery or vein with incomplete transection may bleed massively without clotting.
- In contrast, a blunt wound with *complete transection* and torn, irregular edges often clots because of deposition of platelet thrombi at the end of the vessel and retraction of the divided ends into the surrounding soft tissues.
- A *false aneurysm* is also called a pulsating hematoma. Following injury, the arterial wall tears, and there is leakage of blood. A hematoma forms that is walled off and does not bleed freely. The interior of the vessel is continuous with the hematoma forming an aneurysm. It is described as false because its wall does not contain any of the layers of the vessel wall.
- A *contusion* is a "bruise" on the vessel that is bleeding into the vessel wall.
- If the injury involves the wall of an artery and an adjacent vein, an *arteriovenous fistula* may develop.

PRINCIPLES OF CARE

Care of the patient with a suspected vascular injury must begin at the scene of the accident or as soon as the injury is identified. Patients with major fractures or dislocations must be properly immobilized to lessen the likelihood of blood vessel damage by displaced bone fragments. Consideration must be given to the following:

- The need for life-support measures
- An adequate airway
- Control of hemorrhage
- Establishment of a veinway and restoration of circulating blood volume
- An adequate history of injury with as many details as possible
- Assessment for other injuries
- Establishment of priorities of care of multiple system injuries
- Routine and specific laboratory studies
- Specific adjunct studies, such as noninvasive vascular procedures, angiography

Although they are listed separately, the basic components of care—assessment, resuscitation, and management of the injury—may proceed concurrently.

PREHOSPITAL CARE

The emergency management of a patient with vascular injury includes control of hemorrhage and restoration of circulating blood volume.

Control of Hemorrhage

The best means of keeping bleeding under control are direct pressure, elevation of the part, and use of a tourniquet. The method selected depends on the location and type of vessel injury and the extent of damage. *Under no circumstances should the wound be probed or explored* because a clot may become dislodged, causing further tissue damage and additional blood loss.

Direct Pressure. In a limb, direct pressure over the bleeding site or the major artery supplying the limb may significantly diminish or completely control blood loss. The simplest means is to place several layers of sterile gauze over the wound and apply pressure with the fingers or the heel of the hand. The pressure may be maintained with an outer, circular elastic bandage. Snugly applied, a pressure dressing may function very well in certain areas such as the limbs, scalp, or face. An air splint on the upper limb or pneumatic trousers on the lower limbs may function very well to maintain pressure.

Pressure points in the limbs, the sites where the major arteries lie in a superficial position, can be used to diminish hemorrhage (Chart 17-1). Because of collateral circulation near the major joints, however, this technique may be less

---

Chart 17-1

PRESSURE POINTS

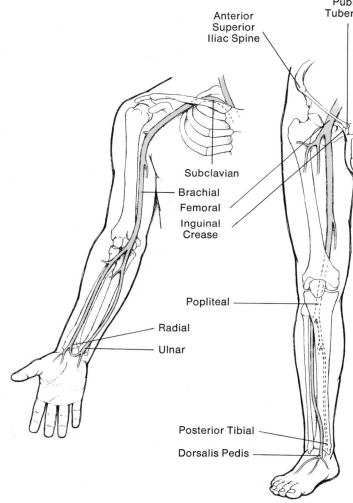

Upper-Limb Pressure Points

BRACHIAL ARTERY

- Palpable on the medial (small finger) aspect of the arm, midway between the shoulder and elbow. The vessel is compressed against the adjacent humerus.
- Palpable on the medial (small finger) side of the antecubital fossa (anterior aspect of the elbow)

RADIAL AND ULNAR ARTERIES

- Palpable on the volar (palmar) side of the wrist on the medial and lateral aspects

Lower Limb Pressure Points

FEMORAL ARTERY

- Palpable on the anterior aspect of the thigh, immediately distal to the inguinal (groin) crease, at a point approximately halfway between the anterior superior iliac spine and the pubic tubercle

POPLITEAL ARTERY

- Palpable on the posterior aspect of the knee joint, in the popliteal space

DORSALIS PEDIS ARTERY

- Palpable on the dorsum (instep) of the foot, approximately at its midpoint. This vessel is normally absent in 10%–20% of the population.

POSTERIOR TIBIAL ARTERY

- Palpable just behind the medial malleolus of the ankle

Drawings indicate the points on major arteries of the extremities where a pulse can be easily palpated and pressure applied.

effective than direct pressure on the bleeding point. Furthermore, it may be difficult to maintain direct finger pressure at a pressure point for any period of time.

Emergency personnel should be familiar with the pressure points used most often and select a point between the wound and the heart.

Elevation of the Part. Elevation of an extremity lessens the pressure in the vessels. This is particularly helpful in patients with damage to the veins, which are low-flow, low-pressure vessels. However, injuries in the limb, especially fractures, may preclude the use of this technique.

Tourniquet. A tourniquet may be used if direct pressure and elevation are ineffective. The use of tourniquets is controversial, most likely because of poor results or tissue damage caused by improper application. Furthermore, vascular reconstruction may be seriously compromised by use of the tourniquet. It will be needed, however, in certain circumstances, and when correctly used can successfully control hemorrhage until definitive measures are instituted.

Points to be stressed in the proper use of a tourniquet are as follows:

- It should be wide and preferably inflatable (pneumatic) so that the desired pressure may be uniformly applied and maintained. An example of an ideal tourniquet is a blood pressure cuff. Narrow straps such as ropes and belts may cause tissue damage.
- Apply only when blood loss is severe and otherwise uncontrollable.
- Peripheral pulses and the appearance of the extremity must be documented before application of the device and during and after its use.
- The tourniquet must be applied between the level of injury and the heart, in a position where it can exert adequate pressure on a major artery. In the upper limb, it should be applied at a point between the elbow and the shoulder, and in the lower limb between the hip and the knee. The artery can be compressed against the humerus in the arm and the femur in the leg. In the distal portion of the limbs, beyond the elbows and knees, the arteries lie between the bones so that adequate pressure cannot be applied.
- The tourniquet must be wrapped firmly and inflated above the level of systolic blood pressure. This point will be marked by disappearance of the distal pulse and slower blood loss. Insufficient pressure will allow continued arterial inflow into the limb and cause venous outflow occlusion, leading to increased pressure in the veins and further blood loss.
- The time of application of the tourniquet is noted by placing a piece of tape on the tourniquet and recording the time. Another site is the patient's forehead, if it is not injured.
- When applied for control of bleeding, it should *not* be deflated except under the supervision of a physician.

Restoration of Blood Volume

A large bore veinway is inserted in an uninjured extremity and Ringer's lactate started intravenously. If necessary, a pressure infusor can be applied to the plastic bag of solution for more rapid delivery. The patient should be readied for transport as soon as possible.

HOSPITAL CARE

ASSESSMENT

History

Once life-saving measures have been initiated and the patient's condition stabilized, a more thorough assessment is needed. Collect as much information as possible from the patient, witnesses, relatives, police officers, and prehospital personnel. If a weapon is involved, details of the type of weapon are helpful. Instruments used in stabbings vary greatly in blade size and length. Firearms have varying muzzle velocity. Low-muzzle-velocity weapons such as small handguns cause considerably less internal tissue damage then do missiles from high-muzzle-velocity weapons, such as a .357 magnum or a military firearm. Shotgun injuries caused by buckshot are much different from those produced by deer slugs.

Whenever possible, a complete history is collected, including past illnesses, associated disease, allergies, metabolic disorders, and current medical therapy.

Physical Examination

Careful physical assessment is needed to determine both the extent of the primary injury and the presence of other injuries. Assessment should be carried out concurrently with resuscitative measures. Move the patient as little as possible. Make an effort to perform as complete an examination as possible without removing any immobilizing devices such as splints or spine board. Have dressings readily available to place immediately on any bleeding wound.

- In penetrating injuries, examine the injuried site for the wounds of entrance and exit. This way you can get some idea of the structures between that could be damaged.
- In limb injuries, compare the damaged limb to its opposite for any alteration in color and temperature.
- Nerves are closely related anatomically to vascular structures and may be damaged at the same time. The patient may complain of sensations varying from paresthesia or numbness to partial or total paralysis of the limb. Sensory and motor function must be tested for sensation by the pin-prick method. Motor activity is evaluated by asking the patient to wiggle his fingers or toes or flex the ankle or wrist. Record these findings because they provide important baseline data.
- The arterial pulses are palpated in each limb to evaluate the circulation. It is especially important to assess the pulses distal to the site of injury. In some patients, a distal pulse may be palpated even though the flow in the major vessel is interrupted proximally, at the level of injury. This is possible because of the redirecting of blood flow through major collateral channels.
- The cardinal findings of acute arterial occlusion are:

  Pain

  Pallor

Pulselessness

Paresthesias

Paralysis

All of these features must be kept in mind in evaluating a patient suspected of having a vascular injury.

- Auscultation at the level of injury may reveal the presence of a bruit, indicating alteration of blood flow.

- A total assessment of the patient must be completed as the patient's condition permits. Concomitant injuries must be evaluated and priorities established.

Adjunct Studies

Vascular injuries require specialized techniques for complete diagnosis. One of the most important advances in this area is the use of ultrasonic monitoring devices. These instruments are noninvasive and are applied to the skin over the course of a vessel. The simplest device in current use is the portable Doppler Flowmeter. It is similar to a stethoscope and is perfectly suited to assessing vascular integrity in the emergency setting. More sophisticated tests include plethysmography and ultrasonic imaging, which are best done in a vascular laboratory by trained personnel.

Single-injection limb angiography, though an invasive procedure, can be performed in most emergency department x-ray units or with portable machines with a minimum of equipment (Fig. 17-1). Selective angiographic studies may be performed in the x-ray department or operating room as conditions require.

MANAGEMENT

Priorities of Care, Continuing Care

This subject is covered in detail in Chapter 10. Ongoing assessment proceeds with therapeutic intervention. Diagnostic studies are not begun until the patient's condition has stabilized.

- Blood pressure, pulse, respiratory rate, and skin color are periodically determined and recorded.

- Bleeding is considered to be major if 30% to 35% of the circulating blood volume is lost. This is equivalent to a loss of 1500 ml to 1800 ml of blood in a 70-kg (150-lb) man and requires treatment by both crystalloid solution (Ringer's lactate) and blood.

- An indwelling catheter is placed and urinary output measured. Urine output should be maintained at a rate of 1.0 ml/kg of body weight per hour in an adult and 0.5 ml/kg/hr in a child.

- A central-vein catheter is inserted to assess central venous pressure (CVP) if indicated.

- Routine laboratory orders include complete blood count (CBC), urinalysis, SMA-18, type and crossmatch, arterial blood gases.

Wound Care

Primary wound care in the emergency department is a minor consideration in the presence of vascular injury. No attempt should be made to probe or explore the wound, lest a clot be dislodged and major bleeding ensue. It is best to apply a sterile pressure dressing if one is not already in place.

Tetanus prophylaxis is given according to established recommendations (see Table 19-3, p 316). Both tetanus toxoid and hyperimmune globulin may be needed, especially when extensive soft-tissue damage is present. Broad-spectrum antibiotic therapy should be initiated in the emergency department. The patient should be prepared for transfer to the operating room.

Treatment

Management of any major vascular injury requires surgical intervention. The level of care required for such a patient is not available in all hospitals with emergency facilities; hence the patient may require transfer to a hospital with broader capabilities, either a secondary or tertiary level facility. Whether definitive care is to be given or transfer undertaken, the following points should be considered.

- The patient's injury

- The availability of support services such as laboratory, blood bank, and diagnostic x-ray, including angiography

- The expertise of the surgical team, including nurses, surgeons, and anesthesiologists

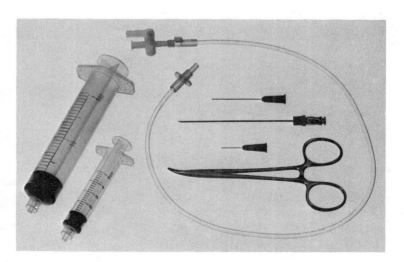

Figure 17-1 *Minimum equipment for the single-injection limb arteriography. Included are syringes (30 ml, 5 ml), needles for local anesthesia (22- and 25-gauge) and for arterial puncture (19-gauge spinal), connecting tubing with 3-way stopcock, clamp. Skin prep, anesthetic solution, and dye are not shown.*

- The availability of trained critical care personnel after surgery
- The proximity of the higher-level facility
- Availability of established transfer protocols

Surgical management is directed toward repair or reconstruction of the damaged vascular segment with the intent of limb salvage and patient survival. The patient and family should be informed of the nature and gravity of the injury and advised frankly of the possibility of amputation if it exists.

OCCULT ARTERIAL INJURY

Occult arterial injuries may follow blunt trauma or occur in association with long-bone fractures. Such injuries may vary from contusion of the vessel wall to complete transection. Although there may be no obvious bleeding, there is invariably a decrease in circulation to the affected part, which can be detected by careful assessment.

Assessment. Diminished arterial circulation is manifested by:
- Pain in the limb
- Lowered skin temperature
- Pallor
- Changes in sensory and motor function
- Diminution or lack of pulses distal to the point of injury
- Slow capillary filling

Management. Patients exhibiting circulatory defects associated with fractures or dislocations require early reduction and immobilization. At times, these maneuvers correct the vascular problem. More often, diagnostic angiography is necessary to identify the site of injury. Corrective surgery is usually carried out by a team that includes both orthopedists and general or vascular surgeons.

VASCULAR PROBLEMS ASSOCIATED WITH DEGENERATIVE DISEASE

Degenerative vascular disease may be classified as follows:
- Acute arterial occlusion due to embolus
- Acute arterial occlusion due to thrombosis
- Abdominal aortic aneurysm

Patients with vascular problems secondary to degenerative disease more often than not have some associated disease such as diabetes, arteriosclerotic heart disease, congestive heart failure (CHF), cardiac arrhythmia, or chronic lung or renal disease.

Usually the patient is older. Serious and complicated diagnostic and therapeutic judgments and decisions by emergency personnel may be required. The number of patients with degenerative vascular disease is increasing as the average life span grows.

ACUTE ARTERIAL OCCLUSION

Sudden occlusion of an artery is accompanied by cessation of major blood flow. Some limited flow may occur through smaller collateral arteries around the site of occlusion. Vascular occlusion is found as a complication of arteriosclerosis or a disturbance in cardiac rhythm, particularly atrial fibrillation.

Primary occlusion by arteriosclerotic plaque formation is a classic example of thrombosis; acute obstruction of flow by a clot displaced from the heart and lodged in a peripheral artery exemplifies arterial embolism. In either case, the patient will demonstrate evidence of vascular compromise and lessened blood flow.

In most patients, one can easily distinguish thrombosis from embolism. Confusion in making the exact diagnosis may result from lack of an obvious source for an embolus, absence of heart disease, and slowly progressing signs and symptoms of ischemia. It is most important to recognize the dissimilarity between thrombosis and embolism since the pathologic conditions found in these forms of acute arterial occlusion are different and different surgical procedures are used to restore blood flow.[1]

Obviously, the primary objective of treatment is the patient's survival, but a secondary objective is to save a functioning limb for the patient. The duration of the occlusion and the condition of the extremity when the patient is first seen will be major factors in limb survival.

Embolic Occlusion

An embolism occurs when a blood clot in one part of the cardiovascular system (usually the heart) breaks off and enters the arterial stream until it reaches a point of luminal narrowing. The embolus lodges at this point and obstructs distal flow, leading to ischemia. Typically, an embolus lodges at the bifurcation of an artery.

The most common sites of embolic occlusion are the following bifurcations (Fig. 17-2):
- Abdominal aorta
- Common femoral artery
- Popliteal artery
- Carotid artery
- Brachial artery
- Mesenteric artery

Assessment. Levels of physiologic changes are usually detectable and serve as a guide to the location of the block. The level of color and temperature change is some distance distal to the actual site of occlusion, since blood flow through collateral channels allows blood to detour around the site of obstruction. (Fig. 17-3).

As the period of occlusion lengthens, pallor changes to mottled cyanosis due to anoxia and decreased tissue perfusion. Motor weakness progresses to complete paralysis.

Definitive Treatment. Time is one critical factor for a successful outcome in the patient with an acute arterial occlusion. Although embolectomy has been successfully accomplished as late as 24 hours after onset, flow is more often restored in patients whose arteries have been occluded for shorter periods.

Definitive treatment is directed toward surgical removal of the embolus and restoration of flow. This can often be performed under local anesthesia, even in patients with a saddle embolus of the aorta. The procedure is facilitated to a great extent by the availability of the Fogarty balloon catheter. This catheter is inserted into a small incision in the artery beyond the point of occlusion, the balloon is inflated, and the catheter is withdrawn, extracting the embolus in the process.

Anticoagulant therapy with heparin is initiated in the emergency department if surgery is to be delayed for any

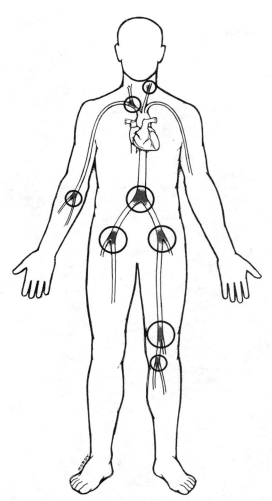

Figure 17-2 *Common sites of embolic arterial occlusion. Bifurcations of major vessels are most commonly involved in occlusions.*

Tenderness is often elicited along the course of the artery at the point of occlusion. Because of diminished arterial flow, capillary filling is slowed and the superficial veins usually collapse. Occlusion of the terminal aorta (saddle embolus) causes these findings to be present in both legs.

Further lengthening of the interval after embolization leads to decreased flow in the artery proximal and distal to the point where the embolus is lodged. This slowing of the circulation leads to thrombosis, additional compromise of the circulation, and eventually gangrene. A patient with frank gangrene usually has a long established obstruction and requires a period of careful study to determine the most beneficial type of operative intervention.

Adjunct Studies. The level and amplitude of arterial pulsations is measured using Doppler techniques. Segmental pressure studies are also helpful in locating the site of occlusion. Angiography may be used to further evaluate the character of the vessels and the level of occlusion.

Other emergency evaluation includes electrocardiogram (ECG), arterial blood gases, type and crossmatch in addition to routine blood studies, and urinalysis.

Figure 17-3 *Temperature and color changes due to occlusive disease. A. In the upper limb, occlusion of the axillary artery results in a level of demarcation in the distal arm. Saddle embolus of the aorta causes change distal to mid-thigh bilaterally. Occlusion of the brachial artery in the right limb causes changes distal to the mid forearm. B. Occlusion of popliteal artery causes change at level of mid-calf. C. Occlusion of common femoral artery produces level of change in distal third of thigh.*

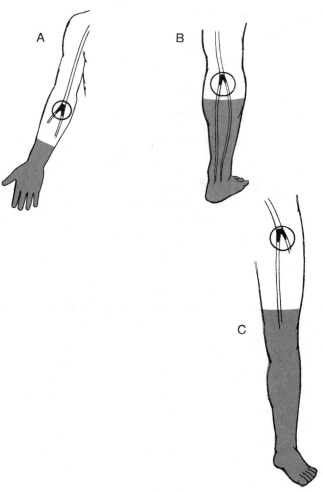

reason. An initial dose of 100 to 150 units/kg of body weight is given intravenously through a heparin trap followed by 5000 units every 4 to 6 hours. Anticoagulation is evaluated by partial thromboplastin times.

Long-term anticoagulant therapy is often necessary, depending on the etiology.

Thrombotic Occlusion

Thrombosis is usually the result of arteriosclerotic vascular disease. As opposed to embolism, thrombosis usually occurs gradually over a varying period of time and is commonly found in the lower extremities. Thrombosis is seen most often in males, smokers, and persons over 60 years of age.

An arteriosclerotic plaque develops on the intima (inner lining) of an artery. These plaques frequently have sharp edges which serve as a nidus for the deposition of platelets. These groups of platelets develop into small thrombi that gradually increase in size as more cells cling to the clot. As the clot enlarges, the lumen of the artery narrows and blood flow diminishes. As the process continues, the clot increases in size until complete occlusion occurs. Since this is a gradual process, collateral vessels develop, to varying degrees. This may be explained schematically as follows:

Arteriosclerotic plaque
↓
Deposition of platelets
↓
Increasing size of platelet thrombus
↓
Narrowing of lumen of artery
↓
Decreased blood flow
↓
Further increase in thrombus
↓
Partial/complete occlusion

Although thrombotic occlusion characteristically develops over a period of time, in some patients the narrowed artery may *suddenly* become completely thrombosed, precipitating an acute vascular episode (Fig. 17-4).

Assessment. The symptoms are those of ischemia (diminished blood flow).

History. Typically, the patient gives a history of crampy pains in the leg(s) with exercise or merely walking (intermittent claudication). The location of the pain is related to the site of occlusion, as follows:

- Terminal portion of abdominal aorta—pain in both hips or lower limbs

- Iliac artery—pain in buttocks or hip on involved side

- Femoral artery—claudication only in the involved leg
  The severity of claudication varies directly with the degree of arterial occlusion and the extent of collateral circulation. For example, some patients may have claudication after walking a quarter of a mile while others have symptoms after walking a block or less. The cramps are relieved after a few minutes of rest, at which time the patient may resume

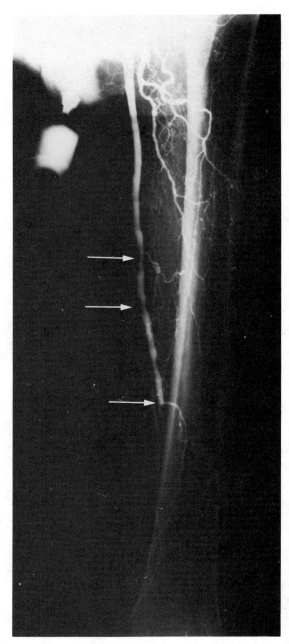

Figure 17-4 X-ray indicating thrombotic occlusion. Eighty-four-year-old woman was admitted to emergency department after her left leg "collapsed" and she was unable to walk thereafter. Leg was cool and pale beyond mid-calf. Arteriogram was done with emergency department x-ray. Note notching of femoral artery (upper 2 arrows), sudden termination of dye column (lowest arrow), and relative lack of collateral circulation. At exploration, a thrombus was extracted. Diagnosis was arteriosclerotic vascular disease with acute thrombotic occlusion.

walking. The common sites of atherosclerotic occlusion are depicted in Fig. 17-5.

Patients seen in the emergency setting are more often in an advanced stage of the disease, with complaints of gangrenous changes in the limb, particularly the toes and foot. The disease is much more common in men and in smokers and is frequently found in diabetics.

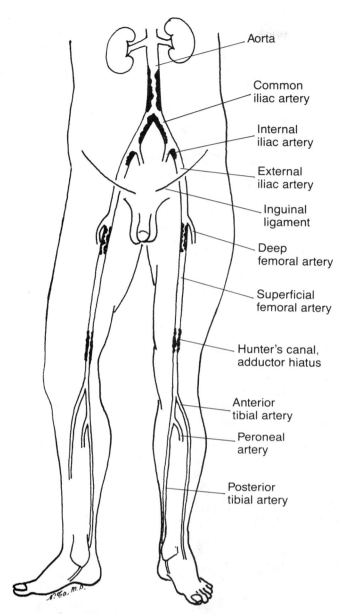

Figure 17-5 *Common sites of atherosclerotic occlusive disease.*

Physical Examination. The physical signs are those of chronic, gradual progressive ischemia:

- Lack of pulses distal to the occlusion
- Coolness of the limb(s)
- Cadaveric pallor when the limb is elevated above heart level
- Dependent rubor when the limb is placed over the side of the examining table
- Shiny appearance of the skin with loss of skin appendages
- Thickening of the nails

In the absence of frank gangrene, it may be difficult to determine the level of occlusion. In the majority of patients, the obstruction is in the lower third of the femoral artery.

Thus, the femoral pulse would be palpable and the popliteal and pedal pulses absent.

Management. Patients with thrombotic occlusion are not candidates for emergency surgery but must be admitted for diagnosis and treatment. However, some patients with a fairly long history of intermittent claudication may develop symptoms of sudden, complete occlusion of the artery. The arteriogram of such a patient is shown in Fig. 17-4. Physician evaluation is necessary to determine whether urgent surgical treatment is indicated. New methods of increasing blood flow to an impaired limb have been developed in recent years. One such method is transluminal dilation of an artery using a reinforced balloon catheter.[3,6] Other methods involve more sophisticated surgical procedures using improved graft materials now available.[4,7–10]

RUPTURED ABDOMINAL AORTIC ANEURYSM

An aneurysm is a local dilatation in an artery, most often secondary to arteriosclerosis. Rupture of an aortic aneurysm is a catastrophic event. An aneurysm occurs most often in the lower portion of the abdominal aorta in men over the age of 60.[12] The types of abdominal aortic aneurysm are illustrated in Fig. 17-6. One is a well-localized dilatation of the aortic wall (saccular), the other a more diffuse widening extending over a considerable length of the vessel (fusiform).

Etiology

The aneurysm develops at a point of weakness in the wall of an artery as a result of degenerative changes in the medial layer (medial necrosis) that accompany arteriosclerosis. The aneurysm is a single manifestation of a generalized disease process of the cardiovascular system that progresses over a period of time. Once the aneurysm has formed, it has a tendency to enlarge over time as the lateral pressure increases in the dilated segment (Fig. 17-7).

Rupture of the aneurysm may begin with a small tear in the intima that allows blood to leak into the wall of the aorta, causing a dissection of the layers. As the process continues, with increasing pressure, the tear may extend through the outer layer(s) of the vessel and cause bleeding into the retroperitoneal space. Since most aneurysms project to the left of the midline, the rupture is usually to the left. Rarely, the aneurysm ruptures anteriorly into the peritoneal cavity or to the right. Subsequent to the rupture, blood extravasates into the retroperitoneal space, and a hematoma forms. To some extent, this limits the amount of blood loss, the peritoneum acting as a restraint. If the rupture opens into the peritoneal cavity, massive and often fatal hemorrhage follows. In either case, major blood loss results, and hypovolemic shock ensues.

Assessment

History. The most common initial symptom of a ruptured abdominal aortic aneurysm is sudden onset of severe, con-

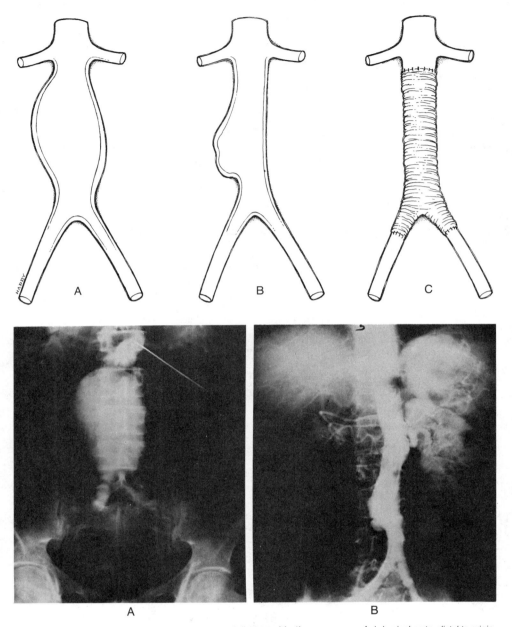

Figure 17-6 *Aneurysms. A. Translumbar aortogram and diagram of fusiform aneurysm of abdominal aorta, distal to origin of renal arteries. B. Retrograde aortogram and diagram of saccular aneurysm of abdominal aorta, distal to origin of renal arteries. C. Aneurysmal segment excised and replaced by prosthetic graft.*

stant pain in the abdomen and back; the pain increases in severity.

- As bleeding continues, vascular collapse due to hemorrhagic shock occurs.
- Syncope may follow as the patient becomes weak and diaphoretic.
- There may be no symptoms that suggest chronic vascular disease.

Physical Examination. The patient usually appears acutely ill. Profound hypotension is usually present; blood pressure is undetectable if extensive blood loss has occurred. Occasionally, the patient is normotensive or only slightly hypotensive.

The most significant findings relate to the abdomen. A pulsatile mass may be noted on inspection. Signs of peritoneal irritation may be present but are not striking in relation to the patient's symptoms (see Chap. 22, Care of the Patient With an Acute Abdomen). A pulsatile, *expansile,* tender mass is usually palpated in the area of the umbilicus, primarily to the left of the midline. The mass should be palpated carefully with both hands to estimate its size and distinguish it from a cystic mass that is transmitting the aortic pulsation (Fig. 17-8). Size may vary but is usually more than 7.0 cm (2.75 inches) in diameter. The femoral pulses are usually palpable. Pulses distal to the femoral may be present or absent, depending on the degree of peripheral vascular disease.

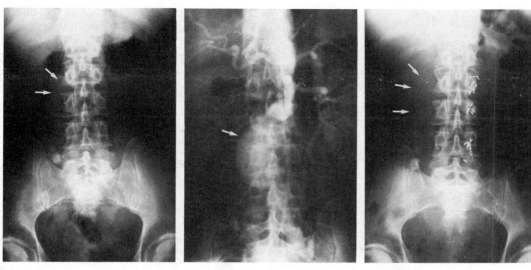

Figure 17-7 *Progressive enlargement of abdominal aortic aneurysm. Left: Flat film, with rim of calcification to right of midline at level of second lumbar vertebra (1979). Center: Aortogram demonstrating aneurysm below renal arteries. Note rim of calcification. Aneurysm is lined with a mural thrombus. Right: Flat film 4 years later (1983). Calcification wider. Patient fainted at home. Ruptured aneurysm found at laparotomy. Aneurysm excised and replaced by Dacron graft.*

Figure 17-8 *Assessment of abdominal aortic aneurysm. Top. A mass overlying a normal aorta may transmit the aortic pulsation, but the pulsation will not be expansile. It will neither enlarge nor contract as does an aortic aneurysm. Bottom. With each pulsation, the aorta enlarges and contracts. This is referred to as an expansile pulsation, which is characteristic of an aneurysm of an artery.*

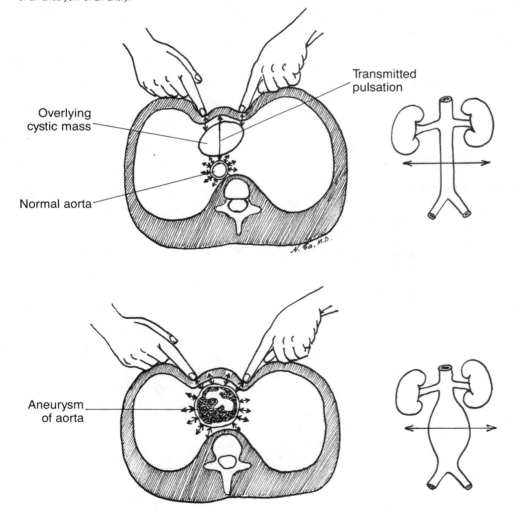

Management

Prehospital care and emergency management of the patient in the hospital are summarized in Chart 17-2. Once the diagnosis is established, the patient should be made ready for transfer to the operating room. In the absence of exten- uating circumstances, the pneumatic trousers should be left in place and remain inflated until the patient reaches the operating room.

Emergency thoracotomy in the emergency department may be indicated in severely hypotensive patients who do not respond to fluid replacement. The left chest is entered

---

Chart 17-2

MANAGEMENT OF THE PATIENT WITH A RUPTURED AORTIC ANEURYSM

Assessment/Signs and Symptoms

- Abrupt onset of abdominal and back pain
- Sharp, constant pain
- Patient is usually male, over age 60
- Hypotension is usually present
- Pulsatile tender mass in the midabdomen
- Peritoneal irritation (see Chap. 22)

Prehospital Care

1. Observe for signs and symptoms listed above.
2. If the diagnosis is suspected, the following measures should be undertaken:
   - Apply pneumatic trousers.
   - Insert a large-bore veinway in the upper limb(s); start Ringer's lactate at rapid rate to restore circulating volume.
   - Give oxygen by mask or nasal cannula.
   - Monitor vital signs.
   - Prepare the patient for transport.

Hospital Care

- Assess patient (ongoing).
- Continue oxygen by mask or nasal cannula.
- Obtain laboratory studies as detailed below.
- Place an indwelling bladder catheter and monitor urinary output.
- Insert a central vein catheter to monitor CVP and use as a route for rapid fluid or blood replacement.
- Administer adequate amounts of type-specific blood as needed. Some patients require as much as 8 to 12 units.
- Apply pneumatic trousers or, if applied previously, leave in place until patient reaches operating room.
- Prepare for early transfer to the operating room.

Laboratory Studies

- CBC
- SMA-18
- Urinalysis
- Blood type and crossmatch
- Arterial blood gas determinations
- ECG (most of these patients have arteriosclerotic heart disease)
- Three-way x-rays of abdomen (Fig. 17-7). These often demonstrate a rim of calcification lateral to the lumbar vertebrae, which is pathognomonic of an abdominal aneurysm and usually confirms this diagnosis when used in conjunction with other findings.

and the thoracic aorta cross-clamped to lessen blood loss at the site of aortic perforation. The time of clamping should be documented.

Definitive Treatment. Urgent surgery is indicated as a life-saving procedure. Without surgery, the disease is invariably fatal. With surgery, the mortality rate varies from 30% to 50%.

The purposes of operative treatment are as follows:
- To control hemorrhage
- To remove the diseased segment of aorta
- To restore vascular continuity with a prosthetic graft
  The procedure is illustrated in Fig. 17-6.

VASCULAR PROBLEMS OF VENOUS ORIGIN

Occlusion in the venous system may result from thrombosis or embolism. Most problems relate to venous thrombosis, and occur most frequently in the lower extremity. The following *factors contribute to venous thrombosis:*
- Trauma
- Sepsis
- Birth control pills
- Varicose veins
- Iatrogenic factors
- Stasis

Anatomically, the network of leg veins consists of a superficial and a deep venous system. Thrombosis can occur in either system. On occasion, the thrombus may fragment and embolize. This is more often associated with deep-vein thrombosis than with occlusion of the superficial system.

SUPERFICIAL-VENOUS OCCLUSION

Occlusion of a superficial vein is most often a minor condition that causes temporary discomfort but few permanent sequelae. It is due to a clot that is firmly adherent to the

---

Chart 17-3

SYMPTOMS AND SIGNS OF SUPERFICIAL VEIN OCCLUSION

- Pain in the limb, varying from mild to severe
- Aggravation of pain in the lower extremity upon walking
- Tender, cord-like thickening of the vein in the involved area
- Swelling and erythema of the overlying skin
- Swelling of the distal limb, especially when the lower extremity is involved
- Low incidence of systemic reaction
- Absence of Homans' sign (see p 284)

TABLE 17-1. FEATURES OF SUPERFICIAL AND DEEP VENOUS OCCLUSION

	Superficial	Deep
Frequency	Common	Common
Serious	Rare	Frequent
Systemic reaction	Rare	Common
Embolization	5% to 10%	10% to 60%
Permanent sequelae	Rare	Frequent
Mortality	Practically nil	Low but significant

vein wall. Embolization may result in 5% to 10% of patients. This condition is called phlebitis.

Assessment

Observe for the signs and symptoms of superficial-vein occlusion, which are listed in Chart 17-3.

Management

Treatment is symptomatic and consists of the following:
- Removal of the offending agent (*e.g.,* birth control pills, intravenous line)
- Rest and elevation of the part
- Warm, moist dressings to relieve discomfort and promote healing
- Analgesics
- Nonsteroidal anti-inflammatory agents (optional), *e.g.,* ibuprofen, sulindac, to reduce local tissue response
- Elective varicose vein removal when etiologically related
  Circumferential elastic (Ace) bandages are poorly tolerated in the acute phase because the compression may cause more pain. Anticoagulants are rarely indicated, and hospitalization is rarely necessary.

DEEP-VENOUS OCCLUSION

Occlusion of the deep veins is a serious, common problem. It is estimated to occur in as many as one-third of hospitalized patients. Deep-vein occlusion may involve any portion of the deep venous system but is much more common in the lower extremities. Unlike superficial vein thrombosis, this disease in the deep veins may leave permanent sequelae and is associated with a significant mortality rate. A comparison of the two problems is noted in Table 17-1.

The condition begins with slowing of blood flow through the veins. Some believe that a change in blood coagulability may influence thrombus formation. Once the clot has formed, there is further slowing of blood flow proximal and distal to the site, causing further clot formation. These clots are not usually attached firmly to the vein wall and are likely to fragment and embolize. The most common site of embolization is the lung; when massive, pulmonary embolism may be fatal.

Clinically, there are two types of deep-vein occlusion, phlebothrombosis and thrombophlebitis. Phlebothrombosis is a bland, often painless process manifested by swelling, calf tenderness, and a positive Homans' sign (pain in the posterior aspect of the calf when the foot is dorsiflexed with the knee extended). See Figure 17-9. In contrast, thrombophlebitis is usually a painful process manifested by swelling and systemic reactions (fever, tachycardia, leukocytosis). As in phlebothrombosis, calf tenderness and a positive Homans' sign may be present. This form of the disease is thus usually associated with a septic process and may present in one of two forms:

1. Phlegmasia cerulea dolens—leg appears hot, red, swollen, and tender.
2. Phlegmasia alba dolens—leg appears cool, pale, swollen and tender owing to a combination of venous occlusion and arterial spasm.

Assessment

Observe for the symptoms and signs of deep-vein occlusion, shown in Chart 17-4.

Adjunct Studies. In overt cases with obvious clinical findings there is reason to be highly suspicious of this diagnosis. However, sometimes it is difficult and often missed, deep-vein thrombosis being clinically detected in 5% to 10% of patients, whereas autopsy studies reveal the incidence to be nearer to 30%.[13-15]

A number of adjunct tests are available to assist in detecting venous occlusion. These include the use of Doppler ultrasound, impedance plethysmography, the ^{125}I-Fibrinogen uptake test, and an isotope venogram. The Doppler device, probably the most readily available of the three mentioned, is portable and can be used in the emergency setting. The fibrinogen uptake test is unsuitable for emergency situations because special preparation is required. However, it is useful for detecting even small thrombi that are less than 7 days

---

> **Chart 17-4**
>
> ## SYMPTOMS AND SIGNS OF DEEP VEIN OCCLUSION
>
> * Swelling and varying degrees of discomfort in the limb
> * Pain that may be aggravated by walking
> * Tenderness along the course of the deep veins
> * Leg may appear hot, red, swollen (phlegmasia cerulea dolens), or
> * Leg may be cool, pale, swollen (phlegmasia alba dolens)
> * High incidence of systemic reaction (fever, tachycardia, leukocytosis)
> * Presence of Homans' sign
> * Regional lymphadenopathy may be found in the inguinal area

---

old. The isotope venogram is a simple and accurate method of identifying the level of occlusion and can be used in the emergency setting. Phlebography is fairly accurate but is rarely used in emergencies.[13]

Management

Patients with deep-venous occlusion require admission to the hospital. Treatment is directed toward prevention of complications during resolution of the process.
* Bed rest is maintained.
* Broad-spectrum antibiotics are used in the presence of sepsis.
* Anticoagulation is the therapy most commonly used. Both heparin and coumadin should be started simultaneously.
* Baseline clotting and partial thromboplastin and prothrombin times are obtained in the emergency setting prior to initiating therapy.
* Heparin is usually started with a dose of 100 to 150 units/kg of body weight, given intravenously as a bolus dose and followed with a continuous infusion at the rate of 750 to 1000 units per hour.
* Coumadin is begun orally and its dosage altered as needed, to maintain the prothrombin times in the therapeutic range of 2 to 2.5 times the control.
* Once the therapeutic range is reached, heparin is discontinued.

Currently, there is great interest in the use of thrombolytic agents, particularly streptokinase and urokinase. These drugs are in lysing clots but must be used with caution since they have significant side-effects. They are usually given by a bolus dose followed by continuous infusion. The patient must be observed for clotting defects. Both are relatively expensive. An investigational drug that may be of value in the future is that derived from snake venom. Such agents

Figure 17-9 *Assessment of deep venous occlusion. A. Homans' sign—pain at the back of the calf or knee when the ankle is forcibly dorsiflexed indicates early or established thrombosis of the deep veins of the leg. B. Compression of the calf reveals tenderness over the area of occlusion.*

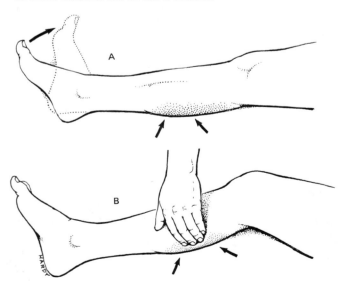

are expected to be particularly useful when they become commercially available.

During treatment, the patient must be observed closely for any complications, the most serious being pulmonary thromboembolism.

In some medical centers, urgent surgery is performed to extract the thrombus (thrombectomy) and restore blood flow immediately. The incidence of recurrent thrombosis is high and the technique is associated with some difficulty; in fact, it may be hazardous if thrombolytic agents have been given. The procedure is not in general use, but one should be aware that the possibility of surgical intervention exists.

VASCULAR PROBLEMS ASSOCIATED WITH EXPOSURE TO COLD

Serious tissue damage may result from exposure to cold. It is common in wartime combat conditions in cold-weather climates. In civilian life, it is seen in construction workers, skiers, outdoorsmen, and derelicts. A combination of temperature, humidity, wind, and exposure time contributes to the process. The damage is thought to result from interference with circulation by sludging of blood in smaller vessels and through changes in the tissue cells due to lowered temperature. This subject is discussed in detail in Chapter 29.

REFERENCES

1. Fogarty TJ: Management of arterial emboli. Surg Clin North Am 59:749–753, 1979
2. Buch WS, Fogarty TJ: Arterial embolism. In Hardy JD (ed): Rhoads Textbook of Surgery, 5th ed, p 1843. Philadelphia, JB Lippincott, 1977
3. Dotter CT et al: Transluminal iliac artery dilatation. JAMA 230:117–124, 1974
4. Veith FJ et al: New approaches to limb salvage by extended extra-anatomic bypasses and prosthetic reconstruction to foot arteries. Surgery 84:764–774, 1978
5. Baron HC: Chronic arterial insufficiency of the lower limbs. Hosp Med 14:33–55, 1978
6. Baron HC et al: Gas endarterectomy in the treatment of the ischemic lower extremity. Arch Surg 98:754, 1969
7. David TE, Drezner AD: Extended profundoplasty for limb salvage. Surgery 84:758–763, 1978
8. Veith FJ et al: Expanded polytetrafluoroethylene grafts in reconstructive arterial surgery. JAMA 240:1867–1869, 1978
9. Piccone VA Jr et al: Limb salvage by inverted Y vein grafts to below-knee arteries. Arch Surg 113:951–955, 1978
10. Blaisdell FW et al: Management of acute lower extremity arterial ischemia due to embolism and thrombosis. Surgery 84:822–834, 1978
11. Darling RC: Arterial embolism. Hosp Med 10:8–32, 1974
12. Hardy JD: Infrarenal aortic and iliac artery aneurysms In Hardy JD (ed): Rhoads Textbook of Surgery, 5th ed, p 1760. Philadelphia, JB Lippincott, 1977
13. Brose NL: Current thoughts on venous thrombembolism. Surg Clin North Am 54:229–238, 1974
14. Bloomfield DA: Axioms on acute pulmonary embolism. Hosp Med 12:6–14, 1976
15. Spittell JA Jr et al: Thrombi and Emboli. Emerg Med 8:140–159, 1976

18
THE COMATOSE PATIENT

DIANN ANDERSON and JAMES H. COSGRIFF, JR.

The patient in coma requires the highest priority of care. Such a patient represents a particular challenge, one that taxes the emergency team's skill and judgment to the greatest extent. In caring for the comatose patient, one must base the approach on maintenance of life and simultaneously initiate a plan of diagnostic measures leading to an early and correct diagnosis. Although the contents of this chapter are presented in a step-by-step manner, it must be stressed that many of these steps must take place concurrently.

SAFE HANDLING OF THE COMATOSE PATIENT

The comatose or unresponsive patient depends entirely for safe handling on those who provide care. It is the duty of all who come in contact with an unresponsive patient to ensure that no further harm or injury results from inappropriate or improper handling. The measures outlined in Chart 18-1 should be carried out to safeguard the patient.

CAUSES OF COMA

There are many causes of coma, but they may be grouped into the following categories:

- *Metabolic coma*—due to diabetic ketoacidosis, hypoglycemia, thyroid crisis, adrenal insufficiency with addisonian crisis

- *Structural coma*—due to cerebrovascular accident, ruptured intracranial aneurysm, neoplasm, trauma, infections, or seizure disorder

- *Intoxication coma*—due to drugs, alcohol, carbon monoxide.

- *Functional coma*—due to psychogenic causes.

The mechanism of coma is not fully understood. Coma ensues as a result of deleterious action on the cerebral cortex and brain stem by a focal or diffuse disease process. The process may be reversible, resulting in partial or total recovery; or it may be irreversible or not treatable, resulting in permanent disability or mortality.

ASSESSMENT OF THE COMATOSE PATIENT

HISTORY

Evaluation and treatment begin the moment the patient comes in contact with emergency personnel. Since the patient is unable to respond to questioning, other sources must be used in obtaining the history, including family, friends, and witnesses. It is helpful to know whether the patient had any condition or habit that might have been a prelude to the unconscious state and whether the onset of the coma was witnessed.

Witnessed Coma

1. Ascertain nature of onset of unconscious state.
   - *Gradual*—as with certain types of metabolic or structural disorders such as a neoplasm or alterations in blood sugar levels
   - *Sudden*—such as might follow a cerebrovascular accident or a ruptured aneurysm
2. Was headache noted before the onset of coma (this often occurs with intracerebral and subarachnoid hemorrhage)?
3. Was there a fall or an injury beforehand?
4. Did the patient have any neurologic abnormalities such as slurred speech, motor weakness, or a seizure before becoming unconscious?
5. Did the patient have any symptoms of neurologic disorder in the days, weeks, or months prior to coma?

Chart 18-1

SAFE HANDLING OF THE COMATOSE PATIENT

1. Immediately correct any airway problems, using the modified jaw thrust or chin lift. Do not extend the neck until cervical spine injury is ruled out.
2. Perform a rapid assessment and take neurologic and vital signs.
3. Palpate spinous processes of the vertebral column and along the extremities to rule out any possible injury to the spine or skeletal structures.
4. If such injuries exist, apply a cervical collar without moving the neck, immobilize patient on a spine board and splint any affected extremity.
5. Move or transfer patient as a unit, taking care to immobilize the cervical spine (see Chart 20-1 and Fig. 20-21) when there is a history of trauma.
6. Ambulance attendants should remain in the emergency department until they have provided full details of the incident from the time of their arrival on the scene until the patient entered the hospital.
7. Detain any relatives, friends, co-workers, etc., until all necessary information has been collected.
8. A staff member should remain with the comatose patient at all times.
9. Ensure that the patient is strapped to the stretcher or examining cart and that padded siderails are in position to avert harm and prevent injury.

6. Does the patient have any medical problems?
7. Had the patient been on any drugs or prescribed medications? If so, what preparations and for what disorders?

Unwitnessed Coma

Ask about the circumstances under which the patient was found.
1. Was there any evidence of urinary or bowel incontinence?
2. Was there any evidence at the scene suggesting trauma (a weapon, broken or displaced furniture)?
3. Were any medications, drugs, or drug paraphernalia found near the patient or in the household?
4. Were any bottles of alcoholic beverages found with the patient?
5. If the victim was found in a home, a garage, or an enclosed area, were any fumes noticed or was there any evidence of improperly vented gas heaters?

Additional Sources of Information

Carry out a careful search of the personal belongings of the patient.
- Look particularly for wallet cards that might contain medical information, physicians' prescriptions, or any materials (jewelry, tags, bracelets) identifying an existing medical condition.
- If the patient is alone, look for names and phone numbers of persons who could provide information.

PHYSICAL EXAMINATION

A rapid general assessment is completed before moving the patient.

Vital Signs

1. Take vital signs and record immediately for baseline information.
2. Repeat at regular intervals (initially every 15 minutes).

Trauma

1. Disrobe patient completely once initial assessment has revealed no fractures and patient is secure on emergency cart.
2. Inspect the body for evidence of trauma.
   - Check for blood in ear canals, nares, and mouth.
   - Note any bruises, abrasions, and bleeding or open wounds.
   - Check tongue for scars or fresh wounds that could indicate a history of seizures.

Breath Odors

Note the presence of any odors.
- Fruity odor on breath—diabetic acidosis due to acetone
- Alcoholic odor—excessive intake of alcohol
- Urine smell on breath—uremia
- Fetid, mousy odor—hepatic failure

Skin Irregularities

Observe the face, trunk, and extremities for:
- Cyanosis—possible respiratory problem, shock
- Pallor—possible bleeding, shock
- Jaundice of skin or sclerae—hepatic failure
- Spider angiomata on upper trunk, sparse axillary hair in male and venous pattern in umbilical area (caput medusa) or flank regions (thoracoepigastric vein) seen in cirrhosis
- Argyria—metallic gray hue to skin from prolonged use of silver preparations as nasal astringents (silver gradually becomes deposited in the skin). It is a rare condition and may be confused with cyanosis.
- Warm, red skin—possible sunburn or heat stroke
- Cherry red color to lips and red skin—carbon monoxide poisoning
- Rashes, petechiae or ecchymoses—possible blood dyscrasia
- Needle marks or "tracks" along course of vein, on forearm, or in antecubital space of elbow—drug abuse.

Respirations

1. Observe rate, depth, and quality of respirations.
   - Central neurogenic hyperventilation (deep, rapid respirations) suggests brain stem involvement (midbrain or upper portion level).
   - Biot's or ataxic respirations (irregularly alternating periods of apnea and hyperpnea) associated with meningitis and disorders causing increased intracranial pressure.
   - Cheyne-Stokes respirations (respirations that gradually increase then decrease in rate and depth, until they cease for 5 to 50 seconds before resuming) occur with increased intracranial pressure, severe cardiopulmonary disease, and terminal stages of illness and in some normal persons during sleep.
   - Kussmaul breathing (deep, rapid respirations)—associated with diabetic acidosis or uremia
2. Auscultate chest for heart and lung sounds.
   - Wheezes and rhonchi (varying-pitched musical sounds) indicate partial obstruction to airflow in respiratory passages narrowed by secretions, swelling, etc.
   - Rales (crackling sounds) occur in conditions that produce moisture in the lungs.

Heart

1. Determine whether apical and radial pulse rates are the same. Difference in rate may indicate apical (auricular) fibrillation.
2. Count the rate to detect any alternation in rhythm.
3. Check for tachycardia or bradycardia.
   - Tachycardia is present in shock states, anxiety states, febrile episodes, cardiac problems, drug overdoses, and poisonings.
   - Bradycardia may be noted in digitalis intoxication, heart block, vasovagal episodes, drug overdose (especially central nervous system depressants), hypothermia, and normally in well-conditioned athletes.

Head and Neck

1. Gently palpate head and neck for swelling, wounds, or depressions.
   - Look for *Battle's sign* (bruise over mastoid area behind ear) resulting from a basilar skull fracture.
   - "Raccoon's eyes" (bilateral black eyes) suggest an anterior basal skull fracture.
2. Inspect nose and ears for damage to tympanic membrane or for drainage of clear, serosanguineous or nonclotting bloody fluid.
   - Drainage that contains glucose and does not clot indicates cerebrospinal fluid (CSF) secondary to a basilar skull fracture.
3. Gently palpate cervical spine. Twenty percent of patients with head injuries also have cervical spine injuries.
4. Once it has been established by examination and cervical spine x-rays that there is no cervical spine injury, test for signs of meningeal irritation, which may accompany subarachnoid hemorrhage or meningitis:
   - *Nuchal rigidity*—with the patient supine, flex the neck by placing the hand behind it and note the presence of pain, resistance, or rigidity.
   - *Brudzinski's sign*—passive flexion of one lower extremity causes a similar movement in the other leg, or flexion of the neck results in flexion of the ankle, knee, and hip.
   - *Kernig's sign*—flex one leg at the hip and knee. Note pain, resistance, and inability to extend the knee.

Note: These findings may be diminished or absent in deeper stages of coma.

Eyes

1. Observe for presence of contact lenses; remove (see Charts 33-1 and 33-2) and store with identification of left and right lenses.
2. Assess size and shape of pupils, their equality and reaction to light. For accuracy, use a pupil-size chart or a pocket ruler in mm and record on the neurologic flow sheet (see Fig. 18-4).
   - Unequal pupils more dilated and sluggishly reactive on one side than on the other—indicate a lesion, usually on the same side of the brain, that is exerting pressure on the oculomotor (3rd cranial) nerve.
   - Pupils that are equal in rate and degree of constriction occur with coma of other origins (metabolic, toxic, or psychogenic causes).
       Dilated pupils—anticholinergic agents (atropine, mushrooms) some barbiturate intoxication (glutethimide; see Chap. 30, Poisoning and Drug Overdose) severe hypoxia, terminal states
       Pinpoint or constricted pupils—opiates, pontine lesions, miotic drops for glaucoma
       Horner's syndrome (constriction of the pupil, partial ptosis, and decreased sweating on same side of face) suggest involvement of the descending sympathetic fibers in the ipsilateral brain stem or upper cord.
   - Test for consensual light reflex—hold both eyelids open, shine light into one eye, and observe the other. If the opposite pupil does not constrict, interruption of nerve connections in brain stem has occurred.

- Be aware that pupil response can mislead the examiner in the presence of eye trauma, blindness, eye prosthesis, and use of eye medications.
3. Assess ocular movements.
   - Determine presence of abnormal eye movements. Deviation of one or both eyes laterally or inferiorly Nystagmus (common with phencyclidine intoxication)
   - *Oculocephalic reflex* (doll's eye movements)—hold the upper eyelids open and quickly turn the head first to one side, then to the other. The fully conscious patient normally moves his eyes unpredictably or slightly in the direction opposite to that of the movement of the head. The comatose patient with an intact brain stem has doll's eye movements: when the head is turned, the eyes remain in their initial position, much as dolls' eyes do. Absence of these movements in the comatose patient suggests a lesion of the midbrain or pons, or very deep coma. This test is best performed by a neurosurgeon, since a spinal cord injury could be produced even if cervical spine x-rays are normal.

Note: Be sure that cervical spine injury has been ruled out first.
   - *Oculovestibular reflex with caloric stimulation*—elevate the head 30 degrees. Instill 1 ml ice water into ear canal. Normally, the eyes flick in the direction opposite to the irrigated ear; in the patient with brain stem damage there is no response.
       Be sure that eardrums are intact and canals are clear. Examiner should wait 5 minutes before performing this test in opposite ear.
       Caloric stimulation normally produces nystagmus.
4. Examine the fundus.
   - Papilledema (swelling about the optic disk) indicates increased intracranial pressure.
   - Hemorrhage or exudates indicate long-standing severe hypertensive or diabetic retinopathy.

Level of Consciousness

The conscious state relies on a network of cells and fibers in the brain stem, called the reticular formation, which sends impulses to the cerebral cortex, keeping the person awake and perceptive. Injuries to the brain, certain hormones, drugs, and levels of oxygen, glucose, and many other substances affect the reticular formation and its ability to send impulses to the cortex. These especially sensitive cells may forewarn of pathophysiology in alterations of consciousness long before it becomes manifest elsewhere in the body.

The level of consciousness (LOC) is routinely assessed on all patients, but in the patient whose function is depressed, it assumes increased importance.
- Avoid labels such as "stuporous," "obtunded," or "semicomatose." Rather, describe the patient's response to specific stimuli, such as voice or pain.
- Serial monitoring of LOC is the most important measurement to be made; interpretations of other neurologic findings and data are made in relation to this parameter. Consciousness is lost in a specific order. By serial determination of specific responses, one can determine whether the patient is improving or worsening.
- The Glasgow Coma Scale (GCS) has become a widely accepted method of recording LOC information over time (Fig. 18-1).

- Assessment of the LOC includes the following:
  1. Ask questions to assess the patient's orientation to:
     - Events—does he remember what happened, what the incident was that caused the present problem?
     - Time—what day of the week is it—morning, afternoon, evening?
     - Place—where is he at present?
     - Person—what is his name?
  2. Observe the patient's activity. Is he restless or somnolent?
  3. Determine the patient's response to verbal stimuli. How loud must one talk to arouse him? Describe his response to the stimuli as follows:
     - Appropriate—patient follows instructions, responds to his name by opening his eyes and saying "What?" or "Yes?"
     - Inappropriate
     - None
  4. If the patient does not respond to verbal stimuli, determine his response to pain. The stimuli should be applied to an uninjured area in a manner that elicits deep pain without tissue injury, such as:

- Rubbing the sternum
- Pinching the trapezius muscle or earlobes
- Applying supraorbital pressure with the index fingers
- Applying pressure to the base of the fingernail with an object such as a pencil (Fig. 18-2). (This may not be useful in the patient with hemiparesis or spinal cord injury)

Describe the patient's response to painful stimuli as follows:

- Appropriate—does he move the examiner's hand away?
- Inappropriate—does he move aimlessly?
- Note whether it is accompanied by decerebrate or decorticate posturing (Fig. 18-3)
- No response

  5. To determine whether coma is of psychogenic origin:
     - Raise the patient's hand over his head and allow it to drop. If it falls away from the face, the patient is protecting himself and the coma is most likely of psychogenic origin. If his hand falls on his face,

Figure 18-1 Glasgow Coma Scale. How to score responses. Scoring of Eye Opening; *4 = if the patient opens his eyes spontaneously; 3 = if the patient opens his eyes in response to speech (spoken or shouted); 2 = if the patient opens his eyes only in response to painful stimuli such as digital squeezing around nail beds of fingers; 1 = if the patient does not open his eyes in response to painful stimuli. Scoring of Best Motor Response: 6 = if the patient can obey a simple command such as "Lift your left hand off the bed."; 5 = if the patient moves a limb to locate the painful stimuli applied to the head or trunk and attempts to remove the source; 4 = if the patient attempts to withdraw from the source of pain; 3 = if the patient flexes only his arms at the elbows and wrist in response to painful stimuli to the nail beds (decorticate rigidity); 2 = if the patient extends his arms (straightens his elbows) in response to painful stimuli (decerebrate rigidity); 1 = if the patient has no motor response to pain on any limb. Scoring of Best Verbal Response: 5 = if the patient is oriented to time, place, and person; 4 = if the patient is able to converse although not oriented to time, place, or person (e.g., "Where am I?"); 3 = if the patient speaks only in words or phrases that make little or no sense; 2 = if the patient responds with incomprehensible sounds such as groans; 1 = if the patient does not respond verbally at all.* (Hickey JV: Clinical Practice of Neurological and Neurosurgical Nursing. Philadelphia, JB Lippincott, 1981)

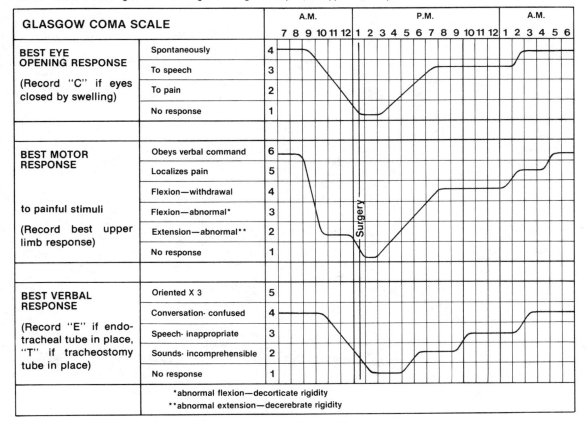

GLASGOW COMA SCALE			A.M. 7 8 9 10 11 12	P.M. 1 2 3 4 5 6 7 8 9 10 11 12	A.M. 1 2 3 4 5 6
BEST EYE OPENING RESPONSE (Record "C" if eyes closed by swelling)	Spontaneously	4			
	To speech	3			
	To pain	2			
	No response	1			
BEST MOTOR RESPONSE to painful stimuli (Record best upper limb response)	Obeys verbal command	6			
	Localizes pain	5			
	Flexion—withdrawal	4			
	Flexion—abnormal*	3		Surgery	
	Extension—abnormal**	2			
	No response	1			
BEST VERBAL RESPONSE (Record "E" if endotracheal tube in place, "T" if tracheostomy tube in place)	Oriented X 3	5			
	Conversation- confused	4			
	Speech- inappropriate	3			
	Sounds- incomprehensible	2			
	No response	1			
	*abnormal flexion—decorticate rigidity **abnormal extension—decerebrate rigidity				

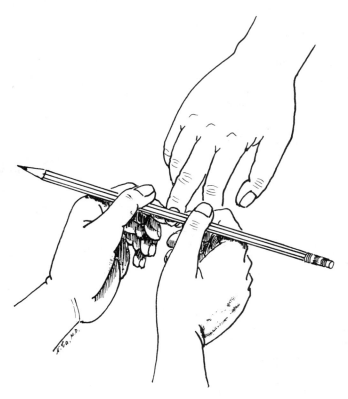

Figure 18-2 *Application of pressure to patient's finger to evoke response to a painful stimulus.*

3. Observe skin for possible causes of coma (*e.g.,* needle tracks indicating drug abuse).
4. Apply a painful stimulus and observe whether active withdrawal occurs and whether the motion is equal on both sides.
5. Raise the arm or leg and allow it to drop.
   - In deep coma, the limb will drop suddenly, in a limp manner.
   - In lighter coma, the limb will fall gradually.
6. Note any resistance to passive motion by the elbow or knee joints. Unilateral rigidity or flaccidity may indicate a neurologic lesion.
7. Compare deep tendon reflexes bilaterally including the biceps, triceps, knees, and ankles. A diminished or hyperactive reflex may indicate neurologic lesion.

Chest

1. Assess respiratory movements. Note rate, depth, and presence of sounds.
2. Note deformity, soft tissue injury, or paradoxical or unequal motion of the chest wall, suggesting trauma.
3. Auscultate lungs to evaluate ventilatory exchange and to note presence of rales, wheezes or rhonchi suggestive of cardiac or pulmonary disease.

Abdomen

1. Inspect for incisional scars, or soft tissue injury suggestive of trauma.
2. Note asymmetry, visceral enlargement, or increasing abdominal girth.
3. Assess femoral pulses.
4. Note abdominal spasm or rigidity (these may be masked by coma).
5. Peritoneal tap or gastric lavage may be indicated.

See Chapters 21, Thoracic and Abdominal Trauma, and 22, The Patient With an Acute Abdomen, for details of abdominal and chest assessment.

Adjunct Studies

The number and types of adjunct studies used vary with the circumstances, the tentative diagnosis, and the hospital set-

the coma state is probably not of psychogenic origin.
   - Gently brush the patient's eyelashes. The patient with psychogenic coma will flinch or move his eyelids in a protective reflex.
6. Record serial observations as in the GCS.

Extremities

1. Evaluate for evidence of deformity or fracture.
2. Observe for spontaneous movements of the limbs.
   - Are the movements unilateral or bilateral?
   - Is one side weaker than the other?

Figure 18-3 Top. *Decorticate rigidity.* In decorticate rigidity the upper arms are held tightly to the sides, with elbows, wrists, and fingers flexed. The legs are extended and internally rotated. The feet are plantar flexed. This posture implies a destructive lesion of the corticospinal tracts within or very near the cerebral hemispheres. When unilateral, this is the posture of chronic spastic hemiplegia. Bottom. *Decerebrate rigidity.* In decerebrate rigidity the jaws are clenched and the neck extended. The arms are adducted and stiffly extended at the elbows, with forearms pronated, wrists and fingers flexed. The legs are stiffly extended at the knees, with the feet plantar flexed. This posture may occur spontaneously or only in response to external stimuli such as light, noise, or pain. It is caused by a lesion in the diencephalon, midbrain, or pons, although severe metabolic disorders such as hypoxia or hypoglycemia may also produce it. (Bates B: Guide to Physical Examination. Philadelphia, JB Lippincott, 1979)

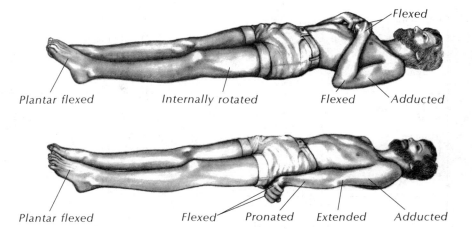

Flexed

Plantar flexed   Internally rotated   Flexed   Adducted

Plantar flexed   Flexed   Pronated   Extended   Adducted

ting. Studies that may be useful in clarifying the diagnosis include blood work, urinalysis, lumbar puncture, echoencephalography, and x-ray studies, which may include the skull and cervical spine, and special radiologic techniques, including brain scan and cerebral angiography.

Blood Studies. Complete blood count (CBC) and glucose and urea studies are done on all comatose patients to reveal possible anemia, infection, hyperglycemia, hypoglycemia, or renal failure. Serum acetone study is indicated if the glucose is elevated. Creatinine and serum electrolyte studies facilitate detection of renal failure or severe metabolic disturbance.

Other studies may include arterial blood gases in suspected respiratory insufficiency, toxicology studies in suspected drug overdose, blood cultures in febrile states, and type and crossmatch for patients with anemia, multiple injuries, or suspected major blood loss.

Urine Studies. Depending on suspected causes of coma, the urine may be analyzed for specific gravity, glucose, ketone bodies, and protein. Microscopic examination, culture and sensitivity studies, or toxicology studies may be indicated.

Radiologic Studies. Since x-ray studies require that the patient be moved to the radiology department, it is essential that a physician or nurse be in attendance at all times to monitor the patient.

Skull X-rays. Anteroposterior and lateral views of the skull and the *entire* cervical spine should be done with minimum movement and can provide much information. Even though a metabolic disorder or drug intoxication may have precipitated the comatose state, structural damage to the skull, brain, or cervical spine could have occurred from a fall.

Other X-ray Studies. Additional studies of other body structures may be clinically warranted, as in possible child abuse, multiple trauma, etc. Angiograms and brain scans are rarely necessary in the emergency setting unless a rapidly expanding lesion, such as an epidural hematoma, is suspected. Computerized tomography (CT) scans allow the direct visualization of intracranial structures and are being used as diagnostic tools with increasing frequency.

Lumbar Puncture. Lumbar puncture is useful in diagnosing viral or bacterial meningitis, chronic central nervous system (CNS) infections, and in subarachnoid or intracranial hemorrhage, tumors, and brain abscesses. However, *lumbar puncture should not be performed if there is evidence of increased intracranial pressure, particularly as manifested by papilledema;* removal of even small amounts of fluid may cause herniation of the brain or brain stem with serious or fatal consequences.

Additional Diagnostic Tests. Depending on the clinical presentation of the patient, other tests may include echoencephalogram, electroencephalogram (EEG), electrocardiogram (ECG), chest x-ray, thyroid function studies, and analysis of gastric contents.

Documentation. All data should be recorded on a neurologic flow sheet (Fig. 18-4).

GENERAL PRINCIPLES OF MANAGEMENT FOR THE COMATOSE PATIENT

Goals for management of the comatose patient include measures to protect and support the unresponsive patient and activities leading to diagnosis so that definitive care can be initiated. Management of the comatose patient is outlined in Chart 18-2.

EMERGENCIES RELATED TO SPECIFIC CAUSES OF COMA

Four main categories and underlying causes of coma have been described. Coma may be associated with metabolic problems, structural disorders, toxic substance ingestion, or psychogenic causes. Emergencies associated with each of these causes will be discussed in turn.

COMA RELATED TO METABOLIC CAUSES

The major causes of metabolic coma are hyperglycemia, hyperosmolar hyperglycemic nonketotic coma, hypoglycemia, myxedema crisis, and uremia. Less common causes are adrenal insufficiency, lactic acidosis, and hepatic failure. Hyperglycemia, hyperosmolar hyperglycemic nonketotic coma, and hypoglycemia are related to diabetes; myxedema crisis is associated with hypothyroidism and uremia with chronic renal dysfunction.

Diabetic Ketoacidosis (Hyperglycemia)

Diabetic ketoacidosis (DKA) results from an absence or an inadequate amount of insulin, the endocrine secretion of the pancreas responsible for transport of glucose across the cell membrane. Insulin, a hypoglycemic factor, functions by:
- Lowering the blood sugar by increasing the utilization of glucose by tissues
- Promoting the storage of glucose as glycogen in the liver and muscles
- Promoting the formation of fat from glucose
- Decreasing the production of glycogen from fats and proteins

When insulin is present in inadequate amounts, the above functions are affected; as a result, there is a decrease in the transport of glucose into cells and an increase in the breakdown of fat and protein. This altered metabolism ultimately results in dehydration; loss of sodium, potassium, chloride, and bicarbonate; and an increase in ketone bodies, leading to the ketoacidotic state.

The precipitating causes of DKA include the following:
- Failure to take insulin or to take it in sufficient quantities
- Resistance to insulin

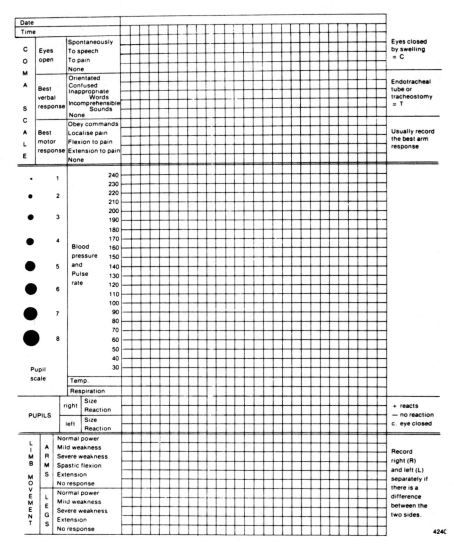

Figure 18-4 *Neurologic flow sheet. (Reproduced with permission of Sisters of Charity Hospital, Buffalo, N.Y.)*

- Presence of infection
- Emotional or physical stress (pregnancy, injury, surgery, anxiety)
- Concurrent use of certain drugs (phenytoin, steroids, phenobarbital)

Assessment. Clinical manifestations of DKA occur *gradually,* secondary to the developing metabolic acidosis, electrolyte imbalance, and dehydration.

The following signs and symptoms may be observed:
- LOC falls gradually.
- Skin is warm, dry, and flushed because of dehydration.
- Tachycardia and hypotension forewarn of hypovolemia.
- Patient resorts to Kussmaul breathing (increased rate and depth of respirations) to compensate for the acidosis.
- Breath has a fruity or acetone odor due to ketosis. Be careful not to assume or confuse with alcohol intoxication.

However, in some instances, both conditions may be present concurrently.
- Signs of infection may be present and suggest a cause for DKA.

Adjunct Studies. These include the following:
1. Blood studies, which show elevated glucose and blood urea nitrogen (BUN), decreased bicarbonate and *p*H, and strongly positive plasma ketones.
2. Urine studies—urine is strongly positive for glucose and ketones and may contain protein.

Management. Because of the altered LOC, the history of diabetes, and the difficulty of distinguishing between DKA and its potentially life-threatening counterpart hypoglycemia, initial management, especially in the field, is directed toward correcting a possibly hypoglycemic state and providing symptomatic support of the patient.

Chart 18-2

MANAGEMENT OF THE COMATOSE PATIENT

Prehospital Care

1. Do a primary survey and manage as appropriate.
   - Protect the spine, especially the cervical spine.
   - Maintain airway, using cervical spine precautions.
   - Provide ventilatory support; assist respirations if depressed; provide oxygen.
2. Complete the secondary survey according to assessment guidelines mentioned previously.
   - Note information provided by observers at scene and appearance of area in which patient found.
   - Bring items at scene (medications, drugs, etc.) that may provide information about patient's history.
3. Monitor vital signs and neurologic signs at frequent intervals.
4. Implement paramedic protocol for unconscious patients, which, in addition to the above, generally includes:
   - Draw blood sample(s) and start IV of D_5W to keep open.
   - Consider glucose 50%, 50 ml IV.
   - Consider naloxone HCl (Narcan), 0.4 mg IV. This is a specific narcotic antagonist. May repeat twice.
   - Place on cardiac monitor.
5. Consider transport on side with suction readied.

Hospital Care

1. Maintain airway, provide ventilatory support as appropriate.
2. Monitor vital signs, neurologic signs, and cardiac activity at frequent intervals. Begin neurologic flow sheet (see Fig. 18-4).
3. Draw blood for analyses and establish veinway if not done in field.
   - Closely monitor infusion rate according to physician's instructions in presence of increased intracranial pressure.
   - IV solution may change as laboratory data become available.
   - CVP line may be indicated in the elderly, those with cardiac compromise and those who require large amounts of IV fluids.
4. Insert nasogastric tube. Aspirate stomach contents for analysis and begin lavage if indicated. A nasogastric tube should not be inserted in the presence of a basilar skull fracture except by the physician.
5. Insert indwelling urinary catheter. Obtain urine specimen.
6. Initiate diagnostic studies as determined by patient history and examination.
7. Administer medications as indicated. See Specific Causes of Coma in the section that follows, and also Chap. 20, Injuries of the Head, Neck, and Spine.

---

1. *Pre-hospital care* is as outlined for the unconscious patient (Chart 18-2). Emergency personnel who are unable to administer an IV bolus of 50% glucose may place sugar, honey, or a specially prepared glucose solution in the cheek or under the tongue of the unresponsive patient, after making sure that the airway is protected by placing the patient on his side. In the hypoglycemic patient, LOC improves, but in the diabetic with DKA, it does not. Insulin is never administered by prehospital emergency personnel.
2. *Hospital care* is directed toward restoring carbohydrate utilization and correcting the fluid and electrolyte imbalance (Fig. 18-5).

In addition to support of the unconscious patient, the following measures are required:
1. Obtain blood samples and a *fresh* urine specimen. (Sugar concentrates in urine that is static in the bladder)
   - Read color changes on chemical test strips in incandescent rather than fluorescent lighting for greater accuracy.
   - Obtain CBC, blood glucose, serum electrolytes, blood pH, and BUN
2. Start intravenous (IV) line of normal or half-normal saline to improve hydration.
3. Insert central venous pressure (CVP) line to monitor fluid administration.
4. Administer regular insulin (crystalline zinc insulin) through IV tubing. IV administration is recommended initially because of dehydration. Subsequent doses may be given IV or subcutaneously (SC) based on the patient's response and changes in blood chemistry and glucose levels.
5. Correct electrolyte imbalance.
   - Potassium chloride, 20 to 40 mEq/L, must be added to the infusion to aid glucose metabolism.
   - Administer after renal function is restored.
   - Closely monitor cardiac status on ECG.
   - When blood glucose reaches desired levels (usually 250–300/100 ml), administer glucose infusion (5% to

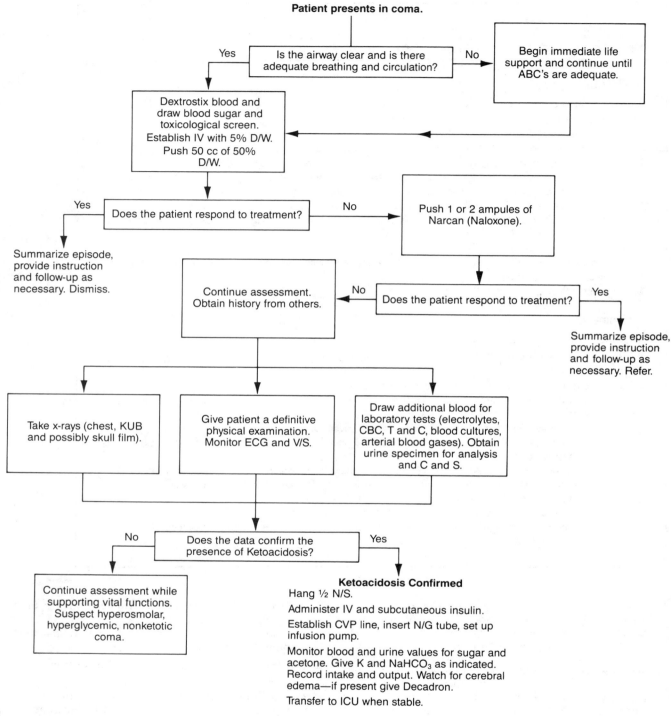

Patient presents in coma.

Is the airway clear and is there adequate breathing and circulation?

Yes → Dextrostix blood and draw blood sugar and toxicological screen. Establish IV with 5% D/W. Push 50 cc of 50% D/W.

No → Begin immediate life support and continue until ABC's are adequate.

Does the patient respond to treatment?

Yes → Summarize episode, provide instruction and follow-up as necessary. Dismiss.

No → Push 1 or 2 ampules of Narcan (Naloxone).

Does the patient respond to treatment?

No → Continue assessment. Obtain history from others.

Yes → Summarize episode, provide instruction and follow-up as necessary. Refer.

Take x-rays (chest, KUB and possibly skull film).

Give patient a definitive physical examination. Monitor ECG and V/S.

Draw additional blood for laboratory tests (electrolytes, CBC, T and C, blood cultures, arterial blood gases). Obtain urine specimen for analysis and C and S.

Does the data confirm the presence of Ketoacidosis?

No → Continue assessment while supporting vital functions. Suspect hyperosmolar, hyperglycemic, nonketotic coma.

Yes →

Ketoacidosis Confirmed

Hang ½ N/S.

Administer IV and subcutaneous insulin.

Establish CVP line, insert N/G tube, set up infusion pump.

Monitor blood and urine values for sugar and acetone. Give K and NaHCO₃ as indicated. Record intake and output. Watch for cerebral edema—if present give Decadron.

Transfer to ICU when stable.

Figure 18-5 *Management of the comatose patient. (Martin P: Is it ketoacidosis? J Emerg Nurs 3:10–14, January–February 1977)*

10% glucose in normal saline) or 50 ml of 50% glucose in water IV push, to prevent precipitant hypoglycemia.

6. Monitor output, sugar, and acetone in urine at hourly intervals.

7. Insert nasogastric tube.

8. Prepare for hospital admission.

Hyperosmolar Hyperglycemic Nonketotic Coma

The comatose patient who is dehydrated and is hyperglycemic with little or no acidosis may be in hyperosmolar hyperglycemic nonketotic coma (HHNC). This condition most commonly occurs in middle-aged or older persons with mild or unknown diabetes. It has been associated with conditions that can lead to fluid imbalances or elevations in blood glucose in susceptible persons.

The precipitating causes of HHNC include the following:

- Infections (especially gram-negative infections), trauma, surgery, or other forms of acute stress that elevate blood glucose through gluconeogenesis (breakdown of proteins or fats to produce glucose)
- Use of steroids, which can increase the body's resistance to insulin as well as promote gluconeogenesis
- Burns, hemodialysis, peritoneal dialysis (in which high sugar concentrations are used as dialyzing fluid and remain long enough for some to be absorbed), hyperalimentation
- Pancreatitis, or pancreatic or other abdominal surgery, which affect insulin availability
- Use of diuretics, especially the thiazides or furosemide
- Cardiovascular or renal disease
- Any variety of problems resulting in a proportionally decreased fluid intake or increased fluid output

Assessment. Clinical manifestations of HHNC are similar to those of DKA, that is, dehydration and hyperglycemia. The distinguishing difference is that acidosis and ketonemia are absent or mild in HHNC, probably because sufficient amounts of insulin are available to prevent fat breakdown.

The following signs and symptoms may be observed:

- Increasing lethargy progressing to coma
- Focal neurologic abnormalities, including seizures (which may confuse the diagnosis with cerebrovascular accident)
- Signs of shock (if the patient is severely dehydrated)
- A history associated with one or more of the above precipitating causes

Laboratory findings help establish the diagnosis; the following are characteristic of HHNC:

1. Elevated blood glucose, often to a level much higher than that found with DKA (greater than 650 mg/100 ml)
2. Elevated serum osmolality (greater than 350 mEq/L)
3. Little or no elevation in serum ketones

HHNC carries a 40% to 70% mortality rate. This high incidence may be due to delayed recognition, advanced age, concomitant medical problems, or other unknown factors.

Management. Management of the patient with HHNC consists of rehydration, correction of electrolyte imbalances, and administration of insulin and glucose. Careful monitoring is essential.

1. Replace fluid volume with 0.45% saline or with normal saline or plasma expanders if profound dehydration with hypotension is present.
   - Half the volume lost should be replaced during the first 12 hours if possible.
   - Monitor CVP carefully to avoid fluid overload.
   - Correct electrolyte imbalances as urinary output is restored.
2. Administer regular insulin, but with cautious monitoring. Responsiveness to insulin varies in these patients. Insulin is usually administered IV and SC in equally divided doses at intervals so that blood glucose levels gradually return

to normal as patient is being rehydrated—usually over 8 to 12 hours.

3. IV administration of glucose may be started when blood glucose concentrations are 250 to 300 mg/100 ml.
4. Closely monitor cardiovascular and neurologic status throughout therapy.

Hypoglycemia

Hypoglycemic reactions may occur when blood glucose falls below 50 mg/100 ml of blood or with higher blood glucose levels when the fall has been rapid. In the diabetic, hypoglycemia may be caused by the following:

- Too much insulin—reactions may occur 5 to 10 minutes after an injection of regular insulin, but may occur later with the intermediate and long-acting forms of insulin. (See Table 18-1 for the peak effects of various insulins).
- Not enough food (a delayed or missed meal)
- Unusual or vigorous physical activity or emotional stress
- Oral hypoglycemic agents (except phenformin, or DBI)

Hypoglycemia can occur in nondiabetic persons and accounts for the bulk of hypoglycemic reactions. Most commonly, hypoglycemia is *functional* and results from an oversecretion of insulin (hyperinsulinism) because of an excessive response to glucose absorption, physical exertion, pregnancy and lactation, or anorexia nervosa. *Organic* hypoglycemia can occur from hepatic insufficiency from any cause (including that caused by chronic alcoholism and drug abuse), resulting in glycogen depletion and impaired glucose production. Pancreatic tumors and numerous other endocrinopathies may be associated with organic hypoglycemia.

Assessment. The early signs and symptoms of hypoglycemia are caused by a reduction in the amount of glucose available to the brain and the body's coping responses. The following may be observed:

- Nervousness or trembling, weakness, and sweating
- Hunger
- Falling LOC (faintness, disorientation, aggressive or erratic behavior)
- Headache
- Tachycardia and palpitations
- Double vision and unsteady gait
- Pallor and chills
- Seizures, usually grand mal seizures, occurring suddenly and without warning

Management. In contrast to the pattern in DKA, the neurologic findings in hypoglycemia occur rapidly, and prompt action is required. Because the brain is deprived of glucose, an essential nutrient, brain damage and sometimes death may occur if the condition is not treated in time.

1. *Prehospital care* for hypoglycemic reactions includes the administration of a glucose source. If the patient is conscious and able to swallow and protect his own airway, give orange juice with sugar, candy, corn syrup, or the like. The less responsive patient may be positioned on his side, and a concentrated sugar solution or paste may

TABLE 18-1.   INSULIN PREPARATIONS COMMERCIALLY AVAILABLE IN THE UNITED STATES, CLASSIFIED ACCORDING TO APPROXIMATE DURATION OF ACTION

Classification	Insulin Preparation*	Action		
		Onset	*Peak*	*Duration*
Rapid	Regular (neutral)	IV:† immediate IM: 5–30 min SC: 30 min	15–30 min 30–60 min 1–2 hr	1–2 hr 2–4 hr 5–10 hr
	Semilente (insulin zinc suspension prompt)	SC: 1 hr	3–4 hr	10–16 hr
Intermediate	Globin zinc insulin	SC: 2 hr	6–8 hr	12–18 hr
	NPH (isophane insulin suspension)	SC: 2 hr	8–14 hr	18–24 hr
	Lente (insulin zinc suspension)	SC: 2 hr	8–14 hr	18–24 hr
Slow	Protamine zinc insulin suspension	SC: 6 hr	16–20 hr	24–30 hr
	Ultralente (insulin zinc suspension extended)	SC: 6 hr	18–29 hr	30–36 hr
Combinations	Regular + NPH	SC: 30 min	2–10 hr	18–24 hr
	Regular + Lente	SC: 1 hr	2–10 hr	18–24 hr
	Semilente + Lente	SC: 1 hr	4–10 hr	18–24 hr
	Semilente + Ultralente	SC: 1 hr	2–24 hr	30–36 hr

* Preparations are available in concentrations of 40, 80, and 100 units/ml in 10-ml vials. Regular, NPH, and Lente insulins are available as beef-pork insulin mixtures and as special monospecies insulins made exclusively from beef or pork pancreas.

† IV, IM, and SC denote intravenous, intramuscular, and subcutaneous routes of administration.

(Owen OE, Boden G, Schuman CR: Managing insulin dependent diabetic patients. *Postgrad Med* 59:128, January 1976)

be placed in the pocket of the cheek for absorption without compromising the airway. (Commercially prepared products are available for this purpose.)

Prehospital personnel authorized to administer IV medications may give 50 ml of 50% glucose solution IV (see Fig. 18–5). When hypoglycemia is the cause of the unresponsive state, a dramatic improvement is observed within seconds to minutes.

2. *Hospital care* includes the following:
   - Obtain a baseline blood sugar and make a Dextrostix determination.
   - Administer 50 ml of 50% glucose solution. (This concentrated solution is irritating to the vein and subcutaneous tissue. Be sure to aspirate before and at intervals during administration.)
   - Provide instruction, follow-up, or referral to prevent recurrent episodes or to treat the underlying problem.

Uremia

Uremia is a less common cause of coma; coma represents the most advanced stage of CNS involvement in uremia. With uremia, a number of acid metabolites increase in the blood, precipitating the comatose state. If a history is available, one may detect a long-standing condition of urinary tract disease. The onset of the coma is gradual; the early phase of uremia is marked by neuromuscular and personality disorders. Seizures may occur. In any comatose patient, particularly the elderly, this cause must be considered.

Assessment.   Assessment may reveal dry, scaling skin (frequently described as "uremic frost"), dehydration, muscle fasciculation, typical Kussmaul respiration, and, at times, a pericardial friction rub. Laboratory work reveals an elevated BUN, potassium, and creatinine. Electrolyte studies and arterial blood gases demonstrate a metabolic acidosis.

Management.   Initial management consists of hydration, correction of the electrolyte imbalance, and stabilization of the patient. Investigative studies are undertaken to identify the underlying cause when the patient's condition warrants.

Myxedema Crisis

The patient who has myxedema in crisis may become comatose as a result of this severe, complicated form of hypothyroidism. It usually results from the body's inability to cope with additional internal or external insults.

Assessment.   Clinical findings that occur with this condition may include the following:
- History of apathy, fatigue, intolerance to cold, anorexia, constipation, menorrhagia, or amenorrhea
- History of thyroid dysfunction, thyroid surgery, or radioactive iodine therapy
- Dry, cool, coarse, and thickened skin
- Hypothermia
- Sinus bradycardia, distant heart sounds, and cardiomegaly
- Increased diastolic blood pressure
- Respiratory depression
- Laboratory findings may show decreased serum thyroxine or increased thyroid-stimulating hormone (TSH).
- Other findings may include elevated cholesterol, triglycerides, sedimentation rate, creatine phosphokinase (CPK), and cerebrospinal fluid protein.

Management.   General supportive measures to treat the manifestations of this illness are applied to treat the problem before laboratory data confirming the diagnosis become available.

1. Treat respiratory depression through assisted ventilation and tracheostomy if necessary.

- Monitor arterial blood gases.
- Avoid sedatives. Drugs are administered in decreased dosages, since they will be metabolized more slowly than normally.
2. Maintain body heat. Avoid exposure to cold and any active external rewarming methods that may move blood away from vital organs to the periphery, producing shock.
3. Establish IV (dextrose solutions are preferred, since hypoglycemia may be present).
4. Administer cortisol, levothyroxine, and other medications as ordered.
5. Monitor cardiac status, vital signs, and neurologic checks.
6. Search for subtle signs of infection, since the hypothyroid patient may not manifest obvious signs and symptoms.

The mortality rate associated with hypothyroidism approximates 50% to 75%. This high incidence of mortality emphasizes the need for early recognition and treatment.

COMA RELATED TO STRUCTURAL CAUSES

Coma due to structural causes represents serious structural change in the CNS. A lesion is present, which may produce localizing neurologic signs.

Cerebrovascular Accident

Apoplexy and stroke occur most commonly in persons over 50. They are due to compromised cerebral blood flow, resulting in damage to brain cells. The most common etiology is cerebral thrombosis; there may be symptoms of "little strokes" for a period of time.

Assessment. The history is significant. A member of the family may say that the patient had a "falling out" spell or recurring episodes of momentary dizziness, loss of balance, or slurred speech for varying periods of time, then was found unconscious. When due to embolus or hemorrhage, the onset is usually rapid, with few or no preexisting symptoms relating to the CNS.

Important points in assessment are as follows:

- History of the presence of risk factors known to cause cerebrovascular accident, such as hypertension, elevated serum cholesterol, cardiac enlargement, congestive heart failure, coronary artery disease, diabetes, and cigarette smoking
- History of impending manifestations of cerebrovascular accident, such as transient ischemic attacks (TIAs), memory impairment, dizziness, syncope, headache, and blurred vision
- Localized neurologic signs

  Hemiparesis

  Hemiplegia

  Facial palsy

  Diminished deep tendon reflexes (on contralateral side)

  Aphasia
- Diminished LOC
- Possibly, bladder or bowel incontinence

Management. Initial care is supportive. An airway must be maintained, ventilations supported, and the cardiovascular status stabilized. The patient is admitted for further care and rehabilitation.

Ruptured Cerebral Aneurysm

Rupture of a cerebral artery aneurysm is most often found in persons below age 40. This condition must be considered in young adults. Such an aneurysm is congenital and may occur anywhere in the cerebral arterial tree but is most commonly seen at the bifurcation of the internal carotid artery, located at the base of the brain. Leaking or rupture causes bleeding into the subarachnoid space.

Assessment. History may reveal that the patient complained of severe headache just before lapsing into coma. Patients in emergency departments who have severe headaches but are fairly alert have been seen to lapse into coma during the course of evaluation. A frank rupture of the aneurysm has a high mortality rate.

Examination reveals nuchal rigidity, but localizing neurologic signs are often absent. Vital signs may be normal, although bradycardia and high blood pressure are frequently present. With lumbar puncture, bloody fluid is recovered.

Management. Early neurosurgical consultation is advisable, to determine whether urgent surgery is warranted. Cerebral angiography will localize the site of the lesion. Supportive measures are necessary until a decision has been made on the course of management. IV fluid therapy is restricted to prevent further increase in intracranial pressure.

Cerebral Neoplasm

Neoplasms of the brain may cause coma as a late manifestation. They may be either primary or metastatic tumors.

Assessment. The history reveals varying periods of neurologic symptoms and personality or neuromuscular disorders. It may also reveal a period of febrile illness, with gradual worsening of the victim's condition, leading to coma. Neoplasm must be considered in patients known to have malignant disease elsewhere. The most common malignant tumors likely to metastasize to the brain originate in the lung, gastrointestinal tract, breast, and kidney.

Assessment usually reveals unilateral localizing signs. Fever, tachycardia, and leukocytosis are common. Blood cultures are taken as indicated. Lumbar puncture is helpful in clarifying the diagnosis. The cerebrospinal fluid protein content may be elevated.

Management. Emergency care is supportive. In the undiagnosed patient, an intensive workup may be necessary to identify the problem. The necessary studies include tests for meningitis, encephalitis, and brain abscess, and if any of these is positive, massive doses of specific antibiotics should be given early in the course of treatment.

Major Seizure Disorder

There are many types of seizures, but the type that most often produces unconsciousness and brings emergency personnel in contact with the patient is a major motor, or grand mal, seizure. Seizure activity is a sign of underlying pathology that mandates investigation when it occurs for the first time, especially in the adult patient.

Causes. The many causes of seizures include the following:
- Congenital anomalies and genetic disorders
- Brain injury (cerebral palsy, posttraumatic states)
- Infection (encephalitis, meningitis, febrile seizures in children, brain abscess, tuberculosis)
- Vascular disturbances (cerebral thrombosis, embolus)
- Metabolic, nutritional disturbances (hypoglycemia)
- Primary or metastatic tumors
- Degenerative diseases
- Idiopathic epilepsy

Assessment. Though each seizure is unique, depending upon the origin and location of seizure activity in the brain, the typical progression of events in the grand mal seizure is as follows:
1. Aura (a sensory perception, usually visual or olfactory, noted by some patients)
2. Complete loss of consciousness, which may be preceded by a cry or followed by bowel or bladder incontinence and amnesia for the duration of the event
3. Tonic contractions in which the body appears to stiffen
4. Clonic contractions that appear as jerking movements

5. The postictal state, in which the patient is somnolent and minimally responsive. This "sleep" may last minutes to hours. The patient usually has no recall of the event.

During the tonic and clonic contraction phase, the muscles of respiration are also affected, so that breathing ceases and the patient becomes pale or cyanotic with time. Excessive salivation and some initial respiratory distress may be noted as breathing resumes.

Management. The primary goal of treatment is to protect the patient from injury during the seizure and to ensure a protective environment in case the seizure recurs. After the seizure, evaluation and treatment of the underlying causes should ensue. The care of the patient who is having a seizure is outlined in Chart 18-3.

Status Epilepticus

Status epilepticus is a series of grand mal seizures that occurs without the patient's regaining consciousness. This condition can be life-threatening because of the effects of prolonged hypoxia on brain tissue.

Management. Prompt management is essential for this condition. The following measures are indicated:
- Support respiratory and cardiovascular functions.
- Draw venous blood samples for analysis.
- Administer 50 ml of 50% glucose solution IV.
- Add IV of D_5W.
- Administer 5 mg diazepam by slow IV push. Additional 5 mg IV boluses may need to be administered until the

---

Chart 18-3

MANAGEMENT OF THE PATIENT IN A SEIZURE

- Protect patient from injury during seizure. Lower patient to ground if standing and provide additional padding of hard objects, but *do not restrain patient.*
- Loosen constrictive clothing.
- Place a soft object that cannot break between teeth if possible, *but do not pry clenched teeth apart.* Do not insert your fingers into patient's mouth during seizure.
- Following seizure, place patient on side for drainage of sputum and mucus and prevention of aspiration of vomitus.
- Administer oxygen to relieve hypoxia.
- Provide privacy and protect from curious onlookers.
- Gather information to help identify cause.
- Attend patient until he is conscious.
- Administer oxygen if available.
- Reassure patient and reorient him to environment when he awakens.
- Record progression of behavior during seizure.
- Search for information and evidence suggesting cause of seizure.
- Handle or transport patient gently.

TABLE 18-2. ALCOHOL INGESTION AND ALCOHOL BLOOD LEVELS*

Amount of Alcohol Ingested	Percent of Alcohol in Blood	Symptoms
2 oz of whiskey	0.05%	Not under the influence, appears normal
4 oz of whiskey	0.10% (common legal limit for operation of motor vehicle)	Beginnings of outward physical symptoms: • Emotional lability (boastfulness, exhilaration, talkativeness, remorse, belligerence) • Slight muscular incoordination such as slowed reaction time, ataxia • Decreased inhibitions
6 oz of whiskey	0.15%	"Under the influence" • Sensory disturbances (decreased pain sense, diplopia, vertigo, slurred speech) • Confusion • Staggering gait • Rapid pulse • Diaphoresis
8 oz (½ pint) of whiskey	0.20%	Acutely intoxicated • Marked decrease in response to stimuli • Muscular incoordination approaching paralysis • Nausea and vomiting • Drowsiness or stupor • Symptoms listed for 0.15%
	0.30%–0.40%	• Complete unconsciousness • Impaired or absent tendon reflexes • Peripheral vascular collapse (hypotension, tachycardia, cold pale skin, hypothermia, slow stertorous respiration) • Seizures (if present may also indicate hypoglycemia)
1½–2 pints whiskey	0.50%	• Death due to cardiac or respiratory arrest or aspiration pneumonitis

* Minimum blood levels that can produce symptoms in an average (160 lb) adult 30 to 45 minutes after ingestion. There is much variability according to an individual's tolerance to alcohol. Other factors to consider are the type and amount of alcohol ingested and the period of time over which it was consumed.

(Ansbaugh P: Emergency management of intoxicated patients with head injuries. J. Emerg/Nursing 3:10, May–June 1977)

longer-acting anticonvulsant has been absorbed at a level to control seizure activity.

- Phenobarbital may be used in lieu of diazepam.
- Administer phenytoin (Dilantin) as a slow, separate IV solution.
- As soon as possible, insert a nasogastric tube to decompress the stomach and prevent aspiration.
- Monitor vital signs and neurologic checks frequently.
- Prepare for hospital admission.

COMA RELATED TO INTOXICATION

Alcohol Intoxication

The effects of alcohol intoxication are so common that they require little elaboration. They consist of varying degrees of exhilaration and excitement, loss of inhibition, behavior aberrations, loquacity, slurred speech, ataxia, irritability, drowsiness, and, in advanced cases, coma. High blood levels of alcohol may produce death from cardiac or respiratory arrest (see Table 18-2). A potent CNS depressant, alcohol can potentiate or produce an additive effect with CNS depressants and other drugs, notably antihistamines and mind-altering drugs, so that toxic or lethal effects may be produced with lower blood levels of alcohol.

Though the recognition and treatment of the alcohol-intoxicated patient is routine to emergency personnel, the identification and management of the intoxicated patient in coma is not so clear. Only after careful exclusion of other causes for the coma can a diagnosis of alcohol-induced coma be made. Alcoholic coma can be life-threatening when accompanied by respiratory depression and loss of corneal and pupillary reflexes. This condition requires prompt intervention, as outlined in Chart 18-4.

Intoxication Due to Drugs and Toxic Substances

A wide variety of drugs and toxic substances can be responsible for producing coma, because of either their primary effects or the effects of withdrawal. Effects from intoxications are detailed in Chapter 30, Poisoning and Drug Overdose. Carbon monoxide poisoning is discussed in Chapter 15, Respiratory Emergencies.

COMA RELATED TO FUNCTIONAL/PSYCHOGENIC CAUSES

Coma of psychogenic origin is probably least frequently seen in the emergency setting. History usually reveals that the patient has been under psychiatric care or has exhibited personality alterations. The coma may have been preceded by a period of apprehension, overactivity, and hyperpnea.

Complete laboratory studies should be done to rule out any of the other more common causes of coma. If it is psychogenic, the pupils usually appear to be dilated and reactive. The patient may be hyperventilating. Deep tendon reflexes are often hyperactive, with no localizing neurologic signs.

Chart 18-4

MANAGEMENT OF THE PATIENT WITH ALCOHOL-INDUCED COMA

- Establish and maintain airway. Protect from aspiration of vomitus.
- Assist ventilations if necessary.
- Obtain blood gas determinations.
- Obtain blood samples for CBC, electrolytes, toxicology screen, and blood alcohol levels.
- Begin IV of D_5W.
- Monitor vital signs and neurologic checks regularly (especially level of consciousness).
- Insert a nasogastric tube to decompress stomach and prevent vomiting. If a large quantity of alcohol was ingested within the past 1 to 2 hours, lavage may be beneficial.
- IV administration of 50% glucose (for hypoglycemia) or naloxone HCl (if concomitant narcotic intoxication is suspected) may be indicated.
- For the chronic alcoholic, thiamine and other B-complex vitamins, vitamin K, electrolytes, and minerals, including magnesium, may be indicated.
- Insert indwelling urinary catheter and monitor output.
- Prepare for admission.

Management consists of close support for these patients, care being taken to ensure that there are no concomitant conditions that may have provoked or influenced the coma state.

BIBLIOGRAPHY

Bickerstaff ER: Neurological Examination in Clinical Practice, 4th ed. Boston, Blackwell Scientific Publications, 1980

Budassi SA, Barber JM: Emergency Nursing: Principles and Practice. St. Louis, CV Mosby, 1981

Haerer AF: Coma: Some differential considerations in the diagnosis and management. Hosp Med 12:68–83, April 1976

Jones C: Glasgow Coma Scale. Am J Nurs 79:1551–3, September 1979

Martin P: Is it ketoacidosis? J Emerg Nurs 3:11–4, January–February 1977

Meyd CJ: Acute brain trauma. Am J Nurs 78:40–4, January 1978

Noble EP: Alcohol and Health, Third Special Report to U.S. Congress. Rockville, MD, National Institute on Alcohol Abuse and Alcoholism, June, 1978

Plum F, Posner JB: The Diagnosis of Stupor and Coma, 3rd ed. Philadelphia, FA Davis, 1980

Schuckit MA: Drug and Alcohol Abuse: A Clinical Guide to Diagnosis and Treatment. New York, Plenum Medical Book Company, 1979

Wilkins EW (ed): MGH Textbook of Emergency Medicine. Baltimore, Wiliams & Wilkins, 1978

Witt K: HHNK: A newly recognized syndrome to watch for. Nursing 76 (6):66–70, February 1976

19
WOUND MANAGEMENT

JAMES H. COSGRIFF, JR. and DIANN ANDERSON

Wounds constitute the most common reason for seeking emergency treatment. In many instances, primary or even total care may be given by nonphysician emergency personnel. This is especially true in smaller emergency departments and in school and industrial health service settings.

PRINCIPLES OF WOUND MANAGEMENT

From a practical standpoint, wounds may be classified according to the following four criteria:

- *Etiology*—surgical, accidental, self-inflicted
- *Appearance*—incised, crushing, abraded
- *Mechanism of injury*—blunt, penetrating, perforating
- *Presence of gross contamination*—clean, dirty, infected

It is important to describe the wound according to these criteria because these characteristics may serve to indicate the therapeutic approach to a specific wound. For example, the management of a blunt, dirty, abraded accidental wound is different from that of an incised, clean, penetrating surgical wound. The principles of wound management do not vary, but the specific details may.

Complete assessment of the patient is an essential component of proper wound management. When indicated, the ABCs of emergency care—*a*irway, *b*reathing, and *c*irculation—should be initiated. Thorough assessment reveals the following factors that influence the specifics of wound care:

- Type and location of the wound
- Degree of wound contamination
- Presence of foreign substances
- Associated injury to other structures—muscles, blood vessels, nerves, and tendons
- General status of the patient

The overall objective of wound care is to achieve primary healing with a cosmetically acceptable scar and a minimum of disability. The prevention of infection is a means to this end.

PHYSIOLOGY OF WOUND HEALING

When a wound occurs, the body's response is an outpouring of tissue fluid and blood cells into the area, forming a fibrin network. Fibroblasts and capillary buds penetrate this network to bridge the defect. As the capillaries increase in number, more blood cells are brought to the wound site, giving the tissue a red color. This combination of fluid, blood cells, and new vessels is called *granulation tissue* and serves as the basic structure in wound repair. Granulation tissue is present to a greater or lesser degree in every wound.

As the healing continues, the granulation tissue undergoes a maturation process; the fibroblasts increase in number, strengthening the healing wound and gradually squeezing out the blood vessels, thus forming *scar tissue*. This process takes place through the entire depth of the wound. While this new tissue bridges the wound, epithelial cells proliferate to cover the surface of the granulation tissue. Depending on the site and depth of the wound, its tensile strength is usually sufficient to allow suture removal in 7 to 10 days; wound healing continues for 6 to 12 months until a mature scar is formed.

Wound healing occurs in one of three ways: by first intention, by second intention, and by third intention (Fig. 19-1). The mechanism of healing by first and second intention is applicable to all body tissues (skin, fat, muscle, bone, tendon, nerve). Variations in the process result from the unique characteristics of each type of tissue.

First-Intention Healing

First-intention (primary closure) healing is the ideal method of wound healing. The best example of primary closure occurs in a surgical incision. A similar process takes place in most clean, incised wounds. In this type of wound, the various layers of tissue are coapted. This ensures that dead space is obliterated, preventing the collection of serum and blood (hematoma) that can interfere with primary wound healing. After closure of the deeper layers, the skin is carefully approximated to restore the damaged tissue to as near normal alignment as possible. In healing by first intention, the least amount of granulation tissue forms because the tissue defect is small and wound healing is most efficient.

Second-Intention Healing

Healing by second intention occurs in wounds in which there is a loss of tissue that prevents the various layers of the wound margins (edges) from being precisely approximated. An example is the exit wound of a gunshot injury in which portions of the skin and underlying tissues are missing.

In this mode of healing, more granulation tissue is needed to bridge the tissue defect in the depths of the wound than in primary closure. As the granulation tissue reaches the surface, the epithelial cells grow over it from the periphery to provide cover. The amount of granulation tissue determines the scar size.

Third-Intention Healing

Wounds allowed to heal for a period of time by second intention and then closed surgically to produce a lesser scar and more rapid healing are examples of healing by third intention. The most common example is a contaminated surgical incision, such as that associated with a perforated appendix. In this instance, the peritoneal and muscle layers are closed, but the subcutaneous fat and skin tissue remain open, allowing for drainage and formation of granulation tissue. These layers are then sutured 5 to 7 days later. This method is also referred to as healing by secondary suture.

INITIAL ASSESSMENT AND CARE OF SURFACE WOUNDS

Assessment and life-support measures are carried out concurrently as required by the circumstances.

First Intention

Second Intention (contraction and epithelialization)

Third Intention (delayed closure)

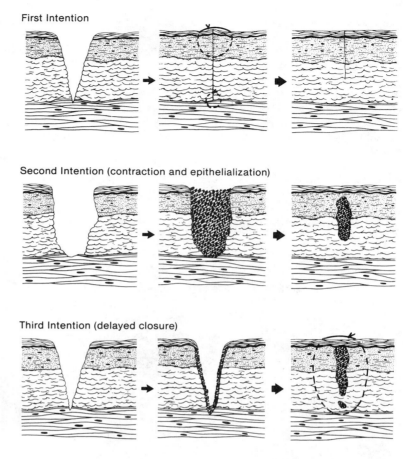

Figure 19-1 *Classification of wound healing. First intention—A clean incision is made with primary closure; there is minimal scarring. Second intention (contraction and epithelialization)—The wound is left open to granulate in with resultant large scab and abnormal dermal-epidermal junction. Third intention (delayed closure)—The wound is left open and closed secondarily when there is no evidence of infection. (Hardy JD: Hardy's Textbook of Surgery, p 109. Philadelphia, JB Lippincott, 1983)*

History

The history of the wound is important in determining the mechanism of injury. An accidental incised wound caused by a clean kitchen knife is very different from a laceration caused by a farm implement; a human bite is usually more serious than a dog bite. A lapse in time of more than 6 to 8 hours between the occurrence of the injury and treatment *usually* contraindicates primary closure.

- Obtain details of how the injury occurred.
- Note any undue delay between occurrence of injury and time when patient appears for treatment.

Physical Examination

1. Carry out rapid assessment of patient, evaluating airway, bleeding, and circulation.

2. Initiate resuscitative measures as indicated: establish airway, control hemorrhage, restore blood volume.

3. Assess patient more fully, especially type and character of wound.

4. In wounds near major blood vessels or nerves, evaluate distal pulses, and motor and sensory function. Loss of motor function in an extremity may indicate muscle, tendon, or nerve injury. A palpable distal pulse does *not* ensure that there is no vascular damage.

5. In extremity wounds, compare the injured limb with its counterpart.

6. Control hemorrhage. Direct pressure is the best method to control bleeding, whether at the accident scene or in the hospital.

- The wound should not be probed until definitive wound treatment is begun.
- Impaled or embedded objects (knife, axe, glass, large splinters, etc.) should not be removed from the wound at the accident scene. Wound closure instruments should be available because major bleeding can ensue following removal.
- An x-ray of the injured part is required when an embedded object is present.
- When there is a large embedded object, angiography may be needed to assess proximity or damage to a major vessel.
- The wound is prepared for closure when the patient has been fully assessed.

Dealing With Anxiety

Most patients who come to the emergency department have a certain degree of anxiety, much of which is based on fear of the injury itself and anticipation of the pain or discomfort that may occur during the course of assessment and treatment. Taking time to explain to the patient what type of pain can be expected, and when, does much to allay his fear and at the same time increases confidence in those who are giving care. Talking to the patient in a calm, reassuring manner while carrying out the assessment and during the process of treatment is most helpful. Tell the patient that the treatment may cause some pain but every effort will be made to minimize it.

If the patient is very young or emotionally unstable, a mild sedative may be prescribed by the physician in attendance. A short-acting barbiturate such as secobarbitol sodium is particularly helpful with children. When prescribed for a child, it is given intramuscularly in the dosage of 1 mg/lb of body weight. Diazepam or a similar preparation is useful in adults. It may be given intravenously, slowly and with caution.

A restraining device can be used for infants and small children. The Papoose Board (Fig. 19-2) is well adapted for

this purpose. When treating pediatric patients, it is helpful to allow a parent to stay with the child during the treatment, to calm him.

The emergency management of wounds is summarized in Chart 19-1.

LOCAL ANESTHESIA

A variety of local anesthetic agents is available. It is not necessary to be familiar with all of these agents, but emer-

Figure 19-2 *Papoose board and various applications. Various sizes are available, depending on patient size and needs. The flaps can be used all together or in any combination, depending on the body area injured and in need of treatment. (Photos courtesy of Olympic Surgical Co., Inc., Seattle, Washington.)*

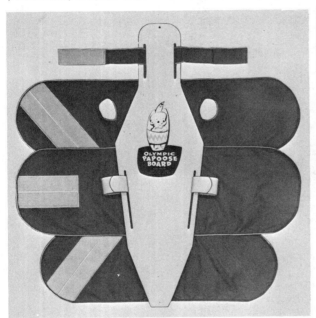
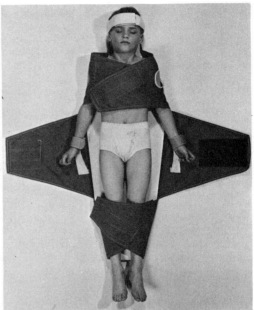
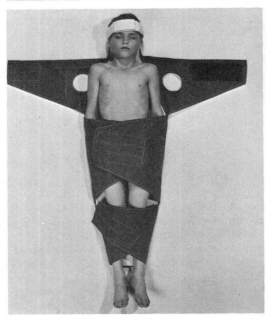
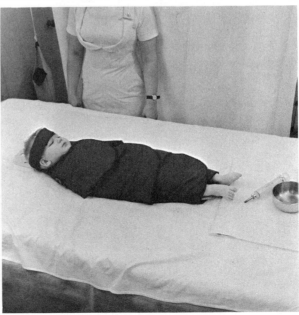

Chart 19-1

EMERGENCY CARE OF WOUNDS

Prehospital Wound Care

- Rapidly assess patient's condition—airway, breathing, and circulation.
- Acquire as many details of history as possible.
- Control hemorrhage by direct pressure, pressure point, or tourniquet.
- Do *not* remove any imbedded objects (knife, glass, etc.) from the wound.
- Do *not* remove tar, grease, etc. from the wound.
- Apply sterile dressing(s).
- Elevate injured part if possible.
- Prepare for transport.
- If injury involves an amputation, make every effort to find the amputated part. Place the part in a sterile bag or towel and bring it to the hospital with the patient.

Wound Care in Emergency Department

- Thoroughly cleanse the injured part with an antiseptic solution, preferably povidone-iodine.
- Use warm irrigating solution. Avoid extremes of temperature.
- Shave excess hair about the wound site. *Note:* Do not shave an eyebrow under any circumstance because it may not regenerate.
- After cleansing, dry the part with a sterile towel.
- A local anesthetic (by field block, regional infiltration, or specific nerve block) may be needed to achieve anesthesia in the area of the wound.
- Explore the wound thoroughly.
- Any devitalized tissue is removed (debridement).
- Bleeding points are identified and controlled.
- Prepare for wound closure and the application of an appropriate dressing.

---

gency personnel should be skilled in the use of one or two injectable agents and a similar number of topical agents. It is important to be familiar with the pharmacologic effects of these drugs.

INJECTABLE ANESTHETIC DRUGS

Injectable anesthetic drugs in common use are listed in Table 19-1. The solutions available in most emergency departments vary in concentration from 0.25% to 2.0%. Thus, each may contain 2.5 to 20 mg/ml of anesthetic. As a general rule, the lowest effective concentration of agent should be used in order to minimize the incidence of reactions, especially when a large volume of drug is needed.

Precautions. The use of injectable local anesthetic agents involves a number of precautions that should be observed by emergency personnel. They may be summarized as follows:

1. Be familiar with the pharmacologic characteristics of the drugs administered—minimal lethal dose (MLD_{50}), diffusibility, duration of action, therapeutic effects, side-effects, contraindications.

2. Be familiar with usual concentrations and dosages.
   - *Concentrations*—the lowest possible concentration is used. Requirements vary. A nerve block requires a more concentrated solution than a field block.
   - *Dosages*—the smallest possible total dose is used.

3. Know the correct mode of administration—subcutaneous, intradermal, etc.; regional or field block, specific peripheral nerve block.
   - *The agent must never be injected into the wound margins*—this may force contaminated material into adjacent noninjured areas.

4. Be aware of variables.
   - *Allergic reactions.* Check with the patient about allergy or sensitivity to specific agents. An agent known to cause reactions is avoided in a patient with a history of sensitivity to the drug.
   - *Sepsis.* The presence of local sepsis may significantly impair the action of a local anesthetic agent.

5. Be aware of *special properties of solutions containing epinephrine.* These solutions are used to prolong duration of drug action and reduce bleeding in highly vascular areas such as the scalp and face. These effects are due to the vasoconstrictive action of epinephrine.

TABLE 19-1. COMMONLY USED INJECTABLE ANESTHETIC DRUGS

Drug	Dosage	Total Dose	Duration of Action
Procaine	14 mg/kg	1000 mg	¾ to 1½ hr
Lidocaine	7 mg/kg	500 mg	1½ to 2 hr
Bupivacaine	3 mg/kg	200 mg	4 to 6 hr
Mepivacaine	7 mg/kg	300 mg	2 to 3 hr

(Cosgriff JH Jr: Atlas of Diagnostic and Therapeutic Procedures for Emergency Personnel, p 180. Philadelphia, JB Lippincott, 1978)

- Solutions containing epinephrine should be used with caution in the elderly and in persons who are hypertensive or have contused wounds.
- *Solutions containing epinephrine should not be used to block the digital nerves of the hands or feet.* Digits are supplied by end-arteries. Vasoconstriction in these areas could result in gangrene of the digits.

Types of Local Anesthesia

Emergency personnel may employ a number of methods to produce local anesthesia, depending on the needs of the patient and the procedure to be performed. The methods most often used in the emergency setting are local infiltration, regional or field block, or block of a specific nerve.

Local Infiltration. Local infiltration involves injecting anesthetic agent directly over or into the surface of the lesion. It is particularly useful in draining infected cysts or abscesses but is to be avoided in dealing with an incised or open wound that requires accurate approximation, because it may distort the tissue. The injection is made into the line of the planned incision. This method requires the weakest concentration of anesthetic agent.

Regional or Field Block. Regional or field block involves injecting anesthetic agent into the normal tissues about the wound without injecting the wound itself. The areas around the margin of the wound and underneath the wound are anesthetized. This technique is useful in accidental wounds that are to be debrided and closed by primary suture. Care is taken not to inject the agent too close to the wound, thus minimizing distortion of tissues.

Specific Peripheral Nerve Block. Specific nerve block involves injecting anesthetic agent about an individual nerve. This provides anesthesia in the area of distribution of the nerve, distal to the point of the block. It is a particularly useful technique when treating lesions or wounds of the face or extremities. A stronger concentration of anesthetic agent is required to achieve such a block.

Technique of Local Anesthesia

The following principles apply to almost all types of local anesthesia, with the exception perhaps of local infiltration technique.

- The type of anesthesia appropriate to the specific patient's wound should be selected.

- The skin should be prepared with a topical antiseptic solution.
- Local anesthesia should be initiated by raising an intradermal skin wheal; a small-bore (25- or 26-gauge) needle is used.
- The anesthetic agent is injected through the skin wheal at a point remote from the wound margins.
- *For a field block,* the agent should be injected in the subcutaneous tissue, completely surrounding the wound and underneath the wound if possible. Technique is illustrated in Chart 19-2.
- *For a peripheral nerve block,* knowledge of the anatomy of the nerve is important. The agent must be injected about the nerve. When the nerve is touched with the needle, a paresthesia will be elicited along the sensory distribution of the nerve, indicating the correct site of injection.

TOPICAL ANESTHETIC AGENTS

This type of anesthesia is used primarily on mucous membranes, but one form, ethyl chloride, can be used when draining a small abscess of the skin. Ethyl chloride is a refrigerant type of topical anesthetic agent sprayed onto the skin at the site of the planned incision.

The agents in common use are cocaine (in a 4% to 10% solution), tetracaine (in a 0.5% to 2.0% solution), and lidocaine (in a 2% to 4% solution) (Table 19-2). They are applied topically with a cotton swab or an atomizer; a prepackaged commercial aerosol dispenser may be used instead. These agents are of great value in examining certain lesions of the mucous membranes, in emergency laryngoscopy or bronchoscopy, and in endotracheal intubation. Further uses include insertion of nasal packing or placement of a nasogastric tube.

Precautions. These drugs provide superficial anesthesia only. They are rapidly absorbed and carry a high risk of toxicity. It is important to know the characteristics of each drug and to be aware of the total dose of the agent used.

WOUND MANAGEMENT AND CLOSURE

Emergency department personnel should be familiar with the following aspects of wound management and closure.

Once anesthesia is effected, the wound is carefully explored with instruments that produce a minimum of trauma to the tissues (Fig. 19-3). Adson-type toothed forceps or skin hooks are ideal for this purpose, and should be available. The full thickness of the wound is checked. If the deep fascia of an extremity has been penetrated, there may be damage to the underlying muscle or tendons. If the patient exhibited motor or sensory loss during assessment, the wound is carefully checked for injury to the tendons or peripheral nerves in the area.

Hemostasis is achieved by pressure or by clamping and tying bleeding points. Devitalized tissue and grossly visible foreign bodies are removed by sharp dissection, using scissors or a scalpel blade (Fig. 19-4). The wound is then irrigated and prepared for closure.

Closure. Closure is performed in layers to obliterate dead space and minimize the possibility of collection of serum (seroma) or blood (hematoma), which could impede wound healing (Fig. 19-5). Muscle, fascia, fat, and skin are closed as single layers.

The smallest suture available for the task at hand is used. *Absorbable sutures* are generally used in the deeper layers. Absorbable suture materials include plain and chromicized catgut and synthetic materials such as polyglycollic acid and polyglactin 910. The synthetics are more consistent in size and tensile strength than the catgut. *Nonabsorbable sutures* are generally used in the skin. These sutures may be made of silk or a variety of synthetic materials (Mersilene, Prolene, Dermalon, Ethiflex, Ethilon), and may be monofilamentous (single strand) or braided. Sutures are not always required. Some wounds on flat surfaces (especially clean, incised wounds with straight, sharp edges) can be closed with Steri-strips.

A drain may be placed in the wound if there is concern that a seroma or hematoma may form. When wound closure is completed, a dry, sterile dressing is applied, as described later in this chapter.

WOUNDS THAT REQUIRE SPECIAL CARE

Wounds of the Eyelids

Wounds that involve the tarsal plate require special closure technique. (See Chap 33, Ocular Injuries)

Penetrating Wounds of the Neck

In many instances, these wounds appear significant. Those that penetrate the platysma layer are more serious and are best explored in the operating room. (See Chap. 20, Injuries to the Head, Neck, and Spine.)

High-Pressure Spray Gun Injuries of the Hand

Although the surface wound often appears innocuous, such a wound is a serious injury. The damage results from the high pressure that these instruments may develop (as high as 2000 psi) and from the chemical accidentally injected into the wound. The chemicals used in these devices contain solvents that cause extensive tissue destruction.

Scalp Wounds

These wounds are unique because of the vascularity of the scalp and their association with skull fracture. Scalp lacerations may result in severe blood loss, enough to produce hypovolemic shock, especially in children. If possible, pressure dressings should be applied to reduce bleeding, and the head should be kept slightly elevated. Except for minor lacerations, all scalp wounds should be explored with the finger, to rule out skull fracture. Early, vigorous, and thorough surgical debridement of such a wound in the operating room is imperative.

Abrasions (Brush Burns)

Abrasions are painful wounds involving the epidermis and upper layers of the dermis. Because of the nature of the injury (a sliding fall), imbedded foreign bodies such as cinders, dirt, and debris may be present. These must be completely removed to prevent tattooing. In abrasions involving a small surface area, debridement may be adequately performed using a sterile needle point, a Number 11 scalpel blade, or an intermittent spurting device such as a Water-Pik. Anesthesia may not be needed for smaller wounds. In more extensive injuries, diazepam or a local or general anesthesia is often required. A surgical hand brush also serves well to scrub the wound and remove the embedded objects.

Puncture Wounds

Puncture wounds occur most often in the extremities. They are a form of penetrating wound in which a sharp and narrow pointed object such as a nail is forced through the skin. Depending on whether the object is clean or contaminated, pathogens may be introduced into the depths of the wound. The surface wound seals readily, and ordinarily little bleeding occurs. If the penetrating object was a rusty nail, complete excision of the wound tract is necessary. The wound is left open to drain and heal by second intention. Thorough cleansing of the site is important.

Embedded Foreign Bodies

Embedded objects often present problems in management because sometimes the patient is not sure that the object is present in the tissue. A history of the direction of entry may be helpful in locating the foreign body when it is not palpable. If the object is metallic or glass with a high lead content, x-rays of the part may identify its location. Objects that lie close to or protrude through the skin may be removed by gentle, careful traction without anesthesia. Those that lie deeper may be difficult to locate and remove. In some patients, it is better to adopt a wait-and-see attitude if one feels that more damage might be done by surgical intervention. Embedded needles are often difficult to extract from the deeper tissues. Many of the objects, if they are close enough to the surface, may be extruded by the body to a level where they are accessible for removal. After a foreign body has been removed, it should be affixed to the patient's chart with transparent tape and remain a permanent part of the record.

Wood Splinters

Wood splinters in the skin or under a fingernail can be removed with a sharp-pointed splinter forceps. Applying gentle pressure on the surrounding skin while placing traction on the splinter may facilitate removal. The same technique applies for splinters lodged beneath the fingernail. If

Chart 19-2

TECHNIQUE OF REGIONAL OR FIELD BLOCK ANESTHESIA

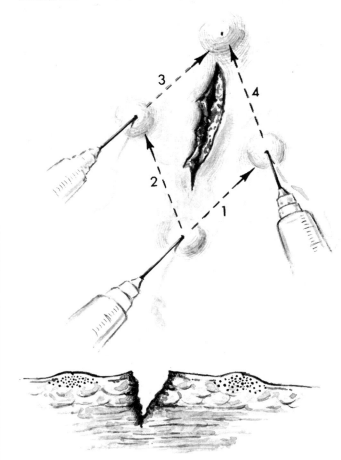

A. Draw an imaginary triangle or diamond about the lesion and, using the 25-gauge ⅝ inch needle attached to the syringe, raise a skin wheal at each point of the geometric figure. Introduce the needle quickly with the face of the bevel down into the dermis (the layer of the skin beneath the epidermis) and parallel to the surface of the skin.

Inject 0.2 ml to 0.3 ml of anesthetic agent until the skin blanches and a small raised area appears which resembles an orange peel. This raised area is the wheal and should measure approximately 1 cm in diameter.

During this portion of the procedure, the patient may experience a rather intense burning sensation at the injection site. Advance preparation of the patient and calm reassurance by emergency department personnel may allay undue fear, apprehension, and pain.

---

the trailing end of the splinter does not project beyond the end of the nail bed, it can sometimes be reached by inserting the forceps in the tract formed by the foreign body. On occasion, the nail may have to be split longitudinally with a sharp pair of scissors and a narrow V-shaped wedge of nail excised to remove the splinter.

Subungual Hematoma

Hematoma under the nail is often seen in the hands or feet. This is secondary to a crush injury, such as might occur when the finger is trapped in a car door. This lesion is marked by a bluish discoloration of the nail due to bleeding from the nail bed. It is often associated with a fracture of the distal phalanx of the involved digit. This condition is very painful. Drainage of the hematoma using a hand or battery operated drill provides immediate relief of pain. If the hematoma extends over the entire length of the nail bed, it may be evacuated with a Number 11 scalpel blade, which is inserted into the hematoma and kept close to the undersurface of

the nail. Most often, no anesthesia, only calm reassurance, is needed.

Fish Hooks

Fish hooks often become embedded in the extremities, particularly the fingers, but may enter any other part of the body. If the barbed end is embedded in the deeper tissue, a small incision should be made over the tip of the barb and the tip forced through. The shaft of the hook is then cut close to the skin with a wire cutter and the remainder of the hook is pulled, barbed end first, through the incision (Fig. 19-6). When both ends of the hook are protruding through the skin, the same technique can be used; it is preferable to cut off the barbed end.

Complicated Wounds

In wounds involving extensive tissue damage or loss of tissue, healing by first intention is not possible. If the defect is

Chart 19-2

TECHNIQUE OF REGIONAL OR FIELD BLOCK ANESTHESIA (*CONTINUED*)

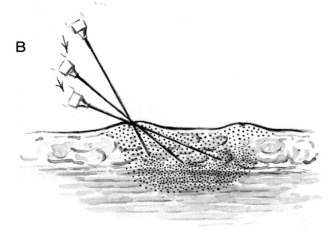

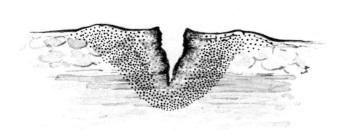

B. After developing the appropriate wheals, replace the 25-gauge, ⅝-inch needle with the 22-gauge 1½-inch needle.

Introduce this syringe-needle assembly into one wheal and penetrate to the subcutaneous tissue at a 45-degree angle. Aspirate in two planes, and, if no blood is recovered, inject a small amount of solution (0.5 ml). Continue to introduce the needle in the direction of an adjacent wheal, alternately aspirating and injecting the solution along this line until the next wheal is reached. As the injection continues, palpate the skin overlying the tip of the needle to identify the solution in the subcutaneous tissue and be sure the lesion is completely surrounded.

To minimize patient discomfort, introduce the larger needle through the skin only at the site of the skin wheal.

C. Upon completion of the ring injection, redirect the needle to the tissues underneath the lesion and deposit some anesthetic agent after aspiration.

When the field block is completed, test the skin within the area for pin prick sensation using the point of the needle. Before proceeding, wait until the pinprick is no longer detected by the patient, usually in 3 to 5 minutes. *Note:* If a large area must be blocked, keep in mind the total dose of anesthetic agent used, to minimize untoward reactions.

(Cosgriff, JH Jr: Atlas of Diagnostic and Therapeutic Procedures for Emergency Personnel, Philadelphia, JB Lippincott, 1978)

---

small and in an unexposed area such as the trunk, arms, or legs, healing by second intention may be acceptable. If an exposed area is involved, such as the face, neck, or hands, immediate coverage of the defect is indicated. For wounds of the face and neck, sliding or rotational pedicle flaps may be used; on the hand, split-thickness grafts are applied immediately. These procedures are best done in the operating room. Emergency management consists of cleansing the wound, covering it with a sterile dressing, and preparing the patient for transfer to the operating suite.

Fingertip Amputations (Loss of Full-Thickness Skin)

This type of wound is a common and potentially disabling injury. These injuries can usually be managed adequately in the emergency department, by application of a full-thickness skin graft. Grafts should *not* be taken from hair-bearing areas because the hair follicles in the transplanted skin will continue to function. Preferably, these grafts are taken from donor sites on the inner aspect of the forearm or arm. Careful

attention to details of application will ensure a high success rate with this grafting technique. Other methods include a cross-finger pedicle flap and a palmar pedicle flap.

Tendon Injuries

Injuries of the tendon constitute a serious problem. A laceration of an extensor tendon of the hand or finger can ordinarily be repaired in the emergency department. Repair

TABLE 19-2. COMMONLY USED TOPICAL ANESTHETIC DRUGS

Drug	Total Dose*	Peak Effect	Duration of Action
Cocaine	200 mg	2–5 min	30–45 mn
Tetracaine	60 mg	3–8 min	30–60 min
Lidocaine	500 mg	2–5 min	30–45 min

* Dosages are for the mythical 70-kg man.

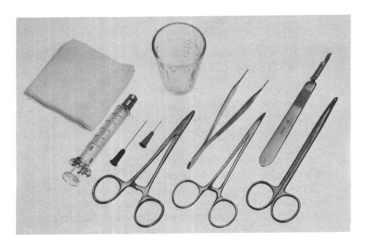

Figure 19-3 *Basic instruments needed for repair of lacerations. Shown above are: medicine glass, syringe (Luer-lok), needles (22- and 25-gauge), needle holder, toothed Adson forceps, curved hemostat, scalpel handle (#3) with #15 blade, small dissecting scissors. A sufficient number of gauze sponges and towels should be included.*

of injury to the flexor tendons of the hand or finger should be performed in the operating room. The indications for primary repair depend on many factors, including the site of the injury, the nature of the primary wound, and the degree of contamination of the wound.

DRESSINGS

Wound care is not complete until a proper dressing is applied. The dressing serves the following purposes:
• Protects the wound from external contamination
• Lessens tension on the suture line
• Immobilizes the part
• Promotes better healing—as a result of these measures

Principles

Dressings should be applied firmly but should not be so tight as to cause constriction. This is particularly true when an extremity is wrapped circumferentially; too tight a dressing may interfere with venous return and cause distal swelling. Joints should be placed in a slightly flexed position before being wrapped. When wrapping a joint, use a figure-8 technique (Fig. 19-7).

Tissues that are elastic and swell readily, such as the eyelid, should be protected with a bulky pressure dressing that includes the following:
1. An inner layer of sterile gauze or nonadherent pad (Telfa)
2. A second layer of folded or fluffed sterile gauze pads or sterile mechanic's waste to provide firm, diffused pressure
3. An outer layer of conforming gauze (Kerlix or Kling)

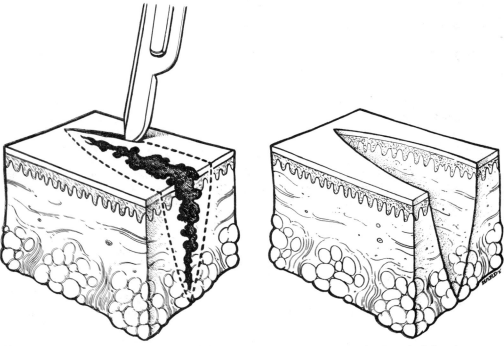

Figure 19-4 *Wound debridement. Jagged tissue edges are excised to provide clean, sharp tissue margins before closure by suture.*

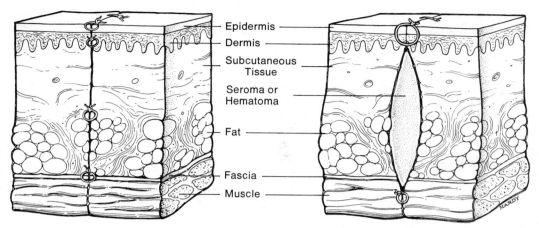

Figure 19-5 *Layered wound closure. Left. Correct method; complete obliteration of dead space. Right. Incorrect method; deeper layer not sutured, with formation of seroma or hematoma to fill the dead space.*

Not all wounds require dressings—for example, a wound that is closed meticulously in layers, such as a facial wound. In other instances, a plastic aerosol dressing, such as Vibesate or collodion applied with a sterile applicator, is sufficient.

Wound Dressing in Specific Areas of the Body

Scalp, Frontal Area, Eyelid, and Ear. Use pressure dressings as needed. To prevent the bandage from slipping off the head, see that the outer layer of the dressing covers the entire outer ear, extending below the lobe. Place a folded gauze pad behind the pinna, next to the mastoid area, to relieve painful pressure on the cartilage of the ear.

Wrist, Hand, Fingers, and Toes. It is usually more comfortable if at least two adjacent fingers are included in the dressing. Thus, if the small finger is lacerated, the ring finger should be included in the dressing. This prevents unnecessary motion of the injured finger and lessens pain.

When more than one finger is to be enclosed in the dressing, place a fluffed gauze pad in the interdigital spaces to absorb perspiration and prevent maceration of the skin.

Figure 19-6 *Ideal method of removing an embedded fish hook. After the part is anesthetized, the barbed point of the hook is pushed through a small incision in the skin (A). A wire cutter is used to cut the shaft of the hook (B). The barbed end may then be pulled through the subcutaneous tissue and removed.*

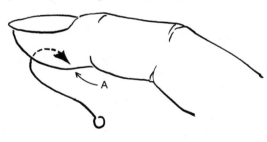

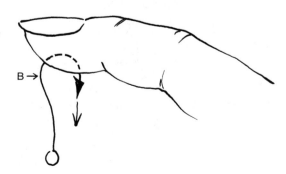

Figure 19-7 *Wrapping a joint. Left. This method of wrapping a joint may be used for the larger joints (elbow, wrist, knee, ankle). (Edge of Ace bandage was colored to indicate method of overlapping.) Right. Joint should be in position of moderate flexion for application of circumferential dressing.*

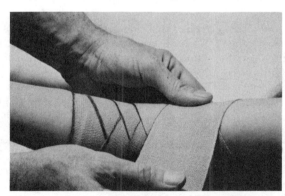

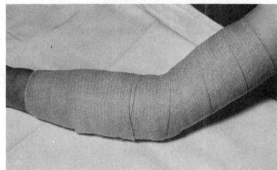

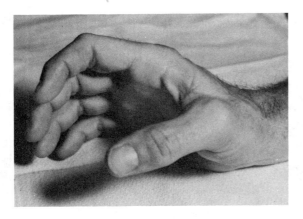

Figure 19-8 "Position of function" of hand. This position is used for occlusive dressings.

In the foot, place a cotton ball between the toes for the same purpose.

When it is necessary to include the entire hand in the dressing, place it in the position of function, that is, with the wrist in midextension and the thumb and fingers in midflexion (Fig. 19-8). A flexible plastic or aluminum splint can be shaped to fit on the volar aspect of the wrist and hand to maintain this position. Pad the splint before application.

If the injury is localized in one finger and immobilization is required, padded aluminum splints are available in varying widths and may be shaped to the desired position of immobilization.

An outer layer of conforming gauze or tubular gauze dressings (available in a variety of sizes) is extremely useful in bandaging digits.

Hair-Bearing Areas. Use inner dressings as needed. If adhesive tape is to be used, shave the skin clean of hair. This allows for better adherence and minimizes discomfort at the time of a dressing change. Check for sensitivity to adhesive tape. The very young and the elderly have delicate skin that may more easily tolerate nonallergenic tape or ordinary Scotch tape. Apply tape so that it is smooth and free of wrinkles.

Apply the tape so as to avoid traction on the skin. Tape pulling on the skin can cause a painful bleb, the equivalent of a second-degree burn, which may heal with a permanent, unsightly scar. If traction is necessary, place a thin layer of tincture of benzoin on the skin before applying the tape. This will provide a protective, adherent surface that is much less likely to blister.

POSTOPERATIVE MANAGEMENT

Following surgery, the part is elevated to minimize swelling and reduce pain. Throbbing pain is not unusual after the anesthesia has worn off, especially when the injury involves an extremity.

For upper extremity injuries, place the part in a sling before discharge from the emergency department. Extend the sling to include the hand. If this is not done, the hand may deviate toward the ulnar side, causing discomfort and some disability.

For severe lower-extremity injuries, provide crutches to prevent full weight-bearing, or at least minimize it, so as to lessen swelling and pain.

Depending on the site and nature of the injury, the dressings need not be changed for 3 to 4 days, barring unforeseen complications. Skin sutures are removed in 7 to 10 days, as determined by the location and severity of the injury.

Provide an instruction sheet for the patient that includes information on follow-up care (Chart 19-3).

PROPHYLAXIS AGAINST INFECTION

Prophylactic Antibiotic Therapy

Because all accidental wounds are contaminated to some extent, antibiotic therapy should be considered as an adjunct to surgical care of the wound. If the surgical principles of wound debridement have been followed—gentle handling of tissues, thorough cleansing of the wound, removal of all foreign bodies, and removal of all devitalized tissue—then theoretically, at least, the wound is clean and can be closed primarily, without antibiotics.

However, patients with extensive wounds and those with vascular disease, diabetes, malnutrition, or general debilitation are likely candidates for prophylactic antibiotic therapy. A broad-spectrum antibiotic that is effective against the common gram-positive or gram-negative organisms should be used alone or in combination with other agents. Penicillin, tetracycline, and the cephalosporins are most commonly employed.

Cultures of the wound may be taken at the time of initial treatment and sensitivity studies may be performed. Should an infection develop, the appropriate specific antibiotic(s) can be prescribed. Antibiotics should not be employed as an alternative to proper surgical care of the wound.

Question the patient carefully about drug sensitivity or idiosyncrasy before an antibiotic is prescribed so that preparations to which the patient is known to be sensitive can be avoided.

Tetanus Prophylaxis

Tetanus is a grave complication of any injury and can occur following seemingly minor wounds. It is caused by *Clostridium tetani,* an anaerobic spore-forming organism that thrives in devitalized tissue and produces a neurotoxin. Even today, this disease, once established, has a 50% mortality rate. The best treatment is prevention. Strict adherence to the proper management of wounds is the best prophylaxis available. Thorough cleansing and complete surgical debridement of devitalized tissue are most effective in preventing tetanus.

In addition to proper surgical technique, biological preparations are available to provide immunity against this or-

---

Chart 19-3

PATIENT EDUCATION FOR WOUND CARE—INSTRUCTION WORKSHEET

Suture Care

1. Sutures should preferably be kept dry and clean.
2. Bandages should be changed if wet or dirty and *at least* every 3 or 4 days.
3. Sutures must be checked for evidence of inflammation, *i.e.,* pus, increase in pain, or increase in redness. If these symptoms or signs occur, notify a physician.
4. If there are sutures in the leg, knee, or foot, elevate that extremity as much as possible during the first week of treatment.
5. Sutures in the mouth or on the lips require special care:
   - Avoid salty, sour, and spicy foods.
   - Rinse area with any mouth wash twice a day.
6. Avoid vigorous bending or stretching at the suture site.

Puncture Wound and Abscess or Infection Care

1. Soak or, preferably, submerge the affected area in warm water and any anti-septic soap. Soak *at least* twice a day, 10 minutes at a time. While soaking, wipe off scab or crusts.
2. Dry thoroughly and apply a thin coat of antibiotic cream, *if prescribed by the physician.*
3. Cover with a clean bandage.
4. *For puncture wounds,* continue this soaking for 2 or 3 days.
5. *For abscess or infections,* continue soaking for entire duration or oral antibiotic prescribed by the physician.

Note: A tetanus immunization is usually effective for 5 years, but to be safe, check with your physician.

Avoid the application of extreme heat or cold to any part of the body, especially a limb, in the elderly, the very young, diabetics, or patients known to have peripheral vascular disease.

Further Steps Necessary for Complete Medical Care (Where Checked)

_____ See personal physician for follow-up care. (If you do not have a personal physician, you may make an appointment for a visit to the Outpatient Department.

_____ Call for appointment in _____ Clinic

_____ Report to Trauma Clinic on _____ at 8:00 A.M.

---

ganism. The two in most common usage today are tetanus toxoid, which provides active immunity, and human immune globulin, which produces passive immunity. Until the 1950s, tetanus antitoxin was the biological agent used almost exclusively for prophylaxis in civilian hospitals. It is prepared from the serum of horses or cows and produces an extremely high rate of sensitivity reactions in humans. Tetanus toxoid was developed and came into wide usage and effectiveness during World War II in the United States armed forces. Only twelve cases of tetanus occurred among 2,500,000 wounded American servicemen. And of these twelve, eight had an incomplete tetanus inoculation series.

It is sometimes difficult to decide what type of immunization therapy should be used. The U. S. Public Health Service Centers for Disease Control (CDC) has recommended several variations in immunotherapy, including the addition of diphtheria and pertussis (DTP) of diphtheria (Td) to the basic adsorbed tetanus toxoid (T).

The tetanus toxoid series consists of an initial intramuscular or subcutaneous dose of 0.5 ml and booster doses 0.5 ml 1 month and 12 months later. For children less than 7 years of age, DTP is preferred unless pertussis vaccine is contraindicated. For patients 7 years old and older, Td is preferred to tetanus toxoid alone. Once the basic immunization has been established, subsequent booster shots are required only at 10-year intervals in the absence of wounding. A booster dose may be given at the time of injury but not within 5 years of a prior injection, except under certain conditions.

In grossly contaminated wounds in which the risk of tetanus is significant or in the absence of prior immunization, 250 units of tetanus immune globulin should be given intramuscularly in addition to 0.5 ml of toxoid, with the restriction noted previously. The globulin provides an immediate protective antibody titer, until the toxoid can produce a recall of antibodies to a protective level. Antibiotics are not generally useful but may be used in special circumstances.

Though reactions to the globulin are rare, incidence of reactions to the toxoid is increasing. Generally, they take

IMMUNIZATION and HEALTH RECORD

Name _____ Phone _____

Address _____

Birth Date _____ Blood Type _____

Family Doctor _____ Phone _____

Notify in an Emergency _____ Phone _____

Served in U. S. Armed Forces from _____ to _____

TETANUS TOXOID IMMUNIZATION DATES			
Initial Series			
Booster Shots			

CARRY THIS CARD IN YOUR WALLET

I AM ALLERGIC TO: Horse Serum ☐ Penicillin ☐

Other _____

I HAVE: Heart Disease ☐ Diabetes ☐ Epilepsy ☐

Other _____

MEDICINES TAKEN REGULARLY: Anticoagulants ☐

Insulin ☐ Other _____

ADDITIONAL MEDICAL INFO: _____

_____

N. Y. STATE HEALTH DEPARTMENT

Figure 19-9 *Immunization card. Front and back sides are shown.*

the form of local erythema and induration at the injection site, often accompanied by a febrile response as high as 40.6°C (105°F). Local applications of cold or ice packs, combined with analgesics and antipyretics, provide symptomatic relief.

Each patient receiving tetanus prophylaxis should be given a wallet-sized immunization card before discharge from the emergency department, as a record of his immune status. Figure 19-9 depicts such a record.

Guidelines recommended for tetanus prophylaxis by the CDC are summarized in Table 19-3.

TABLE 19-3. GUIDELINES FOR TETANUS PROPHYLAXIS

History of Tetanus Immunization (Doses)	Clean, Minor Wounds		All Other Wounds	
	Td	TIG	Td	TIG
Uncertain	Yes	No	Yes	Yes
0–1	Yes	No	Yes	Yes
2	Yes	No	Yes	No‡
3 or more	No*	No	No†	No

* Yes, if more than 10 years since last dose.
† Yes, if more than 5 years since last dose.
‡ Yes, if wound is more than 24 hours old.
(Morbid Mortal Week Rep August 21, 1981)

INFECTIONS

An infection of the integumentary system often brings a patient to the emergency department. The more common types seen are cellulitis; lymphangitis and lymphadenitis; and suppuration and abscess. A primary abscess is exemplified by a carbuncle, paronychia, or felon. A secondary abscess may be located in a prior existing lesion such as a sebaceous cyst or a pilonidal cyst.

Abscesses may occur anywhere on the body. A few of the more common types are discussed below. When an abscess is drained, specimens of the pus are taken for bacteriologic studies, including smear, culture, and sensitivity testing.

Paronychia

Paronychia is a localized infection of the cuticle surrounding a fingernail. It usually follows nail biting or injury to the paronychia when the nails are trimmed. These infections are often painful, and if untreated may extend beneath the nail. Treatment consists of adequate drainage.

Felon

A felon is an infection of the pulp space of the distal phalanx of a finger. It is peculiar to this area. Anatomically, the pulp space is divided into many closed spaces by dense fibrous septa that extend volarward from the phalanx. If it is not recognized early and is left untreated, the abscess may involve the phalanx, causing osteomyelitis. Drainage must be adequate and all the fibrous septa must be incised (Fig. 19-10).

Sebaceous Abscess

A sebaceous abscess results from infection in a sebaceous cyst. These are commonly found on the face, trunk, and back of the neck. The infection follows trauma to the cyst, as in shaving. These abscesses may be very large.

Cellulitis

Cellulitis is an infection of the skin and subcutaneous tissue. It is recognizable by a localized area with the following characteristics: hyperemia (rubor); swelling (tumor); pain (dolor); increased temperature (calor); and interference with mobility or function. Management of cellulitis consists of broad-spectrum antibiotic therapy, rest, and elevation of the part. The patient must be watched closely for spread of the infectious process. Cellulitis is not treated operatively.

Lymphangitis

Lymphangitis indicates a spread of the infection along the lymphatics draining the infected area. It is recognized initially by linear red streaking that extends proximally from the infected site. Lymphangitis most often occurs on an extremity and can extend to the regional lymph nodes that

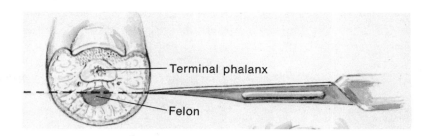

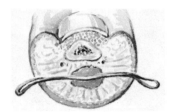

Figure 19-10 *Incision (top) and drainage (bottom) of a felon. (From Cosgriff JH Jr: Atlas of Diagnostic and Therapeutic Procedures for Emergency Personnel. Philadelphia, JB Lippincott, 1978)*

drain the area. In the upper limb it can reach the epitrochlear (elbow) and axillary nodes, and in the lower limb it can extend to the inguinal nodes. *Lymphadenitis,* enlargement of the regional nodes, is also observed. Management is like that for cellulitis: broad-spectrum antibiotics, rest, elevation of the part and close observation for spread of infection.

Suppuration and Abscess

Suppuration and abscess constitute a localized infection characterized by an accumulation of pus; the condition may develop in an area of cellulitis or in a prior existing lesion such as those mentioned above.

Unlike cellulitis, suppuration and abscess are more appropriately treated by surgical drainage. The use of antibiotics as an adjuvant mode of therapy is considered but should not replace evacuation of the pus.

Carbuncle

A carbuncle, also called a boil, is a large, painful abscess that may occur anywhere on the body but is seen more often on the posterior neck. It may follow an abrasion or laceration of the area caused by a barber's errant razor. It may be extremely large and associated with cellulitis, fever, and other systemic symptoms of sepsis.

Pilonidal Abscess

Pilonidal abscess results from secondary infection in a pilonidal cyst. It is located in the upper end of the intergluteal cleft near the lower sacrum. It is identified by the presence of one or more "dimples" in the cleft that are characteristic of a pilonidal cyst and sinus. Pilonidal cysts have a familial tendency. Initial treatment is incision and drainage, but definitive therapy consists of total excision of the cyst. This can be accomplished initially, but must be performed in the operating room.

Perirectal Abscess

Perirectal abscess follows an infectious process in the glands of the anorectal area that ruptures into the surrounding subcutaneous tissue. It is marked by severely painful swelling adjacent to the anal orifice and is easily identified by rectal examination. Once the diagnosis is made, the abscess should be drained in the operating room to prevent serious complications.

BIBLIOGRAPHY

A guide to prophylaxis against tetanus in wound management. Bull. Am Coll Surg, 62, 1979

Cavanaugh CE: Digital replantation. Am J Nurs 64:1433–1436, 1980

Cosgriff JH Jr: Atlas of Diagnostic and Therapeutic Procedures for Emergency Personnel. Philadelphia, JB Lippincott, 1978

Dushoff IM: A stitch in time. Emerg Med 5:1, 1978

Edlich RF et al: Technique of closure: Contaminated wounds. JACEP 3:375, 1974

Flatt AE: The Care of Minor Hand Injuries. St. Louis, CV Mosby, 1972

Gilman AG, Goodman LS et al: The Pharmacologic Basis of Therapeutics. New York, Macmillan, 1980

Hass J: Emergency management of soft tissue injuries. J Emerg Nurs 5:20, 1980

Hentz VR: Common hand problems. Surg Clin North Am 57:1103, 1977

Monroe CW: Basic operative technique. Surg Clin North Am 57:855, 1977

Sabiston D Jr: Davis-Christopher Textbook of Surgery, vol 1. Philadelphia, WB Saunders, 1977

Stephenson KL: Suturing. Surg Clin North Am 57:863, 1977

Worth MH Jr: Emergency treatment of wounds. Hosp Med 16:39, 1980

Zook EG, Kinkead LR: Pressure gun injuries of the hand. JACEP 8:264, 1979

20
INJURIES OF THE HEAD, NECK, AND SPINE

PATRICK J. KELLY, JAMES H. COSGRIFF, JR., and DIANN ANDERSON

Approximately 70% of the 80,000 Americans who lose their lives annually in accidents have sustained injuries to the head and neck.[9,40] A high percentage of these injuries are related to motor vehicle accidents; less frequently, head and neck injuries are caused by falls, penetrating injuries, and blunt trauma. The mortality rate from severe head injury in patients arriving at most hospitals is about 54%.[2,31,34,36,63] However, with aggressive treatment this mortality rate may be lowered to between 30% and 34%.[2,7]

A certain percentage of nervous cellular elements are permanently damaged by the initial impact associated with the traumatic mechanism. In addition, immediately following the injury a series of pathophysiologic processes occur that progressively destroy more brain tissue and thus reduce the patient's chances of a useful recovery.[24,34] Correct and effective management of these patients early in their clinical course can inhibit or impede these pathophysiologic processes and thus improve the likelihood of functional survival following severe central nervous system (CNS) trauma.

Furthermore, head and spine injuries often occur in association with other injuries. Management of patients with nervous system trauma requires vigorous attention to the pulmonary and cardiovascular systems as well. Therefore, a logical, systematic approach to the trauma patient should be employed that encompasses the management of severe head and spine trauma without neglecting the possibility of injury to other organ systems.

In the following section the anatomy and physiology of the intracranial contents as they relate to head injury is discussed first. The emergency and intermediate management of these patients is then described.

HEAD INJURIES

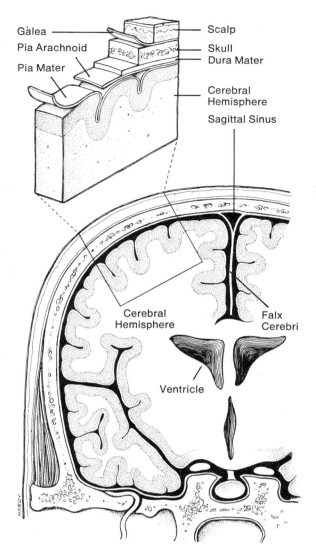

Figure 20-1 Coronal view of the head. The various levels of the scalp, the skull, and the coverings of the brain are depicted.

ANATOMY AND PHYSIOLOGY

The head consists of the skull, the overlying scalp, and the brain (Fig. 20-1). The scalp comprises five layers of soft tissue that cover the skull. The innermost layer of the scalp is the galea, which is composed of coarse connective tissue. The skull is formed by the cranium and the facial bones; the only movable joint is the temporomandibular joint. The cranium itself consists of eight bones that are not joined during the first years of life and later fuse at the suture lines.

The base of the intracranial cavity is divided into three major areas (Fig. 20-2). The anterior or frontal fossa, located above the bony orbit, houses the frontal lobe of the brain. The temporal or middle fossa posterior to the sphenoid ridge is the seat of the temporal lobe. The cerebellum and brain stem reside in the posterior fossa, located behind the petrous ridge. A large opening, or foramen, at the most inferior and midline aspect of the posterior fossa is the foramen magnum, through which the brain stem passes in its descent to the spinal cord in the spinal canal.

Lining the interior of the cranial cavity is the dura mater,

which is attached to the cranium. Reflections of the dura mater subdivide the cranial cavity (Fig. 20-3). The falx cerebri divides the cranial cavity into right and left compartments. The tentorium passes transversely from occipital bone to petrous bone. It divides the cranial cavity into supratentorial and infratentorial compartments. The tentorial notch allows the upper brain stem (midbrain) to emerge from the infratentorial compartment where it connects with deep structures of the cerebrum located above the tentorium. Knowledge of these dural compartments is useful for understanding the mechanism for neurologic deterioration following head injury.

Inside the dura are two other membranes. The outer, the arachnoid, is directly beneath the dura and contains a collection of cerebrospinal fluid (CSF) that bathes the surface of the brain and acts as a shock absorber for minor trauma. The pia mater covers the surface of the brain; through it pass the blood vessels that supply the brain (Fig. 20-1).

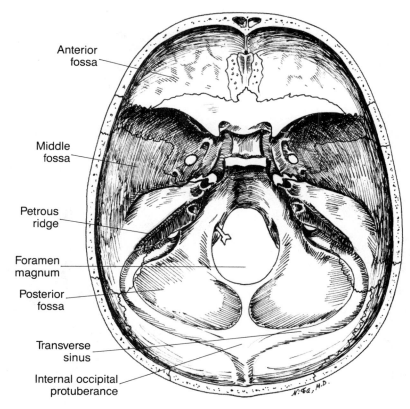

Figure 20-2 *Base of the skull.*

Figure 20-3 *Dural reflections which create sub-divisions of the cranial cavity*

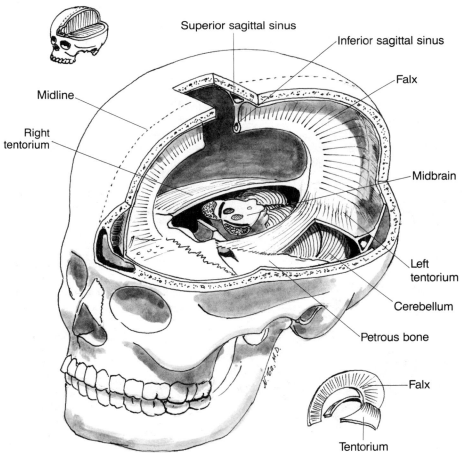

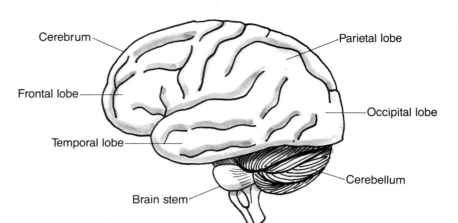

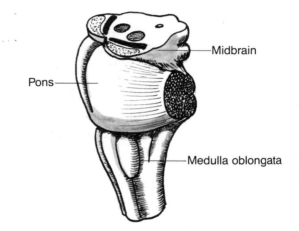

Figure 20-4 Major components of the brain. Top. Cerebral hemisphere, cerebellum, and brain stem. Bottom. Detail of brain stem.

The brain consists of the brain stem, the cerebellum, and the cerebrum (Fig. 20-4). The brain stem is made up of three parts—the medulla oblongata, the pons, and the midbrain. The medulla oblongata controls various vegetative functions, including pulse, blood pressure, and respirations. The pons is a relay station between cerebrum, brain stem, and cerebellum and also contains several cranial nerve nuclei.

The midbrain is of particular importance in head injury (Fig. 20-5) because it lies in a vulnerable position within

Figure 20-5 Horizontal section of the midbrain.

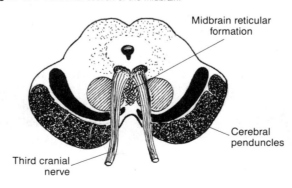

the tentorial notch. The ability to maintain consciousness, the oculomotor (third nerve) nuclei (pupillary light reflex) and the cerebral peduncle containing motor fibers descending from cerebrum to brain stem and spinal cord are located within the midbrain. This is the seat of the ability to maintain consciousness. Damage to the midbrain results in coma, evidenced by fixed, dilated pupils and abnormal motor responses. The medial portions of the temporal lobes lie on either side of the midbrain and the hypothalamus lies directly in front of it.

The cerebrum is the seat of conscious experience, voluntary motor activity, vision, hearing, and somesthetic sensation. It is divided into two hemispheres, right and left. Each hemisphere contains hypothalamus, thalamus, basal ganglia, and cerebral cortex. The hypothalamus has many functions, for example, regulation of temperature control and fluid and electrolyte balance. The thalamus is a relay station that transmits messages from the spinal cord, brain stem, cerebellum, and cortex to the cerebral cortex. The basal ganglia are responsible for fine tuning of voluntary movement.

The cerebral cortex contains multiple layers of nerve cell bodies that send their axons through the white matter and brain stem into the spinal cord or receive input from neurons that are connected to the spinal cord, brain stem, thalamus, basal ganglia, or other areas of the cortex. The cortex has a wrinkled appearance consisting of hills and valleys called gyri and sulci, respectively. Each cerebral hemisphere contains four major lobes—frontal, temporal, parietal, and occipital.

Brain tissue consists of neurons, supporting cells, and blood vessels. The neurons are units that transmit impulses from one portion of the nervous system to another and require supporting cells, or glia, to maintain their physiologic functions. These cells require a constant supply of oxygen and nutrients in order to maintain neurologic function and viability.

PATHOPHYSIOLOGY OF BRAIN INJURY

THE "CLOSED BOX"

Contained within the nondistensible intracranial cavity are three substances that account for 98% of the volume: brain tissue, blood, and water. Brain tissue contains mostly water, both intracellular and extracellular. Blood is contained within the major arteries at the base of the brain, in arterial branches, arterioles, capillaries, venules, and veins within the substance of the brain, and in the cortical veins and dural sinuses. Water is located in the cavities of the brain (ventricular system), in the CSF, and as extracellular and intracellular fluid.

INTRACRANIAL PRESSURE

When brain tissue, blood, and water are in normal proportions, pressure inside the skull is within a few mm Hg above or below atmospheric pressure. Increases in any of these components, such as increases in blood volume due to hematoma or vasodilation of cerebral arterioles, increases in brain water due to swelling of the cells or extracellular space, or enlargement of the ventricular system (hydrocephalus) result in increased intracranial pressure.[39]

Rises in intracranial pressure (ICP) can range from 5 mm Hg to the level of the systolic blood pressure.[48] With mild to moderate elevation of ICP, systemic arterial pressure usually increases in order to maintain a *cerebral perfusion pressure* (mean arterial blood pressure minus ICP) that is adequate to keep brain tissue supplied with blood. As cerebral perfusion pressure falls (when ICP elevations are not offset by corresponding increase in systemic blood pressure), reduction of blood flow to the CNS cellular elements results, and cellular death ultimately occurs.[12,16–18,22,24,25,34,39,57,59]

CAUSES OF BRAIN TISSUE DESTRUCTION

Brain tissue may be injured by forces administered directly to the head (coup) or by rapid deceleration, such as is noted in falls, during which the brain surface strikes the interior wall of the cranial cavity opposite to the site of impact (contrecoup). Shearing forces (twisting) of nerve fibers also damage intracranial cellular elements at the time of impact.[71] In addition, tiny blood vessels are stretched, distorted, and broken, resulting in small hemorrhages into brain tissue.[62] All of these factors destroy a population of nerve cells in proportion to the degree and nature of the traumatic event. Other brain tissue is destroyed by pressure from intracranial hematomas, herniation syndromes, and "brain swelling," or cerebral edema.

Intracranial Hematoma

Hematomas (blood clots) can be located outside the dura (extradural), beneath the dura (subdural), or inside the substance of the brain (intraparenchymal). Bleeding from skull fracture sites or blood vessels results in formation of a clot, which may enlarge progressively. If untreated, hematomas lead to increased intracranial pressure, reduction in cerebral perfusion, and herniations.

Herniation Syndromes

Increased pressure due to hematoma or swelling in one intracranial compartment usually results in herniation. Herniation refers to the protrusion of part of the brain across the falx, the tentorium, or the foramen magnum. Common types of herniation are cingulate (transfalcine, across the falx), transtentorial, and tonsillar (foramen magnum). See Fig. 20-6.

Cingulate Herniation. Protrusion of the cingulate gyrus across the falx produces the following clinical picture: the patient, at first alert, oriented, and readily responsive to questions and commands, becomes disoriented, lethargic, and incontinent of urine. It is important to recognize this herniation syndrome early, before the patient undergoes one of the herniation syndromes described below.

Transtentorial Herniation (Fig. 20-7). Lateral masses result in medial displacement of the temporal lobe (uncus) across the tentorial notch. This compresses the third cranial nerve and results in a substantial dilation of the pupil on the side of the intracranial mass. As the herniation continues, pressure on the cerebral peduncle results in paralysis or abnormal posturing of the opposite side of the body (in 85% of the patients) or the same side of the body as the mass (in 15% of the patients).[66] Abnormal posturing is shown in Fig. 20-8. The patient ultimately becomes comatose from compression of the midbrain reticular activating system.

Central Herniation. Hematomas over the vertex of the brain or generalized brain swelling result in herniation of the hypothalamus downward through the tentorial notch. Early in the course of herniation, examination will reveal a lethargic patient who responds purposefully to pain but whose pupils are small and sluggishly reactive to light. Later in the development of central herniation, bilateral fixed dilated pupils and bilateral extensor (decerebrate) posturing (Fig. 20-8) are observed, and the patient becomes comatose.

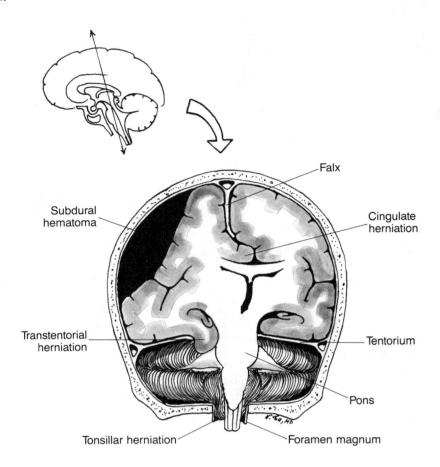

Figure 20-6 *Coronal section of the brain, crossing the pons, medulla oblongata, and foramen magnum. Note cingulate, uncal, and tonsillar herniations.*

Figure 20-7 *Perspective view showing herniation syndromes resulting from displacement of the temporal lobe (uncus) across the tentorial notch. The herniation produces pressure on the ipsilateral 3rd nerve and motor tracts, resulting in a dilated, fixed pupil on the side of the injury and motor paralysis on the side opposite the injury.*

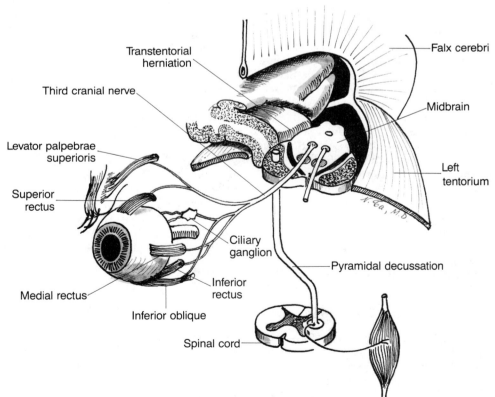

Tonsillar Herniation. Tonsillar herniation indicates protrusion of the cerebellar tonsils through the foramen magnum. This results in compression of the medulla oblongata. Patients experiencing this type of herniation are hypotensive and bradycardic and suffer respiratory arrest.[66] The prognosis is grave.

"Cerebral Edema" and Infarction

Further destruction of brain tissue results from a series of events that begin shortly after CNS injury. A period of apnea is associated with severe head trauma. The resultant respiratory acidosis (manifested by a reduction of arterial oxygen [PaO_2] and elevation in arterial carbon dioxide [$PaCO_2$]) results in reduction of oxygen supply to the surviving cellular elements of the CNS.[10,11,77] These elements shift into anaerobic metabolism.[17,19,41,49,50,51] Brain injury causes blood vessels to dilate in an attempt to reduce resistance to blood flow.[10,16,18,63] This results in an increase in cerebral blood volume,[47] elevation of intracranial pressure, and reduction of cerebral blood flow.[57,73] If these effects are not corrected, cellular brain death—infarction—ultimately occurs.[4,24,25,46,64,74]

MANAGEMENT OF PATIENTS WHO HAVE SUSTAINED HEAD TRAUMA

PREHOSPITAL CARE

1. At the incident site, the first task for emergency personnel is to assess the mechanism of injury quickly; *i.e.,* a fall with direct blow to the head, an automobile crash in which the patient was thrown forward into the windshield, a blunt object striking the head, etc.

2. An assessment should then be made of the patient's level of consciousness.

3. Patients who are awake should be asked whether they have pain in the neck or spine and whether numbness of arms or legs is present. They should then be asked whether they can move their fingers and toes.

4. Always be aware of the possibility of spinal fractures when attempting to move victims of head injury.

5. Vital signs are taken as quickly as possible.

6. Comatose patient
   - The first important step in managing a comatose patient is to establish an adequate airway, *while protecting the cervical spine,* and to ventilate with high-flow oxygen.
   - An airway may be established by inserting a nasal or oral airway device. Esophageal obturator airway insertion, endotracheal intubation, or cricothyroidostomy may be done if the ambulance crew is properly qualified.
   - A portable suction unit for the removal of blood and vomitus from the mouth, pharynx, and upper airway may then be used.
   - Lacerations of the scalp are best gently covered with sterile gauze.

   - Pressure dressings are *not* advisable because of the possibility of depressed skull fracture.

7. In patients with marked initial elevation of intracranial pressure, brain tissue may be noted extruding from the site of a depressed skull fracture. Nothing is to be done about this at the accident site except for the gentle application of a moist sterile dressing.

8. First aid for shock should be instituted when appropriate.

9. Protection of the patient with possible cervical spine injury is a major concern. Emergency personnel should be guided by the following axiom:
   - *Any patient with an injury above the clavicle or a head injury causing unconsciousness should be suspected of having an injury of the cervical spine until a definitive diagnosis can be made.*
   - Management of the patient with suspected cervical spine injury is discussed in detail in the final section of this chapter.

10. Once the victim is fully immobilized against a device that allows no movement of the head and neck, he may be moved to the transport vehicle for transfer to the hospital.

11. During transport, a qualified attendant must be with the patient at all times because the risk of vomiting and airway embarrassment is high.

12. Should the patient begin to vomit, he should be log-rolled to one side with the head and neck supported and the mouth and pharynx cleared of foreign matter. Cervical-spine immobilizing devices permit lateral movement of the patient without motion of the cervical spine.

HOSPITAL CARE

Assessment and Initial Care

1. In the emergency department a brief assessment of level of awareness is conducted in order to decide whether or not the patient is comatose.

2. Pupillary size, equality, and reaction to light are assessed and recorded.

3. Motor responses may be elicited by firm pressure of an instrument on the nail beds (see Fig. 18-2), to determine whether the patient has a purposeful response, an incomplete withdrawal response or an inappropriate response to pain (*i.e.,* decorticate [abnormal flexion] or decerebrate [abnormal extension]), or no response at all (Fig. 20-8).

4. Pulse, blood pressure, and respiratory rate should also be determined. A more detailed assessment is described in Chapter 18, The Comatose Patient.

5. Oxygenation and ventilation
   - *All* comatose head-injured patients require nasotracheal or orotracheal intubation.
   - Cricothyroidostomy or tracheostomy is reserved for patients with severe maxillofacial injuries.
   - It is important to oxygenate and hyperventilate patients to reverse the chain of pathophysiologic events described earlier.

6. Once an airway is established, a large bore veinway should be placed, as well as an indwelling urinary catheter.

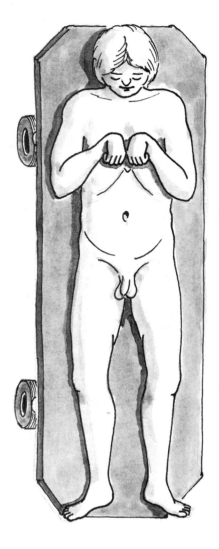
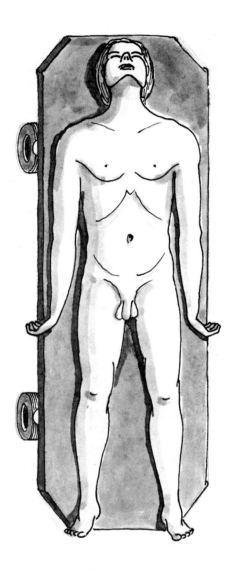

Figure 20-8 *Abnormal posturing. Left. Decorticate rigidity. Right. Decerebrate rigidity.*

7. Central venous lines and a pressure monitor may be useful in patients with coexisting shock.

8. A pneumatic antishock garment (PASG) can be used if necessary.

9. Obtain arterial blood gases as early as possible.

10. Auscultate the chest early to exclude pneumothorax.

11. Hypotension is seen uncommonly after head injuries; if it is present, look for some other etiology. A hypotensive patient has usually sustained significant blood loss and requires the administration of intravenous fluids and blood replacement.

Once the patient is stabilized, a more detailed general physical and neurological examination can be performed before x-ray examinations are ordered.

History. Details of the accident may be obtained from ambulance attendants, police, relatives, or other observers, if not directly from the patient. It is important to know the mechanism of trauma. If injury was sustained in an auto-

mobile accident, the following information should be gathered and recorded:

- Where the patient was sitting in the vehicle at the time of the accident

- The object on which he struck his head

- Mechanisms of spine injury—whether flexion, extension, or lateral flexion

- Knowledge of the type of collision (head-on, rear-end, broadside) and the interior damage to the automobile may help the trauma team piece together the mechanism of injury.

- If the patient arrives conscious, it is important to note whether or not there was a temporary loss of consciousness or whether there is full recall for the traumatic event as well as events immediately preceding or following the incident itself.

- Symptoms such as diplopia, weakness of the extremities, headache, neck pain, and numbness or parasthesias (tingling) in the extremities should be sought and recorded.

Physical Examination. Cervical spine injuries are commonly noted in patients with head injuries. It is imperative to stabilize the neck and render the head motionless until cervical spine injury has been excluded. Cervical spine injuries are discussed in detail in the final portion of this chapter. As stated above, vital signs including pulse, respiratory rate, blood pressure, and temperature should be taken.

1. *Head.* Examination of the head should include the position, length, and depth of scalp lacerations or avulsions. Palpation of the skull through a scalp laceration should be done carefully because of the risk of dislodging a fragment of depressed skull fracture deeper into the brain.

2. *Eyes.* Examination of the eyes for periorbital ecchymoses (raccoon sign) and of the retromastoid area for Battle's sign (ecchymosis of the mastoid area associated with basilar skull fracture) should also be done. The ocular fundi may be examined. A visual field examination should be performed on an awake patient. Pupillary size, equality, and reaction to light and extraocular motions are evaluated. The corneal reflex is tested by touching the cornea with a small wisp of cotton.

3. *Facial movements.* Facial movements can be tested voluntarily in an awake patient or, in patients who are lethargic or somnolent, by the administration of a painful stimulus through the supraorbital nerve by pressure on the supraorbital ridge.

4. *Ears.* Examine the external auditory canals for the presence of blood in the canals behind the tympanic membranes, which is indirect evidence of a basilar skull fracture. The finding of nonclotting blood is often present in basilar skull fracture due to mixture with CSF.

5. *Mouth.* The mouth and pharynx should be inspected for blood, foreign bodies, and the presence of gag reflex. Movements of the tongue to right and left are used to test the hypoglossal nerve.

6. *Caloric testing.* Caloric testing can give very useful information about comatose patients but should be performed only by a neurosurgeon. If cervical spine injury has been excluded, the patient's head is elevated 30 degrees and ice water injected into the external auditory canal to bathe the tympanic membrane. A tonic deviation of both eyes toward the side of the ice water irrigation will result if the neuronal circuit between pons and midbrain is intact. This test is preferably performed by a neurosurgeon. A lacerated eardrum may be a contraindication to this examination.

7. *Sensory and motor responses.* Sensory examination of the arms and legs can be performed by pin prick and light touch. Proprioceptive sensation is tested by moving the fingers or toes up or down and having the patient report his position. Strength in various muscle groups and the flexors and extensors of upper and lower extremities are tested. Mild weakness may be detected by drift or distraction. The patient holds both arms level, with eyes closed, and then is distracted by counting to ten. In a patient with mild weakness, the extremity will drift downward with pronation. Deep tendon reflexes are tested in upper and lower extremities; plantar responses are evaluated by applying a noxious stroking stimulus to the outer sole of the foot. In a normal response, the great toe flexes downward. Dorsiflexion of the great toe (Ba-

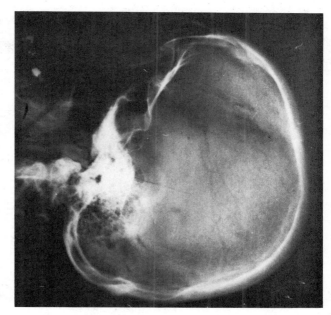

Figure 20-9 *Air fluid level in sphenoid sinus (patient in supine position).*

binski reflex) indicates pyramidal tract damage. The neck is examined by palpation for signs of paracervical muscle spasm. In patients in whom a cervical fracture is suspected, range-of-motion (ROM) testing is not done. Chest, abdomen, and muscular skeletal system examinations are described elsewhere in this book.

Adjunct Studies

Radiologic Examination. Patients with head injuries require x-ray studies of the skull and cervical spine. Skull x-rays consist of standard anteroposterior, Townes, and lateral projections, including cross-table brow-up lateral views to demonstrate air fluid levels in the sphenoid and paranasal sinuses (Fig. 20-9). To be adequate, lateral cervical spine x-ray studies must demonstrate the C7–T1 interspace in order to exclude cervical fracture-subluxation. If there is no evidence of fracture, a more complete series of cervical spine x-ray films may then be obtained.

Plain skull x-rays may demonstrate direct or indirect evidence of fractures. In addition, a shift of the pineal gland, if calcified, on an anteroposterior or Townes projection is an indicator of midline shifts within the cranial cavity due to hematoma or localized brain swelling.

PATIENTS WHO REQUIRE HOSPITALIZATION

Generally, all patients who have sustained a loss of consciousness following head trauma should be admitted to the hospital for at least 24 hours. During this time, no analgesics or sedation are given. Vital signs are checked and a brief neurologic assessment is done at least every 2 hours. This includes assessment of the level of awareness and orientation, pupillary equality and reaction to light and sen-

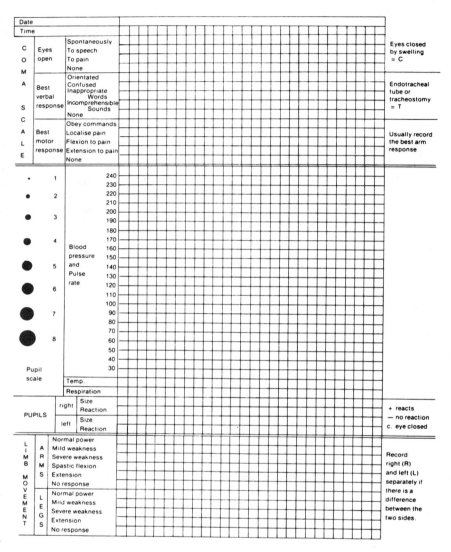

Sisters of Charity Hospital

of Buffalo. N. Y.

NEUROLOGICAL OBSERVATIONS

Figure 20-10 *Neurologic assessment flow sheet. (Reproduced with permission of Sisters of Charity Hospital, Buffalo, New York)*

sation, and movement in upper and lower extremities. The physician should be consulted if any of these parameters change. A neurologic assessment flow sheet, as shown in Fig. 20-10, is a convenient method of monitoring these patients on an ongoing basis.

Neurologically intact patients with skull fractures should also be admitted to the hospital for 3 to 5 days for observation. Patients with head trauma who have never lost consciousness or sustained skull fracture may be monitored by responsible family members. An instruction sheet (Fig. 20-11) must be given to the responsible person.

TYPES OF INJURIES

SCALP INJURIES

Injuries to the scalp include abrasions, lacerations, and avulsions. Laceration(s) of the scalp may result in significant blood loss, enough to produce hemorrhagic shock, especially in children. Abrasions may be cleansed; lacerations should be sutured. All foreign bodies should be removed from such wounds. Complicated surgical techniques, such as rotating a flap of scalp in severe scalp injuries, may be necessary to

---

INSTRUCTIONS: REGARDING HEAD TRAUMA

The examination and treatment you have received in the Emergency Department have been rendered on an emergency basis only and are not intended to provide complete medical care.

The patient has been examined and/or treated in this emergency Department for

_____ .

At this time the history and findings do not indicate a need for hospitalization.

In order for the injured person to be fully cared for, the patient must be carefully observed to determine whether any of the following conditions occur. If they do, the injured person should be returned to the Hospital Emergency Department promptly.

1. *Unconsciousness* (does not answer or respond when you talk to or touch him).
2. *Convulsions* (shaking or stiffening of arms or legs; eyes rolled back or staring into space).
3. *Unequal size of pupils* (different size of black, center part of eyes).
4. *Unusual drowsiness* (unable to be awakened from sleep).
5. *Unusual behavior* (he just does not act right).
6. *Tingling, numbness, or paralysis of face and/or arms and legs* (a funny feeling or no feeling).
7. *Drainage from nose or ears* (blood or other fluid runs from nose or ears).
8. *Unexplained, recurring vomiting* (keeps on vomiting for several hours and cannot keep anything down).
9. *Increased swelling of scalp or face* (the bump gets bigger).
10. *Incontinence of stool or urine* (cannot control his bowels or urine).
11. *Unable to maintain balance* (complains of dizziness).

Further necessary steps required for complete medical care (where checked):

☐ See personal physician for follow-up care.

☐ Call for appointment in _____ Clinic (Tel. _____).

☐ Report to Trauma Clinic on _____ at 8:00 A.M.

It is sometimes impossible to recognize and treat all elements of an injury or an illness in a single Emergency Department visit; therefore, it is important that *you* report any new or continuing problems to your physician. If you do not have a personal physician, you may make an appointment for a visit to Sisters Hospital Outpatient Department (Tel. _____).

Figure 20-11 *Instruction sheet for observing head trauma patient after discharge from emergency department. (Reproduced with permission of Sisters of Charity Hospital, Buffalo, New York)*

cover the exposed cranium in patients who have sustained an avulsion.

FRACTURES OF THE SKULL

Linear Fractures. These are simple fractures of the inner and outer tables of the skull; they are seen as a straight line on x-ray (Fig. 20-12). These fractures are important because they indicate to emergency personnel that the patient has sustained a significant blow to the head. Linear fractures

that cross the middle meningeal groove in the temporal-parietal area, the midline, or the occipital area should alert one to the possibility of extradural (epidural) bleeding from a lacerated middle meningeal artery or dural sinus. All patients with skull fractures should be admitted to the hospital for observation.

Diastatic Fracture. Severe trauma to the skull may separate the coronal, sagittal, or lambdoidal sutures. This is termed a *diastatic fracture.* No specific treatment is indicated

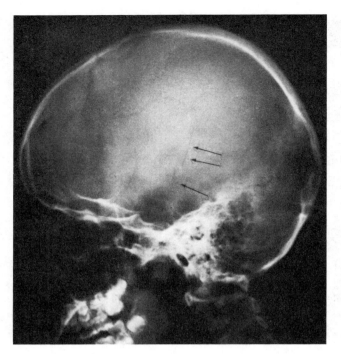

Figure 20-12 *Linear fracture of temporal bone (indicated by arrows).*

except observation of the patient for the development of intracranial hematoma or cerebral edema.

Depressed Skull Fracture. A fracture of the skull in which a loose fragment of bone is driven into the cranial cavity is termed a depressed skull fracture. This type of fracture may be associated with a scalp laceration (compound depressed fracture) or may occur without laceration (simple depressed fracture). If untreated, depressed fractures may lead to intracranial infection or seizures. The management is surgical and requires craniectomy, in which the depressed fragments are removed.

Basilar Skull Fracture. Basilar skull fractures are usually diagnosed by one of the following signs:

- Blood behind the tympanic membrane
- Leakage of CSF from the ears or nose
- Ecchymosis in the mastoid region (Battle's sign)
- Bilateral periorbital ecchymoses (raccoon sign)
- Air fluid levels in the sphenoid, maxillary, or frontal sinuses

There is no specific treatment for basilar skull fracture except bed rest and observation. The use of prophylactic antibiotics is controversial at this time. Nasogastric intubation must be performed with care, especially in patients with fracture(s) of the cribriform plate, because the tube may be inserted through the fracture into the cranial cavity with dire results. If it is absolutely necessary that a nasogastric tube

be used, a precurved silastic nasopharyngeal airway is placed first, and the nasogastric tube is inserted through the airway, which is then removed.

INJURIES TO BRAIN TISSUE

CONCUSSION

Concussion describes a physiologic alteration in the level of consciousness caused by torsional forces on the midbrain, in which the patient loses consciousness but recovers within a few minutes.[29,80] It is the most common and least serious type of brain injury. The patient usually has no recall of events immediately before the injury (retrograde amnesia) and immediately after his recovery of consciousness (anterograde amnesia). Concussion is not typically associated with neurologic deficit. Like skull fracture, a concussion indicates significant trauma to the head. Concussion patients must also be observed for signs of increased intracranial pressure, intracranial hematoma, or brain swelling. The patient who sustains a loss of consciousness should be admitted to the hospital for observation for a period of 24 to 48 hours.

Cortical Contusion

A cortical contusion results from the rupture of tiny blood vessels in the pia mater. If it involves neurologically important brain tissue, an immediate neurologic deficit occurs.

Figure 20-13 *Epidural hematoma. The dark area in the lower left of the drawing represents the hematoma. Note the broken blood vessel and the shift of midline structures.*

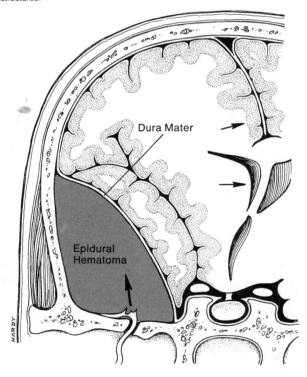

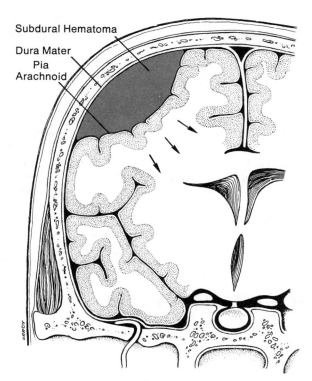

Subdural Hematoma
Dura Mater
Pia
Arachnoid

Figure 20-14 *Subdural hematoma. The dark area in the upper left of the drawing represents the hematoma. Note the shift of midline structures.*

Patients who have cortical contusions are best admitted to the hospital for observation. There is no specific treatment; however, a course of anticonvulsants is recommended to prevent seizures. Glucocorticoids (dexamethasone, 0.004 gm q6h for 4–5 days) may be helpful in reducing brain swelling; criteria for use are strictly empirical.[13,28]

Intracranial Hematomas

Hematomas are classified according to their location as epidural, subdural, or intraparenchymal (within the substance of the brain).

Epidural Hematoma (Fig. 20-13). This is usually a rapidly developing lesion associated with laceration of the middle cerebral artery with hemorrhage as a result of a linear or depressed skull fracture in the temporal bone. Occasionally, bleeding from other fracture sites can also result in epidural hemorrhage. Clinically, the patient has suffered a severe blow to the head, causing momentary unconsciousness followed by a lucid interval that may last minutes or hours and proceed to loss of consciousness and deterioration of vital signs. The pupil on the ipsilateral side (the side of injury) is dilated and nonreactive, and there is paralysis on the contralateral (opposite) side. With injury on the dominant side of the brain (the left side in right-handed persons, the right side in left-handed persons), aphasia, or speech defect may be noted. Skull x-rays may reveal temporal bone fracture

and pineal shift. Computed tomography (CT) scan may localize the hematoma. The appropriate surgical treatment is immediate craniectomy to evacuate the hematoma and control the source of the hemorrhage. The mortality rate is approximately 50%.

Subdural Hematoma (Fig. 20-14). Subdural hematoma is caused by bleeding into the subdural space from ruptured cortical arteries or bridging veins. The hematoma may develop within minutes (acute), hours (subacute), or weeks (chronic) before becoming symptomatic. Subdural hematoma usually indicates a severe head injury; it may occur unilaterally or bilaterally and is often associated with an intraparenchymal injury.

Acute or Subacute Subdural Hematoma. In the acute or subacute type, the patient is unconscious. There may be lateralizing signs that the ipsilateral pupil is dilated and nonreactive, with or without contralateral limb weakness or paralysis. In bilateral or advanced injury, pupillary changes may be seen bilaterally.

Skull x-rays will reveal the fracture or pineal shift. CT scanning will reveal the hematoma and displacement of brain substance.

The need for treatment is urgent and consists of removal of the hematoma, which is usually clotted, by craniotomy or craniectomy. The prognosis is grave, the mortality rate varying between 46% and 90%, but is favorably affected by surgical intervention.

Chronic Subdural Hematoma. Chronic subdural hematomas become manifest weeks to months after injury. They occur more commonly in infants and the aged. The history of injury, being remote, is often forgotten. The mechanism of injury is usually a fall or a blow to the head that is relatively minor. Following injury, bleeding occurs, usually from a torn vein; a hematoma forms and expands over a period of time, causing a gradual increase in intracranial pressure. The patient may complain of nausea and emesis, headache, alteration in consciousness, visual disturbances, and other neurologic deficits.

Skull x-rays and echography will reveal the displacement of midline structures. CT scanning will confirm these findings and the presence of a mass with displacement of brain tissue. Lumbar puncture reveals an increase in spinal fluid pressure; the fluid is yellow-tinged (xanthochromic) because of the breakdown products from the hematoma into the spinal fluid.

The blood in this type of hematoma is liquefied but thick, with the consistency of crankcase oil. It is evacuated by means of two or three burr holes to allow reexpansion of the brain. Unlike that for the acute or subacute forms, the prognosis is excellent, with a 90% survival rate. A neurologic deficit may remain in some patients.

Intraparenchymal Hematoma

Cortical contusions or rupture of blood vessels within the substance of the brain can result in a hematoma, which may enlarge, producing increased intracranial pressure or herniation.

Intracranial hematomas may occur within minutes after head injury or may be delayed, developing slowly over several hours, days, or weeks. In the slower-developing forms, loss of consciousness resulting from concussion is followed by neurologic deterioration. The patient may become lethargic, disoriented, and incontinent (cingulate herniation). Transtentorial herniation usually follows. All intracranial hematomas are diagnosed by CT scanning or cerebral arteriography, which is discussed later in this chapter.

RECOGNIZING THE DETERIORATING NEUROLOGIC PATIENT

Early recognition of neurologic deterioration is necessary for speedy and effective therapy. Patients who are at risk may be monitored clinically by the use of a neurologic grading scale and by measuring intracranial pressure.[14,20]

GLASGOW COMA SCALE

The Glasgow Coma Scale is a uniform grading system for neurologic monitoring.[77,78] Level of awareness, oculomotor findings, and motor responses are determined, and a charted numerical score is given (see Fig. 18-1). A neurologically normal patient has a score of 15, whereas a patient in deep coma with no response to pain has a score of 3. Determining the score every hour is a convenient method of assessing clinical deterioration or improvement.

INTRACRANIAL PRESSURE MONITORING

It is recommended that patients with severe brain injury be monitored clinically and also by measuring (ICP).[68] ICP may be monitored by means of an intraventricular catheter or by a subdural or epidural pressure screw and a calibrated strain gauge connected to a chart recorder or video terminal. The monitoring device is best placed by a neurosurgeon. Normal ICP is below 10 mm Hg. Elevation of ICP due to intracranial hematoma or cerebral edema may be noted and corrective therapeutic measures taken before clinical signs of neurologic deterioration occur.[48,59]

OTHER NEURORADIOLOGIC EXAMINATIONS

Patients who require further neuroradiologic evaluation (CT scanning or arteriography) are those who fail to improve after resuscitation or who demonstrate signs of progressive deterioration.

CT Scanning

Computed tomography (CT scanning) is an x-ray study in which x-ray beam attenuation in many views around the head is reconstructed by computer to produce horizontal slices through the cranial cavity. This allows visualization of the skull and intracranial contents and detection of brain contusion, hematoma (Fig. 20-15), skull fractures, or brain swelling. It is precise and noninvasive.

Cerebral Arteriography

Prior to the availability of CT scanning, arteriography was the major method of diagnosing intracranial hematomas. If CT scanning is unavailable, cerebral arteriography may be necessary to exclude an intracranial mass lesion. Direct needle puncture of the carotid arteries in the neck or transfemoral catheterization for the injection of the cerebral arteries with contrast material will demonstrate displacement of intracranial blood vessels by intracranial mass lesions.

TREATMENT OF CEREBRAL EDEMA

Cerebral edema has two phases; the first involves an increase in cerebral blood volume[42,79] and the second an increase in brain water.[44] The patient with no evidence of intracranial hematoma as determined by CT scanning who has a Glasgow Coma Scale score of 8 or less should be monitored by hourly Glasgow Coma score determinations and, in most cases, by ICP monitoring.

The goal of ICP monitoring is to alert hospital personnel when ICP exceeds 22 mm Hg, at which point cerebral per-

Figure 20-15 *Computed tomography (CT) scan of patient with left subdural hematoma (arrows).*

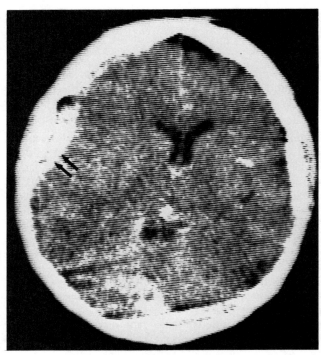

fusion is diminished and treatment is required. Such patients should have ventilatory support by means of endotracheal intubation. Blood gases are measured at frequent intervals. Ideally, the PaO_2 should be above 120 mm Hg; if it is not, oxygen should be administered and a pulmonary evaluation undertaken to determine the cause of the hypoxemia.

If the $PaCO_2$ is above 30 mm Hg the patient should be placed on a ventilator and hyperventilated by increasing the tidal volume and respiratory rate to keep the $PaCO_2$ between 25 and 30 mm Hg.[21,22,69,72]

If the arterial blood gases are within acceptable ranges and ICP still exceeds 22 mm Hg, small doses of hyperosmotic agents such as mannitol (1.5 gm/kg body weight, IV, q4h) may be administered. Serum osmolality must be determined twice daily. If it exceeds 315 mOsm/L, breakdown of the blood-brain barrier occurs, and hyperosmotic agents are counterproductive.

Patients with serum osmolalities above 300 mOsm are best treated by inducing barbiturate coma, which reduces the metabolic demand of the brain and physiologically reduces cerebral blood flow and cerebral blood volume,[6,8,62] resulting in a reduction in ICP.[52-54] Pentobarbital is most commonly used for this purpose. A loading dose of 3 to 5 mg/kg body weight of pentobarbital is followed by frequent intravenous doses in order to maintain a blood level of pentobarbital of 4 mg/dl. Ventilatory assistance is required when barbiturate coma therapy is used.

Cerebral Edema in the Inebriated Patient. If a person whose brain is already depressed by alcohol sustains a brain injury, assessment becomes difficult because the decreased level of consciousness and sensory-motor functioning can be due either to alcohol or cerebral edema secondary to injury. Likewise, bradycardia and vomiting may be caused by either.

In intoxicated patients, the onset of cerebral edema is delayed, possibly because of the antidiuretic effect of alcohol, until the alcohol has been metabolized. The edema may then persist for a longer period of time. Any inebriated patient suspected of having sustained head trauma should be carefully observed for any alteration in neurologic status.

CONCLUSIONS

Head trauma is categorized as either significant or insignificant. Any patient who has lost consciousness or who has a skull fracture or a neurologic deficit has sustained significant head trauma. Patients who become neurologically normal should nevertheless be observed in the hospital for a while to ensure that they do not undergo neurologic deterioration because of intracranial hematoma or brain swelling. Patients with severe head injuries who are deeply comatose because of either herniation syndromes, brain swelling, intracranial hematoma, or primary brain-stem injury require intensive monitoring and treatment. Intracranial hematomas are best

diagnosed by CT scanning and should be evacuated as soon as possible. Patients with cerebral edema require intensive clinical and ICP monitoring. Increased ICP is treated by artificial ventilation and osmotic diuretics or barbiturate coma.

NECK INJURIES

SOFT-TISSUE INJURY OF THE NECK

The soft-tissue structures of the neck may be injured with or without a concomitant injury to the cervical spine. The neck is protected posteriorly and laterally to a great extent by the bulky trapezius muscles and the cervical spine. Anteriorly, the relatively small strap muscles afford little protection, making the underlying structures vulnerable to injury. Almost any of the organs of the neck may be damaged by blunt or penetrating trauma.

The organs in the neck that are potentially subject to injury are the following:
- Airway
   Larynx
   Trachea
- Blood vessels
   Carotid artery and branches
   Jugular vein
   Vertebral artery
- Gastrointestinal tract
   Pharynx
   Esophagus
- Nerves
   Brachial plexus
- Other
   Thyroid gland
   Thoracic duct
   Apex of the lung(s)

BLUNT INJURY OF THE NECK

The more common causes of blunt neck injury are:
- Vehicular accident, especially for occupants of the front seat
- Fall
- Physical assault
- Sports injury

The larynx and trachea are in a relatively superficial, unprotected position and thus are the structures most commonly damaged. In mild injuries, these airway structures may be contused and edematous, with subsequent stridor. In serious injuries, a tear or fracture of the airway may lead to subcutaneous emphysema and potentially serious respiratory embarrassment, which can end in death.

Injury to the larger vascular structures in the neck can cause bleeding deep in the cervical fascia. Over a period of time, a hematoma may form, which can expand, producing pressure on the trachea.

The esophagus may rarely be damaged by blunt trauma that leads to perforation and spillage of saliva into the soft tissues of the neck, and a serious local infection may result.

Brachial plexus injury most often follows a blow, such as a karate chop, to the anterolateral aspect of the cervical area. The most common type of damage is a contusion, rather than a laceration, of the neural structures.

Assessment

It is important in caring for a patient with a blunt injury to suspect and recognize injury to structures in the neck.

1. Symptoms of injuries to neck structures correspond to the organ(s) damaged and include:
   - Pain at the site
   - Dysphonia—difficulty in speaking
   - Dyspnea—difficulty in breathing
   - Dysphagia—difficulty in swallowing
   - Hemoptysis
2. The signs of structural injury are:
   - Loss of palpable landmarks
   - Swelling or tenderness in the neck
   - Contusion or ecchymosis of the skin at the site of injury
   - Subcutaneous emphysema if there is a rupture of the airway or esophagus
   - Varying degrees of respiratory embarrassment, varying from stridor (noisy breathing) to labored respiration marked by supraclavicular tugging, intercostal retraction and apprehension
3. If brachial plexus injury is suspected, careful neurologic examination of the ipsilateral upper extremity is necessary to evaluate motor or sensory loss.

Prehospital Care

1. Apply the ABCs of care. Ensure that the airway is adequate. Stridor may be an early sign of impending airway obstruction.
2. Make the patient as comfortable as possible. Application of a cervical collar may be beneficial.

Note: Keep in mind the possibility of a concomitant cervical spine injury and manage it accordingly (see pp 338–345).

3. Airway obstruction is apt to occur at the level of the larynx or the trachea. Needle or tube cricothyroidostomy is not expected to be beneficial, since it gives access only above the point of obstruction. Under such cicumstances, the preferred method of securing an adequate airway is by endotracheal intubation through the nose (nasotracheal route) or mouth (orotracheal route).
   - If injury to the cervical spine is a significant consideration, the nasotracheal method is preferred to avoid hyperextension.

4. The patient should be transported early to the hospital on a spine board with the neck fully immobilized.

Hospital Care

1. The prime consideration is to establish and maintain an adequate airway. Any compromise of the airway must be managed swiftly. If the endotracheal tube cannot be passed, tracheostomy must be considered and performed early.
2. Intravenous lines should be placed in the lower limbs, because of the possibility of injury to the great vessels of the neck. A nasogastric tube should be inserted.
3. Once the patient's condition has stabilized, x-rays of the neck and chest are taken. The presence of air in the tissues of the neck indicates perforation or rupture of either the esophagus or trachea, or damage to the apex of the pleura or lung.
4. If esophageal injury is suspected, a gastrograffin swallow is helpful in confirming the diagnosis.
5. Laryngoscopy or bronchoscopy is used to identify damage to the airway.
6. The presence of an expanding hematoma in the neck is an indication for appropriate angiographic studies.
7. Early surgical exploration of the neck, repair of the damaged structure, and drainage of the involved area is advisable.

PENETRATING INJURY OF THE NECK

Such injuries may result from:
- Stabbing
- Gunshot wound
- Flying object
- Iatrogenic effect of prior attempt at central-vein catherization

Any or all of the organ structures susceptible to blunt injury may be damaged by penetrating trauma. From the standpoint of management, penetrating wounds of the neck are very similar to those of the peritoneal cavity. The platysma muscle, which extends over the entire anterior and lateral aspects of the neck from the mandibles to the clavicles, is analogous to the peritoneum. Generally, any wound penetrating the platysma mandates surgical exploration to identify and treat injury of the underlying structures. Mortality rates of 6% to 10% have been reported in patients with penetrating neck injuries. Most of the deaths are due to injury of the carotid and subclavian arteries and the jugular and subclavian veins. The remainder follows wounds of the larynx, trachea, and esophagus. Often, the nature of the flesh wound is deceptively insignificant in relation to injury to the deeper structures. One must not be misled by what appears to be an innocuous wound of the skin. Recently, the availability of more sophisticated and precise diagnostic studies has led some to follow a course of selective exploration of penetrating neck injuries. The presence of such modalities in a hospital may suggest such a method of treatment.

Assessment

1. Full assessment of the patient is necessary, starting with a history of the accident. Question the patient carefully about the mechanism of injury.

2. Particular attention is given to vital signs and to the wound itself. One must keep in mind the organ structures that are susceptible to injury and evaluate the patient from this standpoint.

3. In addition to the assessment findings of blunt injury, the patient must be evaluated for evidence of blood loss with resulting hypotension.

4. The ABCs of care are applied. Evaluate the status of the airway, observe any sign of blood loss and circulatory instability.

5. *No penetrating neck wound should be ignored or underestimated.* Palpate the neck carefully to identify any abnormalities such as the following:
   - Tracheal deviation may indicate pressure from an external mass or damage to the apex of the lung or pleura, resulting in pneumothorax.
   - Subcutaneous emphysema indicates an air leak caused by penetration of the esophagus or airway.
   - Pulsatile masses or palpable thrill may indicate damage to a major artery.
   - Nonpulsatile swellings may be secondary to bleeding from venous injury.
   - Auscultatory findings of a bruit may follow trauma to a major artery and vein, resulting in false aneurysm or arteriovenous fistula formation.

6. Ongoing assessment
   - Check for intact peripheral pulses. Absence of the radial or ulnar pulse(s) indicates interruption of flow and suggests proximal arterial injury. The presence of pulses at the wrist does not rule out proximal vascular injury.
   - Take blood pressure recordings in each arm to identify a significant variance that could indicate vascular injury.
   - Check sensory and motor-nerve function of the upper limbs.

Adjunct Studies

1. *Upright chest x-ray.* In reviewing the films, one should look carefully for:
   - Air in the subcutaneous tissues of the neck, indicating penetrating injury to the larynx, trachea, or esophagus
   - Pneumothorax, which may follow penetrating injury to the lung or pleura
   - Retained missiles after gunshot injury

2. *X-rays of the neck* are indicated, especially after a gunshot injury, to locate the retained missile.

3. *Aortic angiography* is necessary when one suspects injury to a major artery. This is more likely to occur in a wound at the base of the neck. Angiography will invariably identify the arterial injury and aid the surgeon in planning the operative approach.

4. Laryngoscopy or bronchoscopy is helpful in ruling out laryngeal or tracheobronchial injury.

A nasogastric tube should be inserted to minimize the chance of aspiration of gastric contents and assist the surgeon in identifying the esophagus at the time of surgical exploration. The finding of injury to the airway, vessels, or esophagus indicates a need for surgical exploration.

Management

Penetrating injuries may cause significant damage to vital structures, which can result in compromise of the airway and hypovolemic shock. Attention must be directed initially to life-support measures following the ABCs of care. An adequate airway must be established and maintained as mentioned earlier. External bleeding is controlled primarily by direct pressure. The circulation is supported by large veinways placed in the lower limb(s). At the outset, Ringer's lactate is used to restore blood volume until type-specific whole blood is available.

The following two axioms are most important in the management of these wounds:

1. No penetrating wound should be ignored or underestimated because wounds that may appear to be innocuous are often associated with major structural damage to the neck.

2. Under no circumstances should the wound be probed in the emergency department. A thrombus could be dislodged, creating the danger of major uncontrollable hemorrhage.

Treatment. Definitive treatment is surgical and is based on the following principles:
- Exploration of the entire neck, entering both sides if clinically warranted
- Thorough debridement of devitalized tissue
- Identification of major structures to establish the presence or absence of damage, including the larynx, trachea, esophagus, major vessels, nerves, and lymph channels
- Surgical repair of identified injuries

INJURIES TO THE VERTEBRAE AND SPINAL CORD

ANATOMY

Spinal Column

The spinal column extends the length of the body from the base of the skull to the perianal area. It consists of seven cervical, twelve thoracic, five lumbar, and five sacral vertebrae and the coccyx. The stability of the spine depends upon the bony articulation of the facet joints and the ligamentous, fascial, and muscular structures that surround the vertebral column throughout its length. Articular facets overlap at the posterior aspect of the spine. The superior facets of the vertebra below articulate with the inferior facets of the ver-

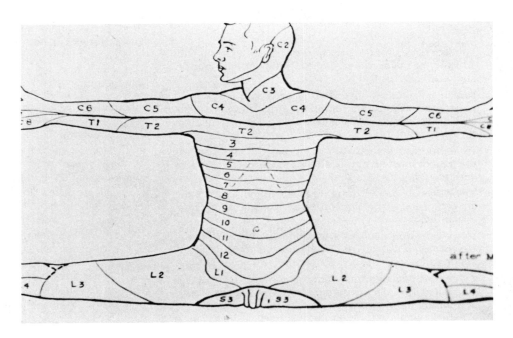

Figure 20-16 Sensory dermatomes.

tebra above. The spinal cord lies protected within the spinal canal, which is a hollow tunnel extending the length of the vertebral column. The spinal cord itself begins superiorly at the foramen magnum in the base of the skull and terminates inferiorly at approximately the level of the 2nd lumbar vertebra, in a structure called the conus medullaris. The

Figure 20-17 *Cross-section of spinal cord showing principal conduction pathways. These tracts are bilateral, but in this diagram ascending tracts are numbered on the right only, and descending on the left only. (Chaffee EE, Lytle IM: Basic Anatomy and Physiology, 4th ed. Philadelphia, JB Lippincott, 1980)*

Descending tracts   **Ascending tracts**

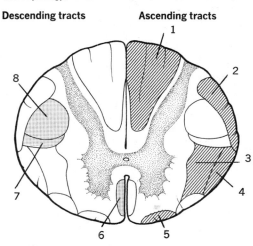

1   Dorsal columns: conscious muscle sense, touch, vibration

2   Dorsal spinocerebellar tract: unconscious muscle sense

3   Lateral spinothalamic tract: pain and temperature

4   Ventral spinocerebellar tract: unconscious muscle sense

5   Ventral spinothalamic tract: light touch

6   Ventral pyramidal tract:voluntary control of skeletal muscle

7   Extrapyramidal tract: automatic control of skeletal muscle

8   Lateral pyramidal tract: voluntary control of skeletal muscle

All tracts are bilateral

TABLE 20-1.   SPECIFIC AREAS OF SENSORY AND MOTOR INNERVATION

Segment	Sensory Area	Motor Distribution
C2	Back of head	—
C5	Shoulder girdle	Shoulder girdle muscles
C6	Thumb	Biceps
C7	Index, middle finger	Triceps
C8	Ring and 5th finger Ulnar border of hand	Intrinsics of hand
T4	Nipple line	—
T6	Lower tip of the sterum	
T10	Umbilicus	Abdominals
L1	Inguinal ligament	Flexors of thigh
L4	Patella	Quadriceps femoris
L5	Medial border of foot	Anterior compartment (dorsiflexors of foot)
S1	Lateral border of foot	Posterior compartments (plantar flexors of foot)
S3–C5	Perineal (saddle area) sacral-sparing	

lumbar and sacral nerves flow from the lower end of the cord in the spinal canal and are referred to as the cauda equina (horse's tail).

Spinal Cord

The spinal cord is a bundle of neurons that connect the brain with the rest of the body. The afferent pathways (leading *to* the cord) carry sensory impulses from receptor organs in the skin, muscle, and viscera by way of peripheral nerves to the spinal cord and thence to the brain. Efferent pathways (leading *from* the cord) carry signals from the brain to effector centers in the spinal cord and thence to effector muscles. The spinal nerves arise from the spinal cord and exit the spinal canal through the intervertebral foramina, which are located in the vertebral interspaces and then extend to the various areas of the body.

The spinal cord is arranged vertically in layers, or seg-

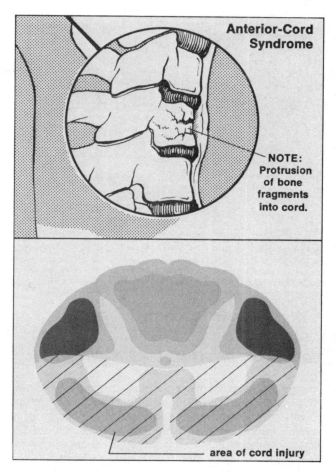

Figure 20-19 *Anterior cord syndrome. This syndrome is seen usually after hyperflexion injuries with protrusion of bone fragments of prolapsed-disk material into the cord or with thrombosis or laceration of the anterior spinal artery. It is characterized by immediate paralysis and hypalgesia below the level of injury but with preservation of posterior-column function (touch, position, vibration, motion). The loss of spinothalamic function (pain and temperature) is the most striking characteristic of the syndrome. There may be some motor sparing, since the corticospinal tracts are somewhat posterior in the cord. (Reproduced from: Emergency Management of Cervical Spine Injuries, by Desmond P. Colohan. Courtesy of Abbott Laboratories)*

Figure 20-18 *Central-cord syndrome. This pattern of cord injury is most common in persons with degenerative arthritis of the neck; a hyperextension injury causes the ligamentum flavum to buckle into the cord. Since the long tracts to the cervical nerve roots are located near the center of the cord and those to the sacral roots near the periphery, with a central-cord injury there will be a greater neurologic deficit in the upper extremities than in the lower extremities. Urinary retention is common, but some saddle sensation is retained. (Reproduced from: Emergency Management of Cervical Spine Injuries, by Desmond P. Colohan. Courtesy of Abbott Laboratories)*

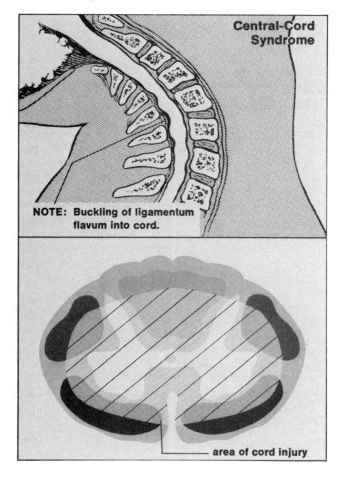

ments, each segment being responsible for a particular band of sensation and specific muscles. The sensory bands, called dermatomes, are shown in Fig. 20-16. Specific areas of sensory and motor innervation are given in Table 20-1.

The spinal cord is made up of three prominent bundles on either side of the midline, posteriorly, laterally, and anteriorly (Fig. 20-17). The posterior bundle (posterior columns) contains sensory fibers that carry proprioceptive, vibratory, and deep-pain sensation to the brain. The lateral column, or gray matter, contains the pyramidal tract and a pathway for pain and temperature sensation (lateral spinothalamic tract). Injury to the lateral spinothalamic tract results in loss of pain and temperature sensation on the opposite side of the body.

The central gray matter is a collection of cell bodies. The dorsal horn contains the cell bodies of sensory neurons. The anterior horn contains motor cell bodies that innervate the muscles of the body.

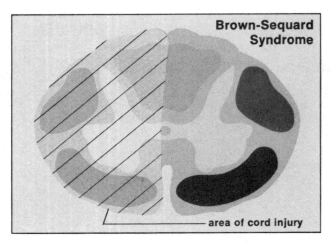

Figure 20-20 *Brown-Sequard syndrome. This syndrome usually results from direct penetrating injuries to the neck. It is characterized by loss of posterior-column function and paralysis on the same side of the body as the injury, and loss of pain and temperature sensation on the other side. (Reproduced from: Emergency Management of Cervical Spine Injuries, by Desmond P. Colohan. Courtesy of Abbott Laboratories)*

MECHANISMS OF SPINAL CORD INJURY

The spinal cord may be injured by a number of mechanisms that compress or impair its blood supply. Specifically, damage may result from a variety of flexion, extension, compression, or rotary forces transmitted through the spinal column. Dislocation (subluxation) of one vertebral element upon another results in narrowing or possibly total obliteration of the spinal canal. If the spinal canal is narrowed beyond a critical level, the spinal cord is compressed. The spinal cord may also be compressed by a ruptured intervertebral disk. Damage to the spinal cord can also occur in the absence of spinal fracture, dislocation, or ruptured disk. An example is a hyperextension injury that compromises the blood supply to the cord. Complete transection of the cord is rare from the anatomic standpoint, but relatively common physiologically.

It is important to have as much information as possible about how the patient sustained the injury. Armed with this knowledge, one can better understand the mechanism of injury and be aware of the potential for further injury.

Because of the risks involved in cervical spine injury, the following important axiom should be applied: *any patient with an injury above the clavicle or a head injury that causes unconsciousness should be suspected of having an injury of the cervical spine until a definitive diagnosis can be made.*

Syndromes of Spinal Cord Injury

Total Transection. This is usually associated with spinal fracture-subluxation. Patients have complete absence of pain, pressure, and joint sensation, and complete motor paralysis below the level of the injury.

Central Cord Syndrome **(Fig. 20-18).** This syndrome is probably vascular in etiology. There is complete sensory loss below the level of the injury, but the sacral dermatomes are usually spared. The arms are weaker than the legs when this injury occurs in the cervical area, as it usually does. There may be bilateral loss of pain and temperature sensation and, in a widespread lesion, impairment of position and vibratory sense. The bladder may be involved in some instances.

Anterior Cord Syndrome **(Fig. 20-19).** This syndrome is frequently caused by pressure on the anterior aspect of the spinal cord by ruptured intervertebral disks or fragments of the vertical body extruded posteriorly into the spinal canal.[3] It may follow an acute hyperflexion injury with damage to the anterior spinal cord or artery. There is complete loss of sensation to pinprick below the level of the injury in all dermatomes, including those of the sacral regions. The upper and lower extremities are equally weak. Deep pain, light touch, and joint sensation are preserved.

Brown-Sequard Syndrome **(Fig. 20-20).** This syndrome is a hemitransection of the cord which may be vascular and may also be associated with a ruptured intervertebral disk or a unilateral encroachment on the spinal cord by a fragment of vertical body, often following knife or missile injuries. Pressure on one half of the spinal cord results in weakness of the upper and lower extremities on the same side as the injury (the ipsilateral side), and loss of pain and temperature on the opposite (contralateral) side of the body.

MANAGEMENT OF PATIENTS WHO HAVE SPINAL CORD INJURY

At the scene of injury, a primary challenge to emergency personnel is to provide life-saving care without further injuring spinal structures. The most important decision is whether or not the patient has a spinal fracture. Emergency personnel should proceed on the assumption that a spinal fracture exists until further examination and a conclusive diagnosis are possible. The spine must be kept immobile in moving these patients. The most critical area for attention is the cervical spine. Thoracic fractures are more stable because they are stabilized by ribs and intercostal musculature. Fractures of the lumbar spine should be immobilized.

PREHOSPITAL CARE

A rapid preliminary assessment and initial care are carried out concurrently as indicated by need.
1. Suspect cervical spine injury with the following:
   - Mechanisms of injury that may have involved flexion, extension, or rotation of the neck and head
   - Presence of head, neck, or facial injury
   - Impaired consciousness

Chart 20-1

MOVING THE PATIENT WITH A POSSIBLE CERVICAL SPINE INJURY

Exteme care must be taken to fully support the neck of anyone suspected of having a cervical spine injury until a rigid immobilization device is applied.

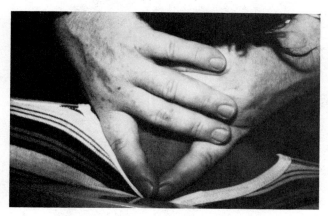

The hand position for supporting the neck is shown at left. • The neck is supported in a neutral position by placing the index fingers just below C7, at the base of the neck. • The thumbs support the mandible (taking care to avoid the area under the mandible, where vessels could be compressed). • The remaining interlocked fingers cradle the occiput and posterior neck. • By keeping the elbows extended outward, the temptation to support the head laterally with the forearm is minimized. Lateral forearm support of the head is inadvisable because inadvertent flexion of the neck could occur during lifting.

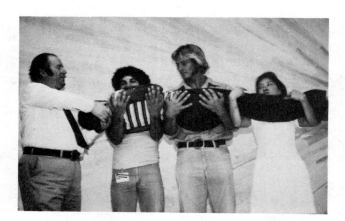

Once the neck is stabilized, assisting personnel can slide their hands and arms under the patient as shown at left. The first arm to go under the patient should be nearest the fracture site. Personnel at the shoulders and neck must coordinate closely and act in unison.

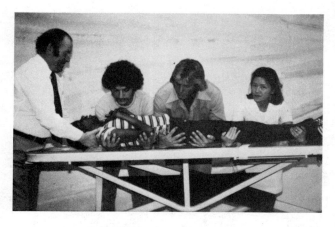

The patient can be lifted and rolled as a unit, if necessary, while the person managing at the head directs each action.

(Courtesy of Conal B. Wilmot, M.D., Chairman, Department of Physical Medicine and Rehabilitation, Santa Clara Valley Medical Center [Northern California Regional Spinal Cord Injury Center], San Jose, California)

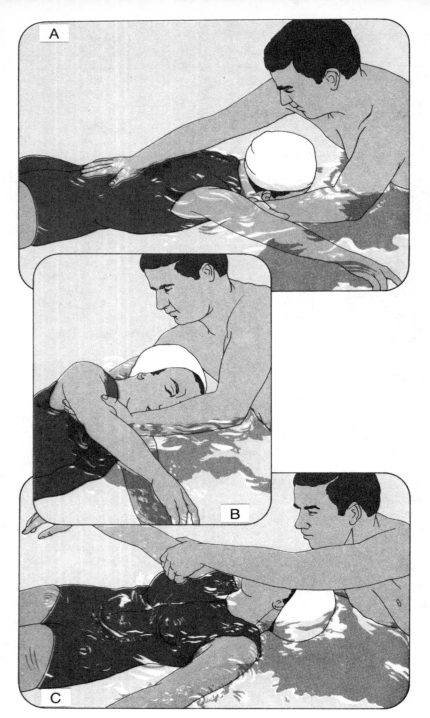

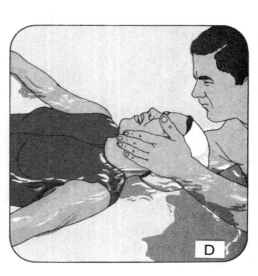

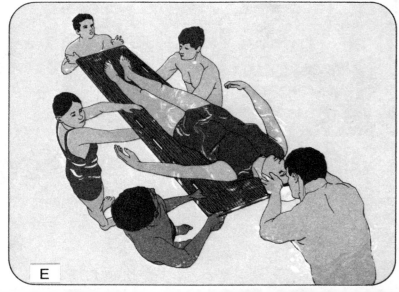

Figure 20-21 Water rescue of the victim with suspected spine injury. (Advanced First Aid and Emergency Care, 2nd ed. Copyright (c) 1979 by the American Red Cross. Reproduced with permission)

A. If the victim is floating face down, turn him over carefully with the least amount of movement, keeping his head and body aligned. Place one of your hands in the middle of the victim's back with your arm right over his head; place your other hand under the victim's upper arm, close to the shoulder, ready to turn him face-up. B,C. Rotate the victim by lifting his shoulder up and over with one hand while your other hand and arm support and maintain his head and body alignment.

The victim can be floated on his back in the water with minimal hand support. His head and neck should always be level with his back (D), his airway must be kept open, and if mouth-to-mouth resuscitation must be administered, use the jaw-thrust maneuver without head tilt. The backboard is placed under the victim by sliding it under the water and letting it float up (E).

Chart 20-2

PRINCIPLES OF APPLICATION OF A SHORT SPINE IMMOBILIZATION DEVICE

A variety of spine immobilizing devices may be used to immobilize the cervical spine. However, for all types the method of application follows a specific order to safely and thoroughly secure the body to the device.

1. Whenever there is doubt about the presence of a cervical spine injury, always secure the victim to an immobilizing device.
2. Before beginning any activity that could cause movement (including entering a vehicle), the patient's head is supported in a neutral position.
   - This support is maintained throughout the entire immobilization process, *including after the cervical collar is applied.*
   - If resistance to movement is noted, support the head in the position in which it was found.
   - When necessary, the airway is maintained with a modified jaw thrust (the mandible only is moved forward).
3. Place a cervical collar around the neck with no movement of the neck. *Note:* Use of a cervical collar is controversial.
4. Slip a short spine board or extrication device behind the patient. Pad all body prominences (coccyx, thoracic spine, occiput).
5. Secure the patient's torso snugly against the board.
6. Immobilize the patient's head against the board.
7. Instruct a helper to release support of the patient's head.
8. Rotate the patient as a unit, *moving the body with the immobilization device.*
   - Do not use the immobilization device as the sole method of moving the patient because traction and movement of the spine may occur.
9. Lay the patient on a long spine board or on a stretcher.
10. Tighten the straps again, since they will loosen when the patient is supine.
11. Secure the patient to the long spine board or the stretcher. Board and patient may be propped to the side for airway protection and maintenance.
12. Transport the patient gently.

- Signs of neurologic deficit in extremities (paralysis, motor weakness, sensory deficit)
- Local tenderness, deformity, or muscle spasm in the neck
- Unexplained hypotension
- Abdominal breathing without chest expansion

2. Suspect thoracic or lumbar injury with the following:
   - Mechanisms of injury involving blunt or penetrating trauma directly to the spine or forces applied to the spine, such as falls from heights, sports injuries, vehicular accidents, etc.
   - Pain or muscle spasm in thoracic or lumbar regions
   - Neurologic deficit in lower extremities

3. Initial care
   - Monitor and treat any alterations in the patient's ABCs.
   - In maintaining a patent airway, use the modified jaw thrust to protect cervical spine area.

4. Extrication and immobilization of victims
   - Victims with spinal injury are often difficult to get to and to extricate from the place where they are found, rendering appropriate application of spine immobilization devices nearly impossible. In such situations, one skilled rescuer must firmly support the cervical spine and must direct the other rescuers in moving the victim to safety and keeping him in a position for im-

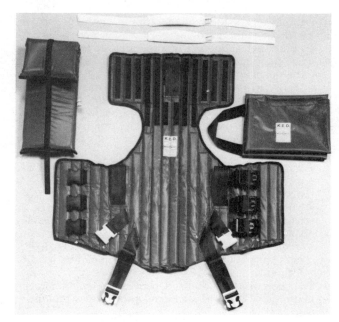

Figure 20-22 *The Kendrick Extrication Device can be used for lifting as well as for cervical spine immobilization. (Courtesy Medi*KED, Inc.)*

Chart 20-3

SUMMARY: CARE OF THE PATIENT WITH KNOWN OR SUSPECTED CERVICAL SPINE INJURY AT THE INCIDENT SCENE*

- Cerivcal spine injury is often associated with injury to the spinal cord.
- The patient should not be moved until he is evaluated for spine and skeletal injury.
- *Stabilize the neck in a neutral position without flexion or extension.* Initially, and until a fixed immobilizing device can be applied, continuous manual support is essential. This can be provided by placing the index fingers against the spinous process of C7 at the base of the neck and the thumbs along the mandible, avoiding compression of the major blood vessels in the neck. The remaining fingers are interlocked to support the occiput and posterior neck while maintaining support of the neck (illustrated in Chart 20-1).
- Ensure an adequate airway and ventilation.
- Immobilize the head and neck using a semirigid cervical collar or similar device.† If the injured person is to be extricated from a vehicle, apply a spine board or an extrication splint (*e.g.,* Kendrick Extrication Device [KED], shown in Fig. 20-22, or Zimmer Extrication Device [ZED])
- After extrication, secure the patient to a long spine board for more complete immobilization before and during transport.
- Continue assessment or resuscitative efforts and prepare the patient for transport.

* Although national minimum standards exist for essential ambulance equipment for spine immobilization, the specific equipment available and the level of expertise of the emergency medical technicians necessarily vary from area to area. As a minimum, an ambulance must carry a cervical collar and spine board. The reader is referred to standard training texts for detailed discussion of immobilization, extrication, and transport techniques.

† The soft cervical collar, the one in most common use, has little or no effect on stabilization of the cervical spine. A semirigid collar (*e.g.,* the Philadelphia collar) provides much better protection by limiting movement of the cervical spine. A semirigid cervical collar is shown in Fig. 20-23.

---

mobilization (Chart 20-1). *Whenever cervical spine injury is suspected, support of the head and neck is essential* prior to *any movement of the patient and throughout the entire immobilization procedure (including after a cervical collar has been applied).*

- This technique is most useful for the victim pinned in a vehicle or for one who is being moved from a stretcher to an x-ray table.
- Whenever the victim is found in a position too difficult to allow for adequate immobilization, providing manual support of the head and neck while moving his body into better alignment is a much safer approach than attempting to immobilize him against a spine board in the position in which he was found.
- If the victim is in water, the rescuer may support the head and neck as illustrated in Fig. 20-21.

5. Spine immobilization devices. Irrespective of the type of device used, the principles of application are standard. These principles are outlined in Chart 20-2. A variety of immobilizing devices are available, for example:

- Wooden short and long boards, scoop stretchers, and patented splints. (Guidelines for applying a short spine-immobilization device are included in Chart 20-2.)
- The Zimmer Extrication Device and the Kendrick Extrication Device (Fig. 20-22) are easily applied cervical spine immobilization devices that are especially useful in the bucket seats of smaller cars. The "KED Sled" is radiopaque and is designed so that it can be used for lifting.

6. Transport the immobilized patient gently, monitoring neurologic and vital signs and providing symptomatic care as necessary.

The principles of care of the patient with known or suspected cervical spine injury at the incident scene are summarized in Chart 20-3.

HOSPITAL CARE

After resuscitation is under way, a lateral x-ray of the cervical spine is taken to identify or rule out cervical spine injury. All seven cervical vertebrae must be visualized on the film before one can ascertain the presence or absence of spinal injury (Fig. 20-24). Experience has shown that failure to visualize the entire cervical spine may lead to an error in diagnosis, mismanagement, and permanent neurologic damage (Fig. 20-25). For a routine lateral cervical spine film, the patient's shoulders should be pulled downward toward the feet to afford a better opportunity to visualize the lowermost cervical vertebrae. If this maneuver is unsuccessful, a lateral Swimmer's view of the lower cervical and upper thoracic area is obtained. Additional x-rays of the cervical spine, including anteroposterior, oblique, and open-mouth odontoid views, can be obtained subsequently. Under no circumstances should the immobilization device(s) be removed from the patient until one is certain that there is no cervical spine damage or until a more permanent form of immobilization is applied.

The thoracic and the lumbar spine are studied by anteroposterior and lateral x-ray films. In the cervical spine, unstable fractures are those with any degree of subluxation, those with separation of the spinous processes, and those involving the pedicle. Patients who have these fractures should be treated with skeletal traction such as Gardner-Wells tongs (Fig. 20-26). Fractures of the thoracic and lumbar spine are treated by immobilization until they can be reduced operatively.

Cervical spine subluxations should be reduced as soon as possible. Reduction is often accomplished by skeletal traction (Gardner-Wells tongs); the procedure should be monitored by serial lateral cervical spine x-ray films. Occasionally a facet joint may be locked; *i.e.,* the inferior facet of the vertebra above is anterior to the superior facet of the vertebra below. If reduction cannot be achieved with traction, an operation to attain the desired alignment may be necessary. A wire and bone fusion of the spine can then be performed conveniently at this time.

Special Considerations

Sacral Sparing. Sacral sparing is a phenomenon that cannot be ignored, because it may serve as an important prog-

Figure 20-23 *Semirigid cervical collar shown in place on patient.*

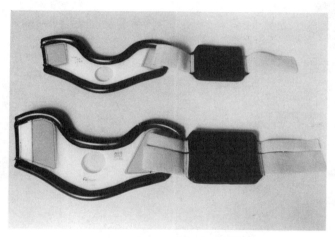

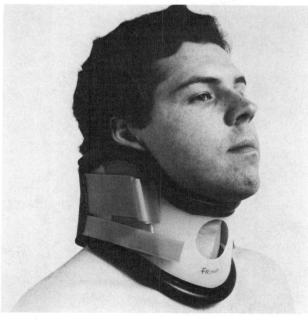

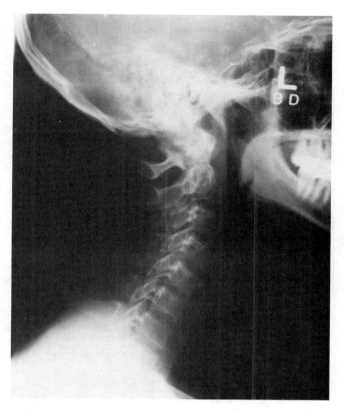

Figure 20-24 *Normal cervical spine; seven cervical vertebrae are shown.*

nostic sign. Sacral sparing indicates that the spinal cord lesion is *incomplete,* and there is a strong chance of functional recovery. This neurologic sign is frequently overlooked in patients with cervical cord injury and serves to indicate that a relatively hopeless situation can be distinguished from a potentially reversible lesion.

Examination for sacral sparing consists of evaluation of anal sphincter tone, perianal skin sensation, and the bulbocavernous reflex. Specifically, anal sphincter tone is checked by digital examination, perianal skin sensation is tested by pinprick stimulation about the anus and observation for the anal wink reflex of the sphincter, and the bulbocavernous reflex is evaluated by squeezing the penis or vulva or pulling on an indwelling catheter and observing for sphincter contraction.

The absence of sacral sparing, especially when spinal shock is present, does not rule out recovery, but when sacral sparing is found, it is a hopeful prognostic sign. When present, it should prompt emergency personnel to take measures to prevent further neurologic damage.

Spinal Shock. Spinal shock refers to the neurologic deficit that occurs immediately after spinal cord injury. Immediately after severe injury to the cord occurs, the following findings are noted distal to the level of injury:

Flaccid paralysis

Flaccid sphincters

Loss of sensation

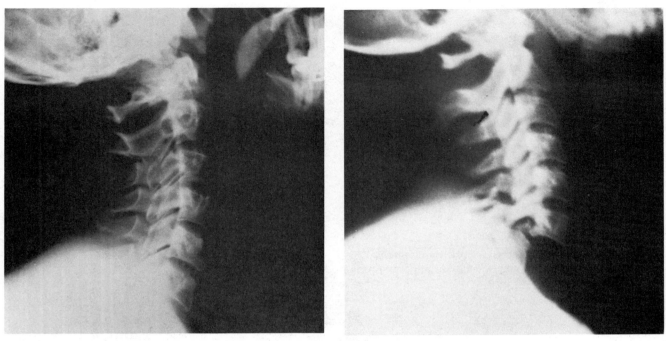

Figure 20-25 Left. Inadequate study of cervical spine; only six cervical vertebrae are shown. Right. Same patient; film shows C6–C7 dislocation.

Figure 20-26 Top. Gardner-Wells tongs used for skeletal traction to stabilize cervical spine injury. Bottom. Gardner-Wells tongs in place. (Courtesy of Dr. W. J. Gardner)

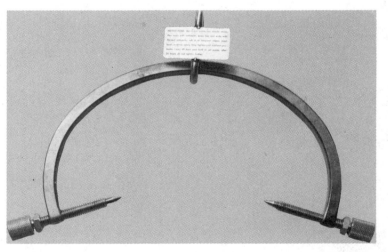

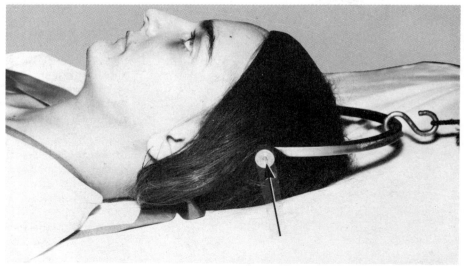

Absent deep-tendon reflexes

Absent pathologic (Babinski) reflexes

Loss of vascular tone

- As a result of blood pooling in the dilated vessels of the viscera, the systolic blood pressure falls to approximately 80 mm Hg and is associated with bradycardia, which helps in distinguishing spinal shock from hypovolemic shock.

- Paralytic ileus may occur along with priapism due to venous engorgement.

- Lack of improvement after 24 hours bodes ill for significant recovery.

- One must be careful to avoid fluid overload in managing a patient with spinal shock.

- The use of vasoconstrictor agents is sometimes of value in increasing vascular tone and raising blood pressure.

Spinal Cord Decompression. Patients whose examinations demonstrate anterior spinal cord syndromes or Brown-Sequard syndromes, should have further studies done after skeletal traction has been instituted and spinal reduction achieved.

- A myelogram (usually performed with a puncture between the first and second cervical vertebrae or a CT scan of the spine) should be performed to exclude the possibility of intraspinal bone fragments or a ruptured disk fragment.

- Both bone and disc should be surgically removed from the spinal canal, usually by anterior decompression.

- Fragments of fractured vertebral bodies posteriorly displaced into the spinal canal in thoracic or lumbar areas can be reduced by a Harrington rod.

- Fragments of bone in the spinal canal are best treated by laminectomy.

- Once the spine has been aligned, the patient is stable in skeletal traction.

- Good nutrition, oxygenation, and intravenous fluid management are conducive to spinal cord recovery, provided the spinal cord has not been irreversibly damaged.

- Dexamethasone, 4 mg q6h, may be of some benefit in promoting spinal cord recovery.

- It is important to realize that patients with spinal cord injuries, especially in the cervical area, have paralysis of the intercostal musculature and must rely on diaphragmatic breathing.

- Thus, it is necessary to institute intermittent positive pressure breathing (IPPB) and frequent changes of position in order to avoid pulmonary complications.

- Patients who have sensory and motor deficits risk pressure sores (decubiti). In order to avoid prolonged pressure on particular areas of skin, especially from the sacrum and hips, patients with spinal cord injuries are usually treated on a circular electric bed or Stryker frame that allows them to be conveniently turned back and forth from supine to prone positions.

- Spine fractures usually become stable with traction and immobilization after 3 months. In some patients it is advisable to begin a rehabilitation program early.

- Operative fusion of an unstable spine fracture is advisable after the patient has stabilized medically in order to begin a rehabilitation program.

INJURY TO THE VERTEBRAE

Injuries to the vertebrae that can result in cord damage are usually caused by acute flexion, as seen in the diving accidents in which the victim strikes his head at the bottom of a shallow depth of water. Similar damage may result from a blocking injury in football when the blocker, in improper position, suffers an acute flexion injury to the neck. This is invariably associated with neck pain and varying alteration in movement and sensation.

CERVICAL SPINE

Palpation of the cervical spinous processes by gentle examination of the posterior midline of the neck may reveal localized tenderness and, sometimes, malalignment. If the spine has been damaged, but no neurologic injury has occurred, the patient must be kept immobile until the extent of injury is determined. Skeletal traction, such as Gardner-Wells tongs, is used to immobilize an unstable injury. This device (shown in Fig. 20-26) is easily applied under local anesthesia, in the emergency department.

THORACIC AND LUMBAR VERTEBRAE

Whereas cervical spine injury is most dramatic because of the associated spinal cord damage and neurologic deficit, the thoracic and lumbar vertebrae are injured more often. Injuries to these vertebrae may occur at any level, but most frequently involve the 12th (last) thoracic and the 1st and 2nd lumbar vertebrae.

The usual mechanism of injury to the thoracic (dorsal) and lumbar vertebrae is acute hyperflexion of the spine as a result of a fall in which the patient lands on his feet or on his buttocks in a sitting position. Because of the sudden deceleration, the weight of the body causes acute flexion of the spine, with compression of the vertebral body. This "wedging" results in a compression fracture (Fig. 20-27), which is most likely to follow a fall from a height or to occur in a patient with bony demineralization (osteoporosis). This type of injury accounts for approximately 60% of all spinal injuries. In the more serious injuries, the vertebral body may actually fragment, so that one vertebra is dislocated onto the adjacent one. In describing dislocations, the process is named according to the uppermost vertebra displaced on the adjacent lower one; *i.e.,* T12–L1 dislocation indicates that the 12th thoracic vertebra is displaced in relation to the first lumbar vertebra.

When a person falls from a height and lands on the feet, great forces are exerted at the point of impact, particularly in the region of the heel. Hence, fractures of the heelbone (os calcis) or lower tibia may be found in association with thoracolumbar spine injury.

OTHER DECELERATION INJURIES

Other deceleration forces may cause vertebral fracture. Lap and shoulder restraints mandated in new cars may be one factor in such injury. With rapid deceleration at impact, the

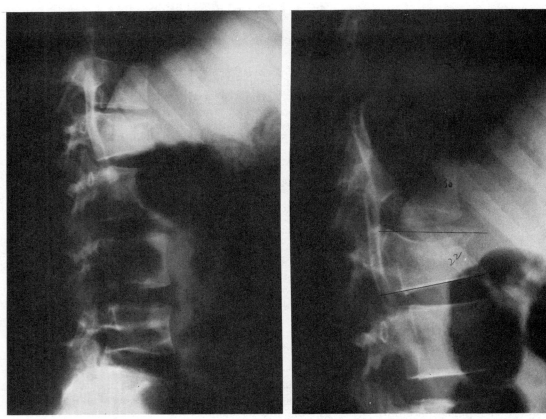

Figure 20-27 *Lumbar vertebra fracture. Left. X-ray shows a compression fracture of the first lumbar vertebra in a patient who fell from a height of three stories, landing on his feet in soft earth. There were no other injuries. Right. In the same patient, spot film shows marked degree of wedging.*

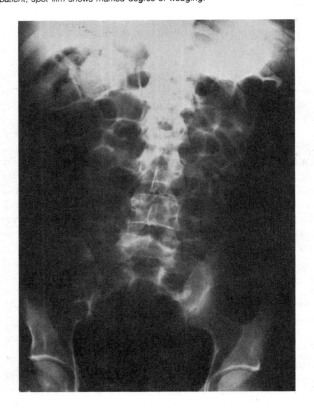

Figure 20-28 *Same patient as in Fig. 20-27. Note large amount of gas scattered throughout both small and large bowel, indicating reflex ileus. The body of the first lumbar segment is narrowed, especially on the right side.*

←

passenger is thrown forward while being restrained by the belt(s), with the result that the upper body may flex sharply over the restraining device, causing a compression fracture. Torsional injury may occur (most likely in the thoracic vertebrae) and is rarely associated with neurologic damage.

Patients with no neurologic injury are admitted to the hospital and treated by bed rest and analgesics until the pain subsides. Abdominal distention due to paralytic ileus may accompany a spinal fracture (Fig. 20-28). Nasogastric intubation and bladder drainage by means of an indwelling catheter are important.

INJURY TO THE PARAVERTEBRAL STRUCTURES

ACCELERATION–DECELERATION INJURY

Whiplash injury is the most common type of injury to the soft tissue structures that surround the cervical vertebrae. It occurs most frequently in an automobile accident, in which the victim is in a vehicle stopped for traffic or at an intersection and is struck in the rear by a second vehicle. Following impact, the first auto is pushed forward and the head and neck of the victim are first extended, then sharply flexed. This extension-flexion injury results in a sprain or strain of the muscular and ligamentous structures that surround the cervical spine. Not uncommonly, but to a lesser extent, the muscles of the lower back are also involved. Symptoms may not occur for 24 hours.

Assessment

Victims of whiplash injury enter the emergency department in varying degrees of distress. Movements of the head, flexion, extension, and lateral flexion and rotation are restricted in all spheres.

- Careful palpation of the neck muscles may reveal spasm of the anterior strap muscles and the trapezius muscles posteriorly.

- Pain and localized tenderness are often present; sensory loss is rare.
- The lower back should be carefully examined to detect injury. The strap muscles of the back (paraspinous musculature) extend the entire length of the vertebral column and can be involved.
- X-rays of the cervical spine are in order to rule out bony injury. The normal lordotic curve of the neck may be absent because of muscle spasm.

Management

Rarely do patients with whiplash injury require admission when this is their only injury. A properly fitted cervical collar combined with analgesics and muscle relaxants is the usual treatment. Physical therapy with ice, followed by range-of-motion and mobilization exercises may help. These patients are often extremely apprehensive and require strong reassurance. The use of a muscle relaxant or tranquilizer such as diazepam (Valium) has been effective in some patients.

REFERENCES

1. Bremer AM et al: Alterations in the distribution of water, sodium, potassium and chloride in brain during the evolution of ischemic cerebral edema. Neurosurgery 3(2):187–195, 1978
2. Becker DP, Miller JD, Ward JD, Greenberg RP, Young HF, Sakalas R: The outcome from severe head injury with early diagnosis and intensive management. J Neurosurg 47(5):491–502, 1977
3. Bricolo A, Turazzi S, Alexandrre A, Rizzuro N: Decerebrate rigidity in acute head injury. J Neurosurg 47(5):681–698, 1977
4. Bronshuag MM: Cellular basis of anoxic ischemic brain injury. West J Med 129(1):8–18, 1978
5. Brown FD, Johns L, Japar JJ, Crockard HA, Mullan S: Detailed monitoring of the effects of mannitol following experimental head injury. J Neurosurg 50(4):423–432, 1979
6. Bruce DA, Raphaely RC, Goldberg AI, Zimmerman PA, Bilaniuk LT, Schut L, Kiehl DE: Pathophysiology, treatment and outcome following severe head injury in children. Childs Brain 5(3):174–191, 1979
7. Bruce DA, Schut L, Bruno LA, Wood JH, Sutton LN: Outcome following severe head injuries in children. J Neurosurg 48(5):679–688, 1978
8. Bruce D, Weeme CT, Ghostine S, Kaiser G: Dynamic studies of the resolution of brain edema. Surg Forum 28:471–474, 1977
9. Caveness WF: Incidence of craniocerebral trauma in the United States in 1976 with trend from 1970 to 1975. Adv Neurol 22:1–3, 1979
10. Cold GE, Jensen FT: Cerebral autoregulation in unconscious patients with brain injury. Acta Anaesthesiol Scand 22(3):270–280, 1978
11. Cold GE: Cerebral metabolic rate of oxygen (CMRO2) in the acute phase of brain injury. Acta Anaesthesiol Scand 22(3):249–256, 1978
12. Cold GE, Jensen FT, Malmros R: The effect of PCO₂ reduction on regional cerebral blood flow in the acute phase of acute brain injury. Acta Anaesthesiol Scand 21(5):359–367, 1977
13. Cooper PR, Moody S, Clark WK, Kirkpatrick J, Maravilla K, Gould AL, Drane W et al: Dexamethasone and severe head injury. J Neurosurg 51(3):307–316
14. Diaz FG, Yock DH, Larson D, Rockswald GL: Early diagnosis of delayed posttraumatic intracerebral hematomas. J Neurosurg 50(2):217–223, 1979
15. Dye OA, Milby JB, Saxon SA: Effects of early neurological problems following head trauma on subsequent neuropsychological performance. Acta Neurol Scand 59(1):10–4, 1979
16. Enevoldsen EM, Jensen FT: Autoregulation and CO₂ responses of cerebral blood flow in patients with acute severe head injury. J Neurosurg 48(5):689–703, 1978
17. Enevoldsen EM, Cold G, Jensen FT, Malmos R: Dynamic changes in regional CBF, intraventricular pressure, CSF pH and lactate levels during the acute phase of head injury. J Neurosurg 44(2):191–214, 1976
18. Enevoldsen EM, Jensen FJ: Cerebrospinal fluid lactate and pH in patients with acute severe head injury. Clin Neurol Neurosurg 80(4):213–225, 1979
19. Fleischer AS, Payne NS, Tindall GT: Continuous monitoring of intracranial pressure in severe closed head injury without mass lesions. Surg Neurol 6:31–34, 1976
20. Frost EA, Arancibia CU, Shulman K et al: Pulmonary shunt as a prognostic indicator in head injury. J Neurosurg 50(6):768–772, 1979
21. Frost EA: Respiratory problems associated with head trauma. Neurosurgery 1(3):300–306, 1977
22. Go KG, Gazendam J, VanZanten AK: Influence of hypoxia on the composition of isolated edema fluid in cold-induced brain edema. J Neurosurg 51(1):78–84, 1979
23. Gilchrist, Wilkinson M: Some factors determining prognosis in young people with severe head injuries. Arch Neurol 36(6):355–359, 1979
24. Graham DI, Adams JH: Ischaemic brain damage in fatal head injuries. Lancet 1:265–266, 1971
25. Graham DI, Adams JH, Doyle D: Ischaemic brain damage in fatal non-missile head injuries. J Neurol Sci 39(2–3):213–234, 1978
26. Grote J, Reulen HJ, Schubert R: Increased tissue water in the brain: Influence on regional cerebral blood flow and oxygen supply. Adv Neurology 20:333–339, 1978
27. Gudeman SK, Miller JD, Becker DP et al: Failure of high-dose steroid therapy to influence intracranial pressure in patients with severe head injury. J Neurosurg 51(3):301–306, 1979
28. Gurdjian ES, Webster JE, Stone NE: Experimental head injury with special reference to certain chemical factors in acute trauma. Surg Gynecol Obstet 78:618–626, 1944
29. Häggendal E, Johansson B: On the pathophysiology of the increased cerebrovascular permeability in acute arterial hypertension in cats. Acta Neurol Scand 48:265–270, 1972
30. Heiskanen O, Sipponen P: Prognosis of severe brain injury. Acta Neurol Scand 46:343–348, 1970

31. Jennett B, Teasdale G, Minderhund J, Heiden J, Kurze T, Brookman R: Prognosis of patients with severe head injury. Neurosurgery 4(4):283–289, 1979

32. Jennett B, Carlin J: Preventable mortality and morbidity after head injury. Injury 10(1):31–39, 1978

33. Jennett B: If my son had a head injury. Br Med J 1(6127):1601–1603, 1978

34. Jennett B, Teasdale G, Galbraith S, Pickard J, Grant H, Braakman R, Avezoot C, Maas A, Minderhaud J, Vecht CJ, Heiden J, Small, R, Caton W, Kurze T: Severe head injuries in three countries. J Neurol Neurosurg Psychiatry 40(3):291–298, 1977

35. Jennett B, Teasdale G, Braakman R, Minderhaud J, Knill-Jones R: Predicting outcome in patients after head injury. Lancet 1:1031–1034, 1976

36. Jennett B, Bond M: Assessment of outcome after severe brain damage: A practical scale. Lancet 1:480–484, 1975

37. Johnston IH, Johnston JS, Jennett B: Intracranial pressure changes following head injury. Lancet 2:433–436, 1970

38. Kalsbeek WD, Hartwell TD: Head and spinal cord injuries: A pilot study of morbidity survey procedures. Am J Public Health 67(11):1051–1057, 1977

39. King LR, McLaurin RL, Knowles HC Jr: Acid-base balance and arterial and CSF lactate levels following human head injury. J Neurosurg 40(5):617–625, 1974

40. Kobrine AI, Timmins E, Rajjoub RK, Rizzoli HV, Davis DO: Demonstration of massive traumatic brain swelling within 20 minutes after injury: Case report. J Neurosurg 46(2):256–258, 1977

41. Langfitt TW: Measuring the outcome from head injuries. J Neurosurg 48(5):673–678, 1978

42. Langfitt TW, Tannenbaum HM, Kassel NF: The etiology of acute brain swelling following experimental head injury. J Neurosurg 24(1):47–56, 1966

43. Levin HS, Grossman RG, Rose JE, Teasdale G: Long-term neuropsychological outcome of closed head injury. J Neurosurg 50(4):412–422, 1979

44. Lewis HP, McLaurin RL: Cerebral blood flow and its responsiveness to arterial pCO_2: Alterations before and after experimental head injury. Surg Forum 23:413–415, 1972

45. Lewis HP, Ramirez R, McLaurin RL: Intracranial blood volume after head injury. Surg Forum 19:433–435, 1968

46. Lundberg N, Troupp H, Lorin H: Continuous recording of the ventricular-fluid pressure in patients with severe acute traumatic brain injury: A preliminary report. J Neurosurg 22(6):581–590, 1965

47. Maas AI: Cerebrospinal fluid enzymes in acute brain injury. 1. Dynamics of changes in CSF enzyme activity after acute experimental brain injury. J Neurol Neurosurg Psychiatry 40(7):655–665, 1977

48. Maas AI: Cerebrospinal fluid enzymes in acute brain injury. 2. Relation of CSF enzyme activity to extent of brain injury. J Neurol Neurosurg Psychiatry 40(4):666–674, 1977

49. Maas AI: Cerebrospinal fluid enzymes in acute brain injury. 3. Effect of hypotension on increase of CSF enzyme activity after cold injury in cats. J Neurol Neurosurg Psychiatry 40(9):896–900, 1977

50. Marshall LF, Smith RW, Shapiro HM: The outcome with aggressive treatment in severe head injuries: I. The significance of intracranial pressure monitoring. J Neurosurg 50(1):20–25, 1979

51. Marshall LF, Smith RW, Shapiro HM: The outcome with aggressive treatment in severe head injuries. II. Acute and chronic barbiturate administration in the management of head injury. J Neurosurg 50(1):26–30, 1979

52. Marshall LF, Smith RW, Rouscher LA, Shapiro HM: Mannitol dose requirements in brain injured patients. J Neurosurg 48(2):169–172, 1978

53. Marshall WJ, Jackson JLF, Langfitt TW: Brain swelling caused by trauma and arterial hypertension: Hemodynamic aspects. Arch Neurol 21:543–553, 1969

54. Meyer JS, Kondo A, Nomura F, Sakamots T, Teraura T: Cerebral hemodynamics and metabolism following experimental head injury. J Neurosurg 32(3):304–319, 1970

55. Miller JD, Sweet RC, Narayan R, Becker DP: Early insults to the injured brain. JAMA 240(5):439–442, 1978

56. Miller JD, Becker DP, Ward JD, Sullivan HG, Adams WE, Rosner MJ: Significance of intracranial hypertension in severe head injury. J Neurosurg 47(4):503–516, 1977

57. Mchedlishki G, Nikolaishvili L, Itkis M: Pathophysiological mechanisms of brain edema development: Role of tissue factors. Stroke 10(1):52–57, 1979

58. Nilsson B, Ponten U: Experimental head injury in the rat. 2. Regional brain energy metabolism in concurrive traumas. J Neurosurgery 47(2):252–261, 1977

59. Nilsson L, Siesjö BK: The effect of phenobarbitone anesthesia on blood flow and oxygen consumption in the rat brain. Acta Anaesth Scand Suppl 57:18–24, 1975

60. Nyáry I, Pásztor E: Reactivity of the cerebral vascular bed to CO_2 in patients with head injury. Adv Neurology 20:517–520, 1978

61. Obrist WD, Gennarelli TA, Segawa H, Dolinskies CA, Langfitt TW: Relation of cerebral blood flow to neurological status and outcome in head-injured patients. J Neurosurg 51(3):292–300, 1979

62. Oppenheimer DR: Microscopic lesions in the brain following head injury. J Neurol Neurosurg Psychiatry 31(4):299–306, 1968

63. Overgaard J, Christensen S, Hvid-Hansen O, Hoose J, Land AM, Hein O, Pedersen KK, Tweed WA: Prognosis after head injury based on early clinical examinations. Lancet 2:631–635, 1973

64. Palmer MA, Perry JF Jr, Fischer RP, Murray KJ: Intracranial pressure monitoring in the acute neurologic assessment of multi-injured patients. J Trauma 19(7):497–506, 1979

65. Piistolese GR, Faraglia V, Agnoli A et al: Cerebral hemispheric "counter-steal" phenomenon during hyperventilation in cerebrovascular diseases. Stroke 3:456–461, 1972

66. Plum F, Posner JB: The diagnosis of stupor and coma. Contemp Neurol Surgery 10:1–286, 1972

67. Rao CJ, Shukla PK, Mohanty S, Reddy YJV: Predictive value of serum lactate dehydrogenace in head injury. J Neurol Neurosurg Psychiatry 41(10):948–953, 1978

68. Saunders ML, Miller JD, Stablein D, Allen G: The effects of graded experimental trauma on cerebral blood flow and responsiveness to CO_2. J Neurosurg 51(1):18–26, 1979

69. Smith DR, Ducker TB, Kempe LG: Experimental in vivo microcirculatory dynamics in brain trauma. J Neurosurg 30(6):664–672, 1969

70. Snoek J, Jennett B, Adams JH, Graham DI, Doyle D: Computerized tomography after recent severe head injury in patients without acute intracranial hematoma. J Neurol Neurosurg Psychiatry 42(3):215–225, 1979

71. Strich SJ: Shearing of nerve fibers as a cause of brain damage due to head injury: A pathological study of 20 cases. Lancet 55:481–505, 1968

72. Teasdale G, Murray G, Parker L, Jennett B: Adding up the Glasgow Coma Scale. Acta Neurochir (Wien) 1979:1(Suppl):28 13–16

73. Teasdale G, Knill-Jones R, VanDerSande J: Observer variability in assessing impaired consciousness and coma. J Neurol Neurosurg Psychiatry 41(7):603–610, 1978

74. Waga S, Tochio H, Sakakura M: Traumatic cerebral swelling developing within 30 minutes after injury. Surg Neurol 11(3):191–193, 1979

75. Walker AE, Kollros JJ, Case TJ: The physiological basis of concussion. J Neurosurg 1(2):103–116, 1944

76. Yen K, Rhodes GR, Baurke RS, Powers SR, Newell JC, Popp AJ: Delayed impairment of arterial blood oxygenation in patients with severe head injury: Preliminary report. Surg Neurol 9(5):323–327, 1978

77. Zupping R: Cerebral acid-base and gas metabolism in brain injury. J Neurosurg 33(5):498–505, 1970

BIBLIOGRAPHY

NECK INJURIES

Ashworth C, Williams LF, Byrne JJ: Penetrating wounds of the neck. Am J Surg 121:387, 1971

Byrne JJ: Neck injuries. Hosp Med 40–53.

Dodson T, Quindlen E, Crowell R, McEnancy MT: Vertebral arteriovenous fistulas following insertion of central monitoring catheters. Surgery 87:343–346, 1980

Flint LM, Snyder WH, Perry MD, Shires GT: Management of major vascular injuries in the base of the neck. Arch Surg 106:407, 1973

Jones RF: Immediate management of penetrating wounds of the neck. Hosp Med 84–92

Lambert GE, McMurry GT: Laryngotracheal trauma: Recognition and management. JACEP 5:883–886, 1974

Meinke AH, Bivins BA, Sachatello CR: Selective management of gunshot wounds to the neck. 138:314–319, 1979

O'Donnell VA, Atik M, Pick RA: Evaluation and management of penetrating wounds of the neck: The role of emergency angiography. Am J Surg 38:309–14, 1979

Penn I: Penetrating injuries of the neck. Surg Clin North Am 53:1469, 1978

Rich NM et al: Traumatic arteriovenous fistulas and late aneurysms: A review of 558 lesions. Surgery 78:817–28, 1975

Rich NM: Missile injuries, Am J Surg 139:414–420, 1980

Sheely CH II, Mattox KL, Beall AC Jr: Management of acute cervical tracheal trauma. Am J Surg 128:805–808, 1974

Sheeley CH IV, Mattox KL, Raul JJ, Beall AC Jr, DeBakey ME: Current concepts in the management of penetrating neck trauma. J Trauma 15:875, 1975

Sher MH: Arteriovenous fistula involving the vertebral artery: Report of three cases. Ann Surg 164:408–13, 1966

INJURIES TO THE VERTEBRAE AND SPINAL CORD

Cloward RB: Treatment of acute fractures and fracture-dislocations of the cervical spine by vertebral body fusion. J Neurosurg 18:201, 1961

Committee on Trauma, American College of Surgeons: Techniques of Helmet Removal from Injured Patients. Bull Am Coll Surg 64:19–21, 1980

Crutchfield WG: Further observations on the treatment of fracture-dislocations of the cervical spine with skeletal traction. Surg Gynecol Obstet 63:513, 1936

Gardner WJ: The principle of spring-loaded points for cervical traction. J Neurosurg 39:543, 1973

Schneider RC: The syndrome of acute anterior cervical spinal cord injury. J Neurosurg 12:95, 1955

Schneider RC: Trauma to the Spine and Spinal Cord: Correlative Neurosurgery. Chap 26, pp 597–648. Springfield, Ill, Charles C Thomas, 1969

Taylor AR: The mechanism of injury to the spinal cord and neck without damage to the vertebral column. J Bone Joint Surg 33-B:543–547, 1951

APPENDIX C

TECHNIQUES OF HELMET REMOVAL FROM INJURED PATIENTS

Victims of trauma to the head, neck, and spine who were wearing a protective helmet at the time can cause confusion for the examining physician or emergency-care technician. In this case the classic findings of face and head injuries, which indicate the need for cervical spine protection, may not exist if the helmet has protected the face and head from such injuries. Therefore, the helmet should be examined for abrasions or other signs of trauma. If they exist, the patient should be treated as if he had a cervical-spine fracture until lateral x-rays rule it out.

The physician, nurse, and emergency-care personnel should understand the mechanisms of helmet removal in order to preserve an open airway, adequately stabilize the head to the short or long backboard, provide in-line traction for moving a patient from automobile to gurney or from gurney to x-ray table, or place Crutchfield or Gardner-Wells tongs. Helmets are easily removed if one understands how they are built and how they conform to the shape of the head. If not, helmet removal can be very frustrating. Inappropriate actions can damage the cervical cord when the overlying bony structure has been fractured.

For these reasons the Committee on Trauma has developed the helmet poster shown in Fig. 20-29.

Types of Helmets

Full face coverage— motorcycle, auto racer

Full face coverage— motocross

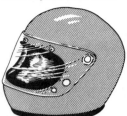 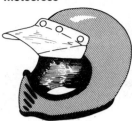

Helmet Removal

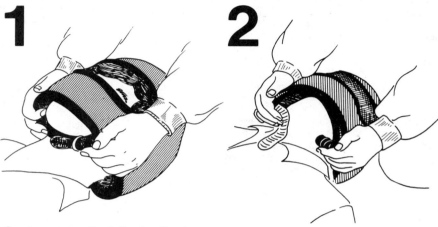

1 One rescuer applies inline traction by placing his or her hands on each side of the helmet with the fingers on the victim's mandible. This position prevents slippage if the strap is loose.

2 The rescuer cuts or loosens the strap at the D-rings while maintaining inline traction.

The varying sizes, shapes, and configurations of motorcycle helmets necessitate some understanding of their proper removal from victims of motorcycle accidents. The rescuer who removes a helmet improperly might inadvertently aggravate cervical spine injuries.

The Committee on Trauma believes that physicians who treat the injured should be aware of helmet removal techniques. A gradual increase in the use of helmets is anticipated because many organizations are urging voluntary wearing of helmets, and some states are reinstating their laws requiring the wearing of helmets.

American College of Surgeons
Committee on Trauma
July 1980

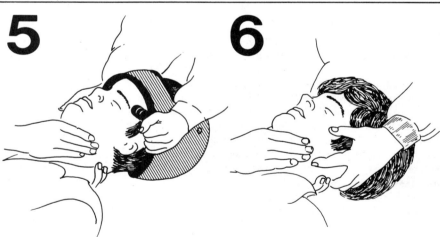

5 Throughout the removal process, the second rescuer maintains inline traction from below in order to prevent head tilt.

6 After the helmet has been removed, the rescuer at the top replaces his hands on either side of the victim's head with his palms over the ears.

Figure 20-29 *Techniques of helmet removal from injured patients. (Reproduced with permission of Committee on Trauma, American College of Surgeons)*

**Partial face coverage—
motorcycle, auto racer**

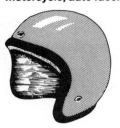

**Light head protection—
bicycle, kayak**

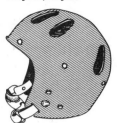

Football

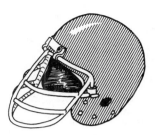

3

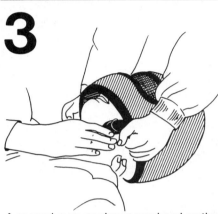

A second rescuer places one hand on the mandible at the angle, the thumb on one side, the long and index fingers on the other. With his other hand, he applies pressure from the occipital region. This maneuver transfers the inline traction responsibility to the second rescuer.

4

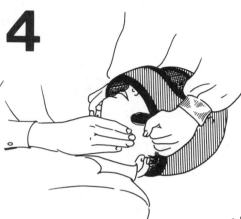

The rescuer at the top removes the helmet. Three factors should be kept in mind:

• The helmet is egg-shaped, and therefore must be expanded laterally to clear the ears.

• If the helmet provides full facial coverage, glasses must be removed first.

• If the helmet provides full facial coverage, the nose will impede removal. To clear the nose, the helmet must be tilted backward and raised over it.

Summary

The helmet must be maneuvered over the nose and ears while the head and neck are held rigid.

• Inline traction is applied from above.

• Inline traction is transferred below with pressure on the jaw and occiput.

• The helmet is removed.

• Inline traction is re-established from above.

7

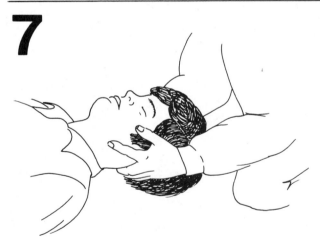

Inline traction is maintained from above until a backboard is in place.

21
THORACIC AND ABDOMINAL INJURIES

JAMES H. COSGRIFF, JR. and DIANN ANDERSON

The incidence of injury and death from accidental causes remains alarmingly high. In 1982 there were more than 175,000 trauma related deaths and many more such injuries. Injuries to the thoracic and abdominal viscera contributed significantly to these numbers and are directly responsible for over 25% of automobile fatalities each year. Mortality related to thoracic or abdominal trauma may be due directly to the severity of injury and thus is inevitable, but in other instances, death may be due to failure to recognize the injury, delays in initiating treatment, or errors in judgment with respect to appropriate management of the patient.

THORACIC INJURIES

Thoracic trauma, in particular, may cause profound disturbances of cardiopulmonary function, which require urgent, decisive therapeutic measures. Often, the treatment needed is not difficult once the correct diagnosis is made.

A patient who has received a severe chest injury should not be considered to be "doing well" until the following criteria, suggested by Scannell, have been met.

1. Resuscitation is taken to the point at which significant hypotension and hypoxia have been relieved.
2. Bleeding is identified and controlled.
3. Severe pain is relieved.
4. Stability of the chest wall is established so that effective cough and ventilation are possible, and a clear airway is established.
5. Pleural cavities are free of any significant blood and air, and the possibility of continuing or recurring pneumothorax is cared for with as complete expansion as possible of both lungs.
6. Recognition is made of any associated visceral injury.
7. Care of any major external wounds is completed.

INITIAL ASSESSMENT AND TREATMENT

Diagnosis and treatment proceed concurrently while a continuing assessment of the situation is being made. As in any injured patient, first attention must be given to establishing a patent airway. This may be merely a matter of adjusting the position of the patient, or may involve using the standard maneuvers of head-tilt, jaw-thrust, or jaw-pull (see Chap. 14, Resuscitation: Principles and Techniques). Noisy or labored respirations indicate respiratory embarrassment. Aspiration of oral and pharyngeal secretions or removal of loosened dentures or foreign bodies in the mouth or throat may be all that is needed. A compromised airway may be due either to aspiration of blood or vomitus or directly to the injury itself.

Note: Failure to recognize a compromised airway and delay in initiating therapeutic measures can contribute to hypoxia and hypotension. This pertains to any phase of the patient's care, whether at the scene of the accident, in transport, or in the hospital emergency department.

In a trauma patient with severe respiratory distress marked by labored breathing, cyanosis, and hypotension, rapid but careful assessment may reveal a tracheal shift that indicates tension pneumothorax requiring immediate insertion of a needle into the thoracic cavity to release the increased intrapleural pressure. This simple maneuver, which can be accomplished by an adequately trained EMT can cause a dramatic reversal of the patient's respiratory distress. Similarly, sucking wounds of the chest, obviously more easily recognized, should be sealed as soon as poossible to restore respiratory mechanics to a more normal state. Flail segments of the chest wall should be immobilized.

Whatever the cause, careful inspection of the chest, with frequent evaluation of respiratory activity and recording of the details, is essential to good, orderly care. Once the emergent problems are attended to, a complete examination can be carried out and appropriate tests ordered, as indicated. Generally, chest and abdominal x-rays should be delayed until emergency resuscitative measures have been initiated and the patient stabilized. If such studies are deemed absolutely necessary for the patient, a nurse or physician should accompany the patient to the x-ray department to monitor the patient's condition, initiate additional emergency measures as needed, and prevent unnecessary delays on the part of x-ray personnel.

Depending on the nature and extent of the injury, a number of parameters should be monitored. These include arterial blood gases, electrocardiogram (ECG), arterial blood pressure, central venous pressure (CVP), hourly urine output, pulse, and respiration. In some centers, patients with severe injuries are taken directly to the operating room for resuscitation, study, and definitive care.

PHYSIOLOGY OF RESPIRATION

The primary object of respiration is to supply oxygen to the blood and tissues and eliminate carbon dioxide. Basically, a functional respiratory system is composed of a complex of pipes and pumps. The pipes are the blood vessels and airway passages that carry blood and air, respectively, through the system. There are two pumps: (1) the heart, which moves blood through the blood vessels (perfusion pipes), and (2) the chest bellows, which moves air in and out of the air passages (the ventilation pipes). Any interference with this basic pump and pipe system may cause varying degrees of compromise to the entire integrated system.

Generally speaking, respiration is referred to as *external* (the mass movement of air—gases—in and out of the lungs to the arterial blood) and *internal* (the exchange of gases between the blood and the tissue at the arteriolocapillary and tissue cell level).

The exchange of gases (ventilation), primarily oxygen (O_2) and carbon dioxide (CO_2), from the atmosphere to the alveoli takes place because of the pressure gradient that exists between atmosphere and alveolar air (Table 21-1).

Similarly, at the tissue level, gas exchange takes place

TABLE 21-1. GAS PARTIAL PRESSURES IN MM HG AT SEA LEVEL

	Dry Air	Tracheal Air	Alveolar Air	Arterial Blood	Tissue Cells	Venous Blood
O_2	159.0	149.0	100	95–100	40	40
CO_2	0.3	0.3	40	40	46	46
H_2O	0.0	47.0	47	47	47	47
N_2	600.7	563.7	573	578–573	573	573
Total	760.0	760.0	760	760	706	706

(Harper, RW: A Guide to Respiratory Care. Philadelphia, JB Lippincott, 1981)

because of the pressure gradient of the gases existing between the arteriolocapillary blood and the cells.

In normal respiration, air is drawn from the atmosphere into the lungs on inspiration through the bronchial system into the alveoli. Inspiration is an active movement caused by contraction of the muscles of the chest wall with elevation of the rib cage and a downward movement (descent) of the diaphragm, similar to the action of a bellows. Expiration, for the most part, is a passive action resulting from the natural recoil or elasticity of the lungs. The lungs are enclosed in the pleural cavities, a closed space. The pressure in the pleural cavity is usually less than, or negative in relation to, atmospheric pressure. This allows the lungs to remain expanded. The intrapleural pressure varies with the phase of respiration, being *more* negative at the end of inspiration and *less* negative at the end of expiration. Airflow in the bronchial system is determined by the magnitude of respiratory movements and the cross-sectional area of the air passages that influences resistance and flow rate.

Injuries to any component of the system, the chest wall, the lungs, pleura, or heart may thus cause alterations that can interfere with the exchange of atmosphere and alveolar gas and with internal respiration as well. For example, pain secondary to a simple rib fracture can restrict chest wall movement and therefore affect ventilation adversely. Multiple rib fractures producing a flail chest can impair respiratory mechanics to the extent that air exchange is limited, depending on the size of the flail segment and the extent of the paradoxical motion. Pneumothorax and tension pneumothorax may be major factors in compromising ventilation and perfusion. Injuries to the lung itself, causing contusion or hematoma, may also interfere with both airflow and alveolar exchange.

Clearly, the fundamentals of treatment of thoracic injuries require one to recognize the pathophysiologic process and restore the respiratory mechanics to a normal state. Important points in the management of a patient with thoracic injury are listed in Chart 21-1.

CLASSIFICATION OF THORACIC INJURIES

Injuries to the chest may be classified in several ways. One such classification divides them into penetrating and nonpenetrating traumas. Perhaps a more functional classification of such injuries relates to structural damage, as follows. This classification system includes injuries to the chest wall, injuries to the intrathoracic viscera, and combined thoracoabdominal injury.

CHEST WALL INJURIES

FRACTURES OF THE RIB CAGE

Fracture of one or more ribs is the most common injury to the chest due to blunt trauma. It is much more common in an adult. The ribs and cartilages in children are much more resilent and thus less likely to break. Rib fracture usually results from direct trauma; however, on occasion, severe coughing may be the causative factor.

Anatomically, the rib cage consists of twelve pairs of bony ribs, attached posteriorly to the articular processes of the thoracic vertebrae and anteriorly by way of intervening costal cartilages to the breastplate or sternum.

Fractures of one or more ribs may greatly interfere with ventilation because of the pain produced by the motion of the chest wall during respiration. Pain and resultant spasm of the thoracic musculature may restrict excursion of the chest wall and make coughing weak and inefficient and thus limit pulmonary exchange. The number of ribs fractured in most instances is directly related to the severity of the trauma. A single rib fracture may be relatively innocuous and require

---

Chart 21-1

KEY POINTS IN THE CARE OF A PATIENT WITH THORACIC INJURY

- Establish and maintain an adequate airway.
- Maintain adequate ventilation, relieve hypoxia.
- Identify and control bleeding.
- Maintain adequate circulating volume, relieve hypotension.
- Stabilize the chest wall when necessary.
- Identify associated organ-system injury.
- Relieve pain.

only relief of pain. In other instances, one or more rib fractures may cause damage to the underlying pleura or lung with serious and sometimes fatal complications. Generally, the greater the number of ribs fractured, the higher will be the incidence of damage to the intrathoracic viscera.

Simple Rib Fracture

Assessment. Careful assessment of the chest by palpation usually localizes the fracture site. Since standard chest x-ray studies may not demonstrate the fracture, a "rib study" should be ordered.

Once the diagnosis is established, the patient should be carefully evaluated for respiratory activity. In an elderly patient or one with chronic pulmonary disease, a single rib fracture may cause severe respiratory embarrassment.

Treatment. Treatment of simple fracture of the rib cage without accompanying pulmonary or pleural injury is directed toward pain relief.
- For many years, adhesive strapping of the rib cage was the method of choice. It is mentioned here only to be condemned. Experience has demonstrated that such strapping decreases respiratory excursion and may lead to progressive atelectasis. Other unpleasant side-effects include skin irritation and blistering from the tape and inability to adjust the binding once applied.
- Elastic rib-belts are available and serve admirably to reduce chest-wall movement and thus lessen pain.
- Mild to moderate chest wall pain may be adequately managed with codeine sulfate in a dosage of 0.030 to 0.060 gm every 3 to 4 hours in conjunction with an analgesic compound such as aspirin, phenacetin, and caffeine (APC) tablets.
- More severe pain is best controlled by intercostal nerve blocks using lidocaine or bupivacaine HCl (Marcaine). The nerve block should be done at the lower margin of the rib, central or proximal to the fracture. Two interspaces above and below the involved rib(s) should be injected for better results. An intercostal nerve block often produces dramatic relief from pain that may last for many hours. If necessary, blocks may be repeated as indicated.
- Since it is easy to puncture the pleura or lung during the course of an intercostal block, an upright chest x-ray should be obtained after the procedure to be sure that pneumothorax has not been produced.
- With pain relief and improved respiratory excursions, motion of the rib at the fracture site may puncture the lung or pleura, causing delayed pneumothorax.
- Rib fractures generally heal in 3 to 6 weeks.

Fractures of the First and Second Ribs

Most rib fractures occur in the middle or lower portions of the rib cage. Fractures of the first and second ribs are rare, primarily because of their guarded location beneath the heavy musculature of the upper chest and back. Isolated fractures of these ribs frequently portend a more serious injury of the thoracic viscera, particularly the thoracic aorta or major bronchi, and are associated with a much higher mortality rate.

Costochondral Fractures

Fractures of the cartilaginous portions of the ribs, the area on the anterior chest wall connecting the bony part of the rib to the sternum, are less common but often more painful and more difficult to manage. These fractures are referred to as costochondral or chondrosternal fractures.

Assessment. Costochondral fractures usually result from direct trauma to the costal cartilage. Palpation usually localizes the site of injury. Delineation of these fractures by x-ray is practically impossible, since the cartilages are not visualized. Because of the relatively poor blood supply to a costal cartilage, healing is frequently delayed and the rate of nonunion is high.

Management/Treatment. Initially, management of a cartilaginous fracture is the same as that for simple rib fracture. In chronic cases with persistent localized pain and tenderness indicating nonunion, excision of the cartilaginous fragments is curative.

COMPLICATIONS OF RIB FRACTURE

Pneumothorax

Single or multiple rib fractures are not usually associated with displacement. On occasion, however, there may be some displacement of the fracture fragments, and under such circumstances a sharp spicule of bone may lacerate the pleura or the lung itself. As described above, it may also occur after intercostal nerve block. As a result, some degree of pneumothorax may develop. Crepitus (subcutaneous emphysema, or air in the tissues) may be palpated at the fracture site and careful examination of the chest by auscultation will reveal signs of a pneumothorax. An upright x-ray will confirm the diagnosis (see Fig. 21-1).

The clinical signs of pneumothorax may be summarized as follows:
- Diminished or absent breath sounds on auscultation
- Diminished vocal fremitus
- Diminished tactile fremitus
- Respiratory distress (not constant)
- Hyperresonant percussion noted on involved side
- Tracheal shift to opposite side (not constant)

Pneumothorax may vary in extent from partial to full collapse of the lung on the involved side and is described by the radiologist as a percentage of collapse. For example, Fig. 21-1 depicts a 90% to 95% right pneumothorax.

Tension Pneumothorax

Tension pneumothorax is a serious problem that usually results from a small tear in the lung produced by a spicule of rib fracture (Fig. 21-2). On inspiration, air is lost into the

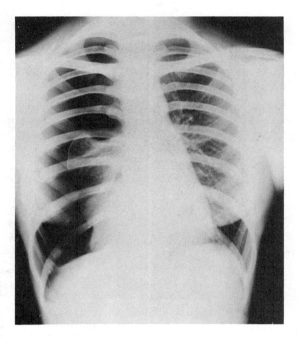

Figure 21-1 *Pneumothorax. Total collapse of right lung is shown. Note the mediastinal structures shifted to the left. Patient was treated by intercostal tube drainage (closed thoracostomy), with full reexpansion.*

Assessment. Dyspnea occurs quickly. Tracheal shift is easily detectable in the suprasternal notch. The involved side is hyperresonant to percussion and there is a considerable loss of chest wall excursion.

Treatment. Immediate treatment is called for and consists simply of inserting a needle in the 2nd and 3rd intercostal space in the midclavicular line anteriorly. When the pleural cavity is entered, there is an audible escape of air from the needle as the pressure is relieved. The patient's respiratory status improves immediately. Any delay by consultation or in obtaining x-rays cannot be countenanced in this emergency, since it may result in fatality.

A simple flutter valve can be devised by attaching a finger cot to the needle (Fig. 21-3), a McSwain dart or a Heimlich valve may be used (Fig. 21-4), or a trap can be established by connecting the needle to an underwater seal, such as a Pleur-Evac (Fig. 21-5). Once a temporary device has been established as a life-saving measure, a more permanent intercostal catheter is inserted and connected to the Pleur-Evac (see Fig. 21-5). In some patients, a thoracic suction pump is needed to better evacuate the air and allow the lung to reexpand.

Emergency management of the patient with tension pneumothorax is summarized in Chart 21-2.

pleural space and trapped. As the amount of intrapleural air increases, the lung collapses. As this increases further, the mediastinum shifts to the opposite side. This results in complete loss of function of the involved side with severe compromise of the contralateral lung. Venous return to the heart is decreased by the shift of mediastinal structures. Cardiac function is diminished and hypotension follows.

Hemothorax

Another common complication of rib fracture is hemothorax, bleeding into the pleural space. It is a result of a laceration of the intercostal vessels that are near the inferior margin of each rib. The degree of hemothorax varies with the number of ribs fractured (Fig. 21-6). Bleeding may also be due to injury to the lung itself.

Figure 21-2 *Left. Tension pneumothorax, right. Note massive collapse of right lung and shift of mediastinum and heart to left. Right. Tension pneumothorax following insertion of chest tube. Note reexpansion of lung.*

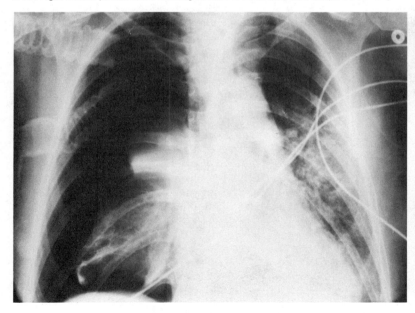
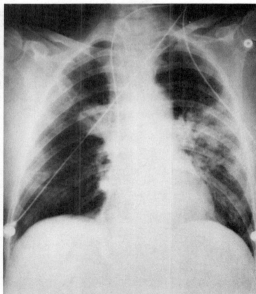

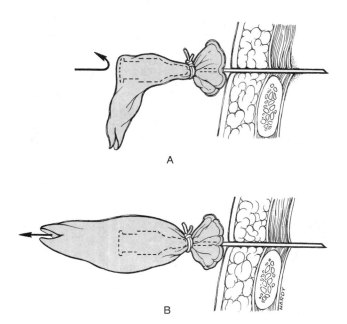

A

B

Figure 21-3 *A simple device for emergency decompression of pneumothorax. A short bevel needle is inserted into an upper anterior intercostal space, just above the upper border of a rib. A finger cot or finger from a surgical glove with a hole in the tip is tied securely to the hub of the needle. A. On inspiration, the finger cot collapses and allows no air into the pleural cavity. B. On expiration, air is forced through the open end of the finger cot.*

The presence of fluid in the chest may be determined by physical assessment and confirmed by an upright chest x-ray. Needle aspiration in a lower intercostal space will confirm the presence of blood, which calls for evacuation of both air and blood from the pleural cavity until the lung is completely reexpanded to fill the pleural space. This can sometimes be accomplished by thoracentesis using a large-bore needle or may require intercostal drainage by means of a closed thoracostomy with underwater seal.

If bleeding into the pleural space recurs or continues in spite of thoracentesis, as indicated by falling blood pressure or rising pulse, emergency thoracotomy should be performed. The usual site of blood loss in such an instance is a torn intercostal artery.

For patients with single or multiple rib fractures in the lower chest, bear in mind the possibility of trauma to upper abdominal viscera lying immediately adjacent to the ribs, namely, the liver, spleen, and kidney. Such injuries are discussed in detail later in this chapter.

Flail Chest

If the stability of the chest wall remains intact, a number of ribs can be fractured without causing serious impairment of pulmonary exchange. When segmental fractures (fracture

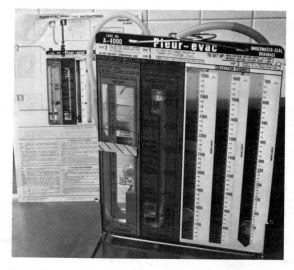

Figure 21-5 *Pleur-evac disposable chest drainage system. (Deknatel Corp.) (Respiratory Care: Concepts and Techniques, an audiovisual publication of JB Lippincott, 1980)*

in two or more sites on the same rib) of three or more adjacent ribs occur, the chest wall becomes unstable, and abnormal excursion of the ribs causing respiratory compromise may result, depending upon the size of the flail segment of chest wall. This is particularly true when the injury is bilateral. Crushing injuries are more likely to lead to flail chest.

Assessment. Flail chest is characterized by an inward movement of the chest wall on inspiration. This is referred to as *paradoxical* motion. As a sequela, ventilatory efficiency is reduced and ventilatory work is increased. This, combined with underlying lung damage, is likely to cause progressive respiratory insufficiency (Fig. 21-7), especially with a large flail segment. Early indications of respiratory embarrassment are dyspnea and cyanosis. Arterial blood gases demonstrate hypercarbia (increased CO_2) and hypoxia (decreased O_2).

In addition to paradoxical motion of the chest wall, air in the bronchi may be moved from the injured side to the contralateral side in a *pendulum* movement. The mediastinum may also shift to the side opposite the injury with each inspiration, causing pressure and diminished ventilation in the uninjured lung and adding further to deranged physiology.

Treatment. Treatment consists of stabilizing the involved segment of chest wall. The easiest method is to hold it in the collapsed position by external pressure. A sandbag serves the purpose well. This is particularly useful at the scene of injury and should be continued until the patient reaches the hospital and even then, until more definitive stabilization

Figure 21-4 *Heimlich valve.*

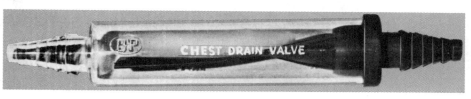

Chart 21-2

MANAGEMENT OF THE PATIENT WITH TENSION PNEUMOTHORAX

Assessment

CLINICAL SIGNS

- Absent breath sounds on auscultation
- Severe respiratory distress
- Hyperresonant percussion note
- Hypotension
- Contralateral tracheal deviation
- Distended neck veins

Emergency Management

- This is an urgent situation. Do not delay for consultation or x-rays.
- Insert large-bore, 16- to 18-gauge needle in 2nd or 3rd anterior intercostal space.
- Attach a temporary flutter-valve device or a Heimlich valve; prepare to establish more permanent chest drainage.
- Insert intercostal catheter and connect to a Pleur-Evac.
- A thoracic suction pump may be needed for some patients in order to assist in evacuating air and reexpanding lung.

can be achieved. When the flail segment is on the posterior aspect of the chest wall, the weight of the patient lying on his back may be sufficient to stabilize the chest wall. Although the use of external pressure may reduce vital capacity, it increases the effective tidal volume and the efficiency of ventilation.

Although stability has been maintained by using external traction, internal fixation as suggested by Avery *et al.* is the

Figure 21-6 Hemothorax. Left. *Hemothorax developed following a simple fracture of the eighth left rib.* Right. *X-ray shows improvement 3 months later, after intercostal tube drainage.*

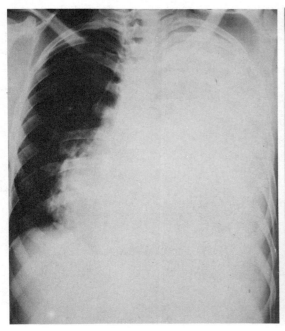
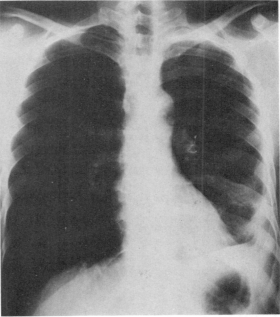

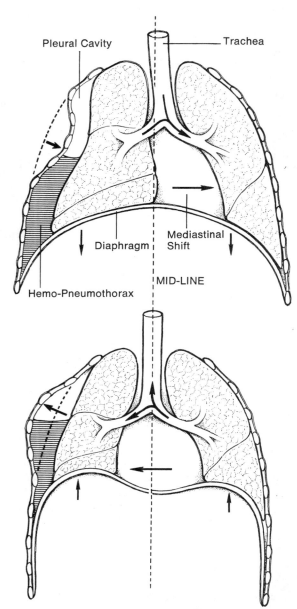

Figure 21-7 *Respiration in a flail chest. Diagram on top shows flail area of right chest wall, which moves in with inspiration. Air moves into the left (normal) lung from the right bronchial tree as well as by normal tracheal inflow. Ventilation of the right lung is compromised. The mediastinum shifts to the uninjured side. On expiration (bottom), air is driven out through the trachea and into the right (injured) side. This movement of air from one lung to the other is known as "pendulum movement," which leads to further deoxygenation. Hemopneumothorax further compromises oxygen exchange.*

most effective method.[2] Immediate tracheostomy or cricothyroidostomy combined with use of a volume-cycled mechanical ventilator is the method of choice. It serves to splint the chest wall internally and maintain optimal lung expansion. To a certain extent, the tracheostomy or cricothyroidostomy in itself will reduce the paradoxical motion by bypassing the upper airway, thus decreasing dead space and lessening respiratory effort. Fig. 21-8 shows the result of such treatment.

Ventilatory Assistance. Ventilatory assistance is deemed necessary if one or more of the following conditions is present: shock, three or more associated injuries, severe head injury, fracture of eight or more ribs, age greater than 65, and previous pulmonary disease (see Chart 21-3).

Continuous monitoring of the patient is necessary. Frequent periodic aspirations of the tracheal tube are needed, care being taken to maintain aseptic technique during the procedure. Ventilatory support is continued until stabilization of the chest wall has occurred and may extend over a 7- to 14-day period. The effectiveness of the therapy can be monitored by periodic arterial blood gas analyses. It has been shown by Nealon *et al.* that the pCO_2 is a more reliable index of when assisted ventilation can be discontinued.[18] Prophylactic ventilatory assistance in patients with flail chest complicating other injuries resulted in a significant reduction in mortality compared to delaying use until there was evidence of respiratory failure.[2]

STERNAL FRACTURE

Fracture of the sternum usually results from a steering wheel injury. Even though the patient may be wearing a seat belt, sudden deceleration may throw him forcefully against the steering wheel, fracturing the sternum. The fracture is usually transverse and often associated with fractures of the costal cartilages and ribs adjacent to the sternum. The fragments are not usually depressed, but may be in more severe injuries.

Assessment

- Assessment reveals tenderness at the site of fracture.
- Ecchymosis or contusion may be noted in the overlying skin. Paradoxical motion is sometimes visible.

Figure 21-8 *Multiple bilateral rib fractures with total flail chest. This x-ray was taken just after initiation of treatment. (Note the airway.) Patient was maintained on a volume control respirator without a tracheal cuff for 3 weeks, then gradually weaned. One year later, patient returned to light work. Pulmonary studies show continued improvement.*

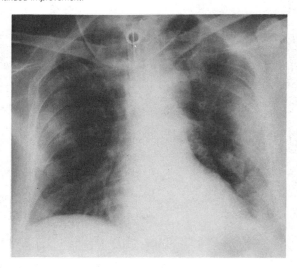

Chart 21-3

CRITERIA FOR VENTILATORY ASSISTANCE WITH FLAIL CHEST

Ventilatory assistance is indicated if one or more of the following conditions are present.
- Shock
- Three or more associated injuries
- Severe head injury
- Fracture of eight or more ribs
- Age greater than 65
- Previous pulmonary disease

(Wilson RF et al: Surg Clin North Am 57:23, 1977)

- X-rays of the sternum may confirm the diagnosis. Special oblique views of the chest are needed to visualize the sternum adequately.
- Because of the position of the heart behind the sternum myocardial contusion is often found accompanying sternal fracture.
- Vascular injury may also occur.
- A myocardial contusion may be manifested by disturbances of cardiac rhythm, hypotension, and electrocardiographic changes.
- Serial ECGs and CPK isoenzyme determinations should be done to rule out myocardial injury.[14]

Treatment

- Treatment consists primarily of medication for relief of pain.
- In severe injury, tracheostomy or cricothyrotomy and the use of a volume ventilator are required.

INJURIES TO THE INTRATHORACIC VISCERA

Injuries to the intrathoracic viscera may occur as a result of either blunt or penetrating trauma. Any structure, singly or in conjunction with other structures, may be damaged. The organ most frequently injured is the lung, probably because of its great size. Less frequently damaged are the great vessels, trachea, bronchi, esophagus, heart, and diaphragm.

INJURY TO THE LUNG

Pulmonary Contusion

Contusion of the lung may follow either blunt or penetrating trauma, but is more likely to be due to the former. It usually occurs secondary to rapid deceleration and is characterized by localized opacification(s) on chest x-ray which in some respects might resemble a tumor. It is accompanied by varying degrees of pain and respiratory distress.

Assessment. Contusion should be distinguished from adult respiratory distress syndrome (ARDS), with which it may be confused. A contusion is more likely to occur soon after injury; it is usually identified on the initial chest x-ray and is apt to progress for 2 to 3 days. ARDS tends to occur later (1 to 3 days after injury), to be diffuse, and to follow vigorous fluid resuscitation. The distinguishing characteristics of pulmonary contusion and ARDS are listed in Chart 21-4.

A contusion is basically a bruise of the lung, in which the pulmonary alveoli are filled with fluid and blood, which compromises pulmonary gas exchange. The degree of respiratory embarrassment is directly related to the size of the contused area.

Treatment. Treatment is directed toward maintaining good ventilation.
1. Monitoring arterial blood gases at intervals is helpful, especially in severe injuries.
2. Broad-spectrum antibiotics are given to prevent secondary infection.
3. Coughing is encouraged, tracheal suction is used as indicated, and oxygen by nasal catheter is also given, if needed.
4. Parenteral fluids are restricted to prevent overhydration. CVP monitoring may be helpful in this regard.
5. In severe injury, tracheostomy and ventilatory assistance are needed to maintain effective ventilatory exchange and complete pulmonary toilet.

Chart 21-4

CHARACTERISTICS OF PULMONARY CONTUSION AND OF ADULT RESPIRATORY DISTRESS SYNDROME (ARDS)

Pulmonary Contusion

- Secondary to direct chest trauma
- Occurs soon after injury
- Usually identified on the initial chest x-ray
- Likely to progress for 2 to 3 days
- Usually appears as a well-localized infiltrate on x-ray.

Adult Respiratory Distress Syndrome

- Not always related to chest injury
- Occurs 1 to 3 days after injury
- Usually follows vigorous fluid resuscitation
- Usually appears as diffuse process on x-ray

Pulmonary Hematoma

Pulmonary hematoma is a serious form of contusion, reflecting a greater disruption of pulmonary tissue. The result is a large extravasation of blood into the lung tissue at the segmental or lobar level. Most hematomas resolve spontaneously over the course of several weeks. Chest x-ray usually reveals a localized infiltrate, although a more diffuse process is present in some patients.

Management is similar to that of pulmonary contusion, namely prophylaxis against complications with antibiotics, maintenance of adequate ventilation, and pulmonary toilet. In long-standing cases without resolution, resectional therapy may be necessary.

Pulmonary Lacerations

A tear in the surface of the lung is rare following blunt trauma and may be due to inward protrusion of a fragment of fractured rib. The patient may have hemoptysis. A hemopneumothorax commonly accompanies a laceration. Insertion of upper and lower chest tubes to evacuate air and blood in the pleural cavity usually resolves the problem. Observe the patient closely for signs of respiratory embarrassment and follow the clinical course with x-rays at intervals.

INJURIES TO THE TRACHEA AND BRONCHI

Injury to the intrathoracic portion of the trachea and bronchi indicates severe trauma and may follow either a blunt or a penetrating wound. Major air leaks may develop in the mediastinum or the pleural cavity. In the latter situation, tension pneumothorax may threaten the patient's life.

Assessment

When the laceration of the trachea causes an air leak into the mediastinum, it may be identified on chest x-ray (mediastinal emphysema). The air may dissect into the neck, so that crepitus is noted in the suprasternal area. Auscultation over the anterior chest often reveals a crunching sound synchronous with the heartbeat (Hamman's sign).

Persistent pneumothorax, subcutaneous emphysema, mediastinal emphysema, and hemoptysis usually suggest an injury to the tracheal or major bronchus.

Management of the patient with an acute tracheobronchial injury is outlined in Chart 21-5.

Management/Treatment

Management consists of a tracheostomy to control further air leakage by reducing intratracheal pressure. Chest tubes may be needed to evacuate the pneumothorax. Bronchoscopy is necessaary to evaluate the tracheobronchial tree and identify the level of injury. If bronchoscopic examination fails to reveal the site of the injury, a bronchogram is indicated.

Sometimes, major tears of the bronchi go unnoticed and are not found until later, after sepsis or atelectasis develops.

Chart 21-5

MANAGEMENT OF THE PATIENT WITH ACUTE TRACHEOBRONCHIAL INJURY

Assessment

HISTORY
- Usually severe trauma to chest
- May be penetrating
- May be blunt, with rapid deceleration

PHYSICAL EXAMINATION
- Crepitus in neck or suprasternal area
- Diminished to absent breath sound on injured side.
- Mediastinal crunch with heartbeat (Hamman's sign)
- Hemoptysis

ADJUNCT STUDIES
- Chest x-ray—pneumothorax, mediastinal emphysema
- Subcutaneous emphysema in neck
- Bronchoscopy and/or bronchogram

Emergency Management/Treatment

- Monitor vital signs
- Tracheostomy or cricothyroidostomy
- Tube thoracostomy if needed, to evacuate pneumothorax
- Bronchoscopy to identify the level of injury
- Bronchogram if bronchoscopy fails to locate site of injury

Less commonly, the lesion may be diagnosed much later, after stenosis of the bronchus occurs at the level of injury.

An uncommon complication of this severe injury is tracheoesophageal fistula. A high index of suspicion aids in the diagnosis.

CARDIAC CONTUSION

Blunt trauma to the heart, as seen in steering wheel injuries, occurs far more frequently than is generally realized and often goes unrecognized. It follows a direct impact of the precordium of the chest onto the steering wheel, compressing the heart between the sternum and the vertebral column.

Cardiac contusion should always be suspected in any patient with a steering wheel injury, especially if there is a major contusion of the sternal area. The injury may affect both normal and diseased hearts, but may be seen more often in the latter. The extent of injury to the heart muscle may vary from a localized contusion to a full-thickness injury of the wall of the heart. A full-blown traumatic myocardial infarction is a severe form of this injury.

Assessment

Clinically, cardiac contusion is usually manifested by tachycardia, less often by varying arrhythmias. An ECG may reveal ST-T wave changes and a current of injury. These are usually temporary. An ECG tracing should be done in the emergency department on any patient with a steering wheel injury or blunt trauma to the anterior chest and should be followed with serial ECGs. Cardiac enzyme studies should also be done.

A distinction has been made between "cardiac concussion" and "myocardial contusion."[14] Myocardial cellular injury may be differentiated from skeletal muscle injury in the presence of severe trauma by creatine phosphokinase (CPK)-isoenzyme determinations. Thus, any patient with suspected blunt cardiac injury should be followed with serial ECGs and CPK-isoenzyme levels. Experience has shown that in actual practice a provisional diagnosis of myocardial contusion should not unnecessarily delay surgical intervention for life-threatening injuries. Therefore, the use of serial CPK-isoenzyme levels, which require 48 to 72 hours for delineation, may not be helpful during the early hours of care.

Treatment

Generally, a cardiac or myocardial contusion should be recognized when present, and any arrhythmia should be treated promptly. The decision to perform or delay major surgery for injuries in such a patient must be made in light of the potential seriousness of the cardiac injury. Cardiologic consultation should be obtained.

CARDIAC TAMPONADE (HEMOPERICARDIUM)

Blood in the pericardial sac is a sequela of either penetrating or nonpenetrating chest trauma. It may also follow perforation of the myocardium by a central venous catheter or a transvenous pacemaker electrode. Following blunt trauma to the anterior chest wall, as in a steering wheel injury, there may be a tear of a coronary vessel that causes bleeding into the pericardial sac around the heart. In penetrating trauma, the blood may arise from a lacerated coronary vessel or from a penetrating wound of one of the chambers of the heart. Since the pericardial sac is a dense structure made up of fibrous tissue that cannot be distended, relatively small amounts of blood, as little as 150 ml, may cause tamponade.

As the blood accumulates in the pericardial sac, external pressure is increased on the heart, interfering with ventricular filling. Venous pressure is thus increased, and cardiac output falls.

Assessment

Clinically, the patient has tachycardia, distended neck veins, decreased arterial blood pressure as cardiac output diminishes, and diminished heart sounds. The triad of arterial hypotension, distended neck veins, and a small, quiet heart strongly suggests tamponade and is called Beck's triad. The urine output is almost always significantly decreased.

Chest x-ray shows the characteristic widening of the cardiac shadow. A "water-bottle" configuration of the heart may be seen. The ECG reveals low voltage with electrical alternans.

Treatment

Treatment consists of early pericardiocentesis under local anesthesia, using the infraxyphoid approach. An 18- to 19-gauge spinal needle is used.

- Constant negative pressure should be applied to the syringe so that the fluid is obtained as soon as the pericardial sac is entered.

- In most instances, the blood recovered does not clot.

- An alligator clip may be applied to the needle and attached to an anterior chest ECG lead. If the needle contacts the myocardium, there will be an alteration of the ECG pattern. The needle should be withdrawn slightly until the electrocardiographic change disappears.

- As much blood as possible should be aspirated. It is of interest that removal of as little as 20 ml to 30 ml of blood may provoke a good clinical response.

- If tamponade recurs, a second tap may be necessary. In such an instance, it is more than likely that operative intervention will be needed to evacuate the pericardial sac. This may be one indication for thoracotomy in the emergency department.

Management of the patient with cardiac tamponade is summarized in Chart 21-6.

AORTIC INJURY

Injury to the major vessels may occur secondary to blunt or penetrating wounds. Aortic rupture is much more common than is generally thought. It is estimated that approximately 12% of deaths due to traffic accidents are associated with rupture of the aorta. Early diagnosis can lead to successful repair. The injury is usually associated with rapid deceleration in a high-speed auto accident. A fall from a height, with crushing injury, may also cause rupture of the aorta.

The usual site of damage to the aorta is in the distal arch just beyond the takeoff of the left subclavian artery and proximal to the ligamentum arteriosum. The ligamentum arteriosum and descending thoracic aorta are relatively fixed, whereas the transverse portion of the arch is relatively mobile. Thus, there is a shearing force at the junction of the mobile and fixed parts with rapid deceleration. The tear is partial, and the adventitia (the outer layer of the aorta) remains intact. A false aneurysm may develop and the patient may survive for a period of time, so that surgical repair may be accomplished. The subclavian artery may be damaged in first or second rib fractures (Fig. 21-9).

Assessment

Clinically, the patient who has aortic injury complains of chest pain, often in the back of the upper chest. The pain usually is not influenced by respiration. Compromise of the left main bronchus by the traumatic aneurysm producing pulmonary complaints may suggest the possibility of such a lesion.

Chest x-ray shows a widening of the mediastinum. Widening greater than 8 cm at the aortic knob is suspicious.

Chart 21-6

MANAGEMENT OF THE PATIENT WITH CARDIAC TAMPONADE

Assessment

HISTORY

- Severe blunt or penetrating thoracic trauma
- Recent intracardiac instrumentation

PHYSICAL EXAMINATION

- Arterial hypotension ⎫
- Distended neck veins ⎬ Beck's triad
- Diminished, distant heart tones ⎭
- Oliguria
- Tachycardia

ADJUNCT STUDIES

- X-ray widening of heart shadow (water-bottle heart)
- Low voltage and electrical changes on ECG.

Management/Treatment

- Monitor vital signs, including CVP and heart rhythm before, during and after needle pericardiocentesis.
- Needle pericardiocentesis is performed to withdraw blood from pericardial sac.*
- If symptoms persist or recur, pericardiocentesis may have to be repeated.
- If patient's condition deteriorates, urgent thoracotomy must be considered, to evacuate the hemopericardium and repair the site of injury.

* A combination needle/catheter device can be used and the catheter left in place to repeat the procedure if needed.

Retrograde aortography should be performed to confirm the diagnosis. Patients who have aortic injury may have unstable vital signs. Early crossmatching of type-specific blood should be done soon after admission to the emergency department.

Treatment

If a partial tear is identified, exploration and surgical repair should be undertaken, provided that the associated injuries offer no contraindication. Repair of this injury requires cardiopulmonary bypass. The patient should be transferred to an appropriate hospital center with this capability once the diagnosis is made. Emergency room thoracotomy has been employed successfully in some centers to establish initial control of the injury before definitive treatment is attempted in the operating room.

Surgical treatment consists of resection of the torn segment of aorta and reconstruction with a prosthetic graft.

Management of the patient with transection of the aorta is summarized in Chart 21-7.

PENETRATING WOUNDS

Penetrating chest wounds may be caused by a number of agents, for example, knives, ice picks, and various missiles. It is worthwhile to find out what the wounding agent was, since this information may offer clues to the nature of the wound itself and the extent of the involvement of the deep structures of the chest.

Wounds caused by ice picks or knives usually relate to the structures underlying the skin in the direction of entry of the weapon. Injuries caused by gunshot wounds vary with the size of the weapon and thus with the size and speed of the missile. Wound ballistic studies indicate that missiles fired from a firearm with a high muzzle velocity produce considerable damage to the viscera as a result of energy waves created by the moving missile. The internal damage is much greater than the wounds of entrance or exit suggest. The path of the missile is usually a straight line unless it is deflected by bone. The wounds of entrance and exit therefore often suggest the nature of the soft tissue involvement in the missile's path. A bizarre pathway is sometimes explained by the position of the patient at the time of wounding. In estimating the extent of the injury, all structures within the thorax and mediastinum must be considered. A line drawn from the wound of entrance to the embedded missile or the wound of exit frequently indicates the organs injured.

At the site of entry of the missile, a persistent defect may be produced in the chest wall. Its size depends on the type and size of the wounding agent. This defect may allow air to move in and out of the pleural cavity (and consequently is called a sucking wound of the chest). The extent to which the underlying lung collapses depends on the size of the opening in the chest wall. In some instances, the nature of

Figure 21-9 Aneurysm. Aortogram was taken because of widening mediastinum following head-on car accident. It shows traumatic aneurysm just distal to left subclavian take-off. Repair by graft was done within 12 hours after injury.

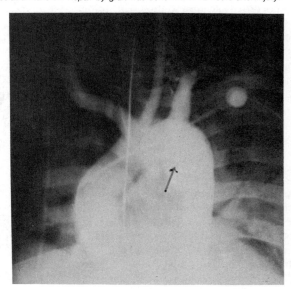

Chart 21-7

MANAGEMENT OF THE PATIENT WITH AORTIC TRANSECTION

Assessment

HISTORY

- Severe injury to chest

PHYSICAL EXAMINATION

- Systolic murmur radiating to back in the area of left 2nd and 3rd rib posteriorly
- Diminished femoral pulses

ADJUNCT STUDIES

- Chest x-ray—consider with fracture of left 1st rib.
- Chest x-ray—left pleural apical cap
- Chest x-ray—widened mediastinum. In supine chest x-ray, if mediastinum is wider than 8.0 cm at the level of the aortic knob, suspect aortic transection.
- Transfemoral aortography will confirm the diagnosis.

Management/Treatment

- Monitor vital signs.
- Place large-bore veinways for volume replacement.
- Surgical repair of aorta is indicated; cardiopulmonary bypass is usually required and should be available.
- If the hospital does not have cardiac bypass capability, the patient must be prepared for transfer to a center that can provide appropriate care.

---

the wound is such that air can flow into the chest on inspiration but is prevented from flowing outward. Air is thus trapped in the chest as with a *tension pneumothorax,* and with each respiratory effort, the mediastinum is shifted to the opposite side, causing progressively severe respiratory embarrassment and reducing venous return to the heart, leading to hypotension.

Prehospital Care

A patient with a sucking wound of the chest should be treated immediately by closure of the wound with an occlusive dressing such as Vaseline gauze. This should be applied at the accident scene by emergency personnel before the patient is transported to the hospital. Another device that is handy in managing these wounds is a temporary colostomy bag which can be applied directly over the wound and serves very well to close it. Either method is only temporary.

When the patient is initially seen with a knife, ice pick, or impaled object protruding from the chest, it is important that the foreign object *not* be removed prior to transportation

to the hospital. Once the patient is in the emergency department, a more complete assessment should be performed before an attempt is made to remove the missile.

Hospital Care

Once the patient is in the hospital, an anterior intercostal catheter in the pleural cavity connected to an underwater seal adds further control until definitive care can be given. Definitive surgical care consists of closure of the wound. Thoracotomy is required when visceral damage is present or when there is persistent bleeding into the pleural cavity.

ESOPHAGEAL INJURY

Rupture of the esophagus from blunt thoracic trauma is rare; indeed, fewer than 50 cases are reported in the literature. It is more likely to occur following penetrating injury.

The danger of this injury lies in contamination of the mediastinum by the saliva contained in the esophagus. Despite its rarity, rupture of the esophagus should be considered in any patient with a severe, crushing injury or a penetrating wound of the thorax.

Assessment

Clinically, the patient complains of pain. In injuries to the upper or middle third of the esophagus, the pain is in the chest, especially posteriorly. In injury to the lower third, the pain may be in the epigastrium. Therefore, any patient being explored for epigastric pain secondary to injury in whom no abnormality is found should have the distal portion of the esophagus evaluated. Fistulae may develop between the esophagus and the trachea and constitute a major complication.

The diagnosis may be confirmed by esophagoscopy or x-ray studies of the esophagus using a water-soluble radiopaque agent.

Treatment

Treatment is surgical and requires drainage of the mediastinum, diversion of the upper gastrointestinal tract, and delayed repair of the damaged esophagus. Antibiotic therapy is important in the management of the patient soon after injury.

INJURY TO THE DIAPHRAGM

The most common cause of rupture of the diaphragm is a rapid deceleration injury characterized by compression of the trunk, particularly by a steering wheel. The usual mechanism is a sharp increase in intra-abdominal pressure. The right leaf of the diaphragm is protected by the mass of the liver and is less likely to be injured. The left leaf of the diaphragm is less well protected and tears more easily. It is often accompanied by injuries to the liver, spleen, and kidneys (Fig. 21-10).

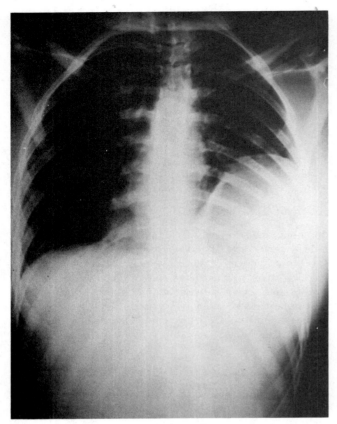
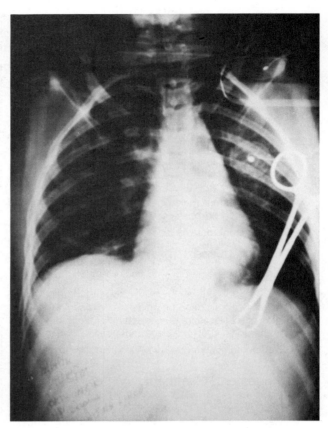

Figure 21-10 *Chest film of patient with combined thoracoabdominal trauma. Left. Traumatic rupture of left diaphragm. Note marked elevation of left diaphragm. Right. Intraoperative radiograph of patient shown at left, following repair of ruptured left diaphragm.*

Assessment

Clinically, the patient may complain of sharp pain in the shoulder with increasing shortness of breath. On examination, the heart may be shifted to the right (the side opposite injury) and breath sounds are distant.

Chest x-ray usually confirms the diagnosis, with elevation of the injured diaphragm and the presence of abdominal viscera, especially the stomach in the chest cavity. It is sometimes better to perform the chest x-ray with the patient in the recumbent position.

Occasionally, the injury may be overlooked on a conventional chest x-ray, only to be identified weeks to years later.

Treatment

Treatment consists of nasogastric decompression, stabilization of the patient, and early surgical repair.

EMERGENCY DEPARTMENT THORACOTOMY

Because of great improvements in prehospital care at the accident scene and during transport to the hospital, many severely injured patients who in the past would not have survived are entering hospital emergency departments in extremis. Patients with severe chest trauma may be candidates for thoracotomy in the emergency department. Admittedly, this group is small, perhaps 1% of such injuries.

Trunkey has stated that the indications for emergency department thoracotomy include penetrating wounds of the heart, pericardial tamponade, air embolism, and hypovolemic cardiac arrest.[3] Other indications include control of intra-abdominal bleeding.

The use of emergency thoracotomy is a controversial issue. Some feel its use should be restricted to major trauma centers,[15] while others claim worthwhile results in a community hospital.[16] A cost benefit analysis of this procedure was reported by Baker *et al.* in which the benefits were shown to be 2.4 times greater than total costs.

In the review by MacDonald and McDowell of 1069 patients from numerous centers, the mortality rate in emergency thoracotomy varied from 10% to 69% and averaged 29%. This factor alone must receive due consideration if this procedure is to be added to the therapeutic armamentarium of a hospital emergency department. Other factors include adequately trained and interested personnel and an appropriately equipped department.

An adjuvant therapeutic modality that has been reported in conjunction with emergency thoracotomy is temporary cardiac pacing.[19]

THORACOABDOMINAL INJURIES

A thoracoabdominal injury is one in which organs in both the thoracic and the abdominal cavities are damaged. Such an injury may follow either blunt or penetrating trauma.

Topographically, the diaphragm rises to the level of the fourth intercostal space on expiration; thus, injuries to the chest at or below this level could potentially damage intra-abdominal viscera. The position of the diaphragm at the time of wounding, especially in penetrating injuries, may determine whether or not both cavities are involved by the wound.

ASSESSMENT

In penetrating trauma, when there is a single wound with a foreign body in place, anteroposterior and lateral x-rays of the chest and abdomen usually give an indication of the presence or absence of a combined thoracoabdominal injury. If wounds of entry and exit are present, projecting a straight line between the two will suggest accurately which organs are involved. Occasionally, the missile associated with a gunshot wound caroms off a bone and is diverted from a straight line course.

On the right side, a wound of entrance above the costal margin that exits posteriorly at the 10th rib involves the diaphragm in two areas and the liver. In this case, no other intra-abdominal organs are injured. On the left side, because of the number of organs in the left upper quadrant, a similar such wound track might involve the spleen, stomach, colon, small bowel, and pancreas. In combined injuries involving the right upper quadrant, abdominal signs may be absent or minimal when the patient is first seen if bleeding from the liver is slight. On the other hand, combined wounds involving the left upper quadrant are much more apt to present striking abdominal signs.

Blunt trauma to the lower ribs posteriorly and laterally, especially with fracture of the 10th and 11th ribs, may cause injury to the kidney, liver, or spleen (Fig. 21-11).

MANAGEMENT

Management of combined thoracoabdominal wounds requires an awareness of the possibility that both the pleural

Figure 21-11 Fracture of right 11th rib and injury to upper pole of right kidney, shown in intravenous pyelogram.

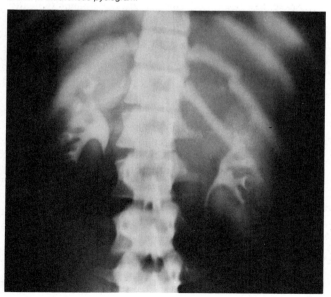

and the abdominal cavities have been violated. In penetrating wounds, an accurate knowledge of the missile path and consideration of the organs that may have been injured is beneficial. Bearing in mind the priorities of care, perform a careful but complete assessment of the patient.

If abdominal findings are not clearly positive or minimal, ancillary studies, particularly peritoneal lavage, may aid in identifying the presence of intraperitoneal injury. The limitations of lavage must be recognized, particularly with regard to retroperitoneal organ damage. Definitive management includes care of the injured organs, repair of the diaphragm, and measures to expand the lung fully. Pulmonary toilet is an important component of care. Adequate volume replacement is important before surgery. Ringer's lactate initially, and later type-specific crossmatched blood, are used. Arterial blood gas determinations should be made at intervals during the resuscitative phase of care in the emergency department. Tube thoracostomy may be required to evacuate fluid or air from the pleural space. All patients with *penetrating* thoracoabdominal wounds require surgical exploration. The use of thoracotomy in the emergency department as a life-saving measure is discussed earlier in this chapter.

ABDOMINAL INJURIES

In civilian life, the majority of abdominal injuries are due to blunt trauma secondary to high-speed automobile accidents and falls from heights. Less commonly, assaults and sports injuries are the causes. Penetrating injuries, although often associated with wartime combat, are being seen with increasing frequency in hospital emergency departments. This is particularly true in the large metropolitan areas of this country with high-density populations. Either mechanism of injury, blunt or penetrating, may cause serious damage to the abdominal organs. Such injuries account for approximately 10% of the trauma deaths that occur annually in the United States. Blunt trauma accounts for the majority of these deaths, probably because damage following such trauma is much more difficult to recognize, so that delay in diagnosis may result. Early recognition of intraabdominal injury is essential to good care. One should recall that the abdomen encompasses a large area of the body, from the diaphragm superiorly to the infragluteal fold inferiorly, including the entire circumference of this region. Thus, penetrating or blunt trauma to the back may result in intraabdominal injury. The importance of repeated assessment of a patient suspected of having intraabdominal injury cannot be overstated. Multiple organ injuries, particularly those involving the central nervous system (CNS), chest, and musculoskeletal system, may obscure damage to the abdominal contents. In instances of multiple-system trauma, in which specialty consultation may be needed, the overall responsibility for treatment must reside with one physician, preferably a general surgeon.

ANATOMIC CONSIDERATIONS

A knowledge of the contents of the abdomen is vital. As mentioned earlier, the abdomen extends from the thoracic diaphragms above to the infragluteal crease below and includes the entire circumference of this region. Assessment of the abdomen is influenced by its anatomic features. For practical purposes, the abdomen may be divided into four areas: the intrathoracic abdomen, the true abdomen, the pelvic abdomen, and the retroperitoneal abdomen. Except for the true abdomen, these areas yield few findings on physical examination.

The intrathoracic abdomen is the portion of the upper abdomen that lies beneath the rib cage (Chart 21-8*A*). Because of the bony and cartilaginous structures, this portion of the abdomen is rather inaccessible to palpation. This area contains the spleen, stomach, liver, and diaphragm, which may be injured when blunt or penetrating trauma is delivered to the rib cage. Peritoneal lavage is useful in identifying organ injury.

The pelvic abdomen lies in the hollow of the pelvis surrounded on all sides by the bony pelvis (Chart 21-8*B*). Contents include the rectum, bladder, urethra, and small bowel and, in females, the uterus, tubes, and ovaries. Trauma to the pelvis, especially fractures, may damage the organs within. Penetrating wounds of the buttocks may injure any one or more of these organs. Injury to these structures may be difficult to diagnose because of the paucity of physical findings. Ancillary studies are helpful, including urethrocystography, sigmoidoscopy, and catheterization.

The retroperitoneal abdomen contains the kidneys, ureters, pancreas, second and third portions of the duodenum, and the great vessels—the aorta and the vena cava (Chart 21-8*C*). Injury to these structures may occur secondary to penetrating or blunt trauma. In the latter instance, the kidneys may be damaged by injury to the lower ribs posteriorly. Any of the structures can be damaged by crushing injuries to the front or sides of the torso. Injury to these structures may result in few physical findings, making evaluation and diagnosis difficult. Peritoneal lavage is of little or no help in the diagnosis of retroperitoneal organ injury. Intravenous pyelography, retrograde aortography, serum amylase, and abdominal x-rays may be valuable.

The true abdomen contains the small and large intestines, the bladder when distended, and the uterus when gravid. Injury to any of these organs is usually manifested by pain and is associated with abdominal physical findings. Peritoneal lavage is a useful adjunct procedure in evaluating suspected injury. Three-way x-rays of the abdomen (flat, upright, and lateral decubitus) are helpful, especially when free air is identified.

PREHOSPITAL CARE

Little can be done for most patients with abdominal injuries at the accident scene. In penetrating wounds, sterile dressing should be applied and the patient carefully monitored. Knives or other foreign bodies imbedded in the trunk should *not* be removed, since major bleeding can ensue. Eviscerations are best left undisturbed except to apply sterile dressing and protect the patient from further injury. Attention should be given to an adequately functioning airway. An intravenous line may be inserted, preferably in an upper extremity, and fluid resuscitation begun.

HOSPITAL CARE

Assessment

Diagnosis and treatment should proceed concurrently, following established principles. (For key points in care, see Chart 21-9.) An isolated organ injury is uncommon in abdominal trauma. One should be more concerned with determining whether the patient has an acute surgical abdomen requiring surgical exploration than with trying to ascertain whether a specific organ is injured. The ABCs of emergency resuscitation—*a*irway, *b*reathing, and *c*irculation—should be initiated.

- A patent functioning airway is of vital importance, especially in a comatose patient.

- If necessary, an endotracheal tube is placed and assisted ventilation begun.

- An upper extremity large-bore veinway is inserted, and fluid volume replacement started using Ringer's lactate.

- At the time of veinway placement, blood samples are withdrawn for basic studies including complete blood count (CBC), electrolytes, amylase, type and crossmatch in the seriously injured patient.

- Arterial blood gases are determined and repeated as indications warrant.

- An early, rapid assessment of the abdomen is performed.

History. If the patient is conscious, a history of the accident should be obtained. In the case of vehicular trauma, essential details include the position of the patient in the car, whether lap or chest restraints were being used, the direction and site of impact (head-on, rear-end, side), whether the patient was ejected, and where the patient was found. Additional information may be obtained from others involved in the accident, witnesses, the police, and ambulance crews. These four sources are extremely important when the patient is unconscious.

Physical Examination. As assessment proceeds, the abdominal examination includes inspection, auscultation, percussion, and palpation.
- Inspect for respiratory movements. Females typically breathe with their intercostal muscles; males are primarily diaphragmatic breathers. Halting, labored breathing may accompany upper abdominal injury.

- Inspect the *abdominal wall* and *back* carefully for any sign of wounding. Ecchymoses of the abdominal wall in the upper half may be due to steering wheel impact, while those in the lower abdomen may be due to the use of lap restraints. Either of these may be associated with serious intra-abdominal injury.

- Auscultation of bowel sounds should precede percussion and palpation. The presence or absence of peristaltic sounds is an important observation in a patient suspected of having an abdominal injury. Peritoneal irritation from blood or intestinal contents causes a diminution in peristaltic sounds.

- Auscultatory findings should be documented accurately at appropriate intervals. Diminished or absent peristalsis over a period of time is an accurate indicator of intraabdominal injury. Palpation may reveal localized tenderness, spasm, or rigidity in the abdominal wall. The finding of

Chart 21-8

CONTENTS OF THE ABDOMEN

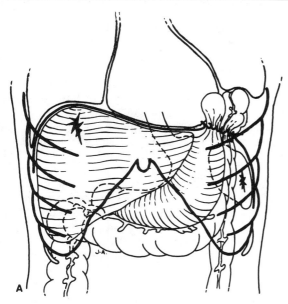

A. Intrathoracic abdomen
   Diaphragm
   Liver
   Spleen
   Stomach

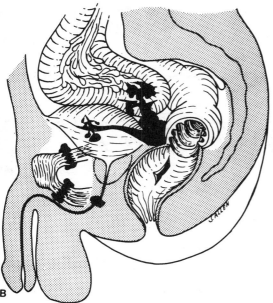

B. Pelvic abdomen
   Urinary bladder
   Urethra
   Rectum
   Small intestine
   Uterus, tubes, ovaries (female)

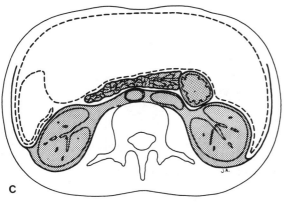

C. Retroperitoneal abdomen
   Kidneys
   Ureters
   Pancreas
   Great vessels
   Duodenum (2nd and 3rd parts)

   True abdomen (not shown)
   Small intestine
   Large intestine
   Distended urinary bladder
   Gravid uterus

Drawings from Hardy JD (ed): Rhoads Textbook of Surgery, 5th ed. Philadelphia, JB Lippincott, 1977

Chart 21-9

KEY POINTS IN CARE OF A PATIENT WITH ABDOMINAL TRAUMA

- Ensure a patent airway and adequate ventilation.
- Control external hemorrhage by pressure.
- Establish a large-bore veinway(s) in the upper extremities and take blood samples for basic laboratory studies, CBC, amylase, type and crossmatch, arterial blood gases.
- Obtain history from patient, witnesses, prehospital care personnel, etc.
- Assess patient briefly.
- Insert a nasogastric tube and send aspirate to laboratory.
- Insert indwelling catheter and maintain output at 0.5 to 1.0 ml/kg/hr. Send urine sample to laboratory for analysis.
- Reassess patient.
- Take x-rays—three-way films of abdomen. Order specific studies as patient's condition warrants.

These procedures should be done in stepwise order but may proceed concurrently.

---

direct or rebound tenderness is another important sign of abdominal injury.

- As assessment continues, an indwelling urinary catheter should be placed and a sample of urine sent to the laboratory for analysis. Microscopic hematuria is perhaps the single most important finding in urinary tract injury. *Note:* If one is suspicious of an injury to the lower urinary tract (the bladder or urethra), particularly in a male, because of an associated pelvic fracture, catheterization should be delayed until urethrography is performed to rule out injury to the urethra. Catheterization in the presence of such an injury is usually unsuccessful, and an attempt to insert a catheter in this circumstance may lead to further damage to the injured urethra, which can result in serious morbidity and permanent sequelae. This is discussed in greater detail in Chapter 24, Genitourinary Emergencies.

- Urinary output is monitored closely because it serves as a guide to the adequacy of volume replacement and thus to the resuscitation process. A urinary output of 1.0 ml/kg/hr is considered adequate. In a child one should strive for an output of 0.5 ml/kg/hr.

- A nasogastric tube is inserted. The aspirate recovered is examined for blood. If there is any suspicion of drug ingestion, toxicology studies are in order.

- Rectal examination is important in assessing a patient with abdominal trauma. The presence of blood (proctorrhagia) usually indicates colon or rectal injury.

The importance of repeated abdominal examinations and accurate documentation of findings cannot be overemphasized. The assessments should be performed by the same individual. If for some reason, there is a personnel change, the new person coming on duty should evaluate the patient

together with the person being relieved. In this way, agreement can be reached on the patient's findings and status in order to provide better continuity of care.

In a conscious patient, major intra-abdominal injuries are almost always accompanied by pain. Other symptoms vary according to the extent of injury and may include nausea, vomiting, thirst, and apprehension. The usual physical signs in such injuries are tenderness, spasm, and diminished or absent bowel sounds. The extent to which these symptoms and signs are present depends in part on how soon the patient is seen after injury. When the interval from injury to examination is short, abdominal complaints and findings may be minimal. This emphasizes the significance of repeated abdominal examinations.

In an unconscious patient, assessment is much more difficult. Once again details of the accident are most important and assume greater importance in such a patient. CNS injury may mask many of the signs of an acute intra-abdominal process. One may then resort to adjunct studies, such as peritoneal tap or lavage, in assessing such a patient.

Adjunct Studies. In addition to history and physical assessment, a number of laboratory and x-ray studies and ancillary diagnostic procedures are useful in evaluating a patient suspected of abdominal injury. These studies are listed in Chart 21-10.

Chart 21-10

ADJUNCT STUDIES FOR ASSESSMENT OF ABDOMINAL TRAUMA

Laboratory Studies

- CBC
- SMA-18 (6 and 12)
- Serum amylase
- Arterial blood gases
- Urinalysis

Radiologic Studies

- Three-way films of abdomen
- Urethrography—cystogram
- Intravenous pyelogram
- Infusion pyelogram
- Radionuclude scan
- Angiography
- Sonography
- CT scan

Special Diagnostic Procedures

- Abdominal paracentesis (peritoneal tap, flank tap, four-quadrant tap)
- Peritoneal lavage

Laboratory Studies. Laboratory studies include CBC, serum electrolytes, SMA-12, serum amylase, and arterial blood gases.

- The CBC may show a decrease in hematocrit and leucocytosis. In patients with blood loss, a certain amount of time must pass before a reduction in the hemoglobin or hematocrit (packed cell volume) is evident. Early on, hemoconcentration may result in normal hematocrit, thus masking an underlying major blood loss. Serial determinations of hemoglobin and hematocrit are needed to identify the presence or absence of major bleeding.

- The serum amylase study is useful in delineating injury to the pancreas.

- Arterial blood gases should be determined in any severely injured patient, at first in the emergency setting and at intervals as the patient's condition indicates.

- Routine urinalysis is an important—and simple—technique of identifying urinary tract injury. Microscopic hematuria is perhaps the single most important finding in urinary tract injury. The patient should be asked to void spontaneously before a catheter is passed, especially when his pelvis is fractured. In an unconscious patient, obviously, this is not possible.

- If the patient is unable to void or a pelvic fracture is noted, and a lower urinary tract injury suspected, perform urethrography before inserting an indwelling catheter.

- The presence of sugar in the urine may identify a diabetic.

X-ray Studies. X-ray studies should be ordered and done as the patient's condition warrants and allows.

- Any severely injured patient who requires x-rays should be accompanied to the radiography department by a physician or nurse whose function is to evaluate the patient's status and initiate any measures necessary to support vital signs.

- Inordinate x-ray studies in a critically injured patient may cause unnecessary delay and may result in death.

- The basic x-ray studies useful in assessing a patient suspected of having an intra-abdominal injury are three-way films of the abdomen (flat, upright, and lateral decubitus).

- Radiographic evidence of free intraperitoneal air indicates a perforated hollow viscus.

Note: Caution is advised in interpreting this finding if the study is done after peritoneal lavage. Free air may be introduced into the peritoneal cavity in the process of lavage.

- Radiographic findings of skeletal injury, particularly involving the lower ribs, the dorsal or lumbar spine, or the pelvis, may give indirect evidence of the extent of injury and offer a clue to the possibility of injury to structures in the retroperitoneal abdomen or the intrathoracic or pelvic portions of the abdomen, which are relatively inaccessible to physical examination (Fig. 21-12).

- Displacement of the gastric air bubble may accompany injury to the spleen.

- In penetrating trauma, a missile or foreign body may be detected on x-ray.

- Intravenous pyelography by single injection can be performed easily in the emergency department radiography unit or by portable technique if necessary. Admittedly, it is only a rough index of renal function, useful in suspected injury to the upper urinary tract. More valuable is infusion pyelography, in which a larger amount of io-

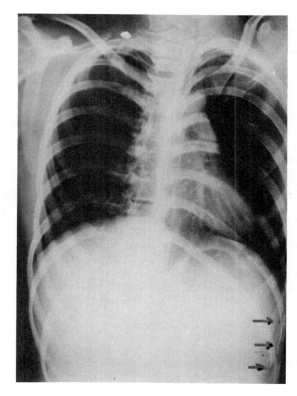

Figure 21-12 Rib fractures. The x-ray shows fractures of the left eighth, ninth, and tenth ribs in a patient who struck his left chest against a gear shift lever. There were also signs of acute abdomen, and a laparotomy revealed rupture of the spleen.

dine dye is given over a period of time and which can better identify disruption of the kidney, ureter, or bladder.

- Urethrography should be performed initially, and if negative, cystography should be performed, especially if a pelvic fracture is present. Injury to the male urethra and urinary bladder often accompanies pelvic fracture.

- Other radiologic studies that may be considered include radionuclide scanning, helpful in suspected occult injury to the solid viscera (liver, kidney, spleen) and angiography using either aortography or selective catheterization techniques.

- Abdominal sonography is of little use in evaluating the acutely injured patient, but may prove valuable later in the patient's course. Computed tomography (CT) scanning of the thorax and abdomen is a useful adjunct in the diagnosis of trauma, particularly trauma to the contents of the retroperitoneal abdomen.

Special Diagnostic Procedures. Abdominal paracentesis (peritoneal tap, flank tap, four-quadrant tap) and peritoneal lavage are very helpful studies in the diagnosis of occult abdominal injury, especially after blunt trauma. Neither study should be performed until after three-way films of the abdomen are completed. Air may be introduced into the peritoneal cavity during the course of the procedure and may serve to confuse the interpretation of the three-way films, with respect to the finding of intraperitoneal air.

1. *Abdominal Paracentesis.* In the past few years, attention has been directed away from paracentesis as the sole assessment of intra-abdominal injury. It is not now used unless free, nonclotting blood is recovered. The accuracy

of peritoneal tap alone is in the range of 60% to 75%. Obviously, it will vary with the experience of the operator. Currently, it is used more often in conjunction with peritoneal lavage. If the tap reveals gross blood, the procedure is considered positive and terminated. If no blood is recovered, the tap is negative and lavage is performed.

2. *Peritoneal lavage.* Peritoneal lavage is a relatively simple procedure in which fluid is introduced into the peritoneal cavity by gravity, recovered by siphon drainage, and then evaluated. The accuracy of peritoneal lavage is much higher than that of a single tap and is estimated to be 95% correct in identifying the presence of intraperitoneal injury. Thus, it is perhaps the best single diagnostic test in assessing otherwise obscure abdominal injury. The finding of a negative tap or lavage does not rule out the presence of an intraperitoneal injury, however, and it must be considered in conjunction with other diagnostic tests and serial physical examination.

   In a patient with injury to the retroperitoneal structures, the lavage usually is negative. Thus a patient with findings of abdominal injury with a negative lavage may have injury to the retroperitoneal abdomen. Not all patients are candidates for peritoneal lavage. The indications and contraindications for peritoneal lavage are listed in Chart 21-11. The technique of peritoneal lavage is simple, and complications are relatively few. The procedure is outlined in Chart 21-11.

3. *Laparotomy.* A positive peritoneal lavage is one indication for exploratory laparotomy. Indications for laparotomy in blunt abdominal trauma are as follows:*

   - Presence of signs of peritoneal irritation
   - Positive peritoneal lavage
   - Persistent unexplained shock
   - Presence of hematemesis or proctorrhagia

Endoscopic visualization of the peritoneal cavity in blunt abdominal trauma has been used, but is not generally accepted.[11]

Prior to laparotomy, certain measures should be undertaken. Preferably, the patient should be stabilized, and a complete assessment should be made. Broad-spectrum antibiotics are started in the emergency department and tetanus prophylaxis is given as indicated. (See Chap. 19, Wound Management.) Adequate amounts of type-specific whole blood or blood components are essential for proper care. Surgical exploration is generally performed under general anesthesia for better control of the patient.

If the patient is first seen in an emergency department and later transferred to another hospital for surgical management, a complete record of his course and therapy must accompany him. Samples of lavage fluid should be sent. All laboratory data and x-rays are sent with the patient to minimize delays and avoid unnecessary duplication. A physician or nurse should accompany the critically injured patient during transfer.

SPECIFIC ABDOMINAL INJURIES

INJURIES TO THE LIVER

The liver, the largest organ in the abdominal cavity, is commonly damaged in blunt and penetrating abdominal trauma

---

* Shaftan G: Personal communication.

and in thoracoabdominal injuries. In some series it is the most frequently injured structure and in others the second most frequently damaged. Injury to the liver must be considered in any patient with a steering wheel injury or a history of epigastric trauma. Following injury, blood and bile escape into the peritoneal cavity, causing signs and symptoms of peritoneal irritation. Hepatic injury is serious and can be life-threatening. It must be considered in any patient with injury to the lower ribs.

The mechanism of injury to the liver directly influences morbidity and mortality. Penetrating wounds from knives, ice-picks, or low-velocity missiles frequently cause minimal devitalization of liver tissue or serious continuing bleeding. On the other hand, blunt trauma or trauma associated with a high-velocity missile, usually results in more extensive liver damage, with greater devitalization of hepatic tissue and more serious bleeding. The more serious the damage to the liver, the greater the likelihood that other organs are damaged. In serious hepatic injury, the major hepatic veins that drain into the inferior vena cava may be lacerated, causing massive blood loss. Generally, morbidity and mortality are directly related to the occurrence of multiple organ injuries.

Assessment

The type and degree of hepatic injury may vary from a relatively minor laceration to extensive crushing injury with extensive fractures of the liver substance. In the latter instance, severe blood loss can result, resulting in unstable vital signs. When less severe hepatic damage is present, abdominal signs may be minimal and the patient may present with a normal blood pressure.

The history is helpful in that there is usually an injury to the lower rib cage on the right side, or to the upper abdomen. Physical findings may vary from minimal to significant signs of peritoneal irritation. The abdomen may or may not be distended, with or without spasm and rigidity in the right upper quadrant.

Laboratory studies are nonspecific in hepatic trauma. X-ray studies are of little help in confirming the diagnosis. Fractures of the lower right rib cage should prompt one to consider liver injury.

If physical signs are equivocal, peritoneal lavage will be helpful in establishing the diagnosis. If lavage is positive, laparotomy is in order.

Management

1. Every attempt should be made to stabilize the patient before surgery.
2. Adequate quantities of type-specific blood should be available for anticipated surgery.
3. The principles of management of liver injuries are the same regardless of the severity of liver damage and are:
   - Control of bleeding
   - Removal of devitalized tissue
   - Establishment of adequate drainage
4. Minor injury such as a laceration may be treated by simple suture.
5. More extensive injury may require varying degrees of liver resection.

The mortality rate varies with the severity of injury to the liver and the number of other organs damaged. In large series, mortality ranges from 4.0% to 70%.

INJURIES TO THE SPLEEN

The spleen, like the liver, is one of the two most frequently injured abdominal organs. In some series it is the intra-abdominal organ most commonly injured by trauma; in other series, it is the second most frequently injured organ. The spleen lies in the left upper quadrant of the abdomen, in the intrathoracic abdomen (see Chart 21-8). It lies to the left of and slightly behind the stomach and to a certain extent is protected by the organs surrounding it medially and anteriorly. Laterally and posteriorly it is protected by the lower portion of the rib cage. Injury to the spleen may follow penetrating or blunt trauma. The latter is more common. Blunt trauma may cause compression of the spleen between the anterior abdominal wall and the posterior rib cage or, by trauma, from a lateral direction compressing the spleen against the vertebral column. A direct blow to the left lower rib cage posteriorly or laterally, such as a kick, or from a thrown ball or other object, may directly damage the spleen. Other common causes include falls and vehicular accidents.

Assessment

The injury to the spleen may vary from a laceration or contusion of the spleen parenchyma without a capsular tear to total rupture and fragmentation of the organ. The spleen is a very vascular structure that bleeds easily when injured. Although most splenic injuries are readily apparent clinically, others, especially when the laceration and initial hemorrhage are minimal, may have few or no clinical signs and symptoms on first examination. A subsequent massive hemorrhage may occur days to weeks or months later. This so-called latent period may be such that the patient cannot recall the initial injury.

History. The history is helpful in that the patient may describe a blow, fall, or sports injury to the lower left chest, flank, or upper left abdomen. In vehicular accidents, the injury may follow contact with the steering wheel or may even be secondary to wearing a seat belt. In penetrating trauma, a wound of entry or exit in this area should make one highly suspicious of splenic injury. The clinical manifestations of splenic damage are those due to acute blood loss and those secondary to peritoneal irritation in the vicinity of the spleen. The patient may complain of pain in the left upper abdominal quadrant that is aggravated by respiration. Pain noted in the left shoulder (Kehr's sign) may be caused by enlargement of the spleen by hematoma or rupture with irritation of the adjacent diaphragm.

Physical Examination. Physical findings include those of shock in a patient with frank rupture of the spleen and abdominal tenderness and spasm, especially in the left upper quadrant. Respirations may be halting and labored because of the pain and diaphragmatic irritation. In less serious splenic injury, the clinical signs may be surprisingly few; however, one must have a high degree of suspicion if details of the trauma support the possibility of damage to the spleen.

Adjunct Studies. Laboratory studies for the most part are nonspecific. Leukocytosis and reduced hematocrit may be evident. Keep in mind, however, that in patients with multiple injuries, hemoconcentration may occur initially, causing the hematocrit to appear normal. If the patient is observed over a period of hours, the hematocrit should fall.

X-rays may be helpful in confirming the diagnosis of splenic injury. Three-way films of the abdomen may show an enlargement of the splenic shadow and medial displacement of the stomach bubble. (Fig. 21-13) Gastrograffin or barium swallow may support this finding (Fig. 21-13 *bottom*). In patients with occult splenic injury, selective splenic or celiac angiography affords a more precise method of demonstrating a tear or rupture (Fig. 21-14). Radionuclide scanning is also useful in patients with few signs or symptoms (Fig. 21-15).

Peritoneal lavage should confirm the presence of blood in the peritoneal cavity. The indications for laparotomy are listed on p 372.

Treatment

In penetrating injury, damage to adjacent structures such as the stomach, pancreas, colon, and diaphragm must be considered and requires laparotomy. In blunt trauma, laparotomy is indicated in patients with frank rupture of the spleen, but may be delayed in those thought to have an intact capsule. Particularly in children, there is a tendency to treat the latter injury expectantly. A number of series have been reported in which treatment is essentially nonoperative. This approach has resulted in some reconsideration by surgeons of the proper management of the injured spleen at the time of operation. Whereas splenectomy was once the recognized treatment of choice for the damaged spleen, a more conservative viewpoint has recently been adopted. At the time of abdominal exploration, the spleen is fully mobilized and examined. If possible, the injured section is removed or the spleen repaired by suture (splenorrhaphy). An attempt is made to conserve as much spleen tissue as possible. Various techniques are employed by the surgeon to achieve this end. It has been found that splenectomy, particularly in the pediatric age group, has a harmful effect on immune response and may make the patient more susceptible to life-threatening sepsis, especially that due to pneumococci. If splenectomy is required, the patient should be given pneumococcus vaccine postoperatively. Close observation of the platelet count is also indicated in the postoperative period when a rise in these cells can be expected.

Management of the patient with an injured spleen is summarized in Chart 21-12.

INJURIES TO THE STOMACH AND DUODENUM

Injuries to the stomach and duodenum are relatively rare, primarily because of their location in the abdomen. The stomach is in the intrathoracic abdomen and is partially protected by the rib cage. Another anatomic feature of the stomach that serves to safeguard it, especially from blunt

Chart 21-11

TECHNIQUE OF PERITONEAL LAVAGE

Indications

- Patient with suspected intraabdominal injury and equivocal physical findings
- Unconscious trauma patient with signs of abdominal injury
- Patient with multiple injuries and unexplained shock
- Patient with thoracoabdominal injuries
- Patient with a spinal cord injury
- Intoxicated patient in whom intraabdominal injury is suspected

Contraindications

- Patient with a history of multiple abdominal operations
- Pregnancy
- Penetrating injury
- Morbid obesity

Equipment

- Local set with prep
- No 3 scalpel handle with No 11 or No 15 blade
- Standard peritoneal dialysis catheter with stylet and connector (Stylocath-Abbott)
- 1000 ml normal saline or Ringer's lactate (for adults)
- Normal saline or Ringer's lactate (for children 10 to 20 ml/kg of body weight)
- One strand 4-O silk suture, swedged needle, needle holder, and scissors
- IV-tubing
- 10-ml syringe
- 0.5% lidocaine with epinephrine

Preliminary Actions

1. The bladder should be emptied by spontaneous micturition or drained by a catheter.
2. Prep the abdomen with providone-iodine and drape the area with sterile towels.

Procedure

1. Infiltrate the midline of the lower abdomen about 3 cm below the umbilicus using 0.5% lidocaine with epinephrine.
2. Make a stab wound at the site of the skin wheal (*A*).
3. Insert the peritoneal dialysis catheter and stylet into the incision and advance with firm pressure in a twisting motion until the peritoneum is entered. There will be a sudden lessening of resistance as the peritoneum is penetrated. Once the peritoneum is entered, withdraw the stylet 1 cm and direct the device at a 45-degree angle toward the lower abdomen (*B*).
4. Remove the stylet and connect the connector.
5. Attach the 10-ml syringe and aspirate the peritoneal cavity. If nonclotting blood is obtained, the study is positive and there is no indication for lavage (see Criteria for Positive Peritoneal Lavage, below). The procedure is then terminated.
6. If no blood is aspirated, attach the IV tubing to the connector and allow 1000 ml of normal saline or Ringer's lactate to infuse into the peritoneal cavity (*D*). (In children use 10 to 20 ml/kg of body weight.)
7. When the infusion is complete, turn the patient from side to side to diffuse the fluid.
8. Place the empty IV bottle on the floor and allow the intraperitoneal fluid to be siphoned (*E*).
9. Bloody fluid indicates positive lavage.
10. All lavage fluid may not be recovered. When the procedure is completed, close the stab wound with a single silk suture and apply a sterile dressing.
11. Analyze the recovered fluid for red blood cell count, amylase, and bile, and culture for bacteria.

Criteria for Positive Peritoneal Lavage

- Grossly bloody fluid
- Red blood cell count of >100,000/m^3
- White blood cell count of >500/m^3
- Amylase greater than 200 units
- Presence of bile, feces, or bacteria

Note: A rough index of the character of the lavage fluid is the ability to read newprint though the fluid. If newsprint can be read, the lavage is considered negative.

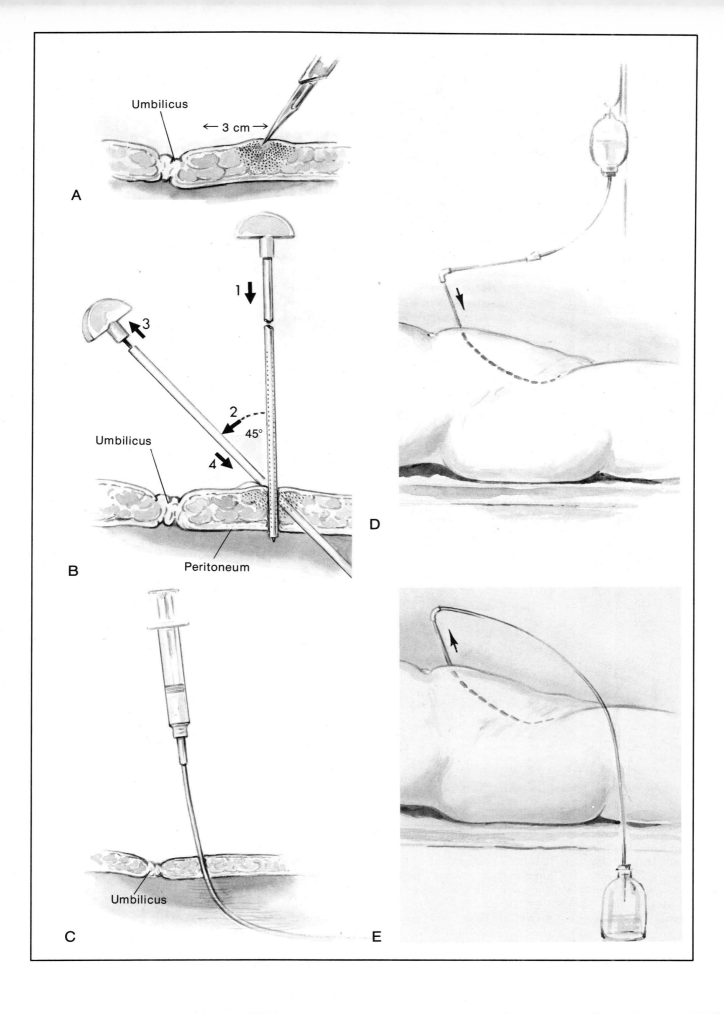

Umbilicus

← 3 cm →

A

1

3

2   45°

4

Umbilicus

Peritoneum

B

D

Umbilicus

C

E

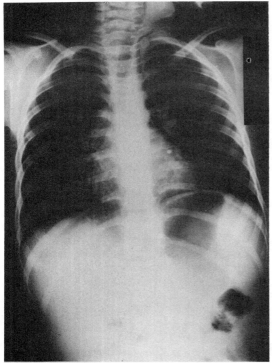

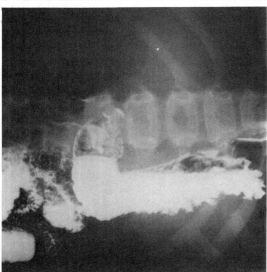

Figure 21-13 *Splenic rupture. Top. Flat film of abdomen of patient who fell, striking lower left chest. Note elevation of left diaphragm and large amount of air in stomach with medial displacement of the greater curvature. Bottom. Lateral decubitus x-ray after barium swallow. Stomach displaced upward by external mass. Patient had intraparenchymal rupture of the spleen.*

injury, is its mobility. For these reasons, perhaps only several hundred such injuries have been reported in the medical literature. The duodenum, on the other hand, is more exposed than the stomach. This is particularly true of its first portion. The second and third portions of the duodenum are in the retroperitoneal abdomen (see Chart 21-8). Most injuries to the organs follow penetrating or perforating wounds such as gunshot wounds. Severe crush injuries to

the upper abdomen may involve either of these organs by trapping them against the vertebral column. In the most severe cases, the stomach or duodenum can be transected. This constitutes a very serious injury, since adjacent structures, especially those in the retroperitoneal abdomen, may also be damaged.

Penetrating wounds invariably involve both the anterior and posterior walls of the stomach.

Assessment

Injuries to these organs are difficult to diagnose for two reasons. First, one does not suspect this rare injury. Second, initial signs and symptoms are misleadingly absent. Physical findings may vary from none to tenderness in the upper abdomen, with or without local spasm.

The most common duodenal injury is an intramural hematoma (a blood clot in the wall of the duodenum). Intramural hematomas vary in size, and if untreated the larger ones may result in obstruction of the upper intestinal tract. This diagnosis should be considered in any patient who has suffered upper abdominal trauma. Most blunt injuries occur in vehicular accidents, but have been seen following falls or sports injuries.

Management/Treatment

1. The management of these patients in the emergency department is directed primarily toward making a correct diagnosis and stabilizing the patient's condition.
2. Repeated observation with documentation of findings is important to proper evaluation of a patient suspected of having such an injury.
3. A nasogastric tube is inserted. The presence of blood in the nasogastric aspirate may point to a gastric or duodenal injury.
4. Blood samples are taken and should include an amylase determination, since the pancreas is frequently injured.
5. Parenteral fluids are started.
6. In patients whose abdominal findings are equivocal, peritoneal lavage is helpful in making a decision with regard to urgent laparotomy.
7. If the patient is stable, and the diagnosis is unclear, a meglumine diatrizoate (Gastrografin) study of the upper gastrointestinal tract is useful in delineating the extent of the injury.
8. Most blunt injuries are handled nonoperatively unless complications occur. Complications include:
   - Bleeding
   - Upper gastrointestinal obstruction
   - Duodenal fistula
   - Pancreatitis
9. Perforating wounds are managed surgically, the objective being to debride and remove devitalized tissue, repair tissue structures to the extent that it is feasible, or resect tissue that is too badly damaged to be reconstructed.

INJURIES TO THE PANCREAS

Injury to the pancreas is usually associated with blunt trauma and results from compression of the upper abdomen. The

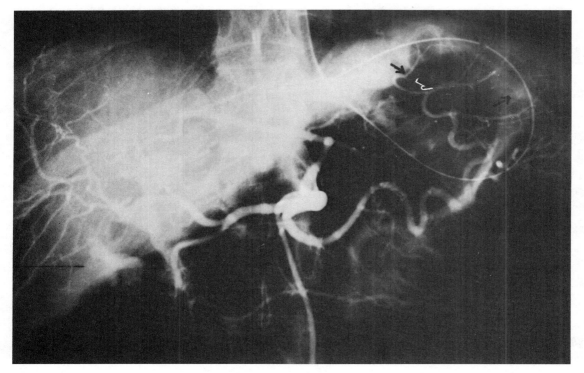

Figure 21-14 *Selective celiac arteriogram. This is an x-ray of the same patient as in Fig. 21-13. The arcuate appearance of splenic vessels (arrows) is abnormal and indicates hemorrhage within the spleen.*

pancreas lies in the retroperitoneal abdomen (Fig. 21-12). An anterior force such as a blow from a steering wheel or a fist, a kick, stomping on the abdomen, or sudden impact to the upper abdomen in a sports event may compress the pancreas against the vertebral column, resulting in a variety of injuries. There may be a simple contusion of the pancreas with rupture of minor branches of the ductal system or complete transection of the pancreas with leakage of pancreatic juice.

The serious nature of pancreatic injury is obvious from the mortality rate.[2] When combined with rupture of the duodenum, the mortality rate exceeds 70%.

Assessment

The diagnosis of pancreatic injury is difficult because of the organ's protected position in the retroperitoneal abdomen. A history of a blow or sudden impact in the upper abdomen should make one suspicious of pancreatic injury. The patient may complain of upper abdominal or epigastric pain.

Physical signs include abdominal tenderness and spasm in the upper abdomen. Peristaltic sounds may be diminished to absent.

The white blood cell count may be elevated. The serum amylase value is often elevated in pancreatic injury. It may

Figure 21-15 *Splenic scan. Lower arrow indicates homogenous density of normal spleen. Upper arrow indicates an area of lesser density, which is found with intraparenchymal hemorrhage of spleen. Hemorrhage was confirmed at laparotomy.*

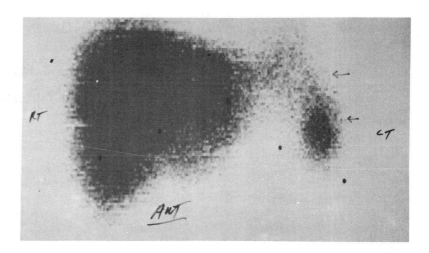

Chart 21-12

MANAGEMENT OF THE PATIENT WITH SPLENIC INJURY

Assessment

HISTORY

- Vehicular accident, fall, assault to abdomen or lower left rib cage
- Thoracoabdominal injury, left side
- Penetrating trauma to left upper quadrant of abdomen
- Pain in upper abdomen aggravated by respiration
- Pain in left shoulder (Kehr's sign)

PHYSICAL EXAMINATION

- Sign of peritoneal irritation, left upper quadrant
- Halting respiration
- Tenderness in left lower rib cage

ADJUNT STUDIES

- Three-way x-ray of abdomen—enlarged splenic shadow, displaced stomach bubble
- Selective splenic arteriogram
- Radionuclide scanning
- Positive peritoneal lavage

Management/Treatment

- Stabilize patient, monitor vital signs.
- Treatment may vary with age of patient.
  Children—many surgeons follow a nonoperative approach if the patient's condition is stable. If unstable, operative intervention is indicated. Every effort is made to preserve as much splenic tissue as possible. *Adults*—the matter of splenic preservation is more controversial. The decision whether to treat by nonoperative means or surgical intervention is left to the judgment and experience of the surgeon.

---

be within normal limits soon after the patient enters the emergency department, but repeat studies should be done 2 to 3 hours later. Gambill and Mason suggested that a determination of amylase in a 2-hour urine sample is a more reliable index of pancreatic injury than serum amylase.

X-ray studies are usually nonspecific, unless there is associated injury to other organs in the upper abdomen. The duodenum and spleen are often involved.

A nasogastric tube should be passed to decompress the upper gastrointestinal tract. Intravenous fluid replacement is begun and the patient carefully evaluated and reevaluated.

Management/Treatment

If the abdominal findings are equivocal, peritoneal lavage is indicated. When the lavage fluid contains amylase greater than 200 units, it is considered a positive lavage and is an indication for laparotomy. If the lavage is negative, a nonoperative approach is taken and the patient reassessed frequently. Should signs progress or the patient's condition deteriorate, surgical exploration is in order. At surgery, contusion of the pancreas may go unrecognized, and later a pancreatic pseudocyst may form.

The most common *major* injury is a fracture of the pancreas at the vertebral body. Complete transection results, and a distal pancreatectomy or drainage procedure into the bowel, such as a pancreaticojejunostomy, is required. For the patient who has an extensive injury involving the head of the pancreas and adjacent structures such as the duodenum, pancreaticoduodenectomy is the procedure of choice. The mortality rate in such injuries is high. An essential feature of any surgery directed at the pancreas is to establish maximally effective drainage of the area of injury. Postoperatively the patient is monitored closely. Management of the patient with an injured pancreas is summarized in Chart 21-13.

INJURIES TO THE SMALL BOWEL

Injuries to the small bowel are most commonly the result of penetrating wounds and are much less commonly associated with nonpenetrating trauma. It is estimated that in a large series of patients with blunt abdominal trauma, only 5% to 10% will have injuries to the small bowel.[20]

The mechanism of blunt injury to the small bowel involves its being crushed against the lordotic curvature of the lum-

---

Chart 21-13

MANAGEMENT OF THE PATIENT WITH PANCREATIC INJURY

History

- History of blunt injury to upper abdomen or back (steering wheel trauma, kick, fist, fall)
- Pain in upper abdomen and back
- Penetrating wound of upper abdomen

  PHYSICAL EXAMINATION

- Peritoneal irritation, especially in upper abdomen
- Diminished or absent peristaltic sounds

  ADJUNCT STUDIES

- Serum amylase usually elevated
- Two-hour urinary amylase elevated
- Peritoneal lavage fluid positive if amylase > 200 units

Management/Treatment

- Stabilize as in any patient with suspected intraabdominal injury.
- Give fluid replacement through large-bore veinways.
- If peritoneal lavage is negative, patient should be observed closely with frequent reassessment.
- Peritoneal lavage fluid containing amylase >200 units is an indication for laparotomy. Management of the injured pancreas depends on the specific nature of the injury to the pancreas and other structures.
- The main principles of surgical treatment of pancreatic injury are hemostasis, debridement, and drainage.

---

bosacral spine. It may follow a hard blow or kick to the abdomen but more often is due to an improperly positioned seat belt. With rapid deceleration, the restraint in effect pinches the small intestine and may actually lacerate the bowel wall or tear the mesentery. The injury often occurs at points of fixation of the intestine such as the ligament of Treitz or the terminal ileum as it attaches to the cecum, or at the point of postoperative adhesions to the anterior abdominal wall or pelvis. The mesenteric injuries may be so severe as to avulse the mesentery from the intestine over a considerable distance. A bursting injury to the intestine is extremely rare. Major vascular injuries to the mesenteric vessels are very unusual but may accompany a severe crushing injury to the abdomen.

Penetrating wounds from knives, ice picks, or guns may damage *any* area of the intestine and its mesentery.

Assessment

Major injury to the intestine or its mesentery causes the usual findings of damage to the abdominal viscera. Signs of peritoneal irritation, tenderness, rigidity, and spasm of the abdomen may be present. The patient usually complains of abdominal pain. Symptoms and signs of hypovolemic shock may also be noted.

Blood studies are rather nonspecific for this injury.

Three-way x-rays of the abdomen may reveal free air in the peritoneal cavity.

Treatment

If the findings on assessment and x-ray are not diagnostic, peritoneal lavage is indicated and, if the findings are positive, operative intervention is indicated. If the findings are negative, the patient should be observed closely for any change in status.

Treatment also consists of nasogastric decompression and intravenous fluid replacement.

At the time of surgery, operative management depends on the exact nature of the injury and varies from repair of a mesenteric defect with control of hemorrhage to resection of irreversibly damaged bowel. In most patients, it is possible to reconstruct the intestinal tract by primary anastomosis, but in rare instances, the ends of the damaged gut have to be brought out to the abdominal wall as a stoma. A secondary closure is performed when the patient's condition allows.

RETROPERITONEAL HEMATOMA

Retroperitoneal hematoma is a common finding in fractures of the lumbosacral vertebrae and pelvis and in injuries to the organs in the retroperitoneal abdomen. It is not usually viewed as a primary injury but as an indication of a serious injury to a retroperitoneal structure. Pelvic and vertebral fractures may account for 50% to 60% of retroperitoneal hematoma. Injuries to the kidney and bladder are next in order of frequency. In addition, injury to the pancreas or duodenum is often associated with a retroperitoneal hematoma. Tears of the major vessels (aorta or vena cava) may cause retroperitoneal hemorrhage and hematoma, but relatively few patients survive to reach the operating room.

Retroperitoneal hematoma signifies that a serious injury has occurred, but does not in itself dictate the need for surgical intervention. The retroperitoneal space extends the full length of the abdomen and can accommodate large amounts of blood, up to several liters. Thus, a patient with this finding may be in hypovolemic shock at the time of entry to the emergency department, or during the time of observation.

Assessment

The patient usually complains of abdominal or back pain. Signs of hypovolemia are often present, along with tenderness, rigidity, and spasm in the area of the hematoma. Peristaltic sounds may be reduced or absent. It is not unusual for a patient with this lesion to develop an adynamic or paralytic ileus. In severe cases, ecchymosis may be found in the flank areas, due to dissection of blood into the soft tissues.

Three-way x-rays of the abdomen usually reveal an absence of the psoas shadow indicative of retroperitoneal hemorrhage. Fractures of the spine or pelvis may be identified and should make one suspicious of this complication. If upper urinary tract damage is considered likely, an excretory urogram is necessary.

Laboratory studies are usually inconclusive, except for the finding of reduced hematocrit in patients with severe blood loss. When pancreatic injury is present, the serum amylase may be elevated. If the upper urinary tract has been damaged, microscopic or gross hematuria is usually found.

Peritoneal lavage, as expected, is negative in a pure retroperitoneal hematoma without soiling of the peritoneal cavity.

Management

The management of retroperitoneal hematoma depends on the type and severity of the associated injury. Those associated with fractures of the lumbar spine alone are not explored. Those associated with injuries of the great vessels, duodenum, or pancreas usually require surgical exploration, as do those related to serious pelvic fracture. The decision to explore or not to explore a retroperitoneal hematoma is usually made by the surgeon at the time of laparotomy. The surgeon faces a dilemma: If the hematoma is not explored, an injury to a major organ or vessel can be missed; however, exploration of the hematoma may disrupt the clot and provoke uncontrollable bleeding.

INJURIES TO THE COLON AND RECTUM

By far the greatest number of injuries to the colon and rectum occur as the result of penetrating or perforating trauma. Such injuries can follow missile injuries of the abdomen, back, or buttocks. Blunt trauma to the colon accounts for only 3 to 5 percent of all blunt abdominal injuries. The amount of blunt force required to damage the colon is considerable and usually causes many other injuries in the process. The colon may be injured by compression, as in deceleration injuries associated with wearing a seat belt. The rectum may be damaged by pelvic fracture or perforated by an enema tip or any number of foreign bodies that might be inserted into the rectum in the course of self-medication or erotic perversion.

Assessment

The history usually involves some injury to the abdomen, be it blunt or penetrating.

The signs and symptoms are not specific for injury to the colon and rectum. Signs of peritoneal irritation, tenderness, rigidity, and spasm may or may not be found. This is particularly true in injuries of the extraperitoneal portions of the colon and rectum.

Laboratory studies are not helpful.

Three-way films of the abdomen may demonstrate free air in the peritoneal cavity.

Peritoneal lavage is of great value in intraperitoneal colon injury. The return fluid may reveal blood or bacteria. If the damage is confined to the extraperitoneal colon or rectum, lavage is of limited value and may be considered negative.

Extraperitoneal colon or rectal injury may be extremely difficult to diagnose. A high degree of suspicion on the part of the examiner is important. Consider the possibility of rectal injury in any patient with penetrating trauma to the lower abdomen or buttocks. Digital examination of the rectum is an important part of the assessment of a patient with abdominal injury and particularly of one suspected of having an injury to the colon or rectum. The presence of blood on the examining finger is strong evidence for colon or rectal injury. Proctoscopic or sigmoidoscopic examination should be performed as well.

Management

The management of injuries to the colon and rectum varies according to the location of the wound, be it intraperitoneal or extraperitoneal.

Intraperitoneal Injuries to the Colon

The management of intraperitoneal wounds of colon is influenced by several factors, especially the nature of the bowel injury itself. Generally, treatment is operative. Perforating or penetrating injuries are more obvious and usually reach the operating room earlier, whereas in blunt injury the problem may not be recognized until later in the patient's course. The time between wounding and surgical exploration influences the severity of the problem and the procedure required. The presence and nature of any associated injury and the general status of the patient must be considered in planning the operative care of such a patient. The colon, more than any other segment of the gastrointestinal tract, has the highest bacteria count among its contents. Soilage of the peritoneal cavity by feces is a serious complication associated with high morbidity and significant mortality.

Large doses of broad-spectrum antibiotics should be given by the intravenous route in the emergency department and at appropriate intervals during the period of observation. Furthermore, antibiotics may be given at the time of surgery, including instillation into the peritoneal cavity.

The general principles of surgical management have been outlined earlier but will be repeated here. Damaged tissue is thoroughly debrided, devitalized tissue is removed, the injured segment of intestine is removed or repaired as conditions allow, and intestinal continuity is restored by primary intestinal anastomosis or the intestine is brought out on the abdominal wall as a stoma. The procedure chosen depends on the findings at the time of exploration.

In injury to the right colon, resection is sometimes feasible and continuity is restored by ileotransverse colostomy. If the reconstruction cannot be accomplished, then the terminal ileum and colon may be brought out as end stomas. Sometimes the injury can be closed by suture and vented by a cecostomy. The fecal stream in the right colon is liquid for the most part, and primary repair can be accomplished with a greater degree of success.

Penetrating wounds of the colon can best be treated by exteriorization of the damaged segment on the abdominal wall. In wounds of the left side of the colon, the principles of care are the same. The fecal stream in this segment of the colon is more formed and solid and presents a more difficult problem. Proximal colostomy must be done in conjunction with any resection or repair of wounds to the left colon. The right side of the transverse colon is the usual site for the colostomy. This is a temporary stoma that is later closed after healing of the colon repair is complete. For patients who may require a colostomy, preoperative explanation of this procedure should be provided to the patient or family, even though the colostomy is only temporary.

Extraperitoneal Injuries to the Rectum

These injuries may present fewer clinical signs than the intraperitoneal variety. The bowel is fixed, and there may be associated injury to other structures in the pelvis such as the urinary bladder. The problem may be complicated when the defect in the rectum is large or displaced fractures of the pelvis are present. The fecal stream in this segment of colon is solid and difficult to manage in surgically unprepared bowel.

Exploration of the damaged segment of bowel is carried out through an abdominal approach. The entire space about the rectum must be evaluated along with the bladder and, in females, the reproductive organs. Foreign bodies, if present, must be removed, the rectum debrided and closed if possible, and a proximal diverting colostomy performed to vent the repair site. The rectum should be cleansed of all stool by manual extraction and irrigation. Adequate drainage of the space behind the rectum must be established by insertion of large rubber tissue drains brought out through the perineum adjacent to the coccyx. The temporary colostomy is closed later, when the rectal wounds have healed. Management of a patient with such an injury is difficult for both the patient and surgeon; months are required before healing is complete.

REFERENCES

1. Ayella RJ, Hankins JR, Turney SZ, Cowley RA: Ruptured thoracic aorta due to blunt trauma. J Trauma 17:199–205
2. Bach RD, Frey CF: Diagnosis and treatment of pancreatic trauma. Am J Surg 121:20, 1971
3. Baker CC, Thomas AN, Trunkey DD: The role of an emergency room thoracotomy in trauma. J Trauma 20:848–855, 1980
4. Collicott P, Gillespie R: A primer in trauma care: Abdominal trauma. Emerg Med 12:93–102, 1980
5. Engrave LH, Benjamin CI, Strate RG, Perry JF Jr: Diagnostic peritoneal lavage in blunt abdominal trauma. J Trauma 15:854–859, 1975
6. Galbraith TA et al: The role of peritoneal lavage in the management of stab wounds to the abdomen. Am J Surg 140:60–64, 1980
7. Grimes OF: Injuries to the chest wall and esophagus. Surg Clin North Am 52:597–610, 1972
8. Hale HW Jr et al: Symposium on blunt abdominal trauma. Contemp Surg 10:39–52, 1977
9. Holmes TW Jr, Netterville RE: Complications of first rib fracture including one case each of tracheoesophageal fistula and aortic arch aneurysm. J Thorac Surg 32:74–91, 1966
10. Layton TR, Dimarco RF, Pellegrini RV: Tracheoesophageal fistula from nonpenetrating trauma. J Trauma 20:802–805, 1980
11. Lindsey D, Navin TR, Finley PR: Transient elevation of serum activity of MB-isoenzyme of creatine phosphokinase in drivers involved in auto accidents. Chest 74:15–18, 1978
12. Lucas CE, Ledgerwood AM: Factors influencing outcome after blunt abdominal trauma. J Trauma 15:839–846, 1975
13. Marleta R, Jones JW: CPK-MB isoenzyme determinations in blunt chest trauma. JACEP 8:304–306, 1979
14. Mattox KL: Diagnosis and management of hepatic trauma. Hosp Med 92–99, 1977
15. Mattox KL: Emergency department thoracotomy. JACEP 7:455, 1978
16. McDonald JR, McDowell RM: Emergency department thoracotomies in a community hospital. JACEP 7:423–428, 1978
17. McSwain NE Jr: Visual examination for blunt abdominal trauma. JACEP 6:56–57, 1977
18. Michelson WB: CPK-MB isoenzyme determinations: Diagnostic and prognostic value in evaluation of blunt chest trauma. JACEP 9:562–67, 1980
19. Millikan JC et al: Temporary cardiac pacing in traumatic arrest victims. JACEP 9:591–593, 1980
20. Orloff NJ, Charters AC: Injuries of the small bowel and mesentery and retroperitoneal hematoma. Surg Clin North Am 52:729–734, 1972
21. Peters RM: The Mechanical Basis of Respiration. Boston, Little, Brown & Co, 1969
22. Sherman R: Perspectives in management of trauma to the spleen: 1979 presidential address, American Association for the Surgery of Trauma. J Trauma 20:1–13, 1980
23. Siemens R, Polk HC Jr, Gray LA et al: Indications for thoracotomy following penetrating thoracic injury. J Trauma 17:493–500, 1977
24. Tibbs PA, Young AB, Bivins BA, Sachatello CR: Diagnosis of acute abdominal injuries in patients with spinal shock: Value of diagnostic peritoneal lavage. J Trauma 20:55–57, 1980
25. Wilson RF, Murray C, Antonenico DR: Nonpenetrating thoracic injuries. Surg Clin North Am 57:17–37, 1977

22
CARE OF THE PATIENT WITH AN ACUTE ABDOMEN

JAMES H. COSGRIFF, JR. and DIANN ANDERSON

ANATOMY AND PHYSIOLOGY

The abdomen is the largest single body cavity. It contains a number of hollow and solid viscera and is lined by a continuous layer of tissue, the parietal peritoneum, that also extends as a cover on the outside of the viscera, the visceral peritoneum. The abdominal cavity is frequently referred to as the peritoneal cavity. Its boundaries are the pleural diaphragm above and the pelvic diaphragm below.

The nerve supply of the visceral peritoneum is derived from the autonomic nervous system; the parietal portion receives its innervation from the peripheral nerves. An understanding of the extent of the peritoneal reflections and their innervation sheds light on the symptom complexes that develop during acute intra-abdominal conditions. Stimulation of the visceral peritoneum occurs with distention of hollow viscera or traction on mesenteric attachments. The resultant pain, conveyed by the autonomic nervous system, is vague and often poorly localized. In contrast, stimulation of the parietal peritoneum by direct contact with an inflamed organ or irritant fluid (blood, pus, gastrointestinal contents) results in pain that is localized to the exact point or area of contact. This pain may move or radiate along the course of the peripheral nerve.

To illustrate this, the pain in early appendicitis is usually poorly localized to the midabdomen and is periumbilical in location, because of an increase in intra-abdominal pressure and distention of the appendix, a hollow organ. As the inflammatory process spreads through the wall of the appendix and reaches the serosal (outer) surface, contact is made with the adjacent parietal peritoneum. The peripheral nerve is thus stimulated and the pain becomes localized to the site of irritation (usually the right lower quadrant).

Innervation of the parietal peritoneum conforms to the distribution of the peripheral nerves. For practical purposes, the umbilicus is located at the level of the 10th intercostal nerve. The innervation of the upper quadrants of the abdomen extends between the 6th and 10th nerves. The superior boundary of the parietal peritoneum, which covers the undersurface (abdominal aspect) of the pleural diaphragm, is innervated by branches of the phrenic nerve, which originates from the 4th, 5th, and 6th cervical nerves.

Because of this nerve distribution, irritation of specific areas of the parietal peritoneum may result in pain at the site; stimulation of the peripheral nerve at this site may extend along the entire length of the nerve, resulting in pain at a remote site—referred pain. A common example of this phenomenon is the frequent association of pain related to inflammatory conditions of the gallbladder arising in the right upper quadrant with radiation along the distribution of the right 8th intercostal nerve to the tip of the right scapula. Fig. 22-1 illustrates common sites of referred pain. Just as pain originating from diseased organs within the abdomen may be referred elsewhere, so may pain arising from other areas, such as the thoracic contents, be referred to the abdomen, because of cross-innervation.

Topography. Knowledge of the location of the organs within the peritoneal cavity is essential for the proper assessment of patients with abdominal pain. Topographically, the abdominal wall is bounded by the costal (rib) margin above and the inguinal ligaments below. The inguinal ligament attaches to the anterior superior iliac spine of the pelvis above and laterally, and to the pubic tubercle in the area of the midline of the symphysis below and medially. This ligament conforms roughly to the inguinal (flexion) crease at the upper end of each thigh. The lateral borders of the abdomen conform roughly to a line extending from the lateral edge of the costal margin in line with the axilla to the lateral border of the pelvis. Internally, the peritoneal cavity actually extends beyond these topographical limits, as do its organs.

The pleural diaphragm separates the peritoneal cavity from the thoracic cavity at approximately the 6th intercostal space. It is divided into a left and a right hemidiaphragm, commonly referred to as the left and the right diaphragm.

Figure 22-1 *Referred pain. A. anterior view; B. posterior view. (Chaffee EE, Lytle IM, Basic Physiology and Anatomy, 4th ed. Philadelphia, J.B. Lippincott, 1980)*

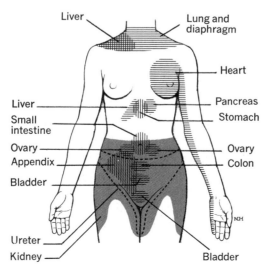

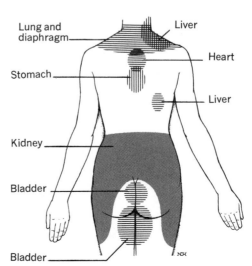

To identify the location of organs within the peritoneal cavity, divide the abdomen into four quadrants by dropping an imaginary vertical line from the xyphoid cartilage to the symphysis pubis (in the midline) and intersecting it with a horizontal line between the iliac crests crossing through the umbilicus (see Chart 22-1).

The upper abdomen contains both solid and hollow viscera. Those in the lower half are hollow. Some organs, the liver for example, are large and extend into two quadrants. The pancreas and kidneys are actually retroperitoneal in location but when inflamed usually produce symptoms of peritoneal irritation.

ASSESSMENT

HISTORY

The history of the illness is vital in assessing the patient with an acute abdominal condition. Careful attention must be given to developing the history in chronologic sequence, with particular stress on the time of onset, and the nature and duration of symptom(s).

Pain is perhaps the most common complaint associated with the abdominal organs. An accurate description of the pain is needed. Elicit information from the patient about the quality of his pain—is it sharp, dull, aching, crampy, burning, pressure-like? Ask whether the pain is continuous, intermittent, or constant intensity, or rising to a crescendo, diminishing, then increasing again. Ask in what part of the abdomen the pain began and whether it radiates or is referred to another area. If the pain moves, does it penetrate (go through) or go around the abdomen to the back? Is it associated with or aggravated by food intake, physical activity, or any increase in intra-abdominal pressure (breathing, coughing, straining, micturition, defecation)? The occurrence of related symptoms (malaise, nausea, vomiting, alteration in bowel or bladder regularity) may be of further assistance in localizing the source of the symptoms to a specific site or organ. Pain patterns associated with acute abdominal disorders are shown in Figure 22-2.

For quick recall of all the parameters of pain assessment, it is helpful to use the PQRST format, in which each letter represents an important measurement.

P	provocation	What initiates or aggravates the pain or makes it worse?
Q	quality	Is is sharp, dull, crampy, heavy, burning, etc. The patient's own description of the quality of pain is significant and should be communicated
R	region radiation referred	Where is the pain felt? Where does the pain go? Is it felt at a distant site?
S	severity	What degree of discomfort is produced by the pain?
T	time	When does the pain occur? How frequently? Is it intermittent or constant?

This format may be used to assess abdominal pain as well as pain elsewhere in the body. A perspective on pain evaluation and management of the patient with pain is presented later in this chapter.

In female patients, a history of menstrual activity is necessary. The date of the last menstrual period and whether it was normal should be noted. If it was abnormal, was this related to duration, time of onset, amount of blood loss, or unusual pain associated with it?

The past history is vital. Information should be sought about any previous illnesses, particularly any abdominal condition or prior surgery or x-rays involving the abdominal organs (*i.e.,* upper gastrointestinal series, barium enema, gallbladder series). Prior x-rays may be valuable in establishing a diagnosis.

PHYSICAL EXAMINATION

The physical assessment of the patient with an acute abdomen should begin when the patient is first seen, continue during the history taking, and be completed with the physical examination itself.

The conditions required for a good abdominal examination include adequate lighting, full exposure of the abdomen, and a relaxed patient. The last condition may be the most difficult to achieve when the patient has acute abdominal pain, since analgesics generally are withheld until the examination is completed. A gentle, reassuring approach will be helpful. To further achieve relaxation, the following guidelines are useful:
- The patient's bladder should be empty.
- A pillow placed under the patient's head and knees will relax the abdominal musculature
- The patient's arms should be folded over the chest or at the side, not under the head.
- It helps if the stethoscope and the examiner's hands are warm and the examiner's fingernails are short.
- Approach slowly and gently, starting from pain-free areas. Palpate tender areas last.
- Distract the patient with conversation or questions.
- If the patient is frightened or ticklish, begin palpation with his hand under your hand.
- Monitor evaluation by watching the patient's face.

Inspection

Initially, observe the patient's position. Frequently the knees will be drawn up to lessen tension on the peritoneum and to decrease intra-abdominal pressure. Next, observe the movement of the abdomen.

Respiration. In males and in infants, respiration is primarily abdominal, by diaphragmatic movement. With inspiration, the diaphragm descends to expand the lung, decreasing the size of the abdominal cavity and increasing intra-abdominal pressure. The anterior abdominal wall protrudes and then falls as the diaphragm rises with expiration. This motion may be sharply curtailed or absent with peritoneal irritation.

Chart 22-1

CONTENTS OF ABDOMEN

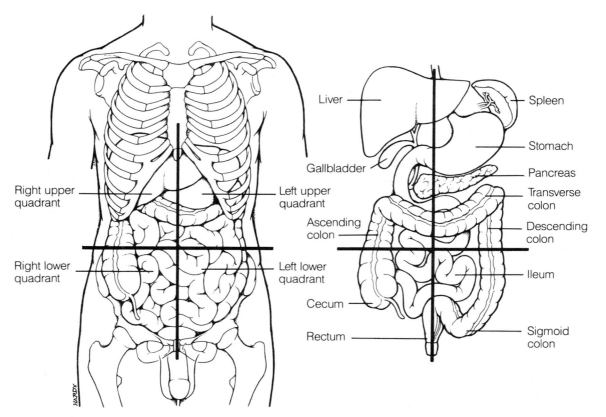

Right Upper Quadrant

- Liver
- Gallbladder
- Extrahepatic bile ducts (cystic, hepatic, common)
- Duodenum
- Head of pancreas
- Right side of transverse colon
- Hepatic flexure of colon
- Right kidney and adrenal

Right Lower Quadrant

- Ascending colon
- Cecum
- Appendix
- Lower small bowel (ileum)
- Right ureter

Lower Midline

RETROPERITONEAL FEMALES

- Urinary bladder
- Uterus, ovaries, fallopian tubes, broad ligaments

Left Upper Quadrant

- Left lobe of liver
- Abdominal portion of esophagus
- Stomach
- Spleen
- Body and tail of pancreas
- Left side of transverse colon
- Splenic flexure of colon
- Left kidney and adrenal

Left Lower Quadrant

- Descending colon
- Sigmoid colon
- Upper portion of rectosigmoid
- Left ureter

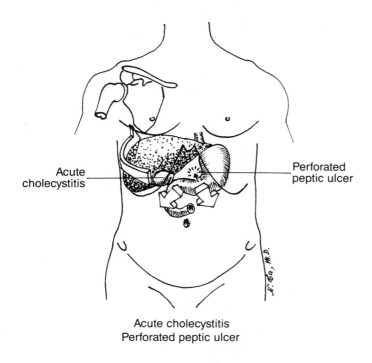

Acute cholecystitis

Perforated peptic ulcer

Acute cholecystitis
Perforated peptic ulcer

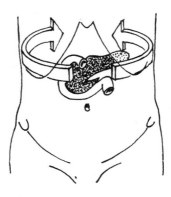

Acute pancreatitis

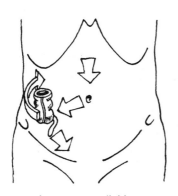

Acute appendicitis

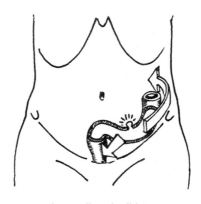

Acute diverticulitis

Figure 22-2 *Pain patterns in acute abdominal disorders.*

In females, respiratory activity is effected primarily by expansion of the chest wall with the thoracic muscles rather than the diaphragm. Respiratory activity during an acute abdominal episode may be described as halting, as the patient takes short, gasping breaths. Similarly, respiratory movements may be restricted by splinting, in which short inspirations are seen.

Peristalsis. Observing for peristalsis may take several minutes; peristalsis may not be visible unless the patient is thin. Peristaltic waves, when observed, may indicate intestinal obstruction.

Pulsations. Pulsations can normally be seen in the epigastrium, corresponding with pulsations of the aorta. When pulsations are increased or are seen elsewhere, an aneurysm or bleeding from an arterial source may be the cause.

Architecture. Observe the contour and symmetry of the abdomen for masses, hernias, ascites, etc.

Skin. Skin overlying the abdomen may yield additional information; check for scars, striae, dilated veins, rashes, or lesions.

Auscultation

Auscultation should precede percussion and palpation of the abdomen: the intestine is sensitive to touch, and these maneuvers may alter the frequency or intensity of bowel sounds.

With the stethoscope, listen in all four quadrants of the abdomen and the epigastrium for 2 to 5 minutes to determine the frequency and character of bowel sounds. The frequency and intensity vary according to the phase of digestion; but typically, clicks and gurgles, occurring from 5 to 34 times per minute, are heard. *Borborygmi*—loud, prolonged gurgles of hyperperistalsis (the familiar "stomach growling")—may be heard.

Bowel sounds may be increased with early intestinal obstruction or conditions causing diarrhea, and may be diminished or absent with peritonitis or paralytic ileus. Abdominal pain, in itself, may cause diminished bowel sounds.

Percussion

Percussion is used to assess the general proportions and distribution of tympany and dullness. Tympany, heard over hollow organs, predominates; dullness is normally heard over solid organs like the liver and spleen. Deviations from the normal air and fluid levels may be helpful in establishing a diagnosis.

Palpation

Palpation is done alternately with percussion by some examiners. Two forms exist: light palpation to identify muscular resistance, abdominal tenderness, and some superficial organs and masses, and deep palpation to delineate less superficial abdominal organs and masses.

Palpation is done with the pads of the fingers in a light, gentle, slightly dipping motion. Palpate smoothly in all four quadrants to identify any masses or areas of tenderness or increased resistance. If *resistance* is present, determine whether it is voluntary (guarding) or involuntary (spasm). Voluntary guarding results from purposeful splinting of the abdominal musculature to avoid additional pain. Relaxation of these muscles normally occurs with expiration. If rigidity persists throughout respiration despite the use of relaxation techniques discussed previously, involuntary spasm probably exists, suggesting peritoneal irritation.

Tenderness. Tenderness may be direct (that elicited in the area being examined) or referred (elicited in an area remote from that being examined). Rebound tenderness is checked by slowly pressing the fingers into the tender area and quickly withdrawing them. Rebound tenderness is noted when pain is felt during the withdrawal maneuver. It is an important sign of peritoneal irritation.

Masses. Evaluate any masses in the abdomen; check size, shape, whether the mass is movable or attached, and whether it moves with respiration (respiratory mobile). Note also whether it pulsates or merely transmits a pulsation. A pulsating mass alternately expands and contracts, whereas one transmitting a pulsation merely moves; it does not expand. (See Fig. 17-8, p 281.)

All operative scars should be palpated to be sure of complete healing. Any defect or mass in the scar may indicate a hernia. Hernias are more evident when a patient is standing or sitting, rather than lying supine.

Pelvic and Rectal Examination

Pelvic examination in the female is useful in assessing abdominal symptoms and is necessary for complete evaluation.

A rectal examination in all patients, including virginal females is also necessary for complete evaluation of abdominal complaints.

ADJUNCT STUDIES

Adjunct studies can be of enormous value in assessing the patient with abdominal pain, but with a few exceptions, they rarely establish a diagnosis. They are also costly and should be selected discriminately. Studies useful in assessing the patient with abdominal pain include the following:
1. *Laboratory*
   - Complete blood count (CBC)
   - Urinalysis
   - Serum electrolytes (SMA-6)
   - Serum amylase and lipase
   - Serum transaminases
   - Arterial blood gases
2. *X-ray*
   - Flat and upright films of the abdomen. In acutely ill or debilitated patients, a lateral decubitus, rather than an upright, x-ray is taken
   - Intravenous pyelogram (IVP)
   - Abdominal angiogram
3. *Other*
   - Peritoneal tap; either a flank tap or a four-quadrant tap of the abdomen
   - Peritoneal lavage
   - Cul-de-sac aspiration

The indications for the use of these adjunct studies will be listed with each disease entity.

PAIN EVALUATION AND MANAGEMENT

Pain is the symptom that most frequently brings the patient to the emergency department; both the patient and the health care team expect it to be alleviated. It is important not only to determine the cause of the patient's pain, but also to identify the best method, or combination of methods, to relieve that pain.

Any attempt to evaluate pain must begin with the recognition that many factors influence the perception, response, and reporting of pain. Pain has at least two identifiable, though interrelated, components: a sensory component and a response component. The sensory component, which includes the location of the pain, its quality, intensity, and chronology, has similarities from person to person, and these commonalities aid in the diagnosis and treatment of the underlying cause.

The response component, however, can vary markedly among individuals and is influenced by psychosocial factors such as personality, cultural background, and prior experiences. Awareness of the patient's responses to his pain is also helpful in determining the best means for alleviating it. The following guidelines may be useful in evaluating and managing pain:
- Accept the patient's perception of pain—that it exists to the degree of discomfort that he says it does. The intensity of the pain may not correspond to the severity of the cause—mild pain may occur with a serious problem, and vice-versa. Whatever the cause, relief from the pain the patient is experiencing is indicated as soon as possible.

- Recognize that responses to pain vary—be sensitive to clues from the patient and to your own intuition. The patient's behavior may belie his words. Frequently, the patient will understate his pain (for fear of hospitalization, surgery, or appearing out of control) only to reveal its severity by his body language—body position, restlessness, facial grimace, quietness and preoccupation with being still, irritability, or emotional lability. Vital signs may become elevated, or with vasovagal stimulation secondary to pain, the pulse and blood pressure may fall, producing syncope.

- Discuss with the patient how the pain has affected him and his activities and how he has coped with it in the past. Information about measures that have been successful or futile and types and amounts of medications taken for past pain may affect his present treatment.

- Discuss with the patient how he feels his pain can best be relieved. His ideas about pain relief may not be consistent with the medical and nursing plan, but exploring them with the patient will lead to a better outcome: pain reduction is more effective when the patient has been involved in decision-making about his pain relief. Discussing his pain and pain-reducing measures also helps reduce the patient's anxiety, which in turn helps him tolerate pain better.

- Let the patient know when and how he can expect relief from pain. Analgesics are often withheld during the diagnostic process, to avoid masking pertinent signs and symptoms. However, knowing that an analgesic *will* be given after the surgeon arrives, or after a specific test or activity, assures the patient that relief *will* come at a specific time.

- Use techniques known to relieve pain—elevation of the part for edema of traumatic injuries, oxygen for chest pain and dyspnea, body positioning, heat or cold, various relaxation techniques, massage, distraction all have a role in pain reduction. The method or combination of methods that the patient has found successful or feels will work, may well be the best choice.

ACUTE AND CHRONIC PAIN

The patient with acute pain is no stranger to the emergency department; but neither is the patient with chronic pain. Though their pain may be equal in intensity, their responses are different.

Persons with chronic pain appear to tolerate pain, although they never become accustomed to it. Chronic pain is wearing, and as physical and mental depletion occurs with time, the smallest amount of additional discomfort may become intolerable. Feelings of depression and increased fatigue are common as the patient's ability to cope with pain reaches its limits. Often, because the cause of the pain is obscure or not amenable to treatment, certain pain-reducing therapies may be indicated, such as hypnotherapy, biofeedback, relaxation techniques, and various modes of physical therapy.

By contrast, the patient in acute pain generally expects complete restoration to his previous pain-free state. He expects total relief, since the cause is usually self-limiting or can be corrected. Acute pain is more frequently accompanied by feelings of anxiety and of urgency to eliminate the pain.

Management of Acute Pain

Acute pain is most effectively relieved by the use of analgesics, usually narcotics. Once the diagnosis is made, an analgesic is prescribed, depending on the nature of the pain and its underlying cause.

A sufficient dose of the selected analgesic must be administered to provide relief from acute pain. Recent studies suggest that patients are commonly undertreated for acute pain: physicians tend to underprescribe by ordering doses that are too low or intervals that are too long, and nurses tend to give less than the amount prescribed. Higher doses may be indicated for the patient with an acute painful episode and for the drug-tolerant person in acute pain.

A history of pain-reducing methods, dose, and degree of effectiveness should be obtained as a baseline. Then the patient is given the dose of narcotic within the recommended range and is monitored to determine effectiveness. An additional dose may be needed to obtain sufficient pain reduction: usually, acute pain is not completely alleviated, but with an adequate dose the patient can be made comfortable. Other considerations to keep in mind when administering narcotics are listed in Chart 22-2.

SPECIFIC CONDITIONS THAT CAUSE AN ACUTE ABDOMEN: ASSESSMENT AND MANAGEMENT

PERFORATED PEPTIC ULCER

Perforation is one of the main complications of peptic ulcer and represents a most urgent indication for treatment.[13] It can occur wherever an ulcer may occur, in the esophagus, the stomach, the duodenum or at the site of a marginal ulcer, which may follow certain types of surgery for peptic ulcer.[10,46]

Rupture of an esophageal ulcer is extremely rare and extremely difficult to diagnose. Symptoms may relate to the upper abdomen or lower retrosternal area, depending on the site of perforation.

Perforations of gastric or duodenal ulcers are much more common, owing to the higher incidence of ulcers in these locations. Most perforations occur in anterior wall ulcers and allow egress of air and gastric and intestinal content into the peritoneal cavity. The highly acid content is extremely irritating to the peritoneum and causes a "chemical" peritonitis, with outpouring of peritoneal fluid.[42] As hours pass, secondary bacterial contamination of the fluid may occur and a purulent peritonitis may develop.

- Contamination of peritoneal fluid is an extremely serious complication, and hypovolemic shock may be produced by the outpouring of body fluid into the peritoneal cavity and subsequent diminution of circulating blood volume.[20]

- Patients in whom this occurs are critically ill on admission to the emergency department, and prompt resuscitative measures to restore circulating blood volume are necessary.

Assessment

History and physical examination are extremely important in diagnosis. The onset of pain is usually sudden. The pain is described as severe, sharp, constant, and located in the

---

Chart 22-2

CONSIDERATIONS IN THE ADMINISTRATION OF NARCOTICS

- Medications administered parenterally relieve pain more rapidly and are absorbed more effectively than those administered orally. With oral administration, codeine is one-half to one-third as effective, meperidine is one-fourth as effective, and morphine is one-sixth to one-fifteenth as effective as the same drugs administered parenterally. Thus, a higher oral dose is needed to produce the same analgesic effect as the parenteral dose of the same drug.

- Intravenous routes are indicated for the patient who is hypotensive or when circulation has been slowed by cold, paralysis, or edema. Once normal circulation has been restored, deposits of im or sc medications could suddenly overload the system, producing toxic or lethal effects.

- The analgesic effect of narcotics is increased when the narcotic is used in combination with other methods known to alleviate pain, such as nonnarcotic analgesics, relaxation techniques, and cutaneous stimulation.

- A repeated dose of analgesic should be administered at once when the pain begins to return, not delayed until it becomes severe. Ask the patient about his pain instead of waiting for him to mention it. Many patients do not speak out until their pain is intense, necessitating a higher dose for adequate pain reduction.

- The duration of action depends on the drug and the route of administration. For example, meperidine has a short duration of action compared with that of morphine and may have to be repeated more often. Drugs administered by oral route generally have a longer duration of action than those given parenterally although onset and peak of action are less rapid.

- Administer narcotics to patients with underlying chronic lung disease with caution: the respiratory depressant effect of narcotics, coupled with the patient's compromised respiratory reserve, may preclude the more aggressive treatment of acute pain advocated above.

- Keep naloxone available for the unforeseen. A small dose (0.1 mg to 0.4 mg) may be administered IV at 2- to 3-minute intervals to offset respiratory depression without altering the analgesic effect. Mechanical ventilation should be used simultaneously.

- Provide a safe environment (bedrails, etc.) because narcotic analgesics induce peripheral vasodilatation and the patient may develop orthostatic hypotension.

- Before administering narcotics, elicit a history of allergies. Anaphylactic reactions are rare but can occur. Allergic reactions generally take the form of urticaria and other types of skin reactions.

  Note. the dose of analgesic and intervals between them must be determined by individual patient response. If the given dose provides inadequate pain relief, generally it should be increased. If the pain is relieved for periods shorter than the prescribed intervals, the interval should be shortened. Periodic assessment of the degree of pain reduction is essential in determining adequate therapy. Patients with chronic rather than acute pain need alternative methods to assist in pain reduction.

(After Goodman, Gilman. In McCafferty M, Hart LL: Am J Nurs 76:1586–1591, 1976)

---

upper abdomen. About 70% of patients give a history of prior ulcer activity or use of antacids; thus, 30% may have no previous ulcer symptoms. These statistics are important; they stress the value of assessment.

Physical examination often reveals restricted diaphragmatic activity. The abdomen demonstrates board-like rigidity due to spasm of the anterior abdominal muscles. The spasm is primarily in the upper abdomen, more often on the right side because of the location of the duodenum. Perforated gastric ulcers in the antral portion of the stomach may also exhibit findings in this area. Peristalsis is diminished or absent.

Vital signs should be noted and recorded, along with evaluation of the patient's general condition. Thirst and poor skin turgor indicate dehydration and a decrease in circulating blood volume. Blood samples are drawn for CBC and electrolyte determination. Baseline arterial blood gas levels may be helpful in future management. Flat and upright x-ray examination of the abdomen may demonstrate free air in 50% to 80% of cases (Fig. 22-3). In the critically ill or debilitated patient, lateral decubitus films taken with the patient lying on the left side will show free air, when present, above the lateral edge of the liver shadow (Fig. 22-4).

Management/Treatment

Preliminary resuscitation in the emergency department is directed toward stabilizing the patient by restoring circulating blood volume. Intravenous fluid replacement should be instituted promptly, using glucose in saline or a balanced salt solution. Antibiotics are not required for chemical peritonitis but are necessary when bacterial contamination is suspected. A nasogastric tube is inserted and, after aspiration of gastric content, placed on intermittent suction to prevent further spillage into the peritoneal cavity. Peritoneal tap is unnecessary, except when the diagnosis is not clear.

The treatment of choice for perforated ulcer is surgery.[7,8,27,43]

The most common surgical procedure is simple closure of the leaking ulcer and cleansing of the peritoneal cavity.[42] Definitive ulcer surgery may not be indicated until several weeks to months after simple closure. Primary gastric resection for perforated ulcer has been performed with an acceptable morbidity and mortality rate.[24,29,38] However, indications for this procedure are limited by strict criteria, including the availability of a capable surgical team.

Care of the patient with a perforated peptic ulcer is summarized in Chart 22-3.

RUPTURE OF THE SPLEEN

Although rupture of the spleen is covered thoroughly in Chapter 21 in relation to trauma, patients with splenic rupture due to other causes may be seen in the emergency department with no history of trauma *per se.*

Diseases causing splenomegaly (enlargement of the spleen) often result in rupture of this organ.[28,34] Delayed rupture (weeks to months after initial trauma) may occur in instances of splenic injury resulting in a splenic hematoma. Internal rupture of the spleen, causing bleeding within an intact capsule, may go unrecognized until rupture of the capsule occurs, with bleeding into the free peritoneal cavity. Spontaneous rupture may also occur, frequently associated with straining or with increases in abdominal pressure.

Assessment

The history often shows that the patient noted a sudden onset of abdominal pain, usually in the left upper quadrant and lower left chest, posterolaterally. Pain may also be referred to the area of the left shoulder because of diaphragmatic irritation (Kehr's sign). In the patient with delayed rupture, the history may not reveal the original trauma.

Clinically, the patient exhibits signs of pain and blood loss, pallor and tachycardia. Abdominal findings relate to peritoneal irritation by blood, primarily including tenderness and spasm, especially in the left upper quadrant area. In the absence of a history of trauma, rupture of the spleen may not be seriously considered, but tests should be performed to confirm any diagnosis.

Peritoneal tap and/or lavage is an easily performed and extremely helpful measure.[3,40] Recovery of fresh blood that does not clot is pathognomonic of intraperitoneal hemorrhage and mandates surgery.

If the peritoneal tap is negative, peritoneal lavage should be performed to confirm the diagnosis. The criteria for positive peritoneal lavage are as follows:
- Grossly bloody return
- Red blood cells > 100,000/mm³
- White blood cells > 500/mm³
- High amylase > 200 units
- Bile or intestinal content in lavage fluid
- Bacteria in lavage fluid

The procedure for peritoneal lavage is outlined in Chart 21-11.

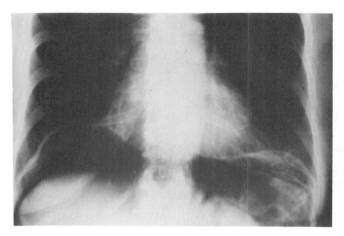

Figure 22-3 *Upright film of abdomen in patient with perforated peptic ulcer. A large amount of free air is seen beneath each diaphragm.*

Management/Treatment

Provision should be made to have an adequate amount of blood available for replacement, and the patient should be prepared for surgery as soon as possible. Emergency resuscitative measures may be initiated to restore circulating blood volume, using Ringer's lactate until type-specific blood is available. In an extreme emergency, type-specific, uncrossmatched blood may be used to correct a volume deficit. The operative procedure employed may vary from splenorrhaphy (surgical repair of the spleen) to splenectomy (removal of the spleen), depending upon the underlying disease process.

ACUTE BILIARY TRACT DISEASE

Acute biliary tract disease includes acute diseases of the gallbladder and bile ducts, which may be difficult to distinguish. It is also important to differentiate inflammatory processes from those due to colic. Acute disease of the gallbladder may be inflammatory (acute cholecystitis) or may

Figure 22-4 *Lateral decubitus x-ray of abdomen. This x-ray demonstrates free air above the liver shadow (arrow).*

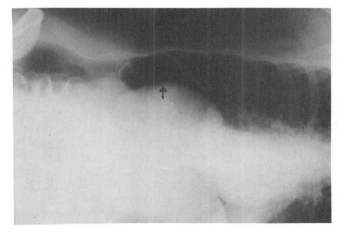

Chart 22-3

MANAGEMENT OF THE PATIENT WITH A PERFORATED PEPTIC ULCER

Assessment

HISTORY

- Sudden onset of severe, constant abdominal pain
- Pain, usually located in upper abdomen
- Prior history of ulcers or use of antacids
- Prior x-rays confirming ulcer

Physical examination

- Board-like rigidity of abdominal wall
- Diminished or absent peristalsis
- Restricted diaphragmatic movement
- Signs of dehydration and hypovolemia (thirst and poor skin turgor)

ADJUNCT STUDIES

- Free air in the peritoneal cavity on x-ray
- CBC, electrolyte determination, arterial blood gases

Emergency Management

- Place large-bore IV lines to restore circulating blood volume. The solution most commonly used is Ringer's lactate or glucose in saline. Electrolytes may be added to the solution as laboratory studies of serum electrolytes (SMA-6) indicate.
- Insert nasogastric tube, evacuate the stomach, and connect tube to intermittent suction.
- Insert indwelling catheter to assess urine output as an indication of fluid replacement.
- Antibiotics are not used routinely.
- Give medication for pain relief as indicated.
- Prepare the patient for surgery.

---

be due to colic (acute biliary colic). Inflammation of the bile ducts is termed acute cholangitis.

Acute Cholecystitis

Acute cholecystitis is invariably associated with gallstones.[1,14] Pregnancy, hemolytic disease, sickle cell disease, and prolonged use of the oral contraceptive pill are predisposing factors to stone formation. Gallstone(s) produce a partial or complete obstruction of the cystic duct (the outflow duct of the gallbladder) causing edema in the area of obstruction with an increase in the intraluminal pressure of the gallbladder. As the process continues, the small veins in the wall of the gallbladder become obstructed, leading to swelling of the gallbladder wall and finally to occlusion of the arterial supply. If the inflammatory reaction is severe enough, frank gangrene (Fig. 22-5) and even perforation of the gallbladder may develop. The incidence of gangrenous cholecystitis is estimated to be 10% to 15%[37,41] and represents a serious, sometimes fatal complication.

Gallbladder disease occurs more frequently in women than in men. Acute cholecystitis can develop in the absence of gallstones (acalculous cholecystitis) but is unusual. When it does occur, it is found more frequently in men than in women. Many texts describe the typical gallbladder patient as "fair, fat, forty, female, and fertile." Nothing could be farther from the truth.

Assessment. Characteristically, the clinical picture of gallbladder disease is one of food intolerance with varying degrees of discomfort, abdominal fullness, and pain in the upper abdomen after a meal. Fatty, greasy, or fried foods are most likely the offending agents. The pain may last for varying periods of time, from minutes to several hours. A history of prior x-ray studies demonstrating abnormal gallbladder function or presence of stones may be obtained.

In acute cholecystitis the pain is typically located at the site of the gallbladder in the right upper quadrant, near the costal margin. Initially, the pain may be colicky in nature and then becomes constant and may be aggravated by in-

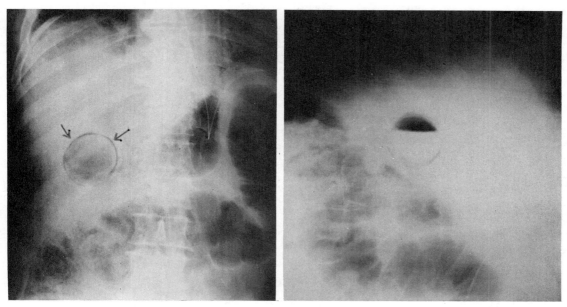

Figure 22-5 *Two x-rays of a patient with gallbladder disease. Left. Abdominal x-ray, showing a "halo" around the gallbladder, characteristic of gangrenous emphysematous cholecystitis. Note also the distended intestine (ileus). Right. Lateral decubitus x-ray showing the air-fluid level in the gallbladder.*

creases in intra-abdominal pressure, as with coughing, straining, and deep breathing. As the serosal surface of the gallbladder becomes involved with the inflammatory reaction, the parietal peritoneum may be irritated and the pain may then radiate around the chest wall to the tip of the right scapula owing to irritation of the 8th intercostal nerve. Less commonly, pain may be referred to the right shoulder when the undersurface of the diaphragm is irritated. Anorexia, nausea, vomiting (less commonly), and mild temperature may be present.

Physical examination may reveal diminished respiratory activity and almost halting respirations, especially on the right side, with diminished sounds over the lower lung field. Significant findings are usually localized to the right upper quadrant with tenderness and muscle spasm on palpation. In 20% to 25% of patients an acutely enlarged, tender globular mass may be felt. The mass is the enlarged gallbladder, and it indicates complete obstruction of the cystic duct leading to hydrops (benign obstruction with "white" bile) or empyema (purulent bile). Fever and leukocytosis are common in empyema, and the patient may appear toxic.

Acute cholecystitis must be distinguished from acute pancreatitis, perforated ulcer, hepatitis, acute appendicitis, and pyelonephritis. Flat and upright x-rays of the abdomen may reveal gallstones. Abdominal sonography of the gallbladder and bile ducts is an excellent noninvasive method of detecting biliary tract stones. CBC, urinalysis and serum amylase are helpful in differentiating acute cholecystitis from other acute upper abdominal disease processes. Amylase levels may be elevated but rarely to a significant degree. Mild icterus can be seen in some patients with acute cholecystitis. To rule out primary liver disease, serum bilirubin and transaminase levels should be obtained.

Treatment/Management. Optimal treatment of patients with acute cholecystitis is surgical removal of the gallbladder.

The decision to operate depends on the general condition of the patient. Once the examination is completed, appropriate prescribed doses of meperidine or morphine should be given for pain relief. Parenteral fluids should be started and a nasogastric tube inserted, especially if the patient has emesis. Urgent surgery is indicated in the presence of a palpable mass in the right upper quadrant, or if gangrene or perforation of the gallbladder is suspected. If the diagnosis is not clear, the patient should be admitted to the hospital for further observation, study, and elective surgery.

Though complete removal of the gallbladder is the definitive treatment of choice (cholecystectomy), in elderly, debilitated, or critically ill patients, simple drainage of the gallbladder (cholecystostomy) may be better tolerated. If necessary, the latter procedure may be done under local anesthesia.

The morbidity and mortality of acute cholecystitis is significant and increases with the severity of the disease and advancing age; interestingly, it is higher for cholecystostomy than for cholecystectomy. This seeming paradox is explained by the fact that drainage procedures are used primarily in more critically ill patients.

Care of the patient with acute cholecystitis is summarized in Chart 22-4.

Acute Biliary Colic

Acute biliary colic is a clinical entity caused by an acute obstruction of the outflow of the gallbladder by a stone caught in the neck or the cystic duct. It is invariably associated with gallstones. The pain of biliary colic is abrupt in onset, sharp and crescendic, and frequently associated with emesis. It is typically located in the region of the gallbladder in the right upper quadrant. It is not necessarily associated with food intake, but may occur at any time, even awakening the patient from sleep. The pain may persist for varying periods

---

Chart 22-4

MANAGEMENT OF THE PATIENT WITH ACUTE CHOLECYSTITIS

Assessment

HISTORY

- Onset of pain in right upper quadrant after a meal
- Possible history of food intolerance
- Anorexia, nausea, vomiting, mild temperature
- Prior x-rays confirming gallbladder dysfunction or gallstones
- Predisposing factors:
  Pregnancy
  Use of the oral contraceptive pill
  Hemolytic disease

PHYSICAL EXAMINATION

- Tenderness, spasm in right upper quadrant
- Restricted respiratory movements
- Palpable mass in right upper quadrant (20%–25% of patients)

ADJUNCT STUDIES

- Gallstones on abdominal x-ray
- Nonfunctioning gallbladder as revealed by oral cholecystography
- Abdominal x-rays to detect gallstones
- Sonography of the abdomen to assess the gallbladder and bile ducts
- Oral cholecystography to determine gallbladder function

Emergency Management

- Place IV lines to restore fluid volume.
- Insert nasogastric tube if patient is vomiting.
- Start broad-spectrum antibiotic IV.
- Give medication for pain relief.
- Prepare patient for further study or surgery as patient's condition indicates.

---

of time, from minutes to hours, and stops as abruptly as it began.

Assessment.   A past history of biliary calculi by x-ray or gallbladder sonography is helpful in identifying this condition. Since the episodes are fleeting, physical examination may reveal surprisingly minimal findings, though tenderness may be present in the right upper quadrant. Frequently, by the time the patient reaches the emergency department he is asymptomatic and examination is completely negative. Routine blood and urine analyses should be ordered as well as abdominal x-rays, which may demonstrate stones in the region of the gallbladder.

Management/Treatment.   Initially, treatment consists of pain relief with appropriate amounts of parenteral narcotics, such as meperidine or morphine. Nasogastric decompression may hasten the dissolution of pain.

The definitive management of acute biliary colic is cholecystectomy. Urgent surgery is rarely needed and under no circumstance should it be recommended until the diagnosis is clear. Admission to the hospital may not be required unless the pain is too severe or unrelieved by the initial dose of narcotic. The frequency and severity of the attacks are unpredictable. The very nature of this condition—sporadic occurrences with bursts of severe pain for varying periods of time—makes it difficult if not impossible to advise the patient when definitive treatment should be provided.

Oral cholecystography or sonography should be scheduled without delay to confirm the diagnosis and elective cholecystectomy planned thereafter.

Acute Cholangitis

Acute cholangitis refers to an inflammation of the bile ducts and is usually associated with a stone in the common bile duct that is obstructing bile flow.[18] It rarely occurs in conjunction with benign duct stricture or obstructing malignant neoplasms. The obstructing process leads to inflammation and secondary infection, usually due to enteric organisms.

Assessment. Clinically, the patient appears acutely ill with right upper quadrant pain accompanied by spiking fever, chills, and some degree of jaundice, a symptom complex referred to as Charcot's Triad. This systemic reaction may cause marked toxicity with a temperature elevation of 40.0°C to 40.5°C (104°F–105°F). If the inflammatory reaction is severe and generalized sepsis has occurred, shock and prostration may be seen. The patient may give a history of prior gallbladder disease proven by x-ray.

Physical examination reveals the patient to be abnormally ill. The sclerae may be icteric. Acute tenderness is noted in the right upper quadrant with spasm or muscle rigidity. At times, the liver is palpably enlarged and tender.

CBC, urinalysis, serum bilirubin, transaminases, and alkaline phosphates must be included in the laboratory studies. The values for the latter three tests are elevated in acute cholangitis. The serum amylase may also be abnormally high. Blood cultures should be drawn and appropriate sensitivity studies ordered. The blood culture is invariably positive; organisms of the coliform group are found most frequently.

Management/Treatment. Initial treatment consists of insertion of a nasogastric tube to effect decompression of the upper gastrointestinal tract. Parenteral fluids are begun and massive doses of antibiotics given intravenously. The antibiotics should be of the broad-spectrum variety effective against intestinal organisms. Once the offending organism is identified by culture, specific antibiotics are given as indicated. When the patient's condition has stabilized, prompt surgical intervention is indicated to relieve the obstruction and decompress the biliary tree.

Care of the patient with acute cholangitis is summarized in Chart 22-5.

ACUTE PANCREATITIS

Acute pancreatitis is an acute inflammatory condition of the pancreas of varying degrees of severity; it is usually associated

---

Chart 22-5

MANAGEMENT OF THE PATIENT WITH ACUTE CHOLANGITIS

Assessment

HISTORY

- Onset of acute right upper quadrant pain
- Shaking chills and fever (possibly as high as 104°F–105°F) ⎫ Charcot's triad
- Varying degrees of jaundice ⎭
- Prior history of gallbladder disease or gallstones

PHYSICAL EXAMINATION

- Acute illness, fever
- Jaundice, icteric sclerae
- Acute tenderness, spasm in right upper quadrant
- Possibly enlarged and tender liver

ADJUNCT STUDIES

- Leukocytosis with shift to the left (immature white cell forms)
- Hyperbilirubinemia
- Elevated serum transaminases, alkaline phosphatase
- Blood cultures usually positive for gram-negative organisms
- Sonography of abdomen to assess the gallbladder and bile ducts may reveal biliary stones or dilated bile ducts.

Emergency Management

- Initiate IV fluid replacement.
- Insert nasogastric tube.
- Give broad-spectrum antibiotic IV.
- Give medication for pain relief as indicated.

with biliary tract disease or alcoholism.[25,31] Less commonly, it may be secondary to mumps, morphinism, or use of certain drugs. The exact cause of acute pancreatitis is unknown, but it appears to be secondary to some form of obstruction of the pancreatic duct. One theory (the common channel theory) postulates that the distal segment of the common bile duct, the ampulla, is blocked by a calculus lodged at this point, causing a reflux of bile into the pancreatic duct.[34] In alcoholics, it is uncertain whether the etiology is due to a direct toxic effect, hypersecretion, or duodenitis with swelling about the ampulla of Vater in the second portion of the duodenum and secondary obstruction. With obstruction, bile regurgitates into the pancreatic duct, activating the enzymes produced by the pancreas. Autodigestion of the pancreas results.

As the pancreas swells, there is an outpouring of fluid into the retroperitoneal space and, as the inflammatory reaction progresses, into the abdominal (peritoneal) cavity. Local digestion and saponification of fat in the omentum and mesentery occur and are seen as areas of fat necrosis. This process binds calcium from the serum and may lead to dangerously low levels of calcium (less than 7 mg/dl) with resultant tetany. The outpouring of fluid contains high concentrations of the pancreatic enzymes amylase and lipase. Acute pancreatitis may be seen as a mild type (acute edematous pancreatitis) and as a more severe, highly fatal form (acute hemorrhagic pancreatitis).

In alcoholic patients and in those with untreated biliary tract disease, acute pancreatitis may recur, leading to scarring and permanent damage to the pancreas. Eventually, this can progress to chronic pancreatitis and pancreatic insufficiency, in which both the exocrine and endocrine functions of the pancreas can be seriously impaired, causing malabsorption, steatorrhea, and diabetes.

Assessment

The history is one of vague indigestion and upper abdominal (epigastric) discomfort but more often a steady, severe epigastric pain penetrating (boring) through to the back. Less commonly, it radiates around one or both costal margins. Nausea and emesis are usually present. In more severe forms, the patient may be in profound, sometimes irreversible, shock. A history of excessive alcoholic intake or dietary excess prior to the onset of symptoms may be obtained. In some patients, symptoms compatible with biliary tract disease or gallbladder dysfunction are present. In others there may be a history of pain associated with jaundice. Acute pancreatitis is seen more commonly in males than in females.

On physical examination, the patient appears acutely ill and is somewhat reluctant to move. In more severe stages of pancreatitis, he may be febrile and toxic, and in peripheral vascular collapse. Palpation of the abdomen reveals acute tenderness, especially in the middle of the upper abdomen, with spasm or rigidity. Pressure in this area may cause pain penetrating to the back. Rebound tenderness is present. Peristalsis is diminished or absent, depending on the degree of inflammation. In instances of hemorrhagic pancreatitis, ecchymoses may be noted in the flanks (Grey-Turner sign) or about the umbilicus (Cullen's sign.) As the pathologic process continues and fluid accumulates in the retroperi-

toneal space and the peritoneal cavity, severe hypovolemia may develop and the patient appears dehydrated and hypotensive.

Laboratory tests should include CBC, serum amylase, lipase, bilirubin, and transaminases. A routine urinalysis and urine levels of amylase and lipase are helpful. Serum electrolyte levels, especially calcium and phosphorous, are ordered; if hypocalcemia is present, replacement therapy must be started. Diabetes is a rare complication of acute pancreatitis; it is seen more often in patients with the chronic recurrent variety. Blood glucose levels, however, should be done routinely.

Peritoneal tap is helpful in confirming the diagnosis of acute pancreatitis, especially if free intraperitoneal fluid is present. In acute edematous pancreatitis, the peritoneal fluid is opalescent and may contain fat droplets. In hemorrhagic pancreatitis, bloody fluid may be recovered. A sample should be sent to the laboratory to test for amylase and lipase levels and another for smear, culture, and sensitivity studies.

Flat and upright x-rays of the abdomen are often nondiagnostic but may exhibit signs of ileus. Occasionally, a so-called sentinel loop may be visualized on x-ray. This is a loop of jejunum in the area of the pancreas that may dilate as a result of the nearby inflammatory process. Calcific densities in the region of the pancreas are strongly confirmatory of the disease. Calculi in the area of the gallbladder suggest a biliary tract component. Pancreatic sonography or radionuclide or computed tomography (CT scanning) may assist in making the diagnosis.

The differential diagnosis includes acute cholecystitis, perforated peptic ulcer, and inflammatory conditions about the kidneys. Significant elevation of the serum amylase, four to five times normal, is an important key in the diagnosis of pancreatitis.

Management/Treatment

Emergency care is directed toward resuscitation and pain relief. Morphine should be avoided, since it is known to cause spasm of the sphincter of Oddi. Meperidine in appropriate dosage is usually adequate. Nasogastric decompression draws off gastric juice and helps to put the stomach at rest, thus reducing pancreatic secretion. Anticholinergic drugs, atropine (0.0004 gm), or probanthine (0.015 gm) are given to reduce pancreatic and gastric secretion.

Parenteral fluid replacement is begun soon after arrival in the emergency department. Ringer's lactate may be used initially to restore depleted blood volume to normal. Calcium gluconate or calcium chloride is added to the intravenous fluid if low serum calcium is found. If the patient's condition requires massive fluid replacement, a central vein catheter should be inserted to monitor the response to fluid therapy. As with any other critically ill patient, baseline determination of vital parameters, including arterial blood gases, is mandatory and should be repeated at intervals as the resuscitation is continued. A broad-spectrum antibiotic may be given prophylactically.

In most instances of acute pancreatitis, the patient is admitted for continuation of fluid replacement, anticholinergic medication, pain relief, and gastrointestinal decompression.

Interval determinations of serum and urinary amylase and lipase levels, combined with repeated examinations of the abdomen, are helpful in assessing the patient's progress. When the acute process has subsided, thorough investigation of the biliary system is indicated. If biliary tract disease is found, surgical intervention is needed to correct the underlying process.

Emergency operative treatment in acute pancreatitis is reserved for patients with jaundice, those with severe hemorrhagic pancreatitis, and those with findings of an acute intra-abdominal process in whom the diagnosis is not clear.[19] Surgical therapy is directed toward decompression of the pancreatic-biliary duct system by cholecystostomy or choledochostomy. When hemorrhagic pancreatitis is found at laparotomy, the pancreas may require decompression by multiple incisions and drainage of the retroperitoneal space. Morbidity and mortality are significant in patients with severe forms of acute pancreatitis.

Pancreatic inflammation secondary to biliary tract disease generally has a favorable prognosis; patients with alcoholic pancreatitis are extremely difficult to cure and have a poor prognosis. Typically, the latter type is seen time and again in the emergency department with recurring episodes of acute pancreatitis. Drug addiction is not uncommon in such patients and admittedly many continue to consume large amounts of alcohol because they find some relief of pain with its use. Generally, alcoholic pancreatitis is refractory to cure.

Care of the patient with acute pancreatitis is summarized in Chart 22-6.

ACUTE APPENDICITIS

Acute appendicitis is the most common cause of an acute abdomen. It is regarded by many as a minor problem, but despite the technical and scientific advances in medicine

---

Chart 22-6

MANAGEMENT OF THE PATIENT WITH ACUTE PANCREATITIS

Assessment

HISTORY

- Steady, boring pain in epigastrium (possibly penetrating to back)
- Nausea and emesis
- History of biliary tract disease or gallbladder dysfunction
- History of prior episodes of pancreatitis

PHYSICAL EXAMINATION

- Acute illness: possible presence of hypovolemia and hypotension: possible shock
- Tenderness in middle of upper abdomen, with spasm and rigidity
- Diminished to absent peristalsis
- In hemorrhagic pancreatitis, ecchymoses in flanks (Grey-Turner sign) or about umbilicus (Cullen's sign)

ADJUNCT STUDIES

- Elevated serum amylase and lipase
- Elevated urinary amylase and lipase
- Opalescent bloody fluid encountered on peritoneal tap
- Positive findings on pancreatic sonogram or CT scan

Emergency Management

- Place large-bore veinways and restore circulating blood volume using Ringers' lactate.
- Insert nasogastric tube. Place patient on intermittent suction.
- Insert indwelling bladder catheter to assess urinary output as a measure of fluid replacement.
- Give anticholinergics IV to lessen pancreatic and gastric function.
- Antibiotics may be used, especially if the etiology of pancreatitis is biliary tract disease.
- Central vein line is placed if significant hypovolemia is present.
- Generally, management is nonoperative unless jaundice is present, in which instance biliary tract decompression may be indicated.

The clinical findings of acute appendicitis relate to the location of the appendix, which may be in one of several positions (Fig. 22-6). It may lie just below the tip of the cecum lateral to it in the colic gutter (retrocecal appendix) or medially behind the terminal ileum, overlying the course of the ureter; or it may fall over the brim of the pelvis, coming in contact with the urinary bladder in the male or the bladder and reproductive organs in the female. Thus, acute inflammatory states in the appendix can mimic a number of other conditions that cause acute abdominal pain. For example, appendicitis must be distinguished from acute gallbladder disease, perforated ulcer, acute pancreatitis, twisted or ruptured ovarian cyst, acute urinary tract disorders, and salpingitis.

The disease may occur at any age and has no predilection for sex.

Assessment

The first and most common symptom of acute appendicitis is pain that begins as a vague discomfort, or "bellyache," in the region of the umbilicus. It is usually accompanied by nausea and anorexia. Anorexia is a very important symptom in acute appendicitis; its absence leaves the diagnosis in doubt. As the disease process continues, emesis occurs and the pain shifts to the area of the appendix in the right lower quadrant. The pain is sharp, constant, and usually aggravated by walking, coughing, or straining. The most common location of pain is known as McBurney's point. It is found by drawing an imaginary line from the right interior superior iliac spine to the umbilicus and locating the junction of the lateral and middle thirds (Fig. 22-7). This anatomic point is of diagnostic value when the appendix lies in juxtaposition to it. However, if the appendix lies in a retrocecal or pelvic position, the pain may be localized to the flank or iliac fossa. This clinical picture evolves in a matter of hours and becomes more severe as time passes. Occasionally, with rupture of the appendix, the patient may note a sudden, temporary lessening of the pain and feel somewhat better, only to develop more severe pain as the inflammatory reaction spreads and peritonitis develops.

In females, it is important to elicit a menstrual history. Pain from a ruptured follicle cyst of the ovary (mittelschmerz) may be indistinguishable from that of appendicitis.

Physical examination must be performed carefully and gently. The patient usually appears acutely ill, especially in the pediatric age group[23] and will be reluctant to move about on the examining table. Not uncommonly the right thigh is flexed in order to lessen intra-abdominal pressure and decrease pain. Evaluation of the abdomen may be particularly difficult in the very young and very old.[23,45,47]

The most common physical findings are tenderness and spasm in the right lower quadrant. Palpation in the left lower quadrant may cause pressure to be transmitted to the right side, causing referred pain (Rovsing's sign). Rebound tenderness and cough pain at the site of the appendix are invariably present. Rectal examination may reveal tenderness in the right lower quadrant. In females, tenderness in the area of the uterine adnexae or on motion of the cervix may indicate primary pelvic disease, and the possibility of an

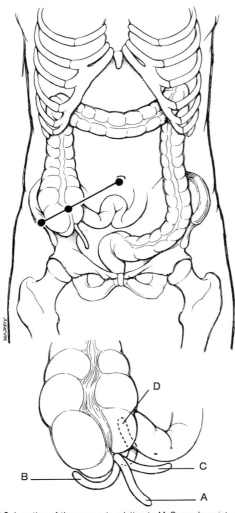

Figure 22-6 Location of the cecum in relation to McBurney's point. Appendix A is in the common location, extending from the cecum. Areas B, C, and D represent other common locations of the appendix, lateral, medial, or retrocecal in position.

and surgery to date, there is an overall mortality rate of slightly less than 0.1%. In gangrenous or perforated appendicitis the mortality rate is significantly higher.[44]

The appendix is attached to the cecum at the lower end of the ascending colon in the right lower quadrant. It is a hollow organ, averaging about 10 cm in length in the adult. Its lumen connects with that of the cecum and its walls contain the various layers of the intestine.

Appendicitis usually results from an obstructive process that blocks the lumen of the organ and initiates an inflammatory reaction characterized initially by swelling and progressing to vascular congestion, impairment of arterial blood supply, and in later stages gangrene and perforation. The perforation may be walled off and form an abscess or rupture into the peritoneal cavity, causing generalized peritonitis. The most common cause of the intraluminal obstruction is a fecalith, or piece of inspissated feces. Less commonly, a foreign body such as a toothpick, chicken bone, or fruit seed may be the offending agent. In a few patients, a benign or malignant neoplasm may be the culprit.

inflamed appendix lying close to the pelvic organs must be kept in mind. In ruptured appendicitis with abscess formation, a mass may be palpated in the right lower quadrant.

Laboratory studies should include a CBC and urinalysis. In more advanced stages of the disease when fever and toxicity are present, serum electrolytes should be measured. Usually, the white blood cell count is elevated with a shift to the left—an increase in the number of immature neutrophils (band forms). Microscopic examination of the urine, though usually negative, is important. When an inflamed appendix overlies the right ureter, red and white cells may be found in the urine. If the organ lies on the dome of the bladder, dysuria and urinary frequency may be present. X-rays of the abdomen are usually nondiagnostic and are rarely needed.

Differential diagnosis includes *any* intra-abdominal condition, including mittelschmerz, pelvic inflammatory disease, ectopic pregnancy, and gastroenteritis. In the pediatric age group, mesenteric lymphadenitis may occur in conjunction with or following an acute upper respiratory infection, and the signs and symptoms may be indistinguishable from acute appendicitis.[26] Mesenteric lymphadenitis involves acute inflammatory changes in the lymph nodes of the mesentery of the small bowel and appendix. Careful attention to the physical examination may allow the examiner to detect more generalized abdominal tenderness (not limited to the right lower quadrant), and when the patient shifts from side to side the pain may also move about.

Treatment/Management

Once the assessment is completed, the patient may be given medication for pain relief and prepared for surgical removal of the appendix. Patients with complicated appendicitis or long-standing symptoms may be toxic and critically ill. Fluid replacement and broad-spectrum antibiotics given intravenously should be initiated to stabilize the patient before surgery is undertaken. The elderly patient may be too ill to undergo surgery, in which case aggressive nonoperative management consisting of fluid replacement, massive doses of antibiotics, and nasogastric intubation may be necessary.

In adolescent girls, when it is impossible to distinguish appendicitis from a ruptured follicle cyst or mesenteric adenitis, a decision whether to operate must be made by weighing the possibility of complications arising from surgery in the face of an incorrect diagnosis as opposed to delaying surgery in acute appendicitis. In most instances, it is much safer to recommend surgery for the patient, taking care to advise both the patient and her family of the possibility that an error in diagnosis may exist but that further delay may be fraught with more danger.

Care of the patient with acute appendicitis is summarized in Chart 22-7.

DIVERTICULITIS

Diverticulitis is a common acute inflammatory condition arising in preexisting diverticula. A *diverticulum* (plural *diverticula*) is an outpouching that develops along the tenia of the colon at the point of entry of the penetrating arterial

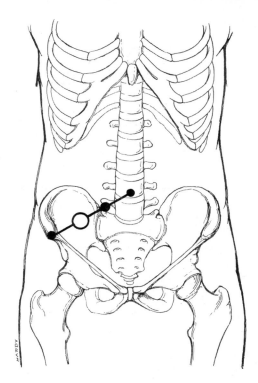

Figure 22-7 *McBurney's point. The characteristic area of tenderness is in the right lower quadrant in a patient with acute appendicitis. This anatomic landmark is located at the junction of the lateral and middle thirds of an imaginary line drawn between the umbilicus and the anterior superior iliac spine.*

branches. The diverticula are more commonly of the *acquired* variety and histologically appear as mucosal outpouchings; in other words, they do not contain all the layers of the wall of the colon. On the other hand, in congenital diverticula, all layers of the bowel wall are present. Diverticula may be found in any portion of the colon. The congenital variety is usually solitary and more often is found in the cecum. The acquired variety is usually multiple and, while it may occur in any portion of the colon, is found most frequently in the sigmoid colon. This relatively asymptomatic, noninflammatory condition is called diverticulosis. It is found in the course of barium enema studies in nearly 50% of patients over the age of 40.[11]

Diverticulitis may occur in any preexisting diverticula. Inspissated feces or food content fills a diverticulum and may initiate an inflammatory reaction with local swelling. If the inflamed diverticulum empties into the lumen of the colon, the reaction subsides, but if not, and inflammation persists, local pain and spasm follow. If the process continues, the inflamed diverticulum may perforate, causing local generalized peritonitis. The perforation may break into the fat about the colon or the mesentery, causing a pericolic abscess. The omentum may attach at the point of inflammation and wall off the process. In advanced stages, a large abscess may develop in the pelvis near the involved area. Such an abscess may contain more than 500 ml of purulent material. In chronic low-grade inflammations, the involved segment of colon may adhere to a loop of small bowel or to the urinary bladder, and in females the vaginal vault may be involved. Abnormal communications (fistulas) may arise

---

Chart 22-7

MANAGEMENT OF THE PATIENT WITH ACUTE APPENDICITIS

Assessment

HISTORY

- Onset of periumbilical pain, shifting to right lower quadrant
- Pain continuous, aggravated by walking, straining, coughing
- Anorexia (if not present, then diagnosis should be reconsidered)
- Pain site varies with location or appendix

PHYSICAL EXAMINATION

- Tenderness, spasm in right lower quadrant (frequently at McBurney's point)
- Variation in location of physical findings according to location of appendix
- Rebound tenderness and cough pain over area of appendix
- Possible flexion of right thigh
- Referred pain in right lower quadrant with palpation in the left lower quadrant (Rovsing's sign)

ADJUNCT STUDIES

- Normal or elevated white blood cell count
- Increase in band forms (immature white cells)

Emergency Management

- Insert nasogastric tube if patient is vomiting.
- Place veinway and start glucose/saline solution with electrolytes added as indicated.
- Prepare patient for surgery.

---

between the organs involved; that is, enterocolic (colon and small bowel), colovesical (colon and urinary bladder), colovaginal (colon and vagina).

In addition to the complications mentioned above, acute diverticulitis may cause a bowel obstruction at the site of the inflammatory reaction.

Complications of diverticulosis-diverticulitis may be summarized as follows:
- Inflammation-diverticulitis
- Intestinal obstruction
- Perforation with abscess formation
- Perforation with fistula formation
- Perforation with generalized peritonitis
- Bleeding

Assessment

The patient usually gives a history of some problems with constipation and may have had a barium enema in the past that demonstrated diverticulosis. Diverticulitis in its acute phase is marked by the onset of dull to sharp constant pain in the area of inflammation, usually the left lower quadrant. It is often referred to as left-sided appendicitis. In milder degrees of inflammation, the patient may notice a cramp; but as the reaction worsens, the pain becomes more severe and constant. Without treatment, the patient may note symptoms of sepsis associated with chills and fever, and as the process continues, the inflammatory swelling may be severe enough to cause bowel obstruction with increasing abdominal distention, constipation, and lack of flatus. (See Large Intestine Obstruction, below.)

If chronic low-grade diverticulitis is present, fistulas involving the bladder or vagina may have developed, in which case the patient may report passing "wind" or stool from the bladder or vagina. Rectal bleeding is uncommon in this condition.[5]

Physical findings vary with the degree of inflammatory reaction. Examination may reveal mild tenderness in the left lower quadrant or iliac fossa or exquisite tenderness with rebound tenderness, spasm, and rigidity, indicating peritoneal irritation. If an obstructive element is present, the abdomen may be distended and tympanitic to percussion, with high-pitched peristaltic sounds. When perforation has occurred and an abscess has formed, in addition to spasm and rigidity, a mass may be palpable at the site of involvement. On rectal or pelvic examination a mass may be outlined in the cul-de-sac, indicating a pelvic abscess. The white blood cell count is usually elevated with a shift to the left. Flat and upright x-rays of the abdomen may be nondiagnostic. However, on an upright film, free air under the diaphragm indicates perforation; the outline of a pelvic mass may be seen, or an enlarged, dilated colon is found when obstruction has occurred. Barium enema may confirm the diagnosis; it should be delayed until the acute inflammatory reaction subsides (Fig. 22-8). Sigmoidoscopy is rarely needed as an adjunct to the diagnosis of diverticulitis in the emergency setting. If it is deemed necessary, the use of air insufflation during the course of the procedure is contraindicated.

The differential diagnosis includes appendicitis, carcinoma of the colon, urinary tract infection, and acute inflammatory conditions of the uterine adnexae. Diverticulitis and carcinoma of the colon both occur most commonly in the sigmoid area. They may present simultaneously, and differentiation may be difficult or impossible.[30] Occasionally, in patients with acute pancreatitis, the intraperitoneal fluid may drain along the left colic gutter and mimic diverticulitis.

Patients with fistula formation secondary to chronic diverticulitis may be seen in the emergency department for treatment of a genitourinary tract infection.

Management/Treatment

Management depends on the severity of the condition. In mild cases with minimal physical findings, the patient may not require admission, but should be treated with analgesics, stool softeners, and an antibiotic effective against enteric organisms. An important part of the treatment plan is a low-residue diet. When the patient is asymptomatic and local tenderness is absent, a barium enema should be performed to confirm the diagnosis. Usually, such patients can be managed nonoperatively but require careful attention to their diets.

In severe cases with evidence of peritoneal irritation, sepsis, obstruction, or perforation, admission to the hospital is indicated and urgent surgery may be necessary.[39] Nasogastric decompression is initiated. If the patient is dehydrated and toxic, parenteral fluid replacement and broad-spectrum antibiotics are given and the patient is stabilized before surgery. Surgical management usually involves a staged procedure with drainage of the abscess, if present, and temporary proximal colostomy to divert the fecal stream. The colostomy is usually made in the colon upstream from the level of inflammation; diversion of the fecal stream prevents continued contamination of the involved segment. At some later date, usually weeks to several months after the colostomy, elective resection of the diseased segment of colon is performed. In the final stage of treatment following the resection, the colostomy is closed to restore intestinal continuity. With the availability of potent antibiotics and improved surgical technique, this classic three-stage procedure has given way in some centers to a two-stage approach in which the diseased segment of colon is removed during the first operation and a temporary colostomy fashioned, which is closed several weeks later. One-stage primary resection is hazardous as an emergency procedure because of the unnecessary risk of morbidity and mortality secondary to sepsis.

OBSTRUCTIONS OF THE GASTROINTESTINAL TRACT

Obstruction of the gastrointestinal tract may occur in any segment. A distinction is made between mechanical obstruction and adynamic or paralytic obstruction, such as par-

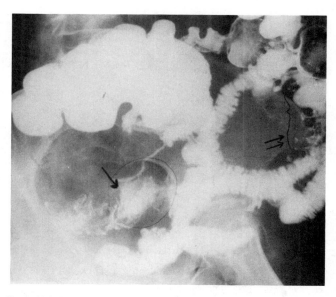

Figure 22-8 Barium enema. Note diverticulitis (single arrow) and diverticulosis (2 arrows).

alytic ileus. Both types produce the same general effects. Etiologic factors include inflammatory or cicatricial scarring, as in peptic ulcer or regional enteritis, adhesion bands, intussusception, and neoplasms of the bowel.[25]

Causes of obstruction of the gastrointestinal tract may be summarized as follows:

- Inflammation: chronic peptic ulcer, regional enteritis, colitis, acute diverticulitis, acute pancreatitis
- Adhesion bands: postoperative, congenital
- Intussusception
- Neoplasms: Carcinoma of stomach, pancreas, small intestine, and colon
- Incarcerated or strangulated hernia: inguinal or femoral hernia
- Sigmoid volvulus
- Paralytic ileus
- Mesenteric vascular occlusion

The level at which obstruction occurs is significant. Common causes of obstruction at various levels in the gastrointestinal tract may be listed as follows:

1. *Stomach-pylorus-duodenum*
   - Chronic, active peptic ulcer
   - Carcinoma of stomach or pancreas
2. *Small intestine*
   - Postoperative adhesions
   - Incarcerated or strangulated hernia
3. *Colon*
   - Acute diverticulitis
   - Carcinoma of colon
   - Sigmoid volvulus

In patients with obstructive disease, severe depletion or alteration of body fluid and electrolytes may develop. These abnormalities result from vomiting of gastric or intestinal fluids and from sequestration of electrolyte-containing fluid in the lumen of the stomach or intestine. Obstruction in the stomach or high in the small bowel causes loss of potassium and chloride ions. Obstruction lower in the small intestine

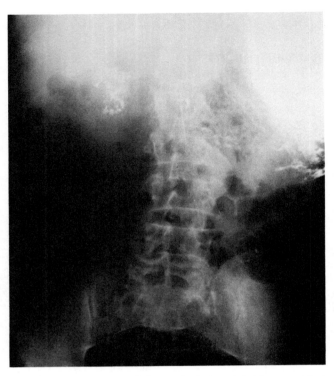

Figure 22-9 *Pyloric obstruction. Barium remains in stomach, in left upper quadrant, 1½ hours after barium swallow.*

may cause depletion of potassium and sodium. The degree of depletion depends to a great extent on the duration of the obstruction.

In addition to loss of electrolytes, mild to severe fluid loss also occurs, resulting in further alterations in acid-base balance. Thus, patients with obstructions are dehydrated, may have scant urinary output and exhibit thirst and poor skin turgor. Severe contraction of circulating blood volume may result in vascular collapse.

Obstructions occurring at different levels of the gastrointestinal tract are discussed in the sections that follow.

Pyloric Obstruction

Pyloric obstruction is obstruction that occurs at the lower end of the stomach or first part of the duodenum. It is most often due to the scarring of chronic active peptic ulcer, but in older patients, especially those over 50 or 60, it may be due to carcinoma of the stomach or, less often, the pancreas.

Assessment. Pain is not common, but the patients relate a history of postprandial fullness, followed by vomiting of undigested food. As the obstruction becomes more long-standing, the stomach compensates by enlarging, and emesis may not occur until several hours after food intake. Weight loss may be noted, especially in neoplastic disease. Careful questioning may elicit a history compatible with ulcer. Prior upper gastrointestinal studies may confirm the diagnosis of preexisting ulcer disease.

Patients with pyloric obstruction usually appear chronically ill and thin. Skin turgor is poor and eyes are sunken.

Physical examination may demonstrate a soft mass in the epigastric area, which is the dilated stomach. With patient observation, peristaltic waves may be seen on the anterior abdominal wall. By placing a stethoscope over the area and gently but firmly shaking the patient from side to side, a "succussion splash" may be heard, due to the splashing of gastric content back and forth within the stomach. Evidence of vascular collapse may be noted.

Electrolyte studies are mandatory in order to establish baseline determinations and evaluate the degree of variation from normal. Hydrochloric acid content of the stomach should be determined. Patients with active ulcer disease ordinarily have a high gastric acidity. The most striking electrolyte deficit will be a marked lowering of the chloride and potassium ions (hypochloremic alkalosis), with an accompanied rise in serum bicarbonate or carbon dioxide ions. Patients in the seventh decade commonly have lower levels of hydrochloric acid in the stomach and may not demonstrate this severe loss of chloride ion. Loss of total fluid will cause contraction of blood volume and evidence of hemoconcentration.

The patient's general status should be evaluated. If the diagnosis is brought into question, an upper gastrointestinal series will be diagnostic (Fig. 22-9).

Management/Treatment. Emergency management consists of decompression of the stomach by continuous nasogastric suction and restoration of circulating blood volume and electrolyte levels to normal limits. The stomach may contain large pieces of undigested food that may plug the nasogastric tube. In such cases, gastric lavage by an Ewald tube, which can be swallowed easily through the mouth, is an effective means of cleansing the stomach.

Further management is directed toward restoring the patient's normal physiology in preparation for early surgery. Surgical treatment should be planned within 48 hours of admission to prevent further depletion of fluids and electrolytes. Nonoperative management results in some improvement, but on discontinuance of nasogastric decompression, recurrent obstruction is common.

Care of the patient with pyloric obstruction is summarized in Chart 22-8.

Small Intestine Obstruction

Obstruction of the small intestine may occur at any site in the small bowel. Obstruction in the proximal small bowel (duodenum or jejunum) is present more often with history of emesis, whereas obstructions lower in the ileum cause distention of the obstructed bowel, with emesis occurring later in the course of the disease. The effects may be the same regardless of the level of obstruction.

Ordinarily, in a healthy individual 7000 to 8000 ml of fluid, rich in electrolytes, enters the gut each 24-hour period. With obstruction, sequestration and vomiting both cause loss of fluid. As the bowel distends, fluid may be lost into the peritoneal cavity, adding to further depletion of extracellular fluid volume. As the obstructive process is allowed to continue, the intestinal wall becomes edematous, and bacteria may proliferate in the gut. This increased intralu-

Chart 22-8

MANAGEMENT OF THE PATIENT WITH PYLORIC OBSTRUCTION

Assessment

HISTORY

- Possible history of peptic ulcer
- Postprandial fullness
- Vomiting of undigested food, sometimes hours after completing a meal
- Demonstration of peptic ulcer in prior upper GI series

PHYSICAL EXAM

- Chronic illness, possible hypovolemia
- Dehydration noted with poor skin turgor, sunken eyes
- Possible soft mass palpated in upper abdomen (dilated stomach)
- Gastric peristaltic wave possibly seen in upper abdomen
- "Succussion splash" may be heard

ADJUNCT STUDIES

- Hemoconcentration, with rise in hematocrit
- Possible decrease in electrolyte K^+ and Cl^- (hypochloremic alkalosis) with an increase in bicarbonate or CO_2
- GI series: demonstrates dilated stomach with partial or complete obstruction at the outlet (pylorus)

Emergency Management

- Place veinway to replace circulating blood volume. Fluid containing electrolytes, especially Na^+K^+ and Cl^-, is necessary to correct the usual hypochloremic alkalosis.
- Insert nasogastric tube, aspirate to empty the stomach, and place patient on intermittent suction.
- Insert indwelling catheter to monitor urinary output as an index of fluid volume replacement
- Insert central vein line to measure central venous pressure, and recheck periodically as a measure of rehydration.
- Admit patient for further study and definitive care.

---

minal pressure may then produce venous and, later, arterial obstruction, which compromise the blood supply and may lead to strangulation of the intestine. Prolongation then causes perforation and spillage of contents into the peritoneum, resulting in a severe chemical or bacterial peritonitis.

Assessment. History includes vomiting or distention. Pain may be noted at the site of obstruction, crampy in nature and marked by crescendos occurring with peristaltic waves. Small bowel obstruction is most often due to adhesion bonds from prior surgical entry into the peritoneal cavity, but there may be other causes, such as acute appendicitis, regional enteritis, complicated hernia, intussusception or mesenteric occlusion.[21]

Physical examination may reveal an incisional scar associated with abdominal distention. Auscultation should be done carefully. Hyperactive bowel sounds may be heard, along with peristaltic rushes and borborygmi, which often can be heard without the aid of a stethoscope. The patient may complain of pain coincident with the peristaltic rush. Severe or generalized tenderness may indicate impairment of blood supply to the intestine (strangulation obstruction).

Serum electrolyte levels should be established on admission. X-rays of the abdomen should be done in the flat and upright or lateral decubitus position. Multiple fluid levels and a characteristic "stepladder" pattern may be seen in the upright or decubitus film. (See Figs. 22-10 and 22-11.)

Management/Treatment. Initial management relates to intestinal decompression by nasogastric or long intestinal tube (Miller-Abbott or Cantor), concomitant with aggressive fluid and electrolyte replacement. Urine output should be monitored. Of singular importance is the determination of vascular occlusion or strangulation obstruction. These conditions require emergency surgical intervention after the patient's condition has stabilized. Their presence is heralded by physical findings of peritoneal irritation, whereas the or-

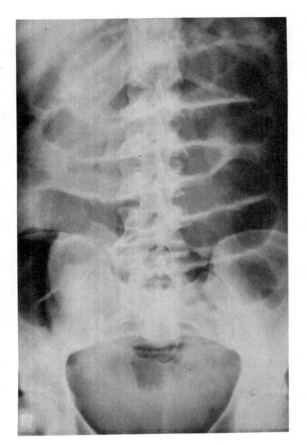

Figure 22-10 *Flat film of abdomen in patient with small bowel obstruction. The small bowel is distended and in the characteristic stepladder pattern of obstruction.*

dinary "bland" mechanical obstruction usually is not. Surgical care involves release of the obstruction. In patients with irreversible damage to the blood supply of the intestine, removal of the involved segment and restoration of intestinal continuity constitute the surgical approach of choice. Antibiotic coverage is indicated in patients with intestinal obstruction.

Paralytic Ileus. Certain disease states (*e.g.,* pneumonia, septicemia, pyelonephritis, renal colic, hip fracture), as well as trauma and abdominal surgery, may affect the autonomic nerves supplying the intestine, leading to decreased or absent peristaltic activity. This condition usually occurs in both the small and large bowels and has a characteristic x-ray pattern (Fig. 22-12).[17] Differential diagnosis is important.

Intussusception

Intussusception occurs when a proximal segment of the bowel telescopes or invaginates into a distal segment. It may be small bowel into small bowel (ileo-ileal), small bowel into colon (ileocolic), or colon into colon (colocolic). The most common is the ileocolic type. This condition usually occurs in the very young, in the first year of life and, less often, in the very old. The cause is not always apparent. Enlarged lymph follicles in the intestinal wall[32] or occa-

sionally a polyp or Meckel's diverticulum may form the starting point for the process.

The history of intussusception in a child is readily characteristic. It is marked by sudden "spasm," with an outcry or screaming. The infant may draw its legs up and emesis may occur. The diaper may be blood-stained and contain stool of the "current jelly" type. Physical assessment may reveal a void in the right lower quadrant and a mass along the course of the colon.

Gentle barium enema is very useful to confirm the diagnosis and is sometimes used therapeutically to reduce the intussusception (Fig. 22-13). It is difficult to be certain that the reduction is complete, though, and operative intervention is usually needed to ensure complete reduction. The in-

Figure 22-11 *Flat and lateral decubitus x-rays of abdomen. Top. Flat film demonstrates large dilated loops of small bowel. Bottom. Lateral decubitus film shows multiple fluid levels in small bowel.*

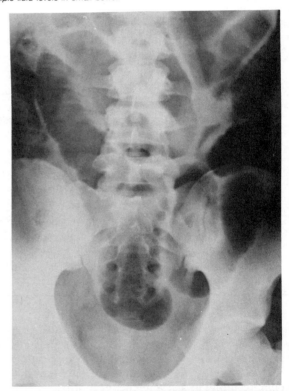

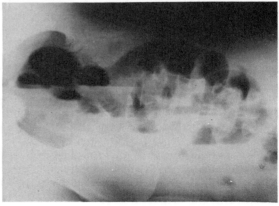

tussusception should be reduced manually and the bowel carefully examined for compromise of blood supply. Recurrence is unusual.

Large Intestine Obstruction

The most common causes of colonic obstruction are neoplasms and inflammatory processes. A much less common etiology is sigmoid volvulus. Inflammatory conditions are primarily related to complications of acute diverticulitis and usually occur in the left side of the colon in the region of the sigmoid. Neoplastic obstruction is most often due to a carcinoma of the colon. The specific lesion is referred to as a "napkin ring" malignant lesion, which grows around the interior circumference of the lumen of the bowel, producing a gradual and eventually complete obstruction. These tumors typically grow in the left half of the colon. Malignant tumors in the right half of the colon are more exophytic, growing into the lumen of the bowel, and rarely obstruct. Sigmoid volvulus is a rare cause of obstruction, accounting for perhaps 3% to 5% of large bowel obstructions. It is due to a torsion or twisting of the sigmoid colon on its mesentery,[16,22] which can result in a closed-loop obstruction.

The history given by the patient varies to a certain extent with the underlying cause of the obstruction. In inflammatory

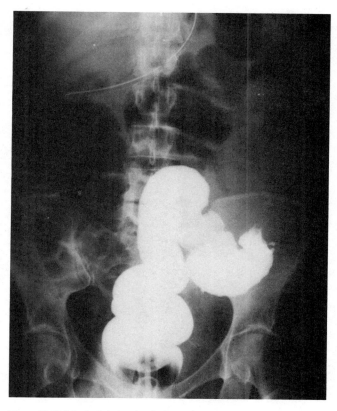

Figure 22-13 *Intestinal obstruction. Barium enema shows obstruction in lower left colon. Intussusception found at operation.*

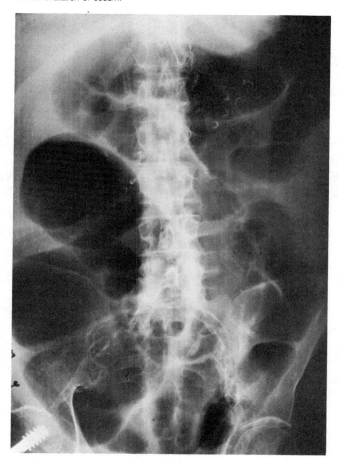

Figure 22-12 *Paralytic ileus. Note distended loops of small and large bowel, as well as dilatation of cecum.*

conditions and volvulus, the most common symptom is pain, which may be constant or crampy and is located in the area of the abdomen where the etiologic process is, usually the lower abdomen (especially the left lower quadrant). In malignant lesions, the patient may give a history of bowel irregularity, with alternating constipation and diarrhea, and a narrowing of stool diameter to the size of a pencil. These are symptoms produced as the tumor grows in the colon.

As the obstructive process continues and becomes complete, the patient notes a lack of flatus and constipation. Both fluid and air may be backed up proximal to the point of obstruction. Intraluminal sequestration of fluid leads to dehydration and electrolyte imbalance. Distention varies, depending on the duration and to some extent the cause of the obstruction, and at times may be massive. This is particularly true if the ileocecal valve is incompetent, allowing the fecal contents to regurgitate into the small intestine. Emesis is not common, but if the patient seeks treatment late in the course of the obstruction, fecal emesis may occur.

Assessment. Physical examination varies according to the duration and cause of the obstruction. Early on, hydration may be adequate and distention minimal. Increased peristalsis with high-pitched sounds may be heard on auscultation. In inflammatory conditions, local tenderness is present in the area of the abdomen where the obstruction is located. In sigmoid volvulus, the lower abdomen is distended with tenderness in the midportion.

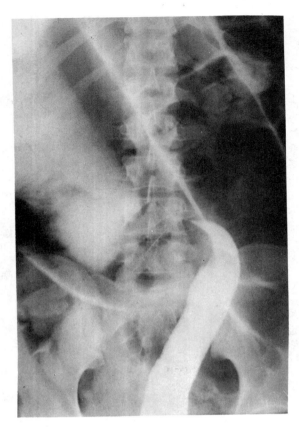

Figure 22-14 *Emergency barium enema in a patient with sigmoid volvulus. Note the typical "bird beak" deformity of the rectosigmoid at the level of obstruction. Patient treated by sigmoid resection after an unsuccessful attempt to reduce by sigmoidoscopy.*

As the obstructive process becomes more severe, abdominal distention increases. With sequestration of fluid in the lumen of the bowel, hypovolemia may result, and the patient may appear dehydrated, with poor skin turgor. In advanced states, hypotension may be found, an ominous sign.

Rectal examination may not be specific unless a low-lying tumor is present. Generally, the tumor must lie within the lowest 8 cm to 10 cm of the anal verge to be palpated, and these tumors are an infrequent cause of colon obstruction. More commonly, the rectal vault is empty.

CBC and electrolyte studies are necessary to assess the patient more adequately. In severely ill patients, arterial blood gases should also be done. Flat and upright x-rays of the abdomen are helpful in establishing the level of obstruction and at times are suggestive of the etiology. On occasion, emergency barium enema may be indicated, especially if the possibility of sigmoid volvulus exists. It may have a characteristic appearance on x-ray (Fig. 22-14). If the cecum appears greatly distended, with a diameter exceeding 8 cm to 10 cm, consider urgent operative intervention. This point will be discussed shortly.

Management/Treatment. The principles of management are directed toward restoration of circulating volume and intestinal decompression. A nasogastric tube should be in-serted and volume replacement initiated with Ringer's lactate or glucose in saline. Electrolytes are added to the intravenous solutions as the baseline studies indicate. Insert an indwelling catheter and monitor urinary output. It should be maintained at adequate levels, usually 0.5 to 1.0 ml/kg/hr. The rate of infusion should be carefully regulated, with particular attention to avoid overloading the patient, especially the elderly or known cardiac patients. A central vein catheter to measure central venous pressure is of some value. Broad-spectrum antibiotics should be initiated early in the course of treatment.

Definitive surgical management to relieve the obstruction depends on several factors. As was indicated earlier, if the cecum is greatly distended (more than 8 cm to 10 cm in diameter; Fig. 22-15) emergency decompression may be needed to avoid perforation. It may be achieved by a transverse loop colostomy, or if the patient's condition is too critical, a tube cecostomy may be performed under local anesthesia. Excessive distention can result in focal gangrenous change, with perforation and massive fecal contamination of the peritoneal cavity.

Following the decompression, delayed *elective* resection of the obstructed segment is done when the patient's condition allows, which may be several weeks to months after the original procedure and following thorough workup of the patient to better identify the site and cause of the obstruction. In some centers, especially in less critically ill patients, the initial procedure may include decompression and resection of the obstructing lesion, especially when it

Figure 22-15 *Upright film of lower colon obstruction. Note the massive enlargement of the cecum on the right side of photo.*

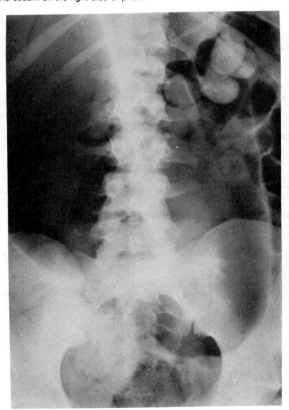

is due to diverticulitis. The final stage of treatment is surgical closure of the colostomy to restore intestinal continuity.

Sigmoid Volvulus. Sigmoid volvulus is a unique lesion that often can be managed in the emergency department by proctoscopy and careful insertion of a well-lubricated large-bore rectal tube. The tube is gently inserted through the proctoscope, and as it reduces the twist in the colon, a sudden release of a large amount of liquid feces occurs, often flooding the operator and his assistants. The tube should be sewn into the perianal skin to prevent premature removal.

If the volvulus cannot be reduced by this technique or if there is clinical evidence of infarction of the bowel, formal operative intervention is required on an emergency basis.

COMPLICATED HERNIAS

A hernia is a protrusion of peritoneal contents through a defect in the abdominal wall. There are numerous types of hernias, but the most common are inguinal, femoral, umbilical, incisional, epigastric, and spigelian.

As a result of the weakness in the abdominal wall, the peritoneum bulges through the defect with increases in intra-abdominal pressure, such as occur with straining, coughing, sneezing, and lifting. As the peritoneum pushes outward through the weakness or defect, a sac is formed into which various organs within the peritoneal cavity may enter. Thus, the hernial sac may contain omentum, small intestine, large intestine, urinary bladder, ovary, and appendix. Generally, hernias are not considered to require emergency treatment unless complications ensue.

In uncomplicated cases, the hernia is reducible; that is, the protruding sac may be replaced into the peritoneal cavity manually by the patient or examiner when intra-abdominal pressure is decreased, as in the recumbent position with the knees flexed.

The most common complications that require emergency care are incarceration and strangulation.

1. *Incarceration*—when incarcerated, the hernia sac is trapped in the abdominal wall defect and cannot be reduced. In this circumstance the patient may have pain, and if the incarcerated sac contains bowel, intestinal obstruction can occur.
2. *Strangulation*—when strangulated, the hernia is not reducible; the blood supply to the contents of the sac, usually the bowel, is compromised, and if left untreated may progress to gangrenous change with its attendant serious implications.

Assessment

Any patient presenting signs or symptoms of an acute abdominal condition must be evaluated for the presence of a complication secondary to a hernia. This possibility must be kept in mind in assessing a patient with intestinal obstruction.

The most common symptom of a complicated hernia is pain at the site of the protrusion. With incarceration, intestinal obstruction may or may not be present. In strangulation, obstruction is more common and is associated with a systemic reaction of fever, leukocytosis, and toxicity. Such a patient may be critically ill and requires complete assessment, including CBC, urinalysis, electrolyte studies, and abdominal x-rays (flat and upright films of the abdomen).

The most common and striking physical finding is a tender mass at the hernia site. The two most common sites of a complicated hernia are the inguinal and femoral regions. It is frequently very difficult to distinguish an inguinal from a femoral hernia because of the proximity of the two sites. The important point is to be able to identify the problem and properly assess whether incarceration or strangulation is present.

Treatment/Management

When an incarcerated hernia is identified, and particularly if it is of recent onset, an attempt should be made to reduce it. This can be done by gentle manipulation of the protrusion, the patient lying on the examining table with the knees flexed to relax the anterior abdominal wall. Inability to reduce an incarcerated hernia is usually an indication for urgent surgery.

If the hernia is thought to be strangulated, an effort can be made to reduce it using the technique described above. It is possible, however, to reduce a strangulated hernia *en masse;* that is, the entire sac and its contents are replaced into the peritoneal cavity as a unit. Thus, the neck of the sac still compromises the blood supply to the hernia contents.

If the hernia is reduced, the patient should be admitted and observed closely to ensure that the acute problem has subsided, and elective repair may be performed during the same hospitalization.

If the hernia is not reduced, or if the acute symptoms do not subside after apparently successful reduction, urgent surgery is necessary. When this judgment is made, fluid replacement should be initiated and the patient prepared for surgery.

MESENTERIC VASCULAR OCCLUSION

Occlusive disease of the blood vessels of the intestine is usually found in patients over the age of 60 and is associated with arteriosclerotic cardiovascular disease. Occlusion may develop in either the arterial or venous mesenteric vessels.[35] Arterial occlusion results from thrombosis or embolism. Venous occlusion follows primary thrombosis. Whether the process starts on the arterial or venous side, the end result, infarction and gangrene of the bowel, is the same.

Thrombotic occlusive disease results from buildup of atheromatous plaque in the lumen of the vessel until complete blockage occurs. In embolic occlusion, the origin of the embolus is usually a mural thrombus in the heart. The cardiac rhythm is typically auricular fibrillation, and a portion of the thrombus breaks off from the left atrium and lodges in the mesenteric artery.

The vessels involved are usually those supplying the small intestine—the superior mesenteric artery or vein. The inferior mesenteric artery, which supplies the left colon, though sometimes occluded in patients with abdominal aortic aneurysm, is much less frequently involved. If involved, it rarely results in infarction of the colon because of good collateral flow through the marginal artery.

Assessment

In acute occlusion of the mesenteric vessels, the most striking complaint is poorly localized pain. The pain is continuous but may be associated with cramps. Constipation or diarrhea may be observed as the process continues. Bleeding from the rectum develops as a result of infarction of the bowel wall. Emesis is not a common finding. The patient may give a history suggestive of mesenteric artery insufficiency or arteriosclerotic heart disease with fibrillation.

The cardiac state is carefully evaluated. Auricular fibrillation in the presence of supportive history and abdominal findings suggests embolic mesenteric artery occlusion. Abdominal findings are often insignificant, especially early in the course of the disease. As the period of vascular occlusion lengthens, gangrenous changes occur in the bowel, resulting in peritonitis. Physical examination may then reveal more striking findings.

Peritoneal tap may be useful. Blood count and urinalysis are not usually abnormal, though leukocytosis can occur. X-rays of the abdomen may reveal a striking absence of gas in the intestinal tract. Arterial blood gases often reveal a significant base deficit and are thus helpful in the diagnosis.

Management/Treatment

Since there may be fluid loss due to peritonitis, fluid replacement is necessary. Early exploration of the abdomen is indicated. In patients who have mesenteric artery occlusion with early ischemic changes, removal of the clot with a Fogarty catheter may restore circulation. Secondary laparotomy may be done 12 to 24 hours later to check on intestinal viability and remove any bowel with impaired blood supply. In instances of frank gangrene, resection of the involved bowel is necessary. At times, massive resection involving almost the entire small bowel may be necessary. In such cases, the prognosis is grave.

SUMMARY

Patients with acute abdominal conditions present a challenge to the knowledge, skills and ingenuity of the emergency nurse.

Familiarity with the anatomy of the abdominal organs and with the pain patterns and clinical pictures of the more common acute abdominal diseases will help determine the cause in the majority of such patients. Laboratory and x-ray studies, as indicated, are helpful in giving additional data to support the diagnosis.

Management in the emergency department is aimed at diagnosis, initiation of measures to correct the altered physiology, control of pain, and preparation of the patient for operative intervention when necessary.

REFERENCES

1. Adams R, Stranahan A: Cholecystitis and cholelithiasis: Analytical report of 1104 operative cases. Surg Gynecol Obstet 85:776, 1947
2. Anderson MC, Scheenfeld FB, Iams WB, Suwa M: Circulatory changes in acute pancreatitis. Surg Clin North Am 47:127, 1967
3. Berne TV, Shore EH: Appraisal of the traumatized abdomen. Surg Clin North Am 48:1197, 1968
4. Brown H, Sass M, Cheng PZ: Infectious mononucleosis and splenic rupture: Report of a case. Ohio Med J 60:954, 1964
5. Byrne JJ, Hennessy VL Jr: Diverticulitis of the colon. Surg Clin North Am 52:991, 1972
6. Carden ABG: Acute large-bowel obstruction: Aetiology and mortality. Med J Aust 1:662, 1966
7. Carnevali JF, ReMine WH: Radical versus conservative surgical management of acute perforated peptic ulcer. Postgrad Med 32:119–126, 1962
8. Ching E, ReMine WH: Surgical management of emergency complications of duodenal ulcer. Surg Clin North Am 51:851–856, August 1971
9. Clark DD, Hubay CA: Tube cecostomy: Evaluation of 161 cases. Ann Surg 175:55, 1972
10. Cleator IGM, Holubitsky IB, Harrison RC: Perforated anastomotic ulcers. Ann Surg 177:436–440, 1973
11. DeBray C, Hardovin JP, Besancon F, Rainibault J: Frequency of diverticulosis of the colon, according to age. Sem Hop Paris 37:1743, 1961
12. Facey FL, Weil MH, Rosoff L: Mechanism and treatment of shock associated with acute pancreatitis. Am J Surg 111:374, 1966
13. Felix WR, Stahlgren LH: Death by undiagnosed perforated peptic ulcer: Analysis of 31 cases. Ann Surg 177:344, 1973
14. Ferris DO, Sterling WA: Surgery of the biliary tract. Surg Clin North Am 47:861, 1967
15. Floyd CE, Stirling CT, Cohn I Jr: Cancer of the colon, rectum and anus: Review of 1687 cases. Ann Surg 163:829, 1966
16. Forward AD: Hypokalemia associated with sigmoid volvulus. Surg Gynecol Obstet 123:35, 1966
17. Gammill SL, Nice CM Jr: Air fluid levels: Their occurrence in normal patients and their role in analysis of ileus. Surgery 71:771, 1972
18. Glenn F, Moody FC: Acute obstructive suppurative cholangitis. Surg Gynecol Obstet 113:265, 1961
19. Gliedman ML, Bolooki H, Rosen RG: Acute Pancreatitis: Current Problems in Surgery. Chicago, Year Book Medical Publishers, 1970
20. Hardy J: Mechanism of shock in peritonitis: Effects upon blood volume, heart action and peripheral vessels. J Surg Res 1:64, 1961
21. Harris S, Rudolf LE: Mechanical small bowel obstruction due to acute appendicitis: Review of 10 cases. Ann Surg 164:157, 1966
22. Hines JR, Geurkink RE, Bass RT: Recurrence and mortality rates in sigmoid volvulus. Surg Gynecol Obstet 124:567, 1967
23. Holder TM, Leape LL: The acute surgical abdomen in children. N Engl J Med 277:921, 1967
24. Jordan GL Jr, Angel RT, DeBakey ME: Acute gastroduodenal perforation: Comparative study of treatment with simple closure, subtotal gastrectomy and hemigastrectomy and vagotomy. Arch Surg 92:449, 1956
25. Lo AM, Evans WE, Carey LC: Review of small bowel obstruction at Milwaukee County General Hospital. Am J S 111:884, 1966
26. McDonald JC: Nonspecific mesenteric lymphadenitis: Collective review. Surg Gynecol Obstet 116:409, 1963
27. McIlrath DC, Larson RH: Surgical management of larger perforations of the duodenum. Surg Clin North Am 51:857–862, August 1971
28. McIndoe AH: Delayed hemorrhage following traumatic rupture of the spleen. Br J Surg 20:249, 1932
29. Maynard AD, Prigot A: Gastroduodenal perforation: A report of

120 cases over a five and one-half year period with consideration of the role of primary gastrectomy. Ann Surg 153:261, 1961

30. Mayo CW, Delaney LT: Colonic diverticulitis associated with carcinoma. Arch Surg 72:957, 1956
31. Nardi GL: Acute pancreatitis. Surg Clin North Am 46:619, 1966
32. Nissan S, Levy E: Intussusception in infancy caused by hypertrophic Peyer's patches. Surgery 59:1108, 1966
33. Opie EL: Diseases of the Pancreas, 2nd ed. Philadelphia, JB Lippincott, 1910
34. Orloff MJ, Peskin GW: Collective review: Spontaneous rupture of the normal spleen. Int Abstr Surg 106:1, 1955
35. Ottinger LW, Austen WG: Study of 136 patients with mesenteric infarction. Surg Gynecol Obstet 124:251, 1967
36. Perry JF, DeMeules JE, Root HD: Diagnostic peritoneal lavage in blunt abdominal trauma. Surg Gynecol Obstet 131:742, 1970
37. Pines B, Rabinovitch J: Perforation of the gallbladder in acute cholecystitis. Ann Surg 140:170, 1954
38. Reimer J: Perforating gastric and duodenal ulcers. Primary resection versus suture: An analysis of two 15-year series. Acta Chir Scand 33:38, 1967

39. Rodkey G, Welch CD: Surgical management of colonic diverticulitis with free perforation or abscess formation. Am J Surg 117:265, 1969
40. Rosoff L, Cohen JL, Telfer N, Halpern M: Injuries of the spleen. Surg Clin North Am 52:667, 1972
41. Rosoff L, Meyers H: Acute emphysematous cholecystitis: An analysis of ten cases. Am J Surg 111:410, 1966
42. Schumer W, Burman SD: The perforated viscus: Diagnosis and treatment. Surg Clin North Am 52:231–237, February 1972
43. Seeley SF, Campbell D: Nonoperative treatment of perforated peptic ulcer. Int Abstr Surg 102:435–446, 1956
44. Talbert JL, Zuidema GD: Appendicitis: A reappraisal of an old problem. Surg Clin North Am 46:1101, 1966
45. Thorbjarnarson B: Acute appendicitis in patients over the age of sixty. Surg Gynecol Obstet 125:1277, 1967
46. Thoroughman JC, Walker LG, Graytaylor B, Dunn T: Free perforation of anastomotic ulcers. Ann Surg 169:790, 1969
47. Williams JS, Hale HW Jr: Acute appendicitis in the elderly. Ann Surg 162:208, 1965

BIBLIOGRAPHY

Bates B: A Guide to Physical Examination. Philadelphia, JB Lippincott, 1983

d'e Lorimier AA: The acute abdomen. In Pascoe D, Grossman M (eds): Quick Reference to Pediatric Emergencies. Philadelphia, JB Lippincott, 1973

Jacox AK: Assessing pain. Am J Nurs 79:895–900, 1979

Jaffe JH, Martin WR: Narcotic analgesics and antagonists. In Goodman LS, Gilman A (eds): The Pharmacological Basis of Therapeutics. New York, Macmillan, 1975

Johnson M: Pain. Nursing '76 6:48–50, 1976

Loebl S et al: The Nurse's Drug Handbook. New York, John Wiley & Sons, 1977

McCaffery M: Nursing Management of the Patient with Pain. Philadelphia, JB Lippincott, 1979

McCaffery M, Hart LL: Understanding of acute pain with narcotics. Am J Nurs 76:1586–1591, 1976

Silen W: Abdominal pain. In Wintrob MM et al: Harrison's Principles of Internal Medicine, 7th ed. New York, McGraw-Hill, 1974

Silman J: The management of pain. Am J Nurs 79:74–78, 1979

Willacker J: Bowel sounds. Am J Nurs 73:2100–2101, 1973

23

CARE OF THE PATIENT WITH GASTROINTESTINAL BLEEDING

JAMES H. COSGRIFF, JR. and DIANN ANDERSON

Patients with gastrointestinal bleeding are frequently seen in emergency settings. Because of the usually sudden onset of symptoms and the nonvisible source, gastrointestinal bleeding can produce a frightening situation for the patient, his family and the uninitiated emergency staff.

Most episodes of gastrointestinal bleeding are minor and, though potentially serious, not life threatening. Less commonly, hemorrhage may be massive and life threatening requiring immediate action. Bleeding from any body orifice, however, presents emergency personnel with a challenging responsibility to evaluate and diagnose the problem and institute prompt and appropriate management. The clinical picture and management are determined by the underlying pathology, the extent of blood loss and the presence or absence of associated disease.

One concept bears repetition: *Massive bleeding may be fatal and requires prompt, definitive treatment.*

Since the early management of the patient with gastrointestinal (GI) bleeding may be handled by emergency personnel, it is necessary that they be familiar with the emergency management of GI bleeding as summarized in Chart 23-1. Although each objective is important in itself, in actual practice, each measure will probably not be achieved singly. It is common in emergency practice to implement several objectives simultaneously.

INSTITUTING LIFE-SUPPORT MEASURES

INITIAL ASSESSMENT AND MANAGEMENT

- Initially, obtain and record the patient's temperature, pulse, blood pressure, and respiratory rate, keeping in mind that the position of the patient and his anxiety level will affect the findings.[11]
- Observe for other signs and symptoms of hypovolemic shock:

  Tachycardia—early in the shock state, tachycardia (usually above 100 bpm) may be the only abnormal vital sign.

  Pallor—especially in the conjunctivae

  Cool, clammy skin.

Chart 23-1

EMERGENCY MANAGEMENT OF THE PATIENT WITH GASTROINTESTINAL BLEEDING

Principles and Objectives

- Assess the need for life-support measures
- Initiate measures to control bleeding and restore circulating blood volume as needed
- Collect and identify pertinent data to establish the bleeding site and determine possible cause
- Prepare the patient and family for definitive treatment, be it surgical or nonsurgical
- Provide comfort and reassurance to the patient and family
- Evaluate the effectiveness of emergency measures at timely intervals

Emergency Management

- Assess and record vital signs
- Treat for shock
- Initiate fluid replacement, using Ringer's lactate through large-bore indwelling veinway
- Obtain blood samples for baseline studies:
  CBC
  Platelet count
  Prothrombin time
  Partial thromboplastin time
  Clotting time
  Type and crossmatch
  Arterial blood gases
- Insert nasogastric sump tube to evaluate stomach contents
- Insert Foley catheter and measure urine output
- Consider continuous iced-saline lavage if upper GI bleeding is present
- Give type-specific blood replacement when available
- Consider preparing the patient for diagnostic upper GI panendoscopy

- Draw venous blood samples immediately for complete blood count (CBC), blood workup, and type and cross-match.
- Use the same veinway to begin fluid replacement with Ringer's lactate until type-specific blood is available.
- Include measurement of arterial blood gases as part of the baseline studies, especially in a patient with massive bleeding or one in frank shock.

While the above measures are being initiated, a brief history and rapid physical assessment should be carried out. Examine for ecchymoses (they could suggest a bleeding tendency), palpate the abdomen for tenderness (ulcer) or masses (enlarged liver or spleen), look for the stigmata of liver disease, check for allergies, and make sure urinalysis is included in the baseline laboratory studies. Information gleaned from this assessment may be helpful in planning the therapeutic program.

Fluid Replacement

The best and most accessible fluid for volume replacement is Ringer's lactate.

The *speed of infusion* depends on numerous factors such as:
- The patient's age
- The presence of cardiac or pulmonary disease
- The amount and duration of blood loss
- The response to infusion as measured by periodic monitoring of vital signs

In elderly or depleted patients or in the young, a central vein catheter should be placed to measure central venous pressure. This is inserted through the jugular, subclavian, or antecubital vein and gives information on the filling pressure of the right heart. This central veinway may provide an index of functional intravascular volume and also serves as a pathway for the rapid infusion of fluids.

The *rate of fluid replacement* should be decided by the physician. In older patients or those with impaired cardiac function, too rapid infusion can result in left heart failure, pulmonary congestion, and frank edema.

The *fluid of choice for replacement* of depleted blood volume, under optimal conditions, is whole blood. In most areas of the country, however, this is no longer available. In its place, packed red cells are used. (See Chapt. 13, Parenteral Fluid Therapy.)
- Although type-specific blood cells are ideal, in an extreme emergency, typed but uncrossmatched packed red cells can be infused with little risk to the patient.
- A specific consent indicating the nature of the emergency and the patient's need for uncrossmatched blood must be signed by the physician.
- In the direst circumstances, universal donor cells (type O) can be given. When these unmatched cells are given, they should be checked by the blood bank against the patient's blood at a later time for incompatibility.

The *amount of blood* needed to restore a patient to a normovolemic state is a critical consideration. First, it must be remembered that in the early hours after onset of bleeding, even massive bleeding, the hemoglobin and hematocrit levels may be near normal or falsely elevated because of vasoconstriction and a decrease in the size of the vascular bed. Between 18 and 24 hours may pass before hemodilution occurs and a more realistic value is obtained. The best indication of adequate replacement is a return of vital signs to normal range and satisfactory serial determinations of hemoglobin and hematocrit at 4- to 6-hour intervals.
- Generally, as a rule of thumb, 1 unit of packed red cells will raise the hemoglobin level 1 gm. Thus, if the patient's hemoglobin on admission was 10 gm and transfusion was necessary, 4 units of packed red cells would be required to raise the hemoglobin to 14 gm.
- Similarly, 1 unit of packed red cells would increase the hemoglobin by 3% to 4%.
- Keep in mind that falsely elevated hemoglobin levels may be found shortly after the onset of bleeding.

Blood Incompatibility (See Table 13-2, p 173)

It is important to be constantly on the alert for any evidence of blood incompatibility. Before initiating blood infusion, properly identify donor blood by its laboratory number, verifying the type and a satisfactory crossmatch. Although reactions due to incompatible blood may not herald a serious outcome, they may produce deleterious effects.

Among the usual reactions of incompatible blood are:
- Urticaria
- Lumbar pain
- Tightness in the chest
- A burning sensation of the face.

There may be some degree of collapse, apprehension, chilling, tachycardia and fever. Although body temperature readings are not routinely taken during blood transfusion, a rise in temperature often occurs before other signs and symptoms; thus, body temperature is worth observing.[2] Hematuria and anuria may also develop, indicating filtration problems in the kidneys.

Observation of any of the aforementioned phenomena requires the following:
- The transfusion should be stopped.
- The physician should be notified.
- Urine output should be measured and the first specimen saved to determine the presence of red cells.
- The remaining blood should be returned to the laboratory to check for type, crossmatching, and bacterial contamination.
- The patient should be observed for further signs of incompatibility.
- Diphenhydramine (Benadryl), given parenterally, is helpful in urticarial reactions.

EVALUATION

During this early phase, close monitoring of vital signs and clinical state is essential to determining the effectiveness of the life-support measures. Although the vital signs are affected by numerous factors, including the patient's age and his usual response to stress, it can be generally stated that additional blood replacement is needed when:

Chart 23-2

ASSESSMENT KEYS IN HYPOVOLEMIA

- Patient apprehensive, restless, may have air hunger
- Skin pale, cool to cold, clammy
- Blood pressure low—in hypertensive patients an otherwise normal blood pressure may be at shock level.
- Tachycardia, pulse rate over 100 bpm.

---

1. The systolic blood pressure falls below 90 to 100 mm. Hg in a previously normotensive person or is significantly lowered in a hypertensive patient.
2. The pulse remains elevated above 100 beats per minute.
3. There are continued signs and symptoms of hypovolemic shock, such as pallor, cold and clammy extremities, restlessness, faintness, dyspnea, thirst, and apprehension (see Chart 23-2).
4. Urinary output falls below 25 to 30 ml/hr.
5. Blood loss continues.
6. Hemoglobin and hematocrit are below normal levels.

ONGOING ASSESSMENT AND MANAGEMENT

Assessment of Hematemesis or Melena

Once life-support measures have been initiated, additional information should be collected to identify the bleeding site and determine the cause. Hematemesis and melena are significant assessment findings. Bear in mind, for practical purposes, that the GI tract may be divided into two main parts (upper and lower) by the ligament of Treitz, a structure supporting the intestine at the junction of the duodenum and the jejunum.

1. The *upper part of the GI tract* consists of the *esophagus, stomach, and duodenum.* Bleeding from the upper portion of the GI tract is manifested by vomiting of blood (hematemesis) and/or passage of bloody or tarry stools (melena). The vomited blood may be unaltered in appearance or may resemble coffee grounds, the latter phenomenon being caused by the action of gastric acid on hemoglobin to form acid hematin. As for melena, experimentally, as little as 50 ml to 80 ml of ingested blood may produce a tarry stool.[7] Blood within the gut tends to stimulate peristaltic activity and speed transit time, which explains the presence of gross blood in the stool from bleeding lesions in the upper tract.

2. The *lower part of the GI tract* consists of the *jejunum, ileum, and colon.* Bleeding from the lower GI tract is manifested by bloody or tarry stools (melena). Although tarry stools more likely indicate bleeding from the upper tract, gastric juices present in the intestine may modify blood loss and produce melena. Gross blood from the rectum, in the absence of blood recovered from the upper tract by the nasogastric tube, usually places the lesion distal to the ligament of Treitz. Bleeding from the upper tract can usually be localized, but it is much more difficult, sometimes impossible, to pinpoint the site of lower tract bleeding.

Management of Gastrointestinal Bleeding

- A nasogastric sump tube should be inserted in any patient with GI bleeding, to provide relief by gastric decompression and assist in determining the severity, nature, and site of bleeding.
- The presence of gross blood may indicate active bleeding and thus requires close observation of the patient.
- If coffee-ground material is recovered, it should be tested for blood by Hematest or some similar method.
- If fresh bleeding is encountered, gastric lavage should be started, using iced saline. Continuous lavage may be initiated in the emergency department and extended to the intensive care unit, if necessary.

Assessment of Drug Effects

A history of the onset of the illness should be obtained from patient or family, including careful questioning about ulcer disease, alcoholism, and ingestion of drugs such as phenylbutazone, aspirin or other salicylates, steroids, and anticoagulants. A tarry stool may be produced by certain foods and drugs, especially iron or bismuth compounds (*e.g.,* Pepto Bismol). A sample of stool obtained by rectal examination may be tested by the Hematest method to establish whether or not blood is indeed present. Commonly used medications that may cause GI bleeding are listed below.

- Anticoagulants—heparin, bishydroxycoumarin, warfarin
- Salicylates—aspirin, salicylate compounds
- Antiinflammatory agents—phenylbutazone, ibuprofen
- Steroids—cortisone, prednisone, prednisolone

EMOTIONAL SUPPORT OF THE PATIENT AND FAMILY

The sight of massive blood loss is a terrifying experience for the patient and family. When the source is not apparent, as in GI bleeding, and the event sudden and unexpected, fear and anxiety are often present. While it is obvious that immediate action must be taken to resuscitate a patient with severe bleeding, it is important not to lose sight of the need for emotional support. For the patient, this can be accomplished by the emergency personnel proceeding in a calm, knowledgeable way and explaining whenever possible what is to be done and why. The patient should be kept warm and in a comfortable position. For the family, providing a quiet room with visits by the nurse or physician to inform them of the progress of treatment and to respond to their questions adds considerably to their support. If urgent surgery is needed, an effort should be made to keep the patient and family fully informed about the nature and purpose of the procedure.

CAUSES OF UPPER GASTROINTESTINAL TRACT BLEEDING

The causes of upper GI tract bleeding are listed in Chart 23-3; common sites are shown in Fig. 23-1. Gastritis, peptic ulcer, and esophageal varices are the conditions most commonly associated with upper GI bleeding. This section discusses the assessment and management of patients with these conditions.

GASTRITIS

Gastritis is an inflammation of the mucosa of the stomach frequently associated with episodes of heavy alcohol intake or prolonged use of aspirin, anticoagulants, phenylbutazone, and related drugs and steroids. Gastritis is the most common cause of upper GI bleeding, although the bleeding is rarely massive.

Assessment

The symptoms of gastritis are of short duration and are not suggestive of ulcer disease. The patient may give a history of heavy alcohol intake or drugs as mentioned above, followed by pain, indigestion, and hematemesis. Physical assessment usually reveals no distinctive signs. Nasogastric drainage contains fresh blood or coffee ground material.

Management

Initial treatment is directed toward:

- Stabilizing the patient
- Obtaining baseline laboratory tests, and

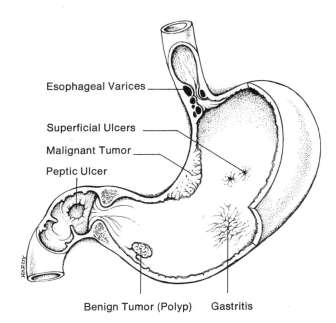

Figure 23-1 *Upper gastrointestinal bleeding. The common sites and causes of massive bleeding are indicated.*

Labels: Esophageal Varices, Superficial Ulcers, Malignant Tumor, Peptic Ulcer, Benign Tumor (Polyp), Gastritis

- Making preparations for emergency diagnostic procedures.

The most useful test is upper gastrointestinal panendoscopy, which can be done by an experienced endoscopist in the emergency department. Once the diagnosis is made, both the patient and family should be advised of the causative factors and properly tutored in dietary and/or medical restrictions.

PEPTIC ULCER

Peptic ulcer is the most common cause of massive upper GI hemorrhage. Although peptic ulcer can occur at any age,[21] it is more common in the fifth through seventh decades. It is estimated that 20% of patients with peptic ulcers bleed, and that 5% bleed massively. The ulcer is most frequently located in the duodenum, less often in the stomach.

Assessment

The history is important. Most patients give a history of prior peptic disease, some identified by previous GI series; others report frequent use of antacids. Perhaps as many as 30% of patients with massive bleeding deny previous symptoms. Bleeding may be in the form of hematemesis or melena. (As previously mentioned, melena alone does not rule out the upper GI tract as a source of bleeding.) At times, the patient may give a history of syncope. When syncope occurs, it usually indicates severe blood loss.

Abdominal findings may be minimal, although tenderness can be found in the area of the duodenal bulb, just above or to the right of the umbilicus. The nasogastric aspirate may contain whole blood or coffee-ground material. It is easy to be misled if only normal-appearing gastric juice is recovered, because in some patients with bleeding from a duodenal ulcer, the pyloric ring may be closed by edema

---

Chart 23-3

CAUSES OF UPPER GASTROINTESTINAL TRACT

Common Causes

- Gastritis
- Peptic ulcer
- Esophageal varices (usually associated with cirrhosis and portal hypertension)

Less Common Causes

- Long-standing use of aspirin or other salicylates, anticoagulants, or steroids, etc.
- Acute pancreatitis with duodenitis
- Focal areas of gastritis in a hiatal hernia
- Linear tears at the gastroesophageal junction (Mallory-Weiss syndrome)
- Benign or malignant neoplasms of the stomach or duodenum
- Congenital malformations of the stomach or duodenum (hemangioma, telangiectasia)
- Stress ulcers associated with severe trauma or underlying disease (burns, central nervous system disorders)
- Esophagitis

surrounding the ulcer, thus prohibiting the regurgitation of duodenal contents into the stomach. For the same reason, bile is not recovered on aspiration. The main symptom in such a patient is *rectal bleeding*.

Management

Initially, treatment follows the principles discussed above: evaluation and stabilization of the patient, use of diagnostic measures to identify the source of bleeding, and initiation of definitive therapy.

Factors that influence the management of a patient with a bleeding ulcer include the physician's preference, the duration and severity of illness, the patient's age, the presence or absence of associated disease, the availability of type-specific blood, and the capability of the surgical team.

- Massive bleeding from a chronic peptic ulcer may be a life-threatening condition, and in a patient with coronary artery disease can precipitate an episode of coronary insufficiency or full-blown infarction.
- Acute ulceration, such as a stress ulcer or one due to medication, also requires special consideration.

The various modes of therapy may be divided into operative and nonoperative approaches.

The *nonoperative approach* includes:
- Diagnostic endoscopy
- Blood volume replacement
- Continuous iced-saline lavage to control bleeding
- Hydrogen-ion suppression with parenteral cimetidine
- Progressive advancement of diet

The *operative approach* to definitive care of the patient with a bleeding ulcer includes blood replacement, diagnostic endoscopy, and urgent surgery. The general principles of transfusion and direct attack on the bleeding site are modified only by the choice of operative procedure.[21]

Definitive surgical procedures for peptic ulcer include subtotal gastric resection, hemigastrectomy and vagotomy, antrectomy and vagotomy, and elective or highly selective vagotomy with suture ligation of the bleeding point and with or without pyloroplasty.

One other mode of therapy should be mentioned; it is referred to as the "test of transfusion." The patient is treated by continuous iced saline lavage, blood replacement, and close observation. If the bleeding ceases in 24 to 48 hours, as evidenced by normal, stable vital signs and rising hemoglobin, nonoperative management is continued. Should bleeding recur, the patient is treated by urgent surgery. The ultimate choice of treatment is made by the physician and the patient, giving due consideration to the factors outlined above.

ESOPHAGEAL VARICES

Esophageal varices are enlarged veins that develop in the portal venous system draining the GI tract (Fig. 23-2). The varices are most prominent in the lower portion of the esophagus and the upper end of the stomach. Other veins involved are those of the omentum, the mesentery, and the diaphragm. The spleen is usually enlarged because of increased pressure in the splenic vein which is a major vessel

Figure 23-2 *Esophageal varices. Such varices usually result from portal hypertension.*

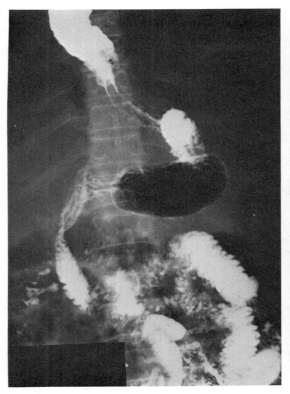
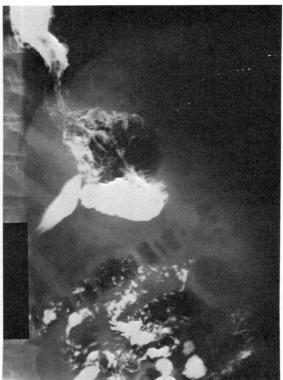

contributing to the portal system. The increased pressure in this system (portal hypertension, Fig. 23-3) is due to a number of factors. In adults, it is usually associated with cirrhosis of the liver secondary to chronic alcoholism (Laennec's type) or following hepatitis (postnecrotic type). It also may be found in children in association with thrombosis of the portal vein (Banti's disease).

Assessment

Variceal bleeding is usually massive. The patient may give a history of hematemesis characterized by blood "welling up" in the throat. One may obtain a history of long-standing alcohol intake.

Cardinal Signs of Chronic Liver Disease. It is most important to be able to recognize the cardinal signs of chronic liver disease on physical assessment: These include the following:

- Spider angiomata of the upper trunk
- Jaundice
- Sparse pubic and axillary hair
- Shoulder-girdle atrophy
- Ascites
- Superficial venous pattern of the trunk and abdomen (thoracoepigastric veins and caput medusa)
- Palmar erythema

It is particularly important to be aware that the incidence of peptic ulcer is 15% to 20% greater in patients with cirrhosis than in the general population. Both the peptic ulcer and varices can thus occur concomitantly, and bleeding may arise from either source.

In variceal bleeding, the nasogastric aspirate is grossly bloody with little significant change. Perhaps the most important means of identifying bleeding varices is endoscopy of the upper GI tract. This can be performed, in the emer-

Figure 23-3 Portal hypertension. The drawing illustrates the abdominal organs and vessels that may be involved in portal hypertension. (After Gray HK, Whitesell FB Jr: Annals of Surgery 132:798–810, 1950)

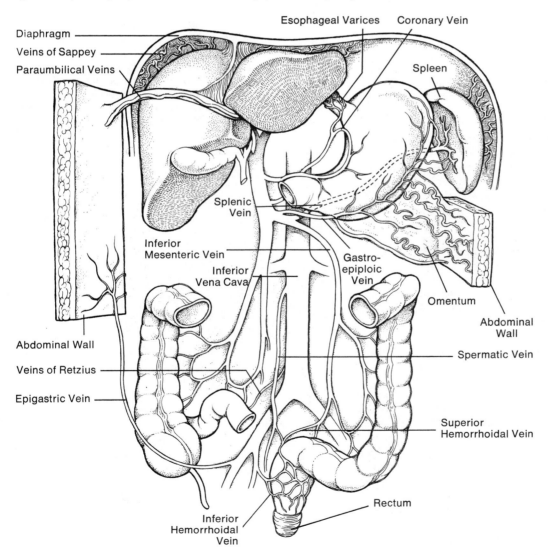

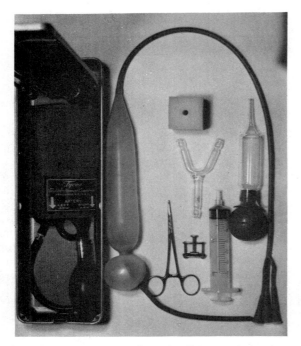

Figure 23-4 *Equipment needed for Sengstaken-Blakemore tube insertion.*

gency department if necessary, by an experienced endoscopist using intravenous and topical analgesia.

Management

Sengstaken-Blakemore Tube. If the bleeding continues and varices are suspected as the cause, the nasogastric tube inserted as part of the routine management for GI bleeding should be removed and a triple-lumen Sengstaken-Blakemore tube inserted. This device has two balloons that, when inflated, provide pressure against the lower portion of the esophagus and fundic portion of the stomach (Figs. 23-4 and 23-5). Successful control of bleeding with this device may serve also as a diagnostic measure. If the bleeding continues when the tube is properly placed, then one must suspect that a bleeding ulcer is present.

Once it has been decided to use the Blakemore-Sengstaken tube, close observation for continued bleeding is necessary, since failure of the tamponade may require some other form of therapy that includes surgical ligation of the bleeding varices or transendoscopic injection of a sclerosing agent into the bleeding vessels.

While the balloons are inflated, oral intake is prohibited. When bleeding ceases, feedings may be given through the gastric lumen of the tube. Parenteral feedings are necessary during the entire period. Tamponade is usually not tolerated for more than 36 to 48 hours. At that time, the esophageal balloon should be slowly deflated first and the gastric balloon left inflated with the traction maintained. During this time, the patient should be observed closely for rebleeding.

Posterior Pituitary Extract. An adjunct measure that may be combined with the Blakemore-Sengstaken tube during the emergency phase of care is the use of posterior pituitary extract (vasopressin or Pitressin).[7,18] Vasopressin causes a fall in portal vein pressure but concomitantly has a vasoconstrictive effect on both peripheral and coronary arteries. It may produce a significant decrease in coronary artery flow and cardiac output and can cause cardiac arrhythmias. It can be given by direct infusion into the superior mesenteric artery at a rate of 0.2 to 0.4 units per minute. The intravenous route has proven effective. A continuous drip is begun at the rate of 0.4 units per minute. If bleeding stops within an hour, the dosage is reduced by one-half. The drug should be used cautiously or avoided in patients with known coronary artery or cerebral vascular disease.

Further management of the patient with bleeding esophageal varices varies and depends in part on the parameters mentioned under the discussion of the patient with a bleeding ulcer. Other considerations are the status of the patient's liver disease and whether the acute hemorrhage can be controlled by tamponade and the patient's condition stabilized with blood replacement.

Liver Function Tests. Basic blood tests should be done on all patients with GI bleeding (see p 412) but in those with bleeding varices, baseline liver function tests should be made (SGOT, SGPT, alkaline phosphatase, bilirubin, total protein). With underlying liver disease, defects in the clotting mechanism may be detected by elevation of the prothrombin time (PT) and partial thromboplastin time (PTT). If a clotting defect is identified, appropriate doses of vitamin K_1 oxide (Aquamephyton) should be given intravenously. Menodione sodium diphosphate (standard vitamin K) is not synthesized by the damaged liver and hence is of no value.

Figure 23-5 *Sengstaken-Blakemore tube in place.*

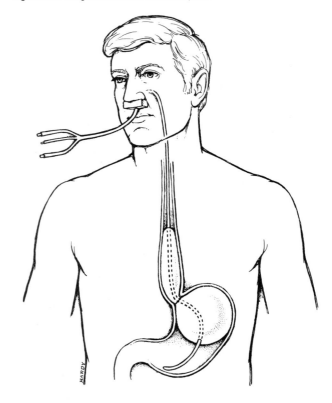

Injection of Sclerosing Agents. Transendoscopic injection of sclerosing agents into the varices has successfully controlled bleeding, but this mode of therapy is presently reserved for high-risk patients who are unacceptable for surgery.

Surgical Procedures. A clinical classification of these patients has been devised by Child by which a better determination may be made as to the mode of treatment that is indicated and that the patient can tolerate.[5] Preferably, surgical decompression is the treatment of choice. Several procedures involving shunting of blood from the high-pressure portal vein to the lower pressure systemic venous system are currently in use, including portocaval, distal splenorenal, and mesocaval shunts.

The operative approach to arrest of acute bleeding from varices includes transesophageal ligation of the varices.

CAUSES OF LOWER GASTROINTESTINAL TRACT BLEEDING

One of the primary considerations in patients with rectal bleeding is determination of the source, keeping in mind the possibility that it may be in the upper tract. The upper tract must first be eliminated as the source of rectal bleeding before causes of lower tract bleeding are considered. Generally, early management of lower tract bleeding is similar to that of bleeding from the upper tract; care is taken to monitor vital signs, obtain baseline hematologic and biochemical data, and assess the patient's clinical state. Replacement of circulating blood volume, observation of urinary output, and initiation of appropriate diagnostic studies are helpful. *Sedatives for such patients should be used with caution and should preferably be administered intravenously.*

Adjunct studies in evaluating a patient with lower tract bleeding include barium enema, upper GI series, sigmoidoscopy, and colonoscopy. Frank rectal bleeding is a primary indication for colonoscopy. Unfortunately, the procedure cannot be adequately performed in the face of active bleeding because visualization will be seriously impaired by the blood.

The most common cause of massive lower GI hemorrhage is diverticular disease. There are two main types, diverticula of the colon and diverticula in the small bowel. Other causes include hemorrhoids, anal fissure, proctitis, ulcerative colitis, intussusception, stercoral ulceration, benign and malignant neoplasms, and certain medications (see Chart 23-4).

COLONIC DIVERTICULA

Diverticulosis of the colon is the most common cause of massive lower GI bleeding and may occur in the absence of detectable secondary inflammation (diverticulitis). Diverticulosis is common beyond age 40. The patient's history may be negative prior to the bleeding episode or may be one of abdominal cramps (caused by the irritating effect of the blood in the colon). Though this type of bleeding may

---

Chart 23-4

CAUSES OF LOWER GASTROINTESTINAL TRACT BLEEDING

Common Causes

- Diverticular disease
  Colon diverticula
  Small bowel diverticula (especially Meckel's diverticulum)
- Hemorrhoids
- Anal fissure

Less Common Causes

- Proctitis
- Ulcerative colitis
- Intussusception
- Stercoral ulceration
- Benign or malignant neoplasms
- Long-standing use of aspirin or other salicylates, anticoagulants, steroids, etc.
- Congenital malformation of the small or large intestine (hemangioma, telangiectasia)

---

be life threatening, it is more likely to stop spontaneously than bleeding from the upper tract.

Sigmoidoscopy can be performed early in the management of the patient. It can be done comfortably with the patient in the lateral (Sims') position but should be undertaken only when vital signs are stable.

Once bleeding has subsided, barium studies of the colon and colonoscopy should be done. Both of these studies require good preparation of the bowel. Urgent surgery is rarely indicated, because bleeding usually stops, and exploratory laparotomy is of little value in identifying and localizing the bleeding site. It is preferable that the patient be stabilized and admitted for evaluation and elective surgery.

SMALL BOWEL DIVERTICULA

This condition is an uncommon cause of rectal bleeding. Small bowel diverticula are outpouchings of the small intestine, and unlike those in the colon, they usually occur singly and are congenital in origin. Diverticula may occur anywhere along the length of the small intestine, but the most common site is that described by Meckel in 1815 and referred to as Meckel's diverticulum. It is found in the lower 12 to 18 inches of the small bowel in 2% to 4% of humans. Bleeding from this source is frequently associated with the presence of ectopic gastric or pancreatic mucosa in the diverticulum.

TABLE 23-1. DIFFERENTIAL DIAGNOSIS OF GASTROINTESTINAL TRACT BLEEDING

Bleeding Etiology	Age	Abdominal Pain	Hematemesis	Rectal Bleeding	Upper GI Endoscopy	Lower GI Endoscopy	Nasogastric Aspirate	Other
Gastritis	Adult	At times	Fresh blood or coffee grounds	Usually tarry	Helpful	Not indicated	Fresh blood or coffee grounds	
Peptic ulcer	Usually adult	At times	Fresh blood or coffee grounds Clots may be present	Tarry or dark blood with clots	Helpful	Not indicated	Fresh blood clots or coffee grounds may be present	30%–50% give history of peptic ulcer

Note: If ulcer is in duoenum with no reflux into stomach, no hematemesis will occur and nasogastric aspirate will resemble normal gastric juice *without* bile.

Bleeding Etiology	Age	Abdominal Pain	Hematemesis	Rectal Bleeding	Upper GI Endoscopy	Lower GI Endoscopy	Nasogastric Aspirate	Other
Esophageal varices	Usually adult age 40 or over	Rare	Fresh blood with or without clots	Dark blood or tarry	Helpful	Not indicated	Fresh blood	Abnormal liver function tests Prothrombin time elevated
Lesion(s) in jejunum or ileum	Usually adult	Rare	Never	Dark blood with or without clots	Not indicated	Not helpful	Gastric juice with or without bile	Selective angiography may identify bleeding site
Meckel's diverticulum	Usually child	Rare	Never	Dark blood may be tarry	Not indicated	Not helpful		Consider technitium 99M scan to identify Meckel's diverticulum with ectopic gastric mucosa
Colonic diverticulosis	Usually adult age 40	Rare	Never	Fresh to dark blood with or without clots	Not indicated	Helpful		Barium enema to identify diverticula
Intussusception	Child	Yes—crampy	Never	Dark blood (currant jelly)	Not indicated	Helpful		Barium enema to identify site of obstruction
Colitis proctitis hemorrhoids	Any age usually adult	No	Never	Usually fresh blood with or without clots	Not indicated	Helpful		Sigmoidoscopy helpful

When the bleeding is massive, it may be manifested clinically by dark red or "currant-jelly" stools. Typically, these lesions are found in the younger age group. Chronic low-grade bleeding is associated with tarry or occasionally bloody stools. The history may include crampy midabdominal or lower abdominal pain that occurs after meals. Physical assessment may be negative except for blood in the rectum.

Resuscitation should be initiated to stabilize the patient. The diagnosis is frequently one of exclusion (*i.e.,* other lesions are ruled out by barium studies of the upper and lower tracts). Transfemoral selective angiography of the superior mesenteric artery is a useful diagnostic test when the patient is actively bleeding. Intestinal scanning using intravenous radioactive technetium has shown some promise in establishing the diagnosis. The radioactive substance is picked up in the diverticulum containing ectopic gastric mucosa.[3,12] The method requires special equipment. Definitive treatment is resection of the involved segment of bowel.

Data required for the differential diagnosis of GI tract bleeding are presented in Table 23-1.

REFERENCES

1. Alvarez AS, Sumerskill WH Jr: Gastrointestinal hemorrhage and salicylates. Lancet 2:920, 1958
2. Beland I, Passos J: Clinical Nursing: Pathophysiological and Psychosocial Approaches, 3rd ed. New York, Macmillan, 1975
3. Berquist TH, Nolan NG, Adson MA, Schutt AJ: Diagnosis of Meckel's diverticulum by radioisotope scanning. Mayo Clin Proc 48:98, 1973
4. Brant B, Rosch J, Krippaehne WM: Experience with angiography in diagnosis and treatment of acute gastrointestinal bleeding of various etiologies. Ann Surg 176:419, 1972
5. Child CG: The Liver and Portal Hypertension. Philadelphia: WB Saunders, 1964
6. Daniel WA Jr, Egan S: Quantity of blood required to produce a bloody stool. JAMA 113:2232, 1939
7. Davis WD, Gorlin R, Reichman S, Storaasli JP: Effect of Pitressin in reducing portal pressure in the human being: Preliminary report. N Engl J Med 256:108, 1957
8. Drapanas T: Current concepts in the surgical management of portal hypertension. Ann Surg 159:72, 1964
9. Drapanas T: Interposition mesocaval shunt for treatment of portal hypertension. Ann Surg 176:435, 1972
10. Foley ML: Variations in blood pressure in the lateral recumbent position. Nurs Res 20:64, 1971
11. Graham LE, Conley EM: Evaluation of anxiety and fear in adult surgical patients. Nurs Res 20:113, 1971
12. Jewett TC Jr, Duszynski DO, Allen JE: The visualization of Meckel's diverticulum with ggm Tc-pertechnetate. Surgery 68:567, 1970
13. Mallory GK, Weiss S: Hemorrhages from lacerations of the cardiac orifice of the stomach due to vomiting. Am J Med Sci 178:506, 1929
14. Margulis AR, Heinbecker P, Bernard HR: Operative mesenteric arteriography in the search for the site of bleeding in unexplained gastrointestinal hemorrhage: A preliminary report. Surgery 48:543, 1960
15. Menguy R, Desbaillets L, Okabe S, Masters YF: Abnormal aspirin metabolism in patients with cirrhosis and its possible relationship to bleeding in cirrhotics. Ann Surg 176:412, 1972
16. Miller AC Jr, Hirschowitz BI: Twenty-three patients with Mallory-Weiss syndrome. South Med J 63:441, 1970
17. Quick AJ: Salicylates and bleeding: The aspirin tolerance test. Am J Med Sci 252:265, 1966
18. Schwartz SI, Bales HW, Emerson GL, Mahoney EB: The use of intravenous pitressin in treatment of bleeding esophageal varices. Surgery 45:72, 1959
19. Sengstaken RW, Blakemore AH: Balloon tamponade for control of hemorrhage from esophageal varices. Ann Surg 131:781, 1950
20. Stanley RJ, Wise L: Arteriography in diagnosis of acute gastrointestinal tract bleeding. Arch Surg 107:138, 1973
21. Stewart JD, Cosgriff JH, Gray JG: Experiences with the treatment of acutely massively bleeding peptic ulcer by blood replacement and gastric resection. Surg Gynecol Obstet 103:409, 1956
22. Sugawa C, Werner MH, Hayes DF et al: Early endoscopy: A guide to therapy for acute hemorrhage in the upper gastrointestinal tract. Arch Surg 107:133, 1973
23. Warren WD, Zeppa R, Fomon JJ: Selective transplenic decompression of gastroesophageal varices by distal splenorenal shunt. Ann Surg 166:437, 1967
24. Wychulis AR, Sasso A: Mallory-Weiss syndrome. Arch Surg 107:868, 1973

Bibliography

Baum S et al: Angiographic diagnosis and control of large bowel bleeding. Dis Col Rect 17:447, 1974
Boley SJ et al: Vascular ectasias of the colon. Surg Gynecol Obstet 149:353, 1979
Cameron AJ: Aspirin and gastric ulcer. Mayo Clin Proc 50:565, 1975
Donovan AJ et al: Selective treatment of duodenal ulcer with perforation. Ann Surg 189:627, 1979
Glickman MG: Angiographic therapy for acute GI bleeding. Consultant 16:79, 1976
Gusberg RJ: Shunts for variceal hemorrhage: Why? When? What? 60:1265, 1980
McGuire HH, Jr, Haynes BW, Jr: Massive hemorrhage from diverticulosis of the colon. Ann Surg 175:547, 1972
Mulholland M et al: Surgical treatment of duodenal ulcer. Arch Surg 117:393, 1982
Myers RT: Esophageal bleeding. Hosp Med 14:80, 1978
Nasbeth DC et al: Bleeding esophageal varices: Treatment by embolization and shunting. Am J Surg 11:8, 1981
Peterson WL et al: Routine early endoscopy in upper gastrointestinal tract bleeding: A randomized controlled trial. N Engl J Med 304:925, 1981
Pitcher JL: Varices among patients with varices and upper gastrointestinal hemorrhage. South Med J 70:1183, 1977
Rosch J et al: Selective arterial infusions of vasoconstrictors in acute gastrointestinal bleeding. Radiology 99:27, 1971
Sack J, Aldrete JS: Primary mesenteric venous thrombosis. Surg Gyn Obstet 154:205, 1982
Veidenheimer MD et al: Colonic hemorrhage. Surg Clin North Am 58:581, 1978
VerSteeg KR, Broders CW: Gangrene of the bowel. Surg Clin North Am 59:869, 1979
Welch CE et al: Hemorrhage from the large bowel with special reference to angiodysplasia and diverticular disease. World J Surg 2:73, 1978
Wright HK: Massive colonic hemorrhage. Surg Clin North Am 60:1297, 1980
Yajko RD et al: Current management of upper gastrointestinal bleeding. Ann Surg 181:474, 1975

24
GENITOURINARY EMERGENCIES

JOSEPH P. GAMBACORTA and MARY C. SAND

Patients with genitourinary problems are frequently seen for the first time in the hospital emergency department. The severe pain of renal colic, inability to urinate, or the sight of gross blood in the urine often prompts patients to seek immediate professional care. These patients deserve a thorough clinical evaluation, an accurate diagnosis, and appropriate definitive treatment and care. The role of emergency personnel in helping to meet these objectives is discussed in this chapter, as well as the various procedures, equipment, and techniques necessary for proper management of the urologic emergency.

ANATOMY AND PHYSIOLOGY

The genitourinary tracts of the male and female differ considerably. In the male, the genitourinary system combines the organs of urine formation and excretion with the organs of reproduction, whereas in the female, the lower portion of the urinary tract is closely related to the reproductive organs but entirely separate from them. Furthermore, in the male, the urinary tract consists of both internal organs and external genitalia (penis, testicles, and scrotum). In the female, the organs that make up the urinary tract are completely within the body and are close to the abdominal cavity. Common to both sexes are the components of the urinary tract; the kidneys, ureters, bladder, and urethra.

The kidneys and ureters are often referred to as the upper urinary tract, the bladder and urethra as the lower urinary tract. The kidneys are paired organs located on either side of the vertebral column, overlying the psoas muscle in the paravertebral gutter. They are located outside the peritoneal cavity in the retroperitoneal space and are surrounded by loose areolar tissue known as the perirenal fat and by a dense layer of fibrous tissue called Gerota's fascia.

Posterior to each kidney are the lowermost rib and the transverse processes of the upper lumbar vertebrae. The angle formed by these bone structures is referred to as the costovertebral angle. Anteriorly, the kidney is next to the abdominal organs. The right kidney is slightly lower than the left, being displaced inferiorly by the liver. In a thin person, the lower pole of each kidney may be palpated by careful abdominal examination during inspiration. The arterial blood supply to the kidneys is derived from the right and left renal arteries, which arise from the abdominal aorta.

The two ureters are fibromuscular tubes that serve as conduits for urine from the kidneys to the bladder. Each extends from the pelvis of the kidney on its medial aspect downward into the paravertebral gutter retroperitoneally. The ureter enters the brim of the pelvis as it crosses over the common iliac artery and enters the bladder at the lower posterior wall.

The bladder is roughly pyramidal in shape, and is positioned so that the apex is at the bottom and the base at the top. From the apex, the bladder empties through the urethra. The superior pole of the bladder is covered by peritoneum. The bladder lies behind the symphysis pubis and is not palpable through the abdomen unless distended with urine.

In the female, the urethra extends from the lower end of the bladder close to the anterior wall of the vagina and reaches its external opening at the meatus just posterior to the clitoris.

In the male, the urethra is longer. Just beneath the bladder apex, the urethra is surrounded by the prostate. The urethra passes through the urogenital diaphragm at the membranous portion and enters the penis. The penile urethra extends the entire length of the penis and ends at the meatus on the glans. The testicles are suspended in the scrotum, which is attached to the posterior aspect of the penis and the perineum.

ASSESSMENT

Evaluation of the patient with suspected urinary tract disease requires a careful history and physical assessment. The most common symptoms are pain and some alteration in urinary habits. In traumatic injuries, urinary tract damage must be suspected in patients with penetrating wounds of the upper abdomen and in those with fractures of the pelvis and ribs.

History, Symptoms, and Signs

The following information should be collected:
- The time of onset and location of the pain
- Description of the type of pain: sharp, dull, aching, burning, stinging, constant, or intermittent
- Does voiding have any effect on the pain?
- Has there been any change in urination? any increase in frequency or variation in amount of urine passed? any nocturia?
- Has there been any unusual color in the urine: clear, cloudy, concentrated ("strong"), bloody?
- Is there a history of chills or fever?

Pain originating from the urinary tract is located at the site of the problem. Lesions of the kidney, infection, or trauma usually produce pain in the area of the costovertebral angle and the upper abdomen (epigastrium). When a ureter is involved, as in calculous disease, pain may be felt in the flank, radiating along the course of the ureter and upward into the kidney or downward and anteriorly into the lower abdomen. In obstructive disease of the lower third of the ureter, the pain may radiate into the labia or testis. Obstruction of the ureter, particularly by calculi, causes a typical colicky pain, which is one of the most severe experienced by humans. The pain cycle is crescendic in manner, reaching a peak that may last for minutes and then gradually subsiding. The cyclic pain is due to the peristaltic activity of the ureter against the obstructing lesion.

Symptoms arising from the bladder are usually localized there, in the lower abdomen, and are frequently associated with pain or burning on urination (dysuria). Patients with chronic urinary retention, either obstructive or neurogenic in origin, usually experience little or no suprapubic pain. The most common cause of bladder pain is infection.

Testicular discomfort may range from a dull ache, as in a varicocele, to the very severe localized pain of testicular trauma, torsion, or epididymitis.

Gastrointestinal symptoms often occur secondary to urinary tract disease. These include anorexia, nausea, vomiting, and abdominal pain and distention. In infectious diseases of the kidney, for example, a reflex intestinal ileus may occur with abdominal discomfort and fullness.

Systemic reactions such as chills, fever, and malaise occur with significant frequency in urinary tract infection, especially when the kidney itself is involved.

Physical Examination

Examination of a patient with complaints referrable to the urinary tract should begin with the vital signs, temperature, pulse, respiration, and blood pressure. Complete physical examination is advisable. The urinary tract can be evaluated to a great extent by careful examination of the abdomen. In renal disease, tenderness may be present on deep palpation in the epigastric region. The kidneys are not normally palpable through the abdomen, except in a thin person or in pathologic conditions associated with enlargement of the kidney. With the patient sitting, percussion or a light punch in the costovertebral angle may elicit pain. With ureteral obstruction, tenderness is often present along the course of the ureter. The physical findings are rarely consistent with the severity of the pain, in that abdominal spasm and rebound tenderness are rarely, if ever, found.

When the bladder is involved, tenderness is usually present in the suprapubic area of the abdomen. The bladder is not palpable unless enlarged because of urinary retention; in this case, a mass may be palpable in the midportion of the lower abdomen. Careful percussion will reveal a dull to flattened note in the area of the enlarged bladder. Bladder enlargement can be confirmed in the female by bimanual and vaginal examination. The urethral meatus should be examined visually.

In the male, the external genitalia should be inspected and the scrotal contents palpated to determine that the testes are completely descended. Each testis is suspended by the spermatic cord, an elastic structure that extends from the testis upward into the inguinal area and enters the abdominal wall at the level of the internal inguinal ring. The structure contains blood vessels, nerves, and the vas deferens (the spermatic duct). In inflammatory conditions of the testes, cord enlargement and tenderness may be present. Transillumination of the scrotum may be useful and indeed should be a routine procedure in patients with a testicular mass. The epididymis should be palpated for induration. Examination of the penis reveals such conditions as syphilitic chancres, the superficial ulcers or vesicles associated with herpes simplex, balanitis, meatal stenosis, and urethral discharge. Rectal examination in males reveals the size and consistency of the prostate gland. Vaginal examination in females is advisable in many instances.

Injuries of the urinary tract should be suspected in penetrating wounds of the abdomen and fractures of the pelvis. When the history or physical findings point to urinary tract involvement, a number of adjunct studies are available and should be used as needed to confirm the diagnosis.

Adjunct Studies

A large number of tests are available to assist in the evaluation of the patient with urinary tract symptoms or injury.

Urinalysis. The test most frequently used is simple analysis of the urine. Gross examination for color, specific gravity, sugar, and protein and microscopic study for blood cells, sediment, and bacteria are extremely helpful. Urine culture and sensitivity studies, although not immediately available to the urologist for diagnosis and treatment, are usually of prime importance. The collection of urine for these laboratory examinations is the responsibility of emergency department personnel. Unless ordered otherwise, a clean voided midstream sample should be collected in a sterile container. Most institutions now use one of the commercially prepared kits for this. These kits include a sterile container, an antiseptic for cleansing the meatus, and instructions for their use.

Occasionally, a catheterized urine specimen is required. In this case, it is mandatory that scrupulous aseptic technique be observed. A tray including sterile gloves, drapes, antiseptic, lubricant, and catheter is needed. A forceps should be used to cleanse the meatal area. The catheter should be well lubricated. The passage of the catheter should be made with a constant, steady, gentle pressure until a free flow of urine is obtained.

The urine specimen should be taken to the laboratory immediately or, if this is not possible, should be refrigerated until it can be transported. After standing for a period of time at room temperature, the urinary sediment is altered, *i.e.,* bacteria multiply rapidly, red blood cells break up, and the urine turns alkaline.

Blood Studies. Blood values are often the key to the physiologic state of the body. A routine complete blood count (CBC) and SMA-18 are done. Of particular importance in evaluating renal disease are the blood urea nitrogen (BUN) and creatinine. The BUN is elevated in volume depletion such as dehydration, low perfusion pressures to the kidney, or an increased catabolic process. The creatinine, unlike the BUN, is practically unaffected by diet and fluid intake. It is a more reliable assessment of kidney function. An indication of homeostasis can be provided by the serum electrolytes—sodium, potassium, chloride, and bicarbonate. Serum acid and alkaline phosphatase may be elevated in cancer of the prostate.

X-ray Studies. X-ray studies available in the emergency department include the kidneys, ureters, bladder (KUB) plate, which aids in identifying the size and location of the kidneys. The film should also be carefully examined for any calcification in the area of the renal shadow and along the course of the ureters, for urinary stones.

Intravenous pyelography (IVP) demonstrates the urinary tract in the most physiologic manner. It consists of the intravenous injection of an iodine-containing contrast material. It is filtered from the blood by the kidneys and excreted in the same manner as urine. While this process is going on, several films are taken at specified times and in specified positions. A variation of this study is the infusion pyelogram, in which a large volume of contrast is infused slowly, rather than the single bolus of dye given in the IVP.

Since the contrast medium contains iodine, a substance to which some individuals are highly sensitive, any history of an allergic reaction to iodine-containing drugs, dyes, or foods should be ascertained. Resuscitation equipment must be available in the event of an anaphylactic reaction.

An IVP is of no value if the patient is in shock. Renal perfusion, and thus perfusion of the contrast material, depends on blood pressure. Renal perfusion is impaired with arterial pressures under 60 mm Hg. An IVP is also dependent on renal function. The kidneys of a patient with significantly elevated BUN and creatinine will not visualize on x-ray. In some cases, an infusion pyelogram rather than an IVP will give satisfactory results. In a patient with renal colic, an IVP can be most helpful in outlining the excretory ducts of the kidneys and the ureters to locate a stone. Any patient with a renal injury that may involve removal of a whole kidney or part of a kidney must have an intravenous pyelogram preoperatively to evaluate the function of both kidneys and assure the physician that both kidneys are indeed present. More involved studies, such as renal scintiscans and renal arteriograms, may be useful in determining renal function, the integrity of the renal parenchyma, or damage, especially in the patient suspected of urinary tract injuries.

Patients with pelvic fracture and blood in the urine must be evaluated for injury to the bladder. A simple technique, which can be carried out in the emergency department, is retrograde cystography (Fig. 24-1). Renograffin or a similar contrast material is injected into the bladder through a catheter, and x-rays of the region are taken (Fig. 24-2). Deformity of the bladder wall may indicate a contusion or hematoma, while extravasation of urine is pathognomonic for perforation of the bladder.

A *urethrogram* may be the procedure of choice in a patient who has sustained a pelvic injury and is unable to void. In this procedure the patient is requested to lie at a 45-degree angle. Contrast material or a mixture of contrast and lubricant is injected into the meatus, and films are taken. Extravasation of the dye is apparent in urethral lacerations (Fig. 24-3).

Important points in the assessment of patients with urinary tract disease are summarized in Chart 24-1.

CALCULOUS DISEASE

Urinary calculi have plagued man from the beginning of recorded history. Despite ongoing research, stone formation is still a common problem, and the cause and prevention

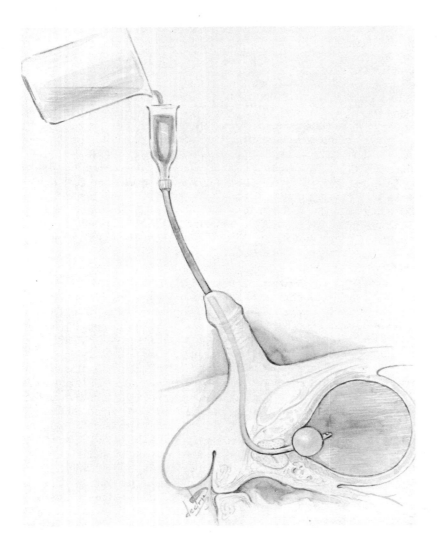

Figure 24-1 *Retrograde cystography. Following placement of a catheter in the bladder, contrast material is allowed to flow into the bladder by gravity drainage until the patient notes slight discomfort. An additional 30 ml of contrast material is then injected through the catheter using a syringe to obtain a "stress" cystogram. (Cosgriff JH Jr: Atlas of Diagnostic and Therapeutic Procedures for Emergency Personnel. Philadelphia, JB Lippincott, 1978)*

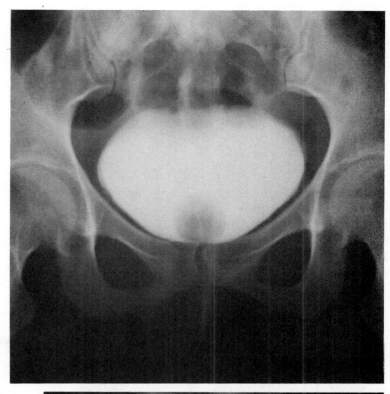

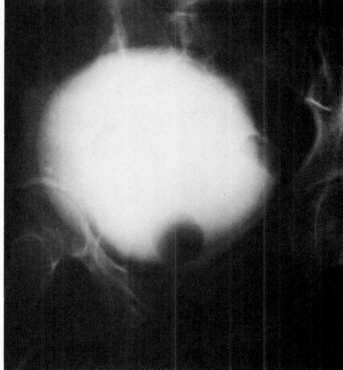

Figure 24-2 *Cystogram x-rays. Anteroposterior (top) and oblique (bottom) views of the bladder are indicated. The latter is helpful in identifying a rupture of the posterior wall of the bladder. (Cosgriff JH Jr: Atlas of Diagnostic and Therapeutic Procedures for Emergency Personnel. Philadelphia, JB Lippincott, 1978)*

of calculi are still undetermined. Calculous disease may occur anywhere in the urinary tract—kidney, ureter, bladder, or prostate. This discussion will be limited mainly to ureteral stones, since this type causes the severe colicky pain that prompts most patients to seek care in the hospital emergency department.

Ureteral calculi occur mainly in middle life; 69% of calculus victims are between the ages of 20 and 50 years. The

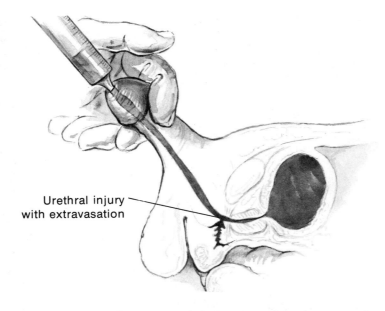

Urethral injury
with extravasation

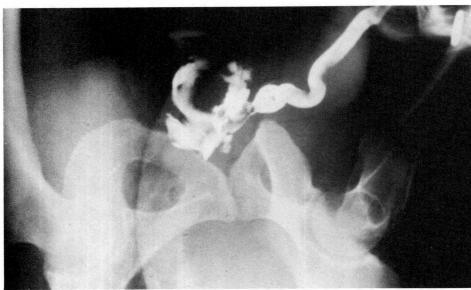

Figure 24-3 Top. *Diagram of urethrogram in male patient revealing an injury to the posterior urethra with extravasation. Bottom. Urethrogram x-ray demonstrating extravasation of contrast material from posterior urethra. (Cosgriff JH Jr: Atlas of Diagnostic and Therapeutic Procedures for Emergency Personnel. Philadelphia, JB Lippincott, 1978)*

condition is seen more often in men than in women and more often in the spring and fall months. Ureteral calculi are formed in the kidneys around a nucleus that may be composed of pus, blood, a crystal, or devitalized tissue. Chemical analysis reveals that 90% of calculi contain calcium in some form, 8% uric acid, and 1% cystine. Thus, some are not radiopaque.

The known causes of urinary calculi are multiple. A urinary tract infection caused by a urea-splitting organism, such as *Staphylococcus* or *Proteus,* seems to predispose to stone formation. Immobilization, which impairs renal drainage, alters the calcium mechanism, and results in skeletal decalcification, is another predisposing factor. Metabolic disorders that result in hypercalcemia or hypercalciuria (such as hyperparathyroidism and hyperthyroidism) are known to cause renal stones. Other metabolic diseases that cause urinary calculi are gout and cystinuria. Some stones are formed secondary to disorders within the urinary tract.

Assessment

The symptoms produced by urinary tract stones are influenced by the presence or absence of obstruction and infection and by local irritation of the renal pelvis or ureter, resulting in edema. Renal stones cause some discomfort or a dull ache in the area of the kidney, which is usually not disabling. Ureteral stones more often cause an acute onset of colic without prodromal symptoms. The pain is severe and intense. It may center in the area of the costovertebral angle, generally radiates down the ureter, and may be referred to the testicle or vulva. The pain may last for hours or may subside within a few minutes.

Chart 24-1

ASSESSMENT OF THE PATIENT WITH URINARY TRACT DISEASE

History

- Pain, usually located in the organs of the urinary tract, *i.e.,*
  Bladder—suprapubic
  Ureter—unilaterally in lower abdomen or flank
  Kidney—epigastric or costovertebral angles
  Prostate—rectal area
- Alteration in urinary habits, *i.e.,* frequency, urgency, burning, stinging, blood in urine, lack of urine
- Trauma to lower ribs, upper abdomen, or pelvis

Physical Examination

- Increased body temperature (not in all patients)
- Tenderness in the area of the organ involved

Adjunct Studies

- Urinalysis may show blood cells or bacteria.
- Blood work may show leukocytosis, changes in electrolytes, increase in BUN or creatinine.
- X-rays
  KUB plate may reveal calculus.
  IVP serves to evaluate kidney function and abnormalities of the renal collecting system.

The patient with ureteral colic is often cold and clammy; his pulse is weak and rapid, and there may be a drop in blood pressure. If the kidney is obstructed and the urine is infected, the patient may have fever and chills. Nausea and vomiting are fairly common, and in some instances all the symptoms may mimic gastrointestinal disease. The stone may pass down the ureter, and as it nears the bladder, the patient may complain of frequency and burning on urination. In most patients with ureteral calculi, there is hematuria, either gross, or, more commonly, microscopic.

A detailed history will reveal the nature of the pain, its location and radiation, and any previous similar episodes or any metabolic disorders, such as gout or parathyroid disease. On physical examination, tenderness can usually be elicited with deep pressure to the renal area anteriorly and gentle percussion in the costovertebral region.

To make a definitive diagnosis of ureteral calculi, laboratory and x-ray studies are necessary. Routine urinalysis should be made and noted for the presence or absence of red blood cells, white blood cells and bacteria. In the female, a clean-catch sample should be obtained. During the menstrual period, catheterization will be necessary. At this time, a culture should be submitted to the laboratory. Blood should be drawn for routine CBC and chemistry profiles, including serum protein, urea, calcium, phosphorus, chloride, CO_2 uric acid, and acid phosphatase.

Perhaps the most helpful diagnostic study for ureteral calculi is x-ray of the abdomen, ordinarily referred to as a KUB, followed by an IVP. In the latter, the renal shadows are outlined, the position of the stone is revealed, any obstruction is evident, the status of the opposite kidney is ascertained, and the status of renal function is indicated. It should be noted that 15% of all renal calculi are not visible on x-ray. Admission is usually required for further workup and treatment.

Electively, a cystoscopy may be performed. If a stone has passed, it will be apparent by the edema about the ureteral orifice. Retrograde pyelograms may be necessary because of incomplete visualization of the entire length of the ureter or poor concentration of the contrast material by the kidney at the time of the IVP. This is done during cystoscopy by passing a fine catheter into the ureteral orifice and injecting contrast material. A complete stone workup is in order to uncover any of the organic or metabolic diseases that are manifested by urinary calculi. Helpful in this respect are urinary excretion studies of calcium, phosphorus, uric acid, oxalate, and cystine, the phosphate reabsorption test, and a parathormone assay.

Management/Treatment

The treatment of ureteral calculi depends on many factors. To be considered are:
- Size of the stone
- Degree of obstruction, if any
- Severity and duration of the symptoms
- Status of the opposite kidney

- Presence or absence of infection
- Occupation, age, and general condition of the patient

Generally, the patient with a small stone that is not accompanied by infection or progressive hydronephrosis and whose colic is not too frequent or disabling may be simply observed, with the hope that it will pass. Of all renal calculi, 90% will pass through the ureters, bladder, and urethra spontaneously.

An intermediate treatment of ureteral stones is ureteral manipulation. This can be done in two ways. At the time of cystoscopy, a wire basket enclosed in a ureteral catheter is passed up the ureter to the stone, the basket is opened and, ideally, the stone engages in the basket and is pulled into the bladder. This treatment is considered only if the stone lies below the pelvic brim. The second method, also done at the time of cystoscopy, involves passing a ureteral catheter up to the kidney and leaving it in place for a time. This relieves any obstruction to the kidney and dilates the ureter, making passage of the stone somewhat easier after the catheter is removed.

Elective surgical intervention is the treatment of choice for stones larger than 1 cm, when renal parenchyma is being destroyed as a result of obstruction of infection or when the symptoms are persistently severe. In all instances of ureteral calculi, individualization of patient treatment is necessary. Sound clinical judgment is required to determine whether to pursue a policy of watchful waiting or intervene surgically.

The long-range treatment of a patient with ureteral calculi depends on the chemical analysis of the stone and the presence of any contributory organic or metabolic disease. Parathyroid adenomas are treated with an appropriate surgical procedure. Gout can be treated with a low purine diet, allopurinol, alkalinization of the urine, and a high fluid intake. Cystinuria can be treated to some extent with D-penicillamine. The vast majority of patients with calculous disease pass calcium-containing stones and have a negative workup for organic or metabolic disease. At present, the long-range regime for these patients is a diet low in calcium, a high fluid intake and, possibly, the administration of ascorbic acid to lower the urinary pH. Management of the patient with calculous disease is summarized in Chart 24-2.

HEMATURIA

Hematuria refers to blood in the urine and may be microscopic or gross in character. It is important to note that hematuria is not a disease but a *symptom;* thus, it is essential that a complete and thorough urologic investigation be undertaken. Such a program consists of cystoscopy with or without retrograde studies, renal scan, and selective renal angiography. With these modalities, a true diagnosis of the etiology of the hematuria can be made in almost all instances.

Causes

The causes of hematuria are numerous; the following are the most common:
- Calculous disease
- Cystitis
- Tumor
- Tuberculosis

Chart 24-2

MANAGEMENT OF THE PATIENT WITH CALCULOUS DISEASE

- *Relieve pain.* The patient typically is walking about, doubled over in pain. Fairly high doses of narcotics may be necessary.
- *Carefully collect laboratory specimens.* Cleanly voided urine is taken unless otherwise ordered. Transport the specimen to the laboratory promptly. If there is to be any delay, refrigerate the urine.
- *Force fluid intake.* 4 L to 5 L in 24 hours is an appropriate amount. It increases urinary output and puts an extra "push" behind the stone. Since many patients with ureteral stone may have nausea and emesis, oral intake may be restricted. In this instance iv fluid therapy is necessary.
- *If the patient is febrile and an infection is present, antibiotics may be ordered.* Determine any drug sensitivity beforehand. An antipyretic may be ordered if the temperature is markedly elevated.
- *Obtain a KUB x-ray.* This may be followed by an IVP. Determine whether any sensitivity to iodine is present in the contrast material. The contrast material acts as an osmotic diuretic and increases urinary output. It may provoke another bout of colic during or just after the IVP.
- *Strain the urine.* This is an important step for any patient with a ureteral stone. A tea strainer lined with a gauze sponge, or a commercially available strainer may be used. *Every voiding must be strained.* If the patient is discharged home, he should be supplied with a strainer and instructed in its use. If the stone is passed and recovered, *it should be analyzed* chemically so that the patient can be put on an appropriate long-range program.
- *If the patient is to be discharged home, give a prescription for pain relief and an antibiotic, if indicated.* Arrange for followup care.

- Benign prostatic hypertrophy
- Polycystic disease
- Trauma
- Anticoagulant therapy
- Glomerulonephritis

When it is associated with renal colic, calculous disease is the primary consideration, although the passage of a clot may cause the same type of pain. Tuberculosis of the urinary tract is not an uncommon cause of hematuria. Studies show a persistent pyuria in the presence of an acid urine, often despite prolonged antibiotic therapy. In this case, a tentative diagnosis of tuberculosis should be made and skin testing and urine cultures for acid-fast organisms should be instituted. Cystitis and bladder stones can cause hematuria; in this case it is accompanied by irritative urinary symptoms. Hematuria without other symptoms may indicate bladder, ureteral, or kidney tumor. Such hematuria is usually intermittent and stops spontaneously. Painless urinary bleeding may also be caused by polycystic kidneys, sickle cell disease, hydronephrosis, glomerulonephritis, or anticoagulant therapy. Once a diagnosis is established, a definitive plan of treatment should be devised, including appropriate follow-up.

Assessment

On admission, record accurate measurement of vital signs, especially blood pressure and pulse. Hematuria, unless it is unusually massive or has been allowed to continue over a long period of time, is rarely an urgent, life-threatening situation. However, careful observation of the patient for signs of shock is important.

A detailed history and thorough physical examination will reveal any preexisting urinary disease, blood disorders, possible injury, recent use of anticoagulants, abnormal bleeding tendencies, or coexisting medical problems. Urinalysis and CBC are the first laboratory studies performed. The CBC reveals whether the amount of blood lost has been significant enough to affect the hemoglobin and hematocrit determinations. Blood for typing and crossmatching may also be drawn at this time. The urine should be examined for color, amount, and presence or absence of clots before transmittal to the laboratory. The method of urine collection, especially in female patients, is an important consideration. In some instances, urine obtained with a catheter will prove the true site of bleeding to be the vagina.

Management/Treatment

Generally speaking, there is no way to stop bleeding from the upper urinary tract, and at this point, there is usually no need to do so. The patient is admitted to the hospital and undergoes a thorough diagnostic evaluation and appropriate treatment.

In contrast, bleeding from the bladder can be controlled in some instances by placement of an indwelling catheter and irrigation, and this procedure is initiated in the emergency department.

Catheterization and Irrigation. Before beginning this procedure, give an adequate explanation, assemble the necessary equipment, and position the patient.

1. *Catheterization equipment.* A routine catheterization tray provides the basic sterile items, such as gloves, drapes, antiseptic prep, and lubricant. Catheter size depends on the physician's preference. Usually, a large size, such as 22 F or 24 F with a 5 ml balloon, has a lumen large enough to permit adequate drainage, irrigation, and passage of clots or other debris.
2. *Irrigation equipment.* Irrigating equipment should include an Asepto syringe, a Toomey syringe (a 50-ml piston syringe with a catheter-adapted tip, shown in Fig. 24-4), and several bottles of irrigating solution, usually normal saline.
3. Once the catheter is inserted, it must be kept patent. Catheter irrigation should be performed as frequently as is necessary and under careful aseptic technique.
4. The Asepto syringe should be used routinely and the Toomey syringe only when the catheter has become obstructed with clots.
5. Once the bleeding is under control, the patient is admitted to the hospital, and a complete urologic investigation is carried out.

Blood in the urine, like bleeding from any body orifice, is a frightening experience for the patient. A small amount of blood in the urine turns the entire urinary output pink or red and seems to the patient much more severe than it actually is. Emotional support, calm reassurance, and skilled, knowledgeable performance of professional duties are vital for the patient and his family.

URINARY RETENTION

Acute urinary retention is a problem very commonly seen in the emergency department. This condition is most often encountered in the 60- to 80-year age group.

Causes

The causes of retention in order of frequency of occurrence are:
1. Benign prostatic hypertrophy
2. Urethral stricture
3. Adenocarcinoma of the prostate

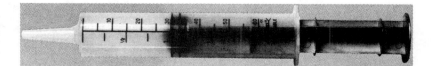

Figure 24-4 *Toomey syringe. Note the conical tip, which inserts easily into a urethral catheter or urethra. (Cosgriff JH Jr: Atlas of Diagnostic and Therapeutic Procedures for Emergency Personnel. Philadelphia, JB Lippincott, 1978)*

4. Calculi
5. Neurogenic bladder
6. Drug induced retention

Assessment

The patient usually gives a history of increased difficulty in voiding manifested by hesitation, straining, voiding with a slow, weak stream and the sensation of incomplete emptying of the bladder. On examination, the patient is usually very restless and in considerable discomfort. He may not have voided at all, or he may dribble constantly or urinate small amounts intermittently. This is usually overflow incontinence, indicating that a much greater amount of urine is retained in the bladder.

Treatment/Management

The most immediate treatment is to establish urinary drainage through urethral catheterization. Occasionally, the urethra cannot be instrumented, and it then becomes necessary to perform a suprapubic cystotomy to establish urinary drainage. In either case, once the bladder has become decompressed, the catheter should be attached to a closed gravity drainage unit.

Much has been said and written about the rate at which the bladder should be decompressed. Studies have shown that although rapid decompression may cause transient hematuria, it does not generally cause hemorrhage or shock. However, experience has shown that *atraumatic* catheterization and rapid decompression cause no ill effects whatsoever.

Once the patient is comfortable, routine laboratory and radiologic data should be obtained. After this, a complete urologic workup is undertaken, including urine for culture and sensitivity, an IVP, and a cystoscopic examination. Following complete medical and urologic studies, a diagnosis is made, and the appropriate treatment is instituted.

Catheterization. After routine laboratory samples are obtained, the patient is prepared for catheterization. An adequate explanation of the procedure should be given him.

1. *Equipment.* A sterile catheterization tray, including gloves, drapes, lubricant, and antiseptic prep, will be needed. The size of the indwelling catheter is determined by the physician. Generally an 18 F catheter with a 5-ml balloon is the size of choice. It is small enough to permit easy passage and large enough to permit adequate flow of urine. Other routine supplies needed at this time are collection containers for urinalysis and culture and sensitivity studies, a closed gravity drainage unit, and possibly an irrigation set. Since the vast majority of patients with retention have a pathologic obstruction either in the urethra or at the vesical neck, a few instruments and catheters unique to the practice of urology should be assembled, as outlined in the following paragraphs.

- *Urethral dilators* (filiforms, followers, LeFort and Van Buren sounds). A filiform is a small plastic catheter with a metal-threaded female tip at one end, used as a guide to bypass urethral strictures. They range in size from 3 F to 6 F. A follower is a plastic catheter with a threaded male tip that can be screwed into the filiform. Followers of increasing sizes are passed to dilate the stricture, from 12 F to 28 F (Figs. 24-5 and 24-6). LeFort sounds are rigid metal instruments with an elbow curve at one end and a threaded male tip. The curve is designed to negotiate the curve of the prostatic and bulbar urethra as it passes under the symphysis pubis. Van Buren sounds are similar to LeFort sounds in size and configuration but without the threaded tip. They are passed as is, without guidance from a filiform (Fig. 24-7).
- *Coudé catheters* are indwelling catheters with a curved tip similar to Van Buren sounds. They are particularly

Figure 24-5 *Filiforms and Philips followers. The filiforms (at bottom) are the straight and spiral type. The followers attach to these and are passed through the urethra in graduated sizes, beginning with the smallest.*

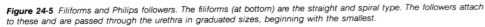

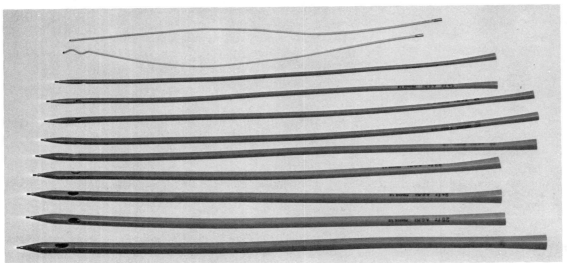

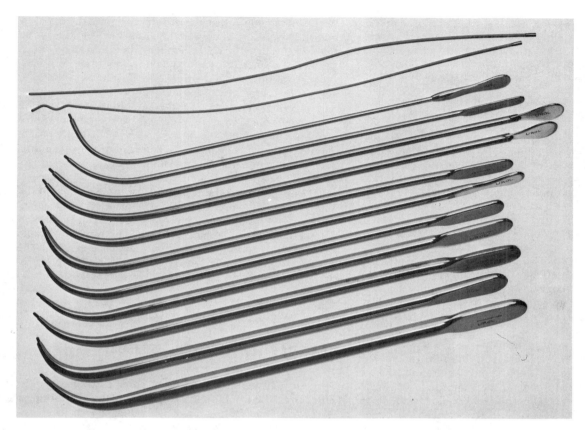

Figure 24-6 *LeFort sounds. These are curved metal dilating instruments with a threaded male tip. They are used in conjunction with filiforms in the same manner as followers. The choice of followers or LeFort sounds depends on the personal preference of the urologist.*

Figure 24-7 *Van Buren sounds. These are smooth metal dilators, available in graduated sizes, from 16 Fr. to 30 Fr.*

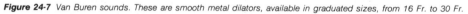

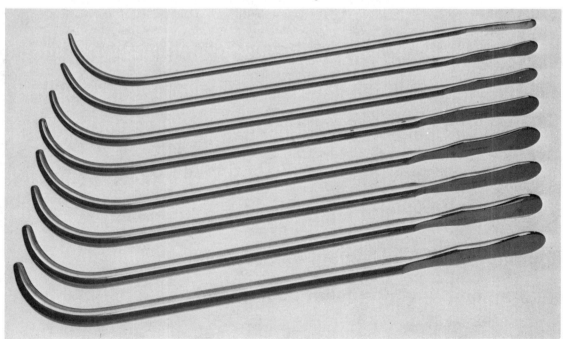

useful for patients with bladder neck elevation due to prostatic hypertrophy (Fig. 24-8).

- A *catheter stylet* is a wire guide, inserted into a catheter to give the tip a curve and some rigidity (Fig. 24-8). This is an extremely dangerous instrument and should be used only by those qualified to do so. It is possible to cause serious injury should the stylet accidentally protrude from the proximal end of the catheter.

2. *Procedure.* The procedure of catheterization is carried out with strict aseptic technique. The patient is draped with a sterile towel, and the meatus is cleansed with a generous amount of antiseptic solution. The catheter is then well lubricated, or the physician may prefer to inject sterile lubricant through the meatus into the urethra. The catheter is passed, using constant, steady, gentle pressure. After a free flow of urine is obtained, the catheter should be connected to a closed drainage unit.

In the rare event that urethral catheterization is impossible, a *suprapubic cystotomy* may be necessary. This can be carried out in the emergency department or the urology department if the urologist uses a trocar or one of the commercially made cystotomy sets such as Cystocath. If it is to be done under direct vision, then the patient goes into the operating room.

The "punch" cystotomy done in the emergency or urology department is considered a surgical procedure and as such requires a written consent. The patient is prepped and draped in a sterile fashion and given a local anesthetic. A small-gauge spinal needle is then passed into the lower abdomen to confirm that the mass is an overdistended bladder. A small incision is made and the Campbell's trocar or the trocar-catheter combination is passed through the abdominal wall. If the Campbell's trocar is used, remove the stylet and pass an 18 F Foley catheter along the sheath and then remove the sheath. If one of the disposable trocar-catheter combinations is used, remove the trocar, leaving the catheter in place. A suture may be placed around the catheter to secure it (Fig. 24-9).

After the catheter has been inserted, either through the urethra or by the suprapubic route, it should be secured by adhesive tape or one of the commercial catheter straps or holders so that it does not pull. The drainage bag should be positioned lower than the bladder to ensure the free flow of urine by gravity. There should be no kinks or coils in the tubing. The bag should be emptied before its capacity is reached. The meatus-catheter junction should be kept scrupulously clean. Catheter irrigations, if ordered, should be conducted under strict aseptic technique.

Following catheterization, the amount of residual urine should be noted. Urine is then sent to the laboratory for analysis, culture, and sensitivity studies. A chemistry profile should be drawn, including blood urea nitrogen, creatinine, sugar, and electrolyte determinations. Occasionally, urinary retention persists for so long that it causes some degree of renal impairment, and this may first become evident in the serum chemistry findings. Some patients are started on antibacterials at this time; therefore, any drug sensitivity should be ascertained. An adequate fluid intake is always important, but especially so to the patient with urinary retention. The patient is often admitted to the hospital for a complete diagnostic workup.

SEXUALLY TRANSMITTED DISEASES

Sexually transmitted or venereal diseases are by far the most common of the communicable diseases of the genitourinary tract. Over 1 million cases of gonorrhea are reported annually, and it is estimated that many more are unreported. As more emergency departments become community health centers, the number of patients with sexually transmitted diseases seen by emergency personnel can be expected to rise.

Patients with sexually transmitted diseases come from all ethnic backgrounds and occupations and range in age from 13 to 70 years. No parental consent is needed to treat sexually transmitted diseases in a minor. Ignorance and fear still surround sexually transmitted diseases, and the attitude of emergency personnel can help bring these diseases and their treatment into proper perspective.

Figure 24-8 *Various catheters. Top to bottom: The stylet is inserted into a catheter, giving it a degree of rigidity. The Robinson catheter is a nonretentive catheter, used for a single insertion. The coudé catheter is a retentive catheter, with a curved tip. The Foley catheter is a retentive catheter with a straight tip.*

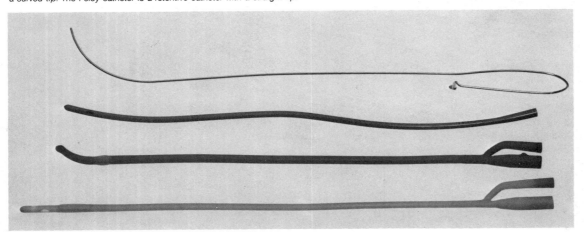

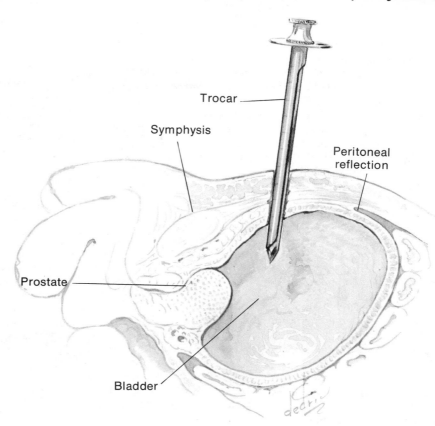

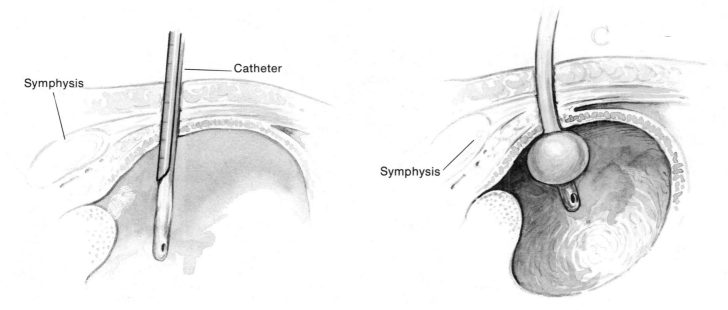

Figure 24-9 *Suprapubic or "punch" cystotomy. Top. This technique may be used to evaluate a distended bladder. Using local anesthesia, a trocar is plunged into the bladder through the abdominal wall. Bottom left. An indwelling catheter is then inserted through the trocar. Bottom right. The catheter in position in the urinary bladder. (Cosgriff JH Jr: Atlas of Diagnostic and Therapeutic Procedures for Emergency Personnel. Philadelphia, JB Lippincott, 1978)*

GONORRHEA

Gonorrhea, the most prevalent of the venereal diseases, is generally seen in the emergency department 2 to 9 days after sexual contact with an infected individual. The presenting symptoms are burning on urination and thick, profuse, purulent urethral discharge. Diagnosis is made from a smear or culture of the exudate; the smear shows gram-negative intracellular diplococci. To obtain a culture, the swab containing the exudate is inoculated on Thayer-Martin or Transgrow medium. It takes at least 24 hours before a culture report is available.

Treatment/Management

Treatment usually consists of procaine penicillin G, 4.8 million units IM divided into two separate doses, one injected into each buttock. Tetracycline may be used for penicillin-sensitive patients. In some areas of the country, ampicillin, 3.5 gm and probenecid (Benemid), 1.0 gm, are given orally.

It is important to obtain a urethral swab prior to urination, when the discharge is most concentrated. Because of the fragility of *Neisseria gonorrhoeae,* the swab should be taken to the laboratory as soon as is feasible. Principal precautions revolve around preventing spread of the infection to the eyes or nasopharynx of emergency personnel and other patients. It is thus important to discard or wash and autoclave anything that comes in contact with the exudate. Careful handwashing is mandatory, since *N. gonorrhoeae* cannot survive soap and water. Because penicillin is the treatment of choice, any history of allergy to this drug must be established. The patient should be observed carefully following injection of penicillin, and emergency resuscitative equipment should be ready in the event of anaphylactic shock. Between 2% and 10% of all patients receiving penicillin have an allergic manifestation.

Follow-up Care. Arrangements should be made for follow-up care, with either a private physician, the hospital clinic, or a community venereal disease treatment center. Patients with gonorrhea rapidly become asymptomatic with medication and because of this may stop taking medication and discontinue medical care. It should be emphasized to them that prompt diagnosis and treatment in most cases prevents complications such as urethral strictures, posterior urethritis, prostatis, epididymitis, and cystitis.

SYPHILIS

Syphilis, caused by the organism *Treponema pallidum,* is transmitted exclusively by sexual contact with a person harboring an open spirochete-containing lesion. After the incubation period of 2 to 4 weeks, the initial lesion, the chancre, appears on the genitalia.

Diagnosis is made from a positive dark-field examination of serous material obtained from a moist lesion or, more commonly, from a serologic response to the infection (VDRL).

Treatment/Management

Treatment consists of benzathine penicillin G, 2,400,000 units, divided into two equal doses, one injected in each buttock. Tetracycline is given to patients who are allergic to penicillin.

Responsibilities in caring for a patient with suspected syphilis are very much the same as for a patient with suspected gonorrhea. They include meticulous attention to handwashing, and proper care of supplies and equipment that come into contact with the lesion, as well as the precautions necessary when administering penicillin. Follow-up care is especially important, and this should be stressed to the patient. Untreated or inadequately treated primary syphilis can proceed to secondary, latent and, finally late syphilis, which ultimately may cause diseases of the heart, arteries, and central nervous system.

HERPES GENITALIS

Genital herpes is becoming one of the most common sexually transmitted diseases seen by physicians today. It is viral in origin and the incubation period is unknown. Frequently it is recurrent. It is due most often to the herpes Type II virus, but Type I is also found. Male patients present with multiple superficial vesicles or pustules on the foreskin or glans penis, usually with local pain or tenderness. Primary herpes may be accompanied by inguinal adenopathy. The lesions are characteristic and easily recognizable. If necessary, the herpes simplex virus can be identified in the laboratory in an appropriately stained scraping from the base of the lesion.

Treatment/Management

A new antiviral agent, acyclovir, has been found effective in primary genital herpes. It is available as an ointment and is applied to the lesions. Local cleanliness should be encouraged and in the acute phase the use of povidone-iodine may help alleviate some of the irritative symptoms. The lesions heal spontaneously and recurrence is common. Genital herpes in women is discussed in detail in Chapter 25, Gynecologic Emergencies.

In dealing with patients with any of the sexually transmitted diseases, evaluation and treatment of all sexual partners of the infected individual are essential. Information about community resources for venereal disease should be given the patient. Often, community clinics provide treatment without cost.

TRAUMA

Patients with genitourinary trauma may present in a variety of ways. Some may have multiple injuries and be in immediate danger of death. Others may have one or two complaints and appear to be in no acute distress. Isolated injuries to the urinary tract are not common and are rarely life endangering.

Immediate Care

The specific needs of each patient must be evaluated and dealt with individually, using basic procedures and techniques, including maintenance of an adequate airway, treatment of hemorrhagic shock with fluid replacement, close monitoring of vital signs, collection of blood and urine samples for laboratory studies, accurate monitoring of intake and output, and, above all, close observation of the patient.

When urinary tract injuries occur in conjunction with trauma to other organ systems, total evaluation of the patient must be made, priorities must be established, and principles of resuscitation followed. Thus, a patent airway must be established and maintained and the cardiovascular system must be stabilized. Initial urinary tract evaluation may be brief, and unless the problem involves major blood loss, the urinary tract is assigned a lesser priority of care.

Two points deserve special mention relative to urologic procedures. First, an IVP is of no value if the patient is in shock. Renal perfusion, and thus perfusion of the contrast material, depends on blood pressure. Renal perfusion is impaired with arterial pressures under 60 mm Hg. However, shock is no contraindication to renal arteriography. Second, it is important to keep a Foley catheter patent. Occasionally, anuria or oliguria can be traced to a nonfunctioning indwelling urethral catheter.

Injuries to the genitourinary tract may be divided into penetrating and nonpenetrating types. Penetrating injuries result from guns, knives, and icepicks, among other instruments. Blunt (nonpenetrating) trauma is more common and most frequently results from automobile accidents. Less often, it follows a fall, a direct blow, or an athletic injury. For clinical evaluation, urinary tract injuries are divided into those involving the upper urinary tract and those involving the lower urinary tract.

UPPER GENITOURINARY TRACT INJURY

Injuries to the kidney occur much more commonly in men than in women (the ratio is approximately 3:1), and are more frequently seen in those below the age of 40. Trauma to the kidney may vary from a mild contusion to complete fragmentation or avulsion from its vascular pedicle. In general, abnormal kidneys are more susceptible to injury than normal ones.

Assessment. Signs and symptoms of renal trauma are hematuria, pain, tenderness, and abdominal rigidity in varying degrees. Renal injury must be considered in blunt or penetrating injury to the upper abdomen or direct blows to the costovertebral area.

After the patient has been assessed, the diagnosis can be confirmed by excretory urogram (IVP). The pyelogram usually shows the extent of injury and allows assessment of the uninjured side. On occasion, renal arteriography is necessary, particularly when major vascular injury is suspected (Fig. 24-10).

Management/Treatment. Management of renal trauma is generally conservative. Rest and observation bring recovery to 80% of patients. Emergency surgery is indicated with evidence of blood loss if the vital signs cannot be stabilized by the transfusion of whole blood or if there is an expansion of the perirenal hematoma. The options for surgery include drainage of the renal area, repair of the damaged kidney and a complete or partial nephrectomy.

LOWER GENITOURINARY TRACT INJURY

Bladder Trauma

Bladder trauma includes contusion, intraperitoneal rupture, extraperitoneal rupture, or a combination of the latter two. It is usually associated with a fractured pelvis. Pelvic fracture

Figure 24-10 *Renal injuries. Left. Flat film of abdomen of young man injured in a motorcycle accident, complaining of abdominal pain. Note gaseous content of small bowel and stomach indicative of ileus (upper right). Note also displacement of loops of bowel to the patient's right side (left side of illustration) by mass in left side of abdomen. Left psoas shadow not visualized. Right. Left renal arteriogram revealing a fracture of the kidney at the junction of its upper and middle thirds. In both fragments, there is extravasation of blood due to damage to the major arteries. Note the sharp kink at the takeoff of the artery supplying the upper pole, indicating partial rupture. Curved radiopaque density in upper right corner of illustration is a nasogastric tube. Patient required nephrectomy.*

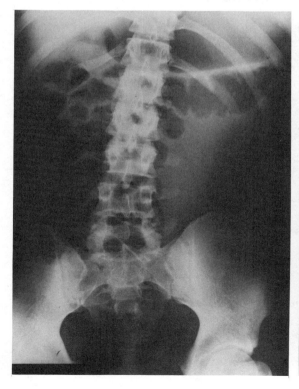
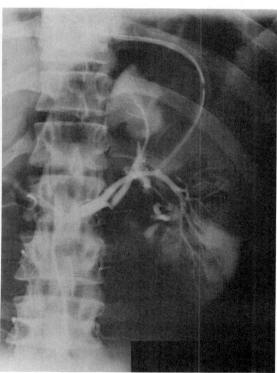

as evidenced by x-ray should raise the suspicion of bladder trauma.

Symptoms of a ruptured bladder are pain over the pubic area, an extreme desire to void (urinary tenesmus) or extreme dysuria, hematuria, shock, and evidence of blood loss. Diagnosis is verified by means of a retrograde cystogram.

Management/Treatment. Surgical treatment is usually necessary to establish suprapubic drainage and thorough drainage of the perivesical area. Immediate diagnosis and treatment are imperative in rupture of the bladder. Deaths have been recorded with delayed exploration.

RUPTURE OF THE URETHRA

Rupture of the urethra almost exclusively results from an automobile accident and is usually associated with a fractured pelvis. As a consequence of trauma, urine extravasates into the tissue at the site of injury, setting up an intensive inflammatory reaction. Injury should be suspected in patients complaining of pain in the bladder area and experiencing urinary tenesmus but unable to void.

Management/Treatment. Diagnosis may be confirmed by insertion of a catheter. In most instances, urine cannot be obtained. If the patient is unable to void, a catheter should not be passed until a urethrogram is performed to rule out urethral injury. Injection of contrast material will confirm the extravasation of urine about the site of injury (Fig. 24-3). The objectives of treatment are to drain the extravesical urine, reestablish urethral continuity, and control hemorrhage.

INJURIES TO THE EXTERNAL GENITALIA

Genital injuries include abrasions, hematomas, and minor lacerations of the penis and scrotum or vulva. Patients with fracture of the penis are occasionally seen in the emergency department. The injury is caused by a direct blow to an erect organ and results in hemorrhage, hematoma, and distortion of the organ.

Management/Treatment. Conservative management of penile fractures consists of splinting the penis, inserting an indwelling catheter, and applying ice packs. Surgical evacuation of the associated hematoma is sometimes required.

Lacerations of the penis or vulva are managed like any similar wound elsewhere on the body. Loss of skin requires immediate coverage, usually by means of split-thickness graft.

TORSION OF THE TESTICLE

Torsion of the testicle is a condition in which a testicle twists on its spermatic cord, disrupting its own blood supply. It may be caused by an injury but more often occurs spontaneously. Torsion causes severe scrotal pain, unrelieved by rest. There is generally a normal urinary sediment. The treatment is surgical exploration of the scrotum and bilateral fixation of both testes. A delay in treatment will result in loss of the testicle; the torsion must be reduced and fixed within a few hours to preserve fertility.

FOREIGN BODIES IN THE GENITOURINARY TRACT

Patients with a foreign body in the genitourinary tract are occasionally treated in the emergency department. The most common predisposing factors for bodily use of foreign bodies, whether internal or external, are abnormal psyche, inebriation, eroticism, and senility.

The bladder and urethra are the most common sites for foreign objects, with one qualification: the object must be small and firm enough to be passed up the urethra. Symptoms center on the associated infection. There may be frequency, dysuria, urethral discharge, and possibly abdominal pain. Occasionally, the foreign body becomes the nucleus around which a stone forms. Diagnosis can be established by urinalysis showing blood and pus, x-ray studies showing a metallic object or encrustation surrounding a nonopaque foreign body, and cystopanendoscopy showing the object under direct vision. Foreign bodies in the urethra and bladder can usually be removed at the time of cystoscopy.

External foreign bodies are most often used to constrict the external genitalia, usually the penis. They can be anything from a thread or hair to a metal ring. The penis becomes swollen and inflamed because of venous congestion and, at times, necrotic up to the point of obstruction. Also accompanying this condition are a purulent discharge and, in extreme cases, urinary retention.

MANAGEMENT/TREATMENT

Patients with internal foreign bodies are usually admitted for an attempt at transurethral removal of the object. Most external foreign bodies can be removed successfully in the emergency department. A minor instrument set-up with sterile towels, sponges, antiseptic prep, scissors, and a hemostat should be prepared. A sedative or tranquilizer is given before the procedure is begun; provisions should be available for administration of local anesthesia. For difficult patients, like children, admission and general anesthesia may be necessary.

Patients with this problem are usually guilt ridden and embarrassed. A matter-of-fact approach by the medical and nursing staff can help allay such feelings. Psychiatric referral may be considered at the completion of surgical treatment.

SUMMARY

Most patients with genitourinary complaints seen in the emergency department are not in an immediate life-threatening condition. They are, however, vitally concerned about their health. Some have additional fears, such as loss of sexual potency, discovery of an incurable disease, or feelings of guilt or embarrassment. Patients with genitourinary problems deserve the utmost privacy. They also need understanding, explanation, reassurance, and sincere interest.

BIBLIOGRAPHY

Beaumont E: Urinary drainage systems. Nursing 74:52, 1974

Bellfly LC: You can improve your catheterized patient's care. RN 77:33, 1977

Brosman SA, Fay R: Diagnosis and management of bladder trauma. J Trauma 13:687, 1973

Brown MS: Syphilis and gonorrhea. Nursing 76:71, 1976

Brown WJ: Acquired syphilis. Am J Nurs 71:713, 1971

Campbell M, Harrison JH: Urology. Philadelphia, WB Saunders, 1970

Cohen S, Gittes R: Patient assessment: Examination of the male genitalia. Am J Nurs 79:689, 1979

DeGroot J: Catheter induced urinary tract infections. Nursing 76:34, 1976

DeGroot J: Urethral catheterization. Nursing 76:51, 1979

Desautels RE: Mismanagement of urethral catheterization. Hosp Med 1:10, 1965

Gault PL: How to break the kidney stone cycle. Nursing 78:24, 1978

Gross M, Arnold T, Waterhouse K: Fracture of the penis: Rationale of surgical management. J Urol 106:708, 1971

Howard J: Tried, true, and new ways to treat and prevent kidney stones. Res Staff Phys 70:67, 1970

Keuknelian JG, Sanders VE: Urologic Nursing. London, Macmillan, 1970

Lauler DP: Venereal disease. New York, Medcom Learning Systems, 1972

Lee R: Genital skin lesions caused by sexually transmitted diseases. Infection Control and Urologic Care 5(1):17–23, 1980

Mathers R: TLC with the penicillin. Am J Nurs 71:720, 1971

McGuckin M: Microbiologic studies: Urine cultures. Nursing 75:10, 1975

Morel AL: Urethral catheters: an ancient device. RN 72:40, 1972

Parker R, Robison J: Anatomy and diagnosis of torsion of the testicles. J Urol 106:243, 1971

Smith DR: General Urology. Los Altos, Lange Medical Publications, 1978

Stark JL: BUN/Creatinine: Your Keys to Kidney Function. Nursing 80:33, 1980

Waterhouse K, Gross M: Trauma to the genitourinary tract: A 5 year experience with 251 cases. J Urol 101:241, 1969

Wiesner PJ, Margolis S: Gonococcal and nongonococcal urethritis. Infection Control and Urologic Care 5(1):3–5, 1980

Winter C, Roehm M: Sawyer's Nursing Care of Patients with Urologic Diseases. St. Louis, CV Mosby, 1968

Woodrow M, Wilsey G, Wiley N: Suprapubic catheters, Part 2. Nursing 76:40, 1976

25
GYNECOLOGIC EMERGENCIES

JOHN D. BARTELS

The majority of women who present themselves to the emergency department with gynecologic problems have some form of vaginal bleeding or abdominal pain. The causes of these symptoms vary tremendously, including aberrations of physiologic menstruation, problems of pregnancy, hormonal imbalance, neoplasm, trauma, infection, and postpartum or postoperative hemorrhage.

ANATOMY AND PHYSIOLOGY

The internal organs in the female pelvis include the female genital tract, consisting of the ovaries, fallopian tubes and uterus, and the urinary bladder, urethra, and rectum. The external pelvic organs in the female include the vagina, the labia, and the clitoris.

The uterus is a thick-walled muscular organ, lying in the midline between the bladder and the rectum. It is roughly pear-shaped and about 3 inches long. The upper portion is called the corpus or body of the uterus; the lower portion, the cervix, protrudes into the vagina. It has a round, smooth surface and a central opening, the external os. The uppermost part of the body of the uterus is the fundus, which is round and smooth. The uterus is supported by a number of ligaments.

From either side of the uterus, just below the fundus, arise the two fallopian tubes, which extend laterally in the uppermost portion of the broad ligament. Each tube is a hollow muscular duct that opens into the uterus medially and laterally broadens into a trumpet-shaped structure with frond-like processes, the fimbriae. The tubes transmit the ova from the ovaries to the uterus.

The two ovaries lie on either side of the pelvis close to the fimbriated ends of the fallopian tubes. Each ovary normally measures about 1½ inches long and ½ inch thick. An ovary produces the ovum (egg) at ovulation in response to hormonal stimulation.

The tubes, ovaries, and broad ligaments are frequently collectively referred to as the uterine adnexae, which literally means "lying next to the uterus."

The vagina is a fibromuscular tube, 3 to 4 inches in length, that opens onto the perineum. Its outlet is bordered by the labia, and in virginal females is partially or wholly closed by the hymen. The uterine cervix protrudes into the upper part of the vagina.

The labia majora and minora are double folds of skin, connective tissue, and glandular tissue on either side of the vaginal orifice. They meet in the midline, posterior to the vagina, to form the posterior fourchette, which lies about 1 inch anterior to the anus. The posterior portion of the labia contains the Bartholin glands, which are usually unrecognized except when diseased. At the anterior end of the labia minora is the clitoris. Posterior to the clitoris and just anterior to the vaginal orifice is the urethral meatus. The urethra extends upward in the anterior wall of the vagina to enter the bladder. Thus, trauma to the vaginal area and pubic bone may damage the urethra.

Blood supply to the female genitalia is derived primarily from branches of the internal iliac vessels. Innervation is through the branches of the sacral plexus.

Between the uterus and the rectum is the cul-de-sac, the lowermost extension of the peritoneal cavity. It comes in contact with the uppermost portion of the vagina, behind the cervix. In diseases of the female genital tract associated with internal bleeding, fluid may be recovered from the cul-de-sac by aspiration (Fig. 25-1). This maneuver may be very helpful in confirming a diagnosis of intraperitoneal hemorrhage, particularly when pelvic in origin.

The pelvic organs are covered by parietal peritoneum. Size and location of the pelvic organs may vary according to whether the woman has borne children. Collectively, the pelvic viscera lie within the peritoneal cavity. The fimbriated ends of the fallopian tubes open into the pelvic portion of the peritoneal cavity, so that blood or pus within the tube drains into the peritoneal cavity. The ovaries discharge the ova into the same area. Similarly, blood or fluid from ruptured ovarian cysts may enter the peritoneal cavity, accounting for abdominal symptoms in gynecologic disease.

As the young girl approaches womanhood, many changes occur—development of the breasts, pubic and axillary hair growth, deposition of fat in both breasts and hips, the beginning closure of the epiphyses, and the maturation of the reproductive organs.

Psychological and behavior changes also occur. There are alterations in mood, awareness of self, and an attraction to the opposite sex.

Associated with adolescence is the appearance of the menarche and an anticipated 35 to 40 years of menstrual function. Early in human history it was recognized that pe-

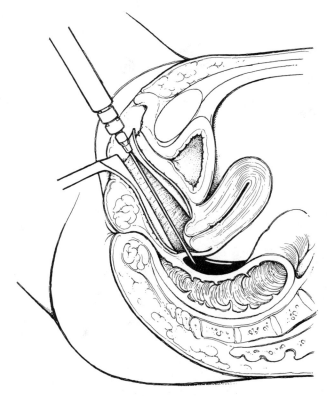

Figure 25-1 *Cul-de-sac aspiration through posterior fornix of the vagina. The vagina is inspected with a speculum in place. The cervix may be grasped by a tenaculum and drawn anteriorly. A 4-inch needle attached to a syringe is inserted through the posterior fornix into the cul-de-sac for aspiration.*

riodic bleeding in women closely followed the phases of the moon, and consequently the name menstrual cycle was applied to the phenomenon. Since many women experienced pain and discomfort at this time, a great deal of negative folklore and religious mythology developed. The woman who was menstruating was considered unclean, possessed, or diseased, and in some cultures was ostracized because it was believed that she could cause the crops to fail or the wine to sour. Even today, with all of our scientific methods and chemotherapeutic ability, it remains somewhat taboo to discuss menstruation, even among women. Therefore, many suffer in silence what can be a debilitating experience for 2 to 5 days of every menstrual cycle.

GYNECOLOGIC ASSESSMENT

Evaluation of a female patient with suspected pelvic disease includes both careful history and physical assessment. Occasionally, particularly in bleeding complications of pregnancy, blood loss can be massive and the patient may be in shock. Naturally, in such patients, initiation of resuscitative and life-support measures takes precedence over complete history and physical data collection.

History

Whatever the complaint, be it pain, vaginal discharge, or bleeding, the history must include time of onset and description of the presenting symptom (color, consistency, amount and odor of vaginal discharge, type of bleeding, presence of clots). The date of the last menstrual period and whether it was considered normal should be established. In traumatic conditions, the mechanism of injury should be determined. History is particularly important in suspected rape cases.

Symptoms relating to other organs are common in many pelvic conditions. With regard to the gastrointestinal tract, nausea is common in association with pelvic disease, but anorexia and vomiting are not. Urinary symptoms are also common, particularly in inflammatory conditions of the female genital tract.

Physical Examination

Basic instruments needed for physical evaluation of gynecologic disease include sterile gloves, various sizes of vaginal specula, and an adequate light source. An examining table with stirrups and clean drapes to protect the patient's privacy are essential. No pelvic examination should be performed without a female employee of the emergency department being present. Additional useful equipment includes:

Sponge forceps with sterile cotton and gauze squares

Uterine dressing forceps for packing

Plain or iodoform- or nitrofurazone (Furacin)-impregnated gauze packing

Uterine tenaculum for grasping the cervix

Cervical punch biopsy forceps

Endometrial aspiration biopsy forceps

A uterine sound can also be useful at times. For cul-de-sac aspiration in order to detect intraperitoneal bleeding, especially when ruptured ectopic pregnancy is suspected, a 4-inch spinal needle and a 10-ml syringe should be available.

The drugs commonly needed in treatment of gynecologic emergencies are listed in Table 25-1.

Complete physical assessment is necessary, the essential points relating to evaluation of the abdomen and pelvis. In the absence of enlargement, the pelvic structures are not palpable through the anterior abdominal wall. However, bleeding or discharge from pelvic structures may cause irritation of the peritoneum, which can be detected by careful assessment of the abdomen.

Vaginal examination of the pelvic organs is one of the most important aspects of the assessment phase. It should be done gently and with a reassuring manner. In children and virginal females, particularly, a pelvic examination may be a painful and very traumatic experience. If it is the opinion of the examiner that the examination is contraindicated, limited evaluation of the pelvic structures may be carried out through the rectum.

Adequate pelvic evaluation includes speculum examination of the vagina and cervix; any discharge is noted. If present, a specimen of the discharge may be taken for culture. The cervix is normally round and pink. In nulliparous females, the external os is round; in parous females, the os is oblong.

Manual examination of the vagina is performed using the index and middle fingers. If the introitus is small, examination may be carried out using one finger. A bimanual examination technique combines intravaginal examination with palpation of the lower abdominal wall (Fig. 25-2). In this manner, the examiner attempts to outline the pelvic contents, evaluate the size of the uterus, and determine whether the adnexae are enlarged. The cervix should be moved from side to side. In inflammatory conditions of the adnexae, particularly in salpingitis, moving the cervix to one side stretches the contralateral salpinx painfully.

Adjunct Studies

Diagnostic Ultrasound. Ultrasound is a new, safe, noninvasive addition to obstetric and gynecologic diagnosis and therapy. It is extremely useful and has found widespread acceptance. Ultrasound instruments do not emit ionizing

TABLE 25-1. DRUGS USED IN GYNECOLOGIC EMERGENCIES

Drug Generic Name	Drug Trade Name
Medroxyprogesterone acetate suspension	Depo-Provera
Sodium warfarin	Coumadin
Heparin	
Clomiphenecitrate	Clomid
Hydroprogesterone caproate injection	Delalutin
Penicillin	
Podophyllin	
Metronidazole	Flagyl
Diazepam	Valium
Oxytocin injection	Pitocin
Probenecid	Benemid
Ampicillin	
Stilbestrol	

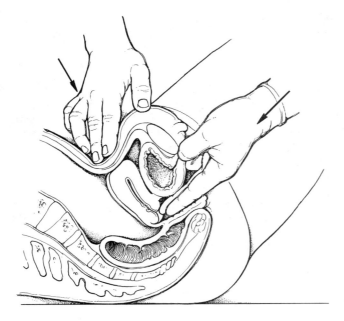

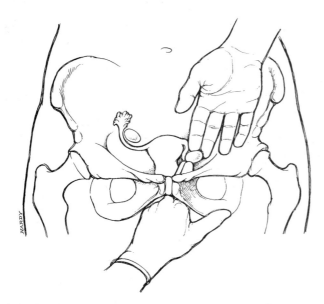

Figure 25-2 *Bimanual examination of the female pelvic organs. Top. The examiner's left hand is inserted into the vagina, and the size of the uterus is evaluated by palpating the organ between the intravaginal hand and the hand on the anterior abdominal wall in the suprapubic area. Bottom. The adnexae (tubes and ovaries) should also be examined in this manner to determine any enlargement, masses, tenderness, or displacement.*

radiation. Sound waves are produced that reflect off the structure being evaluated. No tissue damage has been reported with the energy levels used (5–20 mHz/cm²). Tissue damage has been associated with ultrasound emissions over 1000 mHz/cm². Of course this is hundreds of times more than that used in diagnostic ultrasound.

Since the risk of radiation is not a factor with this technique, it can be used safely even when pregnancy is suspected. It is very useful in diagnosing ectopic pregnancy. Serum pregnancy tests may be used to provide confirmatory data; these tests are very sensitive and are positive in 95% of ectopic pregnancies. With the presence of a positive pregnancy test and no evidence of a fetal sac in the uterus, ectopic pregnancy is a strong possibility. This should alert the physician to the need for further investigation such as culdocentesis or laparoscopy.

In some cases, the unruptured tube in ectopic pregnancy or blood in the cul-de-sac can also be detected by ultrasound. The presence or location of an intrauterine contraceptive device can frequently be determined with the use of ultrasound.

Although most pelvic masses can be felt by a normal bimanual examination, ultrasound evaluation is very useful in distinguishing ovarian cysts from fibroids and in identifying suspected pelvic masses in obese females when examination is difficult or unreliable.

Ultrasound is a safe, valuable tool that can greatly assist in diagnosis but should not replace clinical judgment.

Computed Tomography (CT). Computed tomography (CT scanning) can also be used to evaluate pelvic structures and pathology. The pictures obtained are clearer than ultrasound images, but ionizing radiation is involved. The expense is greater and the technology is not as readily available. Its greatest benefit appears to be in oncology, to detect and follow the extent of tumor growth. The CT scan, of course, should be avoided when pregnancy is a possibility.

Assessment of the patient with a gynecologic problem is summarized in Chart 25-1.

NORMAL AND ABNORMAL MENSTRUATION

The normal menstrual cycle is a delicate mechanism involving the anterior pituitary gland, the ovaries, and the uterine lining. Gonadotropic hormones from the pituitary stimulate primary follicles in the ovarian cortex to develop mature eggs and produce estrogen and progesterone. These hormones stimulate the uterine lining to develop a receptive bed for the potentially fertilized ovum.

The egg is usually released in midcycle. If fertilization by the male sperm does not occur within 36 to 48 hours, the egg undergoes degenerative changes, and the uterine lining is shed, about 2 weeks after ovulation. This release of the uterine lining is accompanied by arterial spasm in the uterine walls and resultant abdominal cramps as the debris and blood are ejected. This constitutes the menstrual period.

Menstrual blood is usually nonclotting and averages 70 ml to 100 ml per period. The discomfort of menstruation is related to the spasm, cramps, pelvic congestion, and smallness of the cervical os, which impedes menstrual flow. The influence of progesterone causes some water retention and the general misery associated with a young girl's periods.

The menstrual cycle varies tremendously, with a range of 20 to 46 days. Most women become fairly regular, varying only 2 to 3 days per cycle. Typically, the menstrual cycle is subject to irregularity mainly early and late in menstrual life, that is, in the young girl and the menopausal woman.

Chart 25-1

ASSESSMENT OF THE GYNECOLOGIC PATIENT

History

- Pain is commonly associated with gynecologic problems, usually in the area of the pelvic organs. Note time of onset.
- Vaginal discharge commonly accompanies infections of the female genital tract. Ask patient about amount, color, consistency, and odor.
- Vaginal bleeding—note amount, time of onset in relation to period, type of bleeding, amount, presence of clots.
- Menstrual period—record date of last menstrual period and prior menstrual periods. Ask about frequency and date of last sexual exposure.
- Urinary symptoms often accompany gynecologic problems. Question patient about any symptoms.

Physical Examination

- Fever may be present.
- Tenderness may be present in the lower abdomen.
- Speculum examination of vagina and cervix, to examine for vaginal discharge or bleeding. Note color, consistency, amount, and odor. If bloody, note presence of clots.
- Bimanual examination of pelvic contents for masses and tenderness on motion of cervix (rectal examination in virginal or prepubertal females)

Adjunct Studies

- Smear and culture of vaginal fluid
- Abdominal x-ray to detect radiopaque lesions
- Urinalysis, culture, and sensitivity
- Cul-de-sac aspiration if intraperitoneal hemorrhage is suspected
- Sonogram of pelvis
- CT scan of pelvis

However, temporary irregularity may occur at any time, for no apparent cause.

Menstrual regularity can be affected by the action of other glands, such as the thyroid and adrenal. Emotional upsets, such as a death in the family, illness, or a drastic change in environment, may cause delayed menses. However, it is important to keep in mind that a missed period in a woman of childbearing age is probably due to pregnancy until proven otherwise.

Dysmenorrhea (painful menses) may consist of abdominal pain, cramps, bloating, and tension. In mild cases, analgesics may be all that is required. Diuretics and tranquilizers can be used to relieve bloating and premenstrual tension. More severe cases of dysmenorrhea respond to prevention of ovulation, which results in development of a thinner uterine lining and, therefore, less debris to be expelled. Ovulation can be prevented by large doses of estrogens, oral progestins (birth control pills), or intramuscular injections of long-acting progestins (*e.g.,* medroxyprogesterone acetate suspension) to produce a pseudopregnancy and amenorrhea for a period of time. Smooth muscle relaxants may also give some relief.

It has recently been established that with the onset of menstruation a powerful substance called prostaglandin is released from the uterine tissue. This chemical causes marked localized and systemic reactions. These include muscular contraction of the uterus and gastrointestinal side-effects such as nausea, emesis, diarrhea, and syncope.

Fortunately, drugs are available that have an antiprostaglandin effect and effectively interfere with the production of this chemical, providing moderate to marked relief of the discomfort associated with dysmenorrhea. Aspirin is now known to work in this fashion, but stronger antiprostaglandins have been developed. Aspirin, besides being a relatively weak antiprostaglandin, can also cause reduced blood coagulability and therefore increase the amount of menstrual flow.

Mefenamid acid (Ponstel), naproxen sodium (Naprosyn), and ibuprofen (Motrin) are three members of this class of prostaglandin synthetase inhibitors.

Maximum relief is obtained if the drugs are begun several days before the onset of the period. Tylenol with codeine may also be added in very protracted cases. In severe dysmenorrhea, thorough evaluation is needed, and surgical treatment may be necessary, including presacral neurectomy or dilatation of the cervix to allow freer uterine flow.

In patients with abnormal bleeding, obviously, the cause must be determined before suitable treatment can be carried out. In the following pages, various types of gynecologic bleeding are discussed, along with typical symptoms and a brief outline of emergency treatment.

DYSFUNCTIONAL UTERINE BLEEDING

PREMENARCHAL ABNORMALITIES

Vaginal bleeding in children has many causes.

Vicarious Menstruation

Vicarious menstruation is seen most commonly in newborn infant girls and consists of a blood-tinged mucous vaginal discharge occurring in the first 2 weeks after delivery.

This is not a pathologic condition; it merely represents withdrawal bleeding from the lining of the infant uterus secondary to cessation of the estrogen which crossed the placenta from the mother's blood during pregnancy. The bleeding is of short duration and requires no treatment except reassurance to the parents bringing the child to the emergency department for assessment.

Premature Menarche

The onset of menses usually occurs between the ages of 10 and 14. However, the first period may normally occur in some children as early as 8 or 9 years. It has even been reported in a girl as young as 5 years of age. However, all children with abnormally early menarche should be investigated to rule out pathologic causes, such as pituitary tumors, certain types of brain tumors, ovarian tumors (such as thecal granulosa cells tumors, which are hormone producing) or the presence of vaginal or uterine neoplasms.

Sarcoma botryoid is a rare vaginal or cervical tumor occurring in young girls or infants that may present with bleeding. It is usually a grape-like growth at the vaginal introitus. However, biopsy is necessary to prove the diagnosis. If confirmed, radical surgery is the treatment of choice.

Infection or Foreign Object in the Vagina

Many children brought to the emergency department present with a bloody, watery discharge secondary to a vaginitis. Before menarche, the vagina is very thin and easily irritated. The cells are not cornified, because there is no estrogen stimulation. Young girls, out of natural curiosity, frequently insert various items into the vaginal introitus. This may cause secondary infection, with discharge and sometimes bleeding. These self-inserted items defy description, varying from small wads of tissue to paper clips and rubber erasers. Speculum examination is difficult. However, an ear speculum, nasal forceps or an x-ray (if the object is radiopaque) will aid in the diagnosis. A minidouche with saline and gentle wash often dislodges small objects. Placing the child in the knee-chest position affords better exposure when examining for the cause of vaginal discharge.

Fifty percent of vulvovaginitis in children is due to non-specific causes such as harsh soaps, suboptimal hygiene, and ill-fitting garments. Specific causes include a foreign body, *Neisseria gonorrhoeae*, β-streptococci, *Candida*, *Trichomonas*, *Hemophilus influenzae,* and herpes simplex Type 2 infection (genital herpes).

Gonorrhea in girls may present as a vaginitis, owing to the lack of protective thickening of the vagina by endogenous estrogen stimulation. This is in contradistinction to women, in whom cervical infection is a result of gonorrhea.

All vaginitis in children should be cultured on chocolate agar in a CO_2 environment or other suitable medium to rule out gonococcus. Gram-stain smears should also be made to detect gram-negative intracellular diplococci. Treatment consists of appropriate antibiotic treatment, as well as investigation for the possible source. Once the diagnosis has been confirmed, local health authorities should be notified so that other contacts may be identified and treated.

Many females, in the same household, regardless of age, exhibit trichomonas vaginal infestation. The typical discharge is watery and yellowish and has a characteristic offensive odor. The diagnosis can be made by detection of motile trichomonads in wet-drop preparations of the vaginal secretion. Treatment for a young child consists of local therapy. In older children and adults, there are many local preparations, as well as an oral medication, metronidazole HCl (Flagyl), that can be used.

Stilbestrol-Related Tumors

Research has shown a significant relationship between the development of vaginal adenosis and clear cell carcinoma in girls whose mothers had diethylstilbestrol therapy during pregnancy. For a period of 10 to 15 years, beginning about 20 years ago, many high-risk pregnancy mothers were treated with stilbestrol in large doses to maintain the pregnancy. A very small percentage of these children have exhibited changes in the vagina and cervix that may develop into very malignant tumors.

The incidence of stilbestrol-related cancers in women remains very low. They are clear-cell carcinomas of the cervix or vagina. It is more common for patients with these cancers to have areas of benign adenosis of the cervix or vagina. Though these areas of adenosis are apparently benign, all daughters of stilbestrol-treated mothers should be followed with vaginal cytology and in some cases with colposcopy.

Many patients do not know whether their mothers took stilbestrol during pregnancy, and in some cases the mothers don't know either. A "cockscomb" cervix or a large congenital erosion should make the examiner suspicious that stilbestrol may be involved, even without a definitive history.

Most of these victims present with vaginal bleeding. Adequate examination and biopsy confirm the diagnosis. It is recommended that all girls whose mothers took stilbestrol during pregnancy have periodic examinations and Papanicolaou (Pap) smears.

Trauma

Penetrating injuries of the vagina may cause vaginal bleeding. Careful exam is necessary. Straddle injuries, such as a fall onto a bicycle crossbar or a fence, can cause large hematomas and lacerations of the perineum. Adequate examination and x-ray studies to rule out intraperitoneal injury are necessary.

Congenital Abnormalities

Imperforate hymen and obliteration of the vagina (partial or complete) may present in an emergency department. The history is typically that a normally developed preteenage girl, with breast development, fat distribution, and hair growth, has not menstruated or has only spotted. The absent or diminished menses is associated with periodic pelvic cramps, which become increasingly severe.

Inspection of the perineum shows a bulging hymen, and a bulging vagina is revealed on rectal examination. Excision of the obstruction under sterile conditions, usually performed in an operating suite, corrects the situation.

MENSTRUAL ABNORMALITIES

Menstrual abnormalities may also be due to defective hormone stimulation of the endometrial lining. It is well-documented that whenever hormone stimulation of the uterine lining is suddenly stopped or fluctuates, withdrawal bleeding occurs. If complete release of the uterine lining occurs, normal menstruation results. However, if irregular shedding occurs, spotting and bleeding result and may continue over a long period of time. On occasion, prolonged estrogen stimulation results in a very thick uterine lining that bleeds readily. Midcycle spotting frequently occurs secondary to a slight hormone drop at the time of ovulation.

Dysfunctional uterine bleeding may be treated in one of several ways. A dilatation and curettage (D & C) will remove the abnormal lining and allow normal rhythmic menstrual growth to occur. Large doses of estrogen will overcome the fluctuations in physiologic hormone levels and stop abnormal spotting and bleeding. Progesterone often produces maturation of the lining, followed 5 to 10 days later by withdrawal bleeding (medical curettage).

Recurrent dysfunctional bleeding often can be prevented by the temporary addition of estrogen and progesterone hormones to mimic a normal cycle. Oral progestins can also be used in this fashion. In most cases, a D & C is done only when the diagnosis is in doubt, the bleeding has not responded to hormone treatment, or the problem is severe.

Dysfunctional bleeding may be associated with physiologic cysts of the ovary, such as a persistent corpus luteum cyst that produces an abnormal amount of hormone and may present a clinical picture suggestive of ectopic pregnancy, appendicitis, or threatened miscarriage.

Anemia in women is most commonly due to chronic blood loss associated with heavy periods over a long period of time. This is especially true in cases of marked hypothyroidism. Many authorities believe that women should receive supplemental iron preparations prophylactically, to replace the body iron stores lost monthly through menstruation. Extremely heavy bleeding or clotting may respond to ergotrate preparations.

Bleeding Associated With IUDs

One of the annoying side-effects of the various forms of intrauterine contraceptive devices (IUDs) is abnormal vaginal bleeding. This is commonly a menorrhagia at the time of normal menstruation or irregular bleeding in the midcycle, which appears to be due to local ulceration of the endometrial lining with associated endometritis. (Other complications secondary to the IUD are detailed in following pages.)

The treatment of menstrual irregularity secondary to an IUD includes vitamin K, vitamin C, and large doses of estrogen or ergotrate preparations to cause uterine muscle contraction and reduction in menstrual flow.

Irregularity Associated With Oral Contraceptives

The physiologic effect of oral progestins, the main component of birth control pills, is to suppress the pituitary gland by increasing hormone levels to inhibit follicle-stimulating hormone (FSH) and thus place the ovaries in a resting state similar to that seen during pregnancy. Since ovulation does not occur, pregnancy cannot result. These pills are given in a cyclic fashion, usually for 20 to 21 days, then discontinued, usually for 7 days, so that withdrawal bleeding and a pseudoperiod may result. These simulated periods are usually lighter in amount and are almost always painless, owing to the reduced thickness of the uterine lining and the decidua-like tissue response.

Although a variety of side-effects may accompany use of the pill, they are usually neither serious nor frequent in occurrence and in part depend on individual tolerance to the medication. Complications that do occur secondary to use of the birth control pill are considered later in this chapter.

If the oral progestins were given alone, there would be a marked degree of "breakthrough" bleeding. To prevent this, varying amounts of estrogen are added. British investigators have shown that it is apparently the added estrogen that is associated with the most serious complications of birth control pills, thrombophlebitis, and embolic phenomena. Therefore, drug manufacturers have reduced the amount of estrogen to 35 μg or less (or its equivalent), in order to reduce the risk. Unfortunately, breakthrough bleeding is now more common.

Vaginal spotting can be dealt with by temporarily increasing the daily dose. Heavier bleeding may require discontinuing the pill for 7 days, even though the monthly supply has not been taken, then restarting another 21-day supply. Often, different combinations of progestins and estrogen or heavier doses will prevent the bleeding side-effect.

POSTMENOPAUSAL BLEEDING

Vaginal bleeding after 6 months of amenorrhea in a menopausal woman is always cause for concern. Gynecologic malignancies reach peak incidence in the 40 to 60 age group. Postmenopausal bleeding must always be investigated to rule out a malignant cause. Cancer of the cervix or endometrium is the most common cause. Rarer tumors of the pelvis associated with vaginal bleeding include primary cancer of the vagina, ovarian tumors that may or may not produce estrogens, and metastatic tumors to the vagina.

Cancer of the Cervix

Carcinoma *in situ* may be present at any age, from 18 to 80. In reality, this is not invasive cancer but a malignant change in the entire upper layer of the epithelium of the cervix or upper vagina. It is completely asymptomatic and can be detected only by Pap test or by use of a colposcope. Iodine solutions in the vagina outline the abnormal areas so that punch biopsy or cone biopsy of the cervix will reveal the lesion. This type of tumor is highly curable and responds to various types of treatment.

Invasive cancer of the cervix almost always presents with vaginal bleeding as the chief complaint. A watery, serosanguineous discharge is often present. Examination shows a polypoid lesion involving the cervix or a firm cervix with an ulcer. Early cases involve the cervix only, whereas in more advanced disease, the vagina, broad ligament, and even the bladder and rectum are involved, sometimes with fistula formation and incontinence.

Emergency treatment of hemorrhage includes transfusion, tight vaginal packing, or hypogastric artery ligation. Treatment of invasive cancer of the cervix includes radical hysterectomy, radium plus cobalt radiation therapy, or pelvic exenteration.

Terminal cases of cancer of the cervix usually present with uremia secondary to obstructive uropathy from tumor compression of the ureters. Distant metastasis with involvement of the lung is not uncommon.

Cancer of the Endometrium

Endometrial cancer usually occurs in menopausal or postmenopausal women. The presenting symptom is almost invariably bleeding. The diagnosis is made by a D & C or endometrial biopsy. It is a highly curable lesion and responds to panhysterectomy, with or without preoperative intrauterine radium. Advanced cases may respond to long-acting progestins in large doses (medroxyprogesterone acetate suspension or hydroprogesterone caproate injection).

Nonmalignant Causes

Postmenopausal bleeding can arise from a number of nonmalignant causes, as follows:

Exogenous Hormones. Many women receive estrogens to combat hot flashes and other menopausal symptoms, and a common side-effect is vaginal bleeding. Endometrial biopsy or curettage is necessary, however, to rule out carcinoma.

Endometrial Polyps. Endometrial polyps can cause vaginal spotting.

Cystic Glandular Hyperplasia. This condition is commonly seen in women undergoing waning ovarian activity.

Bleeding From a Surface Vessel. In some older women, bleeding may occur without evidence of abnormality of the uterine lining. Some physicians have diagnosed this as *uterine apoplexy,* that is, bleeding from a small surface artery, similar to that seen in nosebleed.

Hematometria. This condition is also seen in older women. It usually presents with some vaginal spotting and a great deal of crampy menstrual-type pain. On pelvic examination, a large boggy uterus with a tight or obliterated cervical os is detected. This state is often seen in endometrial cancer but may also be associated with a benign condition or a fibrotic cervix. D & C and drainage through the cervix are both diagnostic and curative.

The symptoms of *pyometria* (uterus full of pus) are quite similar to those of hematometria, although bleeding is rare. Pyometria is usually associated with a uterine malignancy.

Neglected Pessary. Many older women with prolapsed uteri and cystoceles who are poor surgical risks have Gellhorn *pessaries* or *rings* inserted to hold their pelvic organs in place. These devices must be removed and replaced periodically to avoid tissue irritation or overgrowth of tissue, which would fix them firmly in place and make removal difficult. Some patients with pessaries present with vaginal bleeding and discharge. Treatment consists of removal of the pessary and application of local hormone and antibacterial cream to cure the vaginitis and heal the epithelium.

Complete Prolapse. Some older women present with complete inversion of the vagina and prolapse of the uterus, with contact ulcers of the cervix due to abrasion of the prolapsed organ on the underclothing. Treatment is usually surgical, but if the patient is a poor risk (and many are), a vaginal pessary may suffice.

LESIONS OF THE VULVA

Inflammatory lesions of the vulva are the type most often seen in an emergency department. Acute Bartholin's abscess is a common complaint. At one time, these were thought to be gonococcal in origin, but the vast majority encountered today are nonspecific bacterial infections due to coliform organisms.

The patient presents with an acute painful swelling in the midposterior aspect of the vulva, with bulging into the vaginal introitus. Pain is aggravated by sitting or walking. There is considerable soft-tissue swelling. Emergency treatment is incision and drainage, although spontaneous rupture often occurs. The pus should be cultured for predominant organisms and gonococcus. After drainage, antibiotics are rarely necessary. Sitz baths and analgesics relieve the residual inflammation. Recurrences are common. A more permanent cure can be obtained by an operative procedure. The roof of the abscess wall is opened and a wedge of tissue removed. The edges of the wall are then marsupialized to create a new orifice for the Bartholin's gland.

A perirectal abscess can present as a subcutaneous abscess anywhere on the buttock or perineum. The patient complains of a painful swelling in the area. Adequate rectal exam and the lack of bulging into the vaginal introitus can help in distinguishing this condition from Bartholin's abscess. Correct identification is important; the definitive treatment of this lesion is entirely different, since it originates within the anal crypts and requires incision and drainage.

Genital Herpes

There has been an alarming increase in the incidence of genital herpes infection recently; it appears to be as widespread as other sexually transmitted diseases. The lesions are multiple small breaks in the skin and mucous membranes of the vulva and introitus. They may occur singly or in groups and are very painful. Enlarged, tender lymph nodes may be present in the groin. The condition is viral in origin, lasts approximately 10 days, and may recur periodically. Pain and tendency of recurrence are characteristic of genital herpes infection.

Although there is a known relationship between cancer of the cervix and sexual promiscuity, a link between genital herpes and cervical cancer has not been definitively established. It is, however, extremely important that a woman with active herpes lesions of the genital tract, or one with a recent exacerbation, not be allowed to deliver vaginally if her pregnancy comes to term. Herpetic infection of the newborn is associated with a high death rate as well as permanent neurologic damage in surviving infants.

Treatment/Management. Until recently, treatment was symptomatic, consisting of analgesics, sitz baths, and local anesthetic ointments. For initial genital herpes infection a new synthetic antiviral agent, acyclovir, has shown promising results. It is available as a 5% ointment that is applied to the mucocutaneous area of the vulva every 3 hours, 6 times a day for 1 week. Significant side-effects are uncommon. The drug has been of little benefit in patients with recurrent genital herpes infection.

Syphilis

Chancre of the vulva is also being seen with increasing frequency. This is a 1.0-cm to 1.5-cm punched-out ulcer of the skin or mucous membrane, with a grayish, shaggy base. It is only slightly tender and appears 7 to 14 days after infectious sexual contact. A chancrous lesion is highly contagious on contact. It disappears spontaneously in a fortnight, to be followed by the multiple mucous membrane lesions of secondary syphilis.

Blood Wasserman and other serology tests are not positive until 10 to 14 days after the primary lesion appears. When syphilis is suspected, special laboratory tests (dark-field examination) on the scraping from the base of the ulcer are necessary, as well as follow-up serology in 2 to 3 weeks. Inguinal adenopathy may also be detected. Penicillin or broad-spectrum antibiotics in very large doses are the treatment of choice.

Syphilis is a reportable disease—once the diagnosis is confirmed, local health authorities are to be notified so that other patient contacts can be located and appropriate treatment initiated.

Condylomata Acuminata

Venereal warts are now apparent in epidemic form. They are due to a virus and are usually spread by genital contact with an infected partner. They may involve the cervix and vagina but are very common on the labia, perineum, and perianal areas. They occur in groups, some of which follow a linear distribution. The lesions are small, may be single or confluent, and may grow into very large groups.

Treatment. Early lesions respond very well to 25% podophyllin in tincture of benzoin. This solution should be washed off in 4 hours, and abundant analgesic and local anesthetic preparations prescribed, because considerable local tissue reactions occur for about 7 to 10 days. Other forms of treatment include electrocautery, surgical excision, and cryosurgery. Multiple treatments are often necessary to eradicate the lesions.

Furuncles

Many sweat and sebaceous glands are present on the vulva, and infections in them are quite common. Early signs are of cellulitis, with a swollen, red area that is exquisitely tender to the touch. Later, the area becomes fluctuant.

Management/Treatment. In the early phase, local applications of heat or use of sitz baths and antibiotics may be indicated. However, as the area becomes fluctuant, incision and drainage under local anesthesia is the preferred treatment and will give relief. Follow-up care consists of analgesics and sitz baths. If inguinal nodes are involved, specific antibiotics effective against the predominant organism, which is usually staphylococcus, may be prescribed. In recurrent cases, skin care using a hexachlorophene soap should be used prophylactically, and blood glucose tests are in order to rule out diabetes.

VAGINITIS

Monilial (Candidal) Vulvovaginitis

Monilial (or candidal) infection is a very common problem caused by autoinfection from an overgrowth of the yeast organism *Candida (Monilia) albicans.* The patient presents with a discharge and severe burning and itching of the vulvar and vaginal introitus areas. The tissue is reddened and weepy, and on occasion, whitish plaques can be seen. The burning is constant and is aggravated by urination.

This lesion is typical in uncontrolled diabetic patients because the increased sugar content in the tissues and the acid environment predispose to overgrowth of the organism. The organism will grow in brownish-black colonies on Nicholson's culture medium, which is commercially available. Wet smears or gram stains will also show the typical spores and mycelia.

Conditions that predispose to monilial (candidal) infections are pregnancy, oral contraceptives, systemic antibiotic therapy that changes the normal vaginal bacterial flora (particularly tetracycline and penicillin), and diabetes. However, a large number of cases have no predisposing cause.

Treatment/Management. Treatment consists of local medication in the form of vaginal tablets, suppositories, or ointments. The vaginal infestation must be controlled before the vulvitis will respond. Nystatin suppositories are very effective. Alkaline douches, such as 2 tablespoons of bicarbonate of soda in a quart of water, will help relieve the symptoms and restore an alkaline environment to the vagina.

Trichomonas Vaginitis

Trichomonas is the second most commonly occurring vaginitis. The primary symptom is an abundant, yellowish, watery discharge with a slightly disagreeable odor. Itching and severe inflammation may be present. The condition is endemic, and many female carriers are asymptomatic, with the condition detected only on Pap smear. Trichomonas is highly contagious and can infect children; many investigators claim it is a type of venereal diease, but some infections are contracted in a nonvenereal fashion.

Diagnosis is definitive when wet saline drop preparations of the vaginal secretions are examined microscopically for the motile protozoa.

Treatment/Management. For more persistent cases, Flagyl given by mouth will be effective most of the time. In recurrent infections, the male partner should also receive Flagyl, to prevent reinfection. Vinegar douches or commercial acid douches will also help control the condition.

Hemophilus vaginalis Vaginitis

After monilial (candidal) and *Trichomonas* vaginitis, the most common causative organism of vaginal infection is *Hemophilus vaginalis*. Patients with this infection present with a thin, homogeneous, grey, odoriferous, somewhat frothy discharge. The *p*H of the vagina is acid (*p*H 5.0–5.5) and the infection is often confused with trichomoniasis.

Diagnosis is achieved with a wet drop mount and gram stain examined microscopically. The presence of "clue cells," (squamous epithelial cells covered with masses of bacteria) is diagnostic. No Döderlein bacilli are seen.

Treatment. Treatment consists of ampicillin with or without probenecid, or metronidazole (Flagyl) 500 mg bid for seven days. Intravaginal sulfa tablets have also been reported to be effective.

Atrophic Vaginitis

This condition is seen in postmenopausal women who are not taking estrogen replacement therapy. It is in reality a nonspecific bacterial inflammation of the vaginal wall due to estrogen deprivation and thinning of the mucosa with loss of host resistance. The presenting complaint is a foul discharge, yellowish to green or brown in color. Inspection of the vagina shows an almost feces-like exudate in severe cases. Mixed coliform bacteria are found on culture.

Treatment. Local estrogen creams will correct the condition. However, long-term use is often necessary to prevent recurrence.

Forgotten Tampons

Vaginal tampons are being increasingly used by women of various ages. The neglected tampon, inadvertently left in the vagina, produces one of the most foul discharges ever encountered. When, as it sometimes happens, a new tampon is inserted before the used one is removed, the string attached to the first one disappears, and the tampon can then be forgotten. In 3 to 4 days, a foul odor and brownish discharge occur, bringing many women to the emergency department.

Management. Removal of the tampon will cure the condition, but during removal, the atmosphere of the treatment room will become nearly unbearable. Abundant amounts of aerosol spray are necessary. No further treatment is necessary, although sometimes antibiotic vaginal preparations may be prescribed.

OVARIAN DISEASE

In pursuit of its normal functions, both as an endocrine gland producing estrogen and progesterone and as a development site for mature ova, the human ovary during active menstrual life normally produces several types of cystic enlargements which appear and disappear. These include the graffian follicle cyst, which releases the ovum at ovulation, and the corpus luteum cyst, which replaces the graffian follicle cyst at the ovulating site on the cortex of the ovary and produces large amounts of estrogen and progesterone, which mature the endometrium to receive the fertilized egg.

BENIGN DISEASE

Mittelschmerz

Ovulation pain is a common complaint and is often confused with appendicitis if it occurs on the right side. This pain may vary from vague discomfort of short duration to moderately severe pain which persists for several days. Mild pelvic and rebound tenderness may be present. The white blood count is only moderately elevated; temperature readings are 37.5°C (99°F) or less; and there is usually no associated anorexia. The most important sign is the expected date of the next period. This pain is almost always mid-cycle.

Cysts and Tumors

Solid and cystic tumors of the ovary are common. A variety of these benign lesions occur and are discussed in the following paragraphs.

Hemorrhagic Cysts. Hemorrhagic or ruptured corpus luteum cysts occur in the second portion of the menstrual cycle. A very tender, slightly enlarged ovary may be palpated on pelvic examination. Pain and tenderness in the lower abdomen are present. This condition must also be differentiated from appendicitis. Treatment is almost always supportive once appendicitis and ectopic pregnancy are ruled out, merely requiring some form of pain relief and close observation.

Large Cysts. Large benign cysts of the ovary can also occur. Simple cysts are single cell layer cystic enlargements of the ovary. Unless complicated with pain or torsion, most cysts will disappear over a 3- to 4-week period. In fact, many cysts rupture asymptomatically during pelvic exam.

Dermoid Cysts. Dermoid cysts are often found, especially in young women, as asymptomatic pelvic masses, perhaps very large. They contain hair, skin, sebaceous material and, on occasion, even teeth which can be seen on x-ray. If a dermoid cyst ruptures, it can produce a severe chemical peritonitis, but this complication is rare. Torsion of the ovarian pedicle is encountered more frequently. Women with dermoid cysts present with pelvic pain which typically is intermittent but may be constant. Treatment is surgical excision.

Benign Tumors. Benign tumors include Brenner cell tumors, ovarian fibroids, thecomas, endometriomas, cystadenomas, pseudo-mucinous cystadenomas, and many rarer types.

MALIGNANCIES

Malignant tumors of the ovary often reach extensive proportions with very few symptoms; the disease process is insidious. A large proportion of victims of malignant ovarian tumors present with abdominal ascites and palpable lower abdominal masses. Pain is seldom a presenting symptom unless torsion, hemorrhage or bowel obstruction has taken place.

Treatment consists of paracentesis, surgery, radiation treatment and chemotherapy. In the majority of cases, the prognosis is grave.

PELVIC DISEASE

Endometriosis

Pelvic endometriosis is very common, though the cause is unknown. There are two theories on causation. One posits that retrograde menstrual flow occurs through the fallopian tubes, causing random implantation of foci of viable endometrial tissue in the peritoneal cavity. The other theory is that endometrial implants occur in undifferentiated rests of embryonal tissue.

Endometriosis is due to the development of ectopic endometrial tissue, usually limited to the pelvis. This tissue, like the endometrium of the uterus, responds to the hormone cycle and bleeds internally in small amounts during menses. This causes localized blood deposits and tissue reaction. Although the tubes are usually patent and normal ovulation does occur, endometriosis is a leading cause of infertility in women.

The condition may be asymptomatic. However, the typical patient has marked dysmenorrhea, often with rectal pressure and backache. Common sites of endometriosis are the ovary (where rather large, chocolate-like cysts may be produced), the posterior surface of the uterus, the uterosacral ligaments, and the pelvic peritoneum (where small, tender nodules may develop).

Treatment. Treatment of endometriosis may be either medical or surgical. In the presence of large chocolate cysts of the ovary, surgery is the treatment of choice. Conservative surgery is indicated in young women, with meticulous surgical removal of ectopic endometrial tissue and preservation of ovarian and childbearing function whenever possible.

If childbearing function is not important, such as in older women and those who have completed their families, panhysterectomy is indicated when extensive disease is found. It is very important that both ovaries be removed if all the endometrial implants cannot be eradicated. Replacement hormone therapy should not be instituted for at least 6 months if any endometrial implants remain after surgery because reactivation may result.

Medical treatment of endometriosis has improved dramatically with the introduction of danazol (Danocrine). Danazol essentially produces an artificial temporary menopause resulting in regression of the endometrial implants. The drug apparently blocks estrogen receptors, causing hormone starvation of the endometrial implants, with eventual regression and often total disappearance. Very gratifying pregnancy rates have been recorded after its use in women who had no other elicited cause for infertility. The dosage is 400 mg bid for a period of 4 to 6 months. Side effects include water retention, acne, hot flashes, amenorrhea with irregular spotting, and weight gain. It is relatively expensive, costing $5 to $6 per day. The extent of endometriosis should be evaluated by diagnostic laparoscopy before treatment is initiated.

Other medical treatments for endometriosis include the use of oral or injectable progestins (Depo Provera, Delalutin) over long periods of time.

Inflammatory Disease

Inflammatory pelvic disease includes all types of bacterial infections of the pelvis. The most common sites of infection are the cervix, endometrium, and fallopian tubes, although a diffuse infection of the pelvic tissues may occur (pelvic cellulitis).

Tuberculosis. Tuberculosis of the pelvis is still seen, though rarely. It is usually a silent disease, with few symptoms, and is almost invariably associated with pulmonary or renal tuberculosis. Sterility is a common result. The endometrium grows and sheds tubercular infested tissue monthly, so it may be diagnosed by D & C or endometrial biopsy. The tubes are often infected, but pain and fever are not a usual complaint. Treatment consists of prolonged antitubercular drug therapy, although on occasion, pelvic surgery is necessary.

Cervicitis. Cervicitis is an infection of the cervical mucous glands. It is most commonly a low-grade infection, coliform or gonococcal in origin. The symptoms are purulent vaginal discharge and sometimes lower backache. Fever and other constitutional complaints are lacking. A large, boggy, tender cervix with purulent exudate and pseudoerosion are present. Treatment consists of suitable antibiotics followed by electrocoagulation, cryosurgery, or conization of the cervix to correct the pseudoerosion. Hospitalization is not usually required.

Endometritis. Endometritis presents with pelvic pain that is limited to the uterus, often with lower backache and the presence of a tender, swollen uterus. The organism involved is usually *Escherichia coli* or other coliforms. It is secondary to miscarriage, D & C, or intrauterine devices. Treatment consists of bed rest, antibiotics, and removal of the IUD if one is present.

Salpingitis. Salpingitis, inflammation of the fallopian tubes, is a very common pelvic complaint. It is almost always due to gonorrheal or chlamydial infection, although it may be seen after delivery or secondary to other causes of endometritis. *Chlamydia trachomatis* has been implicated in acute salpingitis. This parasite is reaching epidemic proportions and is often involved in nonspecific urethritis in the male. The condition is very difficult to diagnose simply. Chlamydial infections, which are sexually transmitted, do not respond to penicillin but can be treated with Doxycycline, 100 mg daily.

Women with salpingitis will present walking in a doubled-over position. Pain is prominent and usually bilateral (lower abdominal area) and constant, and there is rebound tenderness.

The typical case of salpingitis occurs following a normal menstrual period. About the fourth or fifth day of the period, symptoms of pain develop and become progressively worse. Fever is present up to 40°C (104°F). Pelvic findings in early cases show adnexal tenderness and pain on movement of the uterus; a leukorrhea is often present. Advanced or recurrent cases may show tubo-ovarian pelvic masses or even a pelvic abscess bulging into the cul-de-sac.

Cultures should be taken from the cervix and periurethral glands for detection of gonorrhea and other organisms. Gram stains of the exudate may show intracellular gram-negative diplococci, even when cultures are negative. Even in typical cases, the gonococcus bacteria are not always recovered on culture because secondary invaders, such as enterococci and other coliform bacteria, predominate in cultures. Cervical and vaginal cultures for *Neisseria* species are not always reliable, and many false-negative results occur.

Treatment consists of bed rest, penicillin or broad-spectrum antibiotics, pain medication, and drainage of pelvic abscesses, if any. If bilateral tubal masses remain after treatment, surgical removal of the tubes, ovaries, and uterus should be done. If tubal enlargement persists, the tube is destroyed as an oviduct, and permanent sterility occurs.

Certain strains of *N. gonorrhoeae* have developed penicillin resistance. In areas where these strains are common, gonorrhea should be treated with any of the following; cefoxitin, 2 gm IM; spectinomycin, or 4.8 million units of procaine penicillin G with 1 gm probenecid.

Patients with early symptoms and primary infections will often completely recover with no sequelae after adequate treatment. However, peritubular adhesions, sterility, and ectopic pregnancies are much more common in patients with salpingitis.

Intraperitoneal Rupture. Intraperitoneal rupture of a tubo-ovarian abscess can be a catastrophic event. Peritonitis becomes diffuse, and the patient may go into vascular collapse. Intravenous vasopressors, massive antibiotics, and surgical intervention are necessary if this occurs.

Degenerating Fibroids

Patients may present to the emergency department with pelvic pain secondary to uterine fibroid tumors. Pedunculated fibroids may twist on their stalks; associated pain is due to interference with blood supply and tissue necrosis in the tumor. A tender fibroid tumor is found on examination. Treatment is surgical removal of the fibroid or possibly of the uterus. Large fibroids may undergo degeneration even if they are not pedunculated. The tumor, though benign, may outgrow its blood supply, causing necrosis of tissue, pain, fever, or secondary infection.

Submucous fibroids can develop in the uterine cavity and by uterine contractions deliver through the cervical os. There is usually colicky uterine pain, some bleeding and a necrotic mass protruding through the cervix. These can often be removed with a tonsil snare.

COMPLICATIONS DUE TO BIRTH CONTROL MEASURES

INTRAUTERINE DEVICES (IUDS)

Intrauterine devices (IUDs) are an acceptable, fairly reliable form of contraception. Although there have been few reported deaths (with the exception of Dalkon shield pregnancy-related fatalities), significant side-effects and long term sequelae are associated with their use.

Expulsion remains a problem, and patients may present

to the emergency department with cramps, bleeding and partial extrusion of the device through the cervix. In this instance, the IUD should be removed.

Menorrhagia with clot formation is very common and may be controlled with Methergine or Ergotrate. Vitamin K administration may or may not be of value. In severe cases the IUD should be removed. Bleeding between menstrual periods is often seen because of mechanical erosion of the endometrium by the device. This is usually a self-limited condition that may be controlled with estrogen therapy. The possibility of ectopic pregnancy must always be kept in mind when pain and bleeding are present.

When the patient cannot feel the IUD strings and they cannot be visualized, the problem is determining whether the IUD has been expelled vaginally or whether it has migrated within or even through, the uterus. Probing of the uterine cavity with a uterine sound will often detect the presence of the IUD. Ultrasound is also useful in these cases. A flat plate x-ray film of the pelvis will reveal the presence or absence of the IUD but not necessarily its position. Hysterosalpingoscopy or laparoscopy may be necessary in difficult cases.

Intrauterine and extrauterine pregnancies can occur. In the case of intrauterine pregnancy, when the strings are still visible, the IUD should be gently removed. This can usually be done safely without causing miscarriage, and the pregnancy will progress normally. If the IUD cannot be seen, it may be left *in situ*. Although there is a greater risk of miscarriage, many pregnancies have progressed to term, and the IUD has been recovered in the membranes or placental structures at delivery.

Tubal pregnancies in IUD users are significantly increased. In any case of menstrual irregularity associated with pelvic pain, suitable diagnostic measures must be instituted. Tubal pregnancies are also the most common type of pregnancy after tubal ligation, and this possibility must be borne in mind even though a history of tubal ligation is given.

Infection has been a problem with IUD users. Pelvic inflammatory disease (salpingitis) is seven times more common in women using IUDs than in those using oral contraceptives. Unilateral tubal abscess is sometimes seen. Actinomycosis infections of the uterus and pelvis are being reported in IUD users, especially those who have had their devices for many years. Infertility, probably due to the sequelae of tubal infection, is eight times higher in patients after IUD use than in patients formerly on oral contraceptives.

In cases of severe infection in association with IUD users, the device should be removed and intensive antibiotic therapy should be administered.

BIRTH CONTROL PILLS

Thrombophlebitis is rare, but if the deep veins are involved, it can be a serious side effect of the oral progestins. The symptoms are usually pain and swelling in one or both legs. The posterior aspect of the calf is painful on dorsiflexion of the foot with the knee extended (Homans' sign). Sometimes a tender cord can be palpated behind the knee. Edema of the foot and lower leg may be present and in more serious cases may extend as high as the groin, with tenderness along the course of the femoral vein.

Treatment of severe cases of thrombophlebitis consists of discontinuation of "the pill" and initiation of immediate and long-term anticoagulant treatment, for example, heparin plus warfarin sodium (Coumadin). If embolic events occur while the patient is on therapeutic doses of anticoagulants, ligation of the inferior vena cava may be necessary. Massive thromboembolism to the lungs is often fatal and may occur suddenly, without preexisting symptomatic evidence of thrombus formation in the lower extremities.

Venograms of the legs may be helpful in detecting thrombosis in the deep femoral veins which may not be clearly diagnosed on clinical examination. Acute thrombophlebitis in the superficial veins of the legs occurs more frequently, especially when there are preexisting varicosities. It is usually manifested by localized red and tender areas and usually responds to elastic stockings, local heat, and anti-inflammatory drugs. Although superficial thrombophlebitis has a much less grave prognosis than thrombophlebitis involving deeper veins, these patients should discontinue oral contraceptives and use other forms of birth control.

Other side effects of the pill are signs and symptoms of problems seen in pregnancy, which is understandable, since the two physiologic states are quite similar. These problems include cloasma (the "mask of pregnancy," a brown discoloration of the cheeks and forehead, more prominent after ultraviolet ray exposure); nausea, especially for the first several days of the cycle; transient hypertension (rare); abnormal glucose tolerance (rare); increased ocular pressure, causing discomfort with contact lenses; an increase in occurrence of vascular headaches; and frequently, oligomenorrhea or amenorrhea.

Amenorrhea is fairly common secondary to the use of oral contraceptives; it may be intermittent or persistent but almost invariably disappears after discontinuation of the medication. Frequently, there is a latent period before normal menstruation recurs, after the pills are discontinued, but this seldom lasts more than 6 weeks. On rare occasions, amenorrhea may persist but will usually respond to clomiphene therapy.

Vaginal monilial (candidal) infections are also very common in women on the pill. Despite these side effects, however, the oral contraceptives are by far the most common type of contraceptive used today because of their great efficiency (99% plus effectiveness) and their lack of side effects, compared with other modes of birth control.

Unprotected intercourse during the fertile phase of the menstrual cycle can cause serious concern to the patient at risk. This may be due to a broken condom, rape, or carelessness. Originally, stilbestrol was used to prevent implantation of the potentially fertilized egg. The dose prescribed was 25 mg bid for 5 days. However, because of the slight risk to the embryo of a later stilbestrol-induced genital tumor if the treatment is unsuccessful, other hormone preparations are now being used. Premarin (conjugated equine estrogen) 30 mg/day, in divided doses, for 5 days is effective. Ovral tabs, two every 12 hours for two doses have also been used.

These medications apparently cause the endometrium to become unsuitable for implantation.

The insertion of an IUD for a menstrual cycle also has an excellent success rate. These measures must be initiated within 72 hours of exposure.

TOXIC SHOCK SYNDROME

In the past 2 years there has been a dramatic increase in a previously rare and often unrecognized disease entity now known as toxic shock syndrome. It is a serious disease of acute onset, characterized by sudden high fever with vomiting, diarrhea, and myalgia followed by the development of hypotension and, in some cases, shock. The mortality rate is 8.4%. An erythematous rash is present during the acute phase. After ten days there is desquamation of the skin, especially of the palms and soles.

Cause. The causative organism is always penicillin-resistant *Staphylococcus aureus,* and the disease is related to the absorption of toxins produced by this organism rather than by its direct invasion of the body.

Although toxic shock can occur in men and children with staphylococcal infections, it is much more common in women (95%). What is most significant is that toxic shock is almost always related to menstruation and that an overwhelming majority of these patients used tampons rather than sanitary napkins during their periods.

Apparently the disease can be associated with all makes of tampons. However, in one study, 70% of those affected used superabsorbent tampons (Rely), as opposed to 26% of a control group. Because this tampon is very absorbent and efficient, it is possible that it would tend to be left in place for longer periods of time and thus encourage the growth of staphylococci.

It is advised that the disease can be almost completely eliminated if tampons are avoided. However, women who choose to use tampons should use them intermittently throughout the menstrual cycle (*i.e.,* tampons during the day, napkins at night).

Treatment/Management. Treatment for women suspected of having toxic shock syndrome includes removal of all vaginal tampons, culture of vaginal and cervical secretions for *Staphylococcus aureus,* and aggressive fluid replacement. Beta-lactamose resistant antistaphylococcal antibiotic therapy should be instituted after appropriate cultures are obtained.

BIBLIOGRAPHY

Bhattacharyya MN, Jones BM: *Hemophilus vaginalis* infection: Diagnosis and treatment. J Reprod Med 24:71–75, February 1980

Centers for Disease Control: Epidemiologic Notes and Reports: Toxic shock syndrome: United States, 1970–1980. Morbid Mortal Week Rep 30:25–33, January 1981

Emans SJ, Goldstein DP: Gynecologic examination of prepubertal child with vulvovaginitis: Use of knee chest position. Pediatrics 65:758–760, April 1980

Flesh G, Weiner JM, Corlett Jr RC et al: Intrauterine contraceptive device and acute salpingitis: Multifactor analysis. Am J Obstet Gynecol 135:402–408, October 1979

Furuhjilm M, Karlgren E, Carlström K: Intravaginal administration of conjugated estrogens in premenopausal and postmenopausal women. Int J Gynecol Obstet 17:335–339, January–February 1980

Hibbard LT: Corpus luteum surgery. Am J Obstet Gynecol 135:666–670, November 1979

Kitchin JD III, Wein RW, Nunley WC Jr et al: Ectopic pregnancy: Current clinical trends. Am J Obstet Gynecol 134:870–876, August 15, 1979

McArdle C: Ultrasonic localization of missing intrauterine contraceptive devices. Obstet Gynecol 51:330–333, March, 1978

Notelovitz M: Estrogens and postcoital contraception. Fem Pat 6(7):36–38, July 1981

Photopulos GJ, McCartney WH, Walton LA, Staab EV: Computerized tomography applied to gynecologic oncology. Am J Obstet Gynecol 135:381–383, October 1, 1979

Piver MS, Barlow JJ, Lurain JR, Blumenson LE: Medroxyprogesterone acetate versus hydroxyprogesterone caproate in women with metastatic endometrial adenocarcinoma. Cancer 45:268–272, January 15, 1980

Queenan JT: Diagnostic ultrasound in obstetrics and gynecology. Am Coll Obstet Gynecol Tech Bull 63 October 1981

Reeves RD, Drake TS, O'Brien WF: Ultrasonic Versus Clinical Evaluation of a Pelvic Mass. Obstet Gynecol 55:551–554, May 1980

Rydén G, Fåhraeus L, Molin L, Åhman K: Do contraceptives influence the incidence of acute pelvic inflammatory disease in women with gonorrhea? Contraception 20:149–157, August 1979

Shands KN, Schmidt GP, Dan BB et al: Toxic shock syndrome in menstruating women: Its association with tampon use and *Staphylococcus aureus* and the clinical features in 52 cases. N Engl J Med 303:1436–42, 1980

Smith JP, Day TG Jr: Review of ovarian cancer at the University of Texas Systems Cancer Center, M. D. Anderson Hospital and Tumor Institute. Am J Obstet Gynecol 135:984–993, December 1, 1979

Walton LA, Kernodles W Jr, Hulka B: Factors influencing the occurrence of advanced cervical carcinoma. South Med J 72:808–811, July 1979

26

OBSTETRIC EMERGENCIES

AMBROSE A. MACIE

With few exceptions, pregnancy and childbirth are physiologic processes. Although most pregnancies progress to term uneventfully, various problems may arise during the course of a gestation. The most common symptom is vaginal bleeding. Statistically, there are relatively few obstetric emergencies. When an emergency does occur, it is often serious and may affect the continued progress of the gestation, the well-being of the fetus, and the life of the mother. The major emergencies during pregnancy are hemorrhage, infection, and fetal and maternal death. Because there are two human lives involved when a complication or emergency develops during the course of a pregnancy, prompt assessment and treatment are needed.

PHYSIOLOGY OF PREGNANCY

The average period of gestation, from conception to delivery, is 274 days. Factors that may influence the outcome of a pregnancy include the mother's age, environment, nutrition, and social status. Statistically, less affluent and minority groups show a higher incidence of fetal loss and emergencies during pregnancy. These problems can be traced directly to poor prenatal care, due either to the patient's indifference or to the unavailability of prenatal counseling.

During the entire period of gestation, the mother exhibits a variety of physiologic and emotional changes. Emotional peaks and valley are common and are best countered by an understanding male partner and a supportive, sympathetic obstetrician.

A number of organ systems are altered to a certain extent during pregnancy, and treatment is sometimes required.

Urinary Collecting System.   The kidneys have an extra workload during gestation. A daily urine output of 1500 ml is ideal. Alteration in the configuration of the bladder due to the enlarging uterus and displacement of the bladder and ureters occur as the pregnancy progresses. Urinary frequency, urgency, and dysuria are common and require careful evaluation. A history of prior renal disease is particularly important and should serve as a warning flag if urinary tract symptoms are noted.

Abdominal Wall.   As pregnancy progresses, the muscles of the abdominal wall stretch and thin out, particularly in the region of the umbilicus. This causes the common complaint of umbilical stretching and discomfort. Umbilical hernia may develop.

Breasts.   The breasts increase in size and become turgid. The nipples become erectile and, along with the areola, become darkly pigmented. Cutaneous breast veins are more prominent. Striae (stretch marks) are often noted in the skin. A clear, sticky fluid (colostrum) may be excreted from the nipple. No treatment is indicated.

Weight Changes.   Ideally, the weight gain during the gestational period should be approximately 25 lb, with 11 lb expected in the last trimester. Excessive weight gain in the last few weeks of pregnancy may be an indication of incipient toxemia. Close observation is warranted.

Musculoskeletal System.   As pregnancy progresses, the patient's center of gravity changes, causing the vertebral column to straighten. The shoulders are thrown backward and the head and neck straighten. As a result, backache may be present and is usually more pronounced in multiparous women.

Leg cramps are common, though usually minor. Periods of rest and postural adjustments may alleviate some of the symptoms of backache. Leg cramps may be relieved by calcium supplements and a decrease in whole milk intake.

Skin.   Pigmentation increases in the areola and nipples (as noted above), vulva, umbilicus, abdominal wall, and face. In most patients, the pigmentation disappears following termination of pregnancy.

Vascular System.   Venous problems such as varicose veins, peripheral (dependent) edema, and hemorrhoids are common during pregnancy. It is thought that the *varicosities* are a result of pressure on the intra-abdominal veins by the enlarging uterus. Varicosities may be unilateral or bilateral. Many patients develop none at all, suggesting the possibility of other influences, such as hormonal or hereditary factors. Phlebitis or phlebothrombosis can develop and require specific treatment.

Peripheral edema is common, especially during the later stages of pregnancy and may be related to venous congestion or salt and water retention due to hormonal factors, especially progesterone, which is present during gestation. This may be controlled by one of several methods: elevation, external support stockings, diuretics, and salt restriction.

Symptomatic *hemorrhoids* are relieved by rectal analgesics and proper regulation of bowel habits.

Nosebleeds may be troublesome. Although most are benign, one must be certain that hypertension is not an underlying cause. The patient should be advised about the location of nasal pressure points to control epistaxis. For severe or persistent nosebleeds, nasal packing may be required. Monitor for anemia.

Vaginal Infection.   Vaginitis may occur during pregnancy, and if present, cultures and sensitivity studies should identify the specific organisms and the appropriate antibiotic for treatment.

Miscellaneous.   Headaches, insomnia, fainting spells, and dizziness occur frequently at various stages of gestation. Treatment is usually symptomatic and can maintain the patient comfortably. It consists of mild analgesics, hypnotics, and postural changes.

Recent trends in drug use represent a departure from the routine use of *any* medication during pregnancy. A thorough discussion with the patient about the pros and cons of drug therapy is essential. Generally, required drugs used in moderation and under close supervision are often essential for the physical and emotional comfort of the patient. In severe symptomatic states, hospitalization is often necessary for appropriate treatment.

COMPLICATIONS OF PREGNANCY

Problems that emerge during the course of a pregnancy may be either unrelated or directly related to the pregnancy.

CONDITIONS UNRELATED TO THE PREGNANCY

A woman may develop almost any acute medical or surgical condition during the course of a pregnancy. This includes varying types of trauma, acute intra-abdominal processes such as acute appendicitis, cholecystitis, and ovarian cyst, to name but a few. Generally, the management of the patient, especially when the condition is secondary to trauma or acute surgical processes, is governed by the usual principles outlined in other chapters, depending on the presence and development of the fetus.

The patient must be advised what effect(s), if any, the disease process and the recommended treatment may have on the fetus and the mother, and conversely the effect(s), if any, of not following the recommended treatment. This better-informed patient is better able to make the proper decision about care. Dring the first trimester of pregnancy, both the concurrent disease and treatment, be it medical or surgical, may adversely affect the pregnancy. In the later trimesters, fetal loss is less likely to occur.

Hormonal agents, particularly those related to progesterone, were used widely at one time to minimize the possibility of induced labor, during or after treatment. However, largely because of current controversy and litigation, the trend is to use no adjunctive hormone therapy. If hormone therapy is deemed absolutely necessary, the matter should be discussed in full detail with the patient (and family) and the discussion properly recorded in the hospital record. It is best done in the presence of a nurse or other member of the emergency department staff. In some instances, it may be appropriate to have the patient sign a specific consent if such therapy is indicated and agreed upon by the patient. If there is no anticipated hazard to the mother or the fetus, surgery that is not urgent in certain instances may be delayed until a later stage of pregnancy or until the postpartum period.

The choice of analgesics, narcotics, and other medications may be modified for the pregnant patient, but keep in mind that certain drugs can cross the placental barrier and affect the fetus. If more than one medical discipline is involved in the treatment of the patient, close consultation between the specialty physicians is essential.

X-ray studies of the pregnant patient are ordered cautiously. If they must be done, for example in a patient with extremity or abdominal trauma, every precaution must be taken to protect the fetus from radiation by judicious use of a lead apron or another such device. For the patient who has suffered acute abdominal trauma, priorities must be as-

sessed. If X-ray studies are essential to the pregnant woman because of a life-threatening injury, the risk to the fetus must be of secondary concern. Whenever possible, such decisions should be discussed with the patient and her husband or a close family member. Special studies involving the use of iodine-containing radiopaque dyes may be necessary. It must be kept in mind that these medications may affect the fetal thyroid.

CONDITIONS RELATED TO THE PREGNANCY

ASSESSMENT

Assessment of the patient with a condition related to the pregnancy includes the following:
- A complete history
- Menstrual history, including full details of the present illness, related disease, and estimation of the length of pregnancy
- Past medical history, including prior illnesses, surgical procedures (especially intra-abdominal procedures), pregnancies, and complications, if any
- The prenatal care that the patient is currently receiving
- A complete physical examination with special emphasis on blood pressure
- Stage of gestation
- Pelvic evaluation—pelvic evaluation may be deferred during the later stages of pregnancy if there is excessive vaginal bleeding.
- *Adjunct studies*
  Studies that should be performed routinely:
  Complete blood count (CBC)
  SMA-18
  Urinalysis
  Radiologic studies, especially routine x-ray studies, may be inadvisable, especially during the early stages of pregnancy.
  Sonography to identify fetal size and the locaton of the placenta, when indicated
  Complications related to pregnancy vary greatly, depending on the stage of gestation. Thus it is most useful to consider the complications associated with each of the trimesters of pregnancy.

FIRST TRIMESTER COMPLICATIONS

Nausea and Vomiting

Nausea and vomiting are common during the first 3 months of pregnancy and occasionally persist into the later trimesters. If they become severe or persistent, particularly to the point of dehydration, the patient may seek emergency care. *Hyperemesis gravidarum* is a severe form of this condition.

Management/Treatment. A general appraisal of the patient is indicated following the method previously outlined.

Intra-abdominal disease (*i.e.*, appendicitis, cholecystitis, etc.) must be ruled out. CBC, urinalysis, and serum electrolyte studies are performed as a minimum. Arterial blood gases are drawn in severely ill patients.

Treatment is directed toward fluid replacement by intravenous infusion and correction of any identified electrolyte disturbance. In severe forms, hypokalemic, hypochloremic alkalosis is present and requires the addition of adequate amounts of potassium and chloride to the replacement fluid. Withholding of oral intake and mild sedation until the symptoms are relieved is helpful. In milder cases, antiemetics given orally or by rectal suppository can be used; in the more severe form, parenteral injection is needed.

Spontaneous Abortion

The most common symptom causing a pregnant patient to seek attention in the emergency department is vaginal bleeding. When it occurs early in pregnancy, the continuation of the pregnancy is in jeopardy. Two forms of abortion usually encountered are threatened abortion and incomplete or inevitable abortion.

Threatened Abortion

The symptoms vary from a brown or bloody spotting, to bleeding as heavy as a normal menstrual period, to frank hemorrhage. The patient gives a history of one or more missed periods. Physical examination reveals an enlarged, soft uterus. A speculum examination of the vagina is always indicated to ensure that the bleeding is not from a local lesion of the cervix or vaginal wall. The cervix should be carefully inspected to ascertain whether it is open or closed. If the cervix is closed and no tissue products of conception have been passed, the pregnancy is presumed intact and the patient is treated conservatively.

The above findings may also be present with a missed abortion or a blighted ovum, in which case the pregnancy has ceased and the products of conception will eventually be passed.

Management/Treatment. Primary treatment consists of bed rest. A CBC is done to rule out significant anemia. Vitamin C or vitamin K preparations may be used to assist in the clotting mechanism only when indicated. The use of progestational hormones to bolster inadequate corpus luteum hormone production is controversial at present. Admission is required in severe cases, when blood loss is severe.

Incomplete Abortion

Severe abdominal cramps accompanying vaginal bleeding in the first trimester are more serious. The passage of decidual or placental tissue is diagnostic of an abortion (miscarriage). Placental tissue has a lighter color and contains amorphous fragments resembling hamburger. Blood clots more closely resemble the consistency of liver. On speculum examination, the cervix is dilated and tissue may be seen in the cervical os.

Management/Treatment. CBC is done to identify anemia from excessive hemorrhage. Typed and crossmatched blood should be available for replacement if a transfusion is deemed necessary. The patient is most often admitted for a dilatation and curettage (D & C) to remove the products of conception completely. Further treatment consists of ergot preparations or oxytocin drip.

If seen in the hospital, the patient should be admitted for a D & C. In an early abortion, the patient rarely passes the products of conception completely. Unless all such products are removed, excessive bleeding and menstrual irregularity will be the inevitable result.

Hydatid Mole

Hydatid mole is an uncommon condition of unknown cause that may be associated with alarming hemorrhage. It is a degenerative process of the placenta, causing it to overgrow and eventually destroying the embryo. In addition to vaginal bleeding, a definitive diagnosis is suggested by the passage of tissue resembling clusters of grapes. Spontaneous abortion may occur. On occasion, hypertension and toxemia may be present in the early stages of the pregnancy.

On examination, the uterus is larger than expected and in rare instances may be term-size with huge masses of abnormal tissue present. Speculum inspection of the vagina and cervix reveals the presence of the grape-like clusters. Sonography may demonstrate the absence of a fetus.

Management/Treatment. The patient is admitted for D & C to evacuate the uterus completely. Blood replacement may be required to restore volume lost by hemorrhage. Serum and urinary gonadotropin levels are obtained subsequently, since a mole has the capability of becoming malignant and developing choriocarcinoma. Bimonthly evaluation is adequate.

Ectopic Pregnancy

Ectopic pregnancy is often encountered by emergency personnel, since it occurs once in every 100 to 120 pregnancies. It results when the fertilized ovum becomes implanted outside of the uterine cavity, usually in the fallopian tube and less frequently on the ovary or within the abdomen. Since the fallopian tube is thin walled and cannot stretch sufficiently with the enlarging pregnancy, it ruptures, causing subsequent intraperitoneal hemorrhage.

Assessment. Patients are often young and usually give a history of missing a period or being 2 to 4 weeks late. At the time of tubal rupture and hemorrhage, the patient notes severe lower abdominal pain. There are usually no associated gastrointestinal symptoms. The pain is sudden, sharp, constant, and often accompanied by weakness, dizziness, or syncope due to blood loss. It is felt in the lower abdomen and may be unilateral or bilateral. Less commonly, referred pain may be noted in the shoulder because of diaphragmatic irritation resulting from intraperitoneal blood (Kehr's sign). Vaginal bleeding is not always present, though spotting can and does occur. The temperature is usually normal or below 37.8°C (100°F). The signs and symptoms of ectopic pregnancy are listed in Chart 26-1.

Management/Treatment. *Ectopic pregnancy constitutes a surgical emergency.* The patient appears acutely ill and may be in shock. A CBC, type and crossmatch, urinalysis, and SMA-18 should be taken immediately. Blood volume replacement is initiated immediately with Ringer's lactate and continued with type-specific blood. A serum pregnancy test may be drawn.

Adjunct studies include cul-de-sac aspiration, which is easily performed in the emergency department (Fig. 26-1). Peritoneal tap or lavage may demonstrate the presence of blood in the peritoneal cavity. Colpotomy, culdoscopy, or laparoscopy may be used at times to confirm the diagnosis.

The finding of free blood in the peritoneal cavity is a firm indication for surgical exploration. A negative cul-de-sac aspiration or peritoneal lavage is not of itself a deterrent to laparotomy but must be considered in conjunction with the other clinical findings. Definitive treatment is removal of the products of conception and the ruptured tube (salpingectomy). If the damaged tube can be repaired surgically (salpingoplasty), this approach is preferable.

SECOND TRIMESTER COMPLICATIONS

The middle trimester of pregnancy is invariably the most comfortable for the patient. The physiologic changes taking place are tolerated well. Morning sickness is rare.

Vaginal Bleeding

At this stage of the pregnancy, the placenta is more mature and more secure in its attachment to the endometrium. However, vaginal bleeding may follow any separation of the placenta and indicates a threatening situation. Threatened abortion or premature labor must be considered. The diagnosis may be aided by careful physical assessment, including speculum examination of the cervix. A closed cervix

---

Chart 26-1

SIGNS AND SYMPTOMS OF ECTOPIC PREGNANCY

- History of missed or late menstrual period
- Sudden onset of lower abdominal pain, which may be referred to the shoulder
- Sharp, continuous pain
- Weakness, dizziness, syncope
- Vaginal spotting or bleeding
- Positive cul-de-sac aspiration or peritoneal lavage

---

may herald early labor. The fetal heart tones should be evaluated.

Management/Treatment. Conservative management, bed rest, and continued observation are indicated, especially if the patient is stable. If the cervix is dilated, placement of a suture to prevent further widening may be indicated.

THIRD TRIMESTER COMPLICATIONS

Vaginal bleeding is the most common indication of a complication of pregnancy in the last trimester. It results from separation of the placenta and is usually proportionate to the extent of separation. It may result in premature labor.

Another serious complication at this stage of gestation is toxemia.

Premature Separation of the Placenta

Early separation of the placenta from its attachment to the uterus may vary in degree from minimal to complete; milder forms are mentioned above, under second trimester complications. Extensive or complete separation may be catastrophic; it may result in fetal death and seriously jeopardize the mother's life. Any separation of the placenta is referred to as *abruptio placentae*. The most common symptom is vaginal bleeding, which varies from slight to heavy. Abdominal cramps may be present as a result of uterine contractions. More severe pain indicates a potentially life-threatening condition, especially when associated with an enlarged, tense uterus and absent fetal heart tones (FHTs). Abruptio placentae is invariably accompanied by uterine contractions (labor pains). In instances when the presence or absence of FHTs is uncertain, a fetal monitoring device may be used to identify FHTs and assess fetal distress.

Assessment. Physical assessment is dictated partially by the patient's history. If uterine contractions (early labor) are present, pelvic examination is indicated to determine the dilatation status of the cervix. Vaginal bleedng in the absence of contractions would be an absolute contraindication to the routine pelvic examination. Instead, a pelvic examination should be done under sterile conditions where a cesarean section can be performed. Excessive painless vaginal bleeding in the third trimester is invariably associated with *placenta praevia* (covering of the cervical os by the placenta). A pelvic examination may precipitate even more excessive bleeding; cesarean section delivery is the only solution.

A CBC, SMA-18, blood type and crossmatch, and urinalysis are the minimal laboratory tests to be ordered. Blood clotting studies including prothrombin time, platelet count, and fibrinogen level should be performed as baseline studies in case bleeding persists.

Treatment/Management. The treatment varies with the severity of the placental separation and the degree of hemorrhage. The patient is observed closely for onset of labor.

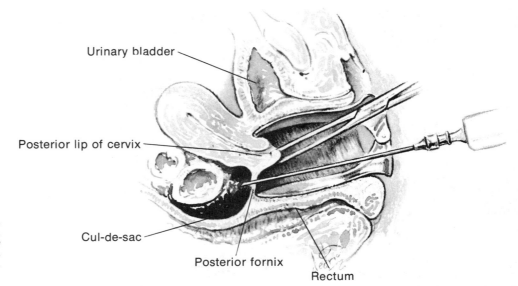

Urinary bladder

Posterior lip of cervix

Cul-de-sac

Posterior fornix

Rectum

Figure 26-1 Cul-de-sac aspiration. The posterior fornix is infiltrated with local anesthetic agent. A 4-inch needle attached to a syringe is inserted into the cul-de-sac parallel with the spine. If nonclotting blood is recovered, the tap is positive.

- When abruptio placentae is suspected, large veinways are placed and volume replacement initiated with Ringer's lactate followed by type-specific blood when available. Emergency cesarean section is required if the cervix is closed and delivery is not imminent or if evidence of fetal distress is apparent (meconium passed vaginally, positive fetal monitor).

- If bleeding continues, certain clotting factors may be depleted, leading to serious problems. Fibrinogen depletion may occur (afibrinogenemia). Thromboplastin substances may be released into the maternal circulation from open placental sinuses, causing a complex reaction to evolve. The mother's blood may fail to clot, causing bleeding to proceed uncontrollably. Disseminated intravascular coagulation (DIC) may follow with its attendant high morbidity and mortality (see Chap. 17).

- Afibrinogenemia should be suspected with bleeding late in pregnancy. Observe the patient's blood for clot development and retraction. Failure to clot is an ominous sign. Afibrinogenemia is managed with heparin to neutralize circulating thromboplastin. Infusion of fibrinogen and fresh frozen plasma with blood replacement should be given. Early termination of the pregnancy should be undertaken.

Placenta Previa

Placenta previa occurs when the placenta encroaches on the internal cervical os. It may be partial or complete.

Assessment. Painless bleeding during the last trimester of pregnancy is pathognomonic. Blood loss may be severe enough to require transfusion and cesarean section. Physical examination is limited. Pelvic examination is contraindicated in any patient with painless bleeding in the third trimester, to decrease the possibility of increasing bleeding until adequate amounts of blood are ready and the operating room is on standby for immediate cesarean section.

Adjunct studies in addition to the routine laboratory work include localization of the placenta by specialized radiologic methods, notably sonography and isotopic modalities.

Treatment/Management. Because the location of the placenta causes an obstruction at the internal os, cesarean section is usually required.

Toxemia of Pregnancy

Toxemia of pregnancy typically occurs in the last trimester of pregnancy. It is unique to humans and its etiology is unknown. Most commonly it occurs in primigravidas, multiple births, and polyhydramnios and is seen in association with preexisting hypertension, diabetes, or renal disease. Two forms of toxemia exist:
1. *Eclampsia*—marked by hypertension (blood pressure $\geq 140/90$), fluid retention with excessive weight gain, and proteinuria
2. *Preeclampsia*—marked by the presence of two of the three findings noted above.

Either form may threaten a pregnancy because preeclampsia may progress to eclampsia, resulting in seizures and a high degree of fetal loss.

Preeclampsia. Preeclampsia is the milder form of toxemia. The patient must be made aware of the complication. Hospital admission is often indicated. Management consists of bed rest, diuretics, restricted salt intake, sedation, and occasionally antihypertensive medical treatment. Medical induction of vaginal delivery or cesarean-section may be required. Fetal monitoring is helpful in assessing the status of the fetus.

Eclampsia. Eclampsia is a much more serious complication, threatening the life of the mother and the fetus. Ominous signs indicating a more serious prognosis include epigastric pain, headache, and convulsions. Convulsions, particularly, are associated with premature separation of the placenta, high fetal loss, and grave maternal risk. Cerebral hemorrhage, renal shutdown, or liver hemorrhage may jeopardize the mother.

Treatment/Management. With the onset of convulsions, diazepam (Valium) is given intravenously along with magnesium sulfate to reduce cerebral edema. Antihypertensive drugs and sedation are useful. Early termination of pregnancy by induction or cesarean section is necessary.

The treatment should be continued after delivery. Since half of all women with eclampsia experience convulsions after delivery, accurate monitoring of intake and output is essential. Peripheral reflexes with the finding of clonus or a hyperactive knee jerk may indicate increasing central nervous system (CNS) irritability.

THE PATIENT AT TERM IN LABOR

Emergency management of childbirth outside the hospital and delivery in the emergency department are discussed in the sections that follow.

CHILDBIRTH OUTSIDE OF THE HOSPITAL

Emergency childbirth outside the confines of the hospital occurs with some frequency. The principle of care is to deliver the mother with a minimum of trauma and without injury to the newborn. The most important decision to be made by out-of-hospital personnel is whether there is sufficient time to transport the mother to the hospital before delivery occurs. One may be guided by the signs and symptoms of imminent delivery.

Signs and Symptoms of Imminent Delivery

- Regular contractions lasting 45 to 60 seconds at 1- to 2-minute intervals
- A feeling by the mother of having to bear down or of having a bowel movement
- A large amount of bloody show
- Crowning
- The mother's saying that the baby is coming
  If, on the other hand, contractions are infrequent, short, and irregular, there is time for transport.

Technique: Delivery and Care of the Newborn

1. *Sterile field.* Once the decision is reached to deliver, make every effort to provide a sterile field. Emergency vehicles should be equipped with a sterile delivery pack (Chart 26-2). Personnel should wear sterile gloves. After positioning the mother for delivery, prep the perineum with povidone-iodine.
2. *Position for delivery.* Place the mother on her back with her knees flexed and widely separated. If the mother is

---

Chart 26-2

EQUIPMENT FOR STERILE DELIVERY PACK

- 3 hemostats or cord clamps
- Scissors
- Umbilical tape
- Rubber bulb-type ear syringe
- Betadine
- 12 4-X-4 gauze sponges
- 4 pairs of sterile rubber gloves
- 6 towels
- Baby blanket
- Sanitary napkins
- Container for placenta

---

in an automobile, have her lie on her back across the seat with one leg flexed on the seat and the other resting on the floorboard. If available, place a pillow beneath her buttocks to facilitate the delivery of the head.

3. *Coaching the mother*
   - Advise the mother to push or bear down during contractions.
   - Encourage the mother to rest between contractions in order to conserve strength. Method: Breathe deeply through the mouth to lessen bearing down and promote rest.

4. *Delivery of the head.* The baby's head should never be held back but should be prevented from "popping out" and possibly tearing the perineum. The delivery of the head may be eased by reaching behind the anal orifice with a sterile towel and lifting and guiding the head through the perineum (Ritgen maneuver). The chin is sometimes caught by the posterior wall of the vagina and may be freed by slipping the index finger under the jaw and sweeping it forward beneath the chin. Once the head is delivered, wipe the mouth and nostrils free of mucus and aspirate with a bulb syringe to clear the remaining mucus.

5. *Check umbilical cord.* Observe closely to determine whether the umbilical cord is wrapped around the neck. If so, release it by lifting it over the infant's head. If this is impossible, the cord may be too tight and could strangle the newborn. In this instance, clamp the cord with two or three hemostats and cut between them to release the pressure.

6. *Completion of delivery.* Once the head is delivered, the baby will rotate so that the shoulders present. Guide the head downward to deliver the anterior shoulder and turn upward to release the posterior shoulder. Once the shoulders have delivered, the remainder of the body should be expelled smoothly by a uterine contraction. Care must be taken in handling the newborn infant, which is very slippery. The umbilical cord should be cut between

hemostats and the baby placed on a flat surface next to the mother.

The baby should be breathing spontaneously at this point and should be placed in a blanket to maintain warmth.

7. *Care of the newborn.* Immediately after delivery the newborn is evaluated according to the Apgar criteria as listed in Table 26-1. Each criterion is rated on a basis of 0 to 2 and the numbers are then added. The higher the total number, the better the prognosis for the infant. Wrap the newborn in blankets to conserve body heat, and transport to the hospital.

8. *Delivery of the placenta.* The placenta (afterbirth) should deliver 10 to 15 minutes after the baby and is usually preceded by a gush of blood from the vagina. Place the placenta in a container and carry it to the hospital for inspection by emergency or delivery personnel. Transport may be initiated once the baby has been delivered and does not necessarily have to be delayed until delivery of the placenta.

Complications

Complications that may occur in the course of delivery include prolapsed cord, unbroken amniotic sac, breech presentation, and multiple births. Chart 26-3 outlines the steps to be taken when these complications occur outside the hospital.

DELIVERY IN THE EMERGENCY DEPARTMENT

A patient may present to the emergency department in active labor. If an obstetric delivery suite is available in the hospital, the patient should be transferred there without delay. If one is not available, or if the labor has progressed too far, the delivery must be completed on the spot. Care should be taken to maintain sterile precautions at all times.

Principles and Procedure

When considering delivery, the following factors are of concern:

Table 26-1. APGAR SCORING METHOD

Criteria	Score		
	0	1	2
Color	Blue; pale	Body pink; extremities blue	Pink all over
Heart rate	Absent	<100	>100
Respirations	Absent	Slow, irregular	Good, crying
Reflex irritability	None	Grimace	Cough, sneeze
Muscle tone	Limp	Some reflex of extremities	Active

The Apgar Score is interpreted as follows:
0–3	severely depressed
4–6	moderately depressed
7–9	slightly depressed or normal
10	normal

- Delivery of the infant without any heroic manipulations
- Elimination of any extensive trauma to the mother
- Establishment of a patent airway for the infant
- Close observation for excessive vaginal bleeding after delivery

Generally, the duration of labor is longer in primiparous women (average 12 to 18 hours) than in multiparous women (average 8 to 12 hours). If labor is advanced, emergency personnel need only provide assistance in the delivery. This is easily done by reaching behind the rectum with a sterile towel (Ritgen maneuver) and helping to lift the baby through the perineum (Fig. 26-2). Injection of a local anesthetic into the midline of the perineum and incision to create an episiotomy facilitate a normal delivery. Care must be taken not to incise the rectal sphincter muscles or the rectum.

Once the head is delivered, check to determine whether the umbilical cord is free or is encircling the infant's neck. If the cord is loose, it can be slipped over the baby's head or shoulder. If the cord is tight about the neck, traction could cause it to tear, with significant blood loss, as delivery progresses. If the cord is tight, place two hemostats on the cord, cut between them, and unwind the loop or loops of cord from the infant's neck. The delivery should then proceed without difficulty.

Care of the Baby. Once delivery is accomplished, direct attention to the infant. Establish a free airway by suctioning the mouth, airway, and nasal passages. The presence of meconium-stained fluid (which is greenish or yellowish and thick in consistency) indicates the need to insert a nasogastric tube as well. Wrap the baby in blankets immediately or, preferably, place him in a heated Isolette to preserve body heat. Ideally, a pediatrician is called when the patient arrives in the emergency department so that he can assume immediate care of the infant.

Immediately upon delivery, and at 5-minute intervals thereafter, the newborn is evaluated using the Apgar scoring method (Table 26-1). The Apgar criteria include heart rate, respirations, muscle tone, reflex irritability, and color. Each criterion is evaluated on a basis of 0 to 2, and the numbers are then added. The higher the total number, the better the prognosis for the infant.

Generally, a slow heart rate (below 80 bpm), poor or labored respirations with "tugging," flaccid or loose muscle tone, poor reflexes and body tone, weak cry, and a color other than pink lead to a low Apgar evaluation and indicate that the newborn's condition is tenuous.

Delivery of the Placenta. Once the delivery is complete and the newborn provided care, attention is directed back to the mother. Delivery of the placenta can be accomplished by gentle traction on the cord combined with gentle massaging action on the fundus of the uterus. Care is taken not to use excessive traction on the cord, in order to prevent tearing. An oxytocic medication (methylergonovine, 0.2 mg IM and/or oxytocin, 10 units IM or IV) is given to stimulate the musculature of the uterus to contract.

A blood loss of 200 ml is expected during this stage. Abnormal bleeding occurs when the loss exceeds 600 ml or 1% of body weight. Following placental extrusion, check the birth canal for any lacerations.

Chart 26-3

PREHOSPITAL MANAGEMENT OF COMPLICATIONS DURING DELIVERY

Prolapsed Cord

1. Observe the perineum to determine presenting part—in this case, a prolapsed cord.
2. Place mother in a knee-chest position if possible.
3. Instruct mother to pant during contractions, breathing normally when each contraction eases.
4. Wrap cord with moist, sterile dressing.
5. Administer oxygen by mask to mother, 10 L/min.

Unbroken Amniotic Sac

1. Observe perineum to determine presenting part—in this case, an unbroken amniotic sac.
2. Puncture amniotic sac with blunt instrument.
3. Strip membrane away from fetal nose and mouth.
4. Continue with steps taken in normal delivery.

Breech Presentation

1. Observe perineum to determine presenting part.
2. Deliver buttocks and legs to the level of fetal umbilicus.
3. Drape fetal legs over your arm.
4. Elevate feet and legs of baby to obtain easier access to airway.
5. Push down on vaginal tissues to gain better access to baby's nose and mouth.
6. Deliver head.
7. Continue with clamping of cord, suction as with normal delivery.

Multiple Birth

1. All criteria apply as for single birth, vertex delivery, and possible breech presentation.
2. Clamp cord of each baby as delivered.
3. Identify time of each birth, label first born.

Complications During Delivery

Complicated Positions of the Fetus. Usually, the normal presentation of the fetus is vertex; that is, the head presents first. Pelvic examination reveals a hard, convex mass in this instance. In the presenting part is soft, with prominences and depressions, one must suspect a breech. If the vagina is empty, a transverse lie is likely. Less frequently, presentation of one arm or one leg can be regarded as either a breech or transverse lie. Significant morbidity and mortality occur with such abnormal presentations. The mother should not be encouraged with labor, and an experienced obstetrician should be consulted without delay.

Prolapse of the Umbilical Cord. Another serious complication is prolapse of the umbilical cord. A pulsating prolapsed cord requires immediate management. Until an obstetrician is available, the patient should be placed in the Trendelenberg position and advised *not* to bear down with contractions. High-flow oxygen is given by mask. With sterile gloves, the examining fingers are placed in the vagina and *the presenting part raised* off the cord to relieve compression until further help arrives.

POSTPARTUM COMPLICATIONS

Bleeding

Alarming hemorrhage may occur after delivery and discharge from the hospital. Normally, all postpartum patients experience a bloody lochia that may persist for 3 weeks, gradually lessening each day. If a patient has a vaginal flow for more than 3 weeks and soaks more than 4 perineal napkins a day, an abnormality should be suspected. This continued bleeding is usually due to uterine relaxation or subinvolution of the uterus. It is most often encountered in women who have

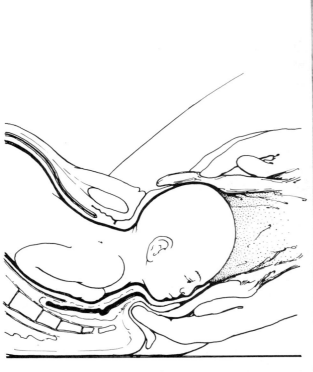

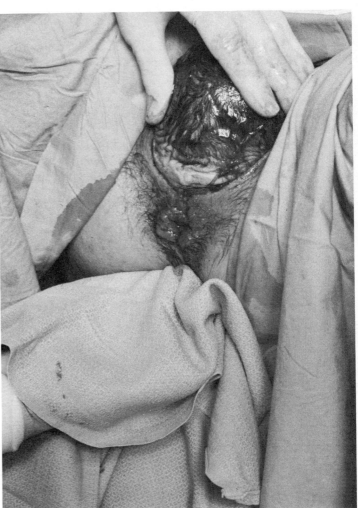

Figure 26-2 *Ritgen maneuver. Pressure is exerted posterior to the rectum to palpate the fetus's chin. A rocking motion of the fingers will thus extend the neck to assist in delivering the head over the perineum. Pressure is exerted with the opposite hand on the fetus's brow to prevent a sudden surge of the head through the vaginal opening.*

had four or more deliveries. Oxytocics given intramuscularly or intravenously will alleviate the problem within 24 hours.

Another common cause of postpartum bleeding is retained secundae (fragments of placenta retained within the uterus). The uterus is usually soft and boggy and does not respond to the oxytocic medication. Careful assessment is required to determine whether excessive blood loss and volume depletion has occurred. If so, a veinway is placed and volume replacement initiated with Ringer's lactate. An emergency D & C is needed to evacuate the uterus, and packing of the uterine cavity is sometimes required. Since this condition can be associated with secondary infection, specimens of the vaginal flow are taken for culture and sensitivity studies.

Infections

Infections may occur in the genitourinary tract during the postpartum period. A temperature higher than 37.8°C (100°F) strongly suggests such a process. Other common causes of postpartum sepsis are salpingitis, endometritis, tubo-ovarian abscess, or breast complications (mastitis).

Infections arising in the genitourinary tract are usually associated with fever and abdominal pain. Assessment reveals a foul-smelling lochia with abdominal and pelvic tenderness and rebound tenderness. A mass may be identified in the pelvis or found bulging into the vagina. The patient is admitted for a course of antibiotic therapy after suitable cervical, vaginal, blood, and urine cultures are taken. When abscess is present, surgical drainage is indicated.

Mastitis is usually manifested by swelling and discomfort of the breasts, with reddening or striae of the overlying skin. Cultures of any nipple drainage are indicated. The treatment of choice is antibiotics with application of local heat. If the patient is nursing, this should be curtailed.

OTHER OBSTETRIC EMERGENCIES

SEPTIC ABORTION

Septic abortion is less common today because of liberalized abortion laws. When an abortion attempt results in incomplete removal of the products of conception, the result is pelvic infection. The patient is most often acutely ill and septic, with high fever, abdominal pain, and foul-smelling lochia.

Assessment. Assessment reveals the patient to be acutely ill with abdominal and pelvic tenderness. Bimanual pelvic examination causes great discomfort, especially with motion of the cervix. Blood and vaginal cultures should be taken. Vital signs are monitored. A catheter is placed to monitor central venous pressure. Arterial blood gases, CBC, SMA-18, and urinalysis are performed for baseline studies.

Management/Treatment. Fluid replacement and massive doses of antibiotics given intravenously are necessary. Since most infections are due to coliform organisms, a broad-spectrum preparation should be chosen. Anaerobic organisms may also play a causative role. Consideration should be given to the use of metronidazole or a similar preparation to cover this eventuality. Vasoactive drugs may be needed to improve and maintain arterial pressure at adequate levels.

DIC may occur as a serious complication. Coagulation studies are indicated to identify any coagulopathy.

Once adequate blood levels of antibiotics are achieved, a D & C is performed.

GENITAL HERPES INFECTION

Herpesvirus infections of the genital tract are becoming more prevalent and constitute a danger in all pregnancies. The disease is caused primarily by herpesvirus type II, although type I organisms may also be found. The patient complains of painful, ulcerating lesions of the vulva and vagina that may spread to involve the thighs, buttocks, or abdomen. The virus resides in the lesions. Genital herpes infections during pregnancy may seriously endanger the newborn. Cesarean section is indicated if herpes is evident during the last 2 weeks of pregnancy. Approximately 80% of newborns

delivered through a herpes-infected vagina are afflicted with brain damage.

Assessment. The lesions are characteristically shallow ulcerations with a weeping, shaggy base. There is a surrounding zone of erythema. The lesions are painful to the touch. Vesicles (blisters) and pustules are often present. Pap smears or scrapings from the cervix or the lesion for virus culture and antibody testing are necessary for ultimate diagnosis.

Management/Treatment. Since the lesions are contagious, the patient should be isolated when herpes is suspected. A new antiviral preparation, acyclovir (Zovirax), has been found effective in the treatment of initial herpes type II lesions. The medication is applied directly to the lesions and appears beneficial in relieving discomfort and healing the lesions. It has been found relatively ineffective in treating recurrent herpes lesions. For the infant who is possibly infected, vidarabine (Vira-A) is used.

TRAUMA IN PREGNANCY

All forms of trauma may occur during the course of a pregnancy. Blunt trauma to the abdomen, such as might be encountered in a fall or motor vehicle accident, can jeopardize the pregnancy if there is direct injury to the uterus. The fetus is usually well enough protected in the uterus, but if the force is severe enough, uterine rupture or premature separation of the placenta may occur.

Penetrating wounds to the abdomen, whether gunshot or stab wounds, should be treated as in any other patient, but keep in mind that two human lives are involved. In either instance, prompt resuscitation and adequate oxygenation following established principles of care will result in salvage of both mother and fetus. If at all possible, the pregnancy should be preserved. If the uterus has been penetrated, hysterotomy is necessary.

BIBLIOGRAPHY

Benson RC: Current Obstetric and Gynecologic Diagnosis and Treatment, 3rd ed. Los Altos, Lange Medical Publications, 1980
Pritchard JA, MacDonald PC: William's Obstetrics, 16th ed. New York, Appleton-Century-Crofts, 1980

Sever JL: Reducing the risk of congenital herpes. Contemp Obstet Gynecol 17(6):191–195, June 1981
Taber B-Z: Manual of Gynecologic and Obstetric Emergencies, p. 847. Philadelphia, WB Saunders, 1970

27
PEDIATRIC EMERGENCIES

MARK SCHIFFMAN

Pediatricians like to say that children are not little adults, meaning that a knowledge of pediatric diseases and, more important, of how to approach children cannot be extrapolated from internal medicine or surgery. Emergency personnel, many of whom are trained primarily in one of the adult specialties, are aware of this fact and thus become anxious when faced with a sick infant or child. There is the added burden of realizing that, although we strive to help all of our patients, the loss of a child is the ultimate disaster in medicine. Nevertheless, we have one important fact on our side: the basic principles of life support are the same for adults and children of all ages, and although certain technical differences exist, in general, the sicker the child, the more one's knowledge and instincts in basic emergency medicine are likely to be relevant.

A special knowledge of pediatrics becomes important when children who are not severely ill arrive in the emergency department. It is here that a knowledge of the difference between benign, self-limited illness and potentially crippling or fatal maladies must be understood. It is the basic purpose of this chapter to identify conditions in pediatrics that must be recognized as potential catastrophes if appropriate intervention is not undertaken and to indicate what this intervention should be.

The exact technical aspects of advanced life support in neonates, infants, and children are explained in full, and certain general areas, such as triage and evaluation, are also explored in this chapter.

ADVANCED CARDIAC LIFE SUPPORT IN CHILDREN

The management of a child in cardiac or respiratory arrest is no different in principle from that of an adult; however, certain technical differences need to be detailed. The etiology of pediatric arrests is also of some interest because most pediatric arrests can, at least theoretically, be anticipated and prevented.

Identification of Cardiopulmonary Arrest

Infants in the early phase of an arrest appear limp, and their color is pale to dusky or frankly cyanotic. Ineffective gasping may be present. In the case of a *cardiac* arrest, pulses and heart sounds are absent as well.

Airway Management

The first step in the management of an arrest is to secure the airway. The mouth, or mouth and nose in the case of a small infant, should be cleared and the neck brought into a neutral position. Hyperextending the neck in small children kinks the airway, as does flexion, so the "sniffing" position is recommended (Fig. 27-1). The sniffing position is attained by starting with the neck in neutral position and lifting the occiput straight up, extending the neck slightly. This results in maximal opening of the airway from the mouth to the larynx. Some children begin moving air just as soon as their

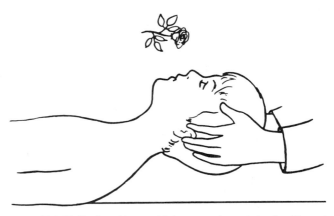

Figure 27-1 *"Sniffing" position to minimize upper airway obstruction. The neck is neither flexed or overextended. The head is lifted as if to help the child sniff an imaginary flower held above his face. (Touloukian R (ed): Pediatric Trauma, p 22. New York, John Wiley & Sons, 1978)*

airways are made patent by these maneuvers, and hence this should always be done first.

If the child does not breathe spontaneously, four quick breaths are delivered mouth to mouth or through a bag-valve mask with 100% oxygen if it is immediately available. While this is being done, another observer should attempt to feel the brachial or femoral pulse. The pulse is frequently difficult to locate in infants even when it is present, and one must therefore sometimes auscultate over the sternum for heart sounds. The presence of heart sounds signifies that the heart is beating and moving blood forcefully enough to open and close the valves. If pulses or heart sounds are absent, closed-chest cardiopulmonary resuscitation (CPR) should begin (see below).

At this time also, the child should be intubated. A good first approximation for selecting an endotracheal tube can be made by finding a tube with a tip diameter the same as the diameter of the tip of the child's little finger. Normal newborns take a 3.5 mm, and older children anywhere from a 4.0 mm to a 7.0 mm size. Laryngoscope blades of all sizes should be available on resuscitation carts.

The most common error in tracheal intubation is inadvertent intubation of the esophagus. A good policy is to concentrate first on locating the epiglottis, which is located at the base of the tongue. The larynx is located just behind the epiglottis. The epiglottis should be elevated to reveal the vocal cords, which give the entrance to the larynx a characteristic appearance, and the endotracheal tube is then inserted. To ensure proper placement, it is essential to see the tube passing between the cords. After it is established that breath sounds can be heard bilaterally, the tube should be secured with tape and the cuff inflated, if a cuffed tube is used.

Following tracheal intubation, positive pressure ventilation with 100% oxygen using an appropriately sized Ambu Bag should commence. An infant can easily develop pneumothorax if too much pressure is applied. Try to estimate the correct volume of delivered oxygen by carefully observing chest wall movements. If a ventilator is available, the tidal volume should be set for 10 to 15 ml/kg, with a ventilatory rate of approximately 20 per minute during an arrest. Naturally, once arterial blood gases are available, adjustments can be made if necessary.

Technique of Closed-Chest CPR

The best place for cardiac compression is directly over the midsternum because of its central location and attachment to other rib cage structures and because rib fractures and liver lacerations are less likely with this technique than with others. In newborns, the preferred method of closed-chest CPR is to encircle the baby's chest with the hands and press both thumbs together over the midsternum. In infants and smaller children it may be possible to achieve good sternal compressions with just a few fingers or one hand. In older children the standard two-handed chest compression technique is most appropriate. These methods are shown in Chapter 14, Resuscitation, in Fig. 14.8. A compression rate of 100 per minute is probably best for all children. Remember that the aim of good CPR is not to follow certain memorized rules about compression rates and ventilatory patterns blindly, but rather to achieve good cardiac output and air exchange. Therefore, the ultimate test of the effectiveness of your efforts is the symmetric rising and falling of the chest with good bilateral breath sounds (and good blood gases when available), and strong peripheral pulses with the cardiac compressions.

Definitive Therapy

Once the airway is secure and chest compressions have been initiated, an intravenous line is established if this has not already been done. In an emergency, look first to the antecubital fossae for an adequate vein. Other good choices for intravenous placement are the external jugular vein and the greater saphenous vein just above the medial malleolus of the ankle.

The decision to use an angiocath rather than a scalp vein needle in this desperate emergency depends on the skill of the operator. If no line can be established, then a cutdown should be done, preferably at the *proximal* greater saphenous vein, high in the medial aspect of the thigh, or a percutaneous cannulation of the internal jugular or subclavian veins attempted.

While an intravenous line is being established, attach ECG monitoring electrodes to the child.

Most cardiac arrests in children are not due to primary cardiac problems, as they are in adults, but are secondary to either respiratory failure or shock. For this reason, the definitive treatment for the majority of children with arrests may already have been accomplished with endotracheal intubation and the initiation of positive pressure ventilations and CPR. However, some children require adrenergic stimulation to restart the heart. Since the heart is usually in asystole, the drug of choice is epinephrine. Depending on the amount of time that has elapsed since the onset of the arrest, sodium bicarbonate is given to correct acidosis, since epinephrine is ineffective in an acidic environment.

Following the administration of epinephrine, one of four situations will prevail, which should be managed as follows:

1. *Return to a stable supraventricular rhythm with good pulses and blood pressure.* Alternatively, the pulses and blood pressure may be somewhat weak at first and may require some support in the form of calcium or dopamine.

2. *Continued asystole or severe bradycardia, with or without pulses.* In this situation the order of drug preference is epinephrine, atropine, and isoproterenol. A temporary artificial pacemaker may be necessary if these measures are ineffective. Attempts are also made to optimize oxygenation and *p*H because most drug therapy is ineffective if these are not corrected.

3. *Electromechanical dissociation.* In this situation a more or less acceptable electrical rhythm is visible on the oscilloscope, but no pulses or blood pressure can be demonstrated. The order of therapeutic priorities in this situation is calcium, dopamine, volume expansion. One must rule out tension pneumothorax and pericardial tamponade.

4. *Ventricular fibrillation or irritability.* The therapy for ventricular fibrillation is immediate direct current (DC) countershock, followed by a bolus of lidocaine to prevent recurrences. If lidocaine does not abolish the ventricular irritability, procainamide may be tried. Bretylium has recently become available for the treatment of refractory ventricular fibrillation. Dosages for medication and defibrillation are outlined in Table 27-1.

Endotracheal Medications

Recently it has been found that many of the drugs used during cardiopulmonary resuscitation can be administered

TABLE 27-1. CARDIAC ARREST MEDICATIONS

Agent	IV Dose
Sodium bicarbonate	1 mEq/kg = 1 ml/kg initially—may be repeated q 10 min or preferably under arterial blood gas guidance
Epinephrine 1:10,000	0.1 ml/kg—may be repeated q 5–10 min if indications still present
Atropine	0.1–0.3 ml/kg—may be repeated once if lower initial dosage is used
Calcium chloride 10%	0.1–0.2 ml/kg
Calcium gluconate 10%	0.3 ml/kg (This preparation has approximately 1/3 the ionic calcium as chloride, which accounts for the difference in dose.)
Dopamine	2–20 µg/kg/min
Isoproterenol	Begin at 0.1 µg/kg/min; generally, dosage must increase to 2–10 µg/kg/min; Titrate to effect.
Lidocaine	1 mg/kg, then 20–50 µg/kg/min drip
Lasix	1 mg/kg as a starting dose
Morphine sulfate	0.1–0.2 mg/kg
Defibrillation	2–4 Watt-sec/kg
Procainamide	2 mg/kg—dose may be repeated in 10 min

by the endotracheal route in addition to the more usual intravenous route. This is especially important in pediatric patients, in whom venous access is often difficult or impossible. The following recommendations can safely be made at this time:

- *Epinephrine*—forcefully inject 1 to 1½ times the usual intravenous dose of the 1:10,000 concentration into the endotracheal tube and immediately deliver several quick bursts of oxygen with the Ambu-Bag to disperse the medication. A rapid onset of action is expected with activity up to four times longer.
- *Atropine*—as with epinephrine, inject about the same or a little more than the usual intravenous dose and forcefully disperse with the Ambu Bag.
- *Lidocaine*—it is recommended that twice the usual intravenous dose be used, but the effect can be expected to last at least twice as long.
- *Narcan,* a preparation of Naloxone HCl, has also been found to be effective when administered by the endotracheal route.
- Unfortunately, sodium bicarbonate cannot be given by this route because of its high osmolarity and alkaline *p*H, which would cause massive tissue injury to the lungs.

Neonatal Aspects of Advanced Cardiac Life Support

Fortunately, most deliveries are uneventful, and the baby is born crying and vigorous. However, emergency personnel should approach any impending delivery, especially in the home setting or in the emergency department itself, as a potential emergency, and the infant should be managed accordingly.

As the head is delivered, the mouth and nose should be gently but thoroughly suctioned with either a bulb suction apparatus or a deLee catheter trap to clear the airway. (Remember that newborns are obligate *nose* breathers.) The umbilical cord should be clamped, leaving approximately a 1½-inch stump or longer with the baby. This stump may prove invaluable later if emergency cannulation of an umbilical vein or artery becomes necessary. Newborns are intolerant of cold temperatures; the baby should be dried and placed in a warm environment at once. If he is not already crying or breathing, he should be stimulated by flicking the soles of the feet. If this fails to stimulate respirations, mouth-to-mouth and nose or bag-valve mask positive pressure ventilations with 100% oxygen should be initiated. An assistant should auscultate the chest for heart tones. A drop in the heart rate to 100 bpm or less signifies critical respiratory insufficiency and is an indication for vigorous manual stimulation of the infant, additional efforts with the bag-valve mask, or immediate intubation.

- *Do not mistake a falling pulse rate in this situation as an indication for atropine!*

Even in older children who are dying of hypoxia the pulse rate begins to fall just before asystole supervenes. The treatment for this condition is assisted ventilation, without which drug therapy is ineffective.

The most common cause of depression in the newborn is mild hypoxic encephalopathy caused by prolonged passage through the birth canal. Most babies with depression from this cause recover quickly after they are given a few assisted ventilations with oxygen. However, some babies are born depressed because they are under the influence of an opioid or other sedative drugs the mother may have taken during labor. The use of neonatal Narcan in this situation can be very helpful diagnostically as well as therapeutically.

Successful resuscitation of the depressed newborn is signaled by a rapid return of the pulse rate to levels approaching 150 and the onset of spontaneous respirations. If the heart rate continues to fall despite adequate air exchange, venous access for the administration of bicarbonate and cardiac stimulant drugs will be necessary. The most rapid method of establishing such access is through an umbilical venous catheter. Many emergency department physicians and nurses are unfamiliar with this technique; however, it is surprisingly easy. The umbilical stump should first be encircled with umbilical tape so that a knot can quickly be tied in case there is spurting from the umbilical artery when the cord clamp is removed. The cord is then cross-sectioned with a scalpel blade. Looking directly at the cross-section you should be able to see three vessels: a central, patulous umbilical vein and, on either side, a relatively muscular umbilical artery. Usually a 5 F polyvinylchloride catheter slips easily into the vein and can be advanced approximately 8 cm to 10 cm into the inferior vena cava. In an arrest, the exact location of the catheter tip is not important, and it is appropriate to secure the catheter as soon as good blood return appears in the catheter. If the catheter is to be left in place for any length of time (for example, if an exchange transfusion is contemplated), the exact location of the catheter tip should be documented radiographically to ensure that it is not in the portal vein or one of the mesenteric or renal veins.

The usual cardiac arrest medications can then be administered according to indication. Since the likely rhythm is slow idioventricular or asystole, the first drug given should probably be epinephrine 1:10,000. Sodium bicarbonate (diluted 1:1 with D_5W to reduce the hyperosmolarity) may be given before the epinephrine to control acidosis. Other drugs that may be useful in the delivery room are atropine, dopamine, isuprel, and Narcan.

RESPIRATORY DISTRESS IN THE NEWBORN

In this situation we are dealing not with a depressed newborn but with a vigorous, active baby who is having rapid, labored respirations. A number of conditions can occur within the first hours of life or even in the delivery room with this syndrome; they are described in the sections that follow.

Congenital Diaphragmatic Hernia. In this condition a developmental defect in the diaphragm has allowed the stomach and other abdominal contents to enter into the left hemithorax, preventing the normal development of the left lung and causing marked respiratory distress beginning at birth. Assisted ventilations with bag-valve mask only makes things worse, because as the stomach becomes filled with air it causes a mediastinal shift and further compresses the normal right lung. It is important to recognize this condition so that endotracheal intubation and immediate surgical correction can be undertaken. Clues to the diagnosis are a very flat or scaphoid abdomen, absent breath sounds (or the presence of bowel sounds) in the left chest, and the immediate onset of respiratory distress. The diagnosis can be confirmed by chest x-ray.

Choanal Atresia. Choanal atresia is another surgical condition presenting with respiratory distress at birth. In this condition the nasal passages are not developed, and since babies are obligate nose breathers, the baby may suffocate simply because he does not know to open his mouth. Interim treatment is an oropharyngeal airway while emergency oropharyngeal consultation is obtained.

Hypovolemic Shock. Hypovolemic shock can present mainly with respiratory symptoms in the neonate, and the diagnosis is not always obvious, especially in the case of a fetal-maternal bleeding. In *vasa previa* in which copious vaginal bleeding from ruptured fetal vessels preceded the delivery, the neonate must be carefully assessed for low blood pressure and possibly anemia, indicating blood loss. The treatment is immediate infusion of whole blood or plasma expanders, usually through an umbilical venous line.

Hypoglycemia. Hypoglycemia is a common and often overlooked cause of neonatal respiratory symptoms. Every neonate with respiratory distress should have a Dextrostix test performed and should be treated with an infusion of 10% dextrose in water if necessary.

Delayed-Onset Respiratory Distress Syndromes. Innumerable conditions such as cyanotic congenital heart disease and idiopathic respiratory distress syndrome of the newborn (hyaline membrane disease) can present with cyanosis and tachypnea beginning hours to days after delivery. A full discussion of this complex situation is beyond the scope of this text; however, one vital point must be made: once surgical and metabolic emergencies have been ruled out and it is determined that a primary cardiorespiratory condition exists, arrangements must be made for the expeditious transport of the sick newborn to a neonatal intensive care center.
- *While awaiting the arrival of the transport team, the baby should be kept warm and well oxygenated.*

Do not let fears of retrolental fibroplasia or pulmonary oxygen damage cause you to allow a sick newborn to remain hypoxic. It is much better in this setting to have too much oxygen than too little, especially for the short period until definitive care can be given.

SUDDEN INFANT DEATH SYNDROME

The leading cause of death in infants 1 week to 1 year of age, sudden infant death syndrome (SIDS), remains a mystery despite years of intensive investigation. The typical example is a baby, often 2 to 4 months old, who is put to bed apparently healthy and is found pulseless and apneic in the morning or at bed check in the middle of the night. Usually no sounds or signs of a struggle can be recalled. Autopsy findings on large series of SIDS babies have failed to show a consistent pathology.

Unfortunately, by the time paramedics arrive, most of these babies are already mottled and the rhythm strip shows a flat line, a sign of prolonged hypoxia (and hence probable brain damage even if the heart could be revived). Nevertheless, in most cases emergency services personnel try to give these babies every chance and proceed with the ACLS protocol as outlined at the beginning of this chapter. These children are good candidates for endotracheal epinephrine, because intravenous lines are very difficult to start in pulseless 3-month-olds.

Following the usually unsuccessful attempt to revive a SIDS baby who has been brought to the emergency department, physicians and nurses have the most difficult job of talking with the parents and siblings. It is essential to emphasize that the parents were *not responsible* for the infant's death. Many hospitals with large pediatric populations have special crisis teams for helping families cope with a SIDS death.

If a SIDS baby has been revived either at the scene by the family or paramedics, or in the emergency department, he must be admitted for close observation and workup to rule out sleep apnea, seizures, sepsis, and dysrhythmias. It is unfortunate that a considerable number of "near miss" SIDS babies ultimately succumb to a second episode following release from the hospital.

RESPIRATORY SYNDROMES IN CHILDREN

Respiratory distress is the most frightening and dramatic emergency encountered in pediatrics. The majority of cardiac arrests in the pediatric age group are preceded by respiratory insufficiency. Respiratory emergencies must be dealt with rapidly and correctly before they degenerate into full cardiac arrests.

Four of the most important conditions that manifest chiefly as repiratory distress are bronchiolitis, asthma, croup, and epiglottitis. Bronchiolitis and asthma are caused by obstruction in the lower airway and therefore present with expiratory difficulty, wheezing being the chief physical finding. Croup and epiglottitis, on the other hand, are associated with obstruction in the upper airway, in the vicinity of the larynx. Upper airway obstruction presents with difficult inspirations, and a crowing sound during inspiration known as *stridor* may be produced.

CONDITIONS ASSOCIATED WITH EXPIRATORY DIFFICULTY AND WHEEZING

Asthma

Asthma refers to a reversible condition of spasm of the small airways brought on by any of a number of inciting conditions:

exposure to allergens, exercise, cold air, infection, emotional upset, and so forth. It may present at any age. The hallmarks of an asthmatic attack are dyspnea, tachypnea, and expiratory wheezing, which may be audible with the aid of the stethoscope or sometimes by the unaided ear. Many children presenting to the emergency department with asthmatic attacks have previously been diagnosed as asthmatic, and in such cases the preliminary diagnosis of acute exacerbation of asthma should be relatively easy; however, the superimposition of inciting conditions, particularly pneumonia, must be considered.

A more difficult problem arises in the case of a child presenting with what appears to be a *first episode of asthma*. In such situations it is wise to remember the adage "all that wheezes is not asthma." Aspirated foreign bodies, pneumonia, and even congestive heart failure can present with tachypnea and wheezing. In patients suspected of having *possible asthma,* a positive family history is important confirmatory evidence. A total absence of asthma or significant allergies from the family history should raise strong suspicions that another process may be responsible for the patient's problem. If there is doubt about the diagnosis, a therapeutic trial with epinephrine and bronchodilators may help to establish the diagnosis as well as alleviate the symptoms. A suggested treatment plan for acute asthmatic attacks is presented in Chart 27-1.

Bronchiolitis

Bronchiolitis is an affliction of infants generally under 1 year old. It occurs in the setting of an upper respiratory infection and presents exactly like asthma, with tachypnea and wheezing. Unlike asthma, bronchiolitis is caused by infection by the respiratory syncytial virus, and the resulting inflammation of the distal airway is seldom responsive to therapy aimed at relieving bronchospasm. Nevertheless, because it is difficult to tell bronchiolitis from a first episode of asthma in a wheezing infant, a therapeutic trial of epinephrine or aminophylline may be warranted. Many children with bronchiolitis do in fact go on to develop true asthma later in childhood.

Other Conditions Associated With Wheezing

Pneumonia. Pneumonia can present quite atypically in childhood, with abdominal pain, back pain, or wheezing as its only manifestations. The key to diagnosis is a high degree of suspicion and careful attention to even minor deviations from the expected history and physical examination.

Congestive Heart Failure. Infants present with tachypnea and wheezing. A clue to this diagnosis is hepatomegaly, which is usually present in these babies, but which might be missed by clinicians without significant pediatric experience. A loud heart murmur is also likely to be present, since most conditions giving rise to early failure are associated with murmurs. The chest x-ray reveals a large heart and pulmonary vascular congestion.

Aspirated Foreign Bodies. The child with a foreign body lodged in the distal pulmonary tree can present with tachypnea and wheezing. This is a rather common cause of repeated pulmonary infections and should be considered in children who present frequently with such a symptom complex. Chest x-ray will reveal an area of atelectasis as well

---

Chart 27-1

MANAGEMENT OF THE CHILD HAVING AN ACUTE ASTHMATIC ATTACK

1. Administer oxygen at 30% to 40% or higher concentrations if the child continues to be cyanotic. Arterial blood gas analysis may be helpful in evaluating the ventilatory status of the child who is more seriously ill.
2. Consider and rule out alternative diagnoses (pneumonia, foreign body aspiration, pneumothorax, etc.)
3. Epinephrine 1:1000, 0.1 ml/kg SC to maximum of 0.4 ml. This dose may be repeated at 15- to 20-min intervals to a maximum of three doses.
4. If this "breaks the attack," administer epinephrine 1:200 (Sus-Phrine), 0.05 ml/kg SC and begin the patient on oral aminophylline as an outpatient.
5. If epinephrine does not relieve the dyspnea and tachypnea, establish an IV line and begin aminophylline infusion, 5–6 mg/kg loading dose over 15 min, followed by 0.9 mg/kg/hr continuous infusion drip. If the patient is already taking an aminophylline preparation at home, the loading dose should be adjusted accordingly. Make liberal use of aminophylline levels in the blood
6. IPPB or hand-held nebulizer treatments with isoetharine HCl (Bronkosol) or isoproterenol (Isuprel) may be helpful in severe cases.
7. A high-dose bolus of corticosteroids (example: 5 mg/kg Solu-Cortef) is mandatory for any steroid-dependent child and optional for children not currently on steroids who continue to do poorly.
8. IV isoproterenol drip at a dose titrated against the heart rate is a last-stand method of avoiding possible endotracheal intubation and assisted ventilation in cases of incipient respiratory failure.

as the foreign body, if it is radiopaque. Treatment is surgical removal, usually by bronchoscopy.

CONDITIONS ASSOCIATED WITH INSPIRATORY DIFFICULTY AND STRIDOR

Croup

Croup, or viral laryngotracheobronchitis, is an inflammation of the paralaryngeal tissues caused by infection with parainfluenza virus and other viruses. It affects infants ranging in age from 6 months to 3 years. Typically, the baby has had a "cold" for a few days and suddenly becomes much worse, usually at night, with noisy stridorous inspirations and a characteristic brassy cough that sounds like the bark of a seal. There may be considerable tachypnea. Despite the often alarming symptoms, these children usually do quite well and are likely to respond to simple treatment in a cool-mist oxygen tent. Admission is not always necessary; sometimes it is sufficient to tell the parents to take the child into the bathroom and turn the shower on full force to create the proper cool, moist, soothing environment for the laryngeal tissues. Some children with croup do require inpatient observation, and additional therapeutic modalities are available for those in need. Nebulized racemic epinephrine (Vaponephrine) is rapidly effective in reducing laryngospasm and edema, but because there is a tendency for marked "rebound" worsening of the stridor as the drug wears off, children administered racemic epinephrine *must* be admitted for further observation. Management of the child with croup is outlined in Chart 27-2. The effectiveness of steroids for viral croup is controversial, but the preponderance of evidence is in favor of using one or two doses of intramuscular dexamethasone for severe cases. Antibiotics are probably worthless.

Epiglottitis

Epiglottitis is the most treacherous condition in children; it can progress from mild to moderate respiratory distress, resembling croup, to a fatal respiratory arrest, without any warning. It is therefore absolutely necessary to have an advance plan for dealing with children who present to the emergency department with symptoms that suggest epiglottitis.

Despite the well-known similarities in presentation between croup, with its usual benign outcome, and epiglottitis, with its marked tendency to rapid progression and sudden death, there are a large number of differentiating features (Table 27-2). Generally, the approach to a young child with stridor is first to determine (on the basis of the features noted in Table 27-2) the likelihood of croup as opposed to epiglottitis. The most helpful features are the characteristic barking cough of croup and the ability of croupy babies to drink; in contrast, children with epiglottitis are unable to handle even their own secretions, and drooling results.

Clinical Differentiation of Croup and Epiglottitis

Initially, one may place these children in one of the three following clinical groups:

- *Group 1: Croup likely.* Obtain a confirming soft-tissue lateral x-ray of the neck (if deemed necessary for diagnosis), and place the child in a cool-mist tent to observe for improvement. The use of steroids or racemic epinephrine is optional and depends on the general condition of the infant. Most of these babies are discharged from the emergency department.

- *Group 2: Diagnosis uncertain.* Children in this group are usually quite ill irrespective of the ultimate diagnosis, and resuscitation equipment should be assembled at once. Equipment includes laryngoscope, several sizes of endotracheal tubes, a large-bore needle for emergency needle cricothyrotomy, and intravenous equipment and arrest medications. Offer oxygen to the child, but if he resists, avoid forcing therapy that may make him more anxious and worsen his general condition. Similarly, it may be necessary to withhold starting an intravenous line at this time. If the child's condition seems fairly stable, he should be offered some water to drink. If he can drink the water, the likelihood is that the diagnosis is croup. Under the direct supervision of a physician, a soft tissue lateral x-ray view of the neck should be taken to clarify the status of the epiglottis and therefore provide the diagnosis. Under no circumstances should attempts be made to visualize the epiglottis directly in the emergency department. Manipulation of the oropharynx can produce enough additional edema of the epiglottis to occlude the airway

---

Chart 27-2

MANAGEMENT OF THE CHILD WITH CROUP

1. Establish the diagnosis
   - Consider and rule out epiglottitis, aspirated foreign body, etc.
2. Administer cool, moist air or oxygen in a croup tent.
3. Administer Vaponephrin 2¼% 0.5 ml in 2½ ml saline through nebulized aerosol for severe cases. Remember that children who have croup must be observed for "rebound" worsening of their symptoms when the Vaponephrin wears off.
4. Dexamethasone (Decadron) 0.3 mg/kg IM is optional and probably advisable for moderately or severely ill children.
5. Antibiotics are not indicated except for infectious complications (*e.g.*, pneumonia, otitis media).

TABLE 27-2. DIFFERENTIAL DIAGNOSIS OF CROUP AND EPIGLOTTITIS

	Croup	Epiglottitis
Age range	6 months–4 yr	3–7 yr
Onset	URI prodrome	Abrupt onset with severe toxicity
General appearance	Appears well, tachypnea of variable severity with substernal and supraclavicular retractions	Appears desperately ill, severe tachypnea with poor color; substernal and supraclavicular retractions
Sounds	Loud stridor, seal-like barking cough. Wheezes in expiration absent.	Stridor may be less prominent (child is moving less air); barking cough absent, voice may be muffled or absent. No wheezes.
Position	Prefers to lie on side.	Sits erect with neck extended into the sniffing position.
Response to offered liquids	Usually drinks unless tachypnea is too severe	Unable to tolerate any liquids including own saliva; drools
Fever	May or may not be present	High fever a regular feature
Lab	WBC nonspecific, blood cultures negative	High WBC with left shift, blood cultures usually positive for *Hemophilus influenzae*.
X-ray	Anteroposterior view of neck may reveal subglottic narrowing; epiglottis will be normal on soft-tissue lateral	Soft-tissue lateral of neck shows markedly enlarged epiglottic shadow.
Pathology	Virus-induced subglottic inflammation	Bacterial inflammation leading to cherry-red, edematous epiglottis
Course	Generally benign and self-limited	Respiratory arrest always a threat; aggressive, *preventative* airway control a must

completely. Direct pharyngeal visualization should be performed only in the operating suite by a qualified physician with the aid of a fiberoptic bronchoscope, and with emergency tracheostomy equipment on standby.

- *Group 3: Epiglottitis likely.* If the child presents *in extremis* with most of the criteria for epiglottitis as outlined in Table 27-2, resuscitation equipment should be readied and a pediatric otolaryngologist or anesthesiologist summoned to aid with airway management. Such children are usually highly anxious and resist any manipulations. They should not be separated from their mothers. Administer oxygen by face mask. Place an intravenous line if the child does not resist too strongly. No further interventions should be undertaken until the specialist arrives. If the child becomes agonal or arrests in the interval, emergency intubation or cricothyrotomy must be undertaken by the most experienced person present.

All Group II and III children are to be admitted, usually to the intensive care unit. If the hospital does not have pediatric intensive care facilities, it is preferable to transport a child with epiglottitis or severe croup to a referral center.

It is extremely unwise to transport a child with probable epiglottitis before the airway has been secured!

Other Conditions That Cause Stridor

An aspirated *foreign body* will cause stridor if it lodges above the thoracic inlet (it will cause wheezing if it passes into the distal pulmonary tree, as discussed above). This possibility should be considered in every case of croup/epiglottitis. Clues to the diagnosis are

1. Atypical or unusually sudden presentation
2. History of foreign body in the mouth shortly before onset of symptoms

All cases of severe upper airway obstruction eventually come to the attention of an otolaryngologist, and hence the diagnosis will be made at the time of laryngoscopy, if not sooner. Radiopaque foreign bodies may be identified on routine chest x-ray.

Severe *tonsillitis* (sometimes caused by mononucleosis), *peritonsillar abscess,* and *retropharyngeal abscess* can all cause upper airway obstruction if tissue edema becomes significant. The first two conditions and sometimes the third are usually apparent from examination of the oropharynx. A lateral soft tissue film of the neck reveals or confirms a retropharyngeal abscess.

Anaphylaxis can occur with severe laryngeal edema, in addition to generalized urticaria, wheezing, and cardiovascular collapse. Emergency management consists of intravenous adrenalin, benadryl, and corticosteroids, as well as other medications for other specific symptoms that may arise.

NEUROLOGIC CONDITIONS

SEIZURE DISORDERS

Epilepsy

The first priority in managing a child having a seizure is to ensure a patent airway and good air exchange by means of an oxygen mask placed around the child's mouth and nose; most children in seizure are already moving enough air and it is unwise to traumatize the oral cavity by attempting to insert an oral airway through clenched teeth. (In certain cases, the use of force or muscle relaxants may be necessary, however.)

The next step is to terminate the seizure itself. Most seizures end spontaneously within a few minutes.

Status Epilepticus. Status epilepticus refers to an exceedingly long grand mal convulsion or a series of grand mal convulsions without intervening periods of normal consciousness. A number of drugs are available for terminating status epilepticus. In adult medicine the overwhelming first choice has been intravenous diazepam (Valium). Diazepam works quickly and is almost always effective, but it is not suitable for maintenance therapy. Another drug generally must be administered concomitantly to prevent additional seizures. Phenytoin (Dilantin) is usually used for this purpose, but it has a number of side-effects that make it unsuitable for prolonged use in children; phenobarbital is the usual first-line maintenance drug in pediatrics. A problem arises because of the inadvisability of mixing parenteral diazepam and phenobarbital, since respiratory arrest can occur. In some centers this problem is circumvented by avoiding diazepam and using phenobarbital as the initial drug for the actual termination of the seizure. Phenobarbital takes longer to work than diazepam, however, and many clinicians still prefer diazepam for this reason. An advantage of phenobarbital is that it can be administered intramuscularly when intravenous access is impossible. Diazepam is erratically absorbed from intramuscular sites and should not be given by this route.

Paraldehyde is a third drug that can be used to terminate status epilepticus. For many years this drug's use was on the decline because of its unpleasant odor and difficulty of administration; however, it is very effective, has few side-effects, and occasionally works when other drugs have failed. Management of the child with status epilepticus is summarized in Chart 27-3.

Febrile Seizures

Febrile seizures are the most common type of seizure encountered among pediatric patients; they affect as many as 5% of all children at one time or another. Children from 3 months to 5 years of age are affected. A febrile seizure is defined as one occurring in this age group for which no cause can be found other than the coexisting presence of a high temperature. The cause of the fever is usually a viral infection such as roseola, but it may be otitis media, gastroenteritis (particularly when caused by *Shigella*), or any other febrile illness. It is mandatory to rule out meningitis as the cause of an apparently febrile seizure, especially in the first such episode in a particular child.

- *A lumbar puncture must be performed!*

Once the diagnosis of febrile seizure is established (*i.e.,* following the receipt of a normal spinal fluid report, and assuming that the child has a normal neurologic examination after the usually brief postictal period), a decision must be made about the use of anticonvulsants. This question has been intensively studied over the past 10 years, and the following conclusions are now established: (1) Children with febrile seizures have a 30% to 40% risk of future febrile seizures. (2) It is possible to prevent these recurrences if *continuous* therapeutic blood levels of phenobarbital are

---

Chart 27-3

MANAGEMENT OF THE CHILD WITH STATUS EPILEPTICUS

1. Oxygen by mask during the seizure and postictal period.
   - Airway and ventilation management if necessary
   - Muscle relaxants as a last resort: anectine, 1 mg/kg IV push
   - Obtain arterial blood gases if ventilation status is uncertain.
2. Use measures to reduce self-injury.
3. Start IV line if possible
4. Medications to control status epilepticus:
   - Diazepam (Valium), 0.3 mg/kg slow IV push, or
   - Phenobarbital 5 mg/kg slow IV push (this dose may need to be repeated), or
   - Paraldehyde, 200 mg/kg (0.2 ml/kg), mixed with an equal volume of vegetable or mineral oil, inserted per rectum, or
   - Paraldehyde, 0.15 ml/kg IV slow drip
5. Be prepared to manage a respiratory arrest when using parenteral diazepam and/or phenobarbital
6. If unable to start IV line, phenobarbital, 10–15 mg/kg IM
7. For seizures associated with fever, begin cooling measures immediately.

maintained. Specifically, this means that the intermittent use of phenobarbital whenever the child becomes ill or febrile is useless. (3) Although there is a slightly increased risk of the development of permanent epilepsy in children with febrile seizures, the febrile seizures themselves do not seem to cause epilepsy but may be its earliest manifestation (*i.e.,* febrile seizures themselves are probably benign). Moreover, there is no evidence that even the correct use of phenobarbital reduces the risk of subsequent epilepsy, although it definitely reduces the risk of subsequent *febrile* seizures. (5) Phenobarbital produces unacceptable behavioral manifestations in up to 40% of the young children in the febrile seizure age group to whom it might be given as prophylaxis against future febrile seizures.

The use of phenobarbital in children who have had a single, simple febrile seizure is on the decline. However, its use is still advisable in certain situations:

1. When the febrile seizure is complicated by excessive length (more than 15 minutes), focal activity, or any neurologic deficit following the seizure
2. When there is a strongly positive family history of epilepsy

In all such cases a pediatric neurologist should be consulted.

Giving a single intramuscular injection of phenobarbital (10 mg/kg) followed by oral therapy at 5 mg/kg/day to all children, even those in the uncomplicated group, seems to control the problem and lessen the frequency of recurrence. It is probably equally important to train the parents of children who have had febrile seizures in the proper methods of fever control, that is, antipyretics and sponge water baths.

Seizures in the Neonatal Period

Seizures in the neonatal period* deserve special consideration because they can be difficult to recognize and they are *always* to be viewed as a symptom, and thus require intensive investigation. As for recognition, emergency department personnel need to be alert to the fact that well-organized grand mal motor activity is comparatively rare in this age group because of the immaturity of neuronal connections. Rather, a wide variety of subtle manifestations such as brief apneic episodes, eye rolling, "turning colors," and multifocal clonic spasms can herald the onset of a serious neurologic or systemic disorder.

A working differential diagnosis of seizures in the neonatal period includes hypoglycemia, hypocalcemia, hypomagnesemia, pyridoxine deficiency, genetic-metabolic defects such as phenylketonuria or maple syrup urine disease, and finally, central nervous system (CNS) birth trauma or congenital malformations. Meningitis must always be considered in any baby or child having a seizure. As the workup proceeds, early attention should be given to life-threatening ongoing processes such as hypoglycemia, hypocalcemia, pyridoxine deficiency, and meningitis, before turning attention to the possibility of CNS malformations, about which relatively little can be done in the emergency setting.

---

* Here and throughout this section, *neonatal* refers to the first 30 days of life.

Altered Level of Consciousness

The child presenting with an altered level of consciousness, including coma, presents the same kind of problem to the emergency department staff as would an adult with the same signs and symptoms (see Chap. 18). First, excellent supportive care is needed to ensure adequate respirations and cardiac output, as well as to prevent pulmonary aspiration of gastric contents. Second, a vigorous search for the etiology of the coma must proceed, with special emphasis on the search for reversible disease.

The most common causes of depressed consciousness in the pediatric age group are as follows:

Postictal States. This can be a confusing diagnosis initially, especially if the seizure was not witnessed and the child is not known to have a seizure disorder.

Trauma. Trauma is not always as obvious as one might imagine. Some battered children present with chronic bilateral subdural hematomas and extremely depressed consciousness without any external signs of trauma. Skull x-rays (and, of course, cervical spine films) should be part of the workup of all children with coma of unknown etiology.

Meningitis/Encephalitis. After intracranial mass lesions are excluded, a lumbar puncture should be performed to rule out these dangerous and potentially treatable causes of depressed consciousness.

Ingestions. Some classic types of pediatric drug overdose, such as aspirin and anticholinergic agents, can present with altered consciousness. Recently, a number of reports linking phencyclidine (PCP) ingestion to unconsciousness and even decerebrate posturing have appeared.

Metabolic Disturbance. Hypoglycemia should always be ruled out in cases of altered consciousness. Occasionally a child will present in coma owing to some other more complex metabolic derangement, such as fulminating hepatic failure.

Reye's Syndrome. This disease occurs mainly in school-aged children, although it has been reported to occur anywhere from 2 months to 19 years. It presents with headache and very pronounced vomiting, progressing rapidly to deep coma and death in severe cases. It occurs in the setting of a viral upper respiratory infection, varicella (chickenpox), or influenza B. The typical story is that as the child is recovering from the prodromal infection, he suddenly becomes much worse, with headaches and continuous vomiting. By the time medical attention is obtained, coma may already have supervened. Physical findings are quite variable but usually include depressed consciousness and hepatomegaly. Jaundice is absent, differentiating this syndrome from acute hepatic encephalopathy. The cause of the alteration in consciousness is a marked increase in intracranial pressure with generalized brain edema, so these children should not undergo routine lumbar puncture; however, should lumbar puncture be done for the purpose of ruling out meningitis in a doubtful case, the fluid will be found to be clear. Laboratory findings are nondiagnostic but frequently show a rise in serum glutamic oxalacetic transaminase (SGOT), serum glutamic pyruvic transaminase (SGPT), and especially serum ammonia. Hypoglycemia may be an incidental finding and should be treated vigorously. The liver biopsy shows a diagnostic pattern of fatty infiltration.

Treatment of Reye's syndrome is directed at reducing brain swelling. The usual methods are employed, such as controlled hyperventilation, mannitol, diuretics, and steroids. Children with Reye's syndrome should be cared for at a tertiary care facility with personnel experienced in this area of medicine.

ABDOMINAL PAIN

Most children who arrive in the emergency department with abdominal pain as a chief complaint have benign, self-limited illness; nevertheless, one must consider and rule out surgical conditions such as appendicitis and incarcerated inguinal hernias; moreover, there are a number of exotic "pediatric" diseases that may present with abdominal signs and symptoms. Certain conditions such as cystitis and lower lobe pneumonia, which have classic presentations in adults, occasionally present mainly with abdominal pain in children. The purpose of this section is to help the reader identify children who may be in need of surgical consultation and to describe briefly the conditions unique to pediatrics that may present chiefly as abdominal pain.

Appendicitis. All emergency personnel are familiar with the usual course of appendicitis in adults. Appendicitis may strike at any age, including early infancy. The significant features are periumbilical pain ultimately localizing in the right lower quadrant, fever, anorexia and possibly vomiting, and abdominal tenderness maximal in the right lower quadrant. Bowel sounds are usually decreased or absent. The white blood count is elevated in the range of 12,000 to 15,000 with a shift to the left, and a fecalith may be visible on abdominal x-ray. No one of these findings is essential for the diagnosis. In doubtful cases it is wise to observe the child for a period of several hours. A repeat physical examination and white blood count will generally clarify the situation. Careful observation of the baby's facial expression and general behavior during abdominal palpation will allow the examiner to identify and localize abdominal tenderness in many cases, even in the youngest infant. Appendicitis in infants often progresses to rupture with peritonitis as a result of delay in bringing the baby for examination. By then, the baby has a persistent fever, refuses to feed, or suffers frank vomiting and a tender, silent, distended abdomen.

The use of barium enema in cases of suspected appendicitis has been advocated by some. Filling of the appendix by barium indicates that it is normal. This method of diagnosis is not yet universally accepted, however.

Intussusception. In this condition, a portion of the bowel (usually the terminal ileum) telescopes into the bowel immediately distal to it, causing intermittent bowel obstruction. Idiopathic intussusception occurs in infants between 1 month and 2 years of age. The clinical picture is that of an infant who periodically becomes extremely irritable and draws up his legs during what appears to be a spasm of colicky abdominal pain. In the pain-free intervals, the child may appear well until late in the course when gangrene of the bowel occurs. A characteristic guaiac-positive stool known as a *currant jelly stool* because of its color and consistency is often passed several hours after the first spasm, clarifying the diagnosis. A sausage-shaped mass, representing the intussusceptum (the intussuscepting segment) may be palpated or seen in the right upper abdominal quadrant; the right lower quadrant is relatively flat and empty. Barium enema examination performed by an experienced pediatric radiologist can be very helpful in establishing the diagnosis as well as occasionally actually reducing the intussusception itself, thus eliminating the need for emergency surgery. Note that in colitis (caused, for example, by *Shigella*), a similar picture of abdominal pain and bloody stools may be seen, but there are no free periods during which the child appears well.

Intussusception may occur in older children as well as infants, but in such cases it is usually due to a mass lesion acting as a leading edge. The lesion is usually a Meckel's diverticulum, but may also be an intestinal wall lymphoma, a section of inflamed bowel wall caused by Henoch-Schönlein purpura, or some other process.

Inguinal Hernia. Inguinal hernia may present at any age with a palpable and visible inguinal mass. The hernia may subsequently become incarcerated (nonreducible), resulting in symptoms of bowel obstruction. It is usually safe for emergency department personnel to attempt manual reduction, sometimes with the aid of a sedative. Of course, surgical follow-up is mandatory to ensure complete reduction. Operative repair on an urgent basis is necessary if the hernia cannot be reduced. If the hernia is reducible, surgical repair may be performed electively.

Mesenteric Adenitis. Mesenteric adenitis often presents the same clinical picture as acute appendicitis. The abdominal pain is usually more generalized, with fewer localizing signs in the right lower quadrant. Often the onset of the abdominal symptoms is preceded by an upper respiratory infection (7–10 days previously). At surgery, enlarged mesenteric lymph nodes are found and the appendix appears normal. Various organisms, notably *Yersinia enterocolitica*, β-hemolytic streptococci, and adenoviruses, have been isolated from these nodes. Mesenteric adenitis is the most common postoperative diagnosis when children who are operated on for presumed appendicitis turn out to have a normal appendix.

Pyelonephritis. Pyelonephritis and even cystitis can be manifested by prominent abdominal pain and fever in young children.

- *It is mandatory to examine the urine of every child with an abdominal condition in order to rule out these medically treatable conditions!*

Pancreatitis. This condition, although rare in pediatrics, can occur, and a test for serum amylase is often justified.

Abdominal Sickle-Cell Crisis. This diagnosis can be difficult if the diagnosis of sickle-cell disease has not yet been made. It is equally important not to neglect to rule out other treatable conditions such as appendicitis or pyelonephritis, even in known "sicklers" who have had repeated abdominal crises in the past. *This* time, they may have something else.

Henoch-Schönlein Purpura. This condition usually begins with an erythematous papular rash (which may be quite evanescent); the rash is most prominent on the extensor surfaces of the limbs, the buttocks, and the back. It may become purpuric or urticarial, and subcutaneous edema may develop. (This condition is also known as *anaphylactoid purpura.*) In addition, abdominal pain with guaiac-positive stools (and possibly even intussusception) may develop because of edema of the bowel wall. Renal manifestations may occur. There is no single test for this disease; the diagnosis is based on the history and physical findings and may be very difficult indeed.

Hemolytic-Uremic Syndrome. As the name implies, this syndrome is mainly characterized by acute hemolysis and renal failure. Fever, abdominal pain, sometimes with bloody diarrhea, and a petechial rash may also be noted. Recent research indicates that the cause of this complex syndrome is probably infectious. Referral to a pediatric nephrologist is urgently required.

Acute Hepatitis. Hepatitis may be anicteric, especially in its early phase, and abdominal pain may predominate. Usually, anorexia is also present. Abdominal examination reveals tenderness in the region of the liver. Liver function tests should establish the diagnosis.

Streptococcal Pharyngitis. For unknown reasons, abdominal pain may become an important complaint in young patients with this disease. Usually, the intense sore throat draws attention to the correct diagnosis.

Diabetic Ketoacidosis. Also for unknown reasons, abdominal pain is sometimes the chief complaint of a patient with incipient ketoacidosis. This is especially insidious because some children who present with ketoacidosis do not even know that they are diabetic. It is absolutely essential at least to check the urine for sugar before submitting a child with a surgical abdomen for appendectomy.

Neonatal Conditions. A number of conditions may present in the first weeks of life that have an obstructive picture in common: progressive abdominal distention, bilious vomiting (*always* a surgical emergency in the neonate), failure to pass stool or meconium (the first stool), and ultimately, as bowel necrosis sets in, heme-positive rectal contents. A list of these conditions would include volvulus, malrotations, intestinal atresias (duodenal, jejunal, and colonic), Hirschprung's disease (aganglionic megacolon), and meconium ileus (always a sign of cystic fibrosis).

These conditions are usually not difficult to identify because the obstructive symptoms rapidly become prominent, especially failure to feed. These symptoms always demand prompt investigation in a neonate.

At 2 to 3 weeks of age a unique condition known as *hypertrophic pyloric stenosis* may occur. The classic case involves a 3-week-old first-born male with unremitting projectile vomiting of non-bile-stained materials. An olive-shaped mass representing the hypertrophied pylorus is occasionally palpable in the right upper abdominal quadrant or epigastrium. It is important not to confuse such a case with simple gastroenteritis for two reasons:

1. Significant fluid and electrolyte disturbance is likely to be present.
2. This condition is not self-limited and requires surgical intervention to relieve the obstruction.

DIARRHEA AND VOMITING

DIARRHEA

In evaluating a patient with acute diarrhea, two key ideas should be kept in mind: (1) although the vast majority of such cases will prove to be benign and self-limited, certain treatable and potentially dangerous conditions can present with diarrhea, and these conditions should be considered and screened for, and (2) even in garden-variety "viral gastroenteritis," the pathophysiologic disturbances of fluid and electrolyte imbalance may require special intervention, including hospitalization in severe cases. Because it is often more important to accurately assess the hydration and electrolyte status of a child with diarrhea than it is to arrive at a specific etiologic diagnosis, a discussion of dehydration and its management is needed, followed by an analysis of the different diarrheal syndromes and their causes.

DEHYDRATION

Dehydration is identified by a combination of features drawn from the history, physical examination, and laboratory tests. For example, a history of numerous liquid stools, perhaps combined with decreased fluid intake (perhaps caused by concomitant vomiting), would alert the clinician to the possible presence of dehydration and lead to a search for confirmatory evidence. Has the child's urine output been abnormally low? Does he seem thirsty? Dry mouth and sunken eyeballs are relatively early physical signs. In young infants in whom the cranial bones have not yet fused, a sunken anterior fontanelle may also be present. Signs of more advanced dehydration are apathy, rapid, thready pulse, decreased blood pressure, and cool extremities with blotchy discoloration.

The laboratory data may reveal an elevated blood urea nitrogen (BUN) and high urine specific gravity. Serum sodium may be low, normal, or high, and potassium may be low or normal. (However, there is undoubtedly a total body sodium and potassium depletion.)

For convenience, the extent of dehydration is estimated as 5%, 10%, or 15%. *Five percent dehydration* means that 5% of the child's weight has been lost acutely, mostly in the form of extracellular fluid. This is a clinical diagnosis based on a history of excessive stool losses. The only signs present at this stage would be thirst and perhaps dry mucous membranes. The diagnosis of *10% dehydration* requires that many of the physical signs discussed in the previous paragraph are present. These children are quite ill and need hospitalization. *Fifteen percent dehydration* implies impending or frank shock and is a critical emergency requiring urgent intervention.

5% Dehydration. The management of a child with diarrhea who is judged to be 5% dehydrated is initially conservative. A clear liquid diet is recommended; one of the commercially prepared oral electrolyte solutions such as Pedialyte or Lytren, or a home substitute such as Gatorade, liquid gelatine desserts, or decarbonated lemon-lime and cola drinks (the latter are perhaps best reserved for older children). After approximately 12 to 24 hours on this diet, a soy-based formula, such as Isomil or Prosobee, diluted 1:1 with water can be tried. The reason for this is that infants with acute diarrhea frequently develop a temporary lactose intolerance, and unlike cow's milk-based formulas, soy formulas do not contain this complex sugar. If the diluted soy formula does not provoke additional diarrhea, it can be offered full strength and the infant gradually returned to a normal diet. It sometimes takes several weeks for the lactose intolerance to resolve, however. Older infants and children whose normal diet does not consist mainly of milk or formula can be offered the BRAT diet following the clear liquid trial. This consists of Bananas, Rice cereal, Apples (be sure to include the peel, which contains pectin), and Toast.

10% Dehydration. The management of a child with 10% dehydration is more urgent. An intravenous line is started and parenteral hydration begun with normal or half normal saline. Potassium probably needs to be added to the infusion, but only after adequate renal function is established by the appearance of fresh urine. The details of parenteral fluid therapy are explained in an appendix to this chapter.

15% Dehydration. Fifteen percent dehydration means clinical shock, and requires urgent volume replacement. It is often difficult to find any veins in which to start an IV because of the extremely low central venous pressure and impending cardiovascular collapse. A cutdown may be necessary, or else a percutaneous central line may be attempted in the most urgent situations. Another technique in a true emergency is *bone clysis,* in which a large-bore needle is thrust directly into the marrow of the tibia and a rapid infusion of fluid made directly into the marrow, where it will be taken up by the bone's ample blood supply.

Etiology of Acute Diarrhea

The majority of cases of diarrhea in infancy and childhood turn out to be "nonspecific"; that is, no exact etiology is determined, and the assumption is that the cause is probably viral or perhaps some enteropathogenic strain of *Escherichia coli.* Usually the patient has passed numerous liquid brown or greenish brown stools, does not appear particularly ill (unless dehydration has supervened), and has a relatively nontender abdomen. Vomiting and fever may or may not be present. Management of this condition should be directed at preventing or treating dehydration. Antimotility drugs such as Lomotil and paregoric probably should not be used in young children, but some authorities feel that Pepto-Bismol or Kaopectate may be of some benefit.

Dysentery. The syndrome of *dysentery* consists of fever, considerable cramping abdominal pain, and the passage of numerous stools laced with mucus and sometimes blood (which may be evident only with the use of guaiac paper or a microscope). Usually, microscopic examination of the mucus reveals numerous pus cells, indicating that the process is inflammatory. Until recently, *Shigella* and *Salmonella* were considered the usual pathogens responsible for acute dysentery, but two newly discovered organisms, *Campylobacter fetus* and *Yersinia enterocolitica,* are appearing more frequently in published reports on the etiology of this syndrome. Stool or rectal swabs from children with dysentery should be sent to the laboratory for culture.

The question of antibiotic therapy arises here. *Shigella* generally responds to ampicillin (but not amoxicillin!) or trimethoprim/sulfamethoxasole; *Campylobacter* responds to erythromycin. The decision to treat these usually self-limited illnesses depends on the severity of the symptoms. Most authorities agree that acute diarrhea caused by *Salmonella* should not be treated with antibiotics, however, because such treatment prolongs the postrecovery carrier state and poses a threat to public health.

Four additional conditions that can occur with the dysentery syndrome, though comparatively rare, should be considered in severe or atypical cases: acute amebic colitis, acute ulcerative colitis or Crohn's disease, and antibiotic-induced pseudomembranous colitis. These diagnoses are usually made by proctosigmoidoscopy and require the consultation of a pediatric gastroenterologist.

Food Poisoning. Finally, diarrheal food poisoning should be mentioned in a discussion of watery diarrhea. The usual cause of this condition is the ingestion of food contaminated with *Salmonella, Clostridium perfringens,* or *Bacillus cereus.* The disease is self-limited and clinically differs little from nonspecific viral diarrhea; the major clue to the diagnosis is the presentation of the child within the context of a single-source outbreak. (Staphylococcal food poisoning presents chiefly with vomiting, not diarrhea.)

VOMITING SYNDROMES

Although diarrhea and vomiting frequently occur together in viral or bacterial enteric infections, vomiting sometimes occurs alone or is so prominent as to be the major manifestation of an illness. Interestingly, the etiology of such illness tends to be different from that of primarily diarrheal disease.

Etiology of Vomiting

Acute illness manifested chiefly by vomiting is generally caused by one of two viruses, the rotavirus and the "Norwalk agent." Among bacteria, some strains of enteropathogenic *E. Coli* seem to cause considerable vomiting as well.

- As was mentioned previously, *staphylococcal food poisoning* presents with vomiting, usually beginning shortly after ingestion of a tainted meal.

- *Intestinal obstruction* ultimately results in significant vomiting, but attention should be drawn to the correct diagnosis by concomitant abdominal pain and distention. One should not overlook the possible diagnosis of pyloric stenosis in a very young vomiting infant who may have no other signs or symptoms. This condition is discussed more fully in the section on abdominal pain.

- Children with *otitis media* frequently vomit for reasons that are unclear. The ears of vomiting infants, in particular, should be carefully examined for evidence of this disease.

- *Increased intracranial pressure* of any cause results in vomiting eventually. Children with this condition usually also complain of headaches and may have papilledema. Another, more benign syndrome of headaches and vomiting occurs in children with *migraine*. Neurologic consultation is frequently advisable.

Management of the Child Who Is Vomiting

Assuming that specific causes of vomiting such as intestinal obstruction and brain tumor have been ruled out, the major problem with a vomiting child is to maintain adequate hydration until the illness passes. It is recommended that a short period, perhaps 4 to 6 hours, of NPO should be observed initially in order to give the stomach a chance to "calm down." Afterward, minute amounts of clear liquids, perhaps as little as a teaspoonful at a time, should be offered to the child. Gradually, tolerance will develop and larger quantities of fluid may be given. Some authorities feel that a teaspoonful or two of Emetrol offered shortly before each attempted feeding increases the chance of its being retained. Other antiemetics, such as Tigan and Compazine, may be useful, but Compazine especially has an unacceptably high incidence of provoking acute dystonic reactions such as spasmodic torticollis and tonic conjugate gaze deviations. Any child who is absolutely unable to tolerate even carefully administered oral liquids, especially a child who also requires medications (such as for an associated otitis media), probably needs to be admitted for a short course of parenteral hydration.

FEVER AND INFECTIOUS DISEASE IN CHILDREN

The majority of fevers in children are caused by self-limited viral infections (examples: viral upper respiratory infections, viral gastroenteritis). However, fever can also be present in many treatable bacterial infections and a few surgical conditions. It is essential to be able to identify these, and it will be found that the history and physical examination yield the most important clues to the etiology of febrile illnesses. On the basis of the history and physical examination, appropriate laboratory tests such as white blood count and differential, urinalysis, and chest x-ray may be ordered.

Normal body temperature is usually defined as 37°C or 98.6°F, measured orally. However, temperature follows a circadian rhythm, peaking in the late afternoon and early evening and reaching its lowest point in the very early morning hours before a person rises.

Another variable in the assessment of a child's temperature is the route by which it is taken. Rectal temperatures are generally 0.5°C higher and axillary temperatures 0.5°C lower than oral temperatures. Finally, infants tend to run higher basal temperatures than older children and adults. In one study, 50% of 18 month olds had daily temperature maxima in excess of 37.8°C (100°F) while remaining well.

TRIAGE

In general, temperatures lower than 38.9°C (102°F) are unlikely to require intervention.* However, children who appear ill and have high fevers should be treated even before a definitive diagnosis has been made. Once a high temperature (say, 39.5°C [103°F] and above) has been documented, it is good practice in many centers to begin applying fever control measures at once, usually after notifying the physician, who may wish to see the child while the high fever is still present. Fever by itself can cause many symptoms that would be considered very serious in its absence, such as lethargy, irritability, tachypnea, and headache. It may be helpful to see the child once the temperature has come down several degrees, so as to assess the respiratory pattern and the level of consciousness and playfulness. For this reason, after initial assessment of a child with a high fever (including a detailed history of recent use of antipyretics at home), the administration of acetaminophen or aspirin in the dose of 1 gr per year of age is recommended. The oral route is preferred unless the child is vomiting, in which case rectal suppositories are available. If the fever is quite high (in the range 40°C [104°F] and above) it is wise to supplement the medication with tepid water sponge baths.

Another important practice that is sometimes neglected is the routine application of urine catching bags to febrile infants at the time of initial assessment. Thus, when the child urinates because of the stimulation of the examination, a ready urinalysis specimen will be available should it be deemed necessary, and much time saved.

Except for very high fevers (greater than 41.1°C [106°F]), fever *per se* is seldom dangerous, although many parents wrongly regard the high temperature as a great emergency. Most febrile seizures will probably already have occurred by the time the child presents to the emergency department. Hence the principal justification for applying fever control

---

* We are speaking only of fever control here. Of course, a child may be quite ill with a temperature below 38.9°C (102°F), and some of the sickest children are in fact hypothermic.

measures in the emergency department is to make the child more comfortable and to provide the examiner with a child whose illness can be viewed clearly, uncomplicated by the additional signs of lethargy, irritability, and tachypnea that fever itself may cause.

CLUES TO THE PRESENCE OF TREATABLE BACTERIAL INFECTIONS

Respiratory Syndromes

These are illnesses characterized by cough, sore throat, runny nose or eyes, ear pain, myalgias, and arthralgias, and fever, either as isolated symptoms or in any combination. Most are due to benign, self-limited viral infections. However, a number of important bacterial infections can present with these symptoms as well.

Streptococcal Pharyngitis, or Strep Throat

The only sure way to diagnose this condition is to obtain a throat culture positive for group A β-hemolytic streptococci. However, it is frequently advisable in the emergency department setting to begin treatment before the results of this culture are known. Clinical clues to the likelihood of streptococcal infection are:

1. A strep epidemic in the community or known exposure of the patient to a documented sporadic case
2. Inflamed pharynx with enlarged tonsils covered with whitish exudate
3. Swollen, tender anterior cervical nodes (this has the best correlation with positive strep cultures)
4. Fever
5. Associated ear pain
6. Abdominal pain

Streptococcal pharyngitis is rare in infants under the age of 2 years. Streptococcal infection is usually manifested as a purulent rhinitis in this younger age group.

While it is sometimes judged more cost-effective to treat certain patients with the above symptoms with penicillin (or erythromycin, if penicillin allergy is present) without even taking a throat culture, children with recurrent episodes of pharyngitis should definitely be cultured because the question of tonsillectomy may hinge on whether repeated streptococcal infections can be *documented*.

- Don't forget to consider infectious mononucleosis in the differential diagnosis of this condition in older children and adolescents.

Otitis Media

Otitis media is probably the most commonly diagnosed bacterial infection in children. This condition results from contamination of the middle ear with microorganisms that are introduced through the nasopharynx and eustachian tube. Consequently, otitis media is frequently superimposed on a viral upper respiratory infection in which the nasopharyngeal-eustachean function is compromised and normal drainage of the middle ear is impaired. It is common for a child who has had a runny nose but who has appeared basically well for 1 to 2 days to suddenly become ill with high fever and irritability, which marks the onset of otitis media. Some children do not demonstrate this upper respiratory prodrome however, and diagnosis depends on the physical examination.

Assessment/Diagnosis. In the history, older children complain of otalgia, but since most children with otitis media are infants, a patient's chief complaint is seldom available. Parents of infants may complain that their child has been irritable, febrile, refusing feedings, possibly vomiting, and pulling at the ears.

On physical examination, the tympanic membranes appear inflamed and occasionally are bulging. Retracted tympanic membranes are sometimes seen. Sometimes tympanic membrane perforation will have occurred and the canal will be filled with purulent debris. The child is usually irritable, but the degree of irritability is less than with meningitis, and he can usually be consoled by holding and rocking, especially after the fever has been brought down with the use of antipyretics and sponging.

Treatment. Treatment of otitis media depends on a knowledge of the bacteria that commonly cause this kind of infection in the various age groups, since infectious material is rarely available for culture except in cases of tympanic membrane perforation or diagnostic tympanocentesis. In the age group most at risk for otitis media (2 months to 5 years) the usual organisms are *Streptococcus pneumoniae* (the pneumococcus), *Hemophilus influenzae,* and, in older children, group A β-hemolytic streptococci. Antibiotic coverage should be arranged for all of these organisms in most cases. Ampicillin or its derivative amoxicillin is usually satisfactory. In certain areas, ampicillin-resistant strains of *H. influenzae* are appearing, and this is an important cause of treatment failures. In such situations, as well as for initial therapy in children allergic to penicillins, a combination of sulfa and erythromycin (available in fixed combination as Pediazole) is useful. Also effective are trimethoprim-sulfamethoxisole combinations (Bactrim, Septra). Cefaclor (Ceclor), a newly introduced cephalosporin antibiotic, also appears to be quite effective for broad-spectrum coverage of middle ear infections.

In neonates, otitis media can be caused by a variety of other organisms such as *Staphylococcus* and gram-negative enteric organisms, as well as by the usual offenders. Any serious infection in the neonatal age group must be managed in consultation with a pediatrician (see discussion below).

Pneumonia

Some children with ''bad colds'' have pneumonia, and it is not always easy to differentiate this group on physical findings alone. Depending on the availability of follow-up, emergency department personnel will have to be more or less liberal in their use of chest radiographs for suspicious cases. Pneumonias in children are most frequently caused by viruses, but *Streptococcus pneumoniae, H. influenzae, Staphylococcus aureus,* and occasionally other organisms can be found. In children over the age of 5 years, *Mycoplasma pneumoniae* is an important cause of pneumonia. Therefore, in younger children, one can generally follow the guidelines for antibiotic therapy for otitis media, whereas in older children erythromycin becomes a more useful drug.

Meningitis

The reason for so much emphasis on the proper diagnosis and treatment of upper respiratory infections in children is the fear that they may spread to involve the CNS in a devastating infection like meningitis. Many children develop meningitis within the context of another infection such as nasopharyngitis or otitis media. However, this is not always necessary or apparent at the time of initial presentation. The cardinal sign of meningitis in children is alteration of the level of consciousness. These babies may be hyperirritable, or alternatively they may be somnolent. Not infrequently, a convulsion heralds the onset of the disease. Most of them are febrile, and beyond 6 months of age, one may hope to find nuchal rigidity, but this is an inconstant and sometimes late sign. Additional signs may include bulging fontanelle in younger infants or papilledema in older ones, both signs of increased intracranial pressure.

Meningitis is a life-threatening infection, and the diagnosis and treatment of this condition constitute top priority in pediatric emergency medicine. The definitive diagnosis can be made only by lumbar puncture and examination of the cerebrospinal fluid. In cases of bacterial meningitis, large numbers of leukocytes will be found, along with smaller numbers of organisms on gram stain. The index of suspicion for meningitis must always be high in an emergency department. One commonly hears the expression, "If you think of doing a spinal tap, do it!" This expression should be modified. When confronted with an irritable, febrile child, one should *always* ask, "Does this child have meningitis?" Then one can specifically examine the child for evidence of excessive irritability and other signs from the history and physical examination that would make him a candidate for a spinal tap. As noted above, this is sometimes made much easier by first taking measures to cool the child and then observing him after the temperature has fallen several degrees. Remember that the child's best interests are always served by having a low threshold for performing a diagnostic lumbar puncture in cases of suspected meningitis.

Beyond the neonatal age group, the usual organisms found in bacterial meningitis are *H. influenzae, Streptococcus pneumoniae,* and *Neisseria meningitidis.* Treatment for suspected cases of bacterial meningitis should be begun as soon as purulent fluid is seen during a lumbar puncture. Ampicillin is usually effective against all three commonly implicated organisms and should be administered intravenously at once. In addition, because of the growing threat of ampicillin-resistant *H. influenzae,* chloramphenicol is administered as well, pending culture and sensitivity testing. A pediatrician or pediatric infectious disease specialist should be consulted if there is any doubt.

In the neonatal age group, bacterial meningitis is caused by a large variety of organisms, principally gram-negative enteric rods, *Listeria,* and group B β-hemolytic streptococcus. Generally a penicillin combined with an aminoglycoside is effective, but a pediatrician should always be consulted in cases of neonatal meningitis.

FEVER ASSOCIATED WITH ABDOMINAL SIGNS

Children with fever and vomiting or diarrhea as the principal symptoms usually have viral acute gastroenteritis, a self-limited illness (management of which has previously been discussed in the section on abdominal pain). However, the following causative factors should be considered and ruled out:

- Bacterial causes of gastroenteritis, such as *Salmonella* and *Shigella.* Bacterial dysentery is an enteroinvasive process, and patients are therefore toxic, often with high fevers. They are quite uncomfortable because of abdominal cramping. The stools are frequently laced with nonbloody or bloody mucus packed with white blood cells. The final diagnosis depends on the results of stool culture.

- Another important cause of fever and abdominal pain that should always be considered and ruled out is acute appendicitis. This condition has been discussed above under the heading abdominal pain.

- Hepatitis and pneumonia (especially lower lobe pneumonia) are two rare causes of abdominal pain and fever that should be considered given the right clinical circumstances.

- Finally, every child with fever and abdominal complaints should have a urinalysis performed to rule out cystitis or pyelonephritis.

FEVER WITHOUT LOCALIZING SIGNS

Not infrequently, a child will present to the emergency department with high fever and the absence of specific, localizing symptoms and signs. Specifically, this means no sign of respiratory infection, including normal tympanic membranes and a normal chest x-ray; a nontender abdomen with a normal urinalysis; and normal skin and extremities. In many cases the etiology of such an illness will declare itself within 1 to 2 days by the appearance of a rash typical of a certain virus. Sometimes the child simply gets well without any specific therapy. Alternatively, the appearance of diarrhea or vomiting may mark this as a case of gastroenteritis. An ear infection may develop, or strep throat, or pneumonia. Septic arthritis or osteomyelitis may be difficult to detect at first. The child should be examined carefully for extremity tenderness and observed for such subtle signs as failure to use an arm or leg normally.

The best course in such confusing cases is frequently to withhold antibiotics until a specific etiology can be determined. This implies the need for careful follow-up. Although this plan is surely ideal and would be supported by infectious disease specialists, in the real world it often happens that a clinician faced with a somewhat ill-appearing child with a high fever and under tremendous parental pressure to "do something" feels compelled to use broad-spectrum antibiotics, not knowing quite what it is he is trying to treat but hoping that if anything is there, he will "hit" it. Recently a new wrinkle has been added to this debate by the emergence in the literature of a newly discovered phenomenon known as *occult sepsis.*

Occult Sepsis in Newborns. It has long been known that infants newly born up to about 2 months of age require special handling at even the slightest hint of infection. In fact, in this special age group few decisions need to be made in the emergency department if fever greater than 38°C (100.4°F) can be documented. It is standard practice in pediatric centers all over the country to admit such babies to the hospital with the intention of ruling out sepsis, pending negative results of blood, urine, and cerebrospinal fluid cultures. Often, treatment with broad-spectrum antibiotics is begun as well. The reason for this is twofold: These babies localize infections poorly and are quite prone to generalized sepsis and they may look remarkably well only hours before going into bacteremic shock. The organisms usually implicated are the same as those for neonatal meningitis, but each geographic area seems to have its own special organisms, so a knowledgeable pediatrician should always be consulted when planning the care of a sick infant. If the baby remains well for two or three days in the hospital and cultures are negative, the child can be released with a diagnosis of probable self-limited viral infection.

Occult Sepsis in Older Infants. Interest has recently been focused on the management of older infants in the age group 3 months to 2 years who present with fever and no localizing signs. It has been discovered that in instances in which the temperature is greater than 39°C (102.2°F), there is a distressingly high incidence of positive blood cultures (usually for *Streptococcus pneumoniae*). In these studies, babies with positive cultures tended to have high white blood counts (greater than 15,000) and elevated erythrocyte sedimentation rates.

Surprisingly, many of these infants do quite well even when treatment is withheld, spontaneously clearing their bloodstreams of the organisms; however, some develop focal infections such as otitis media, pneumonia, or even meningitis.

Although research in this area is continuing, it is likely that we all need to be much more careful with infants in this age group who have high fevers, especially if they appear at all ill or if other laboratory work is abnormal. Blood cultures should be strongly considered and the question of antibiotic therapy should be raised, but bear in mind the apparent degree of illness of the child and the likelihood of good follow-up.

BIBLIOGRAPHY

Biller JA, Yeager AM: The Harriet Lane Handbook, 9th ed. Chicago, Year Book Medical Publishers, 1981

Ferrara A, Anantham H: Emergency Transfer of the High Risk Neonate. St. Louis, CV Mosby, 1980

Fleisher G, Ludwig S: Textbook of Pediatric Emergency Medicine, Baltimore, Williams & Wilkins, 1983

Graef JW, Cone TE (eds): Manual of Pediatric Therapeutics, 2nd ed. Boston, Little, Brown & Co, 1980

Hughes WT, Buescher ES: Pediatric Procedures, 2nd ed. Philadelphia, WB Saunders, 1980

Reece RM (ed): Reece-Chamberlain Manual of Emergency Pediatrics, 2nd ed. WB Saunders, 1978

APPENDIX D: CALCULATING PEDIATRIC FLUID AND ELECTROLYTE REQUIREMENTS

Parenteral therapy becomes necessary when the patient is unable to tolerate oral fluids, perhaps because of vomiting or because he is NPO awaiting or recovering from surgery, or when pre-existing fluid or electrolyte derangements mandate a carefully controlled infusion. The daily fluid requirement for an ill patient must take into account three factors: (1) normal maintenance requirements, (2) pre-existing deficits or excesses, and in some cases (3) ongoing abnormal losses. In the following discussion we will focus on the first two factors in helping us decide how to "hang the first bottle."

MAINTENANCE REQUIREMENTS

The maintenance requirement replenishes the water and electrolytes that are normally lost each day in the urine, stool, and sweat, and through "insensible losses."* Various complicated methods of deriving the daily maintenance requirement are available based on physiologic considerations such as renal function and metabolic rate. Fortunately, a much simpler method, based on the patient's weight, is

---

* *Insensible* refers to water lost mainly by way of exhaled air during respiration.

available that, although only an approximation, is considered accurate for most clinical applications.

For H_2O 100 ml/kg/day for 1st 10 kg of body weight
             50 ml/kg/day for 2nd 10 kg of body weight
             20 ml/kg/day for each additional kg of body weight after 20 kg

For Na   3 mEq/100 ml H_2O calculated
For K   2 mEq/100 ml H_2O calculated

Example: calculate the maintenance requirement for 24 hours for a 25-kg 8 year old.

For H_2O
  100 ml/kg × 10 kg = 1000 ml (for 1st 10 kg)
   50 ml/kg × 10 kg = 500 ml (for 2nd 10 kg)
   20 ml/kg × <u> 5 kg</u> = <u>100 ml</u> (for remaining 5 kg)
           25 kg   1600 ml (total H_2O maintenance
                           requirement for 24 hr)

For Na   3 mEq Na/100 ml H_2O × 1600 ml H_2O = 3 × 16 = 48 mEq Na required

For K   2 mEq K/100 ml H_2O × 1600 ml H_2O = 2 × 16 = 32 mEq/K required

Total is therefore 1600 ml H_2O with 48 mEq Na and 32 mEq K added. This is the same as saying 1600 ml H_2O with NaCl at 30 mEq/L and KCl at 20 mEq/L. D_5 0.2 NS contains Na at 34 mEq/L, which is close enough for most clinical purposes.

Principle: in general, we may use a stock solution of D_5 0.2 NS + 20 mEq KCl/L for normal maintenance requirements. We then need only calculate the volume required based on the patient's weight.

DEFICIT THERAPY

Most pediatric patients requiring intravenous therapy are dehydrated and require that pre-existing deficits be made up at the same time that ongoing maintenance losses are replenished. The calculation of the deficit depends on an estimation of the patients losses based on the history and physical signs. In practice, the deficit is estimated at 5%, 10%, or 15%, as follows:

At *5% dehydration,* physical signs are minimal to absent. This diagnosis is supported by a history of increased output (as in diarrheal stool) or significantly decreased intake (as in vomiting). The child may be thirsty and mucous membranes somewhat dry to the touch.

At *10% dehydration,* the children are already quite ill. They are lethargic with poor skin turgor and possible "tenting." The eyeballs may be sunken and mucous membranes quite dry. Urine output is considerably decreased and has a high specific gravity.

At *15% dehydration* all of the above signs are present with superimposed signs of shock or impending shock, such as weak, thready pulse, fall in blood pressure to the point that it cannot be measured, cool skin, and so forth. Example: calculate the daily fluid requirement for the first 24 hours for a 20-kg child judged to be 10% dehydrated. First, calculate the maintenance requirement.

For H_2O $100 \times 10 = 1000$ (first 10 kg)
                $\underline{50 \times 10} = \underline{500}$ (second 10 kg)
                20   1500 ml (total maintenance H_2O)

For Na $3 \times 15 = 45$ mEq Na required

For K $2 \times 15 = 30$ mEq K required

Next, calculate the deficit. The patient, who weighs 20 kg, is 10% dehydrated, which means that he has lost 10% of the body weight acutely. Ten percent of 20 kg is 2 kg, which translates into 2 L of fluid (1 L H_2O weighs 1 kg by definition).

What is the probable electrolyte composition of this 2 liters of lost fluid? It depends on a number of factors, such as route and rate of loss, recent intake, and the extent of renal Na retention. As an approximation, we can estimate the usual losses due to diarrhea, vomiting, or diabetic ketoacidosis as 110 mEq Na/L of fluid lost. Therefore, the patient's deficit is

H_2O	2000 ml
Na	110 mEq/L $\times$ 2 L = 220 mEq

(We omit a detailed discussion of K losses for the moment. Most of these patients have significant K deficits that must be replenished over a period of several days. It is generally sufficient to supply 30 to 40 mEq/L in the early bottles and watch the serum K carefully). Combining the maintenance and deficit calculations, assuming a complete replacement of the deficit over the first 24 hours, we arrive at a total 24 hour requirement for this patient as follows:

	H_2O	Na
Maintenance	1500 ml	45 mEq
Deficit	2000 ml	220 mEq
Total	3500 ml	265 mEq

3500 ml H_2O with 265 mEq of Na added works out to 3.5 L of H_2O with a final Na concentration of 76 mEq/L. The standard solution 0.45% NaCl, sometimes called half normal saline, contains Na in a concentration of 77 mEq/L.

Principle: in general, we may use a stock solution of $D_5\frac{1}{2}NS + 30$ mEq/L KCl for therapy in children who are judged to be 10% dehydrated.

Sometimes the patient is in such poor condition at the outset of therapy that the foregoing method is too slow. In such cases, one-half of the deficit can be given over the first 8 hours and the remainder over the next 16. In even more severe cases, we can push 10 to 20 ml/kg of an extracellular fluid expander such as normal saline, Ringer's lactate, or even 5% plasma protein fraction (Plasmanate) or Albuminsol.

(For practice, the reader may work out the proper way to manage a child who is 5% dehydrated. It will be found that the solution called for approximates 0.3% NaCl, which contains 46 mEq/L NaCl.)

HYPERNATREMIC DEHYDRATION

This special case calls for great care in the initial stages of therapy because overvigorous rehydration can cause cerebral edema and seizures. Clinical clues to the presence of hypernatremia are
- Occurence in winter
- Relative preservation of the extracellular and intravascular spaces, which leads to better urine output than would be expected for the degree of illness. Also the skin tends not to tent but may have a doughy consistency.
- Extreme irritability.

Of course, the final diagnosis depends on laboratory determination of the serum sodium.

The significance of identifying this condition is that rehydration should proceed *slowly*. In general, it is sufficient to perform the calculations as in the earlier examples, but to replace the deficit over 48 hours rather than 24. This slow rate of replacement is more important than the actual composition of the fluid used. Usually, $\frac{1}{3}$ normal saline will do. Note also that there is a tendency toward significant acidosis and occasional hyperglycemia in this condition. (Therefore, beware the constellation of hyperglycemia, acidosis, and dehydration in a young child who presents with significant diarrhea. You may be dealing with hypernatremic dehydration and not diabetic ketoacidosis!)

28
BURNS

LOUIS C. CLOUTIER and FLORENCE DZIEKAN

A burn is an injury to tissues caused by the application of physical agents. This definition includes frostbite and cold injuries, as well as burns caused by electricity, chemicals, ionizing radiation (x-ray), and heat.

Environmental injuries due to exposure to heat, cold, and radiation are discussed in Chapter 29. The most common burns are those caused by heat applied in the form of solid contact, as from a hot iron or other hot object, by hot fluids, or by flash, most commonly secondary to burning clothing.*

A burn that involves a large percentage of body surface is one of the most severe traumas that can occur to a living organism. The primary organ injured is the skin, which in terms of volume and weight is the largest organ of the body.

The functions of the skin include prevention of invasion of the body by microorganisms, separation of the fluid internal environment from the dry external environment, protection of the deeper structures from trauma, regulation of the body temperature, provision of an elastic covering for the motion of bones and joints, and, not least, beauty or aesthetic value of the individual. All of these functions are compromised by a severe burn, and each of these functions must be considered in the care of the burn.

ASSESSMENT: BURN EVALUATION

The seriousness of the burn is influenced by many factors, including total area and depth, the patient's age and previous medical history, the presence of pulmonary injury, the location of body burns, and associated injuries.

Area of Burn. A general, rapid determination of burn area can be made by using the rule of nines (Fig. 28-1). According to this system, all body areas are divided into percentages or multiples of nine. Figures for each body area are estimated and added to determine the total percentage of body burned. In more extensive burns, one can estimate the *unburned* area and subtract the number from 100% to check the accuracy of the burn area estimate. Overestimation of the extent of injury is common. Smaller burned areas can be estimated with the palm of the hand, which is considered equivalent to 1%.

The rule of nines is adapted for infants and young children with the following changes: the head equals 18%, each leg 14%, and no allocation is made for the genitalia (Fig. 28-2). Surface burn areas according to age can be more accurately calculated as specified in Fig. 28-3. Precise estimates are not necessary in the earliest phases of care: such calculations become more important after initial resuscitation measures have been implemented.

The rule of nines or other surface burn area charts are not helpful for assessing burn extent in electrical burns: surface burn area is small and unpredictable relative to total burn injury.

* Most severe burns are associated with burning clothing. For this reason, the American Burn Association has instituted a program for compiling statistics on the clothes of burn victims, for use in lobbying for legislation to require that clothes be made flame retardant.

Depth of Burn. It may be impossible initially to determine the depth of the burn. Between the extremes of burn depth there is a wide intermediate range where diagnosis is neither possible nor absolutely necessary. The usual classification of depth and burn injury is as follows:
- *First degree*—erythema without actual blistering or desquamation of skin
- *Second degree*—partial-thickness destruction of skin usually with blistering at some time during the course of the wound's history. Variation in depth may be considerable.
- *Third degree*—full-thickness destruction of skin. This may also include a destruction of tissue deep into the skin.

Characteristics of partial- and full-thickness burns are outlined in Table 28-1. Every effort to prevent a partial-thickness burn from becoming a full-thickness burn will considerably decrease the time needed for the recovery and rehabilitation of the patient. Prompt cooling, gentle handling, and the use of aseptic technique are especially important to reaching this goal.

Age. The young and the elderly are subject to higher morbidity and mortality from burns than are young adults. The need for prompt and precise resuscitation is also proportionally greater. Listed in the order of decreasing mortality from burns are the following age groups:
1. 60 years and over
2. 0–1 and 50–59 years
3. 2–4 and 35–49 years
4. 5–34 years

Medical History. The previous medical history is especially significant when the burn injury is complicated by the presence of diabetes or other metabolic diseases, peripheral vascular disease, heart disease, chronic pulmonary disease, or the habitual use of drugs or alcohol. Pertinent information is sometimes provided by family, or by fire department, police, and emergency medical personnel at the scene of injury.

Pulmonary Injury. The presence of pulmonary injury is serious.
1. *Smoke inhalation* is highly probable (97%) when two of the following are present:
   - A fire in a closed space
   - Carbonaceous sputum
   - Blood carbon monoxide greater than 10 mg/dl
2. *Thermal injury to the airway* is likely (95%) when there is:
   - An explosion
   - A flash or steam injury with head and neck burns

Environmental circumstances surrounding the injury should alert emergency personnel to the likelihood of pulmonary injury, as will the physical findings of singed nasal hairs, mucosal burns of the nose or mouth, voice change, and respiratory distress with wheezing and productive cough. (See Chap. 15, Respiratory Emergencies, for assessment and treatment.)

Location of Burn. Even small burns may be serious when they involve the eyes, face, hands, feet, and anal or genital areas. The potential loss of function when such areas are

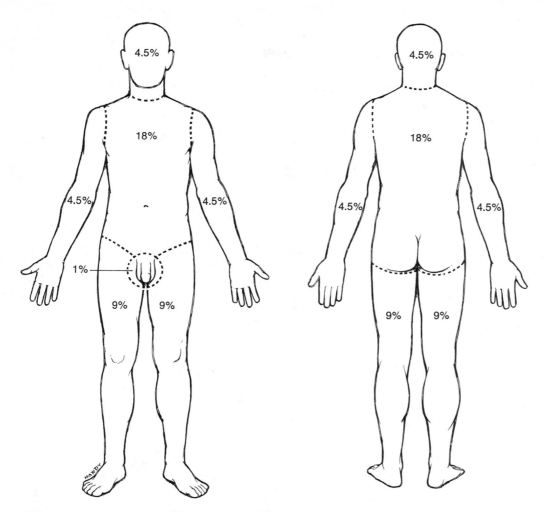

Figure 28-1 *The rule of nines. The diagram of the body surface may be used to estimate the percentage of burned body area.*

Figure 28-2 *Percentage distribution for infant or small child using modified rule of nines. Values for the head and legs are changed from the rule of nines for the adult to reflect proportions in infants and children.*

affected and the need for intensive nursing care may require hospitalization and rehabilitation.

Associated Injuries.   Associated injuries such as fractures, severe trauma, and the systemic effects of electrical injury may further complicate rescue, resuscitation, and recovery.

PREHOSPITAL CARE

Though the burned victim cannot be stabilized in the field, what is done immediately affects patient outcome significantly.

PRIORITIES OF IMMEDIATE CARE

Priorities of immediate care are as follows: (1) stop the burning process; (2) examine the patient and treat injuries;

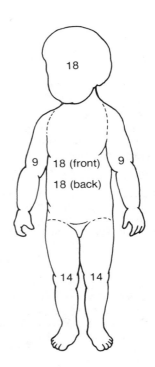

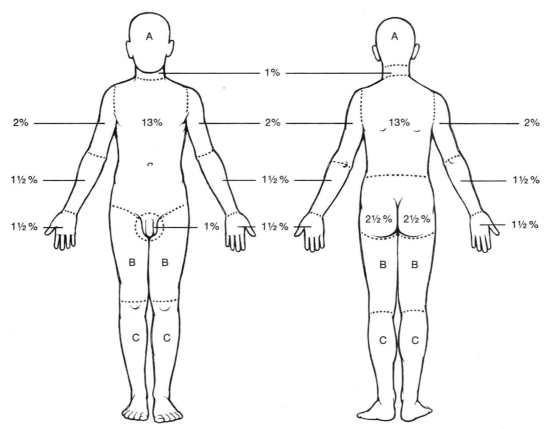

Figure 28-3 The effects of growth on the relative percentages of body surface areas. Areas designated by numbers (reflecting percentage of body area) remain relatively stable throughout life. Areas designated by a letter (A, B, and C) represent percentages of the total body surface area that vary from birth to adult life. The table below indicates the relative percentages of these body surface areas at various stages in life.

| | Age in Years | | | | | |
Area	0	1	5	10	15	Adult
A: ½ of head	9½	8½	6½	5½	4½	3½
B: ½ of one thigh	2¾	3¼	4	4½	4½	4¾
C: ½ of one lower leg	2½	2½	2¾	3	3¼	3½

(3) transport the patient; and (4) assess and treat burn wounds.

1. *Stop the burning process.* (Method varies according to type of burn: thermal, chemical, electrical.)

   • *Thermal burns.* Put the fire out by smothering or drowning it with water. The patient can roll on the ground or on any surface to smother the flames, or he may be wrapped in a blanket or other clothing to extinguish the fire initially. Take care to leave the face exposed so that toxic substances from burning clothes are not inhaled. Avoid contamination from dirt and foreign substances as much as possible, but the first priority always is to extinguish the fire.

   Cool the burn. The burning process must be stopped rapidly to prevent extension of burn area and depth. Immersion in cold water until pain relief occurs or until the burned area feels cool is ideal.

   Avoid overcooling, especially with burns covering a large body area. Once the burning has stopped, the patient's body heat must be maintained to help treat the inevitable shock that occurs with large body burns. After clothing is removed, the victim is wrapped in a clean, preferably sterile, sheet and blanket if necessary or an aluminum blanket (space blanket) to maintain body heat.

   Remove all clothing, including jewelry, belts, shoes, and other items that can become constrictive as edema forms. Cut around clothing that is adhering to the skin but do not attempt to remove it. Adhering clothing can be removed by hospital personnel under better conditions.

   • *Chemical burns.* Chemical burns must be flooded immediately with copious amounts of water until the chemical is removed—15–20 minutes is the general recommended time. Remove clothing during the flushing process. Chemicals in powder form may be brushed off the skin or the clothing removed before flushing. In some instances, water is contraindicated, since some chemicals used in industry react with water; employees can inform emergency responders about treatment for specific chemical exposures. Also contraindicated are neutralizing agents, which produce more heat and subsequent tissue damage through their neutralizing action. A standard hazard signal system has been developed that identifies hazardous materials and indicates numerically and by color the type and degree of envi-

TABLE 28-1. EVALUATION OF DEPTH OF A BURN

Degree	Cause of Burn	Skin Involvement	Symptoms	Appearance	Course
Superficial (First)	Sunburn Low-intensity flash	Epidermis	Tingling Hyperesthesia Painful Soothed by cooling	Reddened; blanches with pressure Minimal or no edema	Complete recovery within a week Peeling
Partial thickness (Second)	Scalds Flash flame	Epidermis and part of dermis	Painful Hyperesthesia Sensitive to cold air	Blistered, mottled red base, broken epidermis, weeping surface Edema	Recovery in 2 to 3 weeks Some scarring and depigmentation Infection may convert to third degree
Full thickness (Third)	Fire Prolonged exposure to hot liquids	Epidermis, entire dermis, and sometimes subcutaneous tissue	Painless Symptoms of shock Hematuria and hemolysis of blood likely	Dry; pale white or charred Broken skin with fat exposed Edema	Eschar sloughs Grafting necessary Scarring and loss of contour and function

(Brunner LS, Suddarth DS: Textbook of Medical-Surgical Nursing, 4th ed. Philadelphia, JB Lippincott, 1980)

ronmental hazard associated with exposure. Methods of handling are specified. The symbols used are shown in Figure 28-4.

- *Electrical burns.* Electrical burns must be stopped by disconnecting the electrical current from the victim. Safety of the rescuer is most important. If the power can be turned off, this is ideal. If not, the rescuer should stand on a dry, non-conductive surface and use non-conductive material (*i.e.,* wood, cloth) to remove the

victim from the source or the source from the victim. Downed electrical wires and other complicated rescue situations may require assistance from the local power company or other public safety agencies to ensure safe rescue.

2. *Examine the patient and treat injuries.*

- Ensure that airway, breathing, and circulation (ABCs) are intact. Respiratory distress may develop rapidly from inhalation of smoke and toxic substances, requiring

Figure 28-4 Standard hazard signal system for identifying hazardous materials. Flammability is indicated by the color red, health by blue, and reactivity by yellow. (Reprinted with permission from NFPA 704-1980, Standard System for the Identification of the Fire Hazards of Materials, Copyright © 1980, National Fire Protection Association, Quincy, Massachusetts 02269. This reprinted material is not the complete and official position of the NFPA on the referenced subject, which is represented only by the standard in its entirety.)

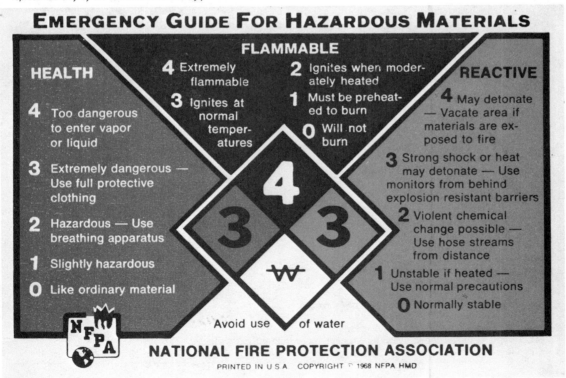

administration of high-flow humidified oxygen. Cardiac and respiratory arrest is a major problem with electrical burns.

- After the patient's ABCs are assessed and treated, obtain baseline vital signs and assess for other injuries—fractures, lacerations, head, chest, or abdominal trauma.
- If the person is unconscious, look for causes other than burns. The victim may have fallen, jumped, or been thrown, producing less obvious but serious injuries.
- Treat injuries appropriately (*e.g.,* splint fractures) and prepare the victim for prompt transport to the appropriate facility.
- When resources are available and the patient has large body burns, begin IV therapy with Ringer's lactate through large-bore catheters.

3. *Transport the patient.*

- Selection of the treatment facility is determined by the extent of injury and by available community resources (Table 28-2).
- Ideally, the patient can be transported to the appropriate facility at once. However, when travel times are longer, and prehospital personnel trained to begin intravenous therapy are not available, the critically burned victim must be taken to the nearest hospital for resuscitation and stabilization.

4. *Assess and treat burn wounds.*

- Make a general assessment of burn area and depth (see Figs. 28-1 through 28-3).
- Burn wounds may be dressed en route, time permitting.
- Thermal and chemical burns are covered with sterile, saline-soaked dressings in order to facilitate ease of removal without further trauma, then dry dressings to prevent contamination.
- Electrical burn wounds are covered with dry, sterile dressings. Since the burned surface area is small, minimal adherence occurs, and dry dressings prevent movement of contamination to the deeper injured structures.
- *No ointments are ever applied* in the prehospital phase of burn wound care.
- Handle burn wounds gently; avoid breaking blisters or manipulating injured part(s).

HOSPITAL CARE

Upon arrival at the emergency department an initial assessment is made of the patient's general status, burn area and depth, and whether definite care can be given at the receiving hospital or the patient will require transfer to a burn facility. When the patient has critical burns, resuscitation measures are promptly instituted and the patient is prepared for transfer to a facility for definitive care as his condition permits.

INITIAL MANAGEMENT OF PATIENT WITH MAJOR OR CRITICAL BURNS

As soon as it is known that a burn victim, especially one with extensive injury, is en route, alert the burn unit to the potential arrival (either locally or at a distant point) of the patient. Have necessary supplies and equipment ready. (Chart 28-1.) Upon the patient's arrival, his assessment and initial resuscitation proceed simultaneously.

1. *Resuscitation measures*

- Sterile technique is mandatory for all personnel in contact with patient; use masks, sterile gowns, and gloves
- Assess ABCs and support as needed.
  Obtain baseline chest x-ray and vital signs.
- Begin fluid resuscitation.
  Establish 1 or 2 large-bore intravenous lines; cutdown may be necessary.
  Avoid areas with circumferential burns, since the developing edema will impede the intravenous flow.
- Administer Ringer's lactate or similar plasma expander.
- Calculate fluid volume by using the following formula: % burned area × patient's weight (kg) × 3 = IV fluid for 24 h
- Administer half of fluid in the first 8 hours and the remaining half in the next 16 hours. (If there has been a delay in starting intravenous fluids, a more rapid rate of infusion for the first hour or two may be necessary.)

2. Obtain blood samples for laboratory analysis before beginning intravenous infusions: complete blood count

---

TABLE 28-2. GUIDE TO SELECTION OF MEDICAL FACILITY FOR OPTIMAL MANAGEMENT OF PATIENT WITH THERMAL INJURIES

Classification	Type and Extent of Burn	Facility for Treatment
Minor	• Second degree less than 10%	Outpatient or general hospital
Major	• Second degree less than 20% • Third degree less than 10% • Minor burns of the hands, feet, face, genitalia • Less than 2 years of age • More than 45 years of age	Community hospital
Critical	• Second degree more than 30% • Third degree more than 15% • Minor burns associated with other traumatic injuries • Burns associated with inhalation injury • Burns in patients with pre-existing disease • Major burns in patients less than 10 years and more than 30 years old • Burns involving muscle, electrical injuries, or chemical injuries	Burn center

(CBC), electrolytes, urinalysis, blood type and cross-match, arterial blood gases, creatinine and blood urea nitrogen (BUN), carboxyhemoglobin.

3. Insert indwelling urinary catheter, obtain specimen for urinary analysis, and monitor urinary output.
   - Output rates should be as follows:
     Adult—30–60 ml/hr
     Child—1 ml/kg/hr
     Cardiac, geriatric patient—15–30 ml/hr

4. Insert nasogastric tube to decompress stomach and connect to low suction. (Most critical burn victims develop ileus and abdominal distention.)

Ongoing Care

- Monitor vital signs, central venous pressure when indicated, and urinary output at regular intervals.
- Consider ECG.
- Weigh patient when feasible.
- Control pain.
  Administer narcotics in small doses and always intravenously. Monitor cardiorespiratory status carefully.
- Administer tetanus immunization.
- Treat burn wounds appropriately.
- Prepare for transport to burn care facility when indicated. In addition to above treatment measures, observe the following:
  See that a nurse or physician accompanies the patient during transport.
  Maintain aseptic technique.
  Avoid extensive burn wound treatment (wrap patient in sterile sheets, blanket).

OUTPATIENT TREATMENT OF MINOR BURNS

Minor burns are second degree burns under 15% in adults and under 10% in children, not involving the face, hands, feet, or perineum. Persons with electrical injuries, complicated injuries, or disease and all poor-risk patients are excluded from this category.

Treatment Measures

- Use aseptic technique throughout.
- Place part in cool saline solution.
- Administer analgesic if necessary.
- *Gently* cleanse with antiseptic solution such as povidone-iodine (Betadine), and thoroughly rinse with saline.
- Remove necrotic tissue, broken blebs, or blebs with cloudy fluid and hair around wound.
- Dress wound (see wound care section).
- Provide for tetanus immunization, and infection prophylaxis.
- Provide instructions for protection of burn wounds at home.
- Provide written and verbal instructions (Fig. 28-5).
- Arrange for follow-up care.

Chart 28-1

SUPPLIES NEEDED FOR INITIAL RESUSCITATION OF BURN VICTIM

Figures in parentheses indicate the number of the specific item needed.

- Large scissors to cut away clothing
- Sterile precaution gowns (6)
- Disposable masks (12)
- Sterile gloves (6 in various sizes)
- Sterile burn linen pack—sheets, gowns, pillow cases
- O_2 with nebulizer, mask, cannula
- Endotracheal set-up, respirator
- Ambu-Bag
- Oral suction machine
- Tracheostomy instruments
- IV solutions with set-ups
- Cutdown instruments
- Blood collecting tubes, urine specimen containers
- Nasogastric tubes, gastric decompression machine
- Foley catheter, catheterization tray, closed drainage system
- Normal saline solution (2)
- Sterile water (2)
- Sterile hand towels
- Sterile basins (2)
- Sterile gauze sponges, small
- Sterile curved scissors (2)
- Sterile forceps (2)
- Cleansing agent, (1 pt)
- Prep razors (sterile)
- Wound culture tubes
- ECG maching
- Medications—narcotics, tetanus toxoid, antibiotics
- Portable lights, extension cords
- Ice and plastic containers (for blood gases)
- Escharotomy equipment
- Topical ointments
- Equipment table (Mayo stand)
- IV poles
- Resuscitation cart

Follow-up Care of Minor Burns

A critical part of the ambulatory care of burns is frequent follow-up. If the patient cannot be re-evaluated frequently, he should not be cared for as an outpatient. The patient or family must be instructed verbally and in writing about ob-

---

Emergency Department

Instructions for Burn Care:

Your wounds do not require hospital admission. To promote healing and avoid complications we recommend:

1. Keep the dressing that has been applied clean and dry.

2. If drainage makes the dressing wet, or

3. If swelling makes the dressing tight, or

4. If pain increases, or

5. If fever occurs,

Seek Medical Care:

Your doctor ☐
The hospital clinic, or ☐
The emergency department ☐

6. If all goes well, the wound should be reexamined in _____ days by _____

_____ .

7. In an emergency, call _____ .

Figure 28-5 *Patient instructions for protection of burn wounds at home. (Reproduced with permission of Sisters of Charity Hospital, Buffalo, N.Y.)*

servation for drainage, fever, and erythema of unburned skin adjacent to the wound, and should also be instructed to return if any of these danger signs is observed.

The patient should be seen 24 to 72 hours after the initial care for further evaluation and dressing changes. Dressing changes are made after the initial dressing is removed by soaking in sterile saline solution in a sterile basin. Further dressing changes are scheduled as often as is needed to prevent infection from bacterial contamination; a dressing wet with wound exudate and dead tissue provides a growth medium for bacteria. Usually, a burn should be seen at least every 3 days until the wound is healed or grafting is obviously needed.

If there is a question of cellulitis or spreading of local infection, cultures are obtained and antibiotics started. Usually, a penicillin or a semisynthetic penicillin effective against penicillinase-producing organisms is given before obtaining the culture and sensitivity reports.

In some instances, when biologic dressings such as heterografts are available, they are applied to obvious partial-thickness burns and dressed into place. The dressings are changed, and the heterografts left in place until healing has occurred or until it becomes apparent that the grafts are not adhering.

After the first 2 or 3 days, it is imperative that joints be routinely moved through their full ranges of motion, especially in older patients who might otherwise develop marked contractures both of small joints in the hand and of larger joints, such as elbows, knees and shoulders.

WOUND MANAGEMENT

Avoiding Sepsis and Promoting Healing

A burn provides an ideal environment for the growth of microorganisms. Necrotic tissue lies next to living tissue, which provides fluid, warmth, and low oxygen tension. It is nearly impossible to prevent bacterial growth in a burn, but the aim must be to decrease this growth so that invasive sepsis does not occur, and to achieve a healed wound without infection in the shortest possible time. Several general measures are used in this effort.

1. Cleansing and debridement are performed. Removal of the necrotic tissue is complicated by difficulty in assessing the exact extent both of the wound (how deep? how wide? where is the edge of nonviable tissue?) and of injury to the intact tissue (anesthesia, blood loss), which should be known before necrotic tissue is removed.

2. Various antibacterial agents are applied topically. These include 0.5% silver nitrate as solution or cream, other silver compounds, mafenide (Sulfamylon), silver sulfadiazine, gentamicin and other antibiotics, and povidone-iodine.

3. Dressings or isolation techniques are used to decrease contamination of the burn wound by the outside environment. However, most of the bacteria arise from the patient himself—from the deep glands of the skin and from the gastrointestinal and respiratory tracts.

4. Systemic measures are taken, including administration of antibiotics, nutrients, vaccinations, and immune sera.

Cleansing and Debridement

Gentle but thorough mechanical cleansing of the burned area is initiated as soon as possible, using a bland soap, such as povidone-iodine scrub, and gauze sponges. The area is well rinsed with sterile saline solution. The detached epidermis is removed with sterile forceps and scissors. Blisters are usually removed by sharp dissection unless they are very firm, as on the soles or palms of the hands. Then they may be left unbroken.

Attentive care must be given to burns involving the head, face, and neck. The singed hair immediately surrounding or adjacent to the burned area must be removed by careful shaving and cleansing, but eyebrows should not be shaved. Copious amounts of sterile saline may be used to irrigate the eyes. Gentle removal of accumulated crust and drainage from the eyes is important.

Care of burned ears includes cleansing, careful debridement, and removal of obviously necrotic tissue. Again, drainage and crusts should be removed by repeated use of saline solutions and cotton-tipped sticks. The application of a topical antibiotic ointment is useful. The mouth must also be examined for possible burns and irritation. The lips should be lubricated with an ointment; frequent oral hygiene is soothing to the patient.

In circumferential burns of the extremities or trunk, the burned skin may act as a tourniquet because it is unyielding to the swelling of tissues beneath it. This may result in difficulty in breathing or obliteration of the pulses, depending on the part involved. Should these occur, an escharotomy is done. This involves cutting through the burn longitudinally on the extremities or chest to relieve constriction.

Full-thickness burns may require grafting to promote healing. Preparation for grafting requires removal of the dead tissue which may be done in a number of ways.

1. Repeated dressing changes to remove dead tissue with the dressing, along with repeated debridement at the bedside or in a Hubbard tank has been used. This debridement should be carried out so as to avoid pain and bleeding.

2. Formal excision of the burn may be carried out if it is clear which areas of the burn wound are full thickness and which are partial thickness. This debridement can include the fascia or subcutaneous tissue. However, excision through the subcutaneous tissue may not be adequate at first try, because it is very difficult to assess the viability of this tissue on immediate cutting.

3. Tangential excision using a dermatome technique has been performed in recent years. Usually, a small hand dermatome is used, and the excision is done under anesthesia. The excision should reach a small capillary bleeding in the viable dermis or subcutaneous tissue. This exposed area should then be immediately covered with a graft or biologic dressing to prevent drying and loss of viability.

4. Various enzymes have been used, most recently sutilains (Travase), in attempts to remove the necrotic tissue without injuring the viable tissue adjacent to or beneath it. This technique involves frequent dressing changes and is incompatible with the use of Sulfamylon or a number of other topical agents.

Topical Antibacterial Agents

Silver sulfadiazine is the most practical topical antibacterial agent for emergency department use. It is painless, has a wide-spectrum antimicrobial action, and is easily removed for later wound inspection. The complications of its use are less common, less varied, or less severe than those associated with other topicals as a group. This agent may, after some time, cause a rash, pruritus, or burning, and it may depress granulocyte formation.

Povidone-iodine has a wide antibacterial spectrum and is available in several forms, but it may cause toxic serum iodine levels. Unless it is cleaned away thoroughly with dressing changes, crusts may form that cause retention of exudate beneath the eschar.

Silver nitrate in 0.5% solution is inexpensive and is easily applied, but its penetration is minimal. Unless it is used from the very beginning, its control of infection may be unsatisfactory. Severe hyponatremia, hypochloremia, and hypocalcemia are a threat, requiring frequent electrolyte checks.

Gentamicin sulfate and *neomycin sulfate,* although effective against many organisms, may cause ototoxicity and nephrotoxicity.

Nitrofurazone, though not absorbed, may cause contact dermatitis. Superinfections have been observed.

Mafenide (Sulfamylon) 10% cream is effective in bacterial control but is painful on application. It carries a 20% to 30% chance of causing an allergic reaction in the unburned skin. By inhibiting carbonic anhydrases it can lead to acidosis, necessitating close monitoring of acid-base balance.

Biologic Dressings

To mimic the functions of the skin that have been lost owing to burning, a number of substances have been used in the treatment of burns. Homografts or skin grafts taken from cadavers are used, although obtaining them is difficult. Porcine heterografts or xenografts can be obtained in an aseptic surgical fashion from the skin of slaughtered pigs. They can be used fresh or kept at refrigerator temperature (4°C) for up to 4 weeks and are available commercially from several firms across the country.

Frozen, as well as dry heterografts, have been used with varying success. The frozen grafts are kept at −50°C and have an unlimited shelf life. Dried grafts are reconstituted by soaking in saline for 30 minutes prior to application. Each of the above substances can be used to cover debrided or partially debrided wounds. In general, biologic dressings must be changed at least every 3 to 4 days. In full-thickness burns, they aid in debridement and act as a test: if the heterograft is apparently "taking" at 3 to 4 days, it is assured that an autograft will take as well.

Attempts to achieve similar results with synthetic skin made of various plastic materials and foams are also being made. Two such commercially available "skin substitutes" are Op-site and Biobrane. These synthetic dressings have a remarkable ability to relieve pain and to permit nearly normal motion of the injured part. They are particularly useful for treatment of superficial partial-thickness burns. They are removed when the wound is healed, eliminating the need for daily or frequent dressing changes. Furthermore, healing is usually more rapid than with older types of dressings. However, care in their application is important: the wound must first be gently but thoroughly cleansed, there should be no necrotic tissue present, and they must be applied so that they remain attached and able to function properly.

EMOTIONAL SUPPORT

Even the most severely burned victim is surprisingly lucid and aware of events and surroundings after sustaining burn trauma. Emergency personnel must be especially careful of verbal and nonverbal communication to the patient and others at this time.

The victim of severe burns suffers profound emotional trauma related to his loss of function and changes in body image. He needs help throughout the grieving process he must inevitably go through to reach a healthy resolution to his loss. Concepts presented in Chapter 6 also apply to the emotional support of the burn victim.

SPECIAL BURNS

Chemical Burns

Chemical burns occur most often in industrial plants and laboratories. Such burns usually result from contact with strong acid or alkali solutions. Less commonly, burns may result from contact with magnesium or phosphorus. Although the skin has a protective layer of keratin and is further protected by surface oils, such strong chemical agents may penetrate or destroy the protective mechanism, with subsequent damage to tissue.

Irrigating the wounds with copious amounts of tap water begins at the scene of the accident and continues at the hospital, either by showering or by submerging the patient in a tub of water. It may be necessary to continue this treatment for 24 to 48 hours to remove all of the offending agent. In general, neutralizing agents have little or no place in the management of chemical burns during the emergency phase of care, since the neutralizing agent may have a more harmful effect than the burning agent.

The wounds of chemical burns are often spotty or scattered, and the pain associated with such an injury may continue for a long period of time. After initial treatment, management is similar to that of a thermal burn.

Electrical Burns

Electrical burns from household voltage (110–220 volts) usually do not cause severe amounts of tissue destruction but may cause death from heart or central nervous system insult. There is a tendency to bleed for about 2 weeks postburn, when the dead tissue separates spontaneously from viable tissue. This bleeding is usually controlled by simple, direct pressure.

High voltage may kill outright, but when it does not, the burns are often very severe and deep, involving vessels, nerves and bones, and frequently require amputations.

Management. Management of electrical burns involves recognition of three unique features:

1. Deep-tissue burn may be much more extensive than the surface wound indicates because heat is generated within the body part by the passage of the electrical current. Nerves, blood vessels, and muscle carry the bulk of current because of lower resistances; they therefore suffer much heavier damage than the overlying skin, except for the areas of skin that are the points of contact with electrical conductors. The need for fluid in resuscitation is often much greater than the area of skin would indicate. Once adequate fluid is being given, according to the usual criteria, add an osmotic diuretic (manitol, 25 gm, IV push) to clear myoglobin rapidly. Check urine for myoglobin, indicated by a port-wine color.

2. Because of the extensive tissue destruction, severe acidosis may ensue. One or two ampules of sodium bicarbonate may be given for each liter of Ringer's lactate until the laboratory data indicate that the acidosis is under control.

3. Severe swelling in the extremities causes vascular compromise in the distal parts. Mere escharotomy such as is done in surface burns will not suffice because the muscles are swollen within their fascial compartments. Fasciotomy is necessary if one is to save the distal part of the involved extremity.

Tar Burns

Tar burns may be treated by applying ice to the affected areas immediately. The tar will harden and may then be easily removed by peeling the crusty surface away from the injured tissue. Then treat as for thermal burns.

BIBLIOGRAPHY

Minar V: Fluid resuscitation of the burn patient. J Emerg Nurs 4:39–43, September–October 1978
Simmons R: Emergency management of electrical burns. J Nurs 3:13–15, March–April 1977
Wagner MM: Emergency care of the burned victim. Am J Nurs 77:788–791, November 1977

29
ENVIRONMENTAL TRAUMA

JAMES H. COSGRIFF, JR. and CAMILLE RATAJCZYK

Since the birth of the nuclear age, specialized applications of nuclear energy have opened new frontiers of diagnosis and therapy using radioisotopes and sophisticated radiation devices. During the same period, there has been a sharp increase in the scope of recreational and industrial activities, which now extend from the depths of the sea to the far reaches of the atmosphere. These changes in the working and leisure-time environments have resulted in a significant number of urgent medical problems, some serious enough to be fatal. The environment is filled with inherent dangers, most of which are avoidable unless one fails to use prescribed safety procedures, protective devices, and ordinary common sense.

Environmental injury may result from exposure to a number of factors and can be classified according to etiology as follows: radiation injury, barotrauma, cold injury, heat illness, submersion injury (near-drowning), and lightning injury.

RADIATION INJURY

Injury secondary to exposure to ionizing radiation occurs infrequently. It is expected that the incidence of radiation injury will increase with the development and expanded use of nuclear medicine studies and commercial nuclear power facilities. In 1978, The Joint Commission on Accreditation of Hospitals (JCAH) promulgated rules and regulations requiring hospitals to establish procedures for dealing with such injury. In areas of the country where industrial plants using radioactive substances are located, radiation treatment centers should be established.

Pathophysiology

A radioactive substance is one that emits ionizing radiation. The four principal types of radiation are:

- *Alpha-particles*—slow moving, heavy particles that usually can penetrate paper. They are a minor hazard when external exposure has occurred, but may produce serious effects if taken internally, by ingestion or inhalation.

- *Beta-particles*—much smaller and weaker than α-particles. They can penetrate air, but are stopped by aluminum and cause less local damage than α-particles.

- *Gamma-rays*—more highly energized and penetrating than α- and β-particles. Their origin is related to that of x-rays. Both γ-rays and x-rays are stopped by lead. Both are more dangerous to tissues than α- or β-particles because of their penetrating manner.

- *Neutrons*—more penetrating than the other types of radiation. This penetrating power causes significant damage to underlying tissue (estimated to be 3 to 10 times greater than that due to γ- or x-rays, but less than the internal hazard associated with ingestion of α- and β-particles).

The most common types of radiation accidents are:

- Those associated with transportation of radioactive substances

- Those occurring at a nuclear facility, in a university, or at a power plant

- Those due to industrial accidents

The amount of radiation is measured by portable instruments.

Following exposure to radiation there is a time of varying length before the first effects are detectable. These biologic effects are described as follows:

Acute—those that appear in a matter of minutes to weeks

Long-term—those that appear years to decades later

When exposed to radiation, the patient is not radioactive and is not a hazard to emergency personnel. But contamination, often referred to as "radioactive dirt," is a hazard. The physiologic responses to short-term radiation exposure are listed in Table 29-1.

Emergency Management

The prehospital and hospital care of victims of radiation injury are summarized in Chart 29-1.

BAROTRAUMA

Barotrauma refers to tissue damage caused by expansion or contraction of gas spaces in the body due to changes in ambient pressure. Such pressure changes may result when one is in an airplane or during descent and ascent in water. It is common in flight crews and passengers with upper respiratory infections, mountain climbers, backpackers, skiers, caisson workers, deep sea divers, and scuba enthusiasts.

TABLE 29-1. RESPONSE TO SHORT-TERM RADIATION EXPOSURE

Dose in Rads*	Response
5–20 Whole body	Asymptomatic. Blood studies normal. Chromosome changes detectable.
20–100 Whole body	Change in the relative numbers of circulating white blood cells. A few may show chromosomal changes occasional nausea, vomiting, fatigue.
200–400 Whole body	Severe reduction in white blood cells. Nausea and vomiting. Loss of hair. Some deaths within 60 days due to altered immune response.
600 Whole body	Bone marrow destroyed. Gastrointestinal disturbance with dysentery and diarrhea. Sterility. Mortality of 50% in 30 days.
1000–2000 Whole body	Destruction of intestinal mucosa, severe diarrhea. Death within 2 weeks.
2000+ Whole body	Severe damage to CNS, fulminating course, death within hours.

The unit of local tissue energy deposition is the *RAD*. The biologic effects of radiation vary with its type. The RADs which refers to the amount of absorbed energy is of somewhat limited value in estimating the extent of biologic injury. The dose equivalent, or REM, provides a gauge of the likely injury to the irradiated part of the organism. The term *REM* stands for *radiation equivalent in man*. For most clinical work, the RAD is equal to the REM. When neutrons or other high energy radiation sources are used, a quality factor (QF) is applied to determine the equivalent dose.

(After Richter LL et al: A systems approach to the management of radiation accidents. Ann Emerg Med 9:303–309, 1980)

Chart 29-1

EMERGENCY MANAGEMENT OF PERSONS WITH RADIATION INJURY

Prehospital Care

- Park rescue vehicles upwind of the accident to minimize contamination.
- Look for signs of radiation exposure. Radioactive packages are marked by clearly identifiable color-coded labels (Fig. 29-1).
- Obtain information about radiation hazards from professional personnel at the scene.
- Use portable instruments to measure the level of radioactivity. If the dose estimates are excessive, rotate rescue personnel. Rescue personnel should wear protective apparel.
- Employ the ABCs of resuscitation.
- Remove the patient's clothing and place in a plastic container.
- Decontaminate the skin by rinsing thoroughly with soap and water.
- Prepare the patient for transport.
- Notify the hospital early during the course of care so that adequate time is allowed for preparations to receive the patient.

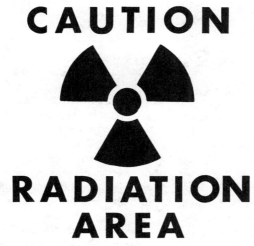

Figure 29-1 Radioactive material warning symbol.

Hospital Care

- Activate the hospital emergency plan for managing radiation injury.
- Take the patient directly to the radiation control area, separate from the main portion of the emergency department.
- Decontaminate the patient further by thorough washing. The staff should be properly gowned and gloved in standard, preferably water-repellent, operating room attire. All washcloths, towels, wash water, and rinse water should be placed in plastic containers for proper disposal. Obtain information for proper disposal from area health officials.
- Continue life-support measures.
- Once the patient is stabilized, check him for contamination using a radiation detector.
- If internal radiation is suspected, obtain swabs of the nose, urine, and feces for evaluation. These samples are placed in plastic containers and evaluated for radioactivity.
- Obtain CBC and platelet count for baseline data.
- Flush all wounds with soap and water to remove any radioactive contamination.
- Obtain medical consultation about radiation injury from the Oak Ridge Methodist Hospital, Oak Ridge, Tennessee, where a 24-hour consultation service is available. (telephone 615-482-2441, beeper 241). Additional assistance may be obtained from the state health department or law enforcement agencies.
- Clean the area properly when emergency care is completed by thoroughly hosing down all used equipment.
- All personnel involved in the care of the patient are surveyed for contamination.

Note. a radiation injury treatment kit can be prepared and stored for handling radiation accidents. It should include disposable surgical garb, yellow rope, plastic garbage bags, garden hose, plastic specimen containers, soap, washcloths, plastic basins, and radiation placards.

Pathophysiology

To better understand barotrauma, one should be familiar with Boyle's law, which states that if the temperature remains constant, the volume of a given gas is inversely proportional to the pressure. Therefore, as the pressure increases, the gas is compressed and its volume diminishes; conversely, as the pressure decreases, the gas expands.

Pressure changes in the atmosphere during high-altitude flying result in expansion of body gases during ascent and contraction during descent. The process occurs in reverse in caisson workers, scuba divers, and deep sea divers. During descent, the gases contract; they then expand during ascent.

Pressure at sea level is equal to 1 atmosphere (ATA) and increases or decreases 1 ATA with each 10-m (33-ft) change in depth or altitude. The contraction and expansion of the gases in the body, as a result of such pressure changes, may cause a variety of symptoms. The body gas most commonly involved is nitrogen, the most abundant gas in the body. The organs most commonly affected are the ear, paranasal sinuses, lungs, teeth, and central nervous system (CNS).

Alterations in pressure in the middle ear (aerotitis) or paranasal sinuses are usually manifested by pain in the involved site.

Gas spaces may be present in decayed teeth or adjacent to dental fillings that have become eroded. Pressure changes in these gaseous spaces may cause severe pain.

Increased pressure on the lung during descent, so-called pulmonary squeeze, may cause a variety of symptoms, including chest pain, hemoptysis, and pulmonary edema. During ascent, overdistention may occur, resulting in pneumothorax and air embolism.

The most serious form of barotrauma is that found in caisson workers, scuba divers, and deep sea divers; it occurs as a result of too-rapid ascent from a depth. During this phase, nitrogen in the body tissues, including the bloodstream, expands as the ambient pressure decreases. Bubbles are formed, which can embolize throughout the body and cause a variety of pathologic changes, some of which may result in permanent disability or death. The air bubbles in the bloodstream interfere with normal circulation to vital organs. This is called decompression sickness. It can be prevented or minimized to a great extent by following a scheduled decompression at a slowed rate of ascent.

Altitude Sickness

Exposure of the human body to high altitudes in excess of 5000 feet above sea level causes a number of adaptive mechanisms to come into play as a result of the decrease in the partial pressure of oxygen (pO_2). Generally, pO_2 is equal to a fixed proportion of the total barometric pressure. At sea level, pO_2 is approximately 160 mm Hg, but at 18,000 feet it is only 80 mm Hg. The result is a significant reduction in the pO_2 in the airway and in arterial and mixed venous blood.

Persons exposed to high altitudes (including mountain climbers, backpackers, hikers, some skiers, and natives of high-altitude communities who descend to sea level for several weeks and then return home) initially experience increased respiratory rate, minute ventilation, and tidal volume and may develop CNS symptoms characterized by headache, nausea, emesis, and alterations in perception and judgment. In those with impaired pulmonary or cardiac function, the changes are more severe. Such symptoms may occur at altitudes of 5000 to 8000 feet and increase considerably at altitudes in excess of 10,000 feet. It is thought that these symptoms are due not only to hypoxia, but also to the physiologic alterations secondary to hypoxia, notably respiratory alkalosis. Sudden loss of consciousness and retinal hemorrhages may follow too-rapid ascent to altitudes of 15,000 to 17,000 feet. Acclimatization may take place as early as 48 to 72 hours after initial exposure and continue over a period of 2 to 6 weeks. The ability to adapt to high altitudes varies greatly from one individual to another.

Although there are a number of clinical conditions that result from exposure to high altitude, those of particular interest to emergency personnel include aerotitis, travel at high altitude, mountain sickness, and high-altitude pulmonary edema.

Aerotitis. Aerotitis occurs primarily during flight and is due to pressure changes in the middle ear. It is manifested by aching or sharp pain in the ear and is relieved by Politzer inflation of the ear, nasal decongestants, and analgesics. Myringotomy (incision of the eardrum) may be necessary to drain any fluid that has collected in the ear.

Travel at High Altitudes. High altitudes generally cause no overt symptoms in normal individuals. Most commercial aircraft in use today have in-flight cabin pressures equivalent to 5000 to 8000 feet. Persons with cardiac or respiratory disease may develop symptoms related to hypoxia, such as weakness, dizziness, and loss of consciousness. The symptoms are alleviated by oxygen. Travelers with moderate to severe cardiopulmonary disease may be given oxygen prophylactically, to minimize the risk of hypoxia. The problem is usually cleared by the time of landing unless more serious sequelae have occurred, such as an acute myocardial infarction. Patients with sickle-cell disease may develop a crisis at high altitudes.

Mountain Sickness. This disorder may occur in persons who have adapted excessively to high altitude. It is characterized by weakness, lethargy, plethora, somnolence, and cardiac failure.

Treatment consists of oxygen therapy and removal of the patient from the high altitude.

High-Altitude Pulmonary Edema. In contrast to mountain sickness, this disorder is usually seen in sea-level inhabitants who ascend to high altitudes and is less common in those who normally reside at high altitude, return to sea level for a few weeks, and reascend to their homes. It is characterized by weakness, tachypnea, dyspnea, nausea, cough, and full-blown pulmonary edema. The mechanism is obscure but appears to be related to changes in the pulmonary vascular bed. It may terminate fatally. Management consists of a return to lower altitude and oxygen.

DECOMPRESSION SICKNESS

This entity is due to the formation of gas bubbles in the tissues and bloodstream. Pain results, particularly in the joints of the extremities. In more severe cases, the bubbles may involve the CNS. Symptoms of decompression sickness may occur during ascent or from minutes to hours later. There are two types of decompression sickness:

- Type I, the less serious form, is referred to as "the bends".
- Type II is much more serious and involves the brain or spinal cord.

Assessment

History. The patient gives a history of working in a caisson or diving. The manifestations observed are as follows:

1. *Type I decompression sickness*
   - Joint pains, stiffness with difficulty in walking
   - Pain may be nagging and gradually increasing over a period of time.
   - Skin rash on the trunk may be present.
   - Swelling occurs in the affected joint(s).
2. *Type II decompression sickness* (in addition to the above)
   - Visual disturbances, blind spots, double vision
   - Headache
   - Confusion
   - Speech disturbances
   - Partial paralysis
   - Numbness, paresthesias of the limb
   - Weakness of the limbs
   - Dizziness

Physical Examination
- Vital signs may be stable
- Varying neurologic findings, including areas of anesthesia, Babinski reflexes, motor weakness, disturbance of balance

Adjunct Studies
- Complete blood count (CBC) may reveal hemoconcentration.
- Chest x-ray may reveal pneumothorax or subcutaneous emphysema of the neck, or may be normal.

Management

Prehospital Care
- Place the patient on the ground, turned slightly toward the left to keep air in the bloodstream in the right heart.
- Follow the ABCs of resuscitation.
- Elevate the hips and feet.
- Give oxygen by mask or nasal catheter.
- Place a veinway using 5% glucose in distilled water or Ringer's lactate.
- Prepare for *rapid* evacuation with the hips and feet elevated.

Hospital Care
- Examine the patient thoroughly to rule out pneumothorax.
- If hemoconcentration is noted, plasma expanders such as low-molecular-weight dextran are useful.

- Prepare the patient for rapid evacuation to a facility with a decompression (hyperbaric) chamber. The U.S. Navy has established a set of treatment tables to be followed for various forms of this disease.

The key to successful treatment is early recognition of the disease with rapid institution of appropriate treatment. The U.S. Navy has not recorded a death from decompression sickness since 1967. A list of locations of hyperbaric chambers is available from the U.S. Government Printing Office (see Bibliography).

COLD INJURY

During wartime combat, cold injury is a common problem, especially in the temperate and subarctic weather zones. It was particularly prevalent during World War II and the Korean conflict, in which 55,000 and 7,000 cases of cold injury, respectively, were recorded. In civilian life, cold injury is seen in the northern parts of the United States and in mountainous regions during winter months. It is particularly prevalent in construction workers, skiers, outdoorsmen, and alcoholics. The very young and the very old are more susceptible to cold injury. It is being seen with increasing frequency in urban areas across the country.

Cold injury may be classified as either core hypothermia or local hypothermia.

- *Core hypothermia* is defined as a body temperature below 35°C (95°F) when measured by an esophageal or rectal probe. It results from (1) exposure to low ambient temperature, with contributing factors such as low environmental temperature, humidity, wind velocity, and exposure time; and (2) immersion in cold water, with or without associated near-drowning.
- *Local hypothermia* is defined as cold injury confined to distal parts exposed to low environmental temperatures and is clinically manifested as chilblains, trench foot, and frostbite.

CORE HYPOTHERMIA

Pathophysiology

The human body normally maintains a core temperature of 37°C (98.6°F). The body temperature varies within a degree or so on a diurnal basis. Maintenance of this temperature is essential to optimal function of vital organ systems of the body. Under ordinary circumstances, the body has adaptive mechanisms to respond to a reduction in ambient temperature.

Initially, as the skin temperature is reduced following exposure to cold, sympathetic stimulation occurs, causing peripheral vasoconstriction, resulting in a decrease in cutaneous blood flow and shunting of blood centrally to vital organs. The blood pressure, cardiac rate, and respiratory rate increase. Shivering or involuntary clonic movements of skeletal muscle occur, increasing metabolic activity and producing heat and blood flow to striated muscle.

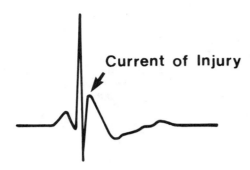

Figure 29-2 *Osborne wave.*

Initially, these responses act to produce an insulating shell to maintain normal core temperature. As exposure to cold continues, the body loses its ability to compensate, and hypothermia results. The ambient temperature itself need not be particularly low, injury being reported at −1.1°C (30°F), but the presence of other contributing factors may be significant. In local cold injury, tissue damage is thought to result from interference with circulation by vasoconstriction, with sludging of blood in smaller vessels and actual changes within the tissue cells as a result of the lower temperature.

As core temperature lowers, progressive cardiac abnormalities that can terminate fatally arise: normal sinus rhythm → sinus bradycardia → T-wave inversion → prolonged PR and QT intervals → atrial fibrillation → ventricular fibrillation. A QRS abnormality, the Osborne wave (Fig. 29-2), is pathognomonic of cold injury. Acid-base disturbances, notably metabolic acidosis, are common. Hypoglycemia may ensue from depletion of glycogen stores by excessive shivering, or hyperglycemia may result from inhibition of insulin action. Blood clotting abnormalities occur frequently. Below 30°C (86°F), the mortality rate exceeds 50%. The physiologic alterations that accompany lowering of core temperature are summarized in Table 29-2 (see also Table 29-3 for Fahrenheit-Celsius conversion).

TABLE 29-2. PHYSIOLOGIC RESPONSES TO LOWERING OF CORE TEMPERATURE

Core Temperature		
(°C)	(°F)	**Responses**
37–34	98.6–93.2	Shivering, confusion, disorientation
34–33	93.2–91.4	Amnesia
33–30	91.4–86	Bradycardia, T-wave inversion, QRS abnormality (Osborne wave), auricular fibrillation, muscle rigidity, metabolic acidosis, loss of consciousness
30–28	86–74.2	Dilatation of pupils, absent deep tendon reflexes, nonpalpable pulse. Ventricular fibrillation
26–24	78.8–75.2	Death (failure to survive)

(After Preston FS et al: Water hazards. Practitioner 211:212, 1973. Reproduced by permission of The Practitioner, London.)

TABLE 29-3. CONVERSION TABLE FOR FAHRENHEIT AND CELSIUS TEMPERATURES

°F		°C
108		42.2
107.6		42
106		41.1
105		40.5
104		40
103.1		39.5
102		38.9
101		38.3
100.4		38
100		37.7
99.5		37.5
98.6	Normal	37
97.7		36.5
96.8		36
95	Core hypothermia	35
93		33.9
92		33.3
90		32.2
88		31.1
86		30
84		28.9
82		27.8
80		26.7
78		25.6
76		24.4
74		23.3
72		22.2
│		│
32		0

To convert °F to °C, subtract 32 and multiply by five-ninths; to convert °C to °F, multiply by nine-fifths and add 32.

Associated factors that may contribute to the hypothermic state include:

- Cerebrovascular accident
- Myocardial infarction
- Myxedema
- Alcoholism
- Trauma
- Drug ingestion
- Hypoglycemia
- Poor physical condition
- Poor judgment
- Limited survival skill
- Overexertion

In the United States, hypothermia is most often seen in the alcoholic population. A lean person may experience a greater fall in rectal temperature than an obese person. Children are more susceptible because of their larger surface area in relation to body mass and their limited amount of fat. Hypothermia is frequently overlooked in the near-drowning victim.

Management

The patient with severe hypothermia may appear dead, because he is cold, pale, and stiff. Resuscitation has been successful from a temperature of 17°C (62.5°F). It is believed that the decrease in core temperature protects the vital body organs (heart, brain, and kidneys) from hypoxia. Thus, life-saving measures should be initiated in all such patients. A patient should not be pronounced dead until he is warmed and still shows the signs of death. Cardiopulmonary resuscitation should be maintained until the core temperature reaches 30°C (86.0°F).

Management of the patient with core hypothermia is outlined in Chart 29-2.

Rewarming Technique

External Warming. External warming is indicated only if core temperature is above 32°C (89.6°F). It may cause vasodilatation, which can lead to hypovolemic pooling shock. Shunting of cold peripheral blood to the core may lead to further chilling of the myocardium and ventricular fibrillation. Be watchful for this "afterdrop" of core temperature.
   Methods and Side-Effects
- Electric blanket—could product thermal burn in under-perfused skin
- Hot water bottles—could cause thermal burn
- Tub bath (40°C–46°C [104.0°F–114.8°F]—may interfere with monitoring
- Heating pads—may produce surface thermal injury

Core Rewarming. This is indicated if core temperature is below 32°C (89.6°F). Many favor this method, since experimentally it has been shown to return cardiovascular function to normal more rapidly. External rewarming may be added after 32°C (89.6°F) has been reached.
   Methods
- Gastrointestinal irrigation
- Inhalation rewarming with oxygen warmed to 42°C–46°C (107.6°F–114.8°F), which is the preferred method
- Peritoneal dialysis using standard potassium-free solution passed through a blood-warming coil heated to 54°C (129.2°F). This gives a dialysate temperature of 43.5°C (110.3°F).
- Hemodialysis requires special equipment. It carries the additional advantage of removing ingested drugs from the blood.
- Extracorporeal blood rewarming through the femoral artery and vein requires a cardiopulmonary bypass device. The blood is warmed by a heat exchanger to 40°C (104°F).

The most readily available and effective methods are inhalation rewarming and peritoneal dialysis. Continuous monitoring of core temperature is essential to good treatment. Frequent determinations of electrolytes and blood gases are needed to identify the ongoing status of acid-base imbalances. Appropriate countermeasures should be initiated as required.

LOCAL COLD INJURY

Local cold injury results when the outer shell tissues (skin, subcutaneous fat, muscles, vessels, and nerves) are exposed to low temperatures. Although local injury may occur in a patient with core hypothermia, most patients with local injury do not have core hypothermia.

The body areas most often involved are the hands, feet, ears, nose, and cheeks.

The severity of injury is frequently classified in a manner similar to that used for burns, from 1st to 4th degree. Clinically, the damaged part may resemble a burn with bleb formation, desquamation, and tissue necrosis.

Pathophysiology

There is some controversy about the exact mechanism by which cold damages the shell tissues. It is thought that as the temperature of the tissue falls, ice crystals form in the interstitial tissues and compress the cells. As a result of this increase in extracellular space pressure, the cell membrane ruptures. The more serious effect of interstitial crystallization is cellular dehydration with concomitant damage or destruction of the cell. The lowering of tissue temperature also causes a decreaase in cell metabolism and anoxia.

Cold causes local vasoconstriction with decreased blood flow to the tissues and hence reduced oxygenation. Precapillary arteriovenous shunts open, shunting blood away from the capillary bed and thus further decreasing blood flow to the damaged part. Damage to the vessel wall causes increased permeability with loss of plasma into the interstitial space and resultant hemoconcentration, clot formation, and obstruction to flow.

Further tissue damage may follow during thawing if refreezing occurs with the formation of larger ice crystals and additional tissue disruption.

Classification

There are three main types of local cold injury: chilblains, immersion foot (trench foot), and frostbite.

Chilblains. *Chilblains* are minor cold injuries resulting from exposure to temperatures varying from 0.55°C to 15.5°C (33°F to 60°F). It most commonly affects the hands and feet. Following the initial response of vasoconstriction, there is a period of vasodilatation, then vasospasm. The injured part is characteristically swollen, with reddish blue patches that burn and itch.
   Treatment. Treatment consists of rewarming by placing the affected part in a warm-water bath. The water temperature should be measured with a thermometer to ensure accuracy; it should not exceed 42.2°C (108°F). Sensory perception in the injured part may be impaired. The heat of the water may increase the severity of burning and itching, and analgesics may be required for relief. The severity of these symptoms is directly proportional to the temperature of the warming bath.

Immersion Foot (Trench Foot). Immersion foot is a more serious form of cold injury caused by prolonged exposure to wetness and cold at temperatures below 10°C (50°F). It most commonly affects the feet because of immobility and dependency. The local changes develop in three phases.
1. *Ischemia and vasospasm*—characteristics of affected part are as follows:
   - Pallor, whiteness, or cyanosis
   - Pulselessness

Chart 29-2

EMERGENCY MANAGEMENT OF THE PATIENT WITH CORE HYPOTHERMIA

Assessment

SIGNS AND SYMPTOMS OF CORE HYPOTHERMIA

- Shallow, slow respirations
- Hypotension
- Confusion ranging to coma
- Shivering ranging to rigor
- Dilated pupils
- Bradycardia or various tachyarrhythmias
- Lowered body temperature
- Generalized edema
- Deep-tendon reflexes absent or delayed

ADJUNCT STUDIES

- Hemoconcentration revealed by CBC
- Platelet count
- Prothrombin time; findings coincide with clotting abnormality
- Fibrinogen level
- SMA-18
- Urinalysis
- Arterial blood gases usually confirm that metabolic acidosis is present, but must be corrected for body temperature (Table 29-4).
- X-rays as indicated to rule out associated trauma; chest x-ray to rule out pneumonia
- Esophageal or rectal temperature monitored continuously
- ECG

TABLE 29-4.   EFFECT OF BODY TEMPERATURE ON ARTERIAL BLOOD GASES

	↑ 1° C (above 37° C)	↑ 1° F (above 98.6° F)	↓ 1° C (below 37° C)	↓ 1° F (below 98.6° F)
pH	0.015	0.008	0.015	0.008
pCO_2 (mm Hg)	4.4%	2.4%	4.4%	2.4%
pO_2 (mm Hg)	7.2%	3.3%	7.2%	3.3%

This table provides the correction factors that must be used to standardize results. The specimen is obtained at core temperature, but laboratory tests are performed at 37°C (98.6° F). Therefore, proper interpretation requires consideration of the deviation with reference to 37° C (98.6° F), as indicated in the table.

(After Reuler JB: Hypothermia: Pathophysiology, Clinical settings and management. Ann Intern Med 89:519–527, 1978)

- Coldness
- Edema

2. *Hyperemia and warming* (lasting 4 to 10 days)—Characteristics of affected part are as follows:

- Redness
- Bounding pulse
- Swelling, pain
- Ulceration or gangrenous changes

3. *Posthyperemia*—characteristics of affected part are as follows:

- Normal color
- Some depigmentation
- Normal pulse
- Hypersensitivity to cold and pain

Treatment. Treatment consists of rewarming with warm baths up to 42.2°C (108°F). The part should be elevated to

Chart 29-2

EMERGENCY MANAGEMENT OF THE PATIENT WITH CORE HYPOTHERMIA (*CONTINUED*)

Management

PRINCIPLES AND GOALS

- Supporting or assisting vital functions
- Rewarming
- Correcting acid-base disturbances, taking care not to overcorrect
- Replacement of depleted circulating volume

PREHOSPITAL CARE

- Remove from insulting environment.
- Initiate ABCs of resuscitation, CPR if needed.
- Give oxygen by mask.
- Remove clothing if wet; place patient in insulated sleeping bag. Handle gently.
- Insert large-bore veinway, give 5% glucose in distilled water.
- Apply warm blankets and cover the head.
- Assess for associated trauma or areas of frostbite. Dress and immobilize as necessary.
- Initiate core rewarming by heating inhaled air using a portable inhalation apparatus, if available.
- Monitor vital signs.

HOSPITAL CARE

- Initiate or maintain cardiopulmonary resuscitation. Do not discontinue until patient is warmed to at least 30°C [86.0° F] and either dead or breathing on his own with spontaneous cardiac activity.
- Give 100% warmed oxygen.
- Monitor ECG continuously, treat cardiac arrhythmias.
- Monitor vital signs.
- Monitor core temperature (rectal or esophageal) continuously (standard oral thermometers record only to 34.4° C [94.0° F].
- Insert central-vein line to infuse fluids. Avoid passing the catheter into the heart, which may be irritable. Fluids may be warmed by passing through a blood-warming coil at 37° C–43° C (98.6° F–109.4° F).
- Insert nasogastric tube, place to suction.
- Monitor arterial blood gases (correct values for core temperature Table 29-4; if the patient is acidotic, give sodium bicarbonate.
- Give broad-spectrum antibiotic to counteract pneumonia.
- Assess for associated injury.
- Initiate rewarming (see Rewarming Technique).

minimize edema. Analgesics are given for pain, which may be more severe with too-rapid warming. During the hyperemia phase, cooling of the part may be needed to lessen pain and reduce the possibility of gangrene. Occlusive dressings are not needed.

Frostbite. Frostbite is the most severe form of local cold injury, causing ice crystals to form in the tissues. Permanent damage may follow vascular occlusion with loss of a part.

The clinical findings depend on the severity of injury. Assess the patient completely for any associated injury. Check the rectal or esophageal temperature to determine whether core hypothermia is present. In superficial frostbite, the part is white, frozen on the surface, and painful. With deeper frostbite, the part is cold, white, solidly frozen, and painless.

Prehospital care consists of splinting or padding the part to prevent further injury. Once the patient has been hospitalized, following thorough assessment, thawing is begun.

In superficial frostbite, gradual rewarming is initiated using a warm water bath starting at 15.5°C (60°F). In deep frostbite, rapid rewarming is started with a water bath of 32.2°C to 42.2°C (90°F to 108°F). Excessive heat (above 115°F) may lead to further tissue damage. The part should be elevated and protected from pressure of bed clothing. Sterile bed linens are preferable, to reduce secondary sepsis. The pathologic process continues for days to weeks after injury with bleb formation, eschar formation, and frank gangrene.

The management is summarized in Chart 29-3.

HEAT ILLNESS

The thermoregulatory mechanism of the body is a complex system that allows the body to maintain a core temperature of approximately 37°C (98.6°F). Aberrations in the function of this mechanism may cause varying degrees of heat illness. There are three types of heat illness: heat cramps, heat exhaustion, and heat stroke.

An estimated 4000 Americans die of heatstroke annually; 80% of victims are over age 50. Heat stroke is the second most common cause of death among high school athletes.

Pathophysiology

The body temperature depends on a system of checks and balances, which include heat production from abnormal metabolic processes or heat dissipation to the environment. Factors contributing to heat illness include the following:

- Exogenous heat gain due to elevated ambient temperature
- Increased heat production due to exercise, infection, and drugs such as amphetamines, phenothiazines, or lysergic acid diethylamide (LSD)
- Impaired heat dissipation due to high ambient temperature with high humidity, failure of acclimatization, heavy clothing, dehydration, and sweat-gland dysfunction.

Environmental heat illness is more likely to develop when the ambient temperature exceeds 32.2°–35°C (90°F to 95°F) and the relative humidity is 70% or more. The clinical findings in heat illness are summarized in Table 29-5.

Heat Cramps

This is the most common and least severe form of heat illness; it is frequently seen in athletes during the summer months before acclimatization. It is due to sodium depletion as a result of excessive sweating associated with strenuous exercise. The sodium loss leads to painful muscle cramps, which often affect the abdominal wall and the extremities. The patient may be agitated because of the cramping. The skin may be warm and moist owing to excessive sweating. Tachycardia and elevated blood pressure are often noted as a result of the exercise.

Management/Treatment. Management consists of removing the patient to a cool, shaded environment and replacing fluid and salt either orally or parenterally. Hospitalization is rarely necessary.

Heat Exhaustion

Heat exhaustion is a more severe form of heat illness associated with more severe water or salt depletion due to sweating. The combined water and salt loss causes the following:

- Muscle cramps
- Nausea, vomiting
- Headache, dizziness
- Weakness, fainting
- Thirst
- Tachycardia
- Hypotension
- Profuse sweating

CBC may reveal hemoconcentration if the body water has been sufficiently depleted. Serum sodium is high or low, depending on the relative amounts of salt and water lost. The urine specific gravity is usually elevated.

Chart 29-3

MANAGEMENT OF THE PATIENT WITH FROSTBITE

- Assess completely, including core temperature.
- Treat any associated injury.
- Start rewarming (gradually in superficial frostbite, rapidly in deep frostbite).
- Provide sterile linens and isolate patient.
- Elevate the part and place cotton between toes.
- Give antibiotics and tetanus propyhlaxis as indicated.
- Give analgesics.
- Avoid rupture of blebs, which are sterile.
- Encourage motion of digits.

TABLE 29-5.   CLINICAL FINDINGS IN HEAT-RELATED ILLNESSES

	Heat Cramps	Heat Exhaustion	Heat Stroke
Temperature	Normal	Usually normal, may be slightly high or subnormal	Increased rapidly may reach 109° F (43°C)
Blood pressure	Normal or decreased	Slightly decreased	Initially increased Later decreased
Respirations	Normal	Rate increased	Decrease in rate, deep; may be Cheyne-Stokes later
Pulse	Rate increased	Increased and thready	Increased and full Later thready
Skin	Pale, moist, cool	Pale, moist, cool	Hot, dry
Diaphoresis	++++	++++	Usually absent
Nausea	Mild	More severe	Usually absent
Vomiting	Rare	More severe	Usually absent
Muscle cramps	Severe, painful	Mild	Severe, may have seizures
Level of consciousness	Normal	Stuporous	Early coma

(After Sturzenberger AJ: J Emerg Nurs 4:25–28, 1978)

Treatment. Treatment consists of rest in a cool environment. Fluid replacement with normal saline is given parenterally. Hospitalization is often required until the patient is stable. Other medical problems that can cause collapse must be ruled out.

Heat Stroke

Heat stroke is the most serious but least common of the various forms of heat illness. It represents a profound disturbance of the heat-regulating system of the body. It is sometimes called sunstroke but is not necessarily related to exposure to the sun. It results in an increase in core temperature due to impairment of the body's heat-dissipating mechanism, associated with dehydration and shutting off of the sweating mechanism.

Mangement/Treatment. Emergency management of the patient with heat stroke is summarized in Chart 29-4.

SUBMERSION INJURY (NEAR-DROWNING)

Water is increasingly popular as a recreational environment. Water sports, skin and scuba diving, water skiing, and surfing are all gaining in popularity each year. In addition, there is an increasing number of private and community swimming pools and beaches. As a result there are approximately 8000 deaths annually in the United States due to drowning. Drowning is among the three leading causes of accidental death. Forty percent of fatalities occur in children under 4 years of age.

Drowning is defined as death within 24 hours after submersion. Near-drowning is defined as survival following submersion. The exact number of near-drowning episodes is unknown, but submersion injuries are being seen with increasing frequency in the emergency department, and this may be due, in part, to an extensive campaign to educate the public in the technique of cardiopulmonary resuscitation.

Drowning occurs in one of two ways:
1. *Dry drowning,* in which no aspiration has taken place
   - It accounts for 10% to 20% of submersion victims.
   - Laryngeal spasm prevents aspiration of fluid.
   - Loss of consciousness occurs and death ensues from asphyxia and cerebral hypoxia.
2. *Wet drowning,* in which aspiration has taken place
   - It accounts for 80% to 90% of submersion victims.
   - Fluid is aspirated through the open glottis.
   - The resultant pulmonary edema causes hypoxemia.

Contributing Factors

Contributing factors associated with drowning include suicide, child abuse, alcohol consumption, hypothermia, seizure, fatigue, diving injury (cervical spine damage), myocardial infarction, and inability to swim.

Pathophysiology

The changes noted depend on several factors:
- The tonicity of the aspirated fluid (fresh water vs. seawater)
- Water temperature
- The duration of exposure and hypoxia
- The presence and nature of any contaminants (sand, algae, vomitus, bacteria, etc.)

The clinical pictures of fresh water and seawater aspiration are remarkably similar.

Fresh Water Aspiration. Fresh water is *hypotonic* to the plasma. When aspirated, it passes from the alveolus into the pulmonary capillaries, causing overload, decreased oncotic pressure and pulmonary edema (Fig. 29-3). It also reduces lung surfactant, thus increasing airway resistance and re-

---

Chart 29-4

MANAGEMENT OF THE PATIENT WITH HEAT STROKE

Assessment

SIGNS AND SYMPTOMS

- Rapid onset
- Fever, usually in the range of 105° F (40.5° C)
- Flushing of the skin
- Anhidrosis (lack of sweating)
- Tachycardia with or without hypotension
- Delirium, psychosis
- Convulsions
- Alteration of consciousness varying from stupor to coma

ADJUNCT STUDIES

- Arterial blood gases—respiratory alkalosis due to excessive bicarbonate in the blood
- SMA-18—low potassium (hypokalemia)

Management

PREHOSPITAL CARE

Treatment is directed toward rapid but closely monitored body cooling.
- Establish and maintain patent airway.
- Check the patient's rectal temperature.
- Remove the patient's clothing.
- Start an IV line of 5% glucose in water or saline before the next step.
- Wrap the patient in wet sheets, packing ice in the neck area, axillae, and ankles, if available.
- Prepare for early transport to the hospital.
- Monitor vital signs, level of consciousness.

HOSPITAL CARE

- Continue the rapid cooling process. Total body immersion in an ice-water bath is ideal. If this is not available, a continuous ice-water sponge bath may be used.
- Endotracheal intubation and ventilatory assist may be needed if the patient is comatose.
- Insert a central-vein line and monitor CVP.
- Insert an indwelling catheter to monitor urinary output.
- Obtain baseline arterial blood gases and repeat as indicated.
- Obtain SMA-18.
- Monitor body temperature by rectal or esophageal probe continuously or at least every 10 minutes.
- Discontinue the cooling process when body temperature reaches 102° F (38.9° C), observing the patient closely to avoid hypothermia.
- Give chlorpromazine, 0.025 gm to 0.050 gm IV if needed to prevent shivering.
- Monitor cardiac rhythm.
- The patient must be closely monitored and transferred to the critical care unit for continuing care.

---

ducing pulmonary compliance. Electrolyte derangements are minimal or absent unless a large amount of water is taken in.

Seawater Aspiration. Seawater is *hypertonic* to the plasma. When aspirated, it draws protein-rich fluid from the plasma of the pulmonary capillary bed into the alveolus (Fig. 29-4). Seawater seems to have little effect on surfactant. Hypoxemia results from perfusion of nonventilated alveoli. Electrolyte derangements are usually insignificant.

The alterations in ventilation-perfusion cause hypoxemia. As this progresses, metabolic acidosis develops. Cardiovas-

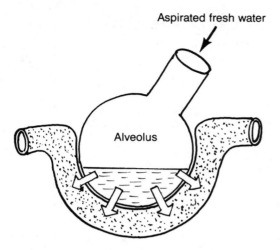

Figure 29-3 *Freshwater aspiration. Fluid passes from the alveolus to the capillary.*

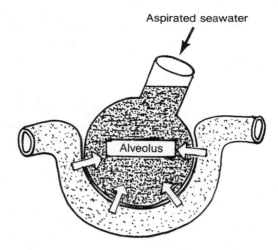

Figure 29-4 *Seawater aspiration. Fluid passes from the capillary to the alveolus.*

cular effects vary from bradycardia to tachycardia. Various arrhythmias may be identified. The blood pressure may be low or elevated. Hypotension is seen more frequently in seawater aspiration.

CNS damage from hypoxia is frequent. Anoxic encephalopathy and cerebral edema follow prolonged submersion. Permanent neurologic sequelae are not unusual. Water temperature, when low, may lead to hypothermia.

Table 29-6 lists the factors considered in a prognostic scoring system. One point is given for each factor identified in a given patient. Patients with scores of 2 or less have a 90% chance of full recovery. Those with scores of 3 or more have only a 5% chance of survival.

Management

Management of the victim of submersion injury is outlined in Chart 29-5.

LIGHTNING INJURY

An estimated 150 to 300 persons are killed by lightning each year in the United States. The exact incidence of lightning injury is unknown, but many more victims survive than is commonly thought.

Pathophysiology

A lightning "bolt," or discharge, results from the passage of electrical current from a cloud to the earth. It possesses two dangerous characteristics—high current and heat production.

When a person is struck by lightning, he becomes electrically charged. If he is grounded, the current passes through his body and exits at the point(s) of grounding. The current may cause violent muscular contractions that throw the victim several feet. As opposed to electrical currents associated with high-voltage sources that cause continuous flow of current until being removed from the source or until the current is discontinued, lightning bolts are instantaneous and ex-

tremely brief. The differences between lightning and high voltage electrical injuries are listed in Table 29-7.

Characteristics of Lightning Injury

1. Lightning produces the following types of injuries:
   - *Electrical current injuries*—damage the CNS and the cardiovascular system
   - *Heat injuries*—burns may occur at the points of entry and exit of the current.
   - *Muscle contractions*—result in a fall and possible accompanying soft tissue injury or fracture
2. The injuries caused by lightning affect the following:
   - CNS
   - Neurovascular system
   - Skin
   - Heart
   - Pregnancy
3. Sudden death by lightning is due to:
   - Paralysis of the respiratory center with apnea
   - Ventricular fibrillation
   - Cardiac arrest
4. Persons who survive may have suffered brief cardiac asystole.
5. The lightning bolt may strike any portion of the body. The prognosis is poorest in those with burns involving the head and scalp and the legs and those with cardiopulmonary arrest.

Clinical Manifestations

The early and late clinical manifestations of lightning injury are listed in Table 29-8.

TABLE 29-6. PROGNOSTIC FACTORS IN SUBMERSION INJURY

Age less than 3 years
Estimated submersion longer than 5 minutes
No attempts at resuscitation for at least 10 minutes after rescue
Patient in coma on arrival at the emergency department
Arterial blood gas $pH \leqslant 7.10$

(Orlowski JP: JACEP 8:176–179, 1979)

Chart 29-5

SUBMERSION INJURY (NEAR-DROWNING): MANAGEMENT OF THE PATIENT

Assessment

HISTORY

- Collect as much information as possible from bystanders or witnesses
- Establish any significant facts about events preceding the submersion injury (diving, running, swimming).
- If possible, determine the length of time of submersion.
- Ascertain water temperature

PHYSICAL EXAMINATION

A broad spectrum of findings is not uncommon:
- The patient may be awake and alert, or obtunded.
- Cardiac arrest may be present owing to asphyxia.
- The patient is cyanotic.
- Rales, rhonchi, or wheezing may be heard.
- Cough and frothy sputum are present.
- Hypothermia may be present.
- Examine carefully for any skeletal injury, especially head and spine trauma.

ADJUNCT STUDIES

- CBC, SMA-18
- Arterial blood gases—may reveal acidosis
- ECG
- Chest x-ray—to identify pulmonary edema, atelectasis
- Urinalysis—check for hemoglobinuria in freshwater submersion.

Management

Early resuscitation is one key to survival.

PREHOSPITAL CARE

- Initiate the ABCs of care.
- Resuscitation efforts should be started in the water after the patient has been evaluated for other injury: immobilize the cervical spine if injury is suspected.
- Initiate CPR.
- Insert an endotracheal tube if available and if the patient is not breathing spontaneously. Initiate assisted ventilation using a tube-valve mask (Ambu-Bag). A mask may be used if an endotracheal tube is not at hand.
- If the patient is breathing spontaneously, give 100% O_2 by mask.
- Insert a large bore veinway and start 5% glucose in dextrose and water or 5% glucose in normal saline.
- Prepare for early transport to the hospital.

HOSPITAL CARE

- Maintain a patent airway and ventilation using a mechanical ventilator with continuous positive airway pressure (CPAP) or positive and expiratory pressure (PEEP).
- Insert central vein line. Monitor CVP.
- Insert nasogastric tube (especially if patient is comatose) to prevent vomiting or aspiration.
- Insert indwelling bladder catheter to monitor urinary output.
- Monitor ABG. Maintain pO_2 at 60 to 90 mm Hg.
- If acidotic, give $NaHCO_3$ IV, 50 mEq of $NaHCO_3$ for each three units of base deficit.
- Use of antibiotics is controversial but may be indicated if the accident occurred in polluted water.
- Use of steroids to reduce pulmonary reaction to aspirated irritants is also controversial.
- All patients are admitted for at least 24 hours.
- Monitor body temperature. If patient is hypothermic, initiate appropriate measures (see p 501).

TABLE 29-7. COMPARISON OF LIGHTNING AND HIGH VOLTAGE ELECTRICAL INJURIES

Factor	Lightning	High Voltage
Time of exposure	Brief, instantaneous	Prolonged, tetanic
Energy level	100 million volts 200,000 amperes	Usually much lower
Type of current	Direct	Alternating
Shock wave	Yes	No
Flashover*	Yes	No

* Flashover is a phenomenon in which the electrical current travels along the external surface of a metal conductor. In lightning injury, the majority of energy may flow around the outside of the body, causing vaporization of perspiration and blasting apart of clothes, thus reducing the energy flowing through the victim.
(After Cooper MA: Ann Emerg Med 9:134–148, 1980)

TABLE 29-8. CLINICAL MANIFESTATIONS OF LIGHTNING INJURY

System	Early Manifestations	Late Manifestations
Central nervous	Coma, convulsions, hysteria, amnesia	Hysteria, psychosis cataracts, hemiplegia
Neurovascular	Intense vasoconstriction, Hypesthesia, paralysis	Neuritis, neuralgia
Skin	Second- and third-degree burns	Scar contracture, Marjolin ulcer
Cardiac	Acute myocardial injury, arrhythmias	Normal ECG
Pregnancy	Fetal maceration and death	

(Apfelberg DB et al: J Trauma 14:453–460, 1974)

In incidents involving more than one victim, primary attention should be directed toward those who are "apparently dead" rather than those who appear alive or are conscious. The reason is that some apparently dead victims may survive with early cardiopulmonary resuscitation, and conscious ones are out of danger.

MANAGEMENT OF THE VICTIM OF LIGHTNING INJURY

Prehospital Care

- In single-victim incidents, perform a rapid assessment.
- If the victim is alive, provide support measures as follows:
  - Establish and maintain a patent, functioning airway.
  - Observe closely for cardiac arrhythmia.
- If the victim is apparently dead (without pulse and respiration):
  - Initiate cardiopulmonary resuscitation (CPR).
  - Maintain CPR during early transport to the hospital.
- In a multiple-victim incident, direct attention primarily to those who are apparently dead. Of lesser priority are those who are conscious; their chance of survival is very good.

- Assess carefully for spinal cord injury: Immobilize and transport.

Hospital Care

- Initiate or maintain CPR.
- Monitor electrocardiogram continuously, treat cardiac arrhythmia as indicated.
- Insert central-vein line.
- Insert indwelling catheter, monitor output.
- Initiate fluid replacement, keeping in mind the extent and severity of associated burns and the possibility of renal shutdown.
- If intense peripheral vasoconstriction is noted, vasodilators are indicated.
- Obtain CBC, urinalysis, SMA-18, arterial blood gases.
- Observe urine for myoglobinuria due to breakdown of muscle tissue, which could lead to renal shutdown. Obtain a sample for laboratory analysis.
- Antibiotics are given depending on the severity of the burn.
- Give tetanus prophylaxis.
- Admit for observation.

BIBLIOGRAPHY

Apfelberg DB et al: Pathophysiology and treatment of lightning injuries. J Trauma 14:453–460, 1974
Bayne CG: Acute decompression sickness: 10 cases. JACEP 7:351–354, 1978
Berrie P: Diving into deep water. Nurs Mirror 15:18–22, 1980
Boswick JA et al: The epidemiology of cold injuries. Surg Gynecol Obstet 149:326–332, 1979
Collins KJ: Oral temperature and hypothermia. Br Med J 1(6167):887–879, 1979
Collins KJ et al: Accidental hypothermia and impaired temperature homeostasis in the elderly. Br Med J 1:353–356, 1977
Conn AW et al: Near-drowning in cold fresh water: Current treatment regimen. Can Anesth Soc J 25:259–265, 1978
Cooper MA: Lightning injuries: Prognostic signs for death. Ann Emerg Med 9:134–138, 1980

DeLapp TD: Taking the bite out of frostbite. Am J Nurs 80:56–60, 1980
Directory of World-Wide, Shore-Based Hyperbaric Chambers, Naviships 0994-010-4011. Washington, DC, U.S. Government Printing Office, January 1971
Editorial: Near-drowning and hypothermia. CMAJ 120:397–400, 1979
Epidemiologic notes and reports: Heat wave related mortality, United States. Morbid Mortal Week Rep 29:357–359, 1980
Fernandez JR et al: Rapid active rewarming in accidental hypothermia. JAMA 212:153–155, 1970
Flanigan WJ et al: The clinical application and technique of peritoneal dialysis. Gen Pract 28:98–109, 1963
Forester D: Fatal drug-induced heat stroke. JACEP 7:243–244, 1978
Guenter CA (Ed): Pulmonary medicine. Philadelphia, JB Lippincott, 1977

Goldfrank L, Osborn H: Heat stroke. Hosp Phys 13:14–18, 1977

Grossheim RL: Hypothermia and frostbite treated with peritoneal dialysis. Alaska Med 15:53–55, 1973

Guild WJ: Rewarming via the airway for hypothermia in the field. J R Naval Med Serv 64:186–193, 1978

Harries MG: Drowning and its treatment. Practitioner 220:771–773, 1978

Hart GB: Treatment of decompression illness and air embolism with hyperbaric oxygenation. Aerospace Med 45:1190–1193, 1974

Hayward JS et al: Accidental hypothermia: An experimental study of inhalation rewarming. Aviat Space Environ Med 46:1236–1240, 1975

Hoff BH: Multisystem failure: A review with special reference to drowning. Crit Care Med 7:310–320, 1979

Houston CS: Acute pulmonary edema of high altitude. N Engl J Med 273:66, 1965

Hudson LD, Conn RD: Accidental hypothermia: Associated diagnoses and prognosis in a common problem. JAMA 227:37–40, 1974

Johnson LA: Accidental hypothermia. Peritoneal dialysis. JACEP 6:556–561, 1977

Kelman GR, Crow TJ: Impairment of mental performance at a simulated altitude of 8,000 feet. Aerospace Med 40:981, 1969

Kleiner JP, Nelson WP: High altitude pulmonary edema: A rare disease? JAMA 234:491, 1975

Knopp R: Near drowning. JACEP 7:249–254, 1978

Lenfant C, Sullivan K: Adaptation to high altitude. N Engl J Med 284:1298, 1971

Lesher DC, Bomberger AS: Experience at Three Mile Island. Am J Nurs 79:1402–1408, 1979

Lloyd EL et al: Accidental hypothermia: An apparatus for central rewarming as a first aid measure. South Med J 17:83–91, 1972

Mettler FA Jr: Emergency management of radiation accidents. JACEP 7:302–305, 1978

Mills WJ Jr: Out in the cold. Emerg Med 11:211–229, 1979

Modell JH et al: Blood gas and electrolyte changes in human near-drowning victims. JAMA 203:99–105, 1968

Morrison JB et al: Thermal increment provided by inhalation rewarming from hypothermia. J Appl Physiol 4G:1061–1065, 1979

Myers RAM et al: Hypothermia: Qualitative aspects of therapy. JACEP 8:523–527, 1979

O'Keeffe KM: Accidental hypothermia: A review of 62 cases. JACEP 6:491–496, 1977

Orlowski JP: Prognostic factors in pediatric cases of drowning and near-drowning. JACEP 8:176–179, 1979

Patton JF et al: Core rewarming by peritoneal dialysis following induced hypothermia in the dog. J Appl Physiol 33:800–804, 1972

Pickering BG et al: Core prewarming by peritoneal irrigation in accidental hypothermia with cardiac arrest. Anesth Analg 56:574–577, 1977

Preston FS et al: Water hazards. Practitioner 211:209–219, 1973

Ravitch MM, Lane R, Safar P: Lightning stroke. N Engl J Med 264:36–38, 1961

Reuler JB: Hypothermia: Pathophysiology, clinical settings and management. Ann Intern Med 89:519–527, 1978

Reuler JB, Parker RA: Peritoneal dialysis in the management of hypothermia. JAMA 240:2289–2290, 1978

Richter LL et al: A systems approach to the management of radiation accidents. Ann Emerg Med 9:303–309, 1980

Rutledge RR, Flor RJ: The use of mechanical ventilation with positive end-expiratory pressure in the treatment of near-drowning. Anesthesia 38:194–196, 1973

Simcock AD: Sequelae of near-drowning. Practitioner 222:527–530, 1979

Speich P: Brought back to life. J Emerg Nurs 4:9–12, 1977

Stine RJ: Heat illness. JACEP 8:154–160, 1979

Strauss RH: Diving medicine. New York, Grune & Stratton, 1976

Sturzenberger AJ: Differentiating among heat syndromes. J Emerg Nurs 5:25–28, 1978

Taussig HB: "Death" from lightning—and the possibility of living again. Ann Intern Med 68:1345–1353, 1968

Thorne IJ: Caisson disease. JAMA 117:585–588, 1941

Trevino A et al: The characteristic electrocardiogram of accidental hypothermia. Arch Intern Med 127:470–473, 1971

Tring FC: Chilblains. Nurs Times 73:1753–5, 1977

Wears RL: Blood gases in hypothermia. JACEP 8:247, 1979

Weiner JS, Khogali M: Heatstroke. Lancet 1:1135, 1979

Whitcraft DD, Karas S: Air embolism and decompression sickness in scuba diving. JACEP 5:355–361, 1978

Wickstrom P et al: Accidental hypothermia: Core rewarming with partial bypass. Am J Surg 131:622–625, 1976

Workman RD: Treatment of bends with oxygen at high pressure. Aerospace Med 39:1076–1083, 1968

30
CARE OF THE POISONED OR OVERDOSED PATIENT

JUDITH STONER HALPERN

All substances are poisons; there is none which is not a poison. The right dose differentiates a poison and a remedy.

Our environment is laden with an infinite number of man-made and naturally occurring poisons. The toxicity of a substance depends on many factors and combinations, such as dose, route of exposure, and species of the victim. Because there are so many variables, poisoning can occur at any time. One can conclude then, that it would be impossible either to be knowledgeable about all aspects of poisoning or to be able to legislate prevention.

Attempts were made to protect the consumer from poisoning as long ago as 1938 when the Federal Food, Drug, and Cosmetic Act was instituted to control drugs and disinfectants intended for use on man or animal. The Federal Hazardous Substances Labeling Act, introduced in 1960, required specific information to be included on labels. The act originally pertained only to a select group of harmful substances but was amended in 1967 to include dangerous toys and other materials that could be labeled to ensure safety. It was not until 1972 that the Consumer Protection Act created an agency to institute and enforce safety standards for consumer products. An example of their efforts is the development of child-proof caps.

The problem of keeping abreast of information about toxic products prompted the United States government to create poison control centers in 1953. Their purpose was to disseminate medical information to health care providers and to the lay public, to collect statistics on toxic substances, and to educate the public on prevention or recognition of toxic exposures. The National Clearinghouse for Poison Control Centers was established in 1957 to distribute data to the centers and to help keep their information current.

Although much has been done to recognize possible hazards and to educate the public on the potentials for poisoning, it has not been sufficient to control the problem. The medical community has a duty to be prepared to recognize and treat toxic emergencies. Because one source cannot be conclusive on all types of poisonings, the health care provider should be familiar with agencies that can provide specific information and guidance, such as poison control centers.

Poisonings are a problem that the emergency care provider encounters frequently. Two million to ten million toxic exposures occur annually in the United States, of which one million are accidental. Nearly 5000 are fatal. It is estimated that one of every ten emergency visits is due to a poisoning.

The intent of this chapter is to address the types of poisoning most frequently encountered and to familiarize the reader with the principles of recognition and treatment. Reference tables have been included to assist the practitioner with specific information. Venomous bites are discussed in Chapter 31, Bites and Stings, and the reader is directed to that section for further information on that topic.

According to statistics from the National Clearinghouse for Poison Control Centers, the ten most common substances involved in poisonings in 1978, for all ages, were (in order of involvement):

1. Plants
2. Combined medications
3. Soap, detergents, cleansers
4. Psychotrophic agents
5. Miscellaneous analgesics
6. Insecticides
7. Antihistamines, cold medicines
8. Miscellaneous internal medications
9. Vitamins, mineral supplements
10. Perfumes, colognes

INITIAL CARE

The victim of poisoning may present with a life-threatening condition and should always be assessed immediately to rule out this possibility. It may be necessary to institute life-support measures before any further definitive care can be started.

The priorities of care are the same for any patient and include establishment and maintenance of ventilation and circulation. Because oxygen is essential for life, the patient must have a patent, open airway. He must be breathing in order to deliver oxygen to the lungs, where it will be exchanged for carbon dioxide. Oxygen diffuses across the alveoli into the pulmonary circulation, where the cardiac system transports it to the tissues.

All patients, particularly the lethargic or unconscious, should be assessed for a functioning airway. Listen or feel for the exchange of air from the mouth or nose. If no exchange can be detected, reposition the patient to promote more adequate respiration. This can be done by moving the tongue from out of the oropharynx, extending the lower jaw, or hyperextending the neck. Rescue breathing should be performed if the patient is not breathing on his own. Mouth-to-mouth breathing or another form of positive pressure ventilation is used to force air into the patient's lungs.

After assessing and beginning ventilations, the patient's circulatory status should be evaluated. If a detectable pulse cannot be heard or felt, artificial circulation should be instituted with closed chest massage. As soon as possible, more specific measures should be instituted to recognize and treat the cause of cardiopulmonary arrest. If the etiology of arrest is poisoning, it is very likely that the patient will not be successfully resuscitated until the toxin is removed, counteracted with an antidote, or symptomatically treated.

GENERAL PRINCIPLES OF ASSESSMENT

Once it has been ascertained that the patient does not have an immediate, life-endangering problem, attention can be directed toward a more thorough assessment and identification of the toxin involved.

History

An accurate history is often the most significant aid in directing care. If the history is unobtainable or uncertain, there are several general guidelines that may prove helpful for the care provider. Chart 30-1 outlines several of the considerations. The possibility of poisoning should always be kept in mind when dealing with a patient who has a sudden-onset, acute illness. If there is a strong suspicion of poisoning, attempt to compare the patient, the suspected toxin and the likelihood of exposure.

Occasionally, the patient or significant other may attempt to treat the poisoning with a home remedy. The first-aid

---

Chart 30-1

GUIDELINES FOR ASSESSING POTENTIAL VICTIMS OF POISONING

The following considerations may be used to help determine the probability or severity of poisoning.

Who

AGE

Accidental poisonings are the most frequent cause of medical emergencies in the pediatric patient population. Childhood ingestions tend to be accidental and involve a single substance. Intentional poisonings occur more often with adults and are more likely to involve multiple substances.

GENDER

Boys are more apt to be the victims of poisoning than are girls. Adult women attempt suicide with poisons more often than men, but men's suicide gestures are associated with a higher mortality rate.

OCCUPATION/PETS/HOBBIES

Industrial chemicals are frequent causes of poisonings and the victim may be exposed unknowingly, such as occurs with bulk transport workers. Exotic pets may be a source of venomous bites.

PREVIOUS HISTORY

Patients with other medical conditions often have multiple medications in the house that could be unintentionally ingested. The use of multiple drugs may cause untoward reactions. The patient with a history of depression may attempt suicide with his psychotropic drugs.

What

CHIEF COMPLAINT

A quick onset and acute illness or condition should make one suspicious of a poisoning, especially if there is no history of previous signs or symptoms that suggest another cause. If a patient presents with a history of poisoning, the benefits/risks of treatment should be compared and therapy given if there is any doubt.

SUSPECTED TOXIN

Rescue personnel should be instructed to bring any container, plant product, or suspected toxin with the patient to the hospital. If multiple plants are growing together, a sample of each should be included. A child's play area should be inspected for possible sources of toxins. It is not unusual for children to retrieve items from garbage containers to use in play.

When

TIME OF POISONING

The history should include time of exposure, onset of symptoms, and time since treatment began. If the toxin was ingested, determine the time since the last meal.

TIME OF DAY

Poisonings in children tend to occur most frequently just prior to mealtimes when they are hungry.

TIME OF YEAR

During the warm months, more poisonings are due to pesticides, plants, and outdoor toxins. In the cold months, there is a higher incidence of ingestions of cold medicines, aspirin, and household poisons.

administered initially may actually present more of a danger than the poison. Table 30-1 lists some of the more popular first-aid practices and explains why they are unsatisfactory. It is important to ask the patient or visitors who accompanied the patient to the hospital if any first-aid attempts were carried out and if so, what was involved.

Physical Examination

Depending on the status of the patient and the reliability of the history, a head-to-toe assessment may prove quite beneficial. Not all patients require total undressing and assessing, but a thorough assessment may provide clues about the unconscious, uncooperative, or suspicious person or the pediatric patient that might otherwise be missed. Needle marks, pill fragments, uneaten leaves or berries, or drug paraphernalia may help to make the diagnosis. The presence of pressure areas on the skin may indicate how long the patient has been unresponsive. Poisoning can be an act of inflicted violence, and the patient may have signs of physical abuse. There have been situations in which, although the reported history for unconsciousness was an overdose, upon closer inspection the patient was found to be a victim of a gunshot or stab wound.

The physical examination should include inspection for respiratory efforts, skin color, pupil size and reactivity, and general status. Auscultation of the lung fields, apical pulse, and bowel sounds will provide a baseline for further assessments and clues to current problems. The blood pressure should be checked as often as necessry to determine cardiovascular stability. Percussion of the thorax and abdomen should be done to detect accumulations of fluid or air.

Odors are important to note. An oily-garlicky smell may be due to pesticides, and the rescuer should take special precautions to protect himself, because these substances can be absorbed through the skin. Other odors may indicate chronic medical disorders (*e.g.,* fruity odor with diabetic ketoacidosis) or neglect of personal hygiene.

Continuous monitoring is crucial to good care. Changes in vital signs, urinary output, response to therapy, and the speed of changes are much more significant when they show a trend than one when they appear as a isolated finding. The patient is an evolving entity and should be observed closely for untoward responses. Sometimes the subtle changes are the most significant.

Adjunct Studies

Toxicology screens are an analysis of serum, urine, or gastric contents to determine whether a substance is present and to what degree. Laboratory levels are helpful but must be considered according to the nature of the substance and its rate of metabolism. Certain substances are sequestered in fatty tissues or are bound to serum proteins, and therefore present with a misleading low serum level.

Studies of serum electrolytes, nonelectrolytes, serum osmolality, arterial blood gases, and urine electrolytes may be used to determine the patient's overall status or ability to respond to therapy. Continuous cardiac monitoring, supplemented with 12-lead electrocardiograms (ECGs), respiratory function studies, intracranial pressure (ICP) monitoring or other invasive monitoring devices may be necessary to help provide symptomatic care.

GENERAL PRINCIPLES OF MANAGEMENT

GOALS OF CARE

In the initial and ongoing care of the victim of poisoning, the following three goals should be kept in mind:
1. Preventing further absorption of the toxin
2. Enhancing elimination of absorbed toxin from the blood
3. Preventing complications by providing symptomatic or specific treatments, including psychiatric management

TABLE 30-1. CONTRAINDICATIONS: COMMON FIRST AID PRACTICES THAT MAY ENDANGER A PATIENT

	Composition of Substance	Dangers of Practice
Universal antidote	A combination of burned toast, milk of magnesia and strong tea.	Has not been shown effective and may be dangerous if allowed to delay appropriate treatment
Commercially prepared antidote	May contain tannic acid and magnesium hydroxide, activated charcoal.	The first two ingredients may interfere with the action of activated charcoal, the only effective ingredient in the preparation.
Saline emetics	1–2 teaspoons of salt in warm water; repeat if ineffective.	Children are especially susceptible to hypernatremia. The salt water does not induce emesis, and repeated doses only increase the sodium intake. Coma, convulsions, and death may occur with the resultant hypernatremia.
Neutralizing caustics	The use of an alkali for an acid substance or vice-versa.	Whenever an acid and an alkali are combined, a chemical reaction may occur. Heat is the by-product of such a reaction and may be sufficient to cause a thermal burn. The chemical by-products of the reactions may also be more dangerous than the original substance (*e.g.*, adding acidic juices to alkaline bleach may release chlorine gas).

Goal #1: Prevent Absorption of Toxin

Ingested Poisons: Considerations for Selecting Therapy. Ingested poisons are best removed while still in the upper gastrointestinal tract. Emesis or gastric lavage is used to empty the stomach; both methods are generally safe, effective, and therapeutic if used in appropriate situations. The overall benefit of gastric emptying for the patient depends on several important considerations, which should be weighed before therapy is initiated.

The goal of any treatment is to help the patient, not to cause further harm, which is certainly possible with emesis or lavage. Before initiating treatment, the patient and the substance should be evaluated for appropriateness of gastric emptying.

Condition of Patient. The patient's general status and ability to vomit should be considered along with the ability to protect his airway from accidental aspiration. If the patient is unconscious, does not have a gag reflex, or is in imminent danger of either development, vomiting should not be induced. Any of the central nervous system depressants is capable of obtunding the protective gag or cough reflex. If the ingested substance has a rapid onset of action, such as some of the barbiturates, it is safer to avoid emetics because of the risk of a sudden decrease in the level of consciousness. Gastric lavage with elective endotracheal intubation would be a more effective choice of therapy.

Patient Cooperation. Willingness to cooperate on the part of the patient should be considered a relative indication for gastric lavage. For adult patients, the desire for treatment is not as important as the manner in which treatment is received. Even though patients may initially refuse care, if approached in a nonthreatening way and given some form of control, they will usually comply. If they are threatened with force or restraints, they are placed in the position of either submitting to coercion or resisting therapy in order to protect themselves.

The pediatric patient may be too young to fully cooperate. Small doses of ipecac are usually not difficult to administer, but making the child drink a large volume of water can be. To remedy this situation, one could pass a small bore lavage tube (small size is preferable because it is less traumatic and will not be used for removal of all stomach contents), aspirate, instill the ipecac and water, and remove the tube before emesis begins. This approach provides the advantages of rapid treatment and greater efficacy of emesis.

Characteristics of Ingested Substance. One must evaluate the substance ingested in order to know which form of gastric emptying, if either, is appropriate. The use of ipecac syrup is generally ineffective against a substance with an antiemetic property, such as the phenothiazines. Waiting for emesis would only cause further delay in care. Other substances have a natural emetic quality if taken in sufficient doses. Hand soaps and liquid soap detergents will produce vomiting when ingested in a large enough quantity. If a natural emetic is ingested, it is not necessary to induce vomiting.

Other substances must be evaluated on an individual basis. Most petroleum distillates, such as furniture polish or cleaning fluids, present a greater hazard for chemical pneumonitis than a systemic intoxication. Even very small amounts can quickly spread over the lung surface if accidentally introduced into the trachea. The general rule is to avoid emesis or lavage in order to reduce the chance of aspiration. There are situations, however, when either the amount, character or additional chemicals present make it necessary to remove the petroleum distillate from the stomach. The choice of emesis or lavage will depend on several factors, including the patient's status and the physician's discretion.

A physical property of the drug may also make it more responsive to a particular type of gastric emptying. Tricyclic antidepressants and phencyclidine (PCP) tend to reenter the acid stomach after being absorbed into the serum. Continuous gastric suction may serve to remove more of the substance than a one-time lavage or emesis.

It is also important to consider the effects of substances on the tissue. Corrosive substances, such as acids, alkalis, and iron supplements, produce irritation and tissue breakdown when allowed to come in contact with the skin or mucous membranes. This becomes important to recognize because therapy may serve to hurt the patient more. Emesis is contraindicated because the substance may cause further injury if reintroduced into the upper gastrointestinal tract. Lavage may be traumatizing because the tube can irritate and possibly penetrate friable tissue.

Occasionally, there may be a question regarding therapy based on the reported amount taken or time since ingestion. The ratio of benefits to risks should be considered in each case. It is not uncommon for the patient to underreport the dosage to avoid an obviously unpleasant experience. Although conservative management with observation is appropriate in certain situations, the risk of not treating might be greater in others. The emergency care provider should consider which would be the greater disservice to the patient and act accordingly.

Time since ingestion is important but should not be used to rule out the benefit of therapy. Again, the patient may choose not to tell the truth, or other factors may affect peristalsis. The stomach tends to empty its contents after one hour, unless a substance that slows gastric motility has been ingested. Narcotics have a tendency to slow peristalsis and may be found in the stomach several hours after ingestion.

If a large number of tablets or pills are consumed at one time, they may clump together in the stomach and form a mass that is too large to pass out of the pylorus. Powdery pills, such as aspirin, have been noted to do this.

It is emphasized that each patient should be evaluated on an individual basis in order to determine how to empty the stomach and prevent further absorption. Chart 30-2 provides a protocol for using emesis or gastric lavage.

Once the substance enters the lower gastrointestinal tract, it can be absorbed through the bowel wall into the rich mesenteric circulation. Because the rate by which this occurs can vary according to substance, rate of peristalsis, and the presence of other substances, it is possible for the poison to be present in the bowel for an extended period of time. If the motility of the intestine can be stimulated or the toxin can be permanently bound to another substance that will be passed out in the stool, further absorption can be greatly reduced.

Chart 30-2

REMOVING INGESTED POISONS

Emesis

1. Administer syrup of ipecac according to age.
   - Ipecac syrup induces vomiting by stimulating the chemoreceptor trigger zone (CTZ) in the brain and by acting as an irritant to the gastric mucosa. Ipecac syrup should not be confused with ipecac fluid extract, a much stronger concentration that can be fatal.

Age	Dose
Under 1 yr	5 ml–10 ml Ipecac syrup
1–10 yr	15 ml
Over 10 yr	30 ml

2. Administer water to distend stomach and induce vomiting.
   - Excessive amounts of water may overdistend the stomach and force gastric contents into the duodenum. Not enough water may fail to induce an immediate response to the Ipecac. Warm water may be more effective in stimulating emesis.
3. If no results are obtained within 20 minutes, a second dose of ipecac may be given. If this still fails to produce vomiting, lavage should be done to retrieve both the poison and the ipecac syrup. It is reported that ipecac has a cardiotoxic effect if allowed to be absorbed.

Gastric Lavage

1. Protect the patient's airway from accidental aspiration.
   - The awake patient should be positioned so as to decrease pooling of secretions or lavage fluids from around the epiglottis. He may be placed in an upright or a head-down position. The patient without a good gag reflex should have an endotracheal tube in place before lavage is begun.
2. Measure length of tube to determine amount to be inserted. A rough estimate of length would be to measure from the tip of the nose to the earlobe and then continue the measurement to the tip of the xyphoid. The tube length is important because a tube introduced too far may kink or be inadvertently introduced into the duodenum. Failure to pass the tube far enough will result in intubation of the esophagus and an inability to suction gastric contents.
3. Introduce an appropriately sized lavage tube into the nares (tube must be large enough to retrieve stomach contents without occluding the lumen). If the patient is alert and cooperative, encourage him to swallow as the tube is being passed. Do not force the tube. If coughing occurs or the patient has trouble speaking, recheck the position of the tube. It may have been accidentally introduced into the trachea.
4. Determine location of the lavage tube. Inspect the back of the mouth to note location and direction of tube. If it extends down the pharynx, aspirate in an attempt to retrieve gastric contents (save contents for gastric analysis). If still uncertain or if no aspirate was obtained, rapidly inject a small amount of air through the tube while auscultating over the gastric region. A bubbling sound should be heard if the tube is in the stomach. If no sound can be heard, attempt to advance or pull back on the tube until it is auscultated.
5. Instill lavage solution in quantities that will not distend the stomach to the point that gastric contents will be forced into the small bowel. An adult can usually tolerate 300 ml at a time. Children have smaller stomachs, and the volume should be titrated to match their body size.
6. Monitor intake and output of gastric lavage volumes to prevent over-filling of the stomach. If fluid is retained, it should be recorded as intake.
7. Continue irrigation/suction process until lavage solution returns clear. This may require several liters of solution.

Administration of Medications

- Activated charcoal may be administered following gastric emptying.
- Some physicians prefer to wait a short time before giving the cathartic because they feel that the charcoal will be carried out of the bowel too quickly if the two drugs are given simultaneously. There is also some question that charcoal may bind some of the carthartic instead of the poisonous substance.
  Note: Refer to the section on acetaminophen for further information about giving charcoal with this drug.

Activated charcoal acts to bind a large number of substances and will enhance elimination. Approximately 15 gm to 30 gm of the powder is mixed with water to form a thick, liquid slurry which is then given to the patient orally or through a nasogastric tube. It is then followed with a cathartic which reduces the time in which the substance or the charcoal is in contact with the bowel wall. Unfortunately, not all poisons that are ingested are bound by charcoal. Table 30-2 lists drugs that are effectively bound and some of the more common ones that are not.

Inhaled Poisons. A patient who has been poisoned by inhalation of toxic gases or powders should be removed from the source as soon as it is safe to do so. No attempt is made to remove the substance, which is usually a vapor or fine particulate matter, from the lung. Removal from the source is the best method of reducing further contact.

Contact Poisons. Contact poisons are dangerous because of their ability to enter the body via the skin or mucous membrane. As long as the substance is in contact with the

TABLE 30-2. EFFECTIVENESS OF ACTIVATED CHARCOAL IN BINDING INGESTED SUBSTANCES

Binds Effectively

Acetaminophen*	Isoniazid
Amitriptyline (Elavil)	Kerosene
Amobarbital (Amytal)	Nicotine
Aspirin	Nortriptyline (Aventyl)
Atropine	Opium
Camphor	Oxalates
Chlordiazepoxide* (Librium)	Paracetamol
Chlorpromazine* (Thorazine)	Paraquat
Cocaine	Parathion
Colchicine	Penicillin
Delphinium	Pentobarbital (Nembutal)
Dextroamphetamine (Dexedrine)	Phencyclidine (PCP)
Diazepam (Valium)	Phenobarbital
Digitoxin	Phenol
Diphenylhydantoin	Probenecid
Ergotamine (Gynergen)	Propoxyphene (Darvon)
Glutethimide* (Doriden)	Propylthiouracil (Propacil)
Hemlock	Secobarbital (Seconal)
Hexobarbital (Sombulex)	Sodium salicylate (Uracel)
Imipramine (Tofranil)	Strychnine
Iodine	Sulfonamides
Ipecac	

Binds poorly

Acetaminophen*	Iron sulfate
Alcohol	Meprobamate (Equanil, Miltown)
Antimalarial drugs	
Boric acid	Methylsalicylates
Chlorpromazine* (Librium)	Mineral acids
Cyanide	Phenylbutazone (Butazolidin)
Glutethimide* (Doriden)	Quinidine
Insecticides	Tolbutamide (Orinase)
DDT	
Lindane	
Malathion	

* These drugs are the subjects of conflicting reports about the effectiveness of charcoal binding.
(Ilo E: Charcoal: Update on an old drug. J Emerg Nurs 8:47, July–August 1980)

TABLE 30-3. ENHANCING RENAL ELIMINATION OF DRUGS

Through Forced Diuresis

Alcohol	Bromide	Quinidine
Amiline	Ethylene glycol	Quinine
Amphetamines	Lithium	Salicylates
Barbiturates	Penicillin	Sulfonamides

Through Acidified Urine

Amphetamines
Phencyclidine
Quinine

Through Alkalinized Urine

Barbiturates
Salicylates

body, it will be absorbed. All clothing and all of the toxic substance should be carefully removed, preferably with an irrigating solution. The rescuer should also take precautions to avoid contact in order to reduce the risk of self-contamination. Clothing may contain significant amounts of the poison and serve as a continuous source of the toxin. Contaminated linen and clothes should be sealed in a sturdy bag or incinerated.

Goal #2: Enhance Elimination of Toxin from Blood

After a substance has entered the serum, it is normally excreted from the body either in an unchanged form or after it has been metabolized by the liver. The liver detoxifies substances present in the blood. The various metabolic by-products are eliminated in the bile or the urine. The bile passes into the intestine and becomes a component of the feces. The kidneys selectively filter, reabsorb, and secrete substances present in the plasma. Elimination of substances in the bile is an unpredictable process and is generally not attempted with severe poisoning.

Urinary excretion of substances, however, can be effectively enhanced by either increasing the filtration process (*i.e.*, by forced diuresis), by inhibiting absorption in the renal tubules, or by stimulating the secretion of substances into the urine.

Forced Diuresis. Forced diuresis is accomplished by giving the patient large volumes of intravenous solutions or diuretics.

TABLE 30-4. USE OF HEMODIALYSIS IN REMOVING SUBSTANCES FROM THE BLOOD

With an Aqueous Dialysate	With a Lipid Dialysate
Barbiturates	Camphor
Borates	Glutethimide
Bromates	Pentobarbital
Ethylene glycol	Phenothiazines
Methanol	Secobarbital
Salicylates	
Sodium chloride	
Thiocyanates	

TABLE 30-5. ANTIDOTE REFERENCE TABLE

This table is intended for informational purposes. Substances are listed in alphabetical order. A reference that is continually kept up to date and is revised annually should be consulted for therapy.

Type of Poisoning	Antidote	Action and Use	General Considerations
Acetaminophen	N-acetylcysteine (Mucomyst) Adult dose: 140 mg/kg po diluted in soft drinks, juice or water. Follow loading dose with 17 additional doses of 70 mg/kg q 4 h (if any dose is vomited within 1 hr after administration, that dose is repeated)	Antidote acts by combining with the toxic metabolite preventing harm to the liver tissue	1. Activated charcoal will absorb the antidote if both are present in the gut. If charcoal is used (*i.e.*, with multidrug ingestions), it must be aspirated before the antidote is given.
Anticholinergic substances *Examples:* Tricyclics—Amitriptyline Atropine Plants—jimson weed, some mushroom species, black nightshade Antihistamines Over-the-counter sleep products	Physostigmine salicylate (Antilirium) Adult dose: 2 mg IV slowly over 2–3 minutes (repeat with a 1–2 mg dose in 20 min if symptoms are still present) (repeat with a 1–4 mg dose if life-threatening symptoms reappear) Pediatric dose: 0.5 mg slow IV over 2–3 min (repeat within 5 min if symptoms recur) (maximum dose: 2 mg)	Physostigmine increases the amount of acetylcholine present at the cholinergic synapses	1. Use is reserved for *severe* poisoning only. This is defined as coma, hallucinations, delirium, tachycardia, arrythmias and hypertension. 2. Rapid IV injection may cause bradycardia, hypersalivation with respiratory difficulties and convulsions. 3. Physostigmine can produce a cholinergic crisis. This is defined as bronchospasm, nausea, vomiting, miosis and abdominal pain. 4. Atropine should be used as an antidote.
Anticholinesterase substances *Examples:* Organophosphate pesticides Carbamate pesticides	Atropine sulfate Adult dose: 2–5 mg IV for pesticides (may repeat every 10–30 min until signs of atropinization appear) Pediatric dose: 0.05 mg/kg for pesticides (may repeat every 10–30 min until signs of atropinization appear)	Interferes with cholinergic stimulation by blocking parasympathetic receptor sites	1. Large doses (2 mg–2000 mg over several hr to several days) may be required to maintain full atropinization (flushed face, fast pulse, dry mucus membranes, dilated pupils) 2. Sudden cessation of Atropine may cause pulmonary edema 3. Maintain adequate ventilation to prevent cardiac arrythmias.
Organophosphate pesticides	Pralidoxine chloride (2-PAM chloride, Protopam chloride) Adult dose: 1.0 gm IV at 0.5 gm/min or diluted in 250 ml saline and given over 30 min (repeat in 3 intervals 8–12 hr apart if muscle weakness is still present) Pediatric dose: 25–50 mg/kg IV (may repeat in 8–12-hr intervals)	Reverses the compound formed by organophosphate and the acetylcholinesterase enzyme. Once the enzyme is free, it can destroy acetylcholine and the cholinergic stimulation will be reduced	1. Use with carbamate type pesticides is contraindicated. Symptoms due to carbamate appear to be aggravated with pralidoxime. 2. Is effective if given up to 36 hr post exposure 3. Pesticide absorption is possible through the skin— wash the patient and remove contaminated clothing as symptoms may reappear again in 48–72 hr.
Anticoagulants *Examples:* Coumadin Warfarin Rat poison	Vitamin K analogue (Aquamephyton) Adult dose: 10 mg IM for large ingestions (can be given po if patient is not vomiting) Pediatric dose: 1–5 mg IM	Anticoagulants in this class act to antagonize vitamin K, a component of the clotting mechanism. Replacing the vitamin restores a physiologic level which allows coagulation.	1. If patient is already using anticoagulants, prothrombin time should be determined and dosage set according to manufacturer's recommendation. 2. Fresh, whole blood may be necessary to stop bleeding. 3. Many drugs potentiate the effect of anticoagulants. A careful history should be done to detect any such drugs.

TABLE 30-5. ANTIDOTE REFERENCE TABLE (*CONTINUED*)

Type of Poisoning	Antidote	Action and Use	General Considerations
Heparin	Protamine sulfate adult dose: 5 ml of a 1% solution slow IV over 10 min (give 1–1.25 mg protamine for each 100 units of heparin thought to be present. Adjustments for time since exposure should be considered since the heparin will be metabolized and the protamine has the potential to act like an anticoagulant.)	Combines with heparin to form a complex that does not have anticoagulant activity.	1. Maximum dose is 50 mg at any one time.
Cyanide	Step I: amyl nitrite inhalants Adult dose: inhale for 30 sec for every 1–2 min while getting IV antidote ready Step II: Sodium nitrite Adult dose: 300 mg in 10 ml solution given IV over 2–4 min (repeat once if symptoms reappear) Pediatric dose: depends upon hemoglobin level Step III: Sodium thiosulfate Adult dose: 12.5 gm in 50 ml solution given IV over 10 min (if symptoms reappear, give sodium nitrite again in half the original dose) Pediatric dose: depends upon hemoglobin level	Converts circulating hemoglobin into methemoglobin which combines with the circulating cyanide. Converts circulating hemoglobin into methemoglobin. Form a nontoxic thicynate compound with the cyanide. The resultant compound can be excreted without further poisoning.	1. Successful resuscitation from cyanide poisoning depends on how rapidly treatment is begun. 1. Nitrites cause vasodilitation. Hypotension is a side-effect.
Heavy metals *Examples:* Iron	Deferoxamine mesylate (Desferal) Dose: 15 mg/kg/hr IV (if not *in extremis*, give 90 mg/kg IM up to a maximum of 1 gm dose q 8 h)	Chelates with free iron and allows for excretion through the urine	1. IV dose given if clinical findings are severe (shock) or serum level exceeds 350 μg% 2. Patient may present with hypotension and acidosis. 3. Renal excretion of compound will cause the urine to be a pink color.
Iron, lead, mercury, copper, nickel, zinc, cadmium, cobalt	Calcium disodium edetate (EDTA, Versene) Adult dose: 75 mg/kg/24 hr deep IM or slow IV infusion given in 3–6 divided doses for up to 5 days (may repeat in a second course after a minimum of 2 days without therapy)	Chelates with heavy metal to allow excretion	1. EDTA should not be started until all lead has been removed from the gut. An abdominal x-ray should be done to check for opacities in the bowel. 2. Rapid injection may precipitate renal failure. If urine flow has not been established in a symptomatic person after 3 hr of fluids, simultaneous hemodialysis should be instituted.
Lead, iron, mercury, copper	D-Penicillamine (Cuprimine) Adult dose: 250 mg qid po for up to 5 days. Do not exceed 40 mg/kg/24 hr Pediatric dose: 24–50 mg/kg/day in 4 doses po	Chelates with heavy metal to allow excretion	1. For use with a patient who has minimal signs and symptoms along with a positive serum lead. 2. Severe symptoms due to lead (encephalopathy) should be treated with BAL and EDTA.
Arsenic, gold, mercury	Dimercaprol (BAL) Adult dose: 3–5 mg/kg deep IM q 4 h for 2 days, then q 4–6 h, for 2 more days, then q 4–12 h up to an additional 12 days	Chelates with heavy metal to allow excretion	1. Must be administered promptly to be effective. 2. Contraindicated with iron poisoning. 3. Requires adequate renal and hepatic function to excrete toxins.

TABLE 30-5. ANTIDOTE REFERENCE TABLE (CONTINUED)

Type of Poisoning	Antidote	Action and Use	General Considerations
Narcotics *Examples:* Morphine Heroin Methadone Merperidine (Demerol) Oxycodone (Percodan)	Naloxone hydrochloride (Narcan) Adult dose: 0.4–0.8 mg IV bolus to reverse the effect of the narcotic (may need to repeat dose every 20–60 min to maintain reversal) Pediatirc dose: 0.01 mg/kg IV bolus	Antagonizes narcotics, pentazocine (Talwin), and propoxyphene (Darvon)	1. Time of action is shorter than the narcotic, therefore, the patient should be observed for return of narcosis (loss of consciousness or depressed respirations). Repeat doses or a continuous infusion may be necessary.

Acidification or Alkalinization of Urine. Manipulation of the absorption or secretion process is done by chemically altering the structure of the substance. All substances will break down into ions in a specific *p*H unique to that substance. Altering the *p*H of the urine with acidifying or alkalinizing drugs allows more of the poison to be forced into the ion state and thus passed out with the urine. This is referred to as "ion trapping." Table 30-3 identifies substances that can be more effectively eliminated with this process.

Renal Hemodialysis. If a dangerous amount of a poison is present or if renal failure is present, renal hemodialysis may be used to promote excretion. Dialysis is only effective in removing substances that are reversibly bound to serum proteins or those that are not stored in the body fat stores. Table 30-4 provides a list of substances that have been reported to be effectively removed with hemodialysis.

Goal #3: Prevent Complications by Providing Specific Symptomatic Care

Use of Antidotes. In some cases, an absorbed toxin can be rendered benign by the use of an antidote. Antidotes act to antagonize, compete with, or override the effects of the poison. In the case of chelating agents, they form a nontoxic compound which is then safely eliminated from the body. Chelate comes from the Greek word "claw," and the literal interpretation is that the antidote forms a grasp which the heavy metal is unable to escape. Table 30-5 is a reference chart of important antidotes.

One should not be lulled into a false sense of security when an antidote has been given. The effect may be temporary if the antidote has a shorter half-life than the poison. If used inappropriately or in wrong doses, the antidotes may actually present more of a danger to the patient. Careful, judicious use of antidotes will prevent these and other problems.

Support of Vital Systems. Symptomatic care involves support of the vital systems. Routine or periodic laboratory and physical assessments should be done to identify potential problems. The patient should be monitored for cardiac rate and rhythm, and for respiratory and renal function. Problems associated with limited mobility should also be anticipated. Frequent turning assists pulmonary and bowel function while also preventing skin breakdown. If large volumes of fluids or drugs that alter serum *p*H are being administered, the patient's electrolyte and acid-base balance must also be monitored.

Emotional Support. Physical support is only half of the care required by a patient who has been poisoned. Any emergency creates a crisis and a need for emotional support. It is not uncommon for the patient to have an underlying emotional conflict, whether the poisoning was intentional or accidental. Parents often feel guilt and shame if their child was the victim. Psychological care will be important if the patient or significant other is to be able to deal satisfactorily with the problem. Many facilities offer the services of a mental health worker while the patient is still in the emergency department. If the problem is minor, the contact has been made and it will be readily apparent that the patient has a good control over events. On the other hand, if the patient is in an emotional crisis as well as a physical emergency, the total patient has been cared for. Victims of abuse, both adults and children, have benefited a great deal from an approach which orients them to counselors.

Goals in the management of poisoning victims are summarized in Chart 30-3. In the sections that follow, these principles are applied to the management of patients who have been exposed to various toxic substances. The goals that are applicable and the order in which they should be implemented are specified for each substance discussed.

CENTRAL NERVOUS SYSTEM DEPRESSANTS

Medications capable of depressing levels of consciousness, thought processes, or important regulatory centers located within the central nervous system (CNS) are discussed in this section. The clinical findings associated with this group can vary a great deal from class to class or within the same drug family because physical effects are dependent on chemical structure of the drug, dose, route of exposure, and rate of metabolism. The chemical structure or purity of clandestine drugs may be affected by variations or deliberate aberrations in the manufacturing process. Drugs discussed in this section are barbiturates, nonbarbiturate sedatives/hypnotics/tranquilizers, and narcotics.

Chart 30-3

GOALS IN THE MANAGEMENT OF POISONING VICTIMS

Goal #1: Prevent Absorption of Toxin.

- *Ingested or Injected Toxins*
  Emesis
  Gastric lavage
  Activated charcoal
  Cathartics
- *Inhaled Toxins*
  Remove victim from source of contamination.
  Administer oxygen or provide fresh air.
- *Contact Toxins* (skin or mucous membranes)
  Remove substance from body surface, preferably with irrigating fluid.
  Remove clothing.
  Use special caution with corrosive materials and pesticides.

Goal #2: Enhance Elimination of the Toxin from the Blood.

- *Ingested or Injected Toxins*
  Forced diuresis
  Acidification or alkalinization of the urine
  Hemodialysis

Goal #3: Prevent Complications by Providing Symptomatic or Specific Treatment.

This goal pertains to all types of exposure.
1. Carefully monitor all life support systems.
2. Continually reassess patient for changes or response to therapy.
3. Administer antidotes as prescribed.
4. Provide symptomatic care as needed for
   - Cardiac dysrthymias
   - CNS depression or stimulation
   - Fluid and electrolyte imbalances
   - Acid/base disturbances
   - Renal function
   - Effects of immobility
5. Provide emotional support to patient and family.

ASSESSMENT

The predominant effect noted in the patient who has been exposed to this group of substances is the altered level of CNS function.

Signs and Symptoms

A spectrum of signs and symptoms is possible because of the selective action of certain drugs on inhibitory or excitatory centers of the brain. Effects may vary a great deal and range from mild euphoria to convulsions or mild sedation to coma. Barbiturates are capable of producing flat electro-encephalograms (EEG), hypothermia, and prolonged unconsciousness. Because of these remarkable qualities of the barbiturates, a negative barbiturate serum level must be established for the patient who is being evaluated for brain death before a legal pronouncement of brain death can be made. Narcotics produce miosis, i.e., constriction of the pupil, and some patients experience nausea and vomiting due to a stimulation of the chemoreceptor trigger zone (CTZ) in the medulla.

The signs and symptoms of a narcotic overdose are usually distinct and help the practitioner to readily identify the substance responsible. The patient has a decreased respiratory rate and tidal volume, miosis, hypotension, and an altered level of consciousness. As obvious as this set of clinical findings may be, it cannot always be relied upon. Other factors may interfere with the usual findings. The decreased respiratory effort may produce hypercarbia, which in turn may cause pupil dilatation. Chronic narcotic users tend to have multiple other problems associated with their drug use or life style; see Table 30-6 for other considerations involved with their care.

When the quantity of CNS depressant has been sufficiently high, depression of vital regulatory centers may be possible. Altered respirations cause hypoventilation, stasis of secretions, and atelectasis. The resultant hypoxia serves to further aggravate the sensorium and cerebral functioning. Narcotics also have the ability to produce idiopathic pulmonary edema.

CNS depressants often possess the ability to cause peripheral vasodilatation with a resultant hypotension and tachycardia. In some cases, the myocardial conduction system can be affected. Dysrhythmias may be due either to this mechanism or, indirectly, to tissue hypoxia.

Patients with an altered level of consciousness are often subject to injury from decreased sensory ability or prolonged immobilization. Reddened areas over boney prominences or pressure points appear within a short time period. Skin blisters are indicative of an altered blood flow, usually due to excessive pressure. Actual skin breakdown can occur in as short a time span as three hours. If external pressure or altered circulation to an extremity is allowed to continue for over four hours, a compartment syndrome may develop.

Effects of Multiple Drug Use. The patient who ingests a combination of drugs may experience a toxicity because of an additive or synergistic effect. Medications known to com-

---

TABLE 30-6.   FACTORS THAT COMPLICATE CARE OF NARCOTIC OVERDOSE PATIENTS

Potential for Multiple Drugs

1. Dealers use substances to dilute or "cut" their drugs to increase the volume of their supply and thus their profit. Examples of other substances found in combination with narcotics are maltose, mannitol, and talcum powder.

2. Users intentionally inject other drugs to modify (prevent too deep a depression) or potentiate the effects of the narcotics. Examples of other drugs:
   Antihistamines
   Amphetamines
   Cocaine

3. Users attempt to reverse the effects of depression by injecting nondrug substances, such as:
   Milk
   Mayonnaise
   Salt
   Coffee

Potential for Acute or Active Infections

1. The use of nonsterile solutions and equipment produces infections. The causative organisms may be those seen only in compromised hosts (i.e., those with overwhelming infections) and are therefore difficult to diagnose and treat. Examples of unusual organisms:
   Aspergillus
   Pseudomonas
   Serratia
   Tuberculosis

2. Frequent exposures and a depressed immune response predispose the patient to severe infections, such as:
   Hepatitis
   Osteomyelitis
   Infective arthritis
   Subacute bacterial endocarditis
   Encephalitis/meningitis

Potential for Life-Threatening Complications
(Presence of Another Severe Disorder)

The presence of another severe disorder may mask signs and symptoms that would be present with narcotic overdose, causing a delay in the treatment of the underlying narcosis.

Respiratory complications—hypoxia, respiratory arrest, pulmonary edema

Cardiovascular complications—cardiac arrest, arrythmias, emboli (air, foreign substances), intra-arterial injections of substances causing local tissue necrosis; microaneurysms

Extremity injury due to prolonged immobilization—if a patient lies on an extremity for a long period of time, excessive pressure may occlude circulation, causing muscle and neurovascular necrosis.

Potential for Danger to Others

Patients consider hospitalization a last resort. They may awaken frightened or angry. They need reassurance that they will not be arrested, that their privacy is protected. If they leave, they may relapse.

plement the action of depressants include antihistamines, phenothiazines, anesthetics, and ethanol. Depressants interfere with the action of other medications, or the concomitant use of multiple drugs may suppress the action of all drugs involved. Occasionally two therapeutic drugs which are given simultaneously have an antagonistic effect on one another. The dosage must be adjusted upward to make up for this effect. If one of the drugs is suddenly discontinued, an overdose of the remaining drug may result. Barbiturates have an inhibitory effect on oral anticoagulants, estrogens, and digitalis. Other CNS depressants are affected by a wide variety of medications, and the reader is referred to a more complete source for further information.

A drug that deserves special consideration is glutethimide (Doriden), a nonbarbiturate sedative. It is erratically absorbed from the bowel and becomes closely bound to proteins and body fats. With an overdose, excessive levels are stored in the bound form and released periodically. This produces an unpredictable clinical picture because the coma can be prolonged or reappear, even after aggressive treatment has been used. Blood levels are misleading because the amount in the serum does not represent total body stores. Elimination normally occurs by way of the hepatic and renal systems, but dialysis is difficult. A lipid dialysate, such as soybean oil, has been used with limited success in some patients.

Effects of Withdrawal. All CNS depressants can produce a physical and psychological dependence. The onset of withdrawal symptoms varies with the type of depressant used. Barbiturates are bound to tissue and serum protein. They are gradually metabolized, which means that withdrawal does not occur until after 12 to 16 hours after the last dose. Symptoms of withdrawal include anxiety, nausea, vomiting, muscle weakness, cramping, and seizures.

Nonbarbiturate sedatives and hypnotics are metabolized quickly and can produce withdrawal symptoms shortly after the drug is discontinued. The nonbarbiturate tranquilizers, however, have a slower rate of elimination than even the barbiturates. Withdrawal effects do not generally occur until 7 to 10 days after cessation of the drug.

Narcotics produce withdrawal within approximately 4 to 12 hours after the last dose. The patient experiences insomnia, yawning, sneezing, vomiting, diarrhea, tremors, sweating, and goose bumps. The patient with signs and symptoms of withdrawal resembles a cold, plucked turkey, hence the source of the term *cold turkey.* Patients may also experience aches, chills, and anxiety.

MANAGEMENT AND TREATMENT

Patients Poisoned With Barbiturate and Nonbarbiturate Sedatives/Hypnotics/Tranquilizers

- *Goal #1: Prevent absorption*
  1. If the substance was ingested, gastric emptying should be done. Ipecac syrup is recommended only if the ingestion was known to have occurred within a relatively short time after treatment. A rapid loss of consciousness may precipitate aspiration with vomiting.

Large doses of barbiturates depress the emetic center in the brain and may prevent a response to ipecac. Gastric lavage may be a safer method of treatment for these reasons.
  2. Activated charcoal and cathartics are given to promote elimination from the bowel before further absorption can occur. CNS depressants can decrease gastric motility, which promotes stasis of the substance in the stomach or intestine.
- *Goal #2: Enhance elimination from the blood*
  1. Forced diuresis has been demonstrated to be helpful in eliminating long-acting barbiturates. Short-acting barbiturates are rapidly bound to tissue and plasma protein and are not readily filtered by the kidney. See Table 30-7 for a listing of short-, intermediate-, and long-acting barbiturates.
     - An additional advantage of diuretic therapy may be related to the effect of barbiturates on antidiuretic hormone (ADH). It is believed that the drug may stimulate the release of ADH. An increase in ADH would cause a reduction in urinary output and consequently, a reduction in urinary excretion of the drug as well.
  2. Alkalinization of the urine is beneficial in increasing the excretion of intermediate and long-acting barbiturates.
  3. Hemodialysis may be required if liver or renal function is impaired or a large dose of barbiturates has been taken.
- *Goal #3: Prevent complications by providing specific and symptomatic care*
  1. There are no antidotes for the barbiturate or nonbarbiturate drugs listed in this group.
  2. *Airway management:* The patient may require endotracheal intubation for ventilation and removal of secretions. Care must be taken when intubating the patient because barbiturates have been noted to precipitate laryngospasm. Arterial blood gas and respiratory function studies are used to determine adequacy of treatment.
  3. *Cardiovascular management:* Hypotension due to hypovolemia or vasodilatation may be present and is best treated with volume replacement. If the hypotension is due to fluid loss through diuresis, electrolyte imbalance is possible and serum levels should be monitored.
  4. *Renal function management:* Any patient who is unable to perceive a full bladder should have an indwelling urethral catheter placed. Hourly urinary output should be monitored because it is a good index of circulating volume, tissue perfusion, and renal performance. The specific gravity should also be monitored to identify the kidney's ability to concentrate urine. Serum creatinine and blood urea nitrogen (BUN) levels are reflective of the filtering function of the kidney.
  5. Maintain normal body temperature: Hypothermia is a common side effect of barbiturate intoxication. External rewarming may be necessary to maintain core body temperature.

Patients Poisoned With Narcotics

- *Goal #1: Prevent complications with specific and symptomatic treatment.*

TABLE 30-7. CENTRAL NERVOUS SYSTEM DEPRESSANTS

Barbiturates

	Ultra-Short	Short	Intermediate	Long
Onset to Recovery:	Minutes	4 hr	4–8 hr	6–10 hr
Use:	Anesthesia	Hypnotic	Hypnotic	Sedation
Drugs:	Methohexital (Brevital), thiamytal (Surital), thiopental (Pentothal)	Hexobarbital (Sombulex), pentobarbital (Nembutal)	Amobarbital (Amytal), aprobarbital (Alurate)	Barbital, mephobarbital (Membaral), phenobarbital (Luminal)

Nonbarbiturate Sedative/Hypnotics

Bromide salts	Flurazepam (Dalmane)
Bromisovalum (Bromural)	Glutethimide (Doriden)
Chloral hydrate (Noctec)	Methalqualone (Quaalude)
Ethchlorvynol (Placidyl)	Methyprylon (Noludar)
Ethinamate (Valmid)	Paraldehyde (Paral)

Nonbarbiturate Tranquilizers

Clonazepam (Clonopin)	Hydroxyzine (Vistaril)
Diazepoxide (Librium)	Oxazepam (Serax)
Flurazepam (Dalmane)	Meprobamate (Miltown, Equanil)

Narcotics

Codeine	
Heroin	Morphine
Hydromorphone (Dilaudid)	Opium
Meperidine (Demerol)	Oxycodone (Percodan)
Methadone (Dolophine)	Oxymorphone (Numorphan)

1. *Airway Management:* A patient with severe depression due to narcotics will have respiratory difficulty. Supplemental oxygen and assisted ventilations should be instituted immediately.
2. *Cardiovascular Management:* Hypotension that accompanies narcotic poisoning is usually due to peripheral vasodilatation and will resolve with the administration of naloxone (Narcan).
3. Administer the antidote naloxone (Narcan). The preferred route for an immediate response is intravenous. It is not uncommon to have difficulty in gaining venous access in a patient with hypotension or sclerotic veins. Sublingual injection into the soft tissue beneath the tongue is an equally acceptable route, as is instillation down the endotracheal tube. Intramuscular injections are reserved for mild depressions or for a long-term effect.
   - The indications for naloxone are respiratory depression, hypotension and depressed level of consciousness due to narcotics, propoxyphene (Darvon), pentazocine (Talwin), or methadone.
   - The patient should be observed closely for the return of symptoms of depresson, since naloxone has a shorter half-life than narcotics. Naloxone tends to lose its effectiveness within one hour.
- *Goal #2: Prevent absorption.*
   1. If the drug was ingested orally, gastric emptying should be performed with the method most appropriate for the patient's level of consciousness. There have been reports of patients who have attempted to avoid arrest for possession of narcotics by swallowing the bags of

drug intended for injection. Once inside the acid environment of the stomach, the bags ruptured and the patient experienced an acute overdose.
   2. Activated charcoal and cathartics may be used to eliminate the drug from the lower gastrointestinal tract. Narcotics do depress bowel motility and may be present for extended periods of time.

Management of the victim of central nervous system depressant poisoning is summarized in Chart 30-4.

CENTRAL NERVOUS SYSTEM STIMULANTS

Many people use some form of central nervous system stimulant in their daily lives. Caffeine is found in coffee, tea, soft drinks, and many nonprescription drugs. Nicotine is present in cigarette, cigar, pipe, and chewing tobacco. Stronger stimulants are available through prescriptions or illegal channels. Commonly used stimulants include amphetamines, caffeine, cocaine, methylphenidate (Ritalin), nicotine, and phenmetrazine (Preludin).

Central nervous system stimulants increase the activity of the reticular activating system, promoting a state of alertness, and the medullary control centers for respiration and cardiovascular function. Patients who use CNS stimulants sense a loss of fatigue, an increased ability to perform muscular activity, and a general sense of well-being. There is

---

Chart 30-4

MANAGEMENT OF THE VICTIM OF CENTRAL NERVOUS SYSTEM DEPRESSANT POISONING

Assessment

- Altered level of consciousness—mild euphoria to coma
- Hypotension
- Constricted pupils (narcotics)
- Reddened pressure points from immobilization
- Withdrawal if drug use not continuous—symptoms depend on drug

Emergency Management

1. *Prevent absorption.*
   - Emesis
   - Lavage
   - Activated charcoal and cathartics
2. *Enhance elimination from blood.*
   - Forced diuresis (see Table 30-3)
   - Alkalinization of urine (see Table 30-3)
   - Hemodialysis (see Table 30-4)
3. *Prevent complications by providing specific and symptomatic care.*
   - Provide airway management for respiratory depression.
   - Provide cardiovascular management for hypotension.
   - Maintain renal function—place indwelling catheter if unconscious.
   - Monitor and maintain body temperature.
   - Give antidote (naloxone [Narcan]) for narcotic overdose.

---

an associated loss of appetite as the person finds he can perform more and tire less while doing so. Therapeutically, stimulants are used to control the sleep states produced by narcolepsy, to overcome depressive disorders, and to assist individuals with weight control. In hyperkinetic children, stimulants have a calming effect.

A stimulant is used by many individuals to reduce fatigue, increase awareness, and improve self-concept. Once on the drugs, the person may find that he is capable of doing more and may continue their use, even to meet unrealistic demands. Inevitably, the effects wear off after the drug is stopped and the patient experiences mental and physical depression. This is referred to as *crashing*. Chronic users regularly readminister a stimulant to avoid the unpleasant effects associated with discontinuing its use.

Those who continue to use the drug for long periods of time will eventually develop a tolerance and will need to periodically adjust the dosage upward to accomplish the same effect. If the drug is acquired through illegal channels, there can be no guarantee of purity or consistency in dosage. The possibility of overdose is always present.

ASSESSMENT

Overdose. CNS stimulants produce both psychological and physical symptoms. The patient may demonstrate repetitive, nonpurposeful movements, grind his teeth, and appear suspicious of others or paranoid. The increased physical stimulation causes an increase in metabolism and the patient appears flushed, diaphoretic, and hyperpyrexic. He may have mydriasis, *i.e.,* dilated pupils, and experience vomiting. It is not unusual for the person to complain of dizziness, loss of coordination, chest pains, palpitations, or abdominal cramps. Death is possible from cardiovascular collapse or as a sequela of convulsions or fever.

Withdrawal. Long-term use of stimulants is believed to produce physical dependency, although this has not been proven. Patients complain of apathy, mental and physical depression lasting several days, and sleep disorders when they discontinue the drug. Sleep patterns can vary from insomnia to sleeping for 20 or more hours per day. The individual may attempt suicide during his depression. Anxiousness and a general state of tension may persist for several months after use of these drugs.

MANAGEMENT AND TREATMENT

- *Goal #1: Prevent absorption.*
  1. If the patient ingested the drug, emesis or lavage may be helpful if the patient is not in immediate danger. This is a situation in which it is necessary to individually evaluate the risk versus benefit. Gastric emptying may precipitate a more severe form of agitation with a concomitant rise in blood pressure, pulse rate, and metabolism.
  2. Activated charcoal and cathartics may be given to promote elimination of the substance from the bowel.

- *Goal #2: Enhance elimination from the blood.*
  Some of the CNS stimulants can be more quickly eliminated from the blood by acidifying the urine. See Table 30-3.

- *Goal #3: Prevent complications by providing specific and symptomatic care.*
  1. There are no antidotes for the CNS stimulants listed in this category.
  2. Provide support of vital functions: The CNS stimulants are capable of stimulating the heart and constricting the blood vessels. The patient should be observed closely for hypertension and tachycardia. Hypermetabolism can occur due to increased activity and the patient may become febrile.
  3. Reduce external stimulation: The patient should be placed in a quiet, nonthreatening environment where a supportive person can attempt to soothe and "talk him down" while observing for untoward reactions.
  4. Sedate when necessary: Although it is not desirable to add more medications in a precarious situation, sedation may be needed to control seizures or keep the patient from doing more self harm.

Management of the victim of CNS stimulant poisoning or overdose is summarized in Chart 30-5.

PHENCYCLIDINE (PCP)

Phencyclidine (PCP) has been a drug of abuse for a number of years but was not recognized as such by the medical community for several reasons. Originally, it was introduced in 1963 as an anesthetic agent. Two years later it was discontinued because of delirium and agitation experienced by the patients who had received it. In 1969, it was reintroduced as an animal tranquilizer, but because of widespread abuse, it has now been completely removed from the market and is available only through illegal home laboratories.

The popularity of phencyclidine has been hard to recognize or predict. Many physicians were unaware of its existence. Patients intoxicated with PCP were labelled psychotic or suicidal. Many were injured and treated only as victims of trauma. In one retrospective study of deaths associated with PCP use, 11 of the 19 had been attributed to drowning only. Federal statistics were originally skewed because PCP was collectively grouped with other hallucinogens and for many years the rapid rise in PCP popularity was hidden because of this method of categorization.

PCP is available on the streets in many forms and is often an unidentified component of illegal psychoactive drugs. A common form of abuse is to sprinkle PCP on marijuana, parsley, or oregano cigarettes and to smoke it. Smoking allows for a better titration and control of effects. The drug can be snorted, ingested, or injected.

ASSESSMENT

PCP intoxication can be identified by the signs and symptoms of the patient. Depending on the dose, route, and time since exposure, the person exhibits characteristic behavioral and physical changes.

High-Dose Intoxication. With a high dose intoxication, the patient has pronounced CNS involvement. He may be comatose, seizuring or have signs of brain stem involvement (posturing, sucking, or loss of protective gag, corneal, and swallow reflex). Multidirectional nystagmus is a classic sign, along with hypertension and an elevated body temperature. One of the distinguishing features of PCP is its ability to produce coma without affecting the respirations. PCP is chemically related to the legal anesthetic ketamine, and the clinical response is very similar in both drugs.

Low-Dose Intoxication. Lower dose intoxications that do not produce unconsciousness typically cause behavioral patterns that reflect depersonalization and distorted perceptions of events or other people. The patient's physical and mental responses may be dulled and slow or abusive and delusional. Suicide may be from overdose, self-mutilation, or dangerous activities such as diving or walking on a freeway. Death can also occur as a result of police action in response to aggressive behaviors like breaking glass or wielding a gun. Table 30-8 presents typical findings of PCP intoxication according to dose.

MANAGEMENT AND TREATMENT

- *Goal #1: Prevent absorption.*
  1. If the drug was ingested, gastric emptying would be effective therapy for decreasing further absorption. Continuous gastric lavage is considered more efficacious than emesis because no matter how it was consumed, PCP can reenter the gastric secretions from the blood and become ionized and "trapped" in the stomach. More of the drug can be removed with ongoing suction than with a one-time emesis. Activated charcoal and cathartics are also used to prevent further absorption.
  2. If PCP was inhaled in smoke or snorted, emesis would not be effective.

Chart 30-5

MANAGEMENT OF THE VICTIM OF CENTRAL NERVOUS SYSTEM STIMULANT POISONING OR OVERDOSE

Assessment

SIGNS AND SYMPTOMS

Overdose
- Complaints of dizziness, chest pains, palpitations, abdominal cramps
- Repetitive, nonpurposeful movements
- Suspiciousness, paranoia
- Flushed skin
- Excessive diaphoresis
- Vomiting
- Mydriasis (dilated pupils)
- Hyperpyrexia
- Death may follow fever, convulsions, cardiovascular collapse.

Withdrawal effects
- Apathy
- Insomnia or excessive sleeping
- Mental and physical depression
- Suicide attempts, high levels of anxiety for several months after cessation of substance use

Emergency Management

1. Prevent absorption.
   - If substance was ingested, prevent further absorption by use of emesis or gastric lavage.
   - Activated charcoal and cathartics may also be used.
2. *Enhance elimination of absorbed toxin from the blood.*
   - Promote urinary loss.
3. *Provide supportive care.*
   - Reduce stimulation and protect from further harm.
   - Be sure to monitor cardiovascular response and body temperature.

- *Goal #2: Enhance elimination from the body.*
  PCP is an alkaline substance and is subject to ion trapping in secretions that can be acidified. Table 30-8 outlines a schematic plan for increasing elimination of PCP by various routes.
- *Goal #3: Prevent complications with specific and supportive care.*
  1. *Psychosis:* PCP affects the person's ability to think rationally or appropriately. Intoxication is marked by paranoid thoughts and the patient responds to therapeutic or friendly gestures with behaviors that range from apprehension to aggressive hostility.
  2. To avoid stimulating the patient and thereby intensifying behaviors, a quiet environment should be provided for his initial assessment and treatment. Because this is often difficult to find in the emergency department, special preparations should be made in ad-

vance. Noises, sights, and sounds only provoke the paranoid ideations and may actually present a risk to the staff and other patients. "Talking down" is usually not successful and probably only serves to make the patient worse.
  3. If the patient is demonstrating hostile or self-abusive forms of behavior, restraints may be needed to protect him and the others present. The use of physical restraints is not without danger and they should never be used as a substitute for a more desirable environment. An agitated patient who has been restrained can exert such an effort to fight the restraints that he accomplishes a type of isotonic exercise which produces muscle injury. Renal failure can be caused by sludging of muscle protein in the renal tubules.
  4. If the threat of danger or psychosis is significant, sedatives may also be necessary to control the patient's

TABLE 30-8. DIAGNOSIS AND MANAGEMENT OF PHENCYCLIDINE TOXICITY: THE METHOD OF CHILDREN'S HOSPITAL OF MICHIGAN, DETROIT

History

Known or reported ingestion of phencyclidine, PCP, tic, tac, animal tranquilizer, pig killer, T, peace, CJ, KJ, supergrass, rocket fuel
Ingestion of substance purported to be THC, cannabinol, LSD, cocaine, mescaline, psilocybin
Smoking or sniffing of angel dust, dust, hog, crystal, pot, snorts, mist, soma, sheets, surfer, cadillac, cyclone

Signs and Symptoms		
Acute High-Dose Intoxication	*Low Dose, Chronic, or Recovery Phase*	**Symptomatic Treatment‡**

	Acute High-Dose Intoxication	Low Dose, Chronic, or Recovery Phase	Symptomatic Treatment‡
Interval			
Since ingestion	Minutes to hours	Hours, days, or weeks	
Dose (serum level)	More than 10 mg (over 100 ng/ml)	Less than 10 mg (0°–100 ng/ml)	
Vital signs			
Blood pressure	Hypotension or *hypertension*†	*Hypertension*	Diazoxide, 2–5 mg/kg by rapid infusion for hypertension
Temperature	*Elevated*	Usually normal	
Respirations	Increased (despite coma), rarely depressed	*Hyperpnea*	Assisted ventilation as needed, intubation (may cause laryngospasm)
Autonomic symptoms	*Diaphoresis, salivation, flushing, lacrimation*		
CNS symptoms (depression or excitation, sometimes *alternating*)	Coma (eyes may be open)	Stupor or *disorientation** *Agitation**	IV fluids and electrolytes as needed
	Convulsions *Rigidity* or flaccidity	*Rigidity on stimulation ataxia** from muscle weakness	Sensory isolation Diazepam (*Valium*) 2–6 mg/m² IV for status epilepticus or
	Purposeless movements, suckling movements	*Repetitive movements*, blank stare, *grimacing*	*smaller doses orally or IM; keep doses low because it may impair excretion of PCP*
	Hyperacusis if conscious	*Hyperacusis*	or paraldehyde, 0.2 ml/kg IM Haloperidol (*Haldol*), administered by psychiatrist, for severe psychosis
	Impaired gag and corneal reflexes		
	Automatic speech (if any), moaning, grunting	Mutism, catatonia, alternating with some responsive, some purposeless talk, often with *profuse obscenity; delusions,** rarely hallucinations; *disordered thoughts** *distorted body images**	Phenothiazines in large doses may be indicated for late recovery-phase psychosis; should be started in hospital. *Avoid:* Force, threatening aura, tight restraints Stimulants Phenothiazines or barbiturates in acute intoxication because they may potentiate depression
	*Impaired pain, touch, and proprioceptive responses; multidirectional** nystagmus		
Tests			
EEG	Delta rhythm, dysrhythmia	Delta rhythm*	
Laboratory	Myoglobinuria, rarely, from severe isometric muscle contractions		

* May occur without other signs in association with low-level toxic psychosis or psychoses precipitated by PCP in susceptible individuals.
† Symptoms in *italics* have particular diagnositic importance.
‡ Toxic manifestations of phencyclidine and its derivatives do *not* respond to the narcotic antagonist naloxone (*Narcan*).
(Done AK, Aronow R, Micell JN: Diagnosis and Management of phencyclidine toxicity. Emerg Med May 1978)

TABLE 30-8. DIAGNOSIS AND MANAGEMENT OF PHENCYCLIDINE TOXICITY: THE METHOD OF CHILDREN'S HOSPITAL OF MICHIGAN, DETROIT (CONTINUED)

Treatment and the fate of PCP in the body

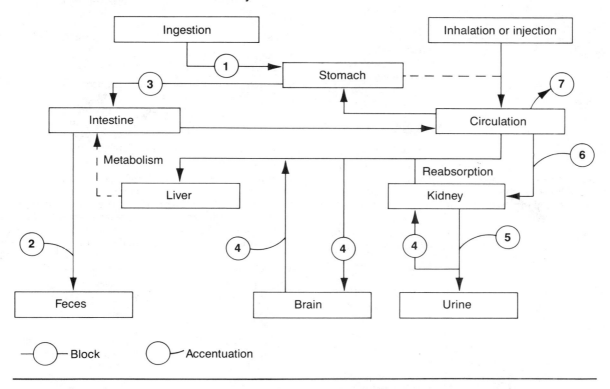

Ion trapping

When blood levels of PCP are observed or expected to be toxic, there are various ways of affecting the drug's distribution and excretion by taking advantage of the fact that PCP (a base) will ionize and be trapped in an acid medium. Acidification both increases urinary excretion of the drug and shifts it from the cells (brain cells, for example) to the extracellular fluid.

The following procedures should be carried out with frequent monitoriing of acid-base status and serum osmolality:

1. Perform gastric lavage *if* patient is seen within 6 hr after ingestion.

2. Instill sodium sulfate, 0.3 gm/kg, by nasogastric tube to promote fecal excretion.
   Wait half an hour to permit passage of the cathartic, then:

3. Begin continuous gastric suctioning and add appropriate isotonic polyionic solution to IV fluids in volume equal to suctioned material.
   If oral route is used for acidification, clamp suction tube for one hour after each installation.

4. Acidify to bring blood *p*H intermittently to 7.2, urine to less than 5:
   Administer:
   ammonium chloride, 2.75 mEq/kg q 6 h by nasogastric tube
   and/or
   IV as 1% or 2% solution in saline
   and
   ascorbic acid, 2 gm q 6 h in IV fluids
   or
   cranberry juice and 1 gm or 2 gm of ascorbic acid po 4 times a day, which may acidify urine rapidly enough if symptoms are mild in low-dose toxicity.
   then:

5. Administer furosemide (*Lasix*), 20 mg to 40 mg IM or IV when urine pH falls below 5.

6. Administer IV fluids in severe cases to enhance excretion.
   In presence of renal insufficiency:

7. Skip steps 4, 5, and 6 and consider hemodialysis or hemoperfusion.

behavior. Chlorpromazine (Thorazine), diazepam (Valium), or haloperidol (Haldol) have been recommended for this purpose.

5. *Seizures:* Diazepam given intravenously has been used to control frequent seizure activity. Rarely, a paralyzing drug has been used to control seizures.

6. *Hypertension:* A significant rise in arterial pressure presents a risk for intracerebral hemorrhage. Diazoxide (Hyperstat) may be needed to treat a hypertensive crisis.

7. *Renal function:* The patient with PCP intoxication may risk renal failure if muscle breakdown has occurred. A high urine output should be maintained and serum BUN and creatinine levels monitored to detect a decrease in renal function.

8. *Fluid/electrolyte and acid-base balance:* The treatment for PCP intoxication involves acidification of body fluids, forced diuresis, and continuous gastric suction. Any of these treatments is capable of producing a significant imbalance which could further jeopardize the patient's recovery.

Management of the patient wih PCP intoxication is summarized in Chart 30-6.

ASPIRIN POISONING

Aspirin is the most common form of salicylate found in the home. In addition to aspirin tablets, it is also in many over-the-counter cold preparations, combination analgesics, and topical ointments. At one time, aspirin was the most common form of poisoning in children. In response to the problem, legislation was implemented to limit the number of tablets in each bottle of baby aspirin to 25 per container, and to package them with child-proof caps.

There are three common causes of aspirin overdose:

1. Accidental ingestion (more common in preschool children)
2. Intentional ingestion (more common in adults)
3. Chronic toxicity (occurs in any age group)

Intentional or accidental ingestions are fairly straightforward in that there is a clear history of poisoning. Chronic toxicity, however, is dangerous because it is not often recognized. Many persons are not aware of correct dosages, may combine multiple drugs that contain aspirin, or may have impaired excretion due to dehydration. The symptoms of aspirin overdose (*i.e.,* dehydration, lethargy, fever) resemble the original problem that is being treated. Chronic toxicity has a higher mortality than acute ingestion.

Aspirin may be ingested orally, absorbed through the rectal mucosa, or applied to the skin in topical preparations. Under normal circumstances, the kidneys serve as the principal organ of excretion.

ASSESSMENT

Aspirin is problematic if present in concentrations of 100 mg/ml of serum or 0.2 to 0.5 gm/kg of body weight. An individual with aspirin toxicity may present with tachypnea, fever, tinnitus, disorientation, coma and convulsions. The clinical picture is due to the systemic effects of aspirin.

- CNS stimulation: Salicylates have a direct stimulatory effect on the respiratory center in the central nervous sys-

tem. The increased rate and depth of respirations cause a decrease in carbon dioxide in the blood which results in respiratory alkalosis. The kidneys respond to alkalosis by eliminating bicarbonate ions in an attempt to compensate. Salicylates also alter metabolic processes, which results in a metabolic acidosis. Blood gases can reflect either acidosis, alkalosis, or a combination of the two.

- Tinnitus, or ringing in the ear, is a symptom of aspirin's effect on the 8th cranial (acoustic) nerve.

- Glucose metabolism: Aspirin interferes with cellular glucose uptake, causing an accumulation in the serum. Eventually the cellular level of glucose will be depleted and the patient may demonstrate tissue effects of hypoglycemic (particularly CNS tissue). The blood level may initially be hyperglycemic. Later, the serum level may be either normal or hypoglycemic.

- Increased metabolism, fluid and electrolyte imbalance: The total body fluid level is adversely affected by the hypermetabolism, which promotes insensible losses and by emesis or renal losses. Electrolytes are also lost via gastrointestinal fluids, renal losses, and, rarely, perspiration. Acid-base disturbances affect serum electrolyte levels and may promote excretion of potassium, sodium, chloride, and bicarbonate.

- Children with therapeutic intoxications may experience a syndrome similar to inappropriate ADH syndrome. They present with oliguria and edema, including cerebral edema.

- Gastrointestinal irritation: Aspirin use is associated with gastrointestinal bleeding, which may be due to local tissue irritation. Patients may be nauseated and vomit after ingestion.

- Coagulopathies: Normal platelet function is altered by aspirin, which may lead to an increased tendency to bleed. This usually does not present a danger to a patient with normal clotting functions, but a person who is taking anticoagulants may be at greater risk for hemorrhage with aspirin ingestion.

Adjunct Studies

To determine if aspirin is present in the urine, a Phenastix can be dipped in a specimen. If it turns purple, *i.e.,* positive, this can be due to aspirin.

Toxicology studies of the blood can detect the presence of aspirin. Tests of salicylate levels should be done 6 hours after reported ingestion. Prior to that, the drug is still being absorbed and blood levels may not be accurate. After 6 hours, the serum level should be compared to a nomogram (Fig. 30-1) to determine if the amount is significant. Repeated levels may be done to determine ability to excrete or if further absorption was prevented. The following levels are general guidelines of toxicity:

Mild:	<150 mg/kg
Mild to moderate:	150–300 mg/kg
Severe:	>300 mg/kg
Fatal:	>500 mg/kg

MANAGEMENT AND TREATMENT

- *Goal #1: Prevent absorption.*

  1. Ingested aspirin should be promptly removed by emesis or gastric lavage. Large numbers of aspirin may

---

Chart 30-6

MANAGEMENT OF THE PATIENT WITH PCP INTOXICATION

Assessment

LOW-DOSE INTOXICATION

- Socially deviant behavior
- Belligerence, agitation, apprehension
- Blank stare
- Multidirectional nystagmus
- Pupils normal and reactive to light
- Poor coordination, increased muscle tone, hyperactive deep tendon reflexes
- Tachycardia, normal to slightly elevated blood pressure

HIGH-DOSE INTOXICATION

- Response to deep pain only
- Coma lasting 4 to 24 hours
- Delirium lasting 2 to 3 days, perhaps a week or longer
- Roving eye movements, disconjugate gaze, multidirectional nystagmus
- Miotic pupils
- Hypertonic muscles, opisthotonus posturing with seizures, tonic/clonic seizures, purposeless movements
- Tachycardia, hypertension (*e.g.,* 180/100)

Emergency Management

1. *Prevent absorption.*
   - If the drug was ingested, begin gastric emptying through nasogastric tube.
   - Activated charcoal and cathartics
2. *Enhance elimination.*
   - Acidify urine to increase renal excretion.
       Mild intoxication—cranberry juice or oral ascorbic acid
       Severe intoxication—gastric tube instillations or IV administration of acidifying agents
   - Continuous gastric suction
3. *Provide specific and supportive care.*
   - Monitor blood pressure and treat hypertensive episodes with diazoxide (Hyperstat).
   - Observe for seizures. If needed, administer diazepam (Valium).
   - Be prepared for psychosis.
       Provide quiet, nonstimulating environment.
       Avoid restraints whenever possible.
       Avoid "talking down."
       Administer sedation as needed.

---

clump together in the stomach, preventing passage through the pylorus.

2. Activated charcoal binds salicylates to prevent further absorption.
3. Cathartics are administered to increase bowel motility and to decrease intestinal absorption.

- *Goal #2: Enhance elimination from the blood.*
   1. Salicylates are weak acids which are excreted by the kidney. Alkalinization of the urine and forced diuresis can significantly increase the elimination of aspirin.
   2. Hemodialysis should be reserved for extreme cases,

such as profound acidosis, high blood levels, persistent central nervous system symptoms, or renal failure.

- *Goal #3: Provide specific and supportive therapy.*
   1. Salicylates have no known antidote.
   2. Prevent dehydration by carefully monitoring fluid output and providing adequate fluid replacement.
   3. Monitor serum electrolytes for imbalance and replace as needed.
   4. Evaluate arterial blood gases to determine if the patient is continuing to have an effect from aspirin toxicity or is not tolerating therapy.

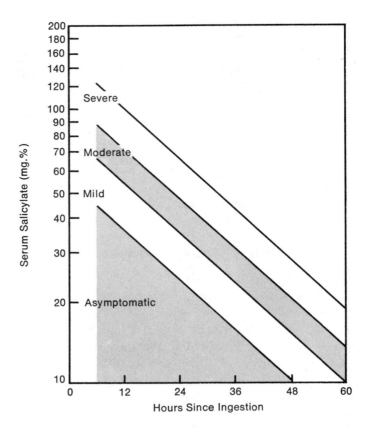

Figure 30-1 *Done's nomogram. The nomogram relates serum salicylate concentrations and expected severity of intoxication at varying intervals following ingestion of one large dose of salicylate. (Arena J: Poisoning: Toxicology, Symptoms, Treatment, 2nd ed. Springfield, Ill, Charles C Thomas, 1975)*

5. Control temperature elevations with sponging. Do not give more aspirin.

The management of the patient who has been poisoned with aspirin is summarized in Chart 30-7.

ACETAMINOPHEN POISONING

The increase in the incidence of acetaminophen toxicity is due in part to its availability and also to a public education campaign that billed it as being "safer than aspirin." In Great Britain, where it is manufactured under the name of paracetamol, deaths were reported in 3% of the overdoses in England and Wales in 1976.

Acetaminophen is an analgesic-antipyretic agent available in many preparations. Phenacetin, a component of Empirin or APC Compound, breaks down into acetaminophen during metabolism. Once the drug is ingested, it is absorbed by the stomach and small bowel. The liver metabolizes nearly 98% of the drug by one of two mechanisms. The greater part of the drug is sent through a pathway that breaks it down into nontoxic by-products. The second hepatic pathway normally handles approximately 4% of the drug and utilizes a process that has a toxic by-product. The liver is capable of detoxifying the toxic by-product by combining it with a naturally occurring substance, glutathione. In the event of an overdose, or in situations in which the minor pathway has already been stimulated (*e.g.,* concomitant use of barbiturates), more of the acetaminophen is sent through the secondary pathway. The toxic by-product accumulates, quickly consumes the available amounts of glutathione, and begins to destroy liver tissue.

ASSESSMENT

The amount of acetaminophen ingested is best determined from the history. Serum levels, although helpful, can be easily distorted. Figure 30-2 is a nomogram that plots measured levels against time post-ingestion. It is a relative indicator of toxicity. A dose of 0.2 to 1.0 gm/kg of acetaminophen is considered to be toxic. Hepatotoxicity occurs after an ingestion of 140 mg/kg or 10 gm in a single dose. Children under the age of 5 years do not appear to suffer the toxic liver damage that is seen with adults. It is considered rare to find even mild hepatic changes in children.

Liver function studies are helpful to recognize hepatic malfunction. These include liver enzymes (SGOT, SGPT), serum bilirubin, protein, prothrombin time, partial thromboplastin time, and platelets.

The pattern of toxicity resulting from an excess of acetaminophen tends to occur over a characteristic three-phase course.

- First 24 hours—vague symptoms of nausea, vomiting, and malaise
- 24–48 hours—vague symptoms subside, but there is an onset of right upper quadrant pain due to hepatic damage. Urine output may decrease as acetaminophen potentiates the effect of antidiuretic hormone. Liver enzymes, bilirubin, proteins, and clotting studies may be abnormal.

Chart 30-7

MANAGEMENT OF THE PATIENT POISONED WITH ASPIRIN

Assessment

SIGNS AND SYMPTOMS OF TOXICITY

- Hyperventilation with respiratory alkalosis
- Metabolic acidosis
- Dehydration
- Tinnitus
- Nausea, vomiting
- Hyperpyrexia
- CNS symptoms of disorientation, coma, convulsions

Adjunct Studies

- Phenastix test of urine
- Arterial blood gas analysis of acid-base balance
- Serum salicylate levels
- Serum glucose levels

Emergency Management

1. *Prevent absorption.*
   - Emesis or gastric lavage
   - Activated charcoal and cathartics
2. *Enhance elimination.*
   - Alkalinization of urine, forced diuresis
   - Hemodialysis if indicated
3. *Provide specific and supportive care.*
   - Provide fluid replacement.
   - Monitor and correct electrolyte disorders.
   - Correct acid-base imbalance.
   - Control fever without aspirin.

- 60–72 hours—liver impairment becomes more obvious and is recognized by the appearance of jaundice, coagulation defects, hypoglycemia, and hepatic encephalopathy. Death from hepatic failure occurs in approximately 10% of severe overdoses. Renal failure or cardiomyopathy may occur.

MANAGEMENT AND TREATMENT

- *Goal 1: Prevent absorption.*
  1. Acetaminophen should be removed from the stomach by emesis or gastric lavage.
  2. If a multidrug overdose occurred, charcoal may be given along with a cathartic.
  3. If acetaminophen was the only drug involved, activated charcoal is not given or is aspirated back from the stomach after 1 hour. The antidote used to treat acetaminophen poisoning is an oral drug. If charcoal is present in the bowel, it will bind the antidote and prevent its absorption along with any other drug that may be present.

- *Goal #2: Enhance elimination from the blood.*
  1. Methods for removing excess acetaminophen from the blood are not very successful. Hemodialysis with a charcoal dialysate has been used in an attempt to remove unchanged acetaminophen from the liver, but nothing removes the toxic by-product which is the major cause of toxic effects. Forced diuresis is not very effective because very little acetaminophen (about 2%) is removed by the kidneys.

- *Goal #3: Provide specific and supportive therapy.*
  1. Acetaminophen is treated with an antidote, *N*-acetylcysteine (Mucomyst). Structurally, it is very similar to

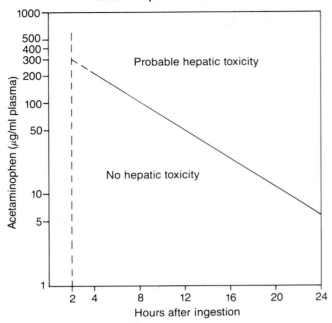

Semi-Logarithmic Plot of Plasma Acetaminophen Levels vs. Time

Figure 30-2 The Rumack-Matthew nomogram for acetaminophen poisoning: a semilogarithmic plot of plasma acetaminophen levels vs time. Cautions for use of this graph: 1. The time coordinates refer to time of ingestion. 2. Serum levels drawn before 4 hours may not represent peak levels. 3. The graph should be used only in relation to a single acute ingestion. 4. A half-life of greater than 4 hours indicates a high likelihood of significant hepatic injury. (Pediatrics 55(6):873, June 1975. Copyright © American Academy of Pediatrics)

glutathione, the substance needed to bind with the toxic by-product. If given within twelve hours of an acute ingestion, it can be effective in preventing hepatic damage. The Rocky Mountain Poison Control Center, Denver, Colorado, has conducted research on the effectiveness of *N*-acetylcysteine and provides the following guidelines for its use:

- The patient should be over the age of 12.
- Therapy should be given for ingestions in excess of 7.5 gm.
- Therapy is effective if begun within 24 hours of ingestion.
  Treatment with the antidote requires 17 oral doses given over a 68-hour time period. The patient may resist therapy because of the taste. No doses should be missed. If a patient vomits within 1 hour of dosing, he should be given a repeat dose equal to the one previously administered.
2. The patient should be observed for hepatic dysfunction, bleeding tendencies, or the effects of low serum protein.

Management of the patient with acetaminophen poisoning is summarized in Chart 30-8.

ENVIRONMENTAL POISONS

CARBON MONOXIDE

Carbon monoxide is a gaseous by-product of incomplete combustion. It may be present anywhere there is a flame

with improper ventilation. Dangerous levels can accumulate rapidly. Common sources of carbon monoxide gas are faulty furnaces, hibachi stoves, radiant heaters, kerosene lamps, cooking stoves, exhaust pipes, and fireplaces. It is estimated that nearly 3000 people die annually from acute carbon monoxide poisoning. With the changes in home heating and more people going toward wood burning stoves and more effective home insulation, carbon monoxide poisoning may become more prevalent.

Assessment

Hemoglobin has a greater affinity for carbon monoxide than for oxygen, and forms a strong compound, carboxyhemoglobin. Because the carbon dioxide displaces oxygen from the red blood cell, the patient experiences hypoxia. Headache, nausea, and vague pains are often noticed. The patient may think that he has a flu syndrome. With a higher level of poisoning, the patient may be tachypneic, have a rapid pulse, or even experience a loss of consciousness. A characteristic red color may be present in the lips or in the skin.

Management and Treatment

- *Goal #1: Prevent absorption.*
  Carbon monoxide is an inhaled toxin. The patient should be removed from the contaminated environment and allowed to breathe fresh air until 100% oxygen can be administered.

- *Goal #2: Provide specific and supportive therapy.*
  1. Hyperbaric oxygenation is used to treat severe cases of carbon monoxide poisoning. Pressurized oxygen treatment effectively reduces the half-life of the carboxyhemoglobin molecule, thereby shortening the duration of effects. Because not every facility has hyperbaric oxygenation available, treatment depends on carboxyhemoglobin serum levels, time since exposure, transport time to the hyperbaric chamber, and the clinical symptoms of the patient.
  2. In rare situations, blood transfusions have been required to supply free hemoglobin capable of carrying oxygen.
  3. Patients should be monitored for adverse effects of hypoxia. They may have convulsions, cardiac dysrythmias, and acid-base disturbances.

Management of the patient with carbon monoxide poisoning is summarized in Chart 30-9.

CORROSIVE CHEMICALS

A number of substances are grouped in this section because of their similar ability to cause local tissue injury. The substances collectively discussed here are listed in Table 30-9.

Ingested corrosives can produce life-threatening complications which may be immediate or late. Swallowing an acid or an alkali can injure the oral and esophageal mucosa, producing ulceration with perforation. Depending on the extent of the tissue penetration, mediastinal structures can be directly affected. Perforation of the upper gastrointestinal tract presents a danger of hemorrhage and mediastinitis. Cardiac arrest can occur as a result of injury or septic shock.

Chart 30-8

MANAGEMENT OF THE PATIENT POISONED WITH ACETAMINOPHEN

Assessment

HISTORY

- Careful history to determine amount ingested

SIGNS AND SYMPTOMS

- First 24 hours
  Vague symptoms of nausea, vomiting and malaise
- 24 to 48 hours
  Vague symptoms subside
  Onset of right-upper-quadrant pain due to hepatic damage
  Decrease in urine output
  Abnormal liver function studies
- 60 to 72 hours
  Signs of liver impairment: jaundice, coagulation defects, hypoglycemia, hepatic encephalopathy
  Renal failure or cardiomyopathy
  Death due to hepatic failure (10% of the cases)

ADJUNCT STUDIES

- Liver enzymes
- Serum bilirubin
- Serum protein
- Clotting studies

Emergency Management

1. *Prevent absorption.*
   - Emesis or lavage
   - Activated charcoal if patient ingested more than one drug
   - Cathartics

   Note: If only acetaminophen was ingested, activated charcoal will be withheld because it binds with the antidote.
2. *Provide specific and supportive care.*
   - Administer *N*-acetylcysteine (Mucomyst) po.

     Follow recommended guidelines for administration.
     Be certain patient receives all of the prescribed doses.
   - Monitor for adverse effects from hepatotoxicity.

The late sequelae of swallowing a corrosive substance involve mucosal scarring with constricture. The scar tissue acts as a mechanical obstruction.

Acids

The acids affect tissue by dissolving it. Hemoglobin is destroyed and vascular tone is impaired, promoting bleeding.

Assessment. The following signs and symptoms are associated with exposure to acids by ingestion, inhalation, or contact.

- Ingestion: Swallowed acids destroy the areas of the upper gastrointestinal tract with which it comes in contact. The patient usually presents with burns in the mouth and pharynx. Complaints include pain, gastric irritation with vomiting, and hematemesis. Hypotension and cardiovascular collapse are also possible.
- Inhalation: Corrosive gases irritate the respiratory system tissues, producing edema as well as alterations in ventilation. The patient may initially experience coughing, choking, gasping for air, and increased secretions. Later, he may experience hypoxia, and pulmonary edema. The late symptoms may take up to 6 to 8 hours to be evident.
- Contact with skin or eyes: Acids begin to destroy as soon as they come in contact with the body surface. Clinical

---

Chart 30-9

MANAGEMENT OF THE PATIENT WITH CARBON MONOXIDE POISONING

Assessment

SYMPTOMS OF HYPOXIA

- Complaints of headache, nausea, vague pains
- Cardiac dysrythmias
- Tachypnea
- Rapid pulse
- Loss of consciousness
- Possibly a red color in lips or skin

ADJUNCT STUDY

- Serum level of carboxyhemoglobin is elevated.

Emergency Management

1. *Prevent absorption.*
   - Remove patient to fresh air.
2. *Provide specific and supportive therapy.*
   - Administer 100% O_2
   - Hyperbaric oxygenation if carboxyhemoglobin levels or patient's symptoms indicate the need

---

findings are similar to other types of burns and include inflammation, pain, ulceration, and involvement of underlying structures. If allowed to remain for a long enough period of time, the acid will cause a sharply defined ulcer.

Management and Treatment
- *Goal #1: Prevent absorption.*
  1. Ingested acid
     - *Do not attempt to induce emesis or lavage.* The substance will cause additional burning when it is ejected from the stomach. A gastric tube could cause structural damage by penetrating or irritating friable tissues.
  2. Acid in contact with skin or eye
     - Begin immediate flushing with a nonreactive liquid and continue to do so for at least 15 minutes to guarantee complete removal.
     - Contaminated clothing should be removed to prevent recontamination.
- *Goal #2: Provide specific and supportive therapy.*
  1. Ingested acid
     - Do not attempt to neutralize the acid.
     - Watch for adverse effects of the acid on tissues: epiglottic swelling, or vital sign changes indicative of hypovolemia or infections.
     - Use caution to prevent further injury. Suctioning of oral secretions should be done carefully and with as much visualization of tissues as possible.
     - The patient may be given water or milk to irrigate the upper gastrointestinal tract.
  2. Inhaled gases
     - The patient exposed to corrosive gases should be evaluated for tissue injury, impaired respiratory

function, and the subsequent effects of hypoxia on the body.
     - Arterial blood gases, ventilation studies, serial chest x-rays and frequent physical assessments are used to monitor for changes.
  3. Acid in contact with skin or eye
     - Contact burns should be protected from potential infection by covering them with a sterile dressing.
     - For hydrofluoric acid burns, a chelating agent, calcium gluconate, may be injected directly into the wound to bind the acid and prevent further injury.

Alkalis

Alkalis produce tissue destruction by interacting with fats and proteins to form a soft, necrotic ulcer. The process continues to destroy and advance deeper as long as the alkali is in contact with the tissue. Erosion of the esophagus and stomach can occur. Peritonitis or mediastinitis are side effects of tissue breakdown with bacteria or gastric juices affecting underlying tissues. Late effects are similar to those produced by acids. Esophageal strictures due to scarring are common. It is estimated that nearly 25% of the patients who ingest a strong alkali will die from the initial insult.

Assessment. Signs and symptoms associated with exposure to alkalis by ingestion or contact are as follows.
- Ingestion: Immediate response to an alkali ingestion is vomiting, pain and possibly diarrhea. The patient may have hemoptysis and increased secretions and may even vomit tissue fragments. Signs of perforation include fever, respiratory difficulty, or peritonitis. Approximately 98% of the patients develop strictures.

TABLE 30-9. CORROSIVE CHEMICALS COMMONLY INVOLVED IN TOXIC EMERGENCIES

Name	Found in Products in the Home	Comments
Acids		
1. Acetic	Vinegar	Generally nontoxic
2. Carbolic	Phenol-disinfectants, -sanitizers	
3. Chlorine	Sanitizing agents, especially water	
4. Hydrochloric (muriatic acid)	Reagents	
5. Hydrofluoric	Germicides Plastic production Semiconductant materials Used to frost glass Used for tannins	
6. Nitric	Commercially used only, as in chemistry labs	
7. Oxalic	Laundry bleach	If absorbed, may decrease serum calcium level
8. Sodium bisulfate	Toilet bowl cleaner	Becomes an acid when added to water
9. Sulfuric	Auto battery acid	
Alkalis		
1. Ammonia	Detergents, inhalants	
2. Cement		
3. Low-phosphate detergents		
4. Sodium carbonate	Electric dishwasher detergent	
5. Sodium hypochlorite	Laundry bleaches	
6. Sodium hydroxide	Lye Clinitest tablets	

- Contact: A chemical burn will develop where the skin has come in contact with the alkali. The slimy, soapy feeling associated with alkalis is due to their effect on tissue fats. Alkalis interact to produce a soap-like substance.

Management and Treatment
- *Goal #1: Prevent absorption.*
  1. Ingested alkali
     - *Do not attempt emesis or gastric lavage.* Because alkalis are neutralized by the gastric acid, there is no need to either treat the substance further or attempt to remove it from the bowel. Lavage tubes may injure the tissue more.
     - The substance can be irrigated with a nonreactive liquid to guarantee that all of the alkali has been removed from the upper gastrointestinal tract.
  2. Contact with alkali
     - Copious irrigation of the point of contact should be done. Continue irrigation for at least 15 minutes,

and in the case of the eye, irrigation may be necessary for up to 30 minutes.
- *Goal #2: Provide specific and supportive therapy.*
  1. Ingested alkali
     - After the initial irrigation, do not allow the patient to eat or drink anything more until an inspection is done to determine amount and extent of burns.
     - Esophagoscopy may be used to identify the degree of injury and to directly irrigate any questionable spots of the mucosa.
     - Alkalis that contain phosphates may produce a systemic hypocalcemia. Intravenous calcium gluconate may be required.
     - Supportive care includes monitoring for systemic effects of perforation or tissue injury.
  2. Contact with alkali
     - Cover all wounds after irrigation.
     - Use sterile dressings to reduce the risk of infection.
     - The patient should be evaluated by a plastic surgeon, or in the case of an eye, an ophthalmologist. Chapter 33 provides detailed information about ocular injuries.

Management of the patient who has been exposed to an acid or an alkali is summarized in Chart 30-10.

PETROLEUM DISTILLATES

Petroleum distillates are very common substances in our environment. They are components of furniture care products, cleaners, solvents, and automotive supplies. Because they are so common, it is not surprising that they are a frequent cause of poisoning. It is estimated that 7% of all poisonings treated each year are due to petroleum distillates.

Some typical petroleum products are benzene, fuel oils, gasoline, kerosene, lacquer diluents, lubricating oil, mineral seal oil, naptha, paint thinners, petroleum spirits, and rubber solvents.

The toxicity of petroleum distillates depends upon several factors.
1. Route of exposure (ingestion versus aspiration)
2. Volatility (ease with which the substance evaporates)
3. Viscosity (density or thickness)
4. Amount ingested
5. Presence of other toxins

Assessment

Obtain an accurate history to identify the substance and mode of exposure. The petroleum distillates present the most serious hazard when accidentally introduced into the respiratory tract. Products with a low viscosity can quickly spread over the lung surface, causing a pneumonitis with low-grade fever, tachypnea, coughing, choking, and gagging. Pulmonary edema is a late effect.

The amount of petroleum distillate necessary to cause pulmonary problems depends on the product. A very small amount (*i.e.,* less than 1 ml) can be very serious if introduced directly into the trachea.

Toxicity with oral ingestions varies with the viscosity and volatility of the substance. The less viscous the substance, the more likely it is to be aspirated. Products that have a low viscosity and high volatility (*e.g.,* benzene, kerosene,

---

Chart 30-10

MANAGEMENT OF THE PATIENT WITH AN ACID OR ALKALI EXPOSURE

Assessment

- Ingestion
  Chemical burns to mouth, pharynx, esophagus
  Gastric irritation with nausea and vomiting
  Systemic effects of hypotension, peritonitis, or mediastinitis with perforation of tissue
- Inhalation
  Coughing, choking, air hunger
  Increased secretions
  Pulmonary edema
- Contact
  Chemical burns on area of contact
  Ulceration at point of contact

Emergency Management

Do not attempt to neutralize the acid or alkali

1. *Prevent absorption*—emesis or lavage is contraindicated. Flush area with nonreactive liquid.
   - Ingested—give patient milk or water to drink.
   - Inhaled—remove from source.
   - Contact—irrigate with copious amounts of fluid.
2. *Provide specific and supportive care.*
   - Use caution with suction tubes, avoid nasogastric tubes if at all possible.
   - Monitor respiratory status to determine whether pulmonary complications have occurred.
   - Protect skin burns with sterile dressing.
   - Hydrofluoric acid—inject calcium gluconate to chelate acid.
   - Perform esophagoscopy to determine extent of injury and for irrigation to remove any remaining substance.

---

turpentine) tend to be poisonous in doses as low as 1 ml/kg. Death has resulted from doses of 10 ml to 250 ml. Mortality is increased if an additional toxic substance is present, or if accidental aspiration occurs.

Petroleum distillates are fat solvents and will rapidly cross the lipid cell membrane. Nerve tissue is especially sensitive to injury. The patient may exhibit local effects, that is, depressed nerve conduction, or central effects, such as altered levels of consciousness, convulsions, and coma. Patients may experience feelings of well-being, headache, tinnitus, dizziness, visual disturbances, or respiratory depression.

Management and Treatment

In a critical patient, supportive care is given as well as treatment specific to the toxin involved. In the awake and alert patient, the decision to treat will be based on the physical properties of the substance, the likelihood of aspiration or other complications, and the amount consumed.

- *Goal #1: Prevent absorption.*
  1. If it has been determined that gastric emptying should be done, emesis is the preferred form of treatment for an awake patient who has a good gag reflex. Table 30-10 lists the indications for emesis on the basis of which product and dose was involved. "Cautious gastric lavage" is not considered desirable for the awake patient because a fair number of patients vomit with nasogastric or endotracheal intubation. This increases the risk of aspiration. Since hydrocarbons may adhere to the tube, an additional risk of aspiration is possible when the tube is removed, if the substance is close to the epiglottis.
  2. If the patient is lethargic or unconscious, an endotracheal tube must be placed prior to lavage.
- *Goal #2: Provide specific and supportive care.*
  1. The patient's respiratory status should be immediately assessed for possible aspiration. If the patient is coughing, has cyanosis or appears hypoxic, he has probably aspirated.
  2. The patient may have cardiac irritability from either the petroleum distillate or the effects of hypoxia. The use of epinephrine for respiratory or cardiac problems should be avoided because catecholamines may precipitate ventricular fibrillation.
  3. If seizures require treatment, diazepam is given intravenously.

TABLE 30-10. INDICATIONS FOR VOMITING WITH PETROLEUM DISTILLATES

Vomiting Recommended	Vomiting Not Recommended
1. If 1 ml/kg or more of the following is ingested: 　Trichloroethane　　Toluene 　Trichloroethylene　Xylene 　Carbon tetrachloride　Benzene 　Methylene chloride　Turpentine 　Charcoal lighter fluid　Kerosene 　Petroleum lighter fluid　Gasoline 　Mineral spirits　　Naphtha	1. The following products are poorly absorbed from the gastrointestinal tract but will cause severe pneumonitis if aspirated: 　Mineral seal oil 　Furniture polish 　Oil polish
2. Any petroleum distillate with any amount of dangerous additives: 　Heavy metals 　Insecticides 　Nitrobenzene 　Aniline	2. These products rarely cause more than a pneumonia if directly aspirated: 　Asphalt or tar 　Lubricants (motor oil, greases, and transmission oil) 　Mineral oil (baby oil, suntan oil, and laxatives) 　Fuel oil (diesel oil)

(After Poisindex J7, 1980)

4. Antibiotics should be reserved for specific infections and should not be given prophylactically.

Chart 30-11 summarizes the care of the victim of petroleum distillate poisoning.

MULTIVITAMINS WITH IRON

An excessive dose of multivitamins is dangerous if vitamin A or iron is involved. Vitamin A is a fat-soluble compound that is stored primarily in the liver. When vitamin A is present in quantities that exceed the liver's ability to store it, it circulates in the blood and is deposited in other tissues.

Iron is unusual in that it has no organ of excretion. After ingestion, ot is bound to transferrin and albumin in the serum. It is eliminated through the skin in perspiration, bile, and the female menses. If an excessive dose is ingested, the capacity of the binding proteins is surpassed and iron will circulate in a free form. The unbound form causes a systemic response and tissue damage. Symptoms may appear when 150 mg/kg of iron is present in the serum. The lethal dose is estimated to be 200 to 500 mg/kg.

Assessment

Signs and symptoms of vitamin A and iron toxicity are as follows.
- Vitamin A. Excessive doses of vitamin A will be stored in fatty non-hepatic tissue. If a large amount is sequestered in the CNS, neurologic disorders may be seen. Patients

---

Chart 30-11

MANAGEMENT OF THE VICTIM OF PETROLEUM DISTILLATE POISONING

Assessment
- Identify what was ingested to determine severity of poisoning.
- Check for respiratory function and accidental aspiration.
　Choking, coughing
　Systemic hypoxia—cyanosis, dysrythmias, altered sensorium
　Arterial blood gases

Emergency Management
1. *Prevent absorption.*
   - Emesis for awake, responsive patients
   - Gastric lavage with endotrachial intubation for unconscious patients
2. *Provide supportive care.*
   - Monitor respirations.
   - Control seizures.
   - Avoid prophylactic antibiotics.

complain of lethargy, headache, nausea, or vomiting. Tinnitus is common. A real danger is present if the stored vitamin can produce a rise in intracranial pressure. Hepatic enlargement and periosteal swelling have also been noticed with excessive vitamin A intake.

- Iron. Ingested iron can be corrosive to the mucosa of the gastrointestinal tract. Bloody vomitus and painless, bloody diarrhea or dark stools have been seen with ingestions. The free form of iron circulating in the blood produces systemic effects. Coma, shock, metabolic acidosis, fever, liver and renal damage may occur. The symptoms of a systemic poisoning tend to be time related. They are

Time after Ingestion	Symptoms
Stage I—30 min–2 hr	Vomiting, diarrhea, abdominal pain, and decreased sensorium
Stage II—6–12 hr	Rapid improvement and a false sense of security that the poisoning was not severe
Stage III—18–72 hr	Cardiovascular collapse, coma, fever, coagulation defects, and death
If the patient survives, Stage IV—4–6 weeks	Gastrointestinal scarring

Management

- *Goal #1: Prevent absorption.*
  1. Gastric emptying is appropriate to remove vitamins or iron tablets from the stomach.
  2. Enteric coated pills may form a mass in the stomach which does not return via a gastric lavage tube. A large bolus may have to be removed through a gastrotomy or gastroscopy.
  3. Cathartics and activated charcoal are also used to decrease bowel absorption.
  4. Iron tablets are radiopaque and can be seen on an x-ray of the abdomen. Flat plate x-rays are helpful in determining if the gastric emptying was successful.
- *Goal #2: Enhance elimination from the blood.*
  Excessive amounts of free iron can be removed from the serum by a chelating agent. Deferoxamine (Desferal) is given if the serum level is above 300 μg/100 ml 6 hours after ingestion, or if a reliable history indicates that a toxic dose has been ingested. Deferoxamine is given until the urine returns to a normal color. If iron is present in the urine, a salmon color is observed. (See Table 30-5 for more information about this drug.)
- *Goal #3: Provide specific and supportive care.*
  1. The patient with vitamin A poisoning should be monitored carefully for increased intracranial pressure. A pressure monitor is used to recognize rising pressures and to monitor the effectiveness of therapy.
  2. The patient who has ingested an excessive amount of iron should be observed for both local and systemic effects. The gastric mucosa may be partially protected by the use of antacids, demulcents, or a bland diet to help reduce irritation. Systemic poisoning presents a danger of hypotension, hypovolemia, bleeding disorders and decreased levels of consciousness.

Chart 30-12 lists the management of a patient who has ingested multivitamins with vitamin A or iron.

FOOD POISONING

The average person consumes a variety of foods that are prepared in many forms and, in today's society, may be handled by many people. Because we eat foods that others have grown or prepared, we may not always be familiar with what they are or how they have been handled. A lack of familiarity with foodstuffs, particularly plants, has caused unfortunate poisoning incidents, such as when an individual ate what he thought was an edible substance. Food handlers can be a source of bacterial contamination if they do not practice good handwashing or cleaning techniques.

In general, food poisoning may result either from the ingestion of substances not meant for human consumption, or from the ingestion of contaminated food. Relatively few people—only a handful of inquisitive individuals—sample products not meant to be eaten. Larger numbers, such as an entire family or restaurant patrons who share a common source, may be exposed to contaminated food. Poisoning caused by plants will be discussed later in the chapter. In the following section, bacterial food poisoning is considered.

Bacterial Food Poisoning

Food contaminated with bacteria may not always poison the person who has consumed it. Depending on the organism and the methods of food storage or preparation, the person may become critically ill or may suffer no consequences at all.

Assessment. If food poisoning is suspected, the following history should be obtained:
- Type of food and its source
- Time of ingestion, and onset of symptoms
- Symptoms experienced, particularly vomiting or diarrhea
- Other unusual symptoms, such as weakness, loss of motor or bleeding disorders
- Effects on others who ate the food

The clinical findings of food poisoning will vary according to the type of bacterial contamination.

Botulism. The term "botulus" is Latin for sausage. During the late 19th century, it was noted that a specific neuroparalytic disorder would appear after people ate blood sausage. They did not know that the sausage had been contaminated with *Clostridium botulinum,* a spore-forming gram-negative bacillus. *C. botulinum* spores are found virtually everywhere.

C. botulinum produces toxins that are poisonous to man. Seven types are produced: A, B, C, D, E, F, and G; types A, B, and E are the most important in terms of toxicity. To produce toxins, *C. botulinum* spores require an anaerobic environment, temperature above 3°C (37.4°F), and a *p*H higher than 4.6. Improperly prepared home-canned meats, fish, and vegetables tend to be the greatest sources of botulism. Cases of botulism acquired from airtight plastic bags have been reported. The toxins are heat labile and can be destroyed if the food is boiled at 100°C (212.0°F), or pressure-cooked for 10 to 15 minutes.

Signs and Symptoms. Botulinus toxin interferes with the release of acetylcholine at the motor end plates of the

---

Chart 30-12

MANAGEMENT OF THE PATIENT WITH VITAMIN A OR IRON POISONING

Assessment

HISTORY

- Obtain history of amount ingested.

SIGNS AND SYMPTOMS

- Vitamin A
  CNS involvement
  Increased intracranial pressure
- Iron—clinical findings appear in stages.
  Stage I—vomiting, diarrhea, abdominal pain, altered sensorium
  Stage II—rapid improvement
  Stage III—cardiovascular collapse, coma, coagulation defects, fever, death
  Stage IV—if patient survives, scarring of gastrointestinal tract

Emergency Management

1. *Prevent absorption.*
   - Emesis
   - Lavage
   - Gastroscopy or gastrotomy if pills have clumped in stomach
     Note: flat plate x-rays of the abdomen can be used to identify any remaining pill fragments in the intestine.
2. *Enhance elimination.*
   - Administer deferoxamine (Desferal) to chelate circulating free iron
3. *Provide specific and supportive care.*
   Vitamin A—monitor for increased intracranial pressure.
   Iron
   - Local effects
     Demulcents, antacids, bland diet
   - Systemic effects
     Maintain intravascular volume and blood pressure
     Monitor and treat coagulation defects
     Protect from complications of coma

---

voluntary and parasympathetic nervous system nerves. Without acetylcholine, muscle paralysis will occur, and a loss of parasympathetic function will be manifested by an unbalanced sympathetic stimulation. The onset of symptoms will vary with the toxin. They may appear within 8 hours or up to 8 days after ingestion.

Symptoms appear in a characteristic head-to-toe progression. Cranial nerves are affected first; the patient complains of ptosis and blurred or double vision and has dilated pupils. As the reaction progresses, the patient has difficulty in swallowing and may feel a soreness in his throat. At this point, symptoms can be easily misidentified as an upper respiratory infection. As the symptoms progress downward, the patient is in danger of respiratory failure due to paralysis of the nerves necessary for breathing. If the paralysis of the

respiratory nerves is not complete, the patient will eventually develop quadriplegia. The toxin does not affect the mental status, and the victim is awake and conscious.

Botulism is fatal in approximately 50% of the patients who contract it; death is due to respiratory failure. If the victim survives, a residual muscle weakness may persist for years.

Management and Treatment. Prompt action to remove residual food is followed by administration of the appropriate antitoxin.

- *Goal #1: Prevent absorption.*

  1. As soon as poisoning is suspected, any residual food in the bowel should be removed. Peristalsis will probably be slowed, and in fact an ileus may be present. The choice between emesis or lavage will depend on

the patient's status and his ability to control his airway. Cathartics will help to eliminate toxins in the bowel.
- *Goal #2: Provide specific and supportive care.*
  1. Antitoxins are administered after the toxin is identified. Since antitoxin is prepared from horse serum, skin testing is recommended prior to administration.

     There are two types of antitoxin, the bivalent (anti A and B toxin), and the trivalent (anti A, B, and E). Antitoxins act to prevent further paralysis, but do not have an effect on already paralyzed muscles. Antitoxin should be given as soon as the need is suspected in order to have an effect on mortality.

Staphylococcus. The staphylococcus organism is found on human skin, in nasal secretions, and in purulent drainage. It is introduced onto food by human contact, commonly from upper respiratory or wound infections.

Staphylococci produce enterotoxins in food that is allowed to be at room temperature. It is particularly apt to grow in dairy foods, creamy desserts, salads, egg preparations, and poultry products. Infection can be prevented by refrigeration of the suspected foods, adequate hand washing, and thorough cleaning of food handling areas. Cooking does not destroy the toxins.

Signs and Symptoms. After the enterotoxin enters the bowel, it produces symptoms within 1 to 6 hours. The gastrointestinal tract is irritated and the patient has profuse vomiting, diarrhea, and abdominal cramping. The severe vomiting and diarrhea can produce a volume depletion that requires parenteral replacement.

Management and Treatment. Therapy includes fluid replacement and correction of electrolyte imbalances.
- *Goal #1: Prevent absorption.*
  1. There is usually little need to induce vomiting or catharsis. Some practitioners feel that the severe diarrhea should be treated with an antidiarrheal drug. This is discouraged because the diarrhea is actually a physiologic response to the enterotoxins and serves to eliminate them from the bowel.
- *Goal #2: Provide supportive care.*
  1. Observe for dehydration and electrolyte imbalances.
  2. Therapy is directed towards replacement and correction.

Salmonella. The salmonella organism is found in the bowel of man and of small animals commonly kept as pets (*i.e.,* turtles, chicks, dogs, cats, and parakeets). Contamination of food occurs when a person with poor handwashing technique carries the organism from the source directly to the food. Occasionally, water supplies are contaminated with sewage. Salmonella may produce local gastrointestinal irritation or a systemic poisoning.

Signs and Symptoms. The patient is observed for gastrointestinal symptoms and possible systemic reactions.
1. Gastrointestinal. The onset of symptoms occurs within 7 to 72 hours after ingestion. The bacteria enters the bowel, multiplies, and begins production of an enterotoxin that inflames and irritates the bowel. Nausea, vomiting, abdominal cramping and a loose, watery diarrhea that may have blood or mucus is noted.

2. Systemic. If the organism invades the mucosal barrier of the bowel and enters the blood stream, it produces a septicemia with fever and chills. This is referred to as the *typhoidal syndrome.* Aside from fever, the patient can have meningeal irritation and splenomegaly. The bacteria can seek out compromised tissue and cause secondary abscesses.

Management and Treatment. In addition to supportive care, antibiotic therapy and fluid and electrolyte replacement are carried out.
1. Gastrointestinal. *Provide supportive care.*
   - Emetics or purgatives are not indicated because of the profound vomiting and diarrhea.
   - Fluid and electrolyte replacement should be provided.
2. Systemic. *Provide specific and supportive therapy.*
   - Parenteral antibiotic therapy is used to control the septicemia. Chloramphenicol or ampicillin is given for a period of several weeks.
   - Close attention should be given to the patient's fluid and electrolyte status, and replacement therapy should be carried out according to losses.

Shigella. Shigella is found only in human feces. It is introduced to food by poor hygiene or sewer contamination of water supplies. It is usually obtained from unwashed fruits, vegetables, or in milk products. Contamination is preventable by adequate sewer systems, treatment of water supplies, pasteurization of milk, and proper handwashing.

Signs and Symptoms. After the microorganism enters the bowel, it incubates for 1 to 3 days. It then begins to irritate the mucosa and causes vomiting, abdominal cramping, diarrhea, and tenesmus. The diarrhea may appear green. Dehydration and fever are secondary symptoms of infection.

Management and Treatment. Supportive care is provided and treatment is directed toward fluid and electrolyte replacement.
- Goal #1: *Provide supportive care.*
  1. Emetics and cathartics are not necessary.
  2. Replace fluid and electrolyte losses with parenteral therapy.
  3. If severe, diphenoxylate (Lomotil) can be used to control abdominal pain or tenesmus; however, it should be remembered that this may prolong the infection and the symptoms.

Management of the patient poisoned with food contaminated with bacteria is summarized in Chart 30-13.

Poisoning Due to Plants

The recent upsurge in the incidence of plant poisoning is a reminder of the prevalence of plants in the home, work place, and recreational areas. Plants are a major source of poisoning in children under the age of 5 years. Although the incidence is high, the fatality rate is fortunately low.

Poisoning caused by plants presents a complex and often difficult situation, mainly in terms of diagnosis. Many people either do not know the correct name of a plant or use a local term. Inability to identify the plant causes a delay in recognition and treatment.

Chart 30-13

MANAGEMENT OF THE PATIENT POISONED WITH FOOD CONTAMINATED WITH BACTERIA

Assessment

HISTORY

1. Type of food and its source
2. Time of ingestion and onset of symptoms
   - Vomiting, diarrhea
   - Unusual—weakness, paralysis, bleeding
3. Effects on other people who ate the same food

SIGNS AND SYMPTOMS (SPECIFIC TO TYPE OF POISONING)

1. Botulism
   - Progressive head-to-toe paralysis
   - Difficulty swallowing, sore throat
   - Respiratory paralysis
   - Quadriplegia
2. *Staphylococcus* infection
   - Profuse vomiting and diarrhea
   - Abdominal cramping
   - Fluid and electrolyte depletion
3. *Salmonella* infection
        Gastrointestinal
   - Nausea, vomiting
   - Loose, watery diarrhea, possibly with blood or mucus
        Systemic
   - Fever, chills
   - Meningeal irritation, splenomegaly
   - Secondary abscesses
4. *Shigella* infection
   - Vomiting, cramping, tenesmus
   - Green diarrhea

Emergency Management

1. *Prevent absorption.*
   - Botulism—emesis or lavage according to patient's respiratory status; ileus may be present.
   - All other forms—emetics and cathartics are not indicated because of the vomiting and diarrhea already present.
2. *Provide specific and supportive care.*
   - Botulism—administer antitoxins (skin test may be needed before use).
   - *Salmonella* infection—administer antibiotics for systemic infection.
     All forms
   - Provide fluid and electrolyte replacement.
   - The choice to treat diarrhea and cramping should be balanced with an understanding that this may prolong the duration of infection.

TABLE 30-11. POISONOUS PLANTS

Plant	Toxic Part and Substance	Symptoms	Treatment
House plants			
Arnica (*Arnica montana, sororia, cordifolia*)	Flowers and roots	GI symptoms, drowsiness, coma	Gastric lavage or emesis; symptomatic
Arum family: calla lily (*Caladium*), dumbcane (*Dieffenbachia*), elephant's ear (*Colocasi*), *Alocasia, Philodendron, Dracunculus, Amorphophallis*	All parts (calcium oxalate, unidentified principles)	Severe burning of mucous membranes with swelling of tongue and throat; nausea; vomiting; diarrhea; salivation; rarely, direct systemic effects	Gastric lavage or emesis; symptomatic
Castor bean (*ricinus communis*)	Seed (ricin, if chewed; if swallowed whole, the hard seed coat prevents absorption and poisoning)	Severe GI symptoms, convulsions, uremia	Immediate gastric lavage or emesis; supportive; 5 gm to 15 gm sodium bicarbonate daily to alkalinize urine
Mistletoe (*Phoradendron flavescens*)	Berries (β-phenylethylamine and tyramine)	GI symptoms and bradycardia similar to digitalis	Gastric lavage or emesis; supportive; potassium, procainamide, quinidine sulfate, or disodium salt of EDTA
Rosary pea, jequirity bean, precatory bean, prayer bean, love bean, or lucky bean (*Abrus precatorius*)	Poisoning unlikely unless bean (abrin) is chewed; if chewed, causes agglutination and hemolysis even in weak dilution	Symptoms may be delayed 1 to 3 days; severe GI symptoms, drowsiness, coma, circulatory collapse, hemolytic anemia, oliguria, fatal uremia	Gastric lavage or emesis; maintenance of circulation; blood transfusions to correct hemolytic anemia; sodium bicarbonate to alkalinize urine
Flower garden plants			
Bleeding heart or dutchman's breeches (*Dicentra pucilla, cucullaria*)	All parts (isoquinoline-type alkaloids such as apomorphine, protoberberine, and protopine)	Trembling, ataxia, respiratory distress, convulsions	Symptomatic
Daphne (*Daphne mezereum*)	All parts (daphnin)	Abdominal pain, vomiting, bloody diarrhea, weakness, convulsions	Gastric lavage or emesis; symptomatic
Foxglove (*Digitalis purpurea*)	Leaves (digitalis glycosides)	Nausea, diarrhea, stomach pain, severe headache, tremors, convulsions, irregular heartbeat and pulse	Gastric lavage or emesis; supportive; atropine, potassium, procainamide, quinidine sulfate, or disodium salt of EDTA
Hyacinth (*Hyacinthus orientalis*)	Bulb	Severe GI symptoms	Gastric lavage or emesis; symptomatic
Indian tobacco (*Lobelia inflata*)	All parts (α-lobeline)	Progressive vomiting, weakness, stupor, tremors, contraction of pupils, coma	Gastric lavage or emesis; artificial respiration; atropine, 2 mg IM as necessary
Jessamine or yellow jessamine (*Gelsemium sempervirens*)	All parts (gelsemine and gelseminine)	Profuse sweating, muscular weakness, convulsions, repiratory depression	Gastric lavage or emesis; atropine, 2 mg IM as necessary; artificial respiration
Lantana, red sage, wild sage (*Lantana camara*)	All parts (lantanin), especially the green berries	Photosensitization with increase in severity from sunlight; acute symptoms resemble belladonna alkaloid (atropine) poisoning	Gastric lavage or emesis; symptomatic and supportive
Lily-of-the-valley (*Convallaria majalis*)	Leaves and flowers (convallatoxin and other glycosides)	Irregular heartbeat, stomach upset	Gastric lavage or emesis; supportive; potassium, procainamide, quinidine sulfate, or disodium salt of EDTA
Narcissus family: daffodil, jonquil (*Narcissus pseudonarcissus, jonquilla*)	Bulb	GI symptoms	Gastric lavage or emesis; symptomatic
Nutmeg (*Myristica fragrans*)	Seeds (myristicin)	Hallucinations and elation, stomach pain, red skin, dry mouth, drowsiness, stupor, double vision, delirium. (Two nutmegs can be fatal)	2 to 4 oz mineral or castor oil, followed by gastric lavage and demulcents

TABLE 30-11. POISONOUS PLANTS (CONTINUED)

Plant	Toxic Part and Substance	Symptoms	Treatment
Oleander (*Nerium oleander*)	Leaves (oleandrin and nerioside)	Nausea, severe vomiting, stomach pain, dizziness, slowed pulse, irregular heartbeat, marked dilation of pupils, bloody diarrhea, drowsiness, unconsciousness, paralysis of lungs. (One leaf can kill an adult.)	Gastric lavage or emesis; symptomatic and supportive; potassium, procainamide, quinidine sulfate, or disodium salt of EDTA
Sweet pea (*Lathyrus odoratus*)	All parts, but especially seeds (β-aminopropionitrile, α-γ-aminobutyric acid)	Paralysis; slow, weak pulse; respiratory depression; convulsions	Gastric lavage or emesis; symptomatic
Vegetable garden plants			
Rhubarb (*Rheum rhaponticum*)	Leaves only (oxalic acid)	Nausea, vomiting, abdominal pain, anuria, hemorrhages	Gastric lavage or emesis with limewater, chalk, or calcium salts; calcium gluconate; forced IV fluids; supportive
Ornamental plants and trees			
Black locust (*Robinia pseudocacia*)	Bark, foliage, and seed (phytotoxin)	Nausea, vomiting, weakness, depression	Symptomatic
Elderberry, black and scarlet elder (*Sambucus canadensis, pubens*)	Leaves, shoots, and bark (sambunigrin, a cyanogenic glycoside)	Nausea, vomiting, diarrhea	Gastric lavage or emesis; commercially available cyanide kit
Heath family: azaleas, *Rhododendron*, laurels (*Kalmia*)	All parts (andromedotoxin)	Salivation, lacrimation, rhinorrhea, vomiting, convulsions, slowing of pulse, hypotension, paralysis	Gastric lavage or emesis; activated charcoal, atropine, hypotensive drugs
Wisteria (*Wisteria sinensis*)	Pods (resin and glycoside, wisterin)	Severe GI symptoms, collapse	Gastric lavage or emesis; symptomatic
Yew (*Taxus baccata*)	All parts (alkaloid taxine)	GI symptoms, dilation of pupils, muscular weakness, coma, convulsions, cardiac and respiratory depression	Gastric lavage or emesis; meperidine to control pain; otherwise, symptomatic
Cherries, wild and cultivated (*Prunus*)	Twigs, foliage, and seeds (cyanide-releasing compound)	Stupor, vocal cord paralysis, tremors, convulsions, coma	Gastric lavage or emesis; use cyanide kit if indicated
Plants that grow in the wild			
Buttercup family: crowfoot or buttercup (*Ranunculus*), cowslip or marsh marigold (*Caltha palustris*), larkspur (*Delphinium*), monkshood (*Acontium*)	All parts; for monkshood, especially roots and seeds	Paresthesia, burning sensation of mouth and skin, nausea, vomiting, hypotension, weak pulse, convulsions	Atropine, 2 mg IM and repeat as necessary; maintenance of blood pressure; artificial respiration
Deadly nightshade (*Atropa belladonna*)	Berries, leaves, and roots (atropine and related alkaloids)	Fever; rapid heartbeat; dilation of pupils; skin hot, flushed, dry	Gastric lavage (4% tannic acid solution) or emesis; pilocarpine for dry mouth and visual disturbances
Laurel: mountain, black, sheep, American. See Heath family, Section IV of Table			
Mushrooms (*Amanita muscaria* and *phalloides*)			
Pokeweed, pokeberry, scoke, or inkberry (*Phytolacca americana*)	All parts, especially root (saponin and glycoprotein); glycoproteins in African species produce lymphocytes that resemble those in Burkett's lymphoma.	Burning bitter taste in mouth, persistent vomiting, amblyopia, slowed respiration, dyspnea, weakness, tremors and convulsions, peripheral blood plasmacytosis (May be fatal)	Gastric lavage or emesis; symptomatic

TABLE 30-11. POISONOUS PLANTS (*CONTINUED*)

Plant	Toxic Part and Substance	Symptoms	Treatment
Poison hemlock (*Conium maculatum*)	All parts (alkaloid coniine)	GI symptoms, necrosis, muscular weakness, respiratory paralysis, convulsions	Gastric lavage or emesis; saline cathartic; maintenance of clear airway; oxygen and artificial respiration; anticonvulsive therapy
Thornapple, jimsonweed, or stinkweed (*Datura stramoniur*)	All parts (atropine and related alkaloids)	Thirst, dilation of pupils, dry mouth, red skin, headache, hallucinations, rapid pulse, high blood pressure, delirium, convulsions, coma	Gastric lavage or emesis; pilocarpine for dry mouth and visual disturbances; barbiturates for convulsions
Water hemlock or cowbane, beaver poison (*Cicuta maculata, virosa*)	Roots (resin cicutoxin)	GI symptoms, convulsions, respiratory depression	Gastric lavage or emesis; symptomatic; parenteral short-acting barbiturates to control convulsions

(Arena JM: The treatment of poisoning. Clin Sympos 30:41, 1978. Copyright © 1978 by CIBA-GEIGY Corporation. Reprinted with permission from Clinical Symposia, by Jay. M. Arena, M.D.)

A desire for a more natural life style has led some persons to harvest plants in the wild. Poisoning occurs because of conflicting information in lay publications on which plants or parts of plants are toxic. Folklore serves to mislead those who hunt the plants or attempt to treat the patient. Table 30-11 lists plants commonly involved in poisonings; toxic parts and substances are identified. The symptoms experienced by the patient and treatment measures are described.

Poisoning Due to Mushrooms

There are old mushroom hunters, And there are bold mushroom hunters, But there are no old, bold mushroom hunters.

Mushrooms have lived in peaceful coexistence with man for centuries. They continue to serve as a source of intrigue and to mystify those who hunt them as food or for their

---

Chart 30-14

COMMON BUT INACCURATE METHODS OF DETERMINING MUSHROOM TOXICITY

Error	Explanation
"Place a silver coin or utensil in the pan when mushrooms are cooked. The coin will turn black if poisons are present."	False. Several very poisonous mushrooms do not tarnish silver, *e.g.,* the death cap, *Amanita phalloides.*
"Caps of edible fungi can be peeled."	False. The cap of the death cap variety does peel easily.
"The color is a safe determinant. The bright ones are poisonous, while the plain ones are edible."	False. Many of the *Amanita* species are yellowish white to completely white.
"Poisonous species change color if cut or bruised."	False. Color changes are due to a chemical reaction and have nothing to do with toxins.
"It is safe to eat what animals eat."	False. Many animals have less sensitive digestive systems than man's. They are able to eat fungi that are poisonous to humans because their digestive systems can neutralize the toxins.
"Poisonous species can be neutralized by soaking or boiling."	False. No method has been found that will effectively neutralize toxins.

TABLE 30-12. TOXIC EFFECTS OF POISONOUS MUSHROOMS ON BODY SYSTEMS

	Destruction at Cellular Level	Toxins Affecting Destruction of Automatic Nervous System	Toxins Affecting Central Nervous System	Toxins Affecting the Gastrointestinal Tract
Mushroom type	Cyclopetides (amanitins) Gyromitrin	Coprine (Antabuse-like) muscarine	Muscimol ibotenic acid (*Amanita muscaria, A. panthenine*) Psilocybin, psilocin	Diverse, mostly unknown
Onset of symptoms	6–24 hr	30 min–2 hr; 30 min after drinking alcohol with Coprine	30 min–2 hr	30 min–2 hr
Signs and symptoms	CNS: faintness, loss of coordination, coma, convulsions; GI: bloated feeling, abdominal pains, nausea, vomiting, diarrhea (watery or bloody); Other: hemolysis, jaundice, muscle cramps	CV: flushed face, distended neck veins, tachycardia, hypotension; GI: metallic taste, nausea, vomiting, salivation, abdominal cramps, water diarrhea; Other: swelling and tingling of hands, sweating, lacrimation, blurred vision	CNS: dizziness, incoordination, staggering, muscle weakness, coma-like sleep, visions, pleasant to apprehensive mood, laughter, drowsiness, convulsions, fever; Other: musle cramps, spasms, hyperkinetic activity	GI: nausea, vomiting, diarrhea, abdominal pain
Mortality	50% mortality for amanitins 25% for Gyromitrin	Rare: unless patient was debilitated	Rare	Rare
Treatment Cyclopetides	Thictic acid, 50 mg–150 mg q 6 h (diluted in 1 L D_5W). May be given up to 2 weeks or until serum liver enzymes return to normal (may cause hypoglycemia). Must be protected from light during storage and administration. Penicillin G, 250 mg/kg/day IV. Vitamin K, 40 mg, IV daily Corticosteroids, e.g., dexamethasone, 20 mg–40 mg IV daily. Observe fluid and electrolyte balance.	Coprine: propranolol may be necessary to control cardiac arrhythmias. Avoid elixirs and tinctures. Muscarine: atropine 1 mg–2 mg IV p.r.n. for symptoms	Muscimol, Ibotenic acid: Physostigmine, 0.5 mg–2 mg slow IV every hour or p.r.n. for anticholinergic symptoms. Do not give unless symptoms are definitely present. Psilocybin and psilocin	Diverse group Supportive care
Gyromitrin, monomethylhydrazine (MMH)	Pyridoxine HCl, 25 mg/kg, IV, titrated to patient's symptoms. Observe methemoglobin and free hemoglobin levels, liver parameters.		Diazepam, 5 mg–10 mg for seizures Chlorpromazine 50 mg–100 mg IM for psychoses	

(After Mitchell D: Mushroom toxicity. Presented at Continuing Medical Education Clinical Toxicology, National Emergency Medicine Service, University of Colorado School of Medicine, Denver, Colorado, March 3, 1977)

Chart 30-15

MANAGEMENT OF A PATIENT POISONED BY A PLANT OR A MUSHROOM

Assessment

- Identify plant or mushroom involved. Be specific; many species may grow together.
- Examine the total patient for signs of systemic response. Signs and symptoms vary according to what has been ingested.
- Ascertain whether other substances have been consumed in addition to the plant or mushroom.

Emergency Management

1. Prevent absorption.
   Emesis
   Lavage
   Activated charcoal and cathartics

2. Provide specific and supportive care.
   Antidotes specific to plant or mushroom
   Monitor respiratory, cardiovascular, neurologic, renal, and hepatic functions.

---

hallucinatory effects. The mystique of the mushroom has also generated numerous problems not only for the one who consumes them, but also for the emergency care providers who have to care for the person poisoned by them.

Of over 200 species in the world, only 50 are considered poisonous. Old wives' tales and superstition are often the only guidelines used to determine if the mushroom is dangerous. Chart 30-14 lists some of the common misconceptions associated with wild mushrooms.

Assessment. There are many reasons why mushroom poisonings are difficult to manage. Clinical findings will depend upon the type of mushroom and the amount ingested, the patient's general state of health, and in some cases, the presence of other substances in the body. The reasons why multiple signs and symptoms can be observed may be listed as follows:
1. Different individuals can respond differently to the same mushroom.
2. The toxicity of a mushroom can vary according to its stage of growth, the soil or climate, and the number of different toxins present in it.
3. The patient may have ingested the mushroom in addition to another substance which then causes a toxic interaction (*e.g.,* the *Gyromitrin* species precipitates an Antabuse effect if alcohol is present in the blood).
4. The uncomfortable effects of overeating or drinking may be misconstrued as a toxic response to mushrooms.
The following factors serve to further confuse the rescuer and distort the understanding of a response to a mushroom:
1. Multiple species of mushrooms may grow together and the wrong mushroom may have been brought in for identification.

2. Mushrooms growing in the wild are subject to environmental pollutants and bacterial contamination.
3. A nontoxic mushroom may be deliberately poisoned in an attempt to commit homicide.

The more severe forms of mushroom poisoning occur with the *Cyclopetides* (amanitins) or *Gyromitrin* species. The high mortality associated with their use is in part due to the severe systemic effects they produce and the inability to prevent fatal complications. The patients have altered levels of consciousness, convulsions, vomiting, diarrhea, and hemolysis. Table 30-12 lists the toxic effects due to various types of mushrooms and indicates antidote therapy.

Management and Treatment. *Remember to treat the patient, not the mushroom.* Let the patient's clinical response to the ingestion be a guide for therapy. In a situation in which it is not possible to identify the type of mushroom, gastric emptying should be done because the risk of nontreatment may be greater.

- *Goal #1: Prevent absorption.*

  1. If vomiting is not already present, initiate emesis or gastric lavage.
  2. Activated charcoal and cathartics are also used, unless diarrhea is present.

- *Goal #2: Provide specific and supportive care*

  1. Table 30-12 outlines antidote therapy for specific types of mushroom poisoning
  2. Supportive care involves monitoring respiratory, cardiovascular, neurological, renal, and hepatic functions.

The care of a patient poisoned with a plant or a mushroom is summarized in Chart 30-15.

BIBLIOGRAPHY

Arena J: Poisoning: Toxicology, Symptoms, Treatments, 3rd ed. Springfield, Ill, Charles C Thomas, 1974

Arena J: The treatment of poisoning. Clinical Symposia 30(2), 1978

Aronow R, Done A: Phencyclidine overdose: An emerging concept in management. JACEP 7(2):56–59, February 1978

Beamon R, Siegel C, Landers G, Green V: Hydrocarbon ingestion in children: A six-year retrospective study. JACEP 5(10):771–775, October 1976

Beede M: Phencyclidine intoxication: Insights into a growing problem of drug abuse. Postgrad Med 68(5):201–209, November, 1980

Breysse P: Carbon monoxide threats never take a vacation. National Safety Council Newsletter, June 1977

Burckhardt D et al: Cardiovascular effects of tricyclic and tetracyclic antidepressants. JAMA 239(3):213–216, January 16, 1978

Burns S, Lerner S: Phencyclidine-related deaths. JACEP 7(4):135–141, April 1978

Domino E: Neurobiology of phencyclidine: An update. In Petersen R, Stillman R (eds): Phencyclidine (PCP) Abuse: An Appraisal. NIDA Research Monograph 21, Stock #017-024-00785-4. Washington, DC: U.S. Government Printing Office, August 1978

Done A: The toxic emergency: Tips and tidbits. Emerg Med 9(6):225–228, June 1977

Done A: The toxic emergency. A phencyclidine pin-up. Emerg Med 10(6):179–182, June 1978

Done A: The toxic emergency: The great equalizers? 1. Insecticides. Emerg Med 11(5):95–107 passim, May 15, 1979

Done A, Aronow R, Miceli J: The pharmacokinetics of phencyclidine in overdose and its treatment. In Petersen R, Stillman R (eds): Phencyclidine (PCP) Abuse: An Appraisal. NIDA Research Monograph 21, Stock #017-024-00785-4. Washington, DC: U.S. Government Printing Office, August 1978

Douglas A, Hamlyn A, James O: Controlled trial of cysteamine in treatment of acute paracetamol (acetaminophen) poisoning. Lancet 1:111–115, January 17, 1976

Dreisbach R: Handbook of Poisoning, 9th ed. Los Altos, Lange Medical Publications, 1977

Erler M: Iron poisoning. J Emerg Nurs 6(2):40–42, March–April 1980

Goldrank L, Osborn H: The barbiturate overdose. Hosp Phys 13(9):30–34, September 1977

Goodman L, Gilman A (eds): The Pharmacological Basis of Therapeutics, 5th ed. New York, Macmillan, 1975

Gross P: Overdose: A time for decision. Emerg Med 9(6):195–198, June 1977

Harace N: Emergency management of mushroom poisoning. J Emerg Nurs 4(3):12–16, May–June 1978

Hollister L: Treatment of depression with drugs. Ann Intern Med 89(1):78–84, July 1978

Holtman D: Acetaminophen overdose. J Emerg Nurs 4(3):50–52, May–June 1978

Hooper R, Conner C, Rumack B: Acute poisoning from over-the-counter sleep preparations. JACEP 8(3):98–100, March 1979

Ilo E: Charcoal: An update on an old drug. J Emerg Nurs 6(4):45–48, July–August 1980

Jelenko C: Chemicals that burn. J Trauma 14(1):65–72, January 1974

Jozwiak J: Acetaminophen overdose: A new and treacherous care problem. RN 41(12):56–61, December 1978

Lerner S, Burns R: Phencyclidine use among youth: History, epidemiology, and acute and chronic intoxication. In Petersen R, Stillman R (eds): Phencyclidine (PCP) Abuse: An Appraisal. NIDA Research Monograph 21, Stock #017-024-00785-4. Washington, DC: U.S. Government Printing Office, August 1978

Loeble S et al: The Nurse's Drug Handbook. New York, John Wiley & Sons, 1977

Lovejoy F: Priorities in poisoning. Emerg Med 11(2):265–277, February 15, 1979

Luisada P: The phencyclidine psychosis: Phenomenology and treatment. In Petersen R, Stillman R (eds): Phencyclidine (PCP) Abuse: An Appraisal. NIDA Research Monograph 21, Stock #017-024-00785-4, Washington, DC: U.S. Government Printing Office, August 1978

Macy A: Preventing hepatotoxicity in acetaminophen overdose. Am J Nurs 79(2):301–303, February 1979

Manoguerra A, Ruiz E: Psysostigmine treatment of anticholinergic poisoning. JACEP 5(2):125–127, February 1976

Mello N: Control of drug self-administration: The role of aversive consequences. In Petersen R, Stillman R (eds): Phencyclidine (PCP) Abuse: An Appraisal. NIDA Research Monograph 21, Stock #017-024-00785-4. Washington, DC: U.S. Government Printing Office, August 1978

Metz V, Hansen I: Management of drug overdose in the adult. J Emerg Nurs 1(6):8–11, November–December 1975

Mitchell D: Mushroom Toxicity. Presented at Continuing Medical Education Clinical Toxicology, National Emergency Medicine Service, University of Colorado School of Medicine, Denver, Colorado, March 3, 1977

Morton J: Plants Poisonous to People in Florida and Other Warm Areas. Miami, Hurricane House, 1971

Muhlendahl K, Krienke E, Bunjes R: Fatal overtreatment of accidental childhood intoxication. J Pediatr 93(6):1003–1004, 1978

Ng R, Darwish H, Stewart D: Emergency treatment of petroleum distillate and turpentine ingestion. CMAJ 111:537–538, September 21, 1974

Pascoe D, Grossman M: Quick Reference to Pediatric Emergencies, 2nd ed. Philadelphia, JB Lippincott, 1978

Petersen R, Stillman R (eds): Phencyclidine: An Overview. Phencyclidine (PCP) Abuse: An Appraisal. NIDA Research Monograph 21, Stock #017-024-00785-4, Washington, DC: U.S. Government Printing Office, August 1978

Pisarcik G: Management of phencyclidine toxicity. J Emerg Nurs 4(5):35–37, September–October, 1978

Poisindex Co, Salicylates, #C-13, 1979

Poisindex Co, Hydrocarbons (Petroleum distillates), #H-I-J 7, 1980

Purin-Parkinson C: Sorting out the adrenergic/cholinergic drugs. RN 42(8):52–54, July 1979

Rappolt R, Gay G: Emergency management of acute phencyclidine intoxication. JACEP 8(2):68–76, February 1978

Rose J: Tricyclic antidepressant toxicity. Clin Toxicol 11(4):391–402, 1977

Santa Clara Valley Medical Center, Department of Emergency Medicine: Nursing Procedures: Ipecac to Water Ratio Protocols, February 1980

Temple A: Acute and chronic effects of aspirin toxicity and their treatment. Arch Intern Med 141(3):364–369, February 23, 1981

Thornton W: Sleep aids and sedatives. JACEP 6(9):408–412, September 1977

Tintinalli J: Hydrofluoric acid burns. JACEP 7(1):24–26, January 1978

Turk S: Houseplant poisoning in children. J Emerg Nurs 5(2):9–13, March–April, 1979

Martin E (ed): Sedative-hypnotic drug use. FDA Drug Bulletin 8(1):5–6, January–February 1978

U.S. Department of Justice Drug Enforcement Administration: Drugs of Abuse, 3rd ed. Washington, DC

Vourakis C, Bennet G: Angel dust: Not heaven sent. Am J Nurs 79(4):649–653, April 1979

Ward D: Danger of saline emetics. Br Med J 2:459, August 13, 1977

31
BITES
AND STINGS

DIANN ANDERSON and JAMES H. COSGRIFF, JR.

Bites and stings are among the most common injuries sustained by humans; they may be inflicted by all kinds of insects, reptiles, and animals, as well as by other humans. Bites can produce both abraded and penetrating wounds, which may be complicated by infection from the bacterial flora of the attacker or by the toxic reaction produced by an injected substance.

Not only are meticulous wound management and repair important, but prophylaxis against infectious substances and neutralization of toxic effects may also be necessary. The assessment of the patient with a bite or sting, and the related emergency management, are discussed in this chapter.

HUMAN BITES

Of all possible bites, a bite by a human is one of the most serious. Human bites may occur in several ways:
- The attacker actually sinks his teeth into the victim's skin, causing a perforating wound or loss of skin.
- A person strikes his fist against another's teeth and incurs a laceration of the knuckles.
- The person bites himself, as in tongue lacerations occurring during an epileptic seizure.

The introduction of bacteria-laden saliva into these wounds, some with crushed or contused tissue, may have serious consequences. Because of the multiplicity of organisms present in the human mouth, these infections are mostly of the mixed type and may be unusually severe. This constitutes the main complication of human bites.

Careful assessment for possible injury to deep structures by evaluating sensory and motor function is most important. In knuckle wounds, the extensor tendon may be divided. The wound can be carefully spread with skin hooks or the patient asked to make a fist and a careful examination made in that position. It is recommended that a culture of the wound be taken and followed by thorough cleansing and debridement of contused or devitalized tissue. Primary closure is usually not recommended. Healing by secondary intention is preferable until evidence of infection is absent; secondary suture of tendons or nerves may then be done. Adequate doses of a broad-spectrum antibiotic should be started immediately.

Self-inflicted bites of the tongue may be deep and tend to bleed profusely. When the injury is deep, suturing is usually required. Because the tongue is very sensitive to injection, use of a topical anesthetic agent, such as tetracaine HCl prior to infiltration is helpful. After closure, the patient should be placed on antiseptic mouthwashes and a liquid or soft diet, as tolerated, until healing occurs.

ANIMAL BITES

A large number of animal bites are recorded annually. When the bite has been inflicted by a domestic animal previously immunized for rabies, the wound can be treated in the usual manner with cleansing and debridement. All devitalized tissue should be excised and the wound allowed to heal by secondary intention. In bites involving exposed areas such as the face, head, neck, and hands, serious consideration must be given to primary suture. Closure of these wounds demands meticulous cleansing and debridement.

The use of prophylactic antibiotics depends on the severity and location of the injury and is not required routinely. Tetanus immunization should be given according to recommendations outlined in Chapter 19, Wound Management.

Emergency management of the victim of an animal bite is summarized in Chart 31-1.

RABIES

Rabies rarely affects humans. Its incidence has decreased from an average 22 cases per year (from 1946 to 1950) to 1 to 5 cases per year since 1960. Rabies vaccination of domestic animals accounts for this decline. However, the disease in wildlife, especially in skunks, foxes, and bats, has become increasingly prominent and now constitutes the most important source of rabies infection in both domestic animals and humans today.

When a bite is made by an animal that may have rabies, special precautions must be taken to prevent this deadly disease in the victim. Children under 12 years of age seem more susceptible to the disease than older children or adults.

Pathophysiology

Rabies is caused by a virus present in the saliva of an infected animal. The infection is transmitted when the infected animal bites another animal or a human. Rabies can also develop following exposure of a fresh skin abrasion or mucous membrane to infected saliva. The virus, which has an affinity for nervous tissue, travels from the site of entry through peripheral nerves to the spinal cord and brain. The virus multiplies in the brain and passes through efferent nerves to the salivary glands and into the saliva.

The incubation period ranges from 10 days to over a year. Victims with extensive bite wounds or wounds of the face, hands, and other vascular areas are at higher risk.

Signs and Symptoms

Signs and symptoms of rabies include the following:
- Fever
- Malaise
- Headache
- Photophobia
- Musculoskeletal pain
- Itching, burning, numbness, or paresthesia around the wound site
- Restlessness progressing to uncontrollable excitement
- Excessive salivation and pronounced spasms of laryngeal and pharyngeal muscles precipitated by the slightest stimuli and causing excruciating pain
- Death usually occurs within 3 to 5 days, from asphyxia, exhaustion, or general paralysis.

Chart 31-1

EMERGENCY MANAGEMENT OF THE BITTEN VICTIM

Prehospital Care

- Maintain ABCs; control bleeding.
- Immediately flush the wound with copious amounts of water and soap or detergent, if available.
- Dress with dry, sterile dressings.
- Transport, while reducing physical and emotional stress of victim.

Hospital Care

- Culture the wound.
- Thoroughly flush and cleanse with soap solution.
- Thoroughly rinse off soap and apply a solution of 1% to 4% benzalkonium chloride (Zephiran), 40% to 70% isopropyl alcohol or povidone-iodine (Betadine).
- Debride devitalized tissue and allow healing by secondary intention. (If wounds are sutured because of cosmetic effect, *i.e.,* face), meticulous cleansing and debridement are mandatory because of high incidence of secondary infection.
- Evaluate need for tetanus and antibacterial prophylaxis and administer as indicated.
- Evaluate need for rabies prophylaxis and provide as appropriate.
- Report bite to local health authorities or to law enforcement agencies as local law indicates.

Because of the high mortality associated with this disease, a careful assessment and appropriate prophylactic measures must be instituted as soon after the injury as possible.

Rabies Prophylaxis

History is of particular importance in determining whether the victim was bitten by a rabid animal and if antirabies treatment is needed. Attention should be given to the following:

- Species of the biting animal—carnivorous animals and bats are more infective than other animals.
- Circumstances of the biting incident—an unprovoked attack is more likely to occur from a rabid animal.
- Type of exposure—since the disease is transmitted by infectious saliva through a break in the skin, the nature of the wounding is important.
- Vaccination status of the biting animal—a properly immunized animal has a minimal chance of developing and thus spreading the disease.
- Presence of rabies in the region—local health officials can provide data about the incidence of the disease and of rabid animals in the locale.

In most localities, animal bites must be reported to local health authorities. The offending animal, if domestic or able to be trapped, is placed under surveillance until the 10- to 14-day incubation period for rabies has passed. If the animal is wild and can be killed, care should be taken to avoid injuring the head, as the brain is examined for evidence of rabies. If the animal is not identified or located or if it is found rabid, antirabies treatment is necessary.

Immunizing Agents

The two commonly used vaccines that provide active immunity are human diploid cell vaccine (HDCV) and duck embryo vaccine (DEV). Passive immunity is provided by one of two globulins—human rabies immune globulin (HRIG) or antirabies serum, equine (ARS). HDCV and HRIG are the substances preferred for use because of their human source and thus their lower incidence of sensitivity reactions. When only DEV or ARS is available, skin testing must be done prior to administration.

Vaccines. HDCV was developed in the 1960s by inactivating a strain of rabies virus grown in human diploid cell tissue culture. Studies using this vaccine show that it yields an antibody titer ten times that of DEV and produces minimal side-effects. No serious anaphylactic, neuroparalytic, or systemic reactions have been reported.

HDCV is administered in five 1-ml intramuscular doses initially and on days 3, 7, 14, and 28. HRIG is administered with the initial dose of HDCV. The vaccine is administered alone only when the individual has been immunized before and has a documented adequate rabies antibody titer. At the conclusion of immunizing therapy or within 2 to 3 weeks of therapy, a serum specimen for rabies antibody testing is collected.

DEV is given in a series of 1-ml subcutaneous doses in one of the two following dosage schedules:
1. 1 ml per day for 21 consecutive days or
2. 1 ml twice daily for 14 days, then 1 ml per day for 7 days.

Booster injections are given 10 and 20 days after the daily injection routine. HRIG is administered with the initial dose of DEV. Since the vaccine causes regional lymphadenitis, it is best given in the anterior abdominal wall, lower back, or lateral aspect of the thighs, varying the site each day.

Globulins. Globulins provide passive immunity and should be administered with the initial dose of vaccine at a separate site. HRIG is administered intramuscularly in the recommended dose of 20 IU/kg, or about 9 IU/lb, of body weight. If possible, up to half the total dose should be thoroughly infiltrated around the wound.

ARS is given only if HRIG is unavailable and only after sensitivity to horse serum is ruled out. (See Table 31-1.) Tables 31-1 and 31-2 outline guidelines for antirabies therapy.

SNAKEBITES

Although snakebite is not considered a common injury, several thousand Americans are bitten each year, of which 10 to 20 die. There are two principal groups of poisonous snakes native to the United States. These are the family Crotalidae (rattlesnake, cottonmouth or water moccasin, and copperhead), also known as pit vipers, and the family Elapidae (coral snake). Coral snakes rarely bite man, accounting for only 1% to 2% of venomous snake bites. By contrast, pit vipers strike promiscuously, often without provocation.

PIT VIPERS

The various species of pit vipers are widely distributed throughout the United States. Identifying characteristics (Fig. 31-1) include:

- A triangular-shaped head with a pit between the eye and the nostril on each side (hence the name "pit viper")
- Elliptical pupils
- One to six fangs (usually two, though they are shed periodically and are replaced by others)
- A single row of plates beneath the tail

Pit viper envenomation and the development of signs and symptoms depend on a number of variables as outlined by Russell:
- Age, size, general health of victim
- Nature, location, depth, and number of bites
- Amount of venom injected
- Species of snake involved
- Condition of the snake's fangs and venom glands
- Victim's sensitivity to the venom
- Pathogens present in the snake's mouth
- Degree and kind of first aid and subsequent medical care
- Factors that motivate the snake to bite
- Length of time snake holds on
- Amount and kind of clothing worn by victim

Pit viper venom is a complex mixture of proteins and enzymes that produce variable effects, depending on the species of snake and on the autogenic responses of the victim. Some common clinical findings follow:

Signs and Symptoms of Pit Viper Envenomation

Local Effects
- Fang marks—one or more puncture wounds varying from 1 mm to 8 mm in depth
- Immediate pain—may be transient or prolonged; pain may be related to edema

---

TABLE 31-1. RABIES POSTEXPOSURE PROPHYLAXIS GUIDE, MARCH 1980

The following recommendations are only a guide. In applying them, take into account the animal species involved, the circumstances of the bite or other exposure, the vaccination status of the animal, and presence of rabies in the region. Local or state public health officials should be consulted if questions arise about the need for rabies prophylaxis.

Animal Species	Condition of Animal at Time of Attack	Treatment of Exposed Person*
Domestic		
Dog and cat	Healthy and available for 10 days of observation	None, unless animal develops rabies†
	Rabid or suspected rabid	RIG‡ and HDCV§
	Unknown (escaped)	Consult public health officials. If treatment is indicated, give RIG‡ and HDCV§
Wild		
Skunk, bat, fox, coyote, raccoon, bobcat, and other carnivores	Regard as rabid unless proven negative by laboratory tests¶	RIG‡ and HDCV§
Other		
Livestock, rodents, and lagomorphs (rabbits and hares)	Consider individually. Local and state public health officials should be consulted on questions about the need for rabies prophylaxis. Bites of squirrels, hamsters, guinea pigs, gerbils, chipmunks, rats, mice, other rodents, rabbits, and hares almost never call for antirabies prophylaxis.	

* All bites and wounds should immediately be thoroughly cleansed with soap and water. If antirabies treatment is indicated, both RIG and HDCV should be given as soon as possible, regardless of the interval from exposure.

† During the usual holding period of 10 days, begin treatment with RIG and vaccine (preferably with HDCV) at first sign of rabies in a dog or cat that has bitten someone. The symptomatic animal should be killed immediately and tested.

‡ If RIG is not available, use ARS. Do not use more than the recommended dosage.

§ If HDCV is not available, use DEV. Local reactions to vaccines are common and do not contraindicate continuing treatment. Discontinue vaccine if fluorescent-antibody (FA) tests of the animal are negative.

¶ The animal should be killed and tested as soon as possible. Holding for observation is not recommended.

(Immunization Practices Advisory Committee: Rabies prevention. Morbid Mortal Week Rep 29(23), June 13, 1980)

TABLE 31-2. RABIES IMMUNIZATION REGIMENS, MARCH 1980

Pre-exposure:

Pre-exposure rabies prophylaxis for persons with special risks of exposure to rabies, such as animal-care and control personnel and selected laboratory workers, consists of immunization with either HDCV or DEV, according to the following schedule.

Rabies Vaccine	No. of 1-ml Doses	Route of Administration	Intervals Between Doses	If No Antibody Response to Primary Series, Give:*
HDCV	3	IM	1 week between 1st and 2nd; 2–3 weeks between 2nd and 3rd†	1 booster dose†
DEV	3	SC	1 month between 1st and 2nd; 6–7 months between 2nd and 3rd† *or* 1 week between 1st, 2nd and 3rd; 3 months between 3rd and 4th†	2 booster doses,† 1 week apart
	or 4			

Postexposure:

Postexposure rabies prophylaxis for persons exposed to rabies consists of the immediate, thorough cleansing of all wounds with soap and water, administration of RIG or, if RIG is not available, ARS, and the initiation of either HDCV or DEV, according to the following schedule.‡

Rabies Vaccine	No. of 1-ml Doses	Route of Administration	Intervals Between Doses	If No Antibody Response to Primary Series, Give:*
HDCV	5§	IM	Doses to be given on days 0, 3, 7, 14, and 28†	An additional booster dose†
DEV	23	SC	21 daily doses followed by a booster on day 31 and another on day 41† *or* 2 daily doses in the first 7 days, followed by 7 daily doses. Then 1 booster on day 24, and another on day 34†	3 doses of HDCV at weekly intervals†

* If no antibody response is documented after the recommended additional booster dose(s), consult the state health department or CDC.
† Serum for rabies antibody testing should be collected 2–3 weeks after the last dose.
‡ The postexposure regimen is greatly modified for someone with previously demonstrated rabies antibody.
§ The World Health Organization recommends a 6th dose 90 days after the first dose.
(Immunization Practices Advisory Committee: Rabies prevention. Morbid Mortal Week Rep 29(23), June 13, 1980)

- Edema formation within 5 to 10 minutes of envenomation
- Ecchymosis around bite area, often involving entire extremity
- Vesiculations, hemorrhagic bullae, and petechiae (in untreated victims) in area of bite. May involve entire extremity in severe envenomations.
- Necrosis—more prevalent in patients who received insufficient or belated antivenin therapy

Systemic Effects
- Weakness, sweating, and chills
- Paresthesias—changes in taste (minty, rubbery, or metallic), numbness or tingling of the tongue and mouth or of the scalp or feet
- Fasciculations may appear early and are most noticeable on the face, back, neck, and involved extremity.
- Nausea and vomiting (may be provoked by administration of narcotics)
- Bleeding phenomena (prolonged bleeding and clotting times, decreased platelet counts or decrease in circulating blood volume and vascular permeability)
- Bleeding problems may result in hypotension and shock, or in hematemesis, melena, hematuria, etc.

- Neurologic deficits, including weakness or paralysis of a part or blurred or yellowed vision

CORAL SNAKES

In the United States, coral snakes can be found in the southeastern states, western Colorado, and Utah southward through Texas and Mexico. Only 1% to 2% of venomous snakebites are caused by the shy, docile coral snake. Physical characteristics of coral snakes are as follows:
- Small, slender bodies with black, red, and yellow bands. Red and yellow bands touch in the venomous coral snake; in nonvenomous species, the red and yellow bands are separated by black bands.
- All rings encircle the body.
- Forepart of bullet-shaped head is black.
- Pupils are round, as in nonvenomous snakes.
- Short, erect fangs are fixed to anterior maxilla

The coral snake has a less efficient method of envenomation than the pit viper. The coral snake must strike and hold so that its chewing action can milk venom from its glands. Because of this, it cannot readily penetrate clothing or grasp any part except the hand or foot.

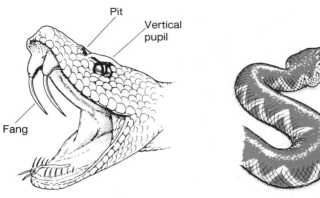

Figure 31-1 *Pit viper. Left. Note the long, hinged pair of fangs, the vertical slit for a pupil, and the pit (the heat-sensing organ) between the eye and the nose. Right. Note the typical flat, triangular head.*

The neurotoxic effects of coral snake venom produce paralysis, though no symptoms may occur for 1½ to 18 hours after the bite. Once symptoms occur, they progress rapidly.

Signs and Symptoms of Coral Snake Envenomation

- Few or no symptoms initially
- Scratch marks or punctures, with or without edema, erythema, or pain
- Numbness, weakness of affected part
- Euphoria, lethargy, drowsiness, apprehension
- Nausea, vomiting
- Excessive salivation
- Fasciculation and tremor of tongue
- Difficulty in swallowing
- Dyspnea
- Possible paresis of extraocular muscles, pinpoint pupils, ptosis of eyelids
- Abnormal reflexes, weakness, or paralysis
- Hypotension and weak, irregular pulse
- Convulsions
- Respiratory paralysis
- Respiratory and cardiac failure associated with death

Because of the high toxicity of coral snake venom, it is wise to initiate antivenin therapy in the absence of initial signs and symptoms simply based on history (identification of snake and its holding onto the victim for a minute or more).

PRINCIPLES OF MANAGEMENT OF SNAKEBITE VICTIMS

Whether the venomous bite was inflicted by a pit viper or a coral snake, the general principles of care are the same. Since the ultimate goals are to neutralize the venom and limit its absorption when possible, these principles also apply to bites and stings of many other venomous insects and animals. Figure 31-2 provides guidelines for the assessment and treatment of the patient with snake venom poisoning.

Management of the patient who has been bitten by a poisonous snake is summarized in Chart 31-2.

Determining Sensitivity to Horse Serum

All patients must be tested for sensitivity to horse serum prior to administration of antivenin or any substance prepared from a foreign protein.
- Evaluate history for

    Asthma, hay fever, urticaria, or other allergic reactions

    Allergic symptoms upon exposure to horses

    Prior injections of horse serum
- Administer skin or conjunctival test.

Skin Test. Inject 0.02 to 0.03 ml of a 1:10 dilution of normal horse serum or antivenin intradermally to raise a wheal. (A 1:100 dilution should be used in patients whose history suggests sensitivity.) A positive reaction occurs within 5 to 30 minutes; it consists of erythema and sometimes an irregular raised projection at the edge of the wheal. Generally, the earlier the reaction, the more sensitive is the individual.

Conjunctival Test. Instill 1 drop of 1:100 or 1:10 of normal horse serum or antiserum into the conjunctival sac. A positive reaction occurs within 10 minutes; it ranges from itching and slight dilatation of conjunctival vessels to marked dilatation of vessels, itching, and edema of the area in more sensitive individuals.
- If the history or skin test is positive or questionably positive, follow the specific instructions in the accompanying antivenin package.
- *Absence of positive findings does not rule out the possibility of a severe, immediate reaction upon administration of the antivenin.*
- Common systemic allergic reactions include restlessness; itching; urticaria; edema of the face, tongue, and airway passages; cough; dyspnea; cyanosis; and collapse
- Prior to administration, have resuscitative equipment, oxygen, a tourniquet, epinephrine (1:1000) and a pressor amine readily available, and have an intravenous line of D_5W or Ringer's lactate established.

Antivenin Therapy

- To be effective, antivenin must be administered within the first few hours after evenomation. It is useless 24 hours after exposure.
- In the patient who is not sensitive to horse serum, there is no limit to the amount of antivenin that can be administered. Some clinicians advocate high initial intravenous doses to neutralize all venom fully. Dosages depend on the severity of the envenomation, *i.e.,* minimal, moderate, or severe.
- In smaller patients, a proportionately higher initial dose must be administered. Children, having less resistance and less body fluid to dilute the venom, may need up to twice the amount that would suffice for an adult.
- Intravenous administration is usually acceptable. Administration around the bite site is not recommended, and some clinicians discourage intramuscular administration.
- Observe the patient's response, giving one vial every half hour if pain and swelling progress.
- Observe for shock, hematemesis, melena, and hematuria, which indicate a hemorrhagic state due to further ab-

sorption of venom and the need for additional doses of antivenin.

- Do not give corticosteroids simultaneously.
- *Serum sickness* is a common sequela in persons receiving foreign proteins, especially in high intravenous doses. Serum sickness is characterized by urticaria, fever, and sometimes lymphadenopathy, splenomegaly, and polyarthritis. It is usually self-limiting and is treated symptomatically with antihistamines, an antipruritic lotion, analgesics, and occasionally corticosteroids. Since serum sickness occurs 10 to 14 days after treatment, the patient should be alerted to the possibility of this event before discharge.

ARTHROPODS

Arthropods constitute about 80% of the animal kingdom. It is fortunate that only a few pose a hazard to man. Only four species of arthropods in the United States possess potentially lethal venoms—the black widow spider, the brown recluse spider, and two species of scorpions, which reside in the Southwest, primarily in Arizona. Others, unless they carry disease (*e.g.,* malaria, Rocky Mountain spotted fever), pose little threat to man, except when the individual is hypersensitive to their venom or to substances in their saliva.

ARACHNIDS (SPIDERS AND SCORPIONS)

In most spider bites one or two small puncture wounds 1 mm to 10 mm apart are present. Multiple bites are not caused by spiders, since they rarely bite more than once. Spiders may bite and not release venom, causing no signs or symptoms.

Black Widow Spider Bites

Black Widow Spiders (*Lactrodectus mactans*) reside in all areas of the continental United States, commonly in wood and brush piles. The female, which bites, is coal black with an orange or red hourglass marking on her abdomen. The potent venom is neurotoxic, producing the effects of ascending motor paralysis. The outcome of her bite is determined by several factors: age, size and health of the victim, amount and potency of venom injected, and location of the bite (absorption is less in extremities than in the trunk or head). There is cause for concern when systemic reactions to envenomation develop within 15 to 30 minutes of the bite.

Signs and Symptoms of Black Widow Spider Bite

1. Local signs and symptoms
   - Pinprick sensation with bite, followed by dull ache or numbness in affected extremity
   - Redness, edema surrounding two tiny fang marks
2. Systemic signs and symptoms
   - Severe abdominal pain when bite is on lower extremity; back, chest, or shoulder pain when bite is on upper extremity. Pain peaks in 1 to 3 hours.

- Vital signs—possible elevation in blood pressure and temperature; weak, slow pulse; and diminished LOC
- Tremor, weakness, sweating, salivation, nausea, vomiting
- Late signs and symptoms include dyspnea, shock, delirium and convulsions.
- Hemolysis and thrombocytopenia

Principles of Management. Treatment objectives are to restrict absorption of the venom, neutralize it, and provide symptomatic relief.

Prehospital Care.
- See Snakebite.

Hospital Care.
1. Establish an intravenous line.
2. Administer intravenous muscle relaxants (diazepam) and 10% calcium gluconate p.r.n. for relief of pain and spasms.
3. Administer narcotics with extreme caution, and only for relief of *severe* pain, since they may potentiate respiratory depression.
4. *Latrodectus mactens* antivenin brings relief from symptoms within 1 to 3 hours.
   - Administer one ampule in 10 ml to 50 ml of saline (following appropriate skin testing).
   - Antivenin is advisable in patients under 16 or over 60 years of age or those with hypertensive heart disease. These patients should be hospitalized for rest and observation.

Brown House Spider Bites

The brown spider (*Loxosceles reclusa*), also known as the brown recluse, is about 2½ inches long and lives in the midwestern and midsouthern states. Its habitat is clothes closets and other dark locations in and around the house. The bite produces a necrotoxin; therefore, the bitten area may develop an ischemic center and ulcerate. Severe local pain, restlessness, and fever may be associated symptoms.

No antivenin is available. However, if the patient seeks treatment within 24 hours, the prognosis is good. Prompt administration of antihistamines and corticotropin will limit the effects of the necrotoxin to the bitten area and reduce systemic reactions. Further management consists of pain control and local wound care. Wide ulceration can result, and in some anatomic areas, such as the pretibial region, delayed healing occurs and secondary grafting may be required.

Scorpion Stings

Scorpions are nocturnal arachnids, lying hidden during the day beneath debris of all kinds, as well as under buildings and lumber piles. Of over 300 known species, only a limited number are considered lethal to man. The poisonous scorpions, which live mainly in the arid southwestern United States, are the *Centruroides sculpturatus* and *Centruroides gertschii.*

The scorpion's venom is present in a bulb-like enlargement at the tip of its tail. Although more toxic than most

LAC-USC Guide for Snake Venom Poisoning

Date: _____

Time: _____

Tissue destruction, hemostatic defects, hemorrhage, cardiovascular and neurological changes, and respiratory distress may result from snake venom poisoning. Immediate or delayed serum reactions and infection may complicate the poisoning. The severity of the injury should be assessed by the degree and rapidity of the onset of symptoms and signs and data from laboratory tests. Continual reevaluation of the poisoning must be made as the response to treatment progresses. Remember, snake venom poisoning is a medical emergency requiring immediate attention, that it is a multiple-type poisoning and, finally, that the fact that the patient has been bitten by a venomous snake does not necessarily mean that he has been envenomated. Twenty percent of all rattlesnake bites seen at this Medical Center show no evidence of poisoning. In cases of a bite by any snake, NOTIFY THE LABORATORY OF NEURO-LOGICAL RESEARCH—4741, 4742, 4743. PLEASE COMPLETE THIS FORM AS COMPLETELY AS POSSIBLE.

ADMITTING DATA: 1. Patient age: _____ 2. Sex: _____ 3. Date/time of bite _____

   4. Location (city, county etc.) _____

   5. Description of snake _____

   6. Species (if known): _____ 7. Identified by: _____

   8. Immediate (<30 min) reactions to bite (circle & comment):

     a. Swelling   0 1 2 3 4 _____

     b. Local pain   0 1 2 3 4 _____

     c. Paresthesias   0 1 2 3 4 _____

     d. Fasciculations 0 1 2 3 4 _____

     e. Ecchymoses   0 1 2 3 4 _____

     f. Nausea   0 1 2 3 4 _____

     g. Weak-paralysis 0 1 2 3 4 _____

     h. Resp. distress 0 1 2 3 4 _____

     i. Other (describe) _____

_____

   9. First aid: yes no Time: _____ Methods: _____

  10. Treatment at other facilities: yes no Time: _____ Describe (include antivenin, dose, route)

_____

_____

     INITIAL LAC-USC FINDINGS Date/time of admission: _____ RR _____ BP _____

  11. Symptoms: _____ Temp _____ HR _____

  12. Describe wound and bitten part: _____

_____

  13. Local sensory-motor exam (pain, pin, range of motion, joint, strength): _____

_____

  14. Edema: 0 1 2 3 4   15. Ecchymoses: 0 1 2 3 4

  16. Petechiae: 0 1 2 3 4   17. Bullae: 0 1 2 3 4

  18. Systemic findings (hemodynamic, hematologic, neuromuscular): _____

_____

  19. Initial lab studies: _____

_____

     FOR ADULTS AND CHILDREN > 35 KG PLEASE OBTAIN 1 RED TOP AND 1 LAVENDER (CBC) TUBE OF BLOOD ON ADMISSION AND Q8H FOR THE INITIAL 48H. LABEL TIME-DATE AND PATIENT NAME. PLACE IN REFRIGERATION ON CD ADMITTING WARD.

  20. INITIAL SEVERITY ASSESSMENT (circle) NO ENVENOMATION MINIMAL MODERATE SEVERE

Figure 31-2 *Guide for snake venom poisoning used by University of Southern California Medical Center, Los Angeles County. (Russell F: Snake Venom Poisoning. Philadelphia, JB Lippincott, 1980)*

21. Comments: _____

_____

_____

_____

_____

_____

_____

_____

Guidelines for Management

By the time the patient arrives at the Medical Center it will be too late for any effective first aid measures. Do nothing but cleanse the wound area at this time.

ANTIVENIN: See brochure in package. If plan to use be sure to skin test. Do not give if lacking evidence of envenomation, give as early as possible, and IV in appropriate vehicle. GIVE ENOUGH. There is a tendency to give too little. Minimal envenomation will require 5–8 vials, moderate, 9–13 and severe, 14–40. Again, DO NOT GIVE WITHOUT SKIN TESTING. Inject all antivenin intravenously. Watch for any reactions, even when skin test has been negative. If skin test is positive and patient requires antivenin, get consultation STAT (4741).

SENSITIVITY TEST: When _____ Where _____
Results _____

ANTIVENIN: Amount _____ When started _____ Dilution _____
When stopped _____ Reactions _____ Additional antivenin,
amount _____ When _____ .

OTHER IMMEDIATE CARE (circle): Immobilization, tetanus, pain medications, Other medications, IV fluids, Oxygen, Burows soaks, debridement, triple dye, antibiotics, p.t., other _____

LABORATORY TESTS: See instructions on board, C.D.2

FOLLOW-UP CARE:

The symptoms and signs of rattlesnake venom poisoning may be relatively minor during the first hour following the bite, in spite of serious envenomation. If swelling progresses rapidly, parasthesias worsen or either fail to respond to initial antivenin administration, anticipate a severe poisoning. Shock may develop in some cases and warrant immediate shock measures. Avoid corticosteroids. Do not perform a fasciotomy. Do not pack in ice. Do not elevate extremity during first 48 hours. If you require consultation, do not hesitate to call 4741. Further instructions and references are on C.D.2 bulletin board. See also J.A.M.A 233(4), 341, 1975.

COMMENTS: _____

_____

_____

_____

_____

_____

_____

_____

_____

_____

_____

_____

_____

_____

Chart 31-2

MANAGEMENT OF THE VICTIM OF SNAKEBITE

Prehospital Care

1. Keep victim physically and emotionally calm.
2. Remove snake from victim, or when possible kill snake (some victims have been bitten more than once).
3. Remove jewelry and loosen clothing because edema will form.
4. Apply a wide constricting band (¾ inch to 1½ inch) above and below the bitten area, to slow lymphatic and venous flow but not arterial flow. Be sure the distal pulse is present.
5. Do not apply constricting bands around a joint.
6. Monitor closely for encroaching edema producing a tourniquet effect, and reposition constricting bands as edema advances.
7. Immobilize and position affected part at the level of the heart.
8. Do not apply cold. The toxins produce tissue ischemia. Cold adds insult to injury.
9. Do not administer vasodilators such as alcohol or stimulants.
10. Carry victim to nearest medical facility; do not allow him to walk.
11. Cleanse bitten area with soap and water.
12. *Incision and suction* to remove venom are highly controversial and generally not recommended. They are indicated only when symptoms appear within the first 30 minutes, when a medical facility is 4 to 5 hours away, and when there is rapid swelling within 15 minutes following the bite.
    - *Note: be aware that this technique could result in permanent injury or deformity, and may not sufficiently remove venom.*
    - Do not delay transport in order to perform incision and suction.
13. *Technique for incision and suction* (Fig. 31-3)
    - Cleanse wound and apply antiseptic.
    - Make a linear (*not cruciate*) cut about ⅛ inch deep and ⅛ inch to ¼ inch long, starting at fang puncture site and extending distally.
    - Using suction cup or mouth, apply suction for 20 minutes.
    - Treat for shock (maintain body heat, reduce physical and emotional stress).
    - Monitor vital signs.
    - Antivenin is not recommended for field use because of risk of anaphylaxis.

Hospital Care

1. Collect samples for type and crossmatch, CBC, hematocrit, platelet count, prothrombin time, clot retraction, bleeding and coagulation time, BUN, electrolytes, and bilirubin, and test for urinalysis.
2. Measure intake and output.
3. Measure circumference of bitten extremity at level of the bite site every 15 to 30 minutes to monitor edema.
4. Administer tetanus prophylaxis and broad-spectrum antibiotic therapy.
5. Establish IV of Ringer's lactate or normal saline for administration of fluid, blood components.
6. Establish IV of normal saline or D_5W for administration of antivenin, when indicated.
7. Determine need for antivenin therapy.
    - Pit viper envenomation is neutralized by Polyvalent Crotalidae Antivenin (Fig. 31-4).
    - Coral snake envenomation is neutralized by North American Coral Snake Antivenin (Fig. 31-4).
8. Do skin or conjunctival testing for sensitivity to horse serum before using either antivenin (see description in text).
9. Administer antivenin according to directions in package insert (see notes on antivenin therapy in text).
10. *Wound management:*
    - Monitor edema, presence of distal pulse, culture wound.
11. Controversy exists regarding fasciotomy. Some feel that higher IV doses of antivenin precludes need for surgical repair.
12. Immobilize affected extremity with bulky dressings in functional position, and dress with bulky dressings.
13. Admit to hospital for observation. (Greatest danger is in first 24 to 48 hours.)

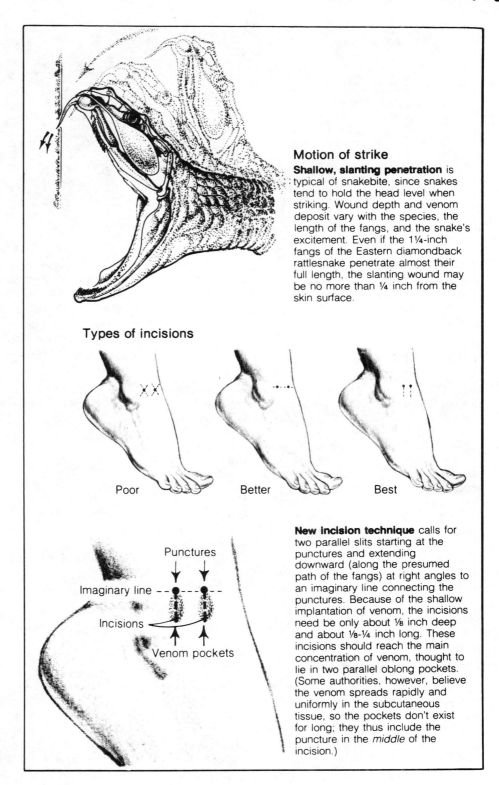

Motion of strike

Shallow, slanting penetration is typical of snakebite, since snakes tend to hold the head level when striking. Wound depth and venom deposit vary with the species, the length of the fangs, and the snake's excitement. Even if the 1¼-inch fangs of the Eastern diamondback rattlesnake penetrate almost their full length, the slanting wound may be no more than ¼ inch from the skin surface.

Types of incisions

Poor Better Best

New incision technique calls for two parallel slits starting at the punctures and extending downward (along the presumed path of the fangs) at right angles to an imaginary line connecting the punctures. Because of the shallow implantation of venom, the incisions need be only about ⅛ inch deep and about ⅛-¼ inch long. These incisions should reach the main concentration of venom, thought to lie in two parallel oblong pockets. (Some authorities, however, believe the venom spreads rapidly and uniformly in the subcutaneous tissue, so the pockets don't exist for long; they thus include the puncture in the *middle* of the incision.)

Punctures
Imaginary line
Incisions
Venom pockets

Figure 31-3 *Incision technique for snakebite. (From Snakebite? Get the facts, then hurry. Patient Care, June 1, 1976, Vol X(11):48–59. Reproduced from Patient Care magazine. Copyright ©1976, Patient Care Communications, Inc., Darien, CT. All rights reserved)*

snake venom, the injected quantity is minute. Thus, fatal scorpion stings occur infrequently; almost all reported deaths from scorpion stings have occurred in children under 6 years of age.

Local evidence of the sting may be minimal or absent. The first symptom is mild tingling or burning at the site. This may be followed by excessive salivation, drowsiness, nausea, vomiting, mydriasis, and photophobia. The poison acts on the nervous system, producing fatality by its effect on the cardiac and respiratory centers. Rapid progression of symptoms within the first 2 to 4 hours indicates a poor prognosis.

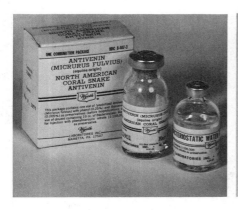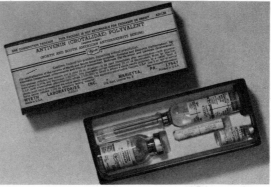

Figure 31-4 *Antivenin kits for coral snake and Crotalidae. (Courtesy of Wyeth Laboratories, Philadelphia, Pa.)*

Emergency measures are as outlined for snakebite. Covered ice packs may be applied for the first few hours to slow absorption. Scorpion antiserum is the specific antidote.

HYMENOPTERA STINGS

In the United States, more people die from allergic reactions to stings from hymenoptera (bees, wasps, hornets, yellowjackets) than from the bites or stings of any other venomous animal. The honeybee accounts for the greatest number of deaths because of its high incidence of exposures, but the yellowjacket is the most likely to produce anaphylaxis. Only female hymenoptera can sting, since the stinging apparatus is a modification of the ovipositor. All except the honeybee have smooth stingers that should be removed from the victim following the sting. The honeybee's barbed stinger and a portion of its abdomen and venom sac remain in the victim; the loss of these structures leads to the bee's ultimate demise. Occasionally, anaphylactic reactions may occur in persons sensitive to substances in the saliva of other biting insects such as deer flies, horse flies, black flies, and kissing bugs, especially when the victim is bitten repeatedly. Hymenoptera venom produces both local and systemic effects.

Local Signs and Symptoms

Hymenoptera venom contains histamine and other chemical substances that, when deposited in the victim, produce local effects such as:
- A pinprick sensation followed by a slight intensity
- Progressive redness, warmth, irritation, and pruritus of the injured part, which subsides in a few hours
- Wheal formation at the bite site, which also subsides in a few hours

Local Treatment of Hymenoptera Stings

- Keep affected part (and victim) at rest.
- Apply constricting bands above and below site (but leave distal pulse intact).
- If stinger is present, remove by scraping off skin in direction opposite to its entry. Avoid squeezing venom sac through use of tweezers or similar device.
- Wash site with soap and water.
- If appropriate, apply a papain-containing meat tenderizer as a paste to inactivate venom.
- Consider applying cool pack for comfort and vasoconstrictive effect.

Systemic Reactions to Hymenoptera Stings

Systemic reactions to hymenoptera venom may include the following:
- Anaphylaxis
- Urticaria and edema remote from the sting site
- Generalized erythema with feelings of flushing and warmth
- Gastrointestinal distress
- Hypotension
- Serum sickness reactions (see p 556)—may occur 10 to 14 days following the sting

Anaphylaxis

Anaphylaxis poses the greatest threat to the victim because it can produce death in highly sensitive victims within minutes.

Treatment/Management. Treatment is aimed at minimizing absorption of the venom and treating the systemic reactions present. When manifestations of anaphylaxis occur, prompt intervention is crucial to avert a fatal outcome. If the victim carries an emergency treatment kit, the first responder should proceed according to the physician's instructions contained in the kit. Such kits commonly contain a preloaded syringe of aqueous epinephrine 1:1000 or a pressurized nebulizer of epinephrine, and an oral antihistamine. Also contained in the kit may be a latex tourniquet and a Medic-Alert tag identifying the patient as allergic to insects. Following initial treatment, the victim is taken to the nearest medical facility for definitive care.

Management of the patient experiencing an anaphylactic reaction is summarized in Chart 31-3.

Chart 31-3

ANAPHYLACTIC REACTION: PATIENT MANAGEMENT

Signs and Symptoms of Anaphylaxis

- Pruritus, urticaria, generalized hives, flushing, feelings of warmth
- Weakness, anxiety, dizziness, disorientation, restlessness
- Nausea, vomiting, abdominal cramps, diarrhea, incontinence
- Respiratory difficulties—dyspnea, retractions of accessory muscles or respiration, hoarseness
- Wheezing
- Hypotension, cardiac arrhythmias, cyanosis
- Collapse, seizures, unconsciousness

Note: anaphylaxis may also occur when the individual is exposed to other substances to which he is sensitive, such as drugs and foods.

Prehospital Care

- Local treatment of affected site (as described in text).
- If emergency treatment kit is available, administer medication(s) according to prescription.
- Reduce physical stress and anxiety.
- Administer high-flow O_2 as needed.
- Establish IV if available.
- Transport to hospital immediately.

Hospital Care

1. Epinephrine 1:1000, 0.3 ml to 0.5 ml for adults and 0.01 ml/kg up to 0.3 ml for children.
   - Administer subcutaneously if patient is not in shock.
   - If patient is in shock, dilute to 1:10,000 and give IV.
   - May administer half the dose intradermally at sting site.
   - May repeat in 20 minutes.
2. Elevate head; administer high-flow oxygen as needed.
3. Establish IV in uninjured limb.
4. Monitor vital signs.
5. Administer antihistamine if indicated.
   - Diphenhydramine chloride (Benadryl), 50 mg to 100 mg, or chlorpheniramine (Chlor-Trimeton), 4 mg to 12 mg (po if symptoms are mild, IV if symptoms are severe)
6. Administer aminophylline, 250 to 300 mg IV over a 10- to 20-minute period for bronchospasm unrelieved by epinephrine.
7. If hypotension persists, establish a metaraminol (Aramine) or levarterenol (Levophed) drip.
8. Administer steroids if reaction is severe or prolonged (100 mg hydrocortisone sodium succinate, Solu-Cortef, over 1 to 2 minutes. Repeat in 20 minutes as necessary).
9. Maintain body heat.
10. Minimize physical and emotional stress.
11. Hospitalize 24 hours to ensure stabilization.

Discharge Instructions and Follow-up Care. Discharge instructions and follow-up care are important in preventing repeated exposure or severe reactions with unavoidable exposures. The following may be indicated:

- A hyposensitization program if the individual's life-style renders him apt to re-exposure

- Advising patient of the possibility of becoming ill 10 to 14 days later (serum sickness)
- The need for an emergency kit, which can be bought at a drug store with the physician's prescription and should be carried whenever the patient is outdoors
- Personal measures to protect the individual from future exposures:

TABLE 31-3. BITES AND STINGS: CLINICAL FINDINGS AND EMERGENCY MANAGEMENT

	Toxin	Signs/Symptoms	Management
Animal Bites	Neurotoxic	• Incubation period—10 days to over a year (avg. 30–50 days) • Fever, malaise, headache, photophobia, musculoskeletal pain • Uncontrollable excitement, excessive salivation, pain with spasms of laryngeal and pharyngeal muscles with slight stimulation • Death within 3–5 days from asphyxia, exhaustion, paralysis	• Thorough wound cleansing, rinsing, then flushing with (Zephiran), alcohol or providone iodine • Evaluation for immunization (see criteria) • Avoid steroids or immunosuppressive agents
Snakes Pit viper (Crotalidae)	Complex mixtures that can produce a varied cardiotoxic, hemotoxic, neurotoxic, and local tissue effect, depending on species.	Fang mark(s) Local—Pain initially followed by paresthesia around wound, edema, ecchymosis formation of vesicles. May progress to petechiae, thrombosis, sloughing and necrosis of injured tissue. General—weakness, sweating, nausea, fainting. Enlarged, tender regional lymph nodes, perioral paresthesia fasciculation, hematemesis, melena, increased or decreased salivation. Laboratory findings—early hemoconcentration, followed by decrease in rbcs and platelets, prolonged bleeding and clotting time, hematuria, glycosuria, proteinuria.	Prehospital care • Minimize physical activity and anxiety. • No alcohol or stimulants; no ice on wound • Position—limb level with heart • Wide constricting band above and below (distal pulse present) • Wash bitten area; incision and suction only as appropriate. • Retrieve dead snake. • Transport immediately, carrying victim. Emergency department care • Establish IV. • Supportive—antibiotics, tetanus, analgesics • Antivenin • Wound care
Coral snake (Elapidae) Black with adjacent red and yellow bands	Neurotoxic	Few or none up to 12 hr. Local—scratch marks or tiny punctures with minimal to moderate edema, erythema, pain, paresthesia General—euphoria, nausea, vomiting, excessive salivation, ptosis of eyelids, dyspnea, seizures, weakness, paralysis (within 7–18 hr), including respiration Once symptoms occur, can progress rapidly.	Treat even though signs and symptoms are absent See treatment for pit viper bite. Coral snake antivenin (*Micrurus fulvis;* Wyeth)
Insect Stings Hymenoptera (honeybee, wasp, hornet, yellowjacket)		Local—pinprick sensation followed by mild to moderate pain. Erythema followed by formation of a wheal. Area may be reddened, warm, and pruritic. Honeybee stinger remains (barbed) while others do not (smooth). Systemic—allergic reactions in sensitive individuals— urticaria, etc.	• Local: Remove honeybee stinger with fingernail or knife blade flat against skin in direction opposite to that of insertion. • Cleanse with soap and water. • Covered cool pack for comfort • Systemic—Constricting bands, rest. • Treat allergic reactions

TABLE 31-3. BITES AND STINGS: CLINICAL FINDINGS AND EMERGENCY MANAGEMENT (*CONTINUED*)

	Toxin	Signs/Symptoms	Management
Arachnid (spiders)	Neurotoxic (ascending motor paralysis)	Local—two small red marks (fangs) with minimal pain initially. Severe local pain develops gradually spreading to abdomen and extremities. General—Sweating, salivation, nausea, vomiting, cramps and rigidity, tremors, severe pain in extremities. Later, bradycardia, feeble pulse, dyspnea, dysphoria, delerium and confusion.	• Establish IV • Administer antivenin after sensitivity testing. • Relieve pain and muscle spasms (IV calcium gluconate, diazepam, curare analgesics)
Brown recluse spider (*Loxosceles Reclusa*)	Necrotoxin	Local—may have no local pain initially. Several hours after envenomation, bitten area becomes congested, swollen, develops ischemic center leading to ulceration and necrosis. Systemic—restlessness, fever.	• Antihistamines, corticotropin to decrease systemic reactions • Analgesics • Wound cleansing, debridement • Antibiotics • Tetanus prophylaxis • No specific antivenin • Use local anesthetics *without* epinephrine.
Scorpions (*Centruroides gertschii, Centruroides sculpturatus*)	Neurotoxic	Local—visual evidence of sting often absent. Initially, tingling, burning at site. Systemic—excessive salivation, drowsiness, mydriasis, photophobia, nausea, vomiting, incontinence, seizures, respiratory, circulatory failure.	• Symptomatic treatment • Restrict absorption as in snakebite. • Apply cool packs. • Scorpion antivenin* • Avoid narcotics that potentiate effects of venom.
Marine Animals			
Seasnake bites Octopus bites	Neurotoxin	Develop within 2–6 hr. Muscle stiffness, myoglobinuria, paralysis, collapse, respiratory arrest.	• Constricting bands • Cardiac/respiratory support • Treat for shock • Antivenin
Coelenterate stings (jellyfish, Portuguese man-of-wars, anemones, corals)	Hematocysts (stinging capsules) may break from organisms and can sting at any time. Mechanical stimulation (rubbing) change in *p*H, exposure to fresh H$_2$O may cause hematocyst to sting. Allergenic toxin.	Allergic reaction, including anaphylaxis, sudden intense pain, sometimes causing collapse. Throbbing headache, cramps, paralysis, feelings of suffocation, nausea, weakness, dizziness.	• Isopropyl alcohol to wounds for 6–8 min (to inactivate hematocysts) • Supersaturated solution of baking soda (to neutralize acid reacting venom) • Analgesic • Severe envenomation and hypersensitivity reactions: constricting bands, rest, no alcohol or stimulants by mouth.
Wounds From Spineous Organisms			
Stingray	Types have not been isolated and identified according to lethal activity.	Usually local reaction: zone blanching around wound followed by erythema and swelling Intense, shooting pain General effects—respiratory distress, cardiac arrhythmias, syncope, peripheral vaso-constriction, tremors, cramps.	• Flush wound with saline to remove toxin, foreign material. • May need to remove stinger • Immerse in hot water (see p 556). • Surgical closure. Tetanus and antibiotic therapy as appropriate. • Elevate.

TABLE 31-3. BITES AND STINGS: CLINICAL FINDINGS AND EMERGENCY MANAGEMENT (*CONTINUED*)

	Toxin	Signs/Symptoms	Management
Scorpion fish (California sculpin, stonefish, lionfish)		Local—immediate, intense pain, swelling and paresthesia. Occasional tissue necrosis. General—with severe envenomation) shock, pulmonary edema, EKG changes, nausea, vomiting.	• Immerse in hot water. • Antivenin • Wound management and supportive care
Catfish		Local—Immediate throbbing pain subsiding in an hour.	• Meticulous wound cleansing • Broad-spectrum antibiotic therapy
Sea urchins	Whether venomous depends on species.	Immediate pain, followed by swelling, erythema, numbness, possible paralysis and respiratory distress.	• Immerse in hot water • Supportive therapy • X-ray examination of spines • Most spines are readily absorbed, though some require surgical removal.

* (Scorpion antivenin) available from Poisonous Animal Research Laboratory; Arizona State University; Tempe, Arizona.

Avoid use of aromatics or clothing that might attract insects such as fragrances and perfumed cosmetics, brightly colored clothing, going barefoot when outdoors.

Avoid flowers, fields, rotting fruit under trees and other areas where insects are likely to be found.

VENOMOUS MARINE LIFE

Some 250 species of marine fishes have been identified as venomous. These can be divided into three categories: those that bite, those that sting, and those that have spines. Each category possesses mechanisms by which venom is transmitted.

1. Animals that bite include sharks, barracudas, moray eels, octopi, sea snakes, sea lions, and killer whales.
2. Stings are inflicted by coelenterates, such as jellyfish, Portuguese man-of-wars, anemones, and corals. Their nematocysts (stinging capsules) contain inverted thread-like stingers that may break loose from the animal and inflict injury to unsuspecting swimmers remote from the animal.
3. Spineous aquatic organisms include the stingray, sea urchin, catfish, and scorpion fish. Barbed spines can transmit venom into the victim through lacerations that can be extensive.

All venoms of known marine life contain substances that produce pain out of proportion to the size or depth of a similar mechanical wound. The poisonous substances are unstable and heat labile. Heat inactivates the venom and relieves the pain as well.

The injured part should be exposed to water as hot as the victim can tolerate 43.3°C to 45.5°C (110°F to 114°F) for 30 to 90 minutes. Immersing the part in very warm water, followed by periodic additions of hot water, permits the patient to acclimate to the higher temperatures. Caution is advised in the very young and very old who tend to dissipate heat less well and blister more easily. Moist heat applications or immersion is indicated each time symptoms return to effect detoxification and pain relief.

Secondary infection is inherent in injuries from marine animals. Considerable bacterial and viral pollution is present in both fresh and salt water. Thus, culture, thorough cleansing, and debridement of wounds is essential. Prophylactic antibiotics are advisable.

Measures to slow absorption of the venom as outlined earlier are applicable to marine life envenomation. Antivenins for sea snake, stonefish, and sea wasp (jellyfish) toxins are available.

Severe envenomation may be accompanied by hypotension and shock and may require ventilatory support, intravenous therapy, and administration of vasopressor drugs.

Principles of Care

The care of the victim of a bite or sting injury centers around a few general principles:
- Ensure meticulous wound management.
- Decrease the absorption of toxic substances.
- Neutralize or inactivate injected toxic substances.
- Provide supportive care as indicated by the patient's signs and symptoms.
- Administer antibiotics and tetanus prophylaxis as appropriate.
- Teach the patient how to avoid future exposures.

Management/Treatment of Marine Bites and Stings.
- Culture wound, then meticulously cleanse it.
- Apply constricting bands as indicated.
- Immerse injured part in water as hot as can be tolerated for 30 to 90 minutes.
- Reduce physical and emotional stress.
- Administer antivenin if available.

- Administer broad-spectrum antibiotic and tetanus prophylaxis as appropriate.

- Provide cardiovascular and ventilatory support as needed.

- Administer analgesic for pain relief as indicated.

In addition to the above, treatment is symptomatic and may be specific to the attacking animal and the known properties of its venom. Table 31-3 outlines the clinical findings and treatment measures for bites and stings discussed in this chapter.

BIBLIOGRAPHY

American National Red Cross: First Aid for Snakebite. Washington, DC, 1978

Anderson GK: Use of human diploid cell vaccine for rabies prophylaxis. USAF Med Serv Dig 30:24–25, November–December 1979

Anderson LI, Wickler WG: Aqueous quaternary ammonium compounds and rabies treatment. J Infect Dis 139:494, 1979

Antivenin (Crotalidae) Polyvalent, Rev ed. Marietta, PA, Wyeth Laboratories, 1968

Arnold R: Controversies and hazards in the treatment of pit viper bites. South Med J 72:902, 1979

Barber JM, Budassi SA: Mosby's Manual of Emergency Care. St. Louis, CV Mosby, 1979

Busse WW: Anaphylaxis: Diagnosis and management. Emerg Med Serv 5:44, 1976

Cromer B: Venomous Hymenoptera: Poison Information. San Diego, San Diego Regional Poison Center, University of California, 1979

Directions for Use of Antivenin (Crotalidae) Polyvalent. Marietta, PA, Wyeth Laboratories, 1968

Frazier CA: Medical emergencies produced by insect bites and stings. Emerg Med Serv 9:9, 1980

Gephardt D: Anaphylaxis from insect stings. J Emerg Nurs 4:19, 1978

Immunization Practices Advisory Committee of CDC: Rabies Prevention. Morbid Mortal Week Rep 29:266, 1980

Miller A, Nathanson N: Rabies: Recent advances in pathogenesis and control. Ann Neurol 2:511, 1977

New rabies vaccine limited to 'no alternative patients.' JAMA 241:870, 1979

New rabies vaccine awaits FDA action. Nat Soc Med Res Bull 31:4, 1980

Orris WL: Aquatic medical emergencies. In Warner CG (ed): Emergency Care: Assessment and Intervention. St. Louis, CV Mosby, 1978

Plotkin SA: Rabies vaccination in the 1980s. Hosp Rev 15:65, 1980

Rabies Vaccine (ADVC) Directions for Administration. Lyon, Institut Merieux, 1980

Recommendation of the Public Health Service Advisory Committee on Immunization Practices: Rabies. Atlanta, Centers for Disease Control, 1977

Russell F: Snake Venom Poisoning. Philadelphia, JB Lippincott, 1980

Russell FE, Van Mierop LHS, Walt CH, Glass TG: Snakebite. The Physician and Sports Medicine. 8:30, 1980

Soldmann WT: Poisonous reptiles and insects. In Warner CG (ed) Emergency Care: Assessment and Intervention, 2nd ed. St Louis, CV Mosby, 1978

Wasnetsky G: Emergency treatment of snakebites. J Emerg Nurs 5:23, 1979

32

INJURIES OF THE BONES, JOINTS, AND RELATED STRUCTURES

JAMES H. COSGRIFF, JR., DIANN ANDERSON, and CARL ANDERSON

Injuries to the bones, joints, and related supporting structures are among those most commonly seen in an emergency setting. Such injuries may occur singly or in association with multiple system trauma. Early, accurate assessment, particularly at the accident scene, and proper immobilization may minimize complications and add considerably to patient comfort.

ANATOMY AND PHYSIOLOGY

Bone is living tissue composed of organic materials (mostly protein), minerals, water, and fatty tissue and located in the marrow cavity. The organic materials account for about 30% of bone weight and the minerals about 45%, including mainly calcium, phosphorus, and magnesium.

Adult bone consists of an inner fatty marrow cavity surrounded by the strong, hard, osseous tissue that constitutes the main structure of the bone. The outer layer is covered by the periosteum, from which new bone cells grow. Vascular supply to bone is derived from blood vessels arising from neighboring arteries that penetrate the bone through small channels called Haversian canals. These vessels are often referred to as nutrient arteries.

The bony skeleton lends structural support to the body. Mobility of the body depends on the joints and their supporting muscles and ligamentous structures. The skeleton is surrounded by varying amounts of soft tissue, which, in addition to muscles and ligaments, include tendons, fascia, blood vessels, and nerves. Injury to a bone involves damage to these many other tissues, which must be taken into consideration in the management of the patient suspected of having a fracture.

Fractures may assume a number of configurations and occur anywhere along the length of the bone: in the shaft, at either end, or extending into the joint. In children, bone growth occurs at ossification centers, usually located near the ends of each bone, called the epiphyseal plate or, more commonly, the epiphysis. Bone growth is completed by approximately age 17. Fractures that occur in the epiphysis before full bone growth has occurred may cause a subsequent failure of growth in the affected bone.

A fracture results from stress applied to a bone or joint. The type of stress may be a direct blow, a penetrating injury (in which a high-energy missile strikes the bone), or ligamentous or muscular stresses about a joint (in which the joint is overflexed or overextended or undergoes torsion).

In joint stresses, type of injury depends on the strength of the structure involved. For example, if a person twists his ankle stepping off a curb, the usual mechanism is to land on the lateral side of the foot so that the foot is inverted. This results in two types of stress. On the lateral aspect of the ankle, the ligamentous structures about the joint are stretched, and this stretching (tensile) force is exerted on the bones at the site of attachment of the ligaments. At the same time, on the medial aspect of the ankle, the bones are curched against each other in another form of stress. The result may be a fracture on the medial side of the ankle

joint and, laterally, a ligamentous tear or avulsion fracture. The ligamentous tear results if the stress is sufficient to pull the ligament apart (often referred to as a sprain). If a ligament holds and pulls the bone away at its site of attachment, it is an avulsion fracture.

Displacement of fracture fragments sometimes results from the mechanism of the causative injury but is more likely due to muscle pull. After disruption of the skeletal structure by fracture, the muscles contract and cause angulation, overlapping, or other deformity of the bone at the fracture site. This assumes great importance, especially if an effort is made at securing a reduction.

Fracture Healing

Physiologically, the healing of a fracture does not vary significantly from the healing of soft tissue wounds. Fracture healing occurs primarily as a local phenomenon at the site of injury. As in other wounds, proper healing depends on accurate apposition of tissue (bone ends), proper immobilization, and adequate blood supply.

After a fracture is incurred, blood and tissue fluid enter the fracture site in a manner similar to that involved in the formation of granulation tissue. As healing progresses, the blood clots and areas of cartilage and calcification develop within the clot as the first stage of callus formation. The amount of callus formed varies in amount, depending on how the bone ends are anatomically approximated. Calcium cells are deposited in the callus, and true bone is then formed. As bone formation progresses, excess callus is resorbed, and periosteum covers the area of the fracture site.

The new shape of the bone after fracture healing depends to a great extent on the initial alignment and subsequent maintenance of the fracture fragments in position. Depending on the site of the fracture and the factors mentioned above (proper reduction, immobilization, and blood supply), healing will occur in 3 weeks (for phalanges) to many months (for femur and hip).

Failure of the fracture to heal is called *nonunion*. Nonunion results from a number of causes:

- Failure to adhere to principles of fracture management
- Inadequate immobilization
- Loss of reduction
- Interposition of soft tissue between the bone ends
- Metabolic diseases
- Infection

In addition, aseptic necrosis of the bone may occur after fractures in which the blood supply to bone ends has been interrupted. It most commonly occurs in the head of the femur following a fracture through the anatomic neck.

TYPES OF INJURIES

The common injuries to the bones, joints and related soft tissue structures are: (1) fracture, (2) dislocation, (3) sprain and (4) strain.

The physical signs merely assist the examiner in making a proper diagnosis by x-ray investigation. The signs and symptoms of these common injuries are outlined in Chart 32-1.

Fracture

A *fracture* is any break in continuity of a bone. Although various types may be described (transverse, oblique, spiral, greenstick, comminuted, or impacted), this is of only relative importance. The diagnosis of fracture type is made by x-ray, since the clinical appearance in many instances is the same (Fig. 32-1).

However, differentiation between so-called closed fractures and open fractures is of primary importance. A closed fracture denotes no direct communication between the fracture and the overlying skin. An open fracture is one in which there is direct communication between the fracture and the overlying skin. Sometimes it is difficult to distinguish the two, such as when a patient has both a laceration and an obvious fracture, although there does not appear to be a direct communication between the two. To avoid such confusion, any patient with an obvious fracture of an extremity and with a wound in the vicinity of the bony injury should be assumed to have an open fracture until proven otherwise.

Dislocation

A *dislocation* is an injury to a joint that involves complete disruption of the contiguous surfaces of the two articulating bones from one another. A *subluxation* of a joint is a lesser, similar injury, in which part of the joint is still articulating.

Symptoms of a dislocation are primarily pain about a joint and complaints of inability to use the extremity. The most common signs of a dislocation are obvious deformity about the joint and lack of motion.

Sprain

A *sprain* is an injury to a ligament that results from incomplete tearing of the ligamentous fibers, involving no loss of continuity to the ligament. There are many degrees of sprain, manifested clinically from very mild pain and swelling about a joint to a more serious disruption of the ligamentous structure. The primary symptom of a sprain is pain in the area of the joint (Chart 32-1). The most obvious physical finding is swelling. It is often extremely difficult to differentiate a sprain from a fracture. A painful swelling about a joint should be considered a fracture until x-ray examination proves it otherwise.

Strain

A *strain* is damage to the muscle or tendinous attachment due to overuse (chronic strain) or overstress (acute strain).

The symptom of a strain is pain in the area of the muscular or tendinous attachment unit that has been traumatized. As opposed to a sprain, the pain is usually away from the joint. The physical sign of swelling is a less constant finding in this injury (Chart 32-1). Pain in the area following trauma,

---

Chart 32-1

SIGNS AND SYMPTOMS OF COMMON INJURIES TO BONES, JOINTS, AND RELATED SOFT TISSUE STRUCTURES

Fracture

- May involve any bone
- Deformity
- Absent or limited motion of the injured part
- Local pain at the site of injury
- False motion at the fracture site
- Crepitation (grating of the bone ends)
- Demonstration of fracture on x-ray

Dislocation

- Involves a joint
- Deformity of the involved joint
- Absent or limited motion of the injured joint
- Pain in the injured joint
- Confirmation of dislocation on x-ray

Sprain

- Usually involves a joint
- Pain at the site of injury
- Swelling above the involved joint
- X-ray negative for fracture or dislocation

Strain

- Usually involves a muscle or its tendonous attachment
- Pain and tenderness at site of injury usually away from a joint
- Swelling may be present but is less constant
- X-ray negative for fracture or dislocation

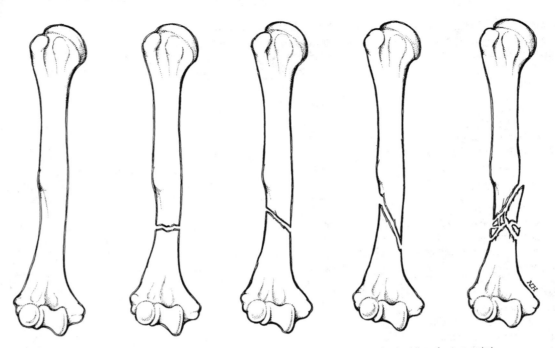

Figure 32-1 *Various types of fractures.* Left to right. *Intact bone, simple transverse fracture, simple oblique fracture, spiral fracture, comminuted fracture.*

along with findings of tenderness and swelling, should suggest a fracture; a fracture must be ruled out before treatment is instituted.

TRIAGE

Emergency personnel must be familiar with triage principles and their application in the management of a patient with a fracture. Generally, fractures occupy a low priority in the overall treatment of the patient with multiple injuries. The exceptions are fractures associated with vascular or neurologic impairment of the injured part. Within the limited category of fractures, a set of priorities does exist. For example, the elderly patient with a fractured hip and stable vital signs is placed lower on the priority list than a young person who has a comminuted fracture of the femur and is in hypovolemic shock.

When a patient has multiple injuries, assess the whole patient. Life-threatening conditions such as airway compromise, hemorrhage, and shock must be identified and treated before turning one's attention to the bone injury. Always be vigilant for associated injuries and for associated disease, especially in the older adult.

ASSESSMENT

Every patient with a fracture perceives the situation as a true emergency, even if this judgment is not substantiated by the presenting symptoms and physical findings. The sudden trauma to bones and joints often leaves the patient stunned and in varying degrees of pain; thus it may be very difficult to elicit an accurate history. A calm approach and emotional support allays anxiety and promotes cooperation.

History

Historical data include the mechanism of injury and the circumstances surrounding its occurrence. Description of a fall or incident may be vague because it occurred too rapidly for the patient to notice details or to have any significant recall of the event. Falls may have been precipitated by momentary loss of consciousness or dizziness, signaling underlying cardiovascular or neurologic disorders. Visual impairment due to glaucoma or cataracts may be the causative factor in the fall or injury but may have been unrecognized and untreated previously because of the insidious nature of these conditions. Many prescription drugs in common use today can cause lack of muscle coordination, disturbances in equilibrium, or changes in the sensorium. Check carefully for a history of drug use.

Use every available source for information pertaining to the injury. Police officers, ambulance personnel, and relatives or friends of the patient at the scene may provide vital facts that will be helpful in assessing the patient.

The extent of the history taken depends on the patient's chief complaint. For example, a young person presenting with pain in the ankle and inability to bear weight does not require the extensive inquiry needed to evaluate the patient with multiple system trauma properly.

Pay attention to every detail when recording the patient's symptoms or complaints. It occasionally occurs that emergency personnel caring for a patient with severe multiple-system injuries attend to the major, life-threatening problems and fail to notice or treat a minor injury that could result in a prolonged occupational disability. For example, a concert violinist in shock with a thoraco-abdominal injury, who complains of pain in his fingers, may not have x-rays taken until the second week of hospitalization, at which time displaced fractures of two fingers are revealed. He recovers uneventfully from his injuries but cannot pursue his chosen profession because of an oversight.

Physical Examination

After the more serious injuries are ruled out, a thorough, gentle examination of the part is done, to determine whether there are any open wounds. Injuries or fractures may occur at sites remote from the fracture site itself. For example, in certain ankle injuries involving the medial malleolus, the upper shaft of the fibula may be fractured. Likewise, in falls in which the patient landed on the feet, fracture of the heel bone, the os calcis, is common, but accompanying compression fractures of the dorsolumbar vertebrae are also frequent occurrences (see Chap. 20, Injuries to the Head, Neck, and Spine). These are primarily at the level of the 12th thoracic and the upper two lumbar vertebrae.

Soft tissue structures in the area of injury must also be evaluated. Loss of motion may be due to major tendon damage. The most commonly injured tendons are the biceps brachii in the upper arm, the quadriceps tendon on the anterior aspect of the knee, and the achilles tendon just above the heel. Rupture of these structures may occur with seemingly little stress, resulting in an inability to use the part.

Circulatory and Neurologic Evaluation. The circulatory and neurologic status of the limb is evaluated by assessing the arterial pulses, motor activity, and sensation distal to the level of injury.

Pain, pallor, pulselessness, paresthesia, paralysis, the five Ps of vascular occlusion, serve as an excellent assessment guide.

Palpate the pulse(s) distal to the fracture site, comparing the findings with the opposite, uninvolved area, if possible. Presence or absence of a pulse cannot be considered sufficient, in itself, to rule out vascular damage. Repeat evaluation at regular intervals.

Ischemia slows metabolic processes so that the involved areas become cooler to the touch. Temperature and color comparisons with an uninvolved area are helpful (Fig. 17-3). Metabolic acidosis occurs as cellular energy sources are rapidly depleted. This may progress until capillary permeability increases, allowing edema to form in the soft tissue. The result is an edematous, cool, and pale extremity, with poor capillary refill in the nail beds.

Although it is common for a patient to complain of pain at the fracture site, pain distal to the level of injury is uncommon, unless the blood or nerve supply is compromised. The pain of hypoxia is burning at first, and progresses to a deep throbbing sensation. Pain produced when the fingers or toes of the injured extremity are passively extended is a reliable sign of early ischemia.

Motor paralysis can accompany or follow loss of sensory modalities, which include touch, proprioception, and temperature. In nerve involvement due to ischemia, loss of deep pain sensory fibers, causing numbness, begins distally, the insensitive area having a glove- or stocking-like distribution. Unlike singular nerve involvement caused by sharp transection or blunt trauma, nerve damage due to ischemia does not correspond to normal anatomic patterns of nerve supply.

Findings indicative of ischemia constitute a true emergency. Comparison with the opposite, uninjured limb is helpful in confirming this diagnosis. Neurologic damage may show up in the form of contusion or partial or complete transection of a nerve. Physician assessment is needed to determine the extent of injury. Contusions of a nerve are usually managed by watchful waiting, while transection of a nerve may require surgical repair at the time of reduction of the fracture.

Basically, management of vascular injury is similar to that for neurologic damage. Any suspicion of impaired blood flow into an injured limb mandates full assessment of the problem, including angiography. In some patients, the vessel may be trapped or angulated by bone ends at the fracture site. Proper reduction of the fracture may alleviate the problem. Transection of a major artery requires immediate surgical attention.

Adjunct Studies

The most helpful and frequently used study of a patient with a suspected bone or joint injury is x-ray of the injured part. Although multiple views are taken, it is not unusual to find the fracture evident in only one view. Most of the splinting devices in popular use today allow complete x-ray study without removing the splint. If the patient's condition is tenuous, a nurse or physician should accompany him to the x-ray area, once it has been established that the study is necessary.

In patients with obvious injury to a joint area but no x-ray evidence of fracture, a ligamentous injury must be considered. If a major ligament supporting a joint has been completely disrupted, significant false mobility of the joint occurs and can be identified by taking special x-ray views of the part while the suspect ligament is stretched (stress films). This process is painful for the patient and usually requires local anesthesia.

Other studies are determined by the seriousness of the injury, the presence of associated trauma or disease, and the mode of anticipated treatment. For example, a patient with a Colles' fracture or ankle injury that is to be reduced under local anesthesia in the emergency department is unlikely to need further tests. A patient with a fracture of the forearm requiring internal fixation under general anesthesia needs a more thorough study. When vascular damage is suspected, emergency arteriography is helpful in localizing the site and delineating the nature of the injury.

Noninvasive vascular studies or vessel imaging may be helpful if these modalities are available However, single-injection limb arteriography is a relatively simple procedure requiring minimal supplies and equipment (Fig. 32-2).

Additional studies include complete blood count (CBC), urinalysis, electrocardiogram (ECG), blood chemistry tests, and any other special tests that may be included.

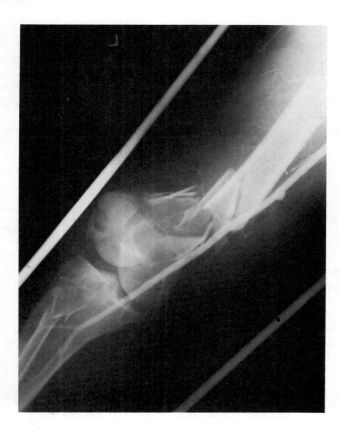

Figure 32-2 Emergency department femoral angiogram of patient with severely comminuted distal femur. The limb was cool below the knee. The femoral artery is intact and there is no evidence of vascular injury.

MANAGEMENT

Severity of injury to an extremity varies widely, from a simple, undisplaced fracture to a badly comminuted open fracture, to multiple injuries with the patient in a life-threatening condition. Early management of lesser injuries is directed toward immobilization of the affected part to minimize discomfort and prevent complications until definitive treatment is given.

Life-Threatening Injuries

In patients with more serious or life-threatening injuries, attention is directed to established principles of care, based on known priorities. These include (1) airway maintenance, (2) control of hemorrhage, (3) management of shock, (4) evaluation of neurologic or vascular complications, and (5) immobilization of the fractures. Then, attention must be given to *every* injury, lest one which is seemingly minor later prove a major source of disability.

Hemorrhage. Control of hemorrhage in the presence of a fracture may be difficult. In closed fractures of the long bones, such as the femur, or in fractures of the pelvis, significant blood loss amounting to several liters can occur into adjacent tissues but exhibit few clinical signs except tachycardia and hypotension. It is impossible to initiate any measures aimed at control of the hemorrhage, since this is usually limited by the confines of the anatomic tissue compartment affected by the injury.

With open fractures, however, extensive external blood loss may occur if a major vessel has been damaged. In this circumstance, control of bleeding is often difficult because of instability at the fracture site. The best initial treatment is application of direct pressure to the bleeding wound. After the skin about the wound is cleansed, sterile dressings are applied with an outer circumferential elastic dressing. No effort should be made to replace protruding bone ends beneath the skin. If the bleeding continues uncontrolled with pressure on the site and at the pressure point, a tourniquet may be necessary, and is applied following principles outlined in Chapter 17, Vascular Emergencies.

Shock. Hypovolemic shock may develop following major blood loss. Replacement of circulating blood volume is often not directed toward restoration of the total lost volume because increase in blood pressure to near-normal levels could cause further hemorrhage. Maintenance of the patient's systolic blood pressure at approximately 90 mm Hg is considered adequate to maintain urinary output until the hemorrhage can be surgically controlled. In patients who are normally hypertensive, adjustments must be made according to clinical signs and symptoms. Initially, circulating volume may be replaced by normal saline or a crystalloid solution without calcium until type-specific whole blood is available.

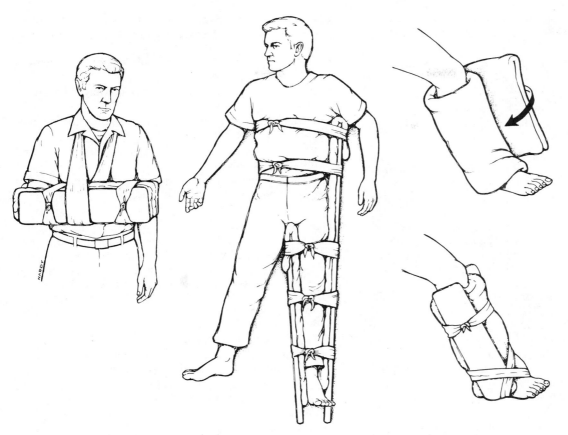

Figure 32-3 *Splinting techniques using padded boards and circular conforming gauze bandage. Patients with a suspected forearm fracture should be immobilized using splints and a simple sling. A lower extremity may be immobilized using longer padded-board splints and circular conforming gauze. The ankle can be splinted by wrapping it in a towel (to keep pressure off bony prominences) and using lightly padded supporting splints exteriorly, maintained in position by circumferential conforming gauze.*

Amputation. Among the more severe forms of soft tissue injury and bone involvement is amputation, whether of a single digit or of a major portion of an extremity. Controversy still continues as to the advisability of replantation, primarily because of the long rehabilitation period, including several stages of operative procedures, and the often uncertain results.

To preserve the integrity of the amputated part, it should be placed in a dry, sterile, plastic bag and placed in a container of ice or iced saline (see Chapt. 19, Wound Management). In the emergency department, x-rays of both the amputated part and the stump of the limb are taken to better assess the extent of injury.

Immobilizing Injured Parts

Once assessment has been completed and the patient's condition is stable, preparation is made for transport and further evaluation. The injured part must be properly immobilized to minimize discomfort and prevent any undue motion and further injury. A wide variety of materals at hand may be used for splinting (Fig. 32-3). Many commercially made splints, such as pneumatic or canvas/Velcro splints are easy to apply and also store compactly.

Most fractures of the upper extremity can be immobilized by a sling and swathe. Femur fractures require application of a traction splint (*e.g.,* a Hare, Thomas, or Sager splint)

to relieve muscle spasms of the quadriceps. Other lower-extremity fractures may be immobilized with long board or cardboard splints. When properly applied, splints are left in place until completion of x-ray studies.

When there is evidence of hypovolemia from fracture(s) of the long bones or pelvis, a pneumatic antishock garment (PASG) may provide both additional stabilization of the fracture and compression of the injury site to control blood loss. It also may be used in conjunction with certain traction splints, such as Sager and Hare splints. After the patient is admitted to the emergency department, the PASG can be deflated sequentially, beginning with the abdominal segment; vital signs should be closely monitored. If the systolic blood pressure falls more than 5 mm Hg, the device should be reinflated.

Principles of Immobilization of Skeletal Injuries. Selection and application of splinting must be done according to established principles of splinting, as follows:
- Evaluate extremity for signs of fracture or dislocation.
- Palpate pulse distal to the level of injury.*
- Test sensory and motor function distal to the level of injury.*

* Compare the pulse and neurologic function on the injured side with that on the uninjured side.

- Place dry, sterile dressings over open fractures before splinting. Do not cover wound area with splinting materials.
- Immobilize at least one joint above and below the level of the injury, taking care to pad all bony prominences. In dislocations, immobilize adjacent bones.
- Palpate distal pulse after immobilizing.*
- Test sensory and motor function distal to injury after immobilizing.*
- Elevate extremity to promote venous return and minimize swelling. Position patient for comfort in relation to total condition.
- Do not remove splint unless it is improperly applied or unless directed to do so by the physician.

All movement of the patient, particularly of the injured part(s) should be performed slowly and cautiously, eliciting the patient's voluntary help when possible. Quick movements, even with an uninvolved extremity or body part, can provoke painful muscle spasms.

Slight muscle tension is desired when the patient is moving his own fractured arm. He should be encouraged to relax the involved muscles only after personnel have supported the limb with their hands or other splinting methods.

The injured part should be firmly supported above and below the fracture site. Once hands have been placed on the patient, they should not be shifted to a different position. This involves planning ahead. Rather than manipulating clothing off the patient's body, quicker access may be gained by cutting it away, preferably along a seam line.

Repositioning. Repositioning at the fracture area may be necessary when:
- Angulation is so great that it is impossible to splint the fracture
- The five Ps are present and repositioning may help reestablish blood flow and neurologic function
- The area to be repositioned *does not* involve a joint

When repositioning, support the fracture site and adjacent joints and apply gentle traction and countertraction to the desired position. Assessment of neurologic and vascular status must be done before and after any repositioning maneuver.

Application of a Sling. A sling can be used singly or in combinaton with other immobilizing materials to stabilize injuries to the upper extremities. The following are principles of application of a sling:
- Support the forearm in a horizontal position or one in which the hand is slightly elevated above the level of the elbow.
- Secure the elbow in the sling, pinning or tying the sling at this area.
- Extend the sling to include the hand at least to the metacarpophalangeal joints to support the wrist and to prevent ulnar deviation.
- Tie the knot away from the bony prominences of the neck or pad well to prevent undue pressure on cervical vertebrae.

Application of Pneumatic Splint. In addition to the above, pneumatic splinting devices (Fig. 32-4) are applied as follows:
- Fully support fracture site and adjacent joints while placing splint in proper position.
- If splint is zippered, place the zipper away from the injured area, if possible.
- Inflate the splint so that its surface slightly dents under pressure of the thumb.
- When possible, place the splint so that distal sensory and motor function can be assessed.
- Monitor for pressure changes in the splint due to changes in ambient temperature or altitude.

Application of Traction Splint. Traction splints help immobilize the fracture site in femur fractures and to relieve the pain associated with muscle spasm and over-riding of bone ends. In addition to the general principles of splinting, these techniques are important in the proper application of traction splints:
- Apply and maintain manual traction on injured leg throughout splinting process.
- Remove shoe and sock if possible.
- Measure and adjust splint so it extends from the bottom of the buttock to approximately 6 inches past the foot.
- Having the assistant support and maintain traction, gently slide splint under the leg (Hare or Thomas) or against the ischial tuberosity (Sager or Conneway).
- Secure thigh strap, then ankle hitch.
- Adjust traction only to where patient feels relief from pain.
- Secure leg support straps.
- Elevate the splint allowing the foot and heel to be freely supported by the ankle and leg straps or cravats.

Removal of a splinting device is not required for routine x-ray studies and should not be done without a physician's order. Indications to remove a splint include evidence of improper application, signs of vascular impairment caused by the splint, initial x-ray studies negative for fracture or dislocation or the need for additional, special x-ray examinations. When a splint is to be removed and a fracture is present, provision should be made for use of other techniques of immobilization. Gentle traction should be applied and the limb carefully removed from the splinting device. This is best done by or under the direct supervision of a physician.

Pain Management

Pain management depends on the type of fracture, the size and age of the patient, any accompanying trauma or complications, anticipated definitive treatment and the final disposition of the patient. To a great extent, pain is caused by muscle spasm; therefore, positioning the patient and appropriate splinting can do much to increase comfort.

Edema at the fracture site adds to discomfort because nerve endings are further stimulated. Applications of covered ice bags or packs during the first hours after fracture will lessen the rate of swelling and increase comfort. Caution should be observed in elderly patients or those with known arterial insufficiency. In those patients whose fractures have occurred more than 12 to 24 hours prior to evaluation, the application of ice is of little value. Positioning the affected part at or above the level of the heart will assist in improving venous return, with reduction of local congestion.

Administration of analgesics is selective. When shock is present, absorption of intramuscular analgesics is impeded and of little immediate value to the patient. Repeated administration of analgesics is also a potential hazard to the resolution of the shock. When sedation or analgesia is necessary, reduced amounts should be administered intravenously over a period of several minutes and timed to have maximum effect during a particular procedure, such as a closed reduction or manipulation of a dislocation. Local anesthesia may be used in the latter situation to afford maximum comfort.

Management of the patient with skeletal or related soft tissue injury is summarized in Chart 32-2.

MANAGEMENT OF INJURIES TO THE UPPER EXTREMITIES

Fracture of the Clavicle

The clavicle is one of the most commonly fractured bones, constituting 5% to 10% of all fractures.

Assessment. The victim will usually give a history of a fall or blow to the shoulder area and subsequent pain and swelling in the region of the clavicle. On examination, swelling and deformity may be noted, and tenderness can be elicited on palpation of the fracture site.

In children, particularly, incomplete fracture of the clavicle may be present although swelling is minimal. Careful palpation of the clavicle will reveal localized tenderness at the area of injury. Typically, the patient will support the affected limb with the opposite one.

The major vessels of the limb, the subclavian and axillary arteries, lie close to the middle third of the clavicle. Careful evaluation of distal pulses is necessary, as well as observation for any significant hematoma of the supraclavicular area which might indicate vascular damage. Rarely is internal fixation necessary.

Management. Following x-ray studies (Fig. 32-5), the management of the fracture involves application of a figure-8 dressing, which is available commercially. The dressing should be applied carefully, with the patient sitting upright on an examining table and the shoulders in the "position of attention" (shoulders squared, chest out). Liberal amounts of powder or cornstarch are placed in each axilla to prevent irritation of the skin from perspiration or rubbing.

Acromioclavicular Separation

This injury occurs to the lateral end of the clavicle, which is attached to the acromion and the coracoid processes of

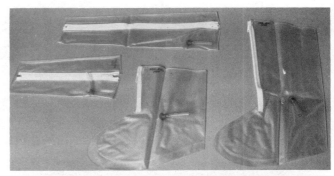
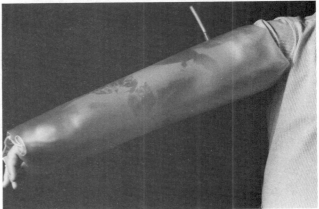
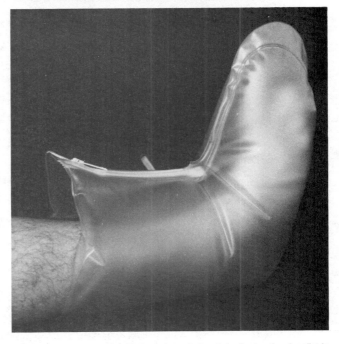

Figure 32-4 *Air splints. Top. Various sizes of air splints. Center. An air splint in place on an arm; note that the fingers are exposed for assessment. Bottom. Air splint for foot or ankle.*

the scapula by strong ligamentous structures appropriately called the acromioclavicular and coracoclavicular ligaments. Separation of the shoulder results from a tear of one or both of these ligaments as a result of a fall directly on the "point" of the shoulder.

Chart 32-2

MANAGEMENT OF THE PATIENT WITH SKELETAL OR RELATED SOFT TISSUE INJURY

Assessment

HISTORY

- How did the fall or incident occur?
- What was the mechanism of injury, the type and extent of forces involved? Be suspicious of concomitant injury.
- Was there dizziness or momentary loss of consciousness (may indicate underlying cardiovascular or neurological condition)?
- Was patient taking medication at the time (Drug effects: muscular incoordination, disturbed equilibrium, changes in sensorium)?
- Is pain present? Absence may indicate neurological injury.
- Where is the pain? What movements cause pain?

PHYSICAL EXAMINATION

- Perform a rapid, *complete* assessment.
- Identify and treat life-threatening conditions—asphyxia, hemorrhage, shock.
- Determine presence of neurological or vascular complications.
- Assess injury or fracture site(s). Consider radiation of forces and mechanism of injury suggesting other areas of injury.
- Evaluate soft tissue structures in area of injury. Assess carefully for nerve or circulatory damage. Check and recheck at intervals the five Ps of vascular occlusion:
  Pain
  Pallor
  Pulselessness
  Paresthesia
  Paralysis
- Physician assesses extent of nerve injury (contusion, partial or complete transection).

ADJUNCT STUDIES

- The following studies are ordered, depending on severity of injury.
- X-ray studies of injured part
- Emergency arteriography or noninvasive vascular study (*i.e.*, Doppler) for suspected vascular damage

---

Assessment. The patient complains of pain and deformity on the point of the shoulder at the lateral aspect of the clavicle. Motion is restricted because of pain. The injured shoulder seems to sag, the clavicle appearing to ride higher and tenting the skin. Palpation over the distal end of the clavicle and the areas of the ligamentous structures elicit tenderness.

A special x-ray technique is used to establish the diagnosis. The x-ray is taken with the patient in the upright position holding a weight in each hand. Both shoulders must be included on a single film to allow comparison between the injured and uninjured sides. As a result of the tearing of the ligamentous structures, there will be widening of the joint between the lateral end of the clavicle and the acromion process which is proportional to the degree of disruption of the ligament(s).

Management. Management of this injury depends on the severity of ligamentous damage and the individual. In lesser injuries, apply adhesive tape over a felt pad to the lateral end of the clavicle and place the arm and shoulder in a sling. In more extensive injuries, especially in an athlete, operative reduction and internal fixation may be necessary.

Anterior Dislocation of the Shoulder

The shoulder is the joint most commonly injured by dislocation, accounting for 50% of all dislocations. It is a serious

---

Chart 32-2

MANAGEMENT OF THE PATIENT WITH SKELETAL OR RELATED SOFT TISSUE INJURY (*CONTINUED*)

Assessment

ADJUNCT STUDIES (CONTINUED)

- Complete blood count
- Urinalysis
- Electrocardiogram
- Blood chemistry tests

Management

PREHOSPITAL CARE

- Maintain airway.
- Control hemorrhage by direct pressure on bleeding wound. Do not replace protruding bone ends. Tourniquet may be needed if bleeding is uncontrolled and development of shock is imminent.
- Immobilize injured part(s) before transporting patient (splint, sling, pneumatic antishock garment [PASG] when there is hypovolemia).
- Splint the injury site in the position in which it is found. *Never reposition a joint.*
- Transport to hospital for further evaluation and treatment.

HOSPITAL CARE

- Deflate PASG as indicated (should be done only by or on the advice of a physician).
- Provide specific treatments as required:
  Reduction of dislocation (operative reduction may be required)
  Special immobilization measures (splints, traction, casts, internal fixation devices)
- Catheterize patient if needed (*e.g.,* in pelvic fracture).
- Admit patient to hospital for surgical procedures as indicated.
- Be careful to treat the *whole* patient.
- If patient is discharged to home, provide cast care instructions, fit with crutches or other assistive devices as required and instruct patient in their use.
- Arrange for follow-up evaluation.

---

injury, in which the head of the humerus is displaced from the shallow articulating surface of the scapula and is associated with a tear in the joint capsule. The humeral head may be dislocated into a number of positions—anterior, inferior, or posterior—in relation to the glenoid fossa of the scapula.

The usual mechanism of shoulder dislocation is a fall on the outstretched (abducted) arm, resulting in severe pain and inability to use the shoulder.

Assessment. The patient ordinarily holds the injured limb with the opposite hand. Any attempt to move the involved shoulder will cause considerable pain.

Physical assessment reveals a bulge over the anterior as-

pect of the shoulder, if the patient is thin enough, and a depression below the point of the shoulder. The patient usually refuses the use of a sling and is reluctant to let go of his arm for fear of increasing the pain.

Management/Treatment. Once the diagnosis has been established by x-ray, reduction should be carried out. If the patient is seen within a relatively short time after injury, muscle spasm may not be a problem, so that reduction can be achieved easily using a minimum of analgesia. Diazepam (Valium), meperidine (Demerol), or morphine, given in appropriate doses intravenously, may be used. If the dislocation occurred many hours previously and muscle spasm is significant, general anesthesia is often necessary to reduce

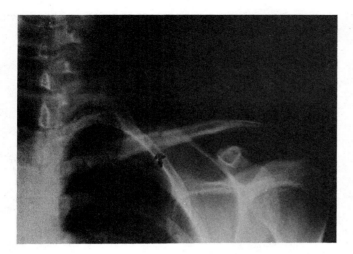

Figure 32-5 *Simple fracture of the clavicle. (arrow) Fragments were stable and in good position in a 30-year-old woman. She was treated by sling only, with good results.*

the dislocation. Postreduction x-rays are advisable to confirm satisfactory position.

In some patients, this injury will recur on numerous occasions, because of permanent stretching of the muscular and ligamentous structures about the shoulder joint. With each recurrence, there may also be damage to the articulating surfaces of the involved bones. In persons with recurrent dislocations, surgery may be necessary as an elective procedure, to shorten the damaged periarticular structure.

In instances in which the dislocation is not confirmed by x-ray, and thus reduction is unnecessary, ligamentous damage is a likely sequela. In such a patient, immobilization of the arm in a sling at the side for at least 3 weeks is advisable, to ensure sufficient ligamentous healing.

Fractures About the Shoulder

Shoulder fractures usually occur as a result of falls.

Assessment. The victim, usually elderly, will have fallen on the outstretched hand or arm and will present complaining of pain or inability to move the shoulder. Often, such persons are not seen until several days after injury. The degree of swelling will vary but is usually present about the area of the shoulder, and in instances where the injury occurred several days previously, the swelling and ecchymosis may extend to the region of the elbow.

Most shoulder fractures involve the neck of the humerus. Careful palpation will elicit tenderness in the upper third of the arm, and x-rays will confirm the diagnosis. The fragments may be impacted or displaced.

Management/Treatment. Management usually consists of application of a sling and analgesics. These patients must be observed closely and need to have physical therapy instituted early, to encourage active motion and prevent a "frozen" shoulder resulting from shortening and scarring of the periarticular structures. In younger patients with dis-

placed fractures, operative reduction may be required to treat the fracture.

Fracture of the Shaft of the Humerus

A fall or direct blow to the arm, with subsequent pain and deformity in the mid-portion of the upper limb often results in fracture of the shaft of the humerus. Assessment will reveal swelling, tenderness and false motion at the humeral area. A grating sensation may be elicited at the fracture site.

The radial artery and nerve lie in close proximity to the middle third of the humeral shaft; thus, vascular and neurologic integrity must be evaluated before any care is provided. The radial pulse at the wrist should be palpated. The radial nerve can be evaluated by asking the patient to dorsiflex the wrist, and sensation may be tested on the dorsum of the hand, in the area of supply of the radial nerve. Radial nerve injury must be considered in the presence of wrist drop and inability to actively dorsiflex the wrist (Fig. 32-6).

The patient may require a sling and swathe, which will fix the arm to the side by means of a circumferential dressing around the chest. Following x-ray confirmation of the diagnosis (Fig. 32-7), management may consist of either application of a cast or open reduction and internal fixation of the fracture fragments.

Fractures of the distal end of the shaft and the supracondylar area of the humerus, just above the elbow joint, are much more serious than those involving the shaft; vascular and/or nerve damage is not uncommon in such fractures. Further, the injury frequently involves the joint surfaces, which constitutes a major complication. Joint injury usually occurs as a result of a fall on the arm or elbow. Internal fixation is often necessary.

Fractures of the Forearm and Wrist

Falls on the outstretched hand may cause injury to the wrist area, fracture of the navicular or radius and ulnar styloid just above the wrist (Colles' fracture, Fig. 32-8) or to the

Figure 32-6 *Wristdrop—radial nerve palsy.*

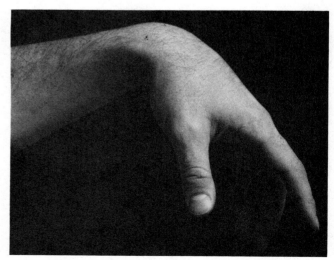

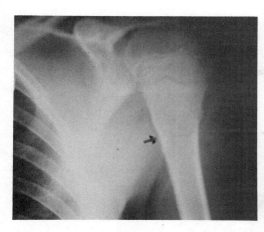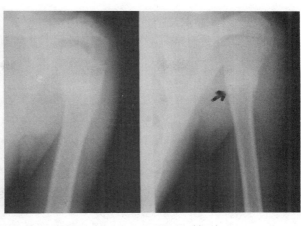

Figure 32-7 *Simple fracture of the humerus. Left. Simple fracture of upper shaft of the left humerus on a 15-year-old male. Fracture was stable; treated with sling and swathe. Right. Good callus formation and partial healing 5 weeks later.*

mid-forearm or elbow area (fracture of the radial head or the humeral condyles). These are more commonly seen in children. There is a history of falling on the outstretched hand, resulting in pain and deformity. Evaluation for Colles' fracture will reveal a typical deformity of the forearm just above the wrist, called a "silverfork deformity." This injury commonly involves both the radius and the ulnar styloid just above the wrist; the degree of deformity varies.

Other fractures about the wrist involve the carpal bones, particularly the navicular, which also results from a fall on the outstretched hand, with subsequent pain and swelling at the wrist. The typical silverfork deformity is not present, however. Careful evaluation of these patients will usually reveal local tenderness at the fracture site. In instances of suspected navicular fracture, pressure may be exerted against the tip of the extended thumb. By pushing this tip of the thumb toward the wrist area, compression of the fracture fragments will occur, and pain can be elicited.

These patients frequently have considerable pain, and a simple padded wooden splint should be applied before x-ray studies. If the films reveal no fracture of the radius or ulna, special studies of the navicular bone should be ordered. Magnified views may be necessary to localize the site of fracture.

In some patients, particularly the young, the fracture line may not be visible immediately after injury. In such instances, the patient should be advised that no fracture can be identified at that time; however, the injury should be managed as a fracture by immobilizing the part, and repeat x-ray studies should be done in approximately 10 days. At that time re-

Figure 32-8 *Wrist fractures. Left. Typical Colles' fracture of the right wrist, involving the distal radius and ulnar styloid. The distal fragment of the radius is displaced dorsally, producing the so-called silverfork deformity at the wrist. Right. Torus fracture of the left wrist of a 5-year-old girl who fell on her outstretched hand 3 days earlier. Note irregularity of the radius (arrow).*

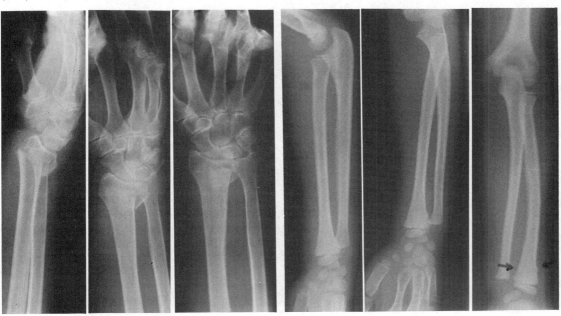

sorption of the bone at the site of fracture can clarify the clinical diagnosis.

Fractures of both bones of the forearm are invariably displaced and unstable. The position and degree of displacement will vary with the level of the fracture and the resultant muscle pull on the fragments, particularly the proximal fragments. This injury is severe. Closed reduction may be attempted; however, if the fragments are not able to be maintained in satisfactory alignment, open reduction and internal fixation is required. (Fig. 32-9.)

On the other hand, greenstick fractures of the mid-portion of the radius and ulna are quite stable. This injury is most common in children. Application of a splint may add to the patient's discomfort; therefore, in this instance, a simple

Figure 32-9 *Displaced fractures of the forearm. Top. Displaced fractures of both bones of the forearm. Position of the fragments is the result of muscle tension in the forearm, causing displacement and overriding of the bone ends (shortening). Bottom. Treatment by open reduction and internal fixation, seen by postoperative x-ray, shows good position of the fragments. The radius was fixed with a side plate and screws, the ulna by means of an intramedullary pin.*

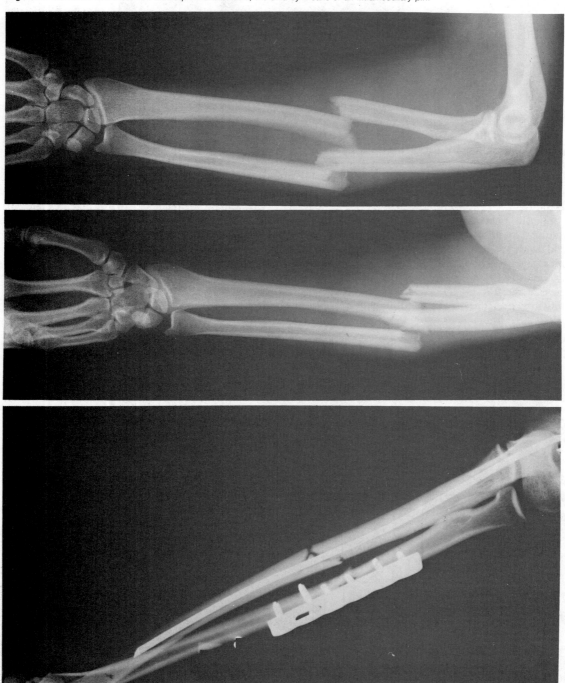

sling might be applied to immobilize the limb until the x-rays are initiated.

Fractures of the Hand

Fractures of the hand represent a common type of open injury to bones and joints. Such injuries usually occur as a result of a direct blow or fall and may represent a complicated injury, particularly when due to an industrial accident.

Assessment will reveal varying bone deformities as a result of muscle pull. Any angulation of metacarpals or phalanges may be quite marked, and motion of the hand or fingers may be painful or limited.

Fracture of the head of the fifth metacarpal is typically incurred by an individual striking his fist against a solid object. (See Fig. 32-10.) Usually the patient will relate a history of being involved in an altercation, in which he swung at an opponent, missed and hit a wall. The distal fragment is typically displaced into the palm. Examination will reveal the knuckle area to be swollen and tender. On palpation the bony projection of the involved knuckle, usually the fifth, will not be felt, and a visible defect is apparent.

Another common injury to the fingers involves the terminal phalanx. The patient will give a history of having been struck on the end of the finger by a ball, with resultant pain and inability to extend the deformed phalangeal joint. The tip of the finger will be in a position of flexion with moderate swelling and tenderness noted on the dorsum of the joint. X-ray studies will reveal a small bone fragment torn away from the dorsal surface of the terminal phalanx. This is a typical example of an avulsion fracture, in which the extensor tendon has remained intact and the site of attachment to the bone has torn away.

After the diagnosis has been confirmed by x-ray, management can proceed in several ways. The most common and conservative method is splinting the finger. It must always be remembered that hand fractures can result in serious disability. Although these injuries may appear minor, adherence to the general principles of fracture management is vital.

MANAGEMENT OF INJURIES TO THE LOWER EXTREMITIES

Fractures of the Pelvis

Fractures of the pelvis rank high as a cause of death after auto accidents. Damage to the bladder, urethra and, in women, the uterus are frequent. Trauma to the sigmoid colon and rectum occurs less frequently. Hemorrhage is the most serious complication. Every cough, sneeze, or movement can cause the unstabilized parts to shift, promoting further bleeding.

Out of the hospital, if the patient is hypovolemic or hypotensive, the pneumatic antishock garment (PASG) should be applied and the patient placed on a spine board for transport. The usual safeguards should be followed after application of the PASG (see Fig. 12-4). The garment should be maintained in position until removed by or on the advice of a physician. The PASG is radiolucent and may be left in position while x-rays are taken.

The most common fracture of the pelvis is fracture of one pubic ramus. Bilateral fractures of the rami have a high incidence of related injuries. They are most dangerous because of associated abdominal injuries, and they tend to cause local and, at times, severe hemorrhage into the extraperitoneal space. Be alert for complaints of abdominal and back pain accompanied by signs of hypovolemic shock, signifying such a hemorrhage. Severe ileus has been noted with fractures of the crest or wing of the ileum. Absent or diminished bowel sounds and vomiting indicate the need to institute nasogastric suction.

Emergency treatment should include evaluation for possible injury to the urinary bladder. The presence of grossly bloody urine or blood at the urethral meatus is presumptive evidence of injury to the lower urinary tract (bladder or urethra). In the male, rectal examination is mandatory. The presence of a high-riding prostate indicates damage to the posterior urethra. Urethral injury in the female is uncommon. Urethrography is necessary to identify the area of injury. Cystography is performed to rule out injury to the urinary

Figure 32-10 Fracture in the hand. Typical displaced fracture of the right fifth metacarpal is seen. (Note displacement into palm.) It was reduced under local anesthesia.

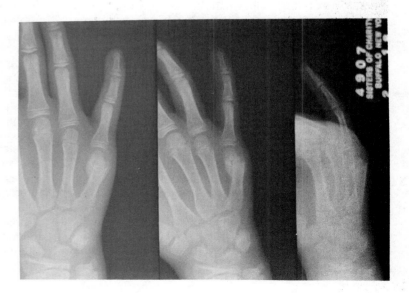

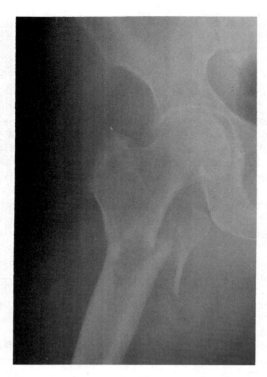

Figure 32-11 Subtrochanteric fracture of the femur. This fracture required internal fixation.

bladder. These studies are easily carried out in the emergency department with portable x-ray equipment. Patients with massive hemorrhage associated with pelvic fracture(s) may be candidates for early angiographic study and embolization of the damaged vessels.

FRACTURES OF THE HIP

Fracture of the hip involves the upper portion of the femur, usually in the trochanteric area or the region of the femoral neck. It is a common injury in the elderly. The usual history is that of an elderly person slipping at home or on the street and incurring severe pain in the hip area. In most instances, hip fracture victims are unable to bear weight following injury, but in the incomplete or impacted fracture, the patient may be able to bear weight, although with considerable pain. The victim may remain in bed for several days after injury before seeking care.

Pertinent physical findings are characteristic; they reveal the injured extremity to be shortened, with the foot in external rotation. There is usually tenderness on palpation about the affected hip.

The patient is preferably examined on the ambulance stretcher prior to removal to the examining table. If the patient is in severe pain, some traction may be applied to the affected extremity by pulling on the ankle. It is rarely necessary to change the rotation of the foot at this time. While traction is being maintained on the leg, the patient may be lifted on to the examining table by a lift team.

The patient with a fracture of the femoral neck or intertrochanteric region should be supported by pillows under the thigh and the lateral aspect of the leg; this reduces muscle fatigue from attempts to hold the limb, already externally rotated, in a position of least tension and pain. Individuals with fractures in this location will also tend to have their buttocks squeezed together, much like an individual anticipating a gluteal injection. Moving the unaffected buttock slightly outward (laterally) will help relieve the tensed position. Attention to the shoulder area will assist in identifying malalignment. With fractures of the pelvis or lower extremities, leverage involved in voluntary movement of the upper part of the body is diminished. Assistance should be offered to the patient to move his torso a few inches to one side or the other.

Appropriate assessment should be carried out and x-rays ordered (Fig. 32-11). To confirm the diagnosis both anteroposterior and lateral x-rays of the hip must be taken. These patients require admission, operative reduction, and internal fixation. Because most are in the older age group, there is a high incidence of associated disease, particularly processes involving the cardiovascular system. The operative procedure is rarely of such an urgent nature that complete preoperative evaluation cannot be carried out. There may be a significant amount of blood loss into the area of fracture, so that blood should be drawn for type and crossmatch. Electrocardiogram and chest x-ray are also indicated.

In some instances, Buck's skin traction is used to maintain limb immobility and provide some measure of comfort for the patient. This type of traction can cause skin necrosis and complicate the postoperative care, however, and proper skin preparation is important.

Dislocation of the Hip

Dislocation of the hip is a serious injury which has become more common as the incidence of automobile accidents has increased. A frequent mechanism is sudden deceleration, which causes the patient to strike his knee on the dashboard. In the sitting position, as in a car, the hip is flexed, and if the blow is severe enough, the head of the femur can be displaced from the acetabulum. In conjunction with this injury, a contusion or fracture of the patella may also be present.

Assessment. The patient will complain of severe pain in the hip and inability to fully extend the hip and knee.

The characteristic position is that of the hip flexed and adducted, so that the knee is toward the midline. The finding is in sharp contrast to a fracture of the hip or femur, in which the hip or leg is usually in external rotation rather than adduction. The patient is unable to move from this position voluntarily, and any attempt to straighten the limb causes extreme pain.

X-ray studies will reveal the dislocation, which may assume a number of positions (Fig. 32-12).

Treatment/Management. If there is no associated fracture about the hip joint, operative reduction can be carried out. These patients are usually admitted to the hospital for reduction under general or spinal anesthesia.

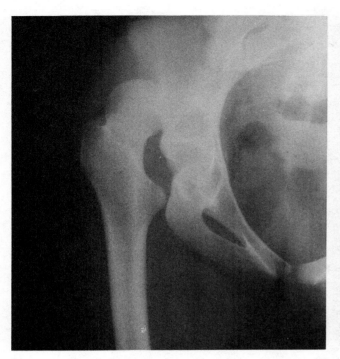 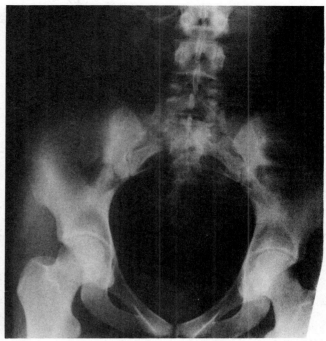

Figure 32-12 *Hip dislocation. Left. Posterior and superior dislocation of right hip. Note femoral head displaced from acetabulum. Right. Postreduction film. Note femoral head replaced in acetabulum.*

Hip dislocation victims must be monitored for a considerable period of time postinjury, since there is a significant incidence of avascular necrosis of the head of the femur as a result of this injury. The blood supply to the head and neck of the femur is derived from three sources. Two of these, the ligamentum teres and the capsule, may be seriously damaged or disrupted as a result of the injury. There is no way in which the outcome can be successfully predicted.

Fracture of the Femur

Of all of the extremity fractures, a fracture of the femur is by far the most important to recognize and manage properly. Although fractures of the extremities are generally not life-threatening and have a low priority of care in a multiple-injury patient, a fracture of the shaft of the femur in an adult can be serious, for it is usually associated with blood loss of 1000 ml to 1500 ml (Fig. 32-13). This loss occurs into the soft tissue structures about the fracture site and is accompanied by massive swelling of the thigh, although it may be quite difficult to estimate the amount of blood lost. The blood loss that occurs can be severe enough to produce severe hypovolemic shock, with no evidence of an external wound. In addition, the neurovascular structures lie in close proximity to the shaft of the femur and may be injured by a fracture.

Assessment. The mechanism of injury is usually a violent incident. The patient will note severe pain, deformity and inability to bear weight on the extremity. Angulation of the fragments results from a pull of the large thigh muscles which attach along the length of the femur.

A traction splint is applied and is left in place while the patient is evaluated in the emergency department. Rapid but thorough physical assessment is carried out, with recording of vital signs and complete examination of the injured extremity, including assessment for distal pulses, intact sensation and motor power of the toes.

A large-bore catheter or needle is inserted into an appropriate vein, particularly one in the upper extremity or the opposite uninjured limb, to draw blood for complete blood count, type and crossmatch. Volume replacement is instituted using normal saline or crystalloid without calcium. After the patient's vital signs have been stabilized and the limb is completely mobilized, the patient may be transferred to the x-ray department for study.

Treatment/Management. Further management of this injury depends on the type of fracture. If the fracture is of the spiral or transverse type without significant comminution, some type of internal fixation, such as the use of an intramedullary rod, is the usual treatment. If there is considerable fragmentation at the fracture site, the injury is managed by the use of balanced traction, using a Steinman pin or Kirschner wire. These devices are inserted under local anesthesia through the femoral condyles or the tibial tubercle and attached to a traction device integrating the principles of a Thomas splint and a Bradford frame.

Fracture and Dislocation of the Knee

Dislocation of the knee typically follows a violent accident: a direct blow, a fall, or a torsional injury involving the knee joint.

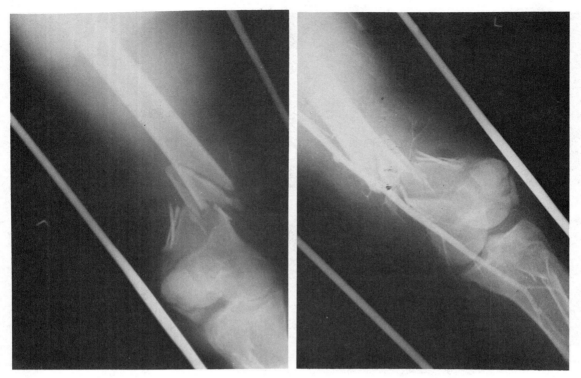

Figure 32-13 Left. *Severely comminuted fracture of the femur. The patient was struck by an auto. The injured leg was swollen, cold, and pale, indicating vascular injury. Right. Arteriogram in emergency department x-ray revealed the intact vessel.*

1. *Torsional injury to the knee,* resulting in damage to both ligamentous and bony structures, is common. Following the episode, the patient will note severe pain, swelling and varying degrees of deformity about the knee. Full assessment of the extremity should be done, including evaluation of both the neurological and vascular status; the popliteal artery and veins and the sciatic nerve are in close proximity to the posterior aspect of the knee joint, in the popliteal space.

   Following assessment, the limb is immobilized in a well-padded gutter splint, for transport. If there is rather marked deformity and angulation or rotation at the knee, it is best to transport the patient without use of an external splint, using sandbags to provide immobilization, or to splint the limb in the position in which it was found.

   After the diagnosis has been established by x-ray, the patient will invariably require admission for surgical reduction.

2. *Fractures of the patella* usually result from a fall with the patient landing on the knee. The patella is anatomically located within the quadriceps tendon overlying the anterior aspect of the knee joint. Injuries to the patella may thus involve varying degrees of damage to the patellar tendon, from tear to complete rupture. The fracture itself may assume a variety of shapes, from a simple transverse type to a comminuted variety with multiple fragments.

   Following injury, the patient complains of pain and difficulty in walking or total inability to walk. Assessment reveals swelling and tenderness about the patellar region. The patient should be asked to actively flex and extend the knee. This can be done by having the patient sit on the examining table with the knee flexed and attempt to straighten out the knee. Success in this maneuver proves the integrity of the quadriceps mechanism. X-ray study will usually confirm the diagnosis.

   The management of the simple transverse fracture of the patella with an intact quadriceps mechanism is obtained by application of a cylinder cast with the knee in full extension or by application of a knee immobilizer. This can be done in the emergency department and the patient can be sent home and ambulated in this manner. In severely comminuted fractures or those involving injury to the quadriceps mechanism, surgical intervention may be necessary. The usual surgical treatment is to excise the fragments of the patella and repair the damage to the quadriceps tendon.

Fractures of the Tibia and Fibula

Fractures of the bones of the lower leg may involve one or both of the bones. Depending on the mechanism of injury, the fractures may occur at the same or different levels, but, because of the application of the forces involved, the fractures usually occur at the same level. The usual mechanism of injury is direct violence. In indirect violence or torsional injury, the tibia is frequently fractured at the middle and distal third and the fibula in the upper third.

Fractures involving the lower third of these bones are serious, since the incidence of non-union is higher in this area than in other portions of the bones. In addition, because of the minimal amount of subcutaneous fat, there is a higher incidence of open fractures in the lower third than in other areas of the tibia.

Physical assessment reveals obvious deformity with tenderness at the level of the deformity. If the fracture is incomplete or undisplaced, the tenderness will be well localized at the fracture site. This can be determined by carefully palpating along the anterior edge of the tibia, usually referred to as the tibial spine. Ordinarily, this should be a continuous, rather sharp edge. A history of injury combined with any disruption or lack of continuity of the tibial spine is good clinical evidence that a fracture may be present. If not already immobilized, the patient's leg should be carefully placed in a gutter type splint and x-rays should be taken (Fig. 32-14).

The management thereafter varies. In incomplete or undisplaced fractures, satisfactory immobilization may be achieved by means of a long leg cast. In displaced, oblique, or comminuted fracture, in which multiple fragments may be involved, an operative approach may be required to maintain the fragments in satisfactory position.

Fractures of the Ankle

Fractures and dislocation about the ankle are commonly seen in adults but are quite uncommon in children.

Assessment. The usual history is that of indirect violence; for example, the patient slips, and severe rotational forces are exerted on the ankle. A common cause of injury is stepping into a hole or walking on uneven surfaces. Following injury, the patient complains of pain, swelling, and difficulty in bearing weight on the injured limb.

Physical assessment reveals swelling and deformity about the ankle site. Careful palpation of the medial and lateral malleoli should be carried out, to ascertain the exact site of fracture. In addition, vascular injuries, though rare in this type of fracture, do occur, and the presence of dorsalis pedis and posterior tibial pulses should be thoroughly evaluated. In some instances, severe swelling and pain may not be due to fracture but to a serious ligamentous injury particularly when the x-ray studies are negative. Further x-rays may be required, using the ''stress'' technique.

Treatment/Management. Management of the fracture depends on the extent of the injury. Simple, isolated fractures of the medial or lateral malleolus may be treated by application of a short-leg walking cast. If there is significant displacement of the fragments, comminution, or serious ligamentous tears, an operative approach is necessary.

Fractures of the Foot and Toes

In the foot region, fractures of the heel bones and the tarsal, metatarsal, and phalangeal bones are possible.

Fractures of the os calcis (the heel bone) constitute one to 2% of all fractures. They result from a fall in which the patient lands on the foot, with varying degrees of injury to the os calcis. Following injury, the patient complains of pain, swelling, and difficulty in bearing weight on the heel or in walking at all. Assessment reveals localized tenderness and swelling, with ecchymoses in the region of the heel and varying degrees of deformity. X-rays confirm the diagnosis (Fig. 32-15).

Forces that result from landing on the heel are transmitted along the shafts of the long bones of the leg and up into the spine, so that it is not uncommon to have os calcis injury associated with fractures of the dorsal and lumbar vertebrae. The vertebral injuries usually occur in the region of the twelfth thoracic and the first or second lumbar vertebrae.

Figure 32-14 *Two lower leg fractures. Left. Isolated fracture of the fibula, from a direct blow in football. Right. Isolated fracture of the tibia.*

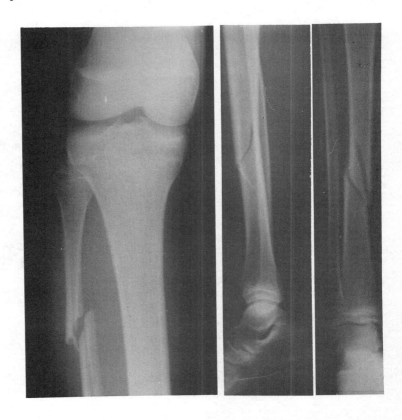

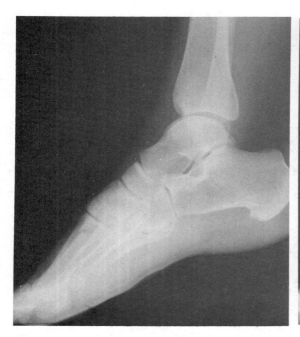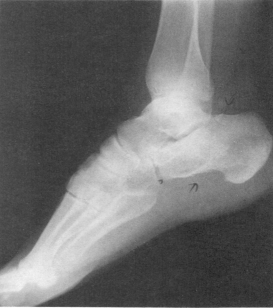

Figure 32-15 The os calcis. Left. Normal os calcis. Right. Fracture of the os calcis, received in a fall from a height.

Management varies. When the injury is only to the os calcis, a good supporting shoe may be effective treatment. At times, swelling, deformity, and discomfort may be significant enough to warrant admission and operative reduction.

Fractures of the tarsals and metatarsals are relatively common and also result from a fall or direct violence. The patient invariably complains of pain and inability to bear weight. Pertinent findings include tenderness, swelling, and ecchymosis of the foot at the area of injury, with varying degrees of swelling of the forefoot. X-rays confirm the diagnosis. Management varies, depending on the degree of injury, from use of a firm shoe to application of a short-leg plaster cast.

Fractures involving the toes are rarely serious, though they may cause considerable discomfort. The usual mechanism of injury is an object dropping on the toes or striking (stubbing) the toe against a rigid object when not wearing shoes. The patient may present for treatment several days after injury because of continued pain, swelling, or inability to walk.

The pain is frequently described as severe and throbbing, worse when the foot is dependent and improved with elevation. Particularly after an object falls on the toe, subungual hematoma (bleeding beneath the nail) is common, and may add considerably to the discomfort.

No splinting is necessary initially. Following x-ray to confirm diagnosis (Fig. 32-16), the treatment of the fracture depends on the type of injury. In transverse fractures of the phalanges, the patient may be able to wear a shoe with comfort and bear weight as long as the normal heel and toe walking gait is altered to that of a flat-footed step. In other instances, the pain may be severe enough to require crutches. Fractures of toes other than the great toe can usually be managed by taping the injured toe to an adjacent one by means of a circumferential adhesive tape wrapping. A piece of cotton or gauze should be placed in the web space be-

tween the toes, to absorb perspiration and prevent maceration of the skin.

Evacuation of the subungual hematoma, when present, provides considerable relief to the patient. This may be accomplished by drilling several holes in the nail, using size 11 scalpel blade or a hand-operated dental drill. In instances where an entire nail bed is involved, an 11 scalpel blade can be gently inserted beneath the nail at its free edge and the hematoma evacuated. Immobilization of the toe is usually necessary for a period of 3 weeks.

CARE OF PATIENTS WITH INJURED EXTREMITIES

One's responsibilities assume different dimensions once the diagnosis has been established and plans for definitive treatment are outlined. Generally, patients who are to be treated in the hospital are transferred to general care areas, the casting room, operating rooms, or an orthopedic clinic. When closed reduction and immobilization necessitating Kirschner wires or Steinman pins for extremity fractures are required, they may be accomplished under local anesthesia in the emergency department.

Complete, balanced traction, under ordinary circumstances, should not be applied in the emergency department, since transporting the patient with traction and weights in place is difficult. Beds with large traction frames rarely fit through doors. And the weights, once applied, should not be lifted.

CASTS

While the principles of cast application remain standard, individual physician preferences for certain materials vary

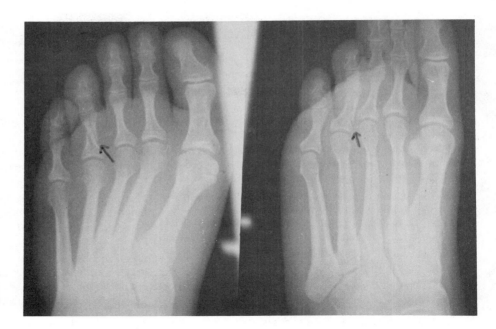

Figure 32-16 *Fracture of the proximal phalanx, fourth toe. The patient was shoeless and stubbed toe on a furniture leg. Treatment consisted of taping fractured toe to adjacent toe.*

widely. The best approach is to maintain a file or reference notebook recording routinely used procedures and preferences of physicians who frequently use the casting facilities.

Participation in casting procedures may include preparing the equipment and providing support and traction for the injured part. Attention should be directed toward observing the tolerance of the patient to the procedure. Weakness, faintness, and nausea may peak during closed reduction and application of the first rolls of plaster. The patient in a sitting position for cast application is especially likely to become light-headed. Sudden movement, as in the case of nausea and vomiting, could prove disastrous.

Once the cast has been applied, it should be handled carefully, with the palms of the hands. The patient should be cautioned not to rest the wet cast on hard surfaces, such as wooden chair arms and coffee tables. A period of 24 hours is sufficient drying time for large leg casts, providing humidity is not high and the cast is not covered. The patient can be taught to test for complete seasoning of the cast by listening for a hollow sound when tapped and feeling the cast for moisture.

Cast Care

An important aspect of treatment is the education of the patient concerning care of the casted extremity. Far too often, the fracture heals well, but loss of functional movement of a shoulder, hips, or fingers results because adequate instruction has not been given the patient concerning range of motion exercises for unaffected joints.

The signs and symptoms of vascular and neurological impairment previously discussed must be explained to the patient at a level commensurate with his understanding. A written list of instructions should be given the patient or his relatives for reference after discharge from the emergency department (Chart 32-3). Reliance on verbal instructions is insufficient. Return appointments can be incorporated into the instructional format, depending upon local protocol.

Children have their own ways of destroying casts, many quite ingenious. The boy in a walking cast may discover that his casted leg kicks a soccer ball much better than it did before. For the smaller child, a lot of fun can be had when sand is put in one end of the cast and allowed to drain out the other. External dirt is of little consequence, however, unless it is moist, like mud. The greater danger lies with children hiding objects in the cast. Unless the child is very young, he will be able to understand the dangers if they are presented well.

The best allies in removing moisture and odors are an old toothbrush and baking soda. The baking soda can be sprinkled on the wet area, allowed to absorb the moisture and brushed away with the toothbrush. Successive applications will return the cast to a fairly odorless and dry state. A hand soap for removing grease or a nonabrasive cleanser and a toothbrush work well for removal of other stains. Use of some of the powdered dry spray deodorants has been suggested for odor removal, but their effects are unsatisfactory in terms of removing moisture. Stockinette may be used to cover the cast and keep it clean. The newer cast materials include a plastic material that is heat-dried and relatively waterproof.

Time must be taken to explain these aspects of cast care before the patient is discharged from the emergency department.

Promoting Joint Mobility and Muscle Strength

Active range of motion exercise for muscles and joints proximal and distal to cast length is important for maintaining mobility and strength of the casted extremity. These exercises should be done at least twice a day and more frequently for optimal results.

The patient with a long arm cast extending beyond the wrist and elbow, should do active range of motion exercises for the shoulder and all noncasted joints of the hand. The patient with a fracture of the tibia or fibula will have a long leg cast, immobilizing all joints of the extremity except the

---

Chart 32-3

CAST CARE INSTRUCTIONS

You have just had a cast applied as part of the treatment of your injury. Because of the nature of your injury and of the plaster of Paris used to make your cast, there are certain precautions you should take to prevent serious problems.

1. Keep the injured limb elevated (propped up) continuously for the next 48 hours. This is to prevent swelling of the limb, and to be effective, your arm (or leg) must be arranged so that your fingers (or toes) are at least 12 inches above your heart.

2. Rarely, there is sufficient swelling within the cast to interfere with the circulation or nerve supply: *Signs you should look out for are excessive blueness, paleness, numbness (loss of feeling), or coldness of your fingers or toes.* This is a serious condition, and it is absolutely necessary that you return to the hospital at once.

3. The pain of your injury should subside rapidly. You may have some mild aching, but this should respond to aspirin. If your doctor feels you need stronger medication, he will prescribe it. If the pain medication does not work within 30 to 45 minutes, you should call your doctor for advice.

4. Do not get your cast wet. If you do, it will only fall apart and no longer perform its proper function.

5. Never, never put anything under your cast. No matter how good it would feel to scratch that itch, you are asking for trouble from infected pressure sores or scratches if you put anything under your cast. If you have trouble with itching, call your doctor. He can prescribe medicine to deal with the problem.

6. Your cast will be set in a few minutes, but it requires 48 hours to harden completely. If it has a walking heel, *do not walk on it* for 48 hours.

7. For proper treatment of your injury, you should come to all your appointments on time.

8. If for any reason you are concerned about your cast or your injury, do not hesitate to call your doctor.

(Orthopedic Service, Emergency Division, Santa Clara Valley Medical Center, San Jose, California)

---

toes and hip joint. "Wiggling" the toes and range of motion exercises at the hip are necessary. Hip abduction is of particular importance in enabling the patient to resume a normal gait pattern when the cast is removed.

Isometric exercises of muscles in casted extremities are effective in maintaining strength and preventing disuse atrophy. Complete instruction in and faithful adherence to an exercise program will result in a stronger and more functional extremity when the cast is removed.

If exercise instructions cannot be accomplished in the emergency department, a referral mechanism for physical therapy is necessary.

CRUTCH FITTING

Patients with lower extremity injuries will need to have crutches fitted and instructions given for safe crutchwalking and transfer techniques before leaving the emergency department.

Many emergency departments use the hospital's physical therapists to fit crutches and instruct patients in safe crutch walking procedures. When this is not possible, emergency personnel should be familiar with the basics of crutch-fitting and physical therapy.

To be capable of walking on standard axillary crutches, a patient should have:
1. Normal upper extremity muscle power (hand grasp, wrist and elbow extension).

2. Normal, uninvolved lower extremity muscle power (hip and knee extension, ankle plantar flexion).

3. Unimpaired balance and coordination.

Measurement for axillary crutches can be done while the patient is supine, with the arms parallel to the side of the body. Crutches can also be fitted with the patient standing erect. But, for safety, the patient must be supported by another person, a walker, or a stationary object during fitting.

Measurement begins one inch inferior to the axillary fold and ends at a point 6 to 8 inches lateral to the inferior aspect of the heel (Fig. 32-17). The patient should be measured while wearing the shoe he will use while a crutch walker. The handpiece should be positioned so that the elbow is flexed 15 to 25 degrees, depending on the patient's comfort.

Crutch tips should be 2 inches in diameter to assure stable crutch positioning during walking. The patient or his family should be instructed to inspect the crutch tips periodically for excessive wear. Padding over the handpiece and axillary bar are not necessary but may be added for comfort. The patient must understand that weight must be borne on the hands, *not* in the axillary region.

CRUTCH WALKING AND MANEUVERS

The gait pattern commonly used by patients with lower extremity injury is a 3-point touch, weightbearing, or nonweightbearing pattern. "Three-point" designation connotes the 2 crutches and the one uninvolved lower extremity. In this pattern, the affected extremity and both crutches advance simultaneously. Then, with the weight borne on the hands, the unaffected extremity follows through. The patient should advance the uninvolved extremity past the point of crutch placement to maintain a tripod stance for stability at each step.

Prior to practicing walking with the patient, a safety belt should be placed around the patient's waist and tightened snugly. A firm hold on the belt while the patient is practicing crutch walking provides him with better balance control and with greater leverage should he start to fall.

Learning the gait pattern is only the beginning, for the crutch walker soon learns there are many environmental objects he has to negotiate with crutches, namely, in and out of chairs, up and down stairs and through doors. The patient needs instruction in these frequently overlooked techniques. The series of figures which follows graphically depicts these techniques. Since instructions in these techniques are time-consuming and require practice, written take-home materials or follow-up physical therapy may be indicated.

From Sitting to Standing

Figure 32-18 illustrates how the crutch user moves from sitting in a chair to standing.
1. The patient moves forward to the edge of the chair and

Figure 32-17 *Fitting axillary crutches. Note that the top of the crutch comes to within an inch of the axillary fold, the bottom of the crutch rests 6 to 8 inches to the side of the heel and the elbow is flexed 15 to 25 degrees.*

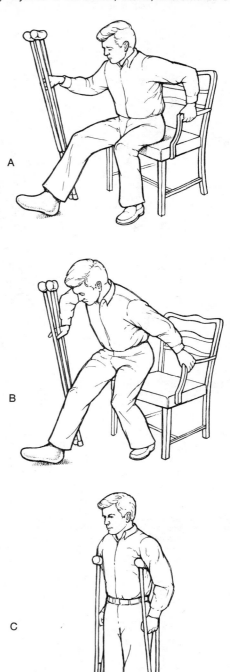

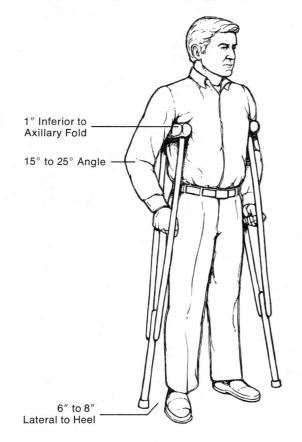

1″ Inferior to Axillary Fold

15° to 25° Angle

6″ to 8″ Lateral to Heel

Figure 32-18 *From sitting to standing with crutches. A. The patient moves forward to the edge of the chair, placing both crutches in the hand on the same side as the affected extremity. The arm and the leg on the unaffected side are readied for standing. B. Patient pushes up with the unaffected leg and both arms. C. The crutches are repositioned for walking.*

places both crutches in the hand on the same side as the affected extremity. The opposite hand is placed on the arm of chair, and the unaffected leg is positioned for standing.

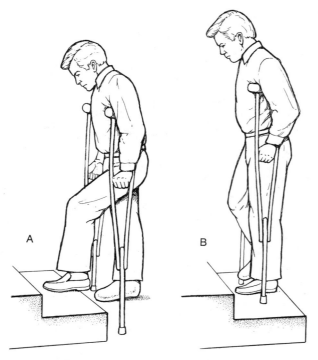

Figure 32-19 *Climbing stairs with crutches. A. Using a three-point crutch gait, the patient bears his weight on his hands through the crutches and steps up with the uninvolved leg. B. The crutches and the involved leg follow.*

2. Patient rises to standing position by pushing up with unaffected leg. Both arms assist in attaining standing position.
3. Patient shifts crutches beneath each arm, to the unaffected side first, and proceeds to ambulate.

To sit, the patient backs up to the chair, feels for the chair with the back of the uninvolved leg, and reverses the sequence outlined in the above list. For safety, all "throw rugs" should be removed from the patient's home. If possible, low chairs and soft sofas should be avoided, since these require additional effort and balance to negotiate. The above pattern can also be applied to the transfer in and out of a car.

Ascending Stairs

Figure 32-19 illustrates the technique of climbing stairs with crutches.
1. The patient uses a three-point crutch gait to ascend stairs by bearing weight on the hands through crutches and steps up with the uninvolved leg.
2. The patient shifts his weight to the uninvolved leg. Crutches and involved leg move up to the next step.

Descending Stairs

Descending stairs is also done in two basic steps. Figure 32-20 illustrates.
1. Crutches and involved leg are lowered to the step below.
2. As the weight is borne on the hands, the uninvolved leg steps down, through the crutches.

When a railing is available, the patient may switch both crutches to one side and hold the railing on the opposite side. The patient then proceeds to descend as outlined above. (Fig. 32-20C)

Doorways

Negotiating doorways is another difficult maneuver on crutches. When the door opens toward the patient, he should

Figure 32-20 *Descending stairs with crutches. A. Crutches and the involved leg are lowered to the step below. B. With weight borne on the hands through the crutches, the uninvolved leg steps down. C. When a railing is available, the patient can transfer both crutches to one side, hold the railing on the other side and proceed as outlined in A and B.*

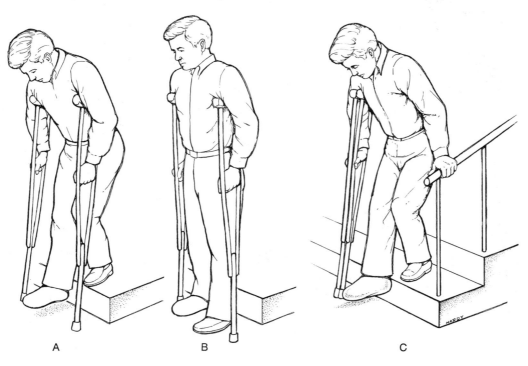

stand almost perpendicular to traffic pattern flow, grasp the door handle, and open the door with the hand opposite the affected leg. (Fig. 32-21*A*)

For doors opening away from patient, he stands directly in front of door, grasps the handle and opens door with hand opposite affected leg (Fig. 32-21*B*). To proceed through the door in either case, the patient places one crutch on the floor next to door to keep it open and advances through (Fig. 32-21*C*).

WALKERS

A patient whose balance and coordination are not adequate to use axillary crutches may be a candidate for a walker. The walker device provides more stability than crutches but limits the places a patient can go (*i.e.,* small spaces and stairs).

1. *Fitting a walker is similar to fitting crutches*
   - The patient should be able to stand erect without slouching.
   - When the patient's hands are on the walker handles, his elbows should be flexed 15 to 25 degrees, depending upon his comfort.
   - With the elbows in that position, the top of the walker will be slightly above the greater trochanter level.
   The sequence for walker walking is similar to that of crutch walking.
2. *Walking forward*
   - The patient moves the walker ahead.
   - He bears his weight through the hands so that he can step with the uninvolved leg into the walker.
   - With each step he should be midway into the walker field of balance.
3. *Turning*
   - The turn should occur with the uninvolved leg on the outer perimeter of the turn radius.
   - The patient should avoid pivoting on the good or uninvolved leg.

- The turning sequence is similar to a forward walking pattern: The first move is with the walker, turning it slightly, then stepping with the uninvolved foot. The sequence is repeated until the patient has turned around.
4. *Walking backward:* The pattern is the reverse of that for walking forward.

CANES

A cane is used when a patient needs lateral support for walking but can bear partial or total weight on an affected leg. The top of the cane should be slightly higher than the patient's greater trochanter. The cane tips, like crutch tips, should be large enough to provide stability.

A cane should *always* be used in the hand *opposite* the affected leg or opposite the side of the body needing additional lateral support. The cane and the feet form a triangular base of support for the walking pattern.

Depending upon the patient's coordination, balance, and strength, either a step-to-cane gait or a step-through-cane gait can be used.

1. The *step-to-cane* gait:
   - The cane is advanced, followed by the involved leg.
   - With the weight on the cane, the good leg is advanced simultaneously.
2. The *step-through-gait:*
   - The cane and involved leg are advanced simultaneously.
   - With the weight on the cane, the uninvolved leg steps past the cane and involved leg.

SUMMARY

Patients with fractures and soft tissue injuries constitute a large proportion of the patients seen in an emergency department. The importance of assessment of their problems,

Figure 32-21 *Negotiating doorways with crutches. A. For doors opening toward the patient, he should stand almost perpendicular to the traffic flow and open the door with the hand opposite the affected leg. B. For doors opening outward, the patient stands in front of the door and opens it with the hand opposite the affected leg. C. The patient places one crutch next to the door, thus keeping it open as he advances through the doorway.*

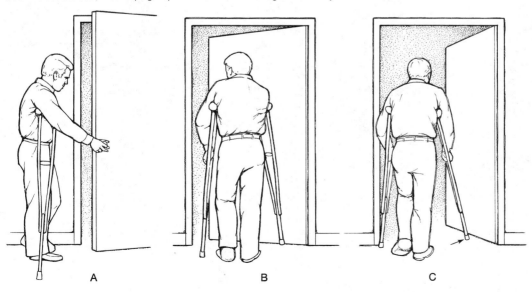

A   B   C

initiation of diagnostic measures, support during treatment and education for rehabilitation cannot be underestimated, considering that the patient's very life-style depends on mobility and a functional skeletal system.

The emergency personnel play a crucial role in each of these important steps in assessment and management, especially in insuring patient well-being in the present emergency situation and in future healing and rehabilitation.

BIBLIOGRAPHY

Abraham EA, McMaster WC, Krijger M, Waugh TR: Whirlpool therapy for the treatment of soft tissue wounds complicating extremity fractures. J Trauma 14:222, 1974

Beck J, Collins J: Theoretical and clinical aspects of post traumatic fat embolism syndrome. In The American Academy of Orthopedic Surgeons, Instructional Course Lectures 22:38–87, 1973

Bennett JE, Hayes JE, Robb C: Mutilating injuries of the wrist. J Trauma 11:1008, 1971

Boucher PR, Morton KS: Rupture of the distal biceps brachii tendon. J Trauma 7:626, 1967

Bredael JJ et al: Traumatic rupture of the female urethra. J Urol 122:560–561, 1979

Cass AS et al: Urethral injury due to external trauma. Urology 11:607–611, 1978

Chan D, Kraus J, Riggins R: Patterns of multiple fractures in accidental injury. J Trauma 13:1075, 1973

Civetta JM et al: Prehospital use of the military anti-shock trouser (MAST). JACEP 5:581–587, 1976

Connally J, Brooks A: Vascular problems in orthopedics. In The American Academy of Orthopedic Surgeons, Instructional Course Lectures 22:12–27, 1973

Emerman CE: Abdominopelvic injury associated with pelvic fracture. JACEP 8:312, August 1979

Eversmann WW: Injuries to the elbow in children. Hosp Med 10:29, 1974

Farrell J: Casts, your patients and you: A review of basic procedures. Nursing 78 8:65, October 1978

Farrell J: Casts, your patients and you: A review of arm and leg cast procedures. Nursing 78 8:57, November 1978

Flint LM et al: Definitive control of bleeding from severe pelvic fractures. Ann Surg 189:709–716, 1979

Gaul JS: Management of acute hand injuries. Ann Emerg Med 9:139, March 1980

Glenn J et al: The treatment of fractures in patients with head trauma. J Trauma 12:958, 1973

Green NE, Allen BL: Vascular injuries associated with dislocation of the knee. J Bone Joint Surg 59A:236–239, March, 1977

Grosz C et al: Volkmann's contracture and femoral shaft fractures. J Trauma 12:129–134, December, 1973

Harris WH, Malt RA: Late results of human limb replantation: Eleven-year and six-year follow-up of two cases with description of a new tendon transfer. J Trauma 14:44, 1974

Heck CC: Sprained ankle. NY State J Med 72:1620, 1972

Levine J, Crampton R: Major abdominal injuries associated with pelvic fractures. Surg Gynecol Obstet 116:223, 1963

Love-Mignogna S: Taping and splinting: Seven common problems. Nursing 80 10:88, April 1980

Lyon LJ, Nevins MA: Nontreatment of hip fractures in senile patients. JAMA 238:1175–1176, September 12, 1977

McAninch JW: Traumatic injury to the urethra. J Trauma 21:291–297, April 1981

McLaughlin HL, Parkes JC III: Fracture of the carpal navicular (scaphoid) bone: Gradations in therapy based upon pathology. J Trauma 9:292, 1969

Makin GS, Howard JH: Arterial injuries complicating fractures or dislocations: The necessity for a more aggressive approach. Surgery 59:203, 1966

Markham DE: Anterior dislocation of hip and diastasis of contralateral sacro-iliac joint: Rear-seat passenger's injury. Br J Surg 59:296, 1972

Mital MA, Patel UH: Fractures and dislocations about the distal forearm, wrist and hand: Progress in treatment in the last decade. Am J Surg 124:660, 1972

Nixon JF: A simple sprained ankle may not be so simple. Consultant 175, 1973

Perry J, McClellan R: Autopsy findings in 127 patients following fatal traffic accidents. Surg Gynecol Obstet 119:586, 1964

Post M, Haskell SB: Reconstruction of the median nerve following entrapment in supracondylar fracture of the humerus: A case report. J Trauma 14:252, 1974

Reckling FW, Peltier LF: Acute knee dislocations and their complications. J Trauma 9:181, 1969

Rosenthal RE et al: Posterior fracture-dislocation of the hip. J Trauma 19:572–581, 1979

Sarmiento A et al: Functional bracing of fractures of the shaft of humerus. J Bone Joint Surg 59A:596–601, July 1977

Schweigel JF, Gropper PT: A comparison of ambulatory versus non-ambulatory care of femoral shaft fractures. J Trauma 14:474, 1974

Sims FH, Detenbeck LC: Injuries of the knee in athletes. Minnesota Med 55:881, 1972

Singh I, Gorman JF: Vascular injuries in closed fractures near junction of middle and lower thirds of the tibia. J Trauma 12:592, 1973

Sladek EC, Kopta JA: Management of open fractures of the tibial shaft. South Med J 70:662–665, June 1977

Smith RF: Fracture of long bones with arterial injury due to blunt trauma. Arch Surg 99:315, 1969

Straight PA: How to help the patient with a dislocated shoulder. Am J Nurs 79:666, April 1979

Taylor AR, Arden GP, Rainey HA: Traumatic dislocation of the knee: Report of 43 cases with special reference to conservative management. J Bone Joint Surg 54B:96, 1972

Waddell JP: Subtrochanteric fractures of the femur. J Trauma 19:582–592, 1979

Wholey MH, Bucher J: Angiography in musculoskeletal trauma. Surg Gynecol Obstet 125:730, 1967

33
OCULAR INJURIES

ARTHUR J. SCHAEFER

Any patient seen in the emergency department with trauma in the facial region must have a careful eye examination and appropriate radiologic studies of the skull and facial bones, including the basic Caldwell, lateral, and Waters projections. Too frequently, patients with other bodily injuries, and in a state of shock, have ocular injuries that are overlooked. One half of all monocular blindness and one fifth of all binocular blindness are due to accidents.[1] The eye occupies only 1/375 of the exposed body surface and 0.27% of the total body surface. Yet from 2% to 2.5% of all World War II casualties, according to Duke-Elder, were ocular.[2] In the Vietnam war, 5% of the total, nonfatal hospitalized casualties, were ocular. Thus, the necessity of checking the eyes carefully in all victims with facial trauma cannot be emphasized too strongly.

Today, automobile accidents contribute greatly to eye injuries. Orbital and ocular injuries account for almost 10% of all automobile injuries, according to a Cornell Medical College research project. In contrast, fewer than 3% of battle casualties in World War II involved ocular injuries, according to Keeney.[3] Eye injuries in racquet sports, especially with the growing popularity of squash and racquetball, have been on the rapid increase. At the National Conference of the National Society to Prevent Blindness in 1980, Dr. Paul F. Vinger of Harvard estimated that there are about 40 million people participating in racquet sports each year in the USA and at least 9000 of them sustain eye injuries.[4] The speed of the ball is 100 miles or more an hour. Therefore, it is imperative that each player take advantage of the newer eyeguards and wear them faithfully to prevent serious eye injury and even loss of the sight of an eye.

ANATOMY AND PHYSIOLOGY

The eyes are paired sense organs that move synchronously to produce binocular vision. Each eyeball, or globe, is roughly spherical. The white portion of the eye, the sclera, surrounds the anterior portion of the globe, the cornea. The cornea is a transparent dome that may be compared to a watch crystal. Behind the protective cornea is the iris, the colored portion of the eye. The iris is an opaque, contractile diaphragm, with a round, regular opening centrally, the pupil, behind which the lens is located.

The interior of the globe contains two fluids, the aqueous humor and the vitreous body. The aqueous humor, a thin fluid, lies in the anterior and posterior chambers of the eye, which are located between the cornea and the lens. These chambers communicate through the pupil.

The dense and jelly-like vitreous body fills the larger, most posterior portion of the globe, which is located between the lens and the retina. The retina forms the inner lining of the posterior portion of the globe and can only be visualized using an ophthalmoscope with special magnification. Figure 33-1 shows two views of the ocular structures discussed above.

Attached to the eyeball are six extraocular muscles that are responsible for the external movements of the eyeball. Anteriorly, the eyeball is protected by the upper and lower eyelids, which involuntarily close over the eye at frequent intervals. This reflex motion, called blinking, serves to moisten the anterior portion of the eye by circulating the tear fluid that flows from the lacrimal (tear) gland located in the lateral anterior aspect of the orbit behind the superior orbital rim. The tear fluid bathes the globe, then exits through the puncta and the lacrimal ducts, located at the most medial end of the upper and lower lid and draining into the nasal cavity.

The eyelids are composed of skin and muscle over a thin layer of dense connective tissue, the tarsal plate, which serves to stiffen them. At the edge of each lid is a fringe of hair, the eyelashes, which are very sensitive to touch and, when stimulated, cause a reflex closure of the lids. Besides this protective action of the eyelids, the eyeball is further safeguarded by the orbicularis oculi muscle, a strong circular muscle surrounding the lids, which can be contracted voluntarily to forcibly close the lids.

Each eyeball rests within an *orbit* surrounded by periorbital fat posteriorly and the eyelids anteriorly. The eyelids are lined by the palpebral conjunctiva, which continues onto

Figure 33-1 Anatomy of the right eye. Top. Anterior view. Bottom. Sagittal view.

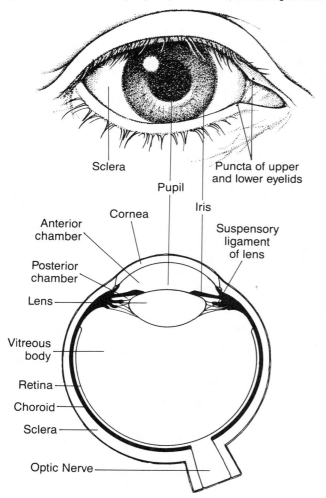

Sclera

Pupil

Cornea

Iris

Puncta of upper and lower eyelids

Anterior chamber

Posterior chamber

Suspensory ligament of lens

Lens

Vitreous body

Retina

Choroid

Sclera

Optic Nerve

the eyeball, covering the anterior portion (the bulbar conjunctiva). The two bony vaults in the cranium, the orbits, which surround and protect the eye, are in direct continuity with the four sinuses: frontal, ethmoid, maxillary, and sphenoidal.

ASSESSMENT OF OCULAR PROBLEMS

History

First, a good history of the injury should be obtained from the patient. If the patient is a child, emergency personnel should obtain the history from the parents or someone else familiar with the accident. It should include the following:

- The time of the injury
- The nature of the injury (scratch, cut foreign body, blunt instrument, or missile)
- The extent of pain
- Any visual disturbance

Careful records must be maintained for the patient's benefit and for medicolegal purposes.

Physical Examination

The following equipment should be on hand for ocular examination and treatment (Fig. 33-2).

- A small flashlight (penlight) or examining light, with a sharp beam of light to aid in critical examination of the eye and its adnexa. A flashlight with a blue beam is needed, as well, for viewing the eye after fluorescein staining.
- A magnifying loupe to visualize minute pathology, such as corneal foreign body or fine corneal abrasion
- A Snellen test card for visual acuity
- A lid retractor or speculum to help hold the lids open if there is swelling or spasm of the lids
- An ophthalmoscope
- A contact lens remover (small rubber suction cup)
- Sterile irrigating solutions
- Sterile cotton applicators
- Fluorescein strips
- Sterile eye pads and tape
- Medications in small, sterile, disposable vials or tubes, including cycloplegics, mydriatics, miotics, anesthetics, and antibiotics. Ocular medications commonly used in the emergency department are listed in Table 33-1.

Note: do not keep atropine or steroid drops on the eye tray because their misuse in some conditions can cause serious problems.

Visual acuity should be recorded for all patients before any examination or treatment is started. If the patient cannot see or read the Snellen test card or is in critical condition, record whether the patient can count fingers or see hand motion with each eye separately and at what distance. If even this is beyond the patient's capacity, record whether he has light perception in each eye.

During an eye examination, the patient is usually frightened, upset, and apprehensive. If he has pain, he will keep

Figure 33-2 *Basic instruments needed for an ocular examination. From left to right: a Snellen test card, an ophthalmoscope, a penlight, a lid retractor, contact lens removers, a magnifying loupe. The cards shown are frequently carried by patients wearing standard or soft contact lenses.*

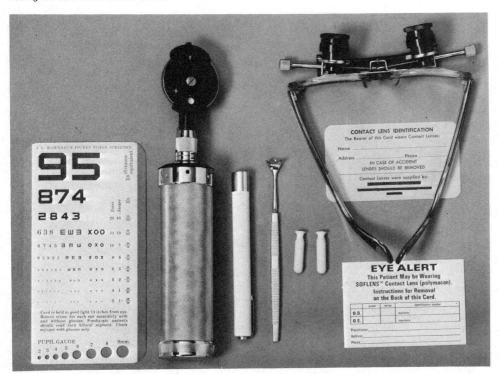

TABLE 33-1. OCULAR MEDICATIONS USED IN THE EMERGENCY DEPARTMENT

Drug Type	Drug Generic Name	Drug Trade Name and Dose
Common mydriatics		
Sympathomimetic ophthalmic solutions	Phenylephrine	Neo-Synephrine, 10%
	Epinephrine	Adrenalin, 1:1,000
	Hydroxyamphetamine	Paredrine Hydrobromide, 1%
	Ephedrine	Ephedrine, 5%
Parasympatholytic ophthalmic solutions (cycloplegics)	Atropine	Isopto Atropine, 0.25% to 0.5%, 1%, 2%
	Homatropine	Homatropine Hydrobromide, 1% to 5%, Isopto Homatropine, 2%, 5%
	Hyoscine (Scopolamine)	Hyoscine (Scopolamine), 0.25% to 0.5%
	Cyclopentolate	Cyclogel, 1%, 2%
	Tropicamide	Mydriacyl, 1%, 2%
Miotics		
Parasympathomimetic ophthalmic solutions	Pilocarpine	Isoptocarpine, Pilocar, P. V. Carpine Liquifilm, 0.25% to 10%
Cholinergic drugs	Carbachol	Isopto Carbachol, P.S. Carbachol Liquifilm 0.25% to 3%
Anticholinesterases	Eserine (Physostigmine)	Eserine, 0.25% to 1%
	Neostigmine	Neostigmine, 3% to 5%
	Echothiophate	Phospholine Iodide 0.03%, 0.06%, 0.125%, and 0.25%
Other glaucoma medications		
Beta-adrenergic receptor blocking agent. New drug used in glaucoma therapy.	Timolol maleated	Timoptic ophthalmic solution, 0.25% to 0.5%
Carbonic Anhydrase inhibitor	Acetazolamide	Diamox 125 mg, 250 mg tablets, 500 mg sequels (sustained release)
		Daranide 50 mg tablets
Prodrug of Epinephrine (diesterification of epinephrine and pivalic acid. New drug used in glaucoma therapy.	Dipivefrin HCl	Propine 0.1% solution
Antibiotics (local)		
	Sulfa	Gantrisin
		Vasosulf, solution and ointment
		Bleph-10 solution
		Isoptocetamide opthalmic solution and ointment
	Neomycin	Neosporin ophthalmic solution and ointment
	Chloramphenicol	Ophthochlor ophthalmic solution (drops)
		Chloromycetin ointment
		Chloroptic drops and ointment
		Econochlor drops and ointment
	Gentamicin sulfate, solution and ointment	Garamycin ophthalmic solution and ointment Genoptic, solution and ointment
Antiviral agents		
	5-Ido 2-deoxyuridine	IDU 0.5% ointment 0.1% solution
	Adenine	Ara-A ointment
	Trifluridine (5-trifluornetteyl) 2-deoxyuridine	Viroptic, 0.1% drops
Antifungal agents		
	Amphotericin B topical solution	2.5 to 10 mg/ml of distilled H_2O or D_5W
	Nystatin	Topical ointment 100,000 μ/gm
	Natamycin	5% topical suspension

his eyes shut tightly as a defense mechanism. He will need reassurance and often a local topical anesthetic to permit adequate inspection of the eye. With the patient's head supported in a head rest, the eye is examined gently and care-fully; special care should be taken not to press against the eyeball at any time.

If the patient has moderate to severe blepharospasm (lid spasm) and cannot voluntarily open his eyelids, the examiner should use one to two drops of a 0.5% topical anesthetic, such as tetracaine HCl (Pontocaine), then wait 30 to 60 seconds before raising the lid. In severe blepharospasm, the dosage of the anesthetic should be repeated in 1 minute, and the lids will relax. The eye can then be examined without force, minimizing the chance of further injury to the eye.

Removal of Contact Lenses. If the patient is wearing contact lenses and is conscious and able to remove them, have him remove them. If the patient is unconscious or incapacitated, remove them as follows.

1. *Hard contact lenses.* Hard contact lenses are removed by applying a small, hard contact suction cup to the lens and extracting the lens with it. The suction cup is pictured on the equipment tray in Figure 33-2. The removal of hard corneal contact lenses is shown in Chart 33-1.

2. *Soft contact lenses.* Soft contact lenses are removed in the following manner. If the lens has been in the eye for some time, it may be difficult to remove if not irrigated well. Therefore, to be sure, irrigate the lens copiously with sterile irrigating fluid directly while it is in the eye. Then slide it gently off the cornea onto the sclera with the index finger. When the lens is over the sclera, gently pick it off by squeezing it between the index finger and thumb. If it does not slide off the cornea easily, the lens must be irrigated again; it will then slide off. If the lens does not slide off the cornea readily, and one persists in trying to slide it off without irrigating it, the whole or part of the corneal epithelium can be denuded in removing the lens. The removal of soft corneal contact lenses is shown in Chart 33-2.

Terminology

For purposes of identification, ocular and adnexal trauma are classified as follows:

* *Anterior segment*—cornea, anterior chamber, iris, and lens
* *Vitreoretinal*—vitreous body and retina
* *Oculoplastics*—lids, lacrimal apparatus, and orbit

COMMON OCULAR INJURIES AND DISORDERS

In the sections that follow, the assessment and management of patients with foreign bodies in the eye, traumatic ocular injuries, infections, and other eye disorders will be discussed. Assessment and management usually proceed concurrently.

FOREIGN BODY IN THE EYE

The most common ocular injury is caused by a simple foreign body, which may be under the upper eyelid or on the corneal or scleral conjunctiva. Corneal abrasions, erosion, or cuts produce the same symptoms as a foreign body in the eye.

Signs and Symptoms

* Sensation of something in the eye on opening and closing the lids.
* Marked increase in tearing

* Diffuse reddening of the conjunctiva
* Fluorescein staining of cornea (with corneal foreign body)

Foreign Body on the Upper Eyelid

1. If a patient has the sensation of a foreign body and if it is difficult for him to open his eye, instill 1 to 2 drops of 0.5% topical anesthetic, such as tetracaine HCl, and wait about 1 minute.

2. The cornea is then inspected carefully with magnification. If no foreign body is seen, evert the tarsal conjunctiva (inner lid). This is where the foreign body is usually lodged.

3. To evert the upper eyelid:
   * The patient looks down toward his feet with both eyes, and the examiner grasps the eyelashes of the upper lid and gently pulls the lid down and slightly outward away from the eye. This step is illustrated in Plate 33-1.
   * While grasping the eyelashes in this downward and outward position, apply gentle pressure directly on the lid (on the upper edge of the tarsus on the skin side, about 10 mm above the upper lid margin), using a small cotton-tip applicator, and simultaneously pull the lashes upward (Plate 33-2). The lid will evert easily (Plate 33-3).

4. Use a sterile cotton-tip applicator, moistened with normal saline or ocular irrigating solution to wipe the foreign body off the upper tarsal conjunctiva (Plate 33-4).

5. When finished, release the upper lid and ask the patient to look up. The will will readily flip back to its normal position.

6. Local ophthalmic antibiotic drops are then prescribed, to be used four times a day for 5 days, to prevent infection.

Foreign Body on the Cornea

1. If a foreign body is not found under the upper lid by the method described above, the next approach is to stain the cornea with a sterile fluorescein strip.

2. Never use fluorescein drops because the solution is easily contaminated with pyocyaneous organisms.

3. Moisten the end of the sterile strip with ocular irrigating solution or sterile normal saline. Then touch the tip of the strip to the inner side of the lower eyelid, remove it, and ask the patient to blink a few times.

4. The fluorescein will mix with the tears and flow over the cornea. A minute corneal foreign body can then be seen in the concentration of fluorescein in the area surrounding it.

5. If a corneal foreign body is present, the patient is given one to two drops of 0.5% topical anesthetic before the particle is swabbed away lightly with a moist cotton-tip applicator.

6. If the particle does not dislodge with this gentle brushing maneuver, stop. The corneal epithelium could be damaged by continued swabbing.

7. Refer the patient to an ophthalmologist for removal.

8. If no immediate help is available, carefully lift the foreign body off the cornea with the point of a sterile No. 25 hypodermic needle, ocular foreign body spud, or a sharp-pointed No. 11 Bard-Parker knife blade.

Chart 33-1

REMOVAL OF HARD CORNEAL CONTACT LENS

Indications

1. Removal of lenses in an unconscious patient.
2. Removal of lenses if the patient is unable to do so.
3. Thorough examination of the globe (eyeball).

Equipment

1. Small vacuum rubber lens remover. (A new suction-type lens remover is available with requires no squeezing. It has a solid stem. When the tip is moistened, sufficient suction is developed to remove the lens.)
2. Sterile isotonic irrigating fluid.
3. Good light source

Anatomical Considerations

1. The corneal lens is correctly placed directly on the cornea.
2. The lens may become displaced from the cornea and lie on the medial or lateral scleral portion of the globe.

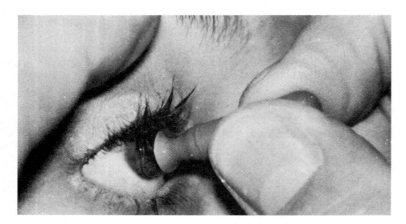

Procedure

1. Examine the eye gently, carefully, and completely to ascertain that a lens is present on the globe. This will require a good light source.
2. Moisten the tip of the vacuum cup with sterile isotonic fluid.
3. Gently spread the lids apart with the thumb and index finger of the left hand, to expose the edges of the contact lens.
4. Squeeze the vacuum device and apply its tip to the contact lens with a minimum of pressure, to get a seal on the lens.

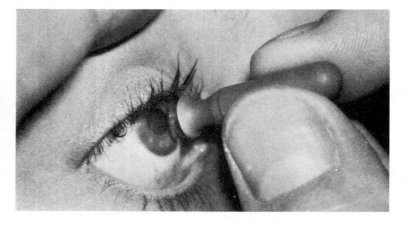

5. Release the pressure on the vacuum device and carefully remove the lens from the cornea.
6. Place the lens in a container with isotonic saline and label with the patient's name for safekeeping.

(Cosgriff JH Jr: Atlas of Diagnostic and Therapeutic Procedures for Emergency Personnel. Philadelphia, JB Lippincott, 1978)

9. An antibiotic ointment and sterile eye pad are applied to protect the eye and lessen discomfort to the patient.

10. Refer the patient to be checked by an ophthalmologist in 1 day.

    Note: if the foreign body was iron in content and a rust ring is present on the eye and does not dislodge easily with the foreign body, the patient should be referred to an ophthalmologist for removal of the rust ring under slit lamp observation. An antibiotic drop is instilled and a sterile eye pad applied before discharging the patient to see an ophthalmologist. Eye pads should be taped with nonallergenic paper tape on a diagonal from above the brow over the malar eminence on the cheek.

Corneal Abrasion, Erosion, or Cut

If no foreign body is present on the cornea, check the cornea with a good focal light; look for a stain on the cornea, indicating an abrasion, erosion, or scratch (cut). These conditions give rise to the same symptoms as a foreign body.

The treatment for corneal abrasion is instillation of an antibiotic ophthalmic ointment and application of a sterile eye pad; instruct the patient to keep both eyes closed. Healing of scratches (cuts), abrasions, and erosions usually occurs in 24 hours, barring infection. The patient should see an ophthalmologist in 24 to 48 hours.

Although these conditions are very painful, never give a topical anesthetic to the patient to take home. Continued use of topical anesthetics promotes further corneal epithelial breakdown and slows the healing process. The patient can take analgesics orally to relieve the pain.

BURNS

Ultraviolet and Flash Burns

Ultraviolet and welder's flash burns (actinic keratitis) are very painful conditions, producing a diffuse, punctate keratitis in the exposed cornea, severe blepharospasm, and sensitivity to light. The patient usually states that he was using a sun lamp or was exposed to direct sunlight, or was welding or near a welder, without proper ocular protection, about 6 to 8 hours before the onset of symptoms.

The following is a history of a patient with typical symptoms of an ultraviolet burn and the typical corneal changes:

> When questioned about her activities for the last 12 hours, the patient stated that she had been outdoors repainting her white patio furniture in direct sunlight. She received enough ultraviolet light from the sun's rays reflecting off the large white table top to produce an ultraviolet burn. She responded rapidly and healed with the usual therapy for flash burns.

To relieve the blepharospasm and facilitate examination, 1 to 2 drops of a 0.5% topical ophthalmic anesthetic should be instilled. The lids relax in 30 to 60 seconds, and the eye can then be examined. The eye is then stained with a fluorescein strip, as described above. A diffuse punctate staining of the cornea can be seen on examination with magnification.

To treat, instill a cycloplegic, cyclopentolate HCl (Cyclogel 1%) or homatropine drops, an antibiotic ointment, and binocular eye pads. Again, give an analgesic and sedation by mouth, and send the patient home for 24 hours of complete rest. These injuries usually heal quickly if treated promptly.

Chemical Burns

Any chemical splashed into the eye should be removed by immediate and copious irrigation with tap water if normal saline or other commercial irrigating solutions are not immediately at hand. Irrigation is continued for at least 10 minutes.

Chemical burns can be caused by acids, alkalis, or organic irritants.

Acid Burns. Acids coagulate a protein barrier on contact and, as a rule, a sharp demarcation of the extent of the burn is immediately visible. If irrigated immediately and properly, acid burns do not penetrate deeply. Their clinical courses are usually predictable within a few hours after injury.

The following history illustrates the importance of prompt irrigation.

> One resourceful patient who splashed acid in his eye was some distance from tap water. He had a full bottle of beer with him, which he poured into his eye to irrigate it when he experienced sudden pain and irritation from the acid. He then went to a tap and irrigated the eye further with water. His fast action, even with beer, probably saved him from more serious corneal damage.

Alkali Burns. Alkali burns are much more serious than acid burns because the causative agents are proteolytic and break down the protein barrier of the eye. The end products of alkali burns are alkaline and are further augmented by the alkaline tears. Alkali particles continue to lyse the corneal protein and burn deeper if not removed. The severity of the burn is determined by the alkali's concentration and the duration of contact. Therefore, it is imperative to irrigate immediately with copious plain tap water at the scene of the accident. A shower can be used if available. The eyelids must be held open to let the stream wash the eye and fornices directly. Then the patient is transported to the nearest emergency facility for further care and evaluation.

At the emergency department, a topical anesthetic is instilled; all foreign particles are removed with a moist cotton applicator or foreign body spud, and the eye is irrigated at frequent intervals. In severe burns, a topical anesthetic should be instilled repeatedly between long courses of irrigation. An ophthalmologist should see the patient as soon as possible if the burn is severe. If many particles of alkali have penetrated the corneal epithelium, the entire corneal epithelium frequently requires debridement to remove all alkali particles and prevent further penetration into the cornea with permanent scarring.

Organic Irritant Burns. Burns caused by organic substances, such as brake fluid, produce a mild reaction, with edema of the conjunctiva and cornea. They are painful but usually do not result in permanent damage.

Chart 33-2

REMOVAL OF SOFT CORNEAL CONTACT LENS

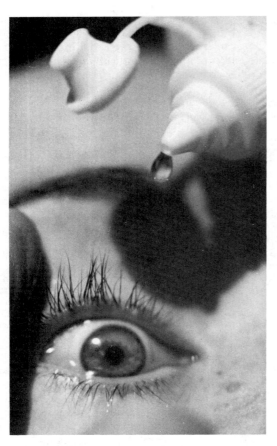

Indications

1. Removal of lenses in an unconscious patient
2. Removal of lenses if the patient is unable to do so
3. Thorough examination of the globe

Equipment

Sterile isotonic irrigating fluid

Anatomical Considerations

1. The soft lens is larger than the cornea and is correctly worn directly on the cornea.
2. The lens may be displaced from the cornea and may lie over the lateral portion of the sclera.

Procedure

1. Examine the eye gently, carefully, and completely to determine where the lens is on the globe. This will require a good light source.
2. Moisten the lens well with sterile irrigating fluid.
3. Ask the patient to turn the eye medially. If the patient is unconscious, omit this step.

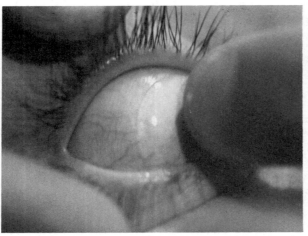
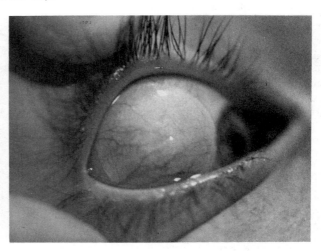

4. Slide the lens from the cornea onto the lateral portion of the sclera using the index finger.

Chart 33-2

REMOVAL OF SOFT CORNEAL CONTACT LENS (*CONTINUED*)

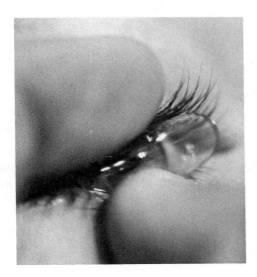

5. Squeeze the lens between the thumb and index finger and it will easily come off the sclera.

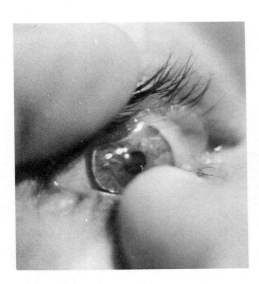 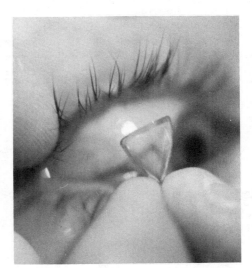

Note: if the lens does not slide easily from the cornea onto the sclera, drop more irrigating solution onto the lens. After removal, place the lenses in isotonic solution to protect them from damage.

(Cosgriff JH Jr: Atlas of Diagnostic and Therapeutic Procedures for Emergency Personnel. Philadelphia, JB Lippincott, 1978)

Tear Gas and Mace. Tear gas and mace injuries to the eye are becoming more common as these products are put to wider use. The treatment is as outlined for chemical burns. In patients with severe injuries requiring admission, 200 mg of hydrocortisone sodium succinate (Solu-Cortef) in 1000 ml of dextrose given daily through a continuous eye lavage unit has been beneficial, in conjunction with the usual medication given in severe chemical burns of the eye.[5]

Treatment and Management of Chemical Burns. Treatment of chemical burns includes irrigation, drug therapy, and immobilization of the eye. Special devices may be used in some instances.

1. *Irrigation.* Treatment of chemical burns begins with immediate copious irrigations with tap water, saline solution, or any available ocular irrigating solution. In severe cases, irrigation should be done every few minutes for several hours. A local anesthetic, such as 0.5 percent Pontocaine should be repeatedly instilled between irrigations to relieve pain and enable the patient to relax the lids for thorough irrigation.

2. *Drug therapy and immobilization.* After irrigation is completed, antibiotic drops are started, and the eyes are patched in patients with corneal involvement. In serious burns, a cycloplegic, such as homatropine or Cyclogel 1%, can also be instilled to relieve ciliary spasm. At night antibiotic ointments and binocular patching are continued, even if only one eye is involved, until the cornea has healed. Binocular patching is necessary to keep both eyes immobile and at rest. Oral medication for pain and sedation for sleep are needed for patients with these painful injuries. Patients with chemical burns should be referred to an ophthalmologist for further therapy and follow-up care as soon as possible.

3. *Special devices.* Success in treating patients with acute chemical burns of the eye using the Water Pic device and distilled water has been reported. It directs a pulsating stream of water to the eye and fornices to thoroughly remove all chemicals. Sterile disposable devices specifically designed for continuous eye lavage and medication are also available (Fig. 33-3). These are plastic units similar to those used in intravenous therapy. On the distal end are plastic scleral-type shells, like scleral contact lenses, which fit under the lids to cover the cornea and through which a constant drip of irrigating fluid or medication can be delivered to the eye. They are used for continuous ocular irrigation in severe chemical burns following emergency treatment and in other conditions of the eye requiring continuous irrigation with local medication or fluids.[6]

Thermal Burns

Thermal burns may be due to either flame or external contact and are similar pathologically, although the flame usually only singes the lashes and lids unless the heat is intense and prolonged. The contact burn involves the eyes directly by the splashing of drops or particles of hot substances into the eye, such as hot lead, tar, water, ashes.

Treatment depends on the degree of injury. Superficial burns require only protection from contamination and the application of local antibiotics. Full-thickness burns of the lids require a new covering with grafted skin and tarsorrhaphies between the upper and lower lids to counteract the vertical contractures that can occur in the healing processes of deep burns of the eyelids. The burned areas must also be cleansed of all foreign material. In severe burns of the eyeball and cornea, a cycloplegic eye drop is used to relieve ciliary spasm, and 0.5% Pontocaine is administered to relieve local pain so that examination and treatment can be carried out. Local antibiotic ophthalmic drops and ointments are also used. The earlier treatment is carried out, the better the prognosis.

OCULAR TRAUMA

Whenever a patient arrives in the emergency department with a history of blunt trauma to the ocular region, he should

Figure 33-3 *Continuous eye lavage. "MedCap" combines a headband with a capacity of 400 ml of irrigating fluid and 2 MorTan therapeutic lenses, which fit under the eyelids. This allows for continuous irrigation of the surface of the eyeball. (Courtesy of MorTan, Inc., Torrington, Wyo.)*

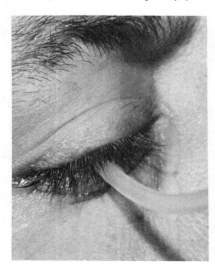
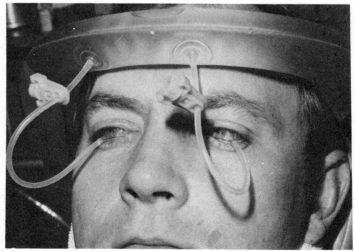

be considered to have a serious injury until all of the previously listed serious lesions have been ruled out. For example, a patient with hyphemia, even without signs of severe ocular trauma, is considered to be in serious condition, since recurrent hemorrhages, absolute glaucoma, and eventual blindness are real possibilities. Emergency personnel must always be on the lookout for these potentially blinding injuries.

Contusions

Superficial Contusions. Superficial contusions may involve only the eyelids; the common "black eye" appearance is characteristic as a result of hemorrhage into the tissues of the lid. Application of cold packs for 20 minutes, four times a day for 2 days is usually adequate therapy; it is followed by warm packs, four times a day thereafter. If marked ecchymosis of the lids occurs, oral administration of a proteolytic enzyme such as Ananase may be helpful.

Moderately Severe Contusions. In moderately severe contusions, the following may be observed in the anterior segment of the eye:

- Traumatic mydriasis (dilation of the pupil)
- Hyphemia (blood in the anterior chamber; note the blood fluid level at the lower part of the cornea in Plate 33-5)
- Small peripheral iris tears or larger tears with separation of the iris from its root (iridodialysis, as illustrated in Plate 33-6)
- Punctate lens opacities and iridodensis (a tremulous iris due to posterior dislocation of the lens, which deprives the posterior iris surface of the support of the lens)
- The posterior segment in moderate contusions may show retinal edema without hemorrhage, choroidal tears or ruptures, and macular changes including edema and holes.

Severe Contusions. Severe contusions involve the eyeball and the orbital bones. Any impact against the eyelids and the eye by blunt force, whether it be a door knob or flying object, can cause a contusion of the eye. Patients with severe contusion should be x-rayed to rule out fractures of the orbital bones and intraocular foreign bodies. In very severe contusions, clinical manifestations of intraocular hemorrhage may occur, including the following:

- Anterior chamber hyphemia
- Hemorrhage in the retina and the vitreous body, or both
- Cataract (opacification of the lens)
- Iris tears
- Gross detachments of the choroid and retina

Management and Treatment of Contusions. Contusions of the eyball, because of their serious nature, demand immediate and proper treatment, which includes the following:

- Admission to the hospital
- Sedation
- Binocular eye pads
- Absolute bed rest (with elevation of the head if hyphemia or vitreal hemorrhage is present)
- Care by an ophthalmologist

Perforating Ocular Wounds

Perforating ocular wounds are more common in children and in victims of automobile accidents. Industrial wounds have been greatly reduced through safety programs. Perforation or rupture of the globe can be seen grossly on examination by lacerations or cuts on the eyeball, with pigment protruding or showing in the lips of the wound (Plate 33-7). If the cornea is perforated, the iris is nearly always prolapsed (Plate 33-8). It may even appear to be a foreign body, since it is black. One must never try to remove it or wipe it away. Be sure also not to press on the globe, since this may cause further injury.

If a perforation is suspected, both eyes are bandaged and *no medications* are instilled. The patient must be admitted to the hospital for complete examination, evaluation, and repair under general anesthesia by an ophthalmologist. More damage, such as severe hemorrhage and increase in tissue prolapse, can be produced in an excited child or adult with marked blepharospasm by trying to examine the eye further after the perforation is seen or is reasonably suspected from other ocular signs.

Blow-out Fracture of the Orbit

A blow-out fracture of the orbit is caused by a sudden increase in intra-orbital hydraulic pressure, resulting from the application of a traumatic force over the orbital area, such as a fist or a baseball. The eye and the orbital contents are compressed into the orbit, an essentially closed area. If the force is great enough, either the eye will rupture or a very thin orbital floor (0.5 mm to 1.0 mm thick) will break and blow out (downward) into the maxillary sinus (Plate 33-9). The compressed orbital contents then herniate into the maxillary sinus. If a patient presents with a history and signs of such an injury and with symptoms of double vision, a blow-out fracture must be considered first.

The ethmoid bone along the medial orbital wall is only 0.25 mm thick and is involved less commonly with a blow-out fracture and entrapment of the medial rectus muscle or its surrounding fascia and fat, thus limiting its motility.

Signs and Symptoms. Blow-out fractures of the orbit produce the following signs and symptoms:

- Pain, swelling, periorbital ecchymosis (sometimes absent)
- Restricted ocular motion
- Diplopia due to entrapment of the extraocular muscles
- Enophthalmos may be seen, but is sometimes masked by edema.
- Areas of altered sensation (infraorbital nerve hypesthesia) along the distribution of the infraorbital nerve
- Crepitus is sometimes palpated about the orbit.
- A rim fracture may be palpable, but not in a pure, simple blowout fracture in which the fracture is posterior to the rim.

Special radiological studies must be made and consultation with an ophthalmologist obtained. General screening tests such as stereo, Waters' and modified Caldwell views are of 50% value. The best tests are polycyclic laminograms and coronal computed tomography (CT) scans. These may show fragments of bone of the orbital floor, prolapse of orbital soft tissue in the maxillary sinus, and even entrapped muscle.

Repair can be done as late as 10 to 14 days after injury, allowing time for adequate and thorough workup and diagnosis and subsidence of the edema and vascular engorgement.

Subconjunctival Ocular Hemorrhage

A common ocular problem, which is also very alarming to the patient, is a subconjunctival hemorrhage on the eyeball (Plate 33-10). The conjunctiva, which lines the eyelids and covers the eyeball, is transparent and not firmly attached to the eyeball. A small hemorrhage appears bright red beneath the conjunctiva. Usually it is a benign, innocuous entity. Rarely, it can be serious when the hemorrhage occurs after a head injury.

Treatment for the common benign subconjunctival hemorrhage is reassurance for the patient that the condition is not serious and that his vision will not be affected.

Lacerations of the Eyelids

Lacerations through the skin of the eyelids, eyebrows, and surrounding tissues should first be checked for associated ocular injury. When serious ocular injury is ruled out (Plate 33-11), the lid lacerations can be closed. Repair of the lid lacerations not involving the lid margins, tear ducts (canaliculus) or levator (elevator) muscles of the upper lids is well within the province of the well-trained general surgeon.

An ophthalmologist should always be called for repair of lid lacerations involving the lid margins, tear ducts, or the levator muscle. Primary repair of these lacerations should be done as soon as an ophthalmologist and an operating suite are available. Emergency management consists of protecting the fresh wound with a sterile dressing and giving appropriate systemic, supportive treatment.

INFECTIONS AND OTHER OCULAR DISORDERS

Conjunctivitis (Redeye)

Conjunctivitis is commonly seen in the emergency department. The conjunctival lining of the lids is usually inflamed, and a purulent or mucopurulent discharge is present in bacterial conjunctivitis. It can also be of a viral, fungal, chemical, or allergic etiology, with different signs and symptoms in each type, as shown in Table 33-2. Treatment consists of local antibiotic drops during the day and ointment at night.

Dendritic Keratitis

Dendritic keratitis is a specific viral infection of the cornea. The eye is injected; photophobia is present; and a foreign body-like irritation is present. When the cornea is stained with a sterile fluorescein strip, a fine lesion can be seen that looks like the branching of a tree.

Steroids must never be given because they lead to rapid

TABLE 33-2. DIFFERENTIAL DIAGNOSIS OF REDEYE

Signs and Symptoms	Acute Glaucoma	Acute Conjunctivitis	Acute Iritis	Corneal Abrasion and Foreign Body
Pain	Usually severe	Minimal or none	Moderate to severe	Moderate to severe
Vision	Poor Usually markedly decreased	Normal	Fair Usually slightly decreased but may be markedly decreased	Variable
Discharge	None	Moderate to copious May be mucopurulent	None	Watery
Cornea	Steamy	Clear	Slightly hazy	Irregular corneal light reflex
Pupil	Middilatation and fixed	Normal	Smaller than opposite side and sluggish	Normal
Conjunctiva	Perilimbal (deep ciliary) injection	Diffuse injection located near fornices (superficial)	Perilimbal (deep ciliary) injection	Diffuse injection
Intraocular pressure	Elevated	Normal	Normal or low	Normal
Emergency treatment	Miotics such as Pilocarpine, Acetazolamide, Admission to hospital	Antibiotic drops	Mydriatic drops Steroids Antibiotics	Removal of foreign body; antibiotic drops or ointment
Onset	Sudden	Gradual	Usually gradual	Sudden

(After A Guide to Emergency Care of Eye Injuries. Committee on Trauma, American College of Surgeons, December 1977)

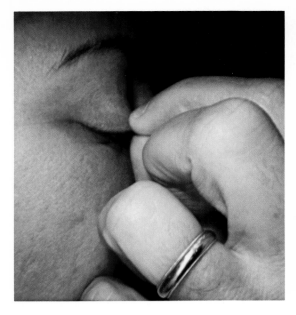

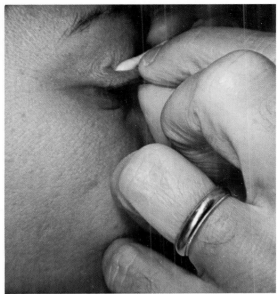

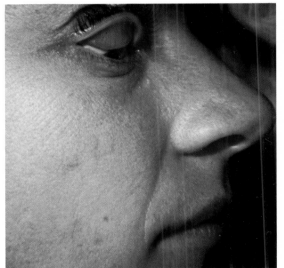

Plate 33-1 Everting the upper eyelid, step one.

Plate 33-2 Everting the upper eyelid, step two.

Plate 33-3 Eversion of the upper eyelid.

Plate 33-4 Foreign body on the upper eyelid.

Plate 33-5 Hyphemia (note the blood fluid level at the lower part of the cornea)

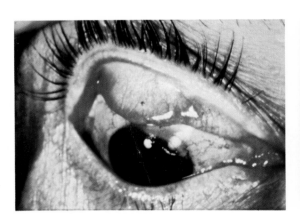

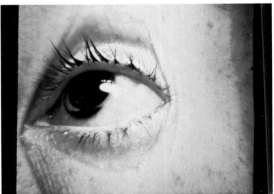

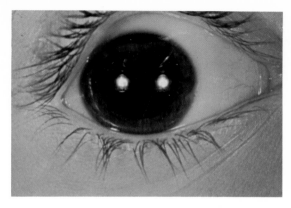

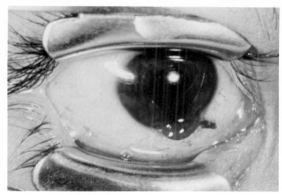

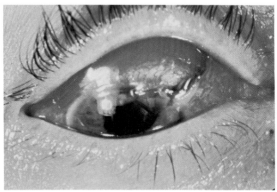

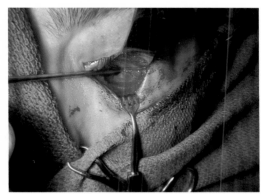

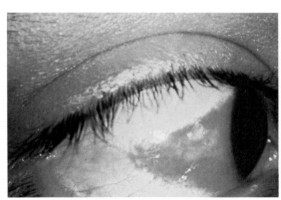

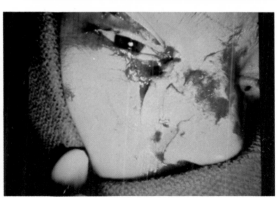

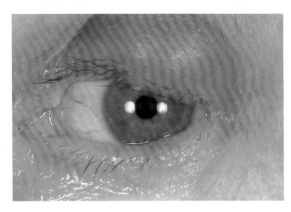

Plate 33-6 Tear of the iris (iridodialysis).

Plate 33-7 Perforation of the cornea with prolapse of the iris.

Plate 33-8 Lacerating wound of the cornea and sclera, with prolapse of the iris and ciliary body.

Plate 33-9 Blow-out fracture of the orbit.

Plate 33-10 Subconjunctival hemorrhage.

Plate 33-11 Multiple lacerations involving the margin of the eyelid and the tear duct.

Plate 33-12 Chalazion.

progression and extension into the depth of the cornea, with permanent scarring and loss of vision. Patients with this condition should be referred to an ophthalmologist.

Chalazion

A chalazion (Plate 33-12) is an infection of one or more of the Meibomian glands in the eyelid. The patient usually complains of a swollen, erythematous, and tender lid. Many times, in the subacute phase, there will be a localized swelling, with point tenderness in the involved area of the lid.

To treat, very warm soaks are applied for one to two hours daily, and local antibiotic drops are instilled. If the chalazion does not improve and a chronic, small localized swelling in the lid forms, the patient is referred to an ophthalmologist for surgical treatment.

Chart 33-3

PRINCIPLES OF MANAGEMENT OF THE PATIENT WITH OCULAR INJURIES

1. Every patient seen in the emergency department with trauma around the facial region requires a careful eye examination. When all life-sustaining measures have been carried out, a careful inspection of the eye by the emergency nurse and physician, if present, will uncover any serious ocular injuries. Institution of prompt and proper treatment will results in saving the sight of many an injured eye.
2. In all eye injuries, the patient is usually frightened, apprehensive, and in pain; characteristically, he keeps his eyes closed tightly as a defense mechanism. He needs and must have reassurance, very gentle care and manipulation, and often local anesthetic drops to permit nontraumatic inspection of the injured eye. The examiner must never press against the eyeball at any time during the examination. It is important to be gentle and reassuring.
3. For all chemical burns, the eye must be irrigated immediately, copiously, and sufficiently long (10 to 15 minutes) with ordinary tap water, unless normal saline or sterile ocular irrigating solutions are immediately available.
4. Ocular medications
   - *Local ocular steroids should not be used in the emergency department, unless prescribed by an ophthalmologist.* They should never be included on an eye tray. They can promote bacterial, viral, and yeast infections, as well as induce glaucoma in susceptible patients. They should never be used in dendritic keratitis (viral ulcer).
   - Ophthalmic antibiotic drops and ointments that should be available in an emergency department are listed in Table 33-1. It must be remembered that ophthalmic ointments are never interchangeable with topical ointments. The mydriatics and cycloplegics are topically applied, autonomic drugs that produce mydriasis (pupillary dilation) and cycloplegia (paralysis of accommodation), respectively. The miotics serve to constrict the pupil.
   - To prevent cross-contamination, it is important that a new sterile bottle of drops or a new tube of ointment be used for each patient. If the medication is not given to the treated patient to take home, it should be discarded.
   - Sterile fluorescein strips, such as Fluor-I-Strips, are preferable to fluorescein liquid drops for staining the eyes because of the danger of pyocyaneous contamination of fluorescein eyedrop bottles on treatment trays in the emergency department. Pyocyaneous infection can cause a rapid fulminating infection, enophthalmitis, and loss of the eye. If fluorescein drops are used, the bottle must be discarded after each use and a new sterile vial of fluorescein opened for each patient.
   - A patient who has had an anesthetic instilled should have the medicated eye patched until the effects of the anesthetic wear off. This precaution protects the eye from foreign body invasion or further trauma. A patient should never be given an anesthetic for outpatient use. Examples of anesthetics are tetracaine, proparacaine HCl (Ophthaine), ophthetic, and butacaine (Butyn).
   - *Instillation of drops.* Drops are properly instilled by having the patient assume a supine or a head-back position while sitting. The patient is instructed to look up while the examiner, using a small piece of gauze, everts the lower eyelid, exposing the conjunctival sac. Any excess splashed onto the face by reflex blinking is removed by the gauze. An ointment is applied similarly, by spreading it from the inner to outer canthus of the conjunctival sac.
   - The eyes, man's windows to the world, are important indeed. Even though an injury to the eye may appear innocuous and nonacute, the very importance of the eyes mandates careful assessment and accurate, complete treatment. Teamwork among alert, well-trained emergency personnel and the ophthalmologist is imperative for the preservation of sight in patients with ocular injuries.

Acute Glaucoma and Iritis

Acute glaucoma or iritis (iridocyclitis) must be ruled out in a patient with acute, severe pain in the eye and around the brow region. The eyeball is usually red and appears very inflamed in both conditions.

Differential Diagnosis. The following observations are useful in distinguishing the two conditions. In glaucoma, the cornea is steamy and with tactile tension (finger tension on the eyeball) feels hard; the pupil is middilated, the vision is poor; and the onset is usually sudden. In iritis, the cornea may be slightly hazy, with a loss of luster, but is not steamy; the tactile tension is normal or lower than normal; the pupil is small (miotic, constricted); the vision is fair; extreme photophobia (sensitivity to light) is present; and the onset is usually gradual. In both glaucoma and iritis, the patient must be referred to an ophthalmologist for care. In both conditions, the affliction can be bilateral. Further details on differential diagnosis are presented in Table 33-2.

Medical management of acute glaucoma consists of constricting the pupil with a miotic, such as pilocarpine, giving acetazolamide (Diamox) or other carbonic-anhydrase inhibitors (which act directly on the ciliary body) and intravenous mannitol if necessary. Oral or injectable medication may be needed for pain. Surgery may be indicated in some patients, to provide a new outflow channel for intraocular fluid.

In iritis, the pupil must be dilated to prevent scarring and adhesions. A mydriatic, such as phenylephrine hydrochloride (Neo-Synephrine) ophthalmic drops, is useful for this purpose. Cycloplegic drops are given concurrently, and oral pain medication may be prescribed. Photophobia can be relieved in part by dark glasses, which are helpful whenever mydriatic drops are instilled. A complete medical workup is needed to determine and treat the underlying cause.

Major considerations in the management of the patient who has sustained ocular injuries are summarized in Chart 33-3.

REFERENCES

1. Dockery RW: Role of the ophthalmologist in acute trauma. J Kentucky Med Assoc 56:449–452, May 1958
2. Duke-Elder S: Textbook of Ophthalmology. 6th ed. St. Louis, CV Mosby, 1954
3. Keeney AH: Ocular injuries in automobile accidents. In Symposium on Industrial and Traumatic Ocular Injuries. New Orleans, New Orleans Academy of Ophthalmology, 1963
4. Vinger PF: Eye injuries in sports: USA. Symposium from National Society to Prevent Blindness, 1980 Nation Conference, New York City, September 22, 1980. Prevent Blindness News 6(1), Fall 1980
5. Forberg PK, Byers LW: Chemical mace: A nonlethal weapon. J Trauma 9:339–342, April 1969
6. Morgan LB: A new therapeutic scleral lens. Rocky Mountain Med J 68:26, 1971

34
EAR, NOSE, AND THROAT EMERGENCIES

JOSEPH C. SERIO

It is an impossible task to include in one chapter all of the emergencies involving the ears, nose, and throat that may be seen in the emergency department. Only the high points and the more common emergencies will be considered. Although each of these systems will be discussed separately, it should be borne in mind that the ears, nose, and throat are anatomically and physiologically related; thus, trauma or disease processes affecting one system often involve one or both of the other systems. To ensure a thorough appraisal of the problem, the examiner should evaluate all three organ systems when a patient complains of a problem with one. Disorders of the nose, the throat, and the ear will be presented in that order; the sequence reflects the frequency with which these conditions are seen in the emergency department. The anatomy and physiology of each system will be reviewed briefly.

THE NOSE AND PARANASAL SINUSES

ANATOMY AND PHYSIOLOGY

The nose is divided into an upper part consisting of nasal bone and the frontal process of the maxilla and a lower part consisting of the cartilages and their skin and connective tissue coverings. The upper part covers the septum and the turbinates. The septum is a dividing bony and cartilaginous partition that creates the right and left chambers (nasal cavities). The lower portion is separated into right and left chambers by the columella, the lowermost portion of the partition formed by the septal cartilage. There are usually three turbinates in number (superior, middle, and inferior). They occupy similar areas in the right and left nasal compartments (Fig. 34-1). These turbinates overhang the meatuses, which are named after turbinates. In the meatus, ostia of sinuses will be found. The *superior* meatus contains openings of posterior ethmoid sinus cells and the *middle* meatus contains the opening (ostia) for drainage of frontal, maxillary, and anterior ethmoid sinuses. The inferior meatus has the ostium for the nasolacrimal duct (Fig. 34-2).

When the sinuses are inflamed or infected, the turbinates may be swollen and infected purulent material may be found in the meatuses with drainage flowing from involved sinuses. The blood supply of the nose is derived from branches of the external and internal carotid arteries. The sphenopalatine branch of the external carotid supplies the turbinates, meatuses, and septum. The anterior and caudal portion of the septum (Kisselbach's triangle) contains a plexus of blood vessels, the most frequent site of nose bleeds (epistaxis).

The roof of the nose is supplied by the anterior and posterior ethmoid vessels (branches of the ophthalmic artery) which also supply the ethmoid and frontal sinuses. The maxillary and sphenoid sinuses are supplied by branches of the internal maxillary artery. The paranasal sinuses include:
1. *Anterior group*—frontal, maxillary, and anterior ethmoids.
2. *Posterior group*—posterior ethmoid and ethmoid and sphenoid sinuses.

Each sinus is named after the bone in which it is found. Sinuses are close to important structures in the skull. The floor of the frontal sinus forms a portion of the roof of the orbit. When the frontal sinus is inflamed, edema and secondary inflammation of the eye may result.

The maxillary sinus forms a part of the floor of the orbit and lies just above the upper teeth; thus toothache may result if the maxillary sinus is involved in acute inflammation, new growth, or trauma.

The lateral border of the ethmoid sinus (lamina papyracea) is part of the inner wall of the orbit which is affected in purulent sinusitis. It may perforate the wall, causing displacement of the eye and possible inflammation of the optic nerve. The roof of the sphenoid sinus is in direct contact with the base of the brain. The roof of the sinuses accommodates the optic chiasm and the sella turcica, which cradles the pituitary gland. The lateral wall of the sphenoid sinus contains the cavernous sinus and the internal carotid artery.

Figure 34-1 Sagittal view of the right naris. This illustration shows the turbinates, which cover the meatuses of the paranasal sinuses.

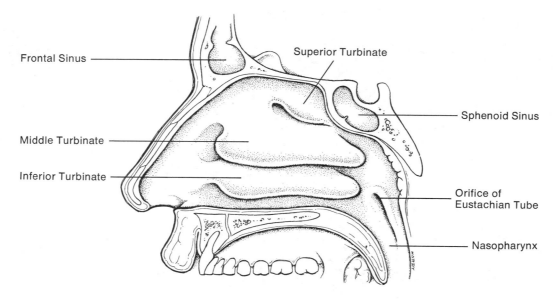

Frontal Sinus

Superior Turbinate

Sphenoid Sinus

Middle Turbinate

Inferior Turbinate

Orifice of Eustachian Tube

Nasopharynx

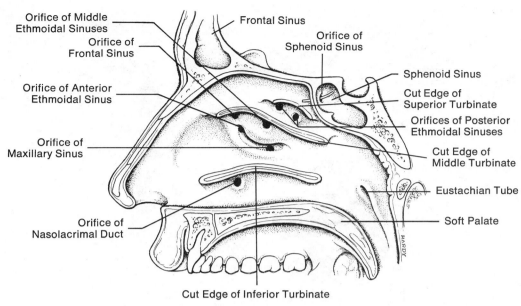

Orifice of Middle Ethmoidal Sinuses
Orifice of Frontal Sinus
Orifice of Anterior Ethmoidal Sinus
Orifice of Maxillary Sinus
Orifice of Nasolacrimal Duct
Frontal Sinus
Orifice of Sphenoid Sinus
Sphenoid Sinus
Cut Edge of Superior Turbinate
Orifices of Posterior Ethmoidal Sinuses
Cut Edge of Middle Turbinate
Eustachian Tube
Soft Palate
Cut Edge of Inferior Turbinate

Figure 34-2 *Internal anatomy of the nose. This is a sagittal view of the right naris with the turbinates removed. The sinus orifices in each meatus are identified.*

The nerve supply of the sinuses arises from the trigeminal (5th) nerve and from the sphenopalatine ganglion. The latter is of clinical importance in that it combines with the autonomic nerve fibers to form the superficial and deep petrosal nerves.

Only the maxillary and ethmoid sinuses are present at birth. The ethmoid sinus is fully developed at birth, but the maxillary is not. Ethmoid sinusitis is a frequent cause of fever in the very, very young. The sinus lining is respiratory epithelium, a special form of psuedostratified columnar ciliated epithelium that moves mucus toward the ostia of the maxillary sinus.

The nose has many functions. It is the organ of smell (olfactory nerve cells); it serves as an air passage, and cleans, humidifies, and warms inspired air. This air-conditioning process is mediated by the septum and turbinates; temperature control and humidification are effected through the nasal mucous membrane. Larger particles in the air are removed by the hairs within the nose; the mucous blanket of the nose, along with its lysozyme, is bactericidal and thus serves to clean the air. The mucous blanket is moved by the cilia.

ASSESSMENT OF THE NOSE

History

The history of the illness is important. In most patients other than small children it can be obtained directly from the patient. The most common symptom is discharge from the nose, which may be watery, bloody, or purulent. Knowing the duration and onset is helpful. One should note any history of nasal obstruction, difficulty in breathing, frequent colds, headaches, or pain with or without fever, chills, or perspiration.

Chronic obstruction, headache, or recurrent pain may indicate chronic sinus disease. In traumatic conditions, the mechanism and time of injury are important. In instances of a blow or a fall, the area involved should be identified.

Physical Examination

Examination begins with careful inspection of the external nose, looking for deformity, recent trauma (abrasions, lacerations), swelling, inflammation, or tumors. Nasal discharge may be noted, dried or fresh blood may be visible. Palpation may reveal false motion of the nasal bones and crepitation. Crepitation (grinding or crunching) may indicate a fractured nose.

The interior of the nose should be carefully examined, using a nasal speculum or an otoscope with a nasal piece attached. Figure 34-3 displays equipment used in examinations of the nose, ears, and throat. Figure 34-4 illustrates speculum examination of the nose. Under normal conditions the septum should be in the midline. Observe for spurs, buckling to one side with narrowing of the nasal passage as the septum contacts the turbinates. The examiner should check for any drainage of the nasal cavity and note whether it is clear, bloody or purulent, and whether there is edema, swelling, unusual pallor, redness, or excessive moisture creating a pathologic situation. The mucous membrane should normally be pink and moist. The turbinates and associated meatuses should be inspected. Involvement of a turbinate reflects a reaction in the sinus that drains into it. Except for the turbinates, the lining of the nose is smooth. Polyps, which are pale and moist grape-like swellings are frequently found. Irritated areas or frank ulcerations may be noted. Transillumination of the paranasal sinuses has limited value in the diagnosis of sinus disease. X-rays are useful in fractures of nasal bones and walls of the paranasal sinuses. Special

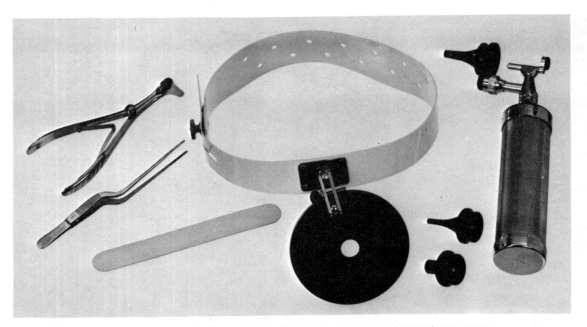

Figure 34-3 Instruments for ear, nose, and throat examination. Left to right. Nasal speculum, bayonet forceps, tongue blade, head mirror, aural and nasal specula with otoscope.

x-rays of the sinuses are helpful in the diagnosis of sinus disease (Fig. 34-5).

MANAGEMENT OF SPECIFIC DISEASES OF THE NOSE

The common cold is a viral infection that is self-limiting and can be associated with a secondary bacterial infection. History includes nasal congestion and stuffiness, sneezing early in the course of the disease, and a burning sensation. Fever is lacking except with a secondary infection. Malaise and anorexia may be noted. Examination reveals hyperemia of the mucous membrane and purulent drainage when secondary bacterial contamination has occurred.

Such patients rarely require hospital admission but should be isolated and given symptomatic care, that is, fluids, rest, aspirin for fever, and vitamin C.

Figure 34-4 Speculum examination of the nose. Middle and inferior turbinates are visualized laterally, the septum medially.

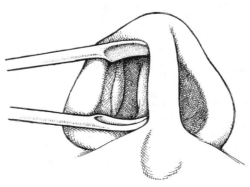

Sinus Disease

Assessment. Involvement of the paranasal sinuses may be acute or chronic. Acute sinusitis may follow a cold or infection of the nose, particularly after swimming. Chronic inflammation of sinuses is frequently seen secondary to allergic condition. The symptoms of sinusitis vary from nasal discharge which is thin and watery to a thick and purulent drainage which enters the postnasal cavity, resulting in sore throat and headache. Pressure may be present in the affected sinus areas. Frontal headache may be associated with disease of frontal sinus, occipital headaches with sphenoid involvement. Pain along the sensory nerve distribution of the involved sinuses is not uncommon.

Maxillary sinusitis results in pain and aching of the face and upper teeth, ethmoid inflammation may cause pain in the region of the eye. Assessment may reveal swelling and tenderness in the involved area. Examination of the nose may reveal a reddened swollen mucosa of the associated turbinate with a mucopurulent or purulent discharge. X-rays may reveal a cloudy sinus. Blood studies may vary and are not specific for sinusitis.

Management/Treatment. Management involves supportive care, increased fluid intake, and analgesic preparations such as aspirin. Local heat and steam inhalation may enhance drainage, providing relief of pain and pressure. Vasoconstrictors and decongestants may be given orally, for example pseudoephedrine (Sudafed, Triaminic, Ornade) along with antihistamines because of possible allergic involvement. Nasal packs of decongestant give some temporary relief. Antibiotics are of value in patients with prolonged purulent drainage as in acute and chronic states of sinusitis.

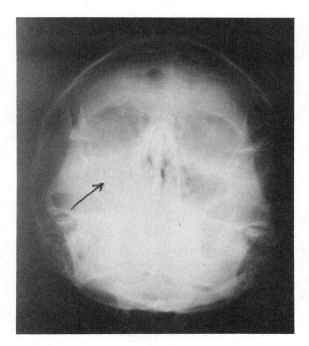

Figure 34-5 *X-ray revealing obliteration of right maxillary sinus. See arrow for location of right maxillary sinus.*

Specimens of the drainage should be taken for culture and sensitivity studies to identify predominant organisms and antibiotic sensitivity. Complications of sinusitis include orbital cellulitis or abscess, brain abscess, osteomyelitis, meningitis, and cavernous sinus thrombosis.

Epistaxis

Nosebleed may be associated with trauma or infections, or may be a manifestation of systemic disease, such as hypertension or coagulation defects and blood dyscrasias. Spontaneous nosebleeds associated with hypertension or anticoagulant therapy may result in massive blood loss.

Assessment. The patient's general condition must be assessed and vital signs recorded. Patients with epistaxis are often apprehensive because of visible blood loss and require reassurance. Tachycardia and hypotension may indicate severe blood loss. A complete blood count should be performed in conjunction with a platelet count and clotting studies such as the prothrombin and partial thromboplastin times. In patients with large blood loss, a type and crossmatch may be needed. Assessment must be careful, gentle, and complete. The patient is preferably examined in a specially designed chair with the head fixed on a headrest. Examination of the exterior and interior of the nose should be done. The internal nose should be examined with a nasal speculum or an otoscope with an adequate speculum. In the young, Kisselbach's area on the anterior portion of the nasal septum should be inspected. Anterior bleeding drains from the external nares. Bleeding from the posterior portion of the nose is more profuse and drains into the pharynx and mouth. If any significant amount of blood has been swallowed, nausea and emesis may occur.

Management/Treatment. Anterior bleeding points are located and pressure is applied by pinching the nostrils between the thumb and index finger for about 5 minutes. This maneuver will usually control a mild hemorrhage. Gentle pressure with a pledget of cotton containing epinephrine will arrest bleeding and allow the bleeding point to be cauterized with a silver nitrate stick. In a child, cotton pledgets moistened with hydrogen peroxide and packed in the anterior nose, assisted by external pressure (squeezing the anterior nares) will control most bleeding points. Vasoconstrictor drugs such as epinephrine should be used with extreme caution in patients with hypertension. Packing of the nose may be required when the bleeding comes from the turbinates or posterior area of the nasal cavity. A petrolatum (Vaseline) gauze may be inserted gently but firmly, using a bayonet forceps. If the bleeding is from the posterior nares and the bleeding point visualized, Gelfoam or Surgicel packing may be inserted to arrest the bleeding.

If the bleeding continues, a posterior nasal pack should be inserted in conjunction with anterior packing (Fig. 34-6). Placing a posterior pack is more traumatic to a patient (Fig. 34-7). A rubber catheter is introduced into each naris until it is visible in the oropharynx. The catheters are pulled out through the mouth and an adequate size pack is tied to them using two pieces of umbilical cord tape. The catheters are then gently withdrawn through the nose until the pack has been pulled upward, above and behind the soft palate. It may be secured in place by a finger or curved hemostat. The umbilical tape is tied across the columella over a wad of cotton or soft cottonoid. A third string attached to the pack is brought out of the mouth and taped to the cheek. This string facilitates removal of the pack after 48 to 72 hours.

The anterior pack is inserted using the posterior pack as an abutment. Analgesics may be necessary while the pack is in place. The anterior packing remains in place for about 5 days. In older patients, it is very important to monitor blood gases, because respiration may be impaired.

Figure 34-6 *Preparation of a posterior nasal pack. A 4 inch × 4 inch gauze is rolled up and cut to size. Three heavy silk sutures are tied around the pack.*

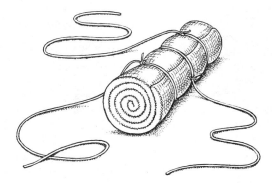

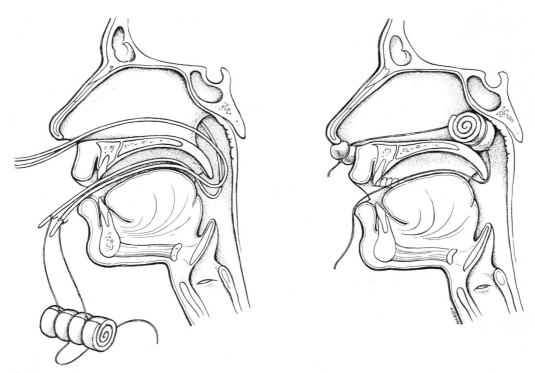

Figure 34-7 *Placing of the posterior nasal pack. Left. The catheters are brought out through the mouth and tied with the lateral sutures on the pack; then the catheters are withdrawn through the nose. These sutures are then tied over a small piece of sponge at the columella. Right. The middle suture is brought out through the mouth and taped to the cheek.*

Pediatric Considerations. Nosebleeds in children require a search for the etiology. Foreign bodies, blood dyscrasias, trauma due to picking the nose and improper wiping of the nose are common causes. X-rays may be of value if a metallic foreign body is present. Caution must be used when extracting a foreign body from the nose. The child should be in the prone position or lying on the side on which the foreign body is lodged, preferably with the head somewhat lowered. The patient should be secured so that he cannot move. The foreign body, when identified, can be removed with an alligator forceps or a hemostat. The position described will help to prevent the foreign body from being aspirated.

Fractures of the Nose

Assessment. Nasal fractures occur as a result of direct trauma. Symptoms may be pain, swelling of the nose, and bleeding. Patients who come to the emergency department hours or days after injury may complain of difficulty in breathing due to a hematoma or abscess of the septum. Examination by inspection may reveal an external deformity of the nose. By careful palpation, one may feel crepitation at the fracture site when gently moving the nasal bones. X-ray of the nasal bones are helpful in confirming the fracture and the position of the fragments.

Management/Treatment. Management consists in reduction of the fragments to a normal or near normal position with or without internal and external splinting. Ice packs applied externally in the first 24 hours will reduce swelling, after which period heat may be helpful. An internal pack and a simple metal splint externally will help to maintain the fragments in position. Nasal fractures are not of high priority in patients with multiple injuries. Satisfactory reduction may be achieved several days after injury.

THE THROAT

ANATOMY AND PHYSIOLOGY

The throat is made up of the nasopharynx, the oropharynx, and the laryngopharynx (hypopharynx). The nasopharynx is the cavity behind the nose. It is bounded posteriorly by the anterior coverings of the vertebral column, inferiorly by the soft palate, and superiorly by the base of the skull. The orifices of the eustachian tubes are located in the fossa of Rosenmüller in the lateral portion of the nasopharynx. These tubes connect to the middle ear and serve as pathways to equilibrate the ambient and internal ear pressures and thus have an effect on the inner ear, accounting for the association of ear involvement with colds and sinus diseases.

In children, the eustachian tube is more horizontal in position; in adults it is more oblique. The fossa of Rosenmüller is an important site because of the relatively high incidence of neoplasms in that area. The oropharynx is visible behind the tongue. Its posterior border is the vertebral column. Laterally its boundaries are the anterior and posterior pillars which contain the tonsils in the tonsillar fossa.

The laryngopharynx lies inferior to the orpharynx and connects with the upper end of the esophagus and with the glottis, which is the opening of the larynx. The glottis contains the vocal cords. The blood supply of the pharynx is derived from the ascending pharyngeal artery (a branch of the external carotid). Innervation is through the pharyngeal plexus from the vagus nerve.

A large amount of lymphoid tissue, known as Waldeyer's ring, is located in the wall of the pharynx.

ASSESSMENT OF THE PHARYNX

Examination of the pharynx is preferably done with the patient in a sitting position. Necessary equipment includes a tongue blade, dental mirror and an adequate light source. A head mirror (Fig. 34-3) will provide excellent illumination of the pharynx and allows excellent light while two hands are free. The mirror should be warmed to prevent fogging. Examination may be difficult if the patient is unable to open the mouth adequately. Initially, inspect the interior of the mouth (Fig. 34-8). The mucous membrane is normally pink. The tonsils are located in their fossae on either side of the oropharynx lateral to the base of the tongue. In the young, the tonsils are frequently enlarged and contain small sacs on their surface (crypts) which may be empty or contain pus. The tonsils may be covered by a purulent exudate when acutely inflamed. The pharynx should be examined for evidence of redness or postnasal drainage. The soft palate forms the posterior portion of the roof of the mouth. Suspended from the middle of it is the uvula, which may assume many shapes. The nasopharynx can be visualized using a dental mirror. To examine the laryngopharynx, grasp the tongue with a gauze sponge and pull it forward gently. The entire laryngopharynx, glottis, and vocal cords may be seen with a dental mirror. The presence of an exudate or membrane in the pharynx should be noted. The examiner should look for growths in the pharynx. The neck should be palpated for swellings, masses, or lymph node enlargement. Note any breathing difficulty through either nose or mouth. The most common diseases of the pharynx seen in the emergency department are inflammatory in nature; trauma is second. The patient may complain of a sore throat, pain in swallowing, an associated cold, fever, chills, and enlarged cervical lymph nodes.

MANAGEMENT OF SPECIFIC PHARYNGEAL DISEASES

Tonsillitis

The most common problem arising in the pharynx for which emergency care is sought relates to the tonsils. Infection of the tonsils may be acute or chronic and recurring.

Assessment. The patient may present with varying degrees of severity. Infections are usually bacterial in origin and associated with symptoms of a cold, malaise, or sore throat. The patient may experience pain on swallowing, referred pain to the ear, fever, malaise, and foul odor of the breath.

Inspection of the pharynx will reveal enlargement of the tonsils, with hyperemia and frequently an exudate on the surface. The oropharynx is reddened and may have a pebble or cobblestone appearance, due to lymphoid hyperplasia; enlarged cervical nodes may be palpable.

Management/Treatment. Management consists of supportive, symptomatic care along with specific antibiotics in the presence of an exudate or a reddened appearance of the tonsils. Culture and sensitivity studies by swabs from the affected areas can direct one to the proper antibiotic for management of the infection.

Peritonsillar Abscess. Peritonsillar abscess occurs with advanced infections of the tonsils. It most commonly involves the superior pole and traps pus, causing local swelling, difficulty in speaking, and inability to open the mouth wide. The patient will speak as if he has a hot potato in his mouth. Temporary relief can be obtained by aspiration of the pus.

Definitive management is incision and drainage of the abscess combined with antibiotic therapy and throat irrigations.

Acute Pharyngitis With Membrane Formation

Acute inflammatory conditions of the oropharynx may be severe and accompanied by systemic reactions of fever, malaise, and anorexia. Severe infections are usually caused by specific organisms and associated with formation of a membrane, which is a film of exudate overlying the mucosa of the pharyngeal structures. The most common types of acute inflammation are:

- Septic sore throat due to streptococcal or mixed infection
- Vincent's angina
- Diphtheria (not common today)
- Blood dyscrasia (leukemia and agranulocytic angina)
- Infectious mononucleosis

Figure 34-8 Anatomy of the mouth, as seen by intraoral examination. When inspecting the oropharynx, the patient should be asked to say "Ah," which causes the soft palate to elevate; thus the pharynx can be better seen.

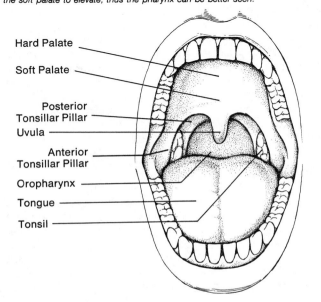

Hard Palate
Soft Palate
Posterior Tonsillar Pillar
Uvula
Anterior Tonsillar Pillar
Oropharynx
Tongue
Tonsil

Assessment. All forms are characterized by sore throat, difficulty in swallowing and talking, fever, malaise, and anorexia. Inspection reveals a membrane which when wiped away leaves a raw area with some bleeding. Cervical lymph node enlargement is common in the submandibular and supraclavicular areas.

Management/Treatment. Management consists of supportive measures and specific antibiotic therapy dependent upon the results of cultures of the membrane. In the case of diphtheria, a specific antitoxin is indicated. The patient should be isolated. The membrane may be widespread beyond the view of the examiner, and may involve the respiratory tract. Breathing may be labored and the patient must be observed closely for respiratory obstruction. Tracheostomy may be necessary.

Retropharyngeal Abscess

Retropharyngeal abscess is usually seen in infants under 3 years of age.

Assessment. Sore throat, difficulty in swallowing, stridor, fever, and malaise are the most common symptoms. Examination of the pharynx reveals reddening and edema of the mucosa of the posterior wall. A bulging mass may be noted. Lateral x-rays of the neck will confirm the presence of the abscess because of the widening of the retropharyngeal space between the pharynx and the cervical vertebrae.

Treatment. Treatment consists of incision and drainage. It must be done with the patient in the Trendelenberg (head down) position using a suction device so that the likelihood of aspiration of pus into the respiratory tract is minimized. A mouth gag is used to keep the mouth open.

Other Pharyngeal Disorders

Less common pathology seen in the pharynx includes carcinoma, syphilis, gonorrheal infection, tuberculosis, and actinomycosis. All may be associated with chronic sore throat. Any ulcerating lesion should be biopsied for diagnosis.

LARYNGOPHARYNGEAL CONDITIONS

Hoarseness

Diseases of the laryngopharynx (hypopharynx) often involve glottic structures (vocal cords) and the upper portion of the trachea. Hoarseness of recent origin may be of an inflammatory, allergic, or neoplastic nature and at times of traumatic origin. Inflammatory conditions can produce edema of the cords. Epiglottic allergic reactions may also cause edematous cords. Neoplastic growth may cause hoarseness early, especially if there is cord involvement.

Trauma may cause damage to the laryngeal and tracheal structures, resulting in hoarseness and respiratory difficulty. Tumors of the larynx and upper mediastinum are not usually encountered in emergency department patients unless airway obstruction is present. The larynx should be examined with a laryngeal mirror to determine if a tumor is present and whether cords are freely movable or thickened or edematous. With the vocal cords in view, ask the patient to say "e." Normally the cords will move to the midline (adduct) with this maneuver. A pathologic process may impair the mobility of the vocal cords.

Allergy

Allergic reactions of the pharynx and larynx result from sensitizing agents such as drugs, pollens and insect venoms.

Assessment. Edema of the larynx associated with difficulty in swallowing or breathing, or both, may occur. Older patients may complain of feeling that the throat is closing up. Allergic reactions in a child may be more serious because in children the larynx contains loose areolar tissue, which can give rise to greater swelling.

Treatment. Rapid relief can be accomplished by spraying with a vasoconstrictor agent such as epinephrine or ephedrine. Antihistamines given by mouth or intravenously and parenteral steroids may reduce the allergic edema. The patient should be observed closely for the possibility of airway obstruction requiring tracheostomy.

LARYNGOTRACHEOBRONCHITIS

Acute laryngotracheobronchitis is a serious condition, particularly in infants and children. It is usually of bacterial origin, the offending organism being B influenza organism or streptococcus.

Assessment. Symptoms are those of an upper respiratory infection with nasal and chest congestion, cough, fever, chills, and respiratory difficulty. If severe, cyanosis of lips, earlobes, and nailbeds may be noted.

Management/Treatment. Management consists of initially taking smears of any drainage for culture and sensitivity studies. The patient should be admitted and placed in a humidified atmosphere with oxygen if cyanosis is present. When respiratory embarrassment is present arterial blood gases should be taken at intervals to monitor the progress of treatment. Tracheotomy may be necessary in instances of severe respiratory problems. Broad-spectrum antibiotic therapy is begun at the time of admission. Modification of the antibiotic selected may be made when sensitivity studies are completed.

FOREIGN BODY IN THE AIR PASSAGE

Sudden respiratory distress may indicate a foreign body in the airway, especially if it occurs while eating. Children commonly put toys and small objects into their mouths, and on occasion one may enter the air passage. When the obstruction occurs in the glottic area, respiratory embarrassment is severe, cyanosis develops rapidly, and death may ensue in a matter of minutes. The patient struggles to take an effective breath and in the process impacts the foreign body. The patient is unable to phonate and typically grasps the throat. An effort should be made to dislodge the object by reaching into the mouth and sweeping the pharynx with the index finger. Currently, the Heimlich maneuver is taught to emergency personnel and the general public. Signs are required in restaurants. The Heimlich maneuver should be done rapidly. If this does not remove the obstruction, cricothyroidotomy should be performed. Some advocate an incision into the cricothyroid membrane; a small opening in this area will permit an airway. Modifications of this will be in order later.

If the aspirated object passes below the vocal cords, it will drop into the trachea and lodge in the right or left main bronchus; or, if the foreign object is small it can lodge in secondary bronchi. When the foreign body has settled in the lower respiratory tract, the patient will complain of cough. At this point, it usually does not create a life-threatening emergency. Partial or complete obstruction may cause emphysema or atelectasis of the involved segment of lung and if it remains for a long period may result in abscess formation. Chest x-rays usually will reveal abnormalities of the area involved. In cases of nonopaque foreign bodies, evidence of altered lung aeration, either atelectasis or emphysema may be seen on x-ray. Metal objects cause little reaction in the bronchi. Organic foreign bodies (*e.g.*, meat, peanuts) may cause severe reactions. Extraction may be done under either local or general anesthesia by bronchoscopy. A variety of special instruments are available to grasp the object. Open thoracotomy may be necessary depending on the severity of the complication.

FOREIGN BODY IN THE ESOPHAGUS

Improper mastication or swallowing too large a piece of solid food (meat, vegetables, or fruit) may result in obstruction. In children coins may pose this danger. The patient will complain of dysphagia and inability to swallow water, even his own saliva. The patient may frequently be able to localize the area of the block. The typical history usually is of sudden onset while eating. Chest x-rays localize a metallic body, while contrast medium (barium or gastrograffin) swallowed under fluoroscopy will demonstrate the area of blockage. Complications may result from perforation of the esophagus by a foreign object or esophagoscopy. Subcutaneous emphysema of the neck region or pneumomediastinum (air in the mediastinum) on chest x-ray are diagnostic. Surgical exploration of the esophagus with drainage and repair of the esophagus are indicated. Large doses of antibiotics are essential.

THE EAR

ANATOMY AND PHYSIOLOGY

The ear is the organ of hearing; it consists of three divisions, the external, middle, and inner ears. The external ear consists of the auricle (pinna), a cartilaginous structure covered by skin and connective tissue, which serves as a baffle to reflect sound. The drum (tympanic membrane) separates the external ear from the middle ear. The canal (external auditory canal) a membranocartilaginous, osseous tunnel about 2.5 cm to 3.5 cm in length, extends obliquely downward and anteriorly to the drum. A narrowing at the junction of the external (cartilaginous) portion and in the internal (osseous) segment can be visualized by direct light (otoscope) or reflected head mirror light. A portion of the parotid gland lies in close proximity to the anterior floor of the canal. The skin of the auricle continues into the canal. The membranocartilaginous portion contains hair follicles and sebaceous and ceruminous glands. Because the skin is densely adherent to the perichondrium and the periosteum, intense pain may result if inflammatory conditions exist.

The middle ear contains the ossicles (the malleus, incus and stapes); the malleus is attached by its handle and connected to the incus and the stapes. The middle ear cavity is bounded by the drum, the inner wall being the outer wall of the inner ear. The middle cranial fossa is above and the jugular bulb below. The upper part of the drum called Shrapnell's membrane, is flaccid. The lower part is the pars tensa. When the ear is examined, a triangle-like cone of light can be seen extending from the lower malleus. This is called the cone of light or light reflex (See Fig. 34-9) usually seen in normal drums. Similarly, Shrapnell's membrane may bulge if fluid or inflammation is present in the middle ear or retract if the eustachian tube is blocked following a cold or other abnormalities.

The internal ear (labyrinth) contains the receptors for hearing (cochlea) and for balance (semicircular canals). The inner ear derives its blood supply from a branch of the basilar artery. The seventh and eighth nerves and the nervus intermedius are contained in the internal auditory meatus; thus, middle ear infections extending to the inner ear may

Figure 34-9 *View of right eardrum through an otoscope. The important anatomic landmarks are identified.*

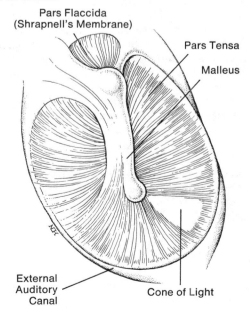

Pars Flaccida (Shrapnell's Membrane)

Pars Tensa

Malleus

External Auditory Canal

Cone of Light

cause labyrinthitis, manifested by dizziness, loss of balance, nausea, vomiting and tinnitus. Examination of the eyes may reveal a jerky motion (nystagmus).

ASSESSMENT OF THE EAR

Examination of the external ear may reveal sebaceous cysts of the ear lobe, infections, and inflammatory problems. Auditory canal examination may reveal swelling, furuncles (boils), narrowing of the canal due to infection or neoplasms. Examination of the external auditory canal may be done with an otoscope or reflected light from a head mirror (see Fig. 34-3). The oblique direction of the canal necessitates pulling the pinna upward and posteriorly to examine for abnormalities. In children, the canal is more horizontal and can be best seen by pulling the pinna posteriorly. Cerumen (earwax) in the canal that obstructs the view of the drum must be removed with a curette or irrigation with (body temperature) water. If the wax is hard, a few drops of sweet oil or hydrogen peroxide will soften the wax. Cautious gentle currettement or washing is necessary to prevent damage to the canal or drum. Redness, bulging, or retraction of the drum is abnormal and should be addressed in proper treatment.

MANAGEMENT OF SPECIFIC DISEASES OF THE EAR

External Ear Disorders

Skin eruptions such as impetigo, furunculosis, herpes simplex, or herpes zoster may occur. Wounds of the external ear, lacerations, or contusions are managed like similar wounds elsewhere. In winter, the pinna may suffer frostbite. The skin is blanched. Slow warming should be done. If blebs occur, puncture under aseptic conditions with application of antibiotic ointments is necessary. Severe frostbite may cause permanent deformity of the cartilage. Diffuse external otitis is manifested by swelling, at times a discharge, tenderness on manipulation causing pain (swimmer's ear). Furuncles (infection of the sweat glands) may be painful, especially when chewing. Management consists of antibiotic drops or neosporin ointment wicks in the canal. Externally applied hot packs may be of value. Analgesics may be required for pain.

Foreign bodies in the external canal may be removed by irrigation, an ear hook, or a curette.

Middle Ear Diseases

Diseases affecting the middle ear are usually associated with pain and hearing loss. Myringitis (inflammation of the drum) may present as infection marked by bullous type elevations and at times a hemorrhagic discoloration. Bullous myringitis is painful. Fever and impaired hearing may be present. On otoscopy, the drum is dull, reddened and inflamed. The blebs may be incised, giving immediate relief of pain. Auralgan ear drops (slightly warm) are also helpful in pain relief. Traumatic rupture of the tympanic membrane may occur as a result of a blow on the ear, explosions, or trauma from a foreign body. It may be associated with pain. Blood is seen on examination and often a perforation of the drum may be observed. It is not advisable to irrigate the ear or instill ear drops in this instance. Rather, a sterile piece of cotton is applied to the orifice of the external canal.

Acute otitis media from bacterial invasion of the middle ear may vary from a catarrhal stage to acute suppuration and perforation. Symptoms may be pain, pressure, some impairment of hearing, and headache. The more severe forms are associated with fever, malaise, and anorexia. On examination, the drum may be red, bulging, or dull with loss of normal landmarks. Tenderness on percussion over the mastoid indicates involvement spreading from the middle ear to the cells of the mastoid cavity. The regional lymph nodes may be palpably enlarged and tender. When the drum is bulging and the above findings are present, a myringotomy (incision into the drum) is necessary to evacuate the fluid. Cultures should be taken of the drainage and will dictate the specific antibiotic to be used when sensitivity studies are complete. Complications may occur, manifested by fever, tenderness, and swelling over mastoid, meningitis, labrynthitis, facial nerve paralysis, lateral sinus thrombosis, and brain abscess. The complication of acute mastoiditis will be manifested by pain on pressure and swelling of the area. Surgical drainage may be necessary and requires otolaryngologic consultation.

Acute salpingitis (eustachian tube) involvement may accompany infections of the throat, nasal allergies, and drainage posteriorly from the paranasal sinuses. In children, adenoid enlargement may cause serous otitis, which should be treated conservatively with steam and decongestants. If this fails, tubes may be required for drainage.

Inner Ear Diseases

Ménière's disease is a pathologic process that involves the inner ear (labyrinth). The patient usually complains of dizziness, unsteady gait, nausea, and vomiting. Examination will reveal nystagmus (jerky movement of the eyes). Hearing may be impaired. Tinnitus (ringing of the ear) may be present. Management is symptomatic. Sedation, Dramamine, Benadryl, or Antivert may have beneficial effects. If Ménière's disease is severe and long lasting, operations on the endolymphatic sac may result in some improvement.

35
DENTAL EMERGENCIES

WILLIAM D. ZITER

In the past decade the distribution of health services in America has clearly been altered. The community hospital, once a storehouse for the hopelessly ill and a treatment center for patients with acute medical or surgical problems, has gradually become a truly comprehensive community health facility.[4] As the center of the community's health resources and services, the hospital seeks to advance the care of the individual as a complete being living in a complex society, taking into account all influences on general health; that is *total health care.*

The obvious relationship between oral/dental health and health in general indicates without question that dentistry plays an important part in a total health plan and should become an integral part of the operation of all community and general hospitals. Naturally, as dental services become available, the emergency department will be faced with an increasing number of patients whose complaints will be primarily dental in origin. It is hoped that the following information will serve to orient emergency department personnel to the needs of these patients.

The dental patient rarely presents to the emergency department with an acute, life-threatening emergency. Occasionally, a patient with serious post-operative hemorrhage is encountered, and uncommonly a patient with a compromised airway as the result of extension of dental infection is seen, but these situations represent rare exceptions. More commonly, dental patients present with a variety of more routine complaints, such as pain and/or swelling related to trauma, oral infection, or previous dental therapy; and although these conditions are not immediately dangerous, they may cause considerable distress to the patient and thus deserve prompt, considerate attention.

It should be noted that the indicated emergency therapy is generally *not* the definitive treatment. Rather, it usually consists of simple procedures that can be carried out quickly to alleviate the patient's immediate problem until a definite diagnosis can be made and a specific treatment plan instituted. With a small amount of indoctrination and experience, emergency personnel can manage many of these emergency measures.

ASSESSMENT

History

When a patient presents with a dental complaint, it is important to obtain as much information as possible about his previous dental experience, in addition to the standard medical history. It should be obvious that a great variety of dental problems may be seen in an emergency department. It is reasonable to assume, therefore, that information about the type and extent of treatment, if any, the patient has previously undergone could be extremely helpful in arriving at a working diagnosis of the problem at hand. This is particularly true when dental procedures have been recently performed. Most patients are well aware of the type of treatment that has been carried out and in many instances can provide valuable insights to the examining emergency personnel.

If sophisticated dental treatment, such as extensive bridgework or multiple root canal procedures, has been undertaken, it is doubtful whether untrained personnel will be able to provide other than symptomatic treatment without potentially doing more harm than good. In such instances, immediate dental consultation is advisable. Conversely, the patient with a toothache who has never been to a dentist and has obvious uncomplicated dental caries probably requires only systemic analgesics as emergency therapy. Subsequent referral to the proper clinic or office for definitive treatment would then be in order.

Physical Examination

To properly evaluate dental patients, however, in addition to the dental history a thorough, carefully performed oral examination is mandatory. In order to accurately perform this exam, only a small amount of special equipment is required, including a dental chair, or a substitute, with a headrest; a source of light that can be focused directly into the mouth, such as a dental light or headlight; an adequate source of suction; and a mouth mirror. The remaining prerequisites include 20/20 vision, probing fingers, and a high degree of suspicion.

The examination of the mouth itself must be detailed and systematic. Each examiner should develop his or her own approach, to be followed each time as a routine, so that no portion of the exam will be omitted. All removable dental appliances, such as complete dentures or removable partial dentures, should be taken out of the mouth before the examination. Inspection and/or palpation of the lips, the labial and buccal mucosa, the hard and soft palates, the tonsillar regions, the floor of the mouth, the tongue, the gingivae, and the teeth must be standard procedure. The examiner should note changes in color, texture, size, position and function of these organs, as well as any indication of overt pathology or trauma. Any abnormal findings should be recorded and the information revealed to the dentist who will ultimately manage the case.

It is particularly important to be thorough when examining a patient who has received oral trauma or has sustained multiple trauma, including trauma to the oral region. Hidden contusions or lacerations, especially of the tongue, floor of the mouth, or oropharyngeal region, could lead to difficulty in breathing or swallowing or to unwarranted blood loss. In addition, foreign particles, such as detached teeth or pieces of teeth, parts of dentures or dental restorations, blood clots and other debris, represent a potential hazard to the airway, particularly in a comatose or semicomatose patient. They should be actively sought and when found, carefully removed. A good source of light and appropriate suction will aid immeasurably in this task.

Adjunct Study

The only study adjunct to history and physical examination commonly used in oral diagnosis is the radiograph. Analysis of the blood or urine and the use of sophisticated electronic equipment is of lesser value in the management of patients with dental emergencies. Therefore, in most cases, when the patient's complaints are related to the teeth or other hard structures of the head and neck, radiographs will be desirable and perhaps should be ordered prior to consultation. Although dental x-rays, such as the periapical and occlusal views, are not routinely taken by medical radiologists, the standard facial series will probably be of value. In the future, it is hoped that dental radiographs will also be available in emergency departments, so that more accurate assessment of the teeth and jaws can be made.

The remainder of the material in this chapter applies to specific problems that may be seen by emergency department personnel. In order to simplify matters, they will be considered under seven main headings:

1. Pain
2. Hemorrhage
3. Swelling
4. Reactions to local anesthesia
5. Trauma to the face, mouth, and jaws
6. Dislocation of the temporomandibular joint
7. Acute oral lesions

Invariably, material will overlap from one category to another. It is hoped, however, that this classification will serve to reduce confusion.

PAIN

Pain is, of course, the most common complaint of dental patients who present to the emergency department of a hospital. The pain is usually related to decayed teeth but may also reflect trauma or pathology in adjacent structures. Because of the wide variety of conditions that are manifest in the oral cavity as pain and because of the frequency of referred pain, the differential diagnosis in these circumstances is often quite confusing and occasionally very difficult. General descriptions of the more common presenting problems follow.

ODONTALGIA

Almost everyone has experienced the distress and discomfort of a toothache and can appreciate why patients sometimes appear in misery at the hospital emergency department in the middle of the night. The usual etiology is dental caries, a disease of the calcified tissues of the teeth, which is unique in respect to all other diseases in that it is *unhealing* and irreversible.[15]

Clinically, in its early stages, dental caries cause the enamel of the crown of the tooth to appear opaque and chalky white. As the process progresses, the lesion discolors to brown or black, and the enamel is soft. As the enamel is completely destroyed, a visible cavity occurs, which has an opaque or whitish periphery. The base of the cavity is composed of brownish, soft, leathery material.

When the etiology is dental caries, the toothache, in its early stages, is best described as a sharp, shooting pain that persists for a short time after removal of the precipitating

stimulus. Later, when damage to the pulp of the tooth is irreversible, the pain becomes more intense and is persistent and more throbbing in character. Heat generally aggravates the pain, whereas cold may relieve it.

The pain can often be accurately localized by the patient to a single offender, but in many instances localization is not possible. Referred pain is very common when dealing with pulpal disease, and the patient may even have difficulty differentiating which jaw the pain is emanating from. At this time, however, the tooth is usually quite sensitive when percussed with a metal instrument, such as the handle of a mouth mirror. When this simple test is positive, it is evidence of probable irreversible pulp damage, and it is likely that endodontic therapy or extraction of the tooth will be indicated.

Toothaches can also be the direct result of inflammation of the gingivae, or gums, a condition which is referred to as periodontal disease. In this chronic disease, the supporting structures of the teeth, both hard and soft tissues, are progressively destroyed. This is a consequence of the irritation of the periodontal tissues by local factors, such as calculus or tartar, and by the action of certain bacteria which accumulate on teeth in a soft, filmy substance, referred to as dental plaque.

Clinically, periodontal disease is characterized by sore, reddened, edematous gingival tissues that bleed freely and easily on provocation. The examiner may also note a purulent exudate around affected teeth, which often become quite loose in the later stages of the disease. "Bleeding gums" and "loose teeth" are almost as common presenting complaints as dental pain.

Although periodontal disease is not always painful, certain periodontal conditions can cause distress. This type of pain can be differentiated from pulpal pain by its character, which is usually dull and gnawing, as compared to the sharp, pulsating pain seen in pulpitis. This is because the inflammation is not confined in any unyielding pulp chamber.[10] The discomfort of periodontal disease is often intensified during function, due to irritation of the tissues by the forceful wedging of food, which results in shifting of mobile teeth.[5] Localization of pain here is much more accurate; the patient can usually point to the etiology of the distress immediately, and no other diagnostic effort is required.[2]

Patients who are in discomfort as the result of recent dental therapy will be also seen periodically. Any one of a number of procedures performed in the dental office can produce lingering oral pain. This list includes dental restorations (fillings), bridges, dentures, root canal or periodontic therapy, surgery, even orthodontic treatment. In such cases, conservative measures should be adopted until the patient's dentist can be contacted.

Management

The management of patients with uncomplicated dental pain in the hospital emergency department is usually quite elementary. In almost all such cases, the definitive treatment that is indicated will require specialized, often sophisticated equipment that is available only in the dental office. Even an experienced dentist will be able to do very little in an emergency department setting. A simple, conservative approach is therefore advocated, consisting primarily of the administration or prescription of systemic analgesics to control the pain until the patient can be seen and evaluated in the proper clinic or office environment.

The drugs that are usually used for pain relief are mild- or moderate-strength narcotics, such as codeine or meperidine, in appropriate doses. The topical administration of commercially prepared gels or drops is usually ineffective, and the topical administration of mild over-the-counter analgesics, such as aspirin, is definitely contraindicated.

If the etiology of the pain is dental caries, and an obvious cavity is present, a sedative dressing, such as zinc oxide and eugenol, can be carefully placed into the cavity and may be successful in controlling the discomfort until definitive treatment can be undertaken. Naturally, common sense instructions regarding oral hygiene, limited activity, and abstention from hot, cold, or sweet foodstuffs or beverages should be stressed.

POSTSURGICAL PAIN

Almost every surgical procedure is associated with some postoperative distress. Oral surgery is no exception; in fact, due to the extremely sensitive nature of the oral area, even minor procedures, such as simple extractions, may produce marked discomfort. The problem is treated with intermittent cold applications to the surgical site during the first 24 hours postoperatively and by the administration of one of the analgesic drugs mentioned above. This simple regimen is followed even when extensive oral surgical procedures, such as the removal of impacted teeth, have been performed.

There is one postsurgical problem that warrants special management. This syndrome is correctly termed alveolar osteitis but is commonly referred to as *dry socket*. The etiology of this condition is unknown, and although it can be seen following the removal of any tooth, the vast majority of cases follow surgical removal of the mandibular third molars (wisdom teeth). Signs and symptoms include severe throbbing pain, often radiating to the ear, which classically begins 2 to 4 days after surgery. The mucosa adjacent to the socket usually appears normal, but the blood clot within the socket is necrotic or absent. The patient complains of a foul taste in his or her mouth, and fetid breath is apparent. Vital signs, including temperature, are generally normal.

Treatment of an alveolar osteitis includes inspection of the wound for the presence of a foreign body, irrigation of the socket with a warm isotonic saline solution, and careful placement of a medicated dressing into the unprotected alveolus. The dressing usually consists of a length of sterile iodoform gauze, with the medication applied in the form of a paste. The medications recommended include anodynes (eugenol or guaiacol), topical anesthetics (butacaine or benzocaine), and antiseptics (iodine). The socket should not be curetted. Antibiotics are not indicated unless concomitant systemic infection exists. Systemic analgesics may be considered, depending on the severity of the pain, but generally the local dressing is more effective than analgesics in controlling the pain of alveolar osteitis.

TOOTH ERUPTION

Pain related to tooth eruption, with one exception, is a problem of very young children.

Children. The pain is frequently accompanied by agitation, a slight elevation of the temperature, and occasionally, rhinitis or nasal discharge. Intraorally, the tissues over the erupting tooth are tender and appear reddened and edematous.

Immediate management of this situation includes application of a topical anesthetic and gentle massage to the overlying tissues. Mild systemic analgesics may be prescribed. The parent should then be instructed to have the child bite on a teething ring to encourage eruption through the mucous membrane, but the tissues should never be incised unless an eruption cyst is present because surgery may predispose to secondary infection.[11]

Adults. The only eruption problem seen in adults involves the eruption of the third molar teeth (wisdom teeth), around the ages of 18 to 20. The clinical situation, termed *pericoronitis,* is most often related to the mandibular third molars. The soft tissues around the crown of the partially erupted tooth are red and inflamed, and suppuration may be seen under the gingival flap. The infection may spread anteriorly and localize as a fluctuant area opposite the first or second molar, or it can spread posteriorly into the masticator space and cause moderate muscle trismus. Tender submandibular lymphadenopathy may also be seen.

The immediate management of this clinical problem includes irrigating under the pericoronal flap with a warm isotonic saline solution to remove accumulated debris and instructing the patient to continue warm saline mouth rinses 4 to 6 times each day. Analgesics should be considered, and if a vestibular abscess is present, it should be drained. Antibiotic therapy is indicated only when there is evidence that the infection is spreading (lymphadenopathy or trismus), or when significant suppuration is present. Ultimately, when the acute symptoms subside and when infection has been controlled, definitive treatment, usually extraction, can be considered.

PAIN OF MAXILLARY SINUS ORIGIN

A brief discussion of maxillary sinusitis is included here because pain associated with infection in the sinus is very often referred to the maxillary teeth in the vicinity and may confuse the clinical picture. Anatomically, the maxillary bicuspids and molars are intimately related to the antrum. Indeed, in many instances, the roots of these teeth project into the sinus, and the two are then separated by only a thin lamina of bone. It is common sense to assume that pathology in one area might well be confused with disease in the other.

Maxillary sinusitis is characterized by a continuous throbbing ache, which is mainly in the infraorbital region, is often bilateral, and may intensify on postural change. The pain can radiate to the maxillary posterior teeth, the cheek, and the frontal region. The infraorbital area is often quite tender when palpated.

The significance of this entity is that it tends to confuse the differential diagnosis of facial pain. The patient is certain that his teeth are the source of his problems, so much so that a great many perfectly good teeth have been sacrificed unnecessarily and unwillingly in a fruitless attempt to alleviate the patient's distress. It is thus important to consider maxillary sinusitis as a potential etiology whenever the presenting complaint is pain in the maxillary posterior teeth. This is particularly important when there is no obvious dental pathology. Once the diagnosis of maxillary sinusitis has been established, the patient should be given systemic antibiotics and analgesics and referred to an otolaryngologist for definitive care.

PAIN IN THE TEMPOROMANDIBULAR JOINT AREA

Patients occasionally present to the emergency department complaining of diffuse pain in the ear and in the preauricular area. Once the presence of pathology in the ear has been ruled out, the examiner should consider the temporomandibular joint and the associated masticatory muscles as potential sources of difficulty. The classical presenting symptoms of this pain dysfunction syndrome include a continuous, dull, diffuse ache in the preauricular region. The pain is usually unilateral, may intensify upon mandibular movement, such as during mastication, and may be referred to the ear, the temporal region or the angle of the mandible.

The etiology of this clinical problem may be related to definitive pathology within the temporomandibular joint. Traumatic, degenerative and rheumatoid changes have been reported.[11] A careful history and precise radiographs will aid in establishing the diagnosis of disease within the joint proper. In such cases, initial management would consist of the administration of systemic analgesics, the application of moist heat to the affected area and restriction to a soft diet.

More commonly, the underlying cause of this clinical syndrome is spasm in one or more of the muscles of mastication. This problem is seen predominantly in women, is related to psychological stress, and is usually associated with some hyperactivity of the masticatory muscles, such as clenching or bruxing. The term presently used to describe this symptom complex is the myofascial pain dysfunction (MPD) syndrome. Symptoms, in addition to those discussed above, include tenderness on palpation of one or more of the muscles of mastication and pain that is either worse on arising in the morning or mild in the morning and gradually worsening as the day progresses. The patient is often unable to open his mouth wide, and the mandible may deviate on opening. Radiographs of the joint are consistently normal.

Emergency department management of the MPD syndrome, in addition to moist heat, soft diet and analgesics, includes the administration of drugs, such as diazepam, to relieve tension and anxiety and provide muscle relaxation.

TRIGEMINAL NEURALGIA

Neuralgias are disturbances of nerves, characterized by paroxysmal pain which extends along the course of the impaired nerve trunk. The pain is usually felt in the terminal peripheral branches of the nerve trunk affected and follows precise anatomical somatic pain pathways. Many varieties of neuralgia have been distinguished, primarily according to the part of the body that is affected. The facial area is no exception, and several facial neuralgias have been described. All are rare, but when they do occur, they are the cause of great distress to the patient and a source of much consternation to the diagnostician. Of the facial neuralgias, the most common and most important is trigeminal neuralgia.

Trigeminal neuralgia, or tic douloureux, is an idiopathic disease most commonly seen in middle-aged and older people. It involves the trigeminal nerve, which supplies the teeth, jaws, face and associated structures, and is characterized by excruciating, paroxysmal, lancinating pain, lasting seconds or minutes. The initiation of the distress is classically related to stimulation of a particular area of the face, that is, a trigger zone. The pain is unilateral in any one paroxysm, is confined to one or more of the branches of the trigeminal nerve, and is associated with no objective sensory loss.[17] The intermissions between paroxysms are generally pain free.[2]

The treatment of trigeminal neuralgia has been extremely varied over the years, and success has not been outstanding. Peripheral and central injections of absolute alcohol have been performed with modest success, as has peripheral surgery. Neurosurgical sectioning of the trigeminal sensory root by any of a number of techniques is recognized by many surgeons as the treatment of choice when attempting a permanent cure.[15] Recently the use of anticonvulsant medications, such as carbamazepine, has been advocated to control the paroxysms rather than destroy the nerve. Success with this approach has been promising, but serious side effects have been reported following prolonged use of these drugs.

Unfortunately, there seems to be no effective emergency treatment for this condition. Patients who report to the emergency department during or just after a bout of pain can only be comforted verbally and directed to where a definitive workup can begin. Systemic analgesics, sedatives and tranquilizers seem to be of little value.[11]

IDIOPATHIC PAIN

Many patients present for treatment complaining of pain for which no immediate cause is apparent. In most instances, the complaint is of long duration, although from the patient's standpoint it has now become so severe or so intolerable that it is considered an emergency. Despite careful search no pathology can be discovered; often the pain does not even follow basic anatomic pathways.

For such persons, an analgesic drug plus a sedative or tranquilizer may provide some comfort during the time necessary for establishing a diagnosis and starting definitive treatment.

HEMORRHAGE

Intraoral hemorrhage is a relatively common occurrence which may follow a surgical procedure or a traumatic accident. When it is encountered, it represents an "honest" emergency, which should be managed quickly and efficiently. The majority of patients who present in pain can be delayed a reasonable period of time prior to definitive treatment, provided adequate systemic analgesics are administered, but the patient with bleeding cannot wait. If simple emergency measures are not effective in controlling the hemorrhage, a dental consultant should be called immediately.

Active hemorrhage in any region of the body is extremely disconcerting to essentially all patients. Bleeding in the mouth, however, is even more likely to produce marked anxiety, for several reasons. The patient cannot see where the blood is coming from and, therefore, tends to exaggerate the extent of the blood loss. Also, the hemorrhage is usually mixed with large volumes of saliva, again distorting the true clinical picture.

Swallowing of some blood is unavoidable, and unfortunately even a modest amount creates distressing nausea and sometimes vomiting. Patients often attempt to clear the mouth through constant expectoration, which not only aggravates the hemorrhage but adds to the thought that blood loss may be reaching serious proportions. The end result is a patient who may be exceedingly apprehensive, a situation which leads to an increase in blood pressure and heart rate, which in turn tends to promote further hemorrhage.

Emergency Management

The emergency management of patients with oral bleeding is not complicated. Once the patient has been reassured, the initial effort should be directed toward application of pressure. Intraoral bleeders can rarely be clamped and tied, and electrocoagulation is of little value. Therefore, time and effort should not be wasted in behalf of these techniques. Rather, all efforts should be extended toward the careful application of pressure directly onto the bleeding site. This is best accomplished by having the patient bite firmly on a large gauze pad. To be effective, however, the gauze must be precisely placed.

First, using adequate light and suction, the mouth should be carefully cleaned of blood, saliva, blood clots and other debris. Then, the exact source of the bleeding can be determined and the gauze pad accurately placed. Firm pressure should be maintained for 20 to 30 minutes while the patient rests comfortably. If at the end of the prescribed period of time the bleeding has been controlled, the patient should sit quietly for an additional 10 minutes before being dismissed, in order to determine if the bleeding will reoccur. If the above regimen is not effective in controlling the hemorrhage, a dentist should be called immediately, who would then under local anesthesia undertake specific measures to control the bleeding. These include the use of hemostatic agents, such as oxidized cellulose, and the placement of sutures.

In addition to directing efforts toward the application of pressure, emergency department personnel should consider the patient's general condition, as well. Vital signs should be taken and recorded, and if the patient shows signs of shock, immediate medical assistance should be obtained.

It is extremely uncommon for hypovolemic shock to result from intraoral bleeding, but it has happened.

If possible, a brief medical history should be taken to determine whether a systemic factor is contributing to the bleeding problem. Previous difficulty with excessive bleeding, a history of a blood dyscrasia, liver disease, anticoagulant therapy, and salicylate therapy are all factors that could seriously complicate oral surgery or facial trauma. If medical problems such as these do exist, medical consultation should be obtained.

SWELLING

The diagnosis of tumors or swellings which affect the soft tissues of the face and mouth is often difficult because of the variety of lesions that manifest themselves in that area. Certainly the swellings most commonly seen in emergency departments are related to bacterial infections, but in order to arrive at an accurate diagnosis, differential diagnosis must include trauma and previous surgery, tumors, systemic diseases, allergies, salivary gland obstructions, and subcutaneous emphysema, in addition to infections.

The principal swellings which affect the face and neck are considered below. Characteristic features and initial management are emphasized.

INFECTIONS

Infections that manifest in and about the face and mouth can be produced by a wide variety of bacterial, viral, and mycotic organisms. Diseases such as tuberculosis, syphilis, cat scratch fever, actinomycosis, and many more can produce infectious swellings and are occasionally encountered in the emergency department. However, the vast majority of swellings related to infections are the direct result of dental pathology, that is, dental caries of periodontal disease.

Acute Alveolar Abscess

The acutely infected tooth, or acute alveolar abscess, is one of the most common dental emergencies encountered. These abscesses are related to a nonvital or degenerative pulp, usually the result of advanced dental caries, and are characterized clinically by a swollen face, an elevated temperature, and varying amounts of pain. The swelling has a relatively distinct outline, and fluctuation can often be elicited. The patient usually has spent one or more sleepless nights, is dehydrated, and may have eaten little since the onset of the condition. Local examination reveals an extremely tender tooth, which the patient can identify with precision.

Initial management of the acute alveolar abscess will vary widely, depending on the individual case. Consideration should be given to antibiotic therapy, incision and drainage, and supportive care.

Systemic antibiotics should be administered if the patient exhibits signs of toxicity, such as malaise, elevated temperature, or leukocytosis. The overwhelming drug of choice for odontogenic infections is penicillin. The drug is exceedingly effective when administered orally in appropriate doses and is associated with very few side effects. For patients who are allergic to penicillin, erythromycin may be substituted. If the patient is nontoxic and the infection is localized, antibiotics may be omitted.

Incision and drainage, with placement of an appropriate sterile drain, should be considered in every case of alveolar abscess where fluctuance is present, denoting an underlying collection of pus. The incision and drainage is indicated whether the patient is toxic or not and may be carried out intraorally or extraorally, as indicated. It may or may not be accompanied by extraction of the offending tooth. The procedure should be performed as quickly as is reasonable, because the problem will not resolve on antibiotics alone, regardless of the dose. Cultures of the exudate should, of course, be taken and sent to the laboratory for examination.

Supportive therapy is critical in managing patients with dental infections. Good nursing care is as important as the pharmacologic or surgical phases of treatment. However, since most patients with dental infections are treated on an outpatient basis, verbal instructions regarding home care must be relied on and, therefore, should be thorough and clearly presented. The following considerations should be included:

1. Complete rest is necessary.
2. Analgesics and sedatives will relieve pain and anxiety and promote sleep.
3. Fluids in several forms should be administered to reverse dehydration.

In severe cases, input-output records should be kept. Adequate nourishment is essential and may be given in liquid or soft form if required. Liquid high-protein dietary supplements may be beneficial.

Cellulitis

The above description of an acute alveolar abscess is obviously based on the classical definition of an abscess, which states that it is a localized collection of pus. The process remains localized because the defensive factors in the region are capable of walling off the infection and preventing it from spreading.[14] Occasionally, the bacterial infection is overwhelming, either because the bacteria are extremely virulent or because the resistance of the host is impaired. The bacterial invasion under these circumstances is unimpeded as it progresses through surrounding tissues to areas remote from the original site of infection. The process is then termed a *cellulitis*.

An acute cellulitis of dental origin is usually confined to the general area of the jaws. The tissues become grossly edematous and firm to palpation. The swelling is diffuse and not sharply demarcated, and no fluctuation is noted. At this stage, suppuration has not occurred.

The patient may show a severe systemic reaction to the infection. The temperature is usually elevated, the white count is increased and the differential count may shift to the left. The sedimentation rate is also increased, and the pulse rate is accelerated. The fluid and electrolyte balance

may be changed, and the patient frequently experiences weakness and malaise. In short, this is an acutely ill patient.

The treatment of an acute facial cellulitis involves the same basic principles as previously enumerated but emphasizes some special considerations. Hospitalization may be indicated. Antibiotic therapy should be aggressive, using parenterally administered drugs. Supportive care must be meticulous. Incision and drainage should be considered in each case but may not be indicated in every case, as suppuration may never occur. Definitive surgery is generally postponed until the patient is nontoxic.

A special cellulitis is classically referred to as Ludwig's angina. This is best described as an overwhelming generalized septic cellulitis of the submandibular region.[14] This infection differs from other types of facial cellulitis in several ways.

Ludwig's Angina

Ludwig's angina is a descending infection, spreading downward from the jaws toward the mediastinum, and is characterized by a board-like, brawny induration of the involved tissues. Three fascial spaces are involved bilaterally: submandibular, submental, and sublingual. If the involvement is not bilateral, the infection is not considered a true Ludwig's angina.

Because of the massive involvement of the sublingual spaces, the floor of the mouth and tongue are markedly elevated toward the palate. This represents a significant threat to the patient's airway, and, therefore, all cases of suspected Ludwig's angina should be treated as distinct emergencies. The patient should be hospitalized and observed closely. Tracheostomy must be considered if there is the slightest hint of respiratory embarrassment. Massive antibiotic therapy, usually administered intravenously, is indicated. Despite the fact that the involved tissues are board-like, incision and drainage, performed intraorally, may be productive. Nursing care should be as intense as with any other life-threatening emergency.

POSTSURGICAL SWELLING

Postoperative edema following oral surgery is quite common. This is particularly true following the surgical removal of impacted teeth, when moderate facial swelling is the rule rather than the exception. Patients are generally warned of this occurrence, but occasionally one will become alarmed and present as an emergency.

Substantial facial edema, either unilateral or bilateral depending on the surgery, will be immediately apparent, and a history of recent surgery will be obtained. Although this situation is generally not serious, it is important to differentiate between postsurgical edema and a postoperative infection. Both entities will cause pain, swelling, and limitation of function, but the infectious process will, in addition, be characterized by the classic signs of abscess or cellulitis previously discussed, including malaise, increased temperature, leukocytosis, fluctuation.

Management of this patient includes reassurance that the

swelling is to be expected, that it may not reach its maximum until 48 to 72 hours following surgery, and that it will resolve in 5 to 7 days. Intermittent cold applications to the operative site (30 minutes per hour) should be used during the first 24 hours after surgery to limit the degree of edema. After the first day, intermittent moist heat (30 minutes per hour) is used to increase circulation and aid in dissipation of the edema. Intraorally, heat is achieved by the use of hot isotonic saline rinses.

The various enzyme preparations and antihistamines suggested for the treatment of postoperative swelling should not be used routinely. Enzymatic agents do not prevent edema but rather redistribute the fluid over a wider area by breaking down connective tissue and fibrin barriers. Some degree of localized swelling may be a desirable physiological response to tissue injury; in addition, disturbance of the tissue barriers can predispose to the spread of infection.[11]

SALIVARY GLAND OBSTRUCTION

Diseases of the salivary glands may affect an individual gland or may involve several at one time. Enlargement may be due to an inflammatory process, a degenerative process, a cyst, a neoplasm or the obstruction of a duct.[8] A brief discussion of salivary gland enlargement resulting from obstruction is included here because it may appear quite similar to many dentally related conditions and, therefore, must be considered in the differential diagnosis of facial and oral swellings.

The location of the swelling is often helpful in making the diagnosis of major salivary gland enlargement. The parotid, submandibular, and sublingual glands have distinct anatomic locations that are not easily confused. Occasionally, however, an enlarged lymph node can be mistaken for a swollen submandibular gland.

When duct obstruction is present, it is related to a stone (sialolith), a mucous plug, cell debris, or a foreign body. Obstruction is generally followed by varying degrees of infection, resulting in signs and symptoms including pain and swelling, which usually increase at mealtime, and the absence of salivary flow from the affected duct. Pus may be excreted if the gland and duct are milked, and signs of systemic involvement, such as an increased temperature, may also be noted.

Minor salivary gland obstructions can occasionally occur on the palate, cheek, lip or floor of the mouth. They are usually asymptomatic unless traumatized and should not be confused with intraoral swellings related to infected teeth.

If obstruction of a major salivary gland is suspected, the gland should be examined roentgenographically for the presence of a sialolith. Anteroposterior and lateral views are used for visualization of the parotid gland, an occlusal view is used for the sublingual gland and anterior extension and duct of the submandibular gland, and a lateral oblique view is used for the main portion of the submandibular gland.[13]

If a stone is present within the duct and is readily accessible and if the patient is having considerable discomfort, the surgical removal of the stone can be considered an emergency measure; consultation is urged. When the stone is within the gland or if the obstruction is due to other causes, the immediate treatment consists of analgesics for pain, belladonna drugs to diminish salivation and relieve the distention, and a broad spectrum antibiotic to combat infection. The patient may then be referred for definitive workup.

NEOPLASMS

Neoplasia is a poorly understood biologic phenomenon which, in some instances, cannot be clearly differentiated from other processes or tissue reactions. Though no precise definition of neoplasia exists, a neoplasm is often considered to be an independent, uncoordinated new growth of tissue which is potentially capable of unlimited proliferation and which does not regress following removal of the stimulus which produced the lesion.[15]

Neoplasms of the oral cavity and adjacent structures are important in the dental profession because of the role the dentist plays in the diagnosis and treatment of these lesions. While tumors do not make up a majority of the pathologic conditions seen in the dental office, they are of great significance, since they have the potential to jeopardize the life, health, and well-being of the patient. For this reason, a brief description of serious neoplasms that may be discovered during oral examination follows.

Squamous cell carcinoma of the oral mucosa is a relatively common lesion, which comprises over 95% of oral malignancies and approximately 10% of all malignant tumors affecting the body. Because of its frequency of occurrence, clinical variability, and potential danger, carcinoma must always be considered in the differential diagnosis of swellings and lesions of the oral cavity.

Clinically, in its early stages, epidermoid carcinoma presents as one of three general patterns: (1) a papillary or verrucous lesion, which is an exophytic growth; (2) an ulcerative type, which has a raised, indurated margin; or (3) a white, raised plaque, which represents a degeneration of the premalignant lesion leukoplakia.

As an oral cancer progresses, the pattern becomes more irregular, and surface trauma and infection invariably complicate the lesion. Oral carcinoma is easily traumatized, and hemorrhage of varying degrees is a relatively common sign. In larger lesions, tissue necrosis may be an obvious feature.

Symptoms of oral carcinoma are of little clinical significance. The lesions are not painful unless ulcerated and infected, and in this condition are not more painful than other oral ulcerations. Lesions of the tongue tend to cause some abnormality of function in this highly active and motile organ. The patient may complain of difficulty in normal speech, and the infiltration of the lingual musculature by carcinoma may also result in symptoms of burning as well as abnormalities of taste sensation.[12]

Oral cancer is seen predominantly in males and is generally a disease of the sixth and seventh decades. Poor oral hygiene and abuse of tobacco and alcohol are common associated findings. Although lesions of carcinoma can be seen affecting all areas of the oral mucosa, certain sites, such as the lip and tongue, are more common than others.[15]

The treatment of oral carcinoma at present involves surgery, radiation, chemotherapy, or combination therapy. The success of the treatment depends upon the differentiation of the tissue and the extent of the tumor. As with malignant disease in other parts of the body, the survival rate following therapy for oral cancer is highest for small lesions detected early in development.

It is crucial, therefore, that all personnel, professional and paraprofessional, who are engaged in oral examination for any reason be aware of the presenting signs and symptoms of this disease and be highly suspicious of *any* intraoral abnormality. Since lesions in the mouth are generally superficial and accessible to examination, it should be possible to discover a great many early lesions. Referral for consultation and perhaps biopsy of such lesions might well be a life-saving procedure. Indeed, biopsy should be seriously considered in every case when an abnormal lesion, especially an ulcer, has been present for 2 weeks and does not show signs of improvement.

There are, of course, a great many benign tumors and tumor-like conditions that present as swellings of the face or mouth. They may be seen in all parts of the oral cavity and generally produce no interruption in function. Nevertheless all such pathology should be properly evaluated by professional personnel, and referral in *all* cases is indicated.

SUBCUTANEOUS EMPHYSEMA

Submucosal or subcutaneous emphysema is an uncommon condition in which air is present in the subcutaneous tissues. It most frequently accompanies fractures of the zygoma or maxilla when the maxillary sinus is involved. Air may also be forced through a surgical incision or intraoral laceration by sneezing with the mouth closed or by forceful blowing, such as is seen when certain musical instruments are played. In addition, the condition may be iatrogenically produced if the air syringes commonly used in dentistry are not used with caution.

Clinically, a swelling of the face or neck of rather sudden onset will be seen. The tissues affected will have a spongy, crepitant feeling on palpation. The process is nontender, and systemic signs and symptoms are absent.

No treatment is necessary for this condition, as the air in the tissues will be absorbed spontaneously within a few days. A few words of reassurance to the patient would, of course, be in order.

REACTIONS TO LOCAL ANESTHESIA

Local anesthetics are the most commonly used drugs in dentistry. Literally hundreds of injections are given weekly by the average practitioner, with unbelievably few complications. In fact, the use of local anesthetics has become such a routine procedure in office practice that one is apt to ignore the possible hazards in their employment. However, complications do occasionally occur and may present as emergencies to the hospital. Some of the more common problems are discussed below. Discussions of systemic reactions, such as allergy and toxicity, will be omitted so that complications

unique to local anesthetic injections in dentistry can be emphasized.

FACIAL PARALYSIS

Penetrations of the anesthetic solution into the parotid gland after a misdirected mandibular block can produce facial nerve paralysis, similar in appearance to Bell's palsy. This condition is characterized by inability to close the eyelid, obliteration of the nasolabial fold, dropping of the corner of the mouth and deviation of the mouth to the unaffected side.

This is a temporary condition, requiring no treatment except covering the eye to prevent corneal abrasion when the lid cannot be closed. The patch should remain in place for the duration of the paralysis.

VISUAL DISORDERS

Temporary loss or blurring of vision (amaurosis) can follow any one of several different injections and results when anesthetic solution diffuses into the orbit and affects the optic nerve. The patient can be assured that the condition is transient, not serious and will subside when the effects of the anesthetic have worn off.

Transient paralysis of one or more of the extraocular muscles can follow some maxillary injections if the anesthetic solution diffuses into the orbit to affect the oculomotor nerve. This results in asynchronous ocular movements and temporary diplopia. No treatment other than reassurance is indicated.

HEMATOMA

Extravasation of blood into the tissues can result when a blood vessel is damaged during injection. This problem usually follows a posterior superior alveolar block, which is used to anesthetize maxillary molar teeth; it results from damage to the posterior superior alveolar artery or the pterygoid venous plexus. Clinically, this hematoma presents as a rapidly enlarging swelling in the cheek.

If recognized quickly, excessive bleeding can be prevented by firm pressure over the region, along with use of ice packs. Otherwise, the condition is self-limiting, and the hematoma requires no immediate treatment. After 24 hours, hot, moist applications may aid in resolution of the swelling, which usually takes 3 to 5 days. Antibiotics are used only if signs of secondary infection appear. The patient should be advised that the tissues in the area of the hematoma will change color as resolution occurs and that, despite a rather ominous appearance, the condition is not serious.

TISSUE SLOUGHING AND ULCERATION

Sloughing and ulceration of the tissues are rare complications which may result from injecting excessive amounts of an anesthetic agent under a firmly attached mucosa or from the use of too high a concentration of vasoconstrictor in the anesthetic solution. Occasionally, especially in children, the lip or cheek may be chewed while anesthetized.

If painful, the lesions can be coated with tincture of benzoin, or a topical anesthetic can be applied. The healing area should be kept meticulously clean, but the use of irritating mouthwashes or antiseptics should be avoided. Antibiotic therapy is generally not indicated.

TRISMUS

Muscle soreness and difficulty in opening the mouth are commonly seen after an inferior alveolar nerve block, which is used to anesthetize mandibular teeth. This is usually caused by trauma to the medial pterygoid muscle, resulting in spasm of the muscle, or by the accidental injection of an irritating solution. Delayed trismus generally is the result of a needle tract infection.

These conditions are treated by hot saline mouth rinses and external hot, moist compresses. Antibiotics are used only if there are overt signs of infection. Gentle jaw exercise is helpful in limiting fibrosis and in reestablishing normal opening. In instances of infection, however, motion should be limited until the inflammatory process has been controlled.

PROLONGED ANESTHESIA OR PARESTHESIA

Persistent loss or alteration of sensation after a nerve block may be caused by trauma from the needle, hemorrhage into the neural sheath or, rarely, from a contaminant in the anesthetic solution.

There is no treatment for this condition. The patient should be advised that in most instances nerve regeneration will occur, although this may take 6 months or more.

TRAUMA TO THE FACE, MOUTH AND JAWS

Emergency treatment of patients with maxillofacial trauma is an important aspect of hospital practice. Professional personnel, including physicians, dentists and nurses, who are called on to evaluate and treat such patients must cooperate and work together so that a broad range of knowledge and experience will be available and correct therapy will be administered.

The treatment of traumatic injuries of the face, teeth, and facial bones should be directed toward restoration of occlusion of the teeth, normal function of the jaws and normal appearance of the face. Careful attention must be given to every injury in this region, to minimize subsequent deformity. In few other injuries is the result so dependent on proper early care and meticulous attention to detail.[16]

GENERAL PATIENT CARE

Unless associated with fractures of the skull, intracranial injuries or serious injuries to other parts of the body, even severe facial injuries are usually not life threatening. Although definitive care of facial trauma should be instituted as soon as possible, management of this trauma should never take precedence over the general care of the patient. Therefore, initial attention should be directed to any concomitant condition, which if uncorrected might have serious or fatal consequences.

First priority must be given to establishment and maintenance of a patent airway, control of hemorrhage, management of shock and recognition and treatment of severe head injuries and trauma to the thorax or abdomen. Airway maintenance and control of hemorrhage are considered below. All other associated injuries are covered in other chapters in this text. The reader is particularly advised to consult Chapter 10 on triage, Chapter 12 on shock, Chapter 19 on wound management and tetanus prophylaxis, Chapter 18 on the comatose patient and the chapters covering the specific injuries encountered.

Airway Maintenance

Since injuries about the face and jaws are likely to produce an obstruction of the upper airway, conditions that interfere with patency of the airway should be sought out and corrected without delay. Blood, in the form of active bleeding or blood clots in the oropharynx, must be controlled. The tongue may also be a threat to the airway, because in an unconscious patient, it may fall against the posterior pharyngeal wall. Foreign bodies, such as dentures, broken teeth, mucus, vomitus, are common causes of obstruction. Lastly, fractures of the maxilla can be displaced posteriorly and interfere with the airway, and mandibular fractures may result in loss of support for the tongue, permitting it to fall back into the oropharynx.

The most important sign of a compromised airway is labored, noisy respirations. For all intents and purposes, noisy breathing is obstructed breathing. Other signs of airway obstruction include gasping for breath, laryngeal stridor, restlessness and apprehension, cyanosis, and circumoral pallor.

When signs of airway problems are encountered, immediate measures must be taken to relieve the obstruction. The tongue should be grasped and pulled forward, and the pharynx should be cleared of all foreign material. This may be done manually or with the use of forceps and suction. Once the airway has been cleared, it can be maintained by positioning the patient on his side, with the face up and the chin extended. The tongue can be held forward with an oral or nasal airway; then oxygen can be administered. If the above measures do not relieve the obstruction, consideration must be given to a cricothyroidostomy, tracheostomy, or the insertion of an endotracheal tube.

Control of Hemorrhage

Hemorrhage associated with facial injuries is seldom a serious problem. Although the blood vessels of the facial areas are numerous, they are small and well supplied with elastic fibers. When severed, they normally retract within bony canals and are occluded by thrombosis.[16] Thus, bleeding related to facial injuries usually stops spontaneously.

When bleeding does persist, it may be extraoral or intraoral. Since most extraoral hemorrhage is of the "seeping" or "oozing" type, the application of a firm pressure dressing over the involved region is usually all that is necessary to control the bleeding. If pressure dressings are ineffective, the margins of the wound must be retracted and the bleeding points identified, clamped and tied.

Intraoral bleeding is generally controlled by applying pressure with gauze to the bleeding area. When hemorrhage from fracture sites is extensive, it is managed by reducing the bony fragments which are then maintained in position with circumdental wires.

CARE OF SOFT TISSUE INJURIES

Although the management of facial fractures may be delayed, wounds to the soft tissues of the face should be treated, whenever possible, within a few hours after the injury. The patient is seldom injured so severely that early closure of facial lacerations cannot be accomplished. Early primary closure stimulates prompt healing, limits the degree of inflammatory reaction and minimizes subsequent development of scar tissue. In addition, such closure seals off avenues of contamination and therefore assists in the prevention and control of infection.[3]

When the general condition of the patient permits, reduction of facial fractures should be carried out prior to closure of the soft tissue wounds. If the soft tissues are closed first, the subsequent manipulative procedures necessary for reduction of the fractures frequently cause disruption of the wounds.[9] It is, therefore, imperative that oral surgical consultation be obtained at the outset of treatment.

Management of soft tissue injuries involves, first, proper cleansing and debridement of the wound. The area around the wound is scrubbed with surgical detergent soap and a brush. Then the area should be thoroughly lavaged with copious amounts of sterile saline. All hematomas should be removed. Radical debridement is not indicated; however, all necrotic and devitalized tissue should be meticulously removed, along with all foreign material. Rough, irregular, ragged, or lacerated margins are then removed, and following complete hemostasis, the wound is closed in layers. Larger wounds are then completely covered by a firm pressure dressing.

Since all major maxillofacial wounds are contaminated, every effort must be made to prevent infection. Prevention is accomplished for the most part by strict adherence to sterile technique, thorough cleansing of the tissue, complete hemostasis, and conservative but adequate debridement and wound closure that eliminates all dead spaces.[16] In addition, antibiotics are generally indicated in major trauma, especially if there is a communication with the oral cavity, which is, of course, contaminated. Penicillin in appropriate doses is generally the drug of choice. Naturally, a negative history of sensitivity must be obtained before administration.

FRACTURED OR AVULSED TEETH

Patients with fractured or avulsed teeth should generally be seen immediately by a member of the dental service. The sooner the injured teeth are treated, the better the prognosis.[1] If only the enamel of the tooth is fractured, the patient is usually asymptomatic. The treatment is to smooth off the sharp edges, to prevent laceration of the tongue or lips. This is not necessarily an emergency.

If, however, the fracture of the crown of the tooth involves the dentin or the pulp, the tooth will be sensitive to touch and thermal changes, such as air passing over the tooth. In such cases, desensitization and restorative procedures must be carried out as soon as is reasonable.

Displaced or avulsed teeth will need substantially more treatment, including realignment or replacement with adequate splinting to stabilize the tooth for 6 weeks. This will require local anesthesia, professional attention, and prolonged follow-up. Avulsed teeth should be kept moist in a clean handkerchief until the patient arrives at the hospital. Then the tooth should be placed in sterile saline.

No attempt should be made by nondental personnel to remove dirt or debris, as critical periodontal fibers still attached to the cementum of the tooth may be destroyed. Attention should be given to controlling hemorrhage in the mouth and to calming and reassuring both the patient and the family until professional help arrives.

FRACTURES OF THE FACIAL BONES

After the patient's general condition has been deemed satisfactory, a detailed examination is indicated to determine the extent of the facial injuries. Diagnosis of fractures is made from the information obtained from the history, clinical examination, and roentgenographic studies. (See also Chap. 32, Injuries to Bones, Joints, and Related Structures.)

The history should include information regarding the time of injury, the type of accident, any loss of consciousness, prior treatment, and associated medical problems. This information can be valuable in assessing the patient's general condition and in planning therapy.

Visual examination will often reveal conditions suggestive of a fracture. Edema, ecchymosis, obvious deformity, limited opening or deviation of the mandible on opening, obvious malocclusion and pain on movement of the jaws are suggestive signs and symptoms.

Intraoral examination will also reveal telltale signs of fracture, including lacerations of the oral mucosa, abnormal alignment of teeth, inability to bring the teeth into occlusion and independent movement of fragments when the patient attempts to bring the teeth into occlusion.

Digital examination yields additional information. Extreme tenderness, inability to manually move the mandible through its normal excursions, palpable fracture lines, abnormal mobility of fragments, and crepitus are indications of possible fracture.

Radiographs are reliable aids in the diagnosis of fractures. They must be adequate in quality and quantity to clearly demonstrate all fracture lines. To describe mandibular fractures, in addition to the standard facial series, the exaggerated Townes' position and temporomandibular joint films are often needed. Intraoral and occlusal views are also of value in certain cases. In maxillary and zygoma fractures, the Waters and vertex-submental views are most frequently used.

It should be noted that radiographs in general are not as helpful in diagnosing maxillary and zygomatic fractures as they are in evaluating mandibular trauma. This is related to the amount of superimposition in this area. To compensate, clinical evaluation must be that much more astute.

MANDIBULAR FRACTURES

The lower jaw is the second most commonly fractured facial bone following the nasal bone. Its prominent position on the face renders it vulnerable to traumatic incidents such as a blow from a fist or a club or to automotive or industrial accidents. Although fractures of the mandible may occur anywhere, they are most commonly seen at the angle of the mandible, especially through an impacted third molar tooth, through the mental foramen area, or through the temporomandibular joint. Because it is a U-shaped bone and will radiate traumatic forces around its curvatures, the mandible is susceptible to multiple fractures. More than 50% of mandibular fractures are multiple, so that if one obvious fracture is noted, the patient and the radiographs should be carefully examined for evidence of additional injuries.

Unlike the patient with a nasal bone fracture, who frequently does not seek treatment, patients with fractures of the mandible seldom go untreated because of the marked pain and discomfort that is experienced, especially during function. Patients also commonly complain that their teeth do not fit together properly, suggesting that the very sensitive relationship between upper and lower jaws may have been altered, however minimally, as by a fracture (Fig. 35-1).

Figure 35-1 Mandibular fracture.

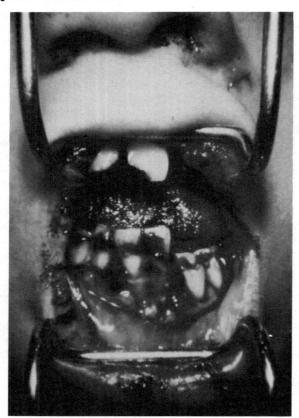

Clinical signs and symptoms of mandibular fractures, in addition to pain and malalignment of the teeth, include contusions and lacerations over affected areas of the mandible, paresthesia or numbness of the lower lip from damage to the inferior alveolar nerve, swelling of the side of the face, and ecchymosis in the floor of the mouth, a sign which is almost pathognomonic of a mandibular fracture.

MAXILLARY FRACTURES (MIDFACE FRACTURES)

Midface fractures may involve the maxilla alone or may include the naso-orbital complex and the zygomatic bones. As a general rule, total fractures of the midface are less common than mandibular fractures because they require severe extraoral trauma. Segmental fractures of the upper jaw, which usually include teeth, however, are quite common.

Major midface fractures are categorized according to the LeFort classification:

1. A LeFort I or horizontal fracture is a transverse detachment of the entire maxilla above the apices of the teeth at the level of the nasal floor. This injury often produces a single, quite mobile free-floating segment.

2. The LeFort II or pyramidal fracture is a fracture of the central portion of the face that includes the maxilla, a medial portion of both maxillary sinuses, infraorbital rims and orbits, and the nasal bones.

3. The LeFort III fracture or craniofacial dysjunction includes fractures of both zygomatic bones in addition to the classic LeFort II. This injury results from extreme forces directed at the face. Extensive comminution, airway obstruction, intracranial injuries, and cerebrospinal fluid leakage are often associated with this massive traumatic injury.

The most obvious sign of a midface fracture is a distortion of normal facial symmetry. The face appears lengthened or flattened or "dished-in" (Fig. 35-2). Often the patient will exhibit an open bite anteriorly, and with the LeFort II or III fracture will show distinct periorbital edema and ecchymosis. Other clinical signs and symptoms include pain, swelling, infraorbital paresthesia, and intraoral ecchymosis.

Confirmation of fractures of the maxilla may be gained using facial radiographs, but more information will usually be gleaned through careful examination. Palpation at the naso-orbital area, the frontozygomatic area, and the infraorbital rims while grasping the maxillary anterior teeth and gently moving the upper jaw will aid immeasurably in confirming the presence of a fracture and in establishing the extent of the injury.

ZYGOMATIC COMPLEX FRACTURES

Fractures of the zygomatic complex usually occur as the result of a direct force striking the prominence of the zygoma, or cheek bone. The zygomatic complex consists of the zygomatic bone and its articulation with several other bones of the face. Since the zygomatic bone forms a major portion of the lateral and inferior rim of the orbit, fractures of this complex very often affect the eye.

Periorbital ecchymosis and subconjunctival hemorrhage are the most frequent clinical signs associated with zygomatic

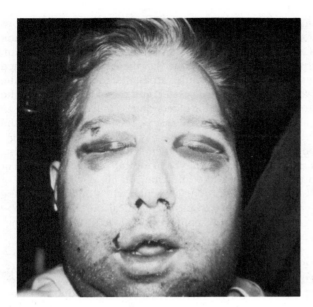

Figure 35-2 Midface fracture.

fractures. (Fig. 35-3) On the affected side, the palpebral fissure may appear canted, and the globe may be displaced downward.

Ocular and visual disturbances are common with fractures of the zygomatic complex and deserve ophthalmologic consultation. Diplopia is common and limitation of the movements of the eye may be seen. Other serious ophthalmologic injuries include retinal detachment, lens dislocation, and hyphemias.

Other clinical signs of zygomatic complex fractures include flatness of the cheek, limited movement of the lower jaw due to impingement of the displaced zygomatic bone on the coronoid process of the mandible, and paresthesia of the molar area and the upper lip on the affected side. Unilateral nosebleed on the injured side may be seen as a result of bleeding from the maxillary sinus into the nose. Step defects at the infraorbital rim and in the zygomaticofrontal suture area are usually palpable.

Clinical Signs of Fractures

The signs that indicate facial fractures are summarized below.

Pain. After trauma, a fracture should be suspected when pain is elicited as the jaw is moved. However, pain is not always a reliable sign, since fractures of the maxilla and zygoma are accompanied by little or no pain.

Swelling. Swelling is not a completely reliable sign of fracture, even though most traumatic injuries producing fractures are accompanied by swelling. Many traumatic injuries, however, produce swelling without concomitant fractures.

Hemorrhage. When bleeding from the nose is encountered after an injury, suspicion of a fracture of the maxilla, zygoma, or nasal bones is warranted.

Ecchymosis. Ecchymosis is not constantly associated with fracture. However, when ecchymosis follows a traumatic injury, a thorough examination to determine whether a fracture has occurred is justified. Ecchymosis behind the ear over the mastoid process is known as Battle's sign and is usually associated with a basal skull fracture.

Crepitus. The grating sound or sensation that is heard or felt when the ends of a fractured bone are brought into contact with each other is a reliable sign of fracture. However, manipulation of the fractured bone is usually accompanied by considerable pain, and since other less traumatic tests for fractures are available, the manual movement of fractured bones as a diagnostic procedure is seldom necessary.

Loss of Function. Inability to move the mandible through its normal excursions, as well as trismus and altered occlusal relationships, is a reliable sign of fracture.

Abnormal Movement. Mobility in any part of the facial bones other than at the temporomandibular joint is a reliable indication of fracture.

Displacements. Grossly displaced fragments often produce facial deformities that are pathognomonic of fractures.

Malpositions. Disruption of normal occlusion or malposition of various segments in the same arch are reliable signs of fracture.

Paresthesias. After trauma, altered sensation is a suspicious sign. Paresthesia of the lower lip suggests a fracture of the body of the mandible, and infraorbital numbness is suggestive of a maxillary or zygomatic fracture.

Fluid Seepage. Loss of cerebrospinal fluid from the nose or ear is pathognomonic of fracture of the facial bones.

Other Signs. Periorbital edema, periorbital ecchymosis, subconjunctival hemorrhage, and impaired ocular move-

Figure 35-3 Zygomatic fracture.

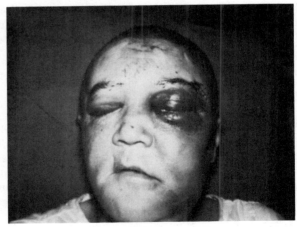

ments should arouse suspicion of zygomaticomaxillary complex fractures.[16]

When a facial fracture has been diagnosed, one should attempt to make the patient comfortable, and immediate oral surgical consultation should be requested. Generally, the swelling and muscular trismus that frequently accompany fractures of the facial bones are very effective in limiting movement and, hence, tend to minimize pain. Manipulation of the fractures or attempts at mastication generally stimulate considerable pain and should be avoided.

Sedation is to be avoided until the condition of the patient is determined and an accurate diagnosis has been made. Heavy sedation will often mask signs of increased intracranial pressure. In the presence of associated head injuries, strong narcotics are to be avoided. Chloral hydrate may be used if sedation is necessary, and codeine sulfate is usually sufficient to control pain.[16]

Antibiotics should be considered in all cases, since most facial fractures are compounded into the mouth or the paranasal sinuses. Penicillin is generally the choice.

DISLOCATION OF THE TEMPOROMANDIBULAR JOINT

Dislocation of the temporomandibular joint occurs with relative frequency when the capsule and the temporomandibular ligament are sufficiently relaxed to allow the condyle to move anterior to the articular eminence during opening. Muscle contraction and spasm then lock the condyle into this position, so that it is impossible for the patient to close his jaws to their normal occluding position. Dislocation may be unilateral or bilateral and may occur spontaneously following stretching of the mouth to its extreme open position, such as during a yawn or a routine dental operation.

Dislocations can usually be reduced by inducing downward pressure on the posterior teeth and upward pressure on the chin, accompanied by posterior displacement of the entire mandible. It is preferable for the operator to stand in front of the patient. Generally, reduction is not difficult. However, muscle spasm may occasionally be sufficient to prevent simple manipulation of the condyle back to its normal position, and it becomes necessary to obtain muscle relaxation to allow proper reduction of the condyle. This can be accomplished by the administration of a general anesthetic, supplemented, if necessary, by a muscle relaxant.[6]

ACUTE ORAL LESIONS

Acute lesions of the oral mucosa are not seen routinely, either in dental practice or in the hospital emergency department. When they do present, they must initially be recognized as such, so that they can be evaluated intelligently. The patient, at such time, may be in acute distress, and efforts must be extended to first relieve discomfort and then to begin the process of diagnosis.

There are, indeed, a great variety of conditions that present as an acute stomatitis. Burns, drug idiosyncrasies, infectious processes, dermatologic disorders, and oral manifestations of systemic diseases can all present with a chief complaint of a "sore mouth." Common initial symptoms, in addition to pain, include a tender mucosa which is generally reddened but may also exhibit whitish areas, due to necrosis of tissue, swollen and perhaps ulcerated gums, and in many cases the presence of vesicles or ulcers on the mucosa.

Burns may be thermal, that is, related to hot foods (the hot pizza syndrome), or they may have a chemical etiology. One of the most common chemical burns seen by dentists is caused when aspirin has been topically applied by a patient to the mucosa next to an aching tooth. A whitish area of tissue necrosis is produced, which will slough off, leaving a reddened, ulcerated base. Chemical burns may also be produced by phenol, commercial toothache drops, and other caustic agents.

Local reactions to drugs or materials used in contact with the oral mucosa are termed *stomatitis venenata.* These reactions are occasionally related to mouth washes, dentifrices, lozenges, and acrylic, the plastic material used to construct dentures. "Stomatitis medicamentosa" refers to the oral mucosal reaction related to drugs administered systematically. Antibiotics, sulfonamides, salicylates and halogens have all been causative in this type of reaction.[7] The oral mucosa and gingivae may become ulcerated, swollen and very painful.

Viral, bacterial and fungal diseases can all produce disabling oral infections. Such systemic diseases as herpes simplex, tuberculosis, syphilis, histoplasmosis, moniliasis, and others can be associated with serious oral lesions, in addition to systemic manifestations. Vesicles and ulcers are the most common oral signs.

Acute necrotizing gingivitis, also known as Vincent's infection or trench mouth, is a common local bacterial infection of the oral cavity. It is a nontransmissible inflammatory disease of the gingivae, caused by a combination of lowered resistance of the patient and local irritation, with superimposition of Vincent's organisms (fusiform bacilli and spirochetes) normally found in the oral cavity. In the acute phase, there is swelling, ulceration, bleeding, and pain primarily in gingival tissues. Systemic signs of infection may be noted.

Aphthous stomatitis (canker sores) may occur in any area of the mouth. The lesions are the most painful ulcerations of the oral cavity. Typically, they vary in size and are yellow-white in color; their margins are erythematous and indurated. The ulcers are present for about a week and heal completely in 10 to 14 days without scarring. The etiology of the condition is speculative.

Dermatological disorders, such as erythema multiforme, pemphigus vulgaris, lupus erythematosus, and others, may affect the oral mucosa in addition to the skin. Clinically, in the oral cavity, they present as vesicles, bullae, or ulcers that are prolonged and associated with systemic signs of infection and generalized disease.

Oral manifestations can be noted with a number of systemic diseases, such as diabetes mellitus, vitamin deficiencies, blood dyscrasias, and renal failure. The lesions are nonspecific; they do not heal unless the primary disease is controlled and are frequently accompanied by spontaneous bleeding from the gums and other parts of the oral mucosa.

It should indeed be obvious that a great variety of conditions can present as a "sore mouth," and making a definitive diagnosis in many instances is a significant task. Emergency management, however, is less complicated. The patient should be treated with sympathy and reassurance. Mild analgesics and topical anesthetics may be utilized to reduce pain. A soft, bland diet should be suggested and fluids encouraged. Bed rest is indicated, along with warm saline mouth rinses, which of necessity must be substituted for normal oral hygiene. Consultation or referral should then be undertaken.

Acute lesions of the oral mucosa usually heal completely in 2 weeks' time. If this does not happen, further investigation, including biopsy, will probably be in order.

SUMMARY

The modern general hospital is faced with an amazing variety of urgent situations. Dental emergencies are not the most glamorous or dramatic, but they do occur with monotonous regularity. Unfortunately, hospital physicians and nurses generally have little orientation toward dentistry and are able to do little in behalf of these patients.

In this chapter, information regarding many phases of dentally related problems has been presented. It is hoped that it will aid in the management of emergency patients and that it will promote consultation and a sincere spirit of cooperation between dentists and emergency personnel.

REFERENCES

1. Andrews R: Injured anterior teeth. In F. McCarthy (ed): Emergencies in Dental Practice, 2nd ed. Chap. 18 Philadelphia, WB Saunders, 1972
2. Bell W: Synopsis of Oral and Facial Pain and the Temporomandibular Joint. Dallas, published by the author, 1967
3. Chipps J, Canham R, Makel H: Intermediate treatment of maxillofacial injuries. US Armed Forces Med J 4:951, 1953
4. Friedrich R, Gambuti G, Linz A: Role of the hospital in the future of dental education. Journal of Oral Surgery 25:47, 1967
5. Glickman I: Clinical periodontology, 4th ed. Philadelphia, WB Saunders, 1972
6. Henry F: The temporomandibular joint. In Kruger G (ed): Textbook of Oral Surgery, 4th ed, Chap. 20. St. Louis, CV Mosby, 1974
7. Huebsch R: Acute oral lesions. In McCarthy F (ed): Emergencies in Dental Practice, 2nd ed, Chap. 21 Philadelphia, WB Saunders, 1972
8. Irby W, Baldwin K: Emergencies and Urgent Complications in Dentistry St. Louis, CV Mosby, 1965
9. Kruger G: Fractures of the jaws. In Kruger G (ed): Textbook of Oral Surgery, 4th ed, Chap. 19. St Louis, CV Mosby, 1974
10. Kruger G, Reynolds D: Maxillofacial pain. In McCarthy F (ed): Emergencies in Dental Practice, 2nd ed, Chap. 20. Philadelphia, WB Saunders, 1972
11. Laskin D: Treatment of common emergencies of the hospital dental patient. In Douglas B (ed): Introduction to Hospital Dentistry, 2nd ed, Chap. 12. St. Louis, CV Mosby, 1970
12. McCarthy P, Shklar G: Diseases of the Oral Mucosa. New York, McGraw-Hill, 1964
13. Mandel L: Salivary gland disease. paper read at St. John's Hospital, Queens, NY, April 19, 1974
14. Moose S: Acute infections of the oral cavity. In Kruger G (ed), Textbook of Oral Surgery, 4th ed, Chap. 11. St. Louis, CV Mosby, 1974
15. Shafer W, Hine M, Levy B: A Textbook of Oral Pathology, ed. 2 Philadelphia, WB Saunders, 1963
16. Shira R: Emergency treatment of patients with facial trauma. In Douglas B (ed): Introduction to Hospital Dentistry, 2nd ed, Chap. 13. St. Louis, CV Mosby, 1970
17. Sweet W: Trigeminal neuralgias. In Alling C (ed): Facial Pain. Philadelphia, Lea & Febiger, 1968

Index

Numbers followed by an *f* indicate a figure; *t* following a page number indicates tabular material; *c* following a page number indicates charted material.